Kanerva's Occupational Dermatology

Thomas Rustemeyer, Peter Elsner, Swen Malte John and
Howard I. Maibach (Eds.)

Kanerva's Occupational Dermatology

Second Edition

Volume 1

With 780 Figures and 514 Tables

Springer

Editors
Thomas Rustemeyer
Department of Dermatology and Allergology
VU University Medical Center
Amsterdam
The Netherlands

Peter Elsner
Department of Dermatology
University Hospital Jena
Jena
Germany

Swen-Malte John
Department of Dermatology, Environmental Medicine
and Health Theory
University of Osnabrück
Osnabrück
Germany

Howard I. Maibach
Department of Dermatology
University of California
San Francisco, CA
USA

ISBN 978-3-642-02034-6 ISBN 978-3-642-02035-3 (eBook)
DOI 10.1007/978-3-642-02035-3
ISBN 978-3-642-02036-0 (print and electronic bundle)
Springer Heidelberg New York Dordrecht London

Library of Congress Control Number: 2012935015

Printed on acid-free paper

Springer is part of Springer Science+Business Media (www.springer.com)

Preface to the Second Edition

The knowledge of occupational Dermatology has expanded – vibrantly – in the decade since the first edition.

The field is far more multidisciplinary – including numerous industrial hygienists, occupational physicians, dermatologists, allergologists, chemists of many types, modellers, and many other health care professionals including nurse practitioners and physician assistants. Prevention more and more may become a stronghold for dermatology: by their specific knowledge and competence – in cooperation with other disciplines – dermatologists can save their patients' health and jobs, and thus also save expenses for tax-payers and insurance systems. Undoubtedly however, awareness to occupational skin diseases, their pathogenesis, and prevention by those at risk has, as yet, to be improved in all countries. Furthermore, preventive intervention needs to be accompanied by global regulatory efforts to limit exposure to hazardous substances, including evidence-based standards for adequate manufacturing and use of gloves, protective creams, and after-work skin care.

Although we look forward to the science and techniques of delivery of health care and prevention to the day when occupational dermatology is no longer necessary, we have much work to do before this can be seriously envisioned. Nevertheless the increased support and work in the last decade should lead all to be optimistic that this will occur – within the century.

The field is far more evidence-based than before – perhaps leading the dermatologic sciences in the rapid progress in this technique and philosophy. We hope this textbook will provide you with all practical as well as background information needed. It may become a resilient support in your daily care for patients.

We are saddened by the loss of Professor Jan Wahlberg and the illness of Professor Lasse Kanerva. Both played a major role in the First Edition and the development of the field Sui Generis. Fortunately their work, their colleagues and students, have continued many of their intellectual and practical endeavours.

The current editors (from the First Edition – Peter Elsner and Howard Maibach) and the new arrivals (Thomas Rustemeyer and Swen Malte John) welcome your criticisms and suggestions.

For the legal implications of occupational skin diseases in the various countries and social insurance systems please refer to: International legal aspects of workers' compensation for occupational contact dermatitis. In: Duus Johansen J, Frosch PJ, Lepoittevin JP (eds.) Contact Dermatitis. Springer Berlin, Heidelberg, (2011), 5th edition, 1029–1051.

The Editors
Thomas Rustemeyer (t.rustemeyer@vumc.nl)
Peter Elsner (elsner@derma-jena.de)
Swen-Malte John (johnderm@uos.de)
Howard I. Maibach (maibach@derm.ucsf.edu)

Preface to the First Edition

The Field of occupational dermatology has been well served by textbooks. The twentieth giants in this field have produced books that are universally accepted. These include Schwartz, Tullipan, and Birmingham, as well as Fousseau and Adams.

What then is the need in terms of the next generation of textbooks in this rapidly evolving and complex clinical research area? The varied complexity an inordinate detail of information makes it difficult for any one individual to cover this huge expanse of knowledge. The present volume stresses individual excellence and scholarship covering the various areas. It is not meant to be a static book. If the readership finds it as interesting as the editors and authors have, this should evolve over generations. The information in the various chapters includes nineteenth century approaches, such as morphology and histology, but is amply supplemented by late twentieth and early twenty-first century clinical bioassays.

Although the field is served by general dermatologists, occupational physicians, and occupational dermatologists, other health workers are also frequently involved. For this reason, we have deliberately included a number of redundancies in an attempt to make it easier for the reader. Whenever possible, we have emphasized evidence-based dermatology, and the authors were chosen on the basis of both their scientific approach and clinical good sense.

Hopefully, a second edition will benefit by increased controlled experimentation currently under way, so that there will be even more hard data included. The editors welcome your comments for the proposed second edition.

The Editors

Editors-in-Chief

Thomas Rustemeyer
Department of Dermatology and Allergology
VU University Medical Center
De Boelelaan, 1117
1081 HV Amsterdam
The Netherlands

Peter Elsner
Department of Dermatology
University Hospital Jena
Erfurter Strasse 35
07743 Jena
Germany

Swen-Malte John
Department of Dermatology, Environmental Medicine and Health Theory
University of Osnabrück
Sedanstraße 115
49090 Osnabrück
Germany

Howard I. Maibach
Department of Dermatology
University of California
Medical Center Way 90
San Francisco, CA 94143-0989
USA

Table of Contents

Section 2 Occupational Skin Diseases: Clinical

Section 3 Causative Factors

Volume 2

[†]Deceased.

Section 4 Diagnosis

Section 5 Therapy

Section 6 Prognosis

Section 7 Prevention

Volume 3

Section 8 Job Descriptions

Section 9 Chemistry and Concentrations of Patch Test Allergens

List of Contributors

Kristiina Aalto-Korte
Health and Work Ability, Control of Hypersensitivity Diseases Team
Finnish Institute of Occupational Health
Helsinki
Finland

Keith William James Adam
Medibank Health Solutions
and
Faculty of Health Sciences
The University of Queensland
Brisbane
Australia

Kerry E. Adam
Occupational Therapist, Clinical Educator, Faculty of Health Sciences, School of Health and Rehabilitation Sciences
The University of Queensland
Brisbane
Australia

Tove Agner
Department of Dermatology
Bispebjerg Hospital
University of Copenhagen, Faculty of Health Science
Copenhagen, NV
Denmark

Kristiina Alanko
Finnish Institute of Occupational Health
Helsinki
Finland

Iris S. Ale
Department of Dermatology
Republic University of Uruguay
Montevideo
Uruguay

Henning Allmers
Department of Dermatology, Environmental Medicine and Health Sciences
University of Osnabrueck
Osnabrueck
Germany
and
Department of Occupational Medicine
University of Osnabrueck
Osnabrueck
Germany

Firas A. Al-Niaimi
Department of Dermatology
Cumberland Infirmary
Carlisle
UK

Agustin Alomar
Servicio de Dermatología
Hospital de la Santa Creu i Sant Pau
Barcelona
Spain

Klaus E. Andersen
Department of Dermatology and Allergy Centre
Odense University Hospital, University of Southern Denmark
Odense
Denmark

Savina Aneja
Department of Dermatology, Desk A-61
Dermatology-Plastic Surgery Institute, Cleveland Clinic
Cleveland, OH
USA

Dimitar Antonov
Department of Dermatology
University Hospital Jena
Jena
Germany

Christian Apfelbacher
Medizinische Soziologie, Institut für Epidemiologie und Präventivmedizin, Fakultät Medizin
Universität Regensburg
Regensburg
Germany
and
Abteilung Klinische Sozialmedizin
Universitätsklinikum Heidelberg
Heidelberg
Germany

Matthias Augustin
Institute for Health Services Research in Dermatology and Nursing (IVDP) and Hamburg Center for Health Economics (HCHE)
University of Hamburg
Hamburg
Germany

Christian Avnstorp
Dermatology Clinic
Rødovre
Denmark

Ângelo Azenha
Department of Dermatology
Hospital Privado da Trofa
Trofa
Portugal

Lynn A. Baden
Centre Dermatology and Aesthetic Medicine
Newton, MA
USA

Robert Baran
Nail Disease Center
Cannes
France

David A. Basketter
DABMEB Consultancy Ltd
Sharnbrook, Bedfordshire
UK

Andrea Bauer
Department of Dermatology
University Hospital Carl Gustav Carus
Technical University of Dresden
Dresden
Germany

Mike H. Beck
Department of Occupational and Environmental Health
Contact Dermatitis Investigation Unit
University of Manchester Dermatology
Hope Hospital
Salford, Lancashire, Manchester
UK

Detlef Becker
Department of Dermatology
University Medical Center
Mainz
Germany

Donald V. Belsito
Department of Dermatology
Columbia University
New York, NY
USA

Viswanath Reddy Belum
Wexner Medical Center at The Ohio State University
Columbus, OH
USA

Andreas J. Bircher
Allergy Unit, Department of Dermatology
University Hospital
Basel
Switzerland

B. Mary E. von Blomberg
Department of Pathology
VU University Medical Center
Amsterdam
The Netherlands

Edith M. de Boer
Department of Dermatology
VU Medisch Centrum
Amsterdam
The Netherlands

Anders Boman
Department of Occupational and Environmental
Karolinska Institutet
Institute of Environmental Medicine, Occupational and Environmental Dermatology
Stockholm
Sweden

Ronald R. Brancaccio
New York
USA

Richard Brans
Department of Dermatology
Environmental Medicine and Health Theory
University of Osnabrueck
Osnabrueck
Germany

Randolf Brehler
Department of Dermatology
University of Muenster
Muenster
Germany

Kristine Breuer
Department of Allergology and Occupational Dermatology
Dermatologikum Hamburg
Hamburg
Germany

Horst C. Broding
Head Exposure Laboratory, Consultant Dermatology - Allergology Occupational & Environmental Medicine
Institute for Prevention and Occupational Medicine of the German Social Accident Insurance – Institute of the Ruhr-University Bochum (IPA)
Bochum, NRW
Germany

Derk P. Bruynzeel
Abcoude
The Netherlands

Magnus Bruze
University of California Medical School
San Francisco, CA
USA
and
Department of Occupational and Environmental Dermatology
Skåne University Hospital Malmö, Lund University
Malmö
Sweden

Letiţia Bucur
Department of Occupational Health
Belsana Grup LLC
Bucharest
Romania

Gheorghe Bucur
Dermato-venereologist
Morarilor Medical Center
Bucharest
Romania

Desmond Burrows
Queens University
Belfast
UK

Jennifer Cahill
Occupational Dermatology Research and Education Centre
Skin and Cancer Foundation
Carlton South, Melbourne, VIC
Australia

Audris Chiang
University of California Medical School
San Francisco, CA
USA

David H. Chu
Scripps Clinic Medical Group
Division of Dermatology
LaJolla, CA
USA

Pieter J. Coenraads
Department of Dermatology
University Medical Centre Groningen, University of Groningen
Groningen
The Netherlands

David E. Cohen
Department of Dermatology and Allergic
Occupational and Environmental Dermatolo
NYU Langone Medical Center
New York University School of Medicine
New York, NY
USA

Luis Conde-Salazar
Servicio de Dermatología Laboral
Escuela Nacional de Medicina del Trabajo
Madrid
Spain

Emanuela Corsini
Department of Pharmacological Sciences
Università degli Studi di Milano
Milan
Italy

Christophe J. Le Coz
Unite Dermato–Allergologie
Hopitaux Universitaires de Strasbourg
Strasbourg
France
and
Cabinet de Dermatologie
Strasbourg
France
and
Laboratoire de Dermatochimie
Strasbourg
France

Thomas L. Diepgen
Department of Clinical Social Medicine
Occupational and Environmental Dermatology
University of Heidelberg
Heidelberg
Germany

Thomas F. Downham
Department of Dermatology
Henry Ford Health System
Taylor, MI
USA

Hans Drexler
Institute and Outpatient Clinic for Occupational
Social and Environmental Medicine
Friedrich-Alexander-University
Erlangen
Germany

Peter Elsner
Department of Dermatology
University Hospital Jena
Jena
Germany

Patricia G. Engasser
Department of Dermatology
University of California
San Francisco, CA
USA
and
Department of Dermatology
Stanford University
Menlo Park, CA
USA

John S. C. English
Department of Dermatology
Queen's Medical Centre Nottingham
Nottingham University Hospital
Nottingham
UK

Tuula Estlander
Terveystalo Healthcare Oyj
Helsinki
Finland

Manigé Fartasch
Department for Clinical and Experimental
Occupational Dermatology
Institute for Prevention and Occupational Medicine of
the German Social Accident Insurance
Institute of the Ruhr-University, Bochum (IPA)
Bochum, NRW
Germany

James Ferguson
Photobiology Unit
Ninewells Hospital and Medical School
Dundee
Scotland, UK

Sara K. Flores
Rush University
Chicago, IL
USA

Mari-Ann Flyvholm
National Research Centre for the Working Environment
Copenhagen
Denmark

Iain S. Foulds
Institute of Occupational and Environmental Medicine
University of Birmingham
UK

Undine Frank
Department of Dermatology and Allergology
University Hospital
Jena
Germany

Sigfrid Fregert
Department of Occupational and Environmental Dermatology
Skåne University Hospital Malmö, Lund University
Malmö
Sweden

Malin Frick-Engfeldt
Department of Occupational and Environmental Dermatology
Skåne University Hospital (SUS), Lund University
Malmö
Sweden

Peter J. Frosch
Klinikum Dortmund gGmbH, Hautklinik
Lehrstuhl Dermatologie der Universitat
Witten/Herdecke
Dortmund
Germany

Menno T. W. Gaastra
Outpatients Clinic for Dermatology and Flebology
Centrum Oosterwal
Alkmaar
The Netherlands

Seema Garg
Department of Dermatology
Rotherham District General Hospital
Rotherham
UK

David J. Gawkrodger
Department of Dermatology
Royal Hallamshire Hospital and University of Sheffield
Sheffield
UK

Matthias Gebhardt
Department of Dermatology
University Hospital Jena
Jena
Germany

Johannes Geier
Information Network of Departments of Dermatology (IVDK), Department of Dermatology
University of Goettingen
Goettingen
Germany

Susan Gibbs
Department of Dermatology
VU University Medical Centre
Amsterdam
The Netherlands

Chee Leok Goh
National Skin Centre
Singapore

Margarida Gonçalo
Clinic of Dermatology, Unit of Skin Allergy
University Hospital and Faculty of Medicine
University of Coimbra
Coimbra
Portugal

An Goossens
Department of Dermatology
University Hospital K.U. Leuven
Leuven
Belgium

Anton C. de Groot
Acdegroot publishing
Wapserveen
The Netherlands

Birgitta Gruvberger
Department of Occupational and Environmental Dermatology
Skåne University Hospital Malmö, Lund University
Malmö
Sweden

Michael Haeberle
Dermatological Office
Kuenzelsau
Germany

Wolfgang Harth
Chefarzt
Klinik für Dermatologie und Allergologie Vivantes Klinikum Spandau
Berlin
Germany

B. M. Hausen
Netherlands Center of Occupational Diseases
Amsterdam
The Netherlands

Uwe-Frithjof Haustein
Department of Dermatology, Venerology and Allergology
University of Leipzig
Leipzig
Germany

Pirji Heikkila

Felipe Heras
Servicio de Dermatología Laboral
Escuela Nacional de Medicina del Trabajo
Madrid
Spain

Rudolf A. Herbst
Klinik für Hautkrankheiten und Allergologie
HELIOS Hauttumorzentrum Erfurt, HELIOS Klinikum Erfurt
Erfurt, Thüringen
Germany

Philip Hewitt
UK and Eurotox Registered Toxicologist Head of Molecular and Cellular Toxicology (MS-DDT-EMT)
Early, Genetic & Molecular Toxicology, Toxicology Merck Serono R&D Merck KGaA
Darmstadt
Germany

P. Heydari
Department of Dermatology
Republic University of Uruguay
Montevideo
Uruguay

Uwe Hillen
Klinik für Dermatologie
Universitätsklinikum Essen
Essen
Germany

Monica Hindsén
Department of Occupational and Environmental Dermatology
Malmö University Hospital
Malmö
Sweden

J. Hobson
Occupational Physician
Michelin Tyre Plc
Stoke-on-Trent
UK

Daniel J. Hogan
Bay Pines VA Healthcare System
Bay Pines, FL
USA

Linn D. Holness
Department of Occupational and Environmental Health
St Michael's Hospital
University of Toronto
Toronto, ON
Canada

Erhard Hölzle
Department of Dermatology and Allergology
Klinikum Oldenburg
Oldenburg
Germany

Bernhard Homey
Department of Dermatology
University Hospital Duesseldorf
Duesseldorf
Germany

Ingrid M. W. van Hoogstraten
Department Pathology
VU University Medical Center
Amsterdam
The Netherlands

Jurij J. Hostynek
Department of Dermatology
University of California
San Francisco, CA
USA

Arieh Ingber
Department of Dermatology
Hadassah University Hospital
Ein-Karem, Jerusalem
Israel

Marléne Isaksson
Department of Occupational and Environmental Dermatology, Department of Clinical Sciences Malmö
Lund University, Skane University Hospital
Malmö
Sweden

Swen-Malte John
Department of Dermatology
Environmental Medicine and Health Theory
University of Osnabrueck
Osnabrueck
Germany

Riitta Jolanki
Control of Hypersensitivity Diseases
Finnish Institute of Occupational Health (FIOH)
Helsinki
Finland

Anneli Julander
Institute of Environmental Medicine
Karolinska Institutet
Stockholm
Sweden

Frank H. W. Jungbauer
Department of Dermatology
University Medical Centre Groningen, University of Groningen
Groningen
The Netherlands

Jakob Mutanu Jungersted
Department of Dermatology
University of Copenhagen, Faculty of Health Science
Copenhagen, NV
Denmark

Lasse Kanerva
Section of Dermatology
Finnish Institute of Occupational Health
Helsinki
Finland

Ann-Therese Karlberg
Dermatochemistry and Skin Allergy, Department of Chemistry and Molecular Biology
University of Gothenburg
Gothenburg
Sweden

Olaf Kaup
Department of Dermatology, Environmental Medicine and Health Theory, Laboratory of Dermatological Microbiology
University of Osnabrueck
Osnabrueck
Germany

Alastair C. Kerr
Photobiology Unit
Ninewells Hospital and Medical School
Dundee
Scotland, UK

Sanja Kezic
Coronel Institute of Occupational Health
Academic Medical Center
University of Amsterdam
Amsterdam
The Netherlands

Mirja Kiilunen
Finnish Institute of Occupational Health
Biomonitoring Laboratory
Arinatie 3
Helsinki
Finland

Nikolaus Knoepffler
Department of Applied Ethics
Friedrich-Schiller-Universität
Jena
Germany

Peter Knuschke
Department of Dermatology
Medical Faculty Carl Gustav Carus
Technische Universität Dresden
Dresden
Germany

David Koh
Saw Swee Hock School of Public Health
National University of Singapore
Singapore
Republic of Singapore

Andrea Krautheim
Information Network of Departments of Dermatology (IVDK)
Georg-August-University
Goettingen
Germany

Jean-Marie Lachapelle
Unit of Occupational and Environmental Dermatology
Catholic University of Louvain
Montigny-le-Tilleul
Belgium

A. Lahti
Department of Dermatology
University California Medical School
San Francisco, CA
USA

Kaija Lammintausta
Department of Dermatology
Turku University Hospital
Turku
Finland

Lilla Landeck
Department of Dermatology
Environmental Medicine Health Theory
University of Osnabrueck
Osnabrueck
Federal Republic of Germany

Antti Lauerma
Control of Hypersensitivity Diseases
Finnish Institute of Occupational Health
Helsinki
Finland
and
Professor of Applied Dermatology and Allergology Skin and Allergy Hospital
Helsinki University Central Hospital
Meilahdentie
Helsinki
Finland

Aneta Lazarov
Tel Aviv University
Tel Aviv
Israel
and
Contact Dermatitis Service
Meir Hospital Sapir Medical Center
Kfar Saba
Israel

Adriene Lee
Department of Dermatology
Monash Medical Centre and St Vincent's Hospital
Melbourne, VIC
Australia

Gerda J. Lensen
Department of Dermatology
University Medical Centre Groningen
University of Groningen
Groningen
The Netherlands

Jean-Pierre Lepoittevin
Laboratoire de Dermatochimie
University of Strasbourg
Strasbourg cedex
France

Holger Lessmann
Information Network of Departments of Dermatology (IVDK), Department of Dermatology
University of Goettingen
Goettingen
Germany

Carola Lidén
Institute of Environmental Medicine
Karolinska Institutet
Stockholm
Sweden

B. Lietzberg
Department of Dermatology
Venerology and Allergology
University of Leipzig
Leipzig
Germany

Markku Linnainmaa
Material and Particle Research
Finnish Institute of Occupational Health
Kuopio
Finland

Christopher R. Lovell
Kinghorn Dermatology Unit
Royal United Hospital, Combe Park
Bath (Somerset)
UK

Calum C. Lyon
Department of Dermatology
York Hospitals NHS Foundation Trust, York Hospital
York
UK

Chuan Ma
Department of Dermatology
Peking University Third Hospital
Beijing
China

Jakob T. Madsen
Department of Dermatology and Allergy Centre
Odense University Hospital, University of Southern Denmark
Odense
Denmark

Vera Mahler
Department of Dermatology
University Hospital of Erlangen
Erlangen
Germany

Howard I. Maibach
Department of Dermatology
University of California
San Francisco, CA
USA

Stefan F. Martin
Allergy Research Group
Department of Dermatology
University Freiburg Medical Center
Freiburg
Germany

Birgitta Meding
Unit of Occupational and Environmental Dermatology
Institute of Environmental Medicine
Karolinska Institutet
Stockholm
Sweden

Torkil Menné
Department of Dermato-Allergology
National Allergy Research Centre, Gentofte Hospital
Hellerup
Denmark

Matthias Moehrle
Praxisklinik Tübingen – Haut und Venen
Tuebingen
Germany
and
Department of Dermatology
Universitaets–Hautklinik
Tuebingen
Germany

Sonja C. Molin
Department of Dermatology and Allergology
Ludwig-Maximilian-University
Munich
Germany

Megan Morrison
Bay Pines VA Healthcare System
Bay Pines, FL
USA

Rodrigo da Mota
Department of Dermatology
University Hospital Duesseldorf
Duesseldorf
Germany

Frank O. Nestle
St. John's Institute of Dermatology, King's College London and NIHR Biomedical Research Centre, Guy's and St. Thomas' Hospitals
London
UK

Mai A. Ngo
California Department of Pesticide Regulation
California Environmental Protection Agency
California, CA
USA

Rosemary Nixon
Occupational Dermatology Research and Education Centre
Skin and Cancer Foundation
Carlton South, Melbourne, VIC
Australia

Fanchon Noël
Laboratory of Skin Bioengineering and Imaging
Department of Dermatopathology
University Hospital of Liège, CHU Sart Tilamn
Liège
Belgium

Michael O'Malley
University of California
Davis, CA
USA

Anthony D. Ormerod
Department of Applied Medicine, Department of Dermatology
University of Aberdeen
Aberdeen
UK

Christopher L. Packham
EnviroDerm Services
North Littleton, Evesham
UK

Philippe Paquet
Laboratory of Skin Bioengineering and Imaging
Department of Dermatopathology
University Hospital of Liège, CHU Sart Tilamn
Liège
Belgium

Marcel C. Pasch
Department of Dermatology
Radboud University Nijmegen Medical Centre
Nijmegen
The Netherlands

Anand N. Patel
Department of Dermatology
Queen's Medical Centre Nottingham University Hospital
Nottingham
UK

Stefanie E. Pentinga
Department of Dermatology and Allergology
VU University Medical Center
Amsterdam
The Netherlands

Pirkko Pfäffli
Helsinki
Finland

Gérald E. Piérard
Laboratory of Skin Bioengineering and Imaging
Department of Dermatopathology
University Hospital of Liège
CHU Sart Tilamn
Liège
Belgium

Jana Präßler
Department of Dermatology and Allergology
Friedrich Schiller University
Jena
Germany

Lorine Preudhomme
Laboratory of Skin Bioengineering and Imaging
Department of Dermatopathology
University Hospital of Liège
CHU Sart Tilamn
Liège
Belgium

Claire Quah
Occupational Safety and Health Division
Ministry of Manpower, Singapore
Singapore
Republic of Singapore

Pascale Quatresooz
Laboratory of Skin Bioengineering and Imaging
Department of Dermatopathology
University Hospital of Liège, CHU Sart Tilamn
Liège
Belgium

Hanspeter Rast
Division of Occupational Medicine
Suva (Swiss Accident Insurance Fund)
Luzern
Switzerland

R. Riala

Thomas Rustemeyer
Department of Dermatology/Allergology
VU University Medical Center
Amsterdam
The Netherlands

Thomas Ruzicka
Department of Dermatology and Allergology
Ludwig-Maximilian-University
Munich
Germany

Carmen Maria Sălăvăstru
Colentina Clinical Hospital
"Carol Davila" University of Medicine and Pharmacy
Bucharest
Romania

Rik J. Scheper
Department Pathology
VU University Medical Center
Amsterdam
The Netherlands

Sibylle Schliemann
Department of Dermatology
University Hospital Jena
Jena
Germany

Anne Schmidt
Büro für Berufsdermatologie
Nürnberg
Germany

Jochen Schmitt
Medizinische Fakultät, Institut und Poliklinik für Arbeits– und Sozialmedizin
TU Dresden
Dresden
Germany
and
Universitäts AllergieCentrum
Universitätsklinikum Dresden
Dresden
Germany

Claudia Schröder-Kraft
Institute for Interdisciplinary Dermatologic Prevention and Rehabilitation (iDerm) at the University of Osnabrueck and Dermatologic Centre, Trauma Hospital
Hamburg
Germany

Nana Y. Schuerer
Department of Dermatology, Environmental Medicine and Health Theory, Laboratory of Dermatological Microbiology
University of Osnabrueck
Osnabrueck
Germany

Geetanjali Sethi
Wexner Medical Center at The Ohio State University
Columbus, OH
USA

Mili Shah
Department of Dermatology
Royal Hallamshire Hospital and University of Sheffield
Sheffield
UK

Christoph Skudlik
Department of Dermatology
Environmental Medicine and Health Theory
University of Osnabrueck
Osnabrueck
Germany

V. Smith
Department of Dermatology
Queen's Medical Centre Nottingham
Nottingham University Hospital
Nottingham
UK

Retno W. Soebaryo
Department of Dermato-venereology Disease
University of Indonesia
Jakarta
Indonesia

Stephanie Soost
Department of Dermatology and Allergology
Charité– Universitätsmedizin Berlin
Berlin
Germany

Aieska De Souza
Department of Dermatology and Allergic
Occupational and Environmental Dermatolo
NYU Langone Medical Center
New York University School of Medicine
New York, NY
USA

Peter H. Soyer
Dermatology Research Centre, School of Medicine
The University of Queensland
Brisbane, QLD
Australia
and
Dermatology Department
Princess Alexandra Hospital
Brisbane
Australia

Radoslaw Spiewak
Department of Experimental Dermatology and Cosmetology
Jagiellonian University Medical College
Krakow
Poland
and
Instytut Dermatologii
Krakow
Poland

Markus F. C. Steiner
Environmental and Occupational Medicine
Department of Child Health
University of Aberdeen
Aberdeen
UK

Harma Stenveld
Centrum voor Huid en Arbeid
Velp
The Netherlands

K. Sugiura
Department of Environmental
Dermatology and Allergology Daiichi Clinic
Nagoya, Aichi
Japan

Päivikki Susitaival
Department of Dermatology
North Carelia Central Hospital
Joensuu
Finland

Katri Suuronen
Occupational Medicine
Finnish Institute of Occupational Health
Helsinki
Finland

Christiane Szliska
Department of Dermatology
Bethesda Hospital
Freudenberg
Germany

Kyllikki Tarvainen
Helsinki
Finland

Helen Taylor
EnviroDerm Services
Mitcheldean, Gloucestershire
UK

James S. Taylor
Department of Dermatology, Desk A-61
Dermatology-Plastic Surgery Institute Cleveland Clinic
Cleveland, OH
USA

Hermann-Josef Thierse
Laboratory of Immunology & Proteomics, Department of Dermatology
University Medical Centre Mannheim, Ruprecht Karls University of Heidelberg
Mannheim
Germany

Jacob P. Thyssen
Department of Dermato-Allergology
National Allergy Research Centre, Gentofte Hospital
Hellerup
Denmark

Tam Tiet
Ross University School of Medicine
Brooklyn, NY
USA

George-Sorin Ţiplica
Colentina Clinical Hospital
"Carol Davila" University of Medicine and Pharmacy
Bucharest
Romania

Akiva Trattner
Department of Dermatology
Rabin Medical Center
Petah Tiqwa
Israel
and
Tel Aviv University
Tel Aviv
Israel

Ron A. Tupker
Department of Dermatology
St Antonius Hospital
Nieuwegein
The Netherlands

Jukka Uitti
Team of Occupational Medicine
Finnish Institute of Occupational Health
Tampere
Finland

Wolfgang Uter
Department of Medical Informatics
Biometry and Epidemiology
University of Erlangen/Nürnberg
Erlangen
Germany

Kim Vander Hulst
Department of Dermatology
University Hospital K.U. Leuven
Leuven
Belgium

Markku Vanhanen
Finnair Health Services
Helsinki
Finland

J. P. Wietze van der Veen
Netherlands Institute for Pigment Disorders and
Department of Dermatology
Academic Medical Centre University of Amsterdam
Amsterdam
The Netherlands

Niels K. Veien
The Dermatology Clinic
Aalborg
Denmark

Juan Vilaplana
Barcelona
Spain

Jan E. Wahlberg

Penpun Wattanakrai
Division of Dermatology
Department of Medicine
Mahidol University, Ramathibodi Hospital
Bangkok
Thailand

Elke Weisshaar
Department of Clinical Social Medicine
University of Heidelberg
Heidelberg
Germany

Thomas Werfel
Department of Dermatology and Allergy
Hannover Medical School
Hannover
Germany

Aaron Wiener
University of California (UCSF)
Menlo Park, CA
USA

Annika Wilke
Department of Dermatology, Environmental Medicine and Health Theory
University of Osnabrueck
Osnabrueck
Germany

Mark S. Wilkinson
Dermatology Department
The General Infirmary
Leeds
UK

Jason D. L. Williams
Contact Dermatitis Investigation Unit
Salford Royal NHS Foundation Trust
University of Manchester Dermatology, Hope Hospital
Salford, Lancashire, Manchester
UK

Marjolein Wintzen
Department of Dermatology
VUmc Medical Center
Amsterdam
The Netherlands

Catriona I. Wootton
Department of Dermatology
Queen's Medical Centre Nottingham
Nottingham University Hospital
Nottingham
UK

Margitta Worm
Department of Dermatology and Allergology
Charité– Universitätsmedizin Berlin
Berlin
Germany

Britta Wulfhorst
Department of Dermatology
Environmental Medicine Health Theory
University of Osnabrueck
Osnabrueck
Federal Republic of Germany

Ian Yamaguchi
Department of Dermatology
University California Medical School
San Francisco, CA
USA

Maryam Yazdani
Netherlands Institute for Pigment Disorders and Department of Dermatology
Academic Medical Centre University of Amsterdam
Amsterdam
The Netherlands

Mirjana Ziemer
Department of Dermatology, Venerology and Allergology
University of Leipzig
Leipzig
Germany

Erik Zimerson
Department of Occupational and Environmental Dermatology
Malmö University Hospital
Malmö
Sweden

Section 1

General Aspects of Occupational Dermatology

1 Immunology and Barrier Function of the Skin

Thomas Rustemeyer[1] · *Manigé Fartasch*[2]
[1]Department of Dermatology/Allergology, VU University Medical Center, Amsterdam, The Netherlands
[2]Department for Clinical and Experimental Occupational Dermatology, Institute for Prevention and Occupational Medicine of the German Social Accident Insurance, Institute of the Ruhr-University, Bochum (IPA), Bochum, NRW, Germany

Core Messages

- A disturbed epidermal barrier may lead to irritant contact dermatitis.
- An enhanced penetration through skin barrier may facilitate sensitization.
- Immunological effects induced by pre-irritation and barrier alteration may further lead to the induction of allergic Typ IV-contact dermatitis and Type I (immediate type reaction) reactions or aggravate allergic reactions.

1 Introduction

The cutaneous permeability barrier largely resides in the outer layers of the epidermis, the stratum corneum (SC). The SC forms an effective barrier between the organism and the environment preventing invasion of pathogens and fending off chemical and physical assaults, as well as the unregulated loss of water and solutes.

It is both metabolically active and interactive with the underlying epidermal cell layers. Hence, it is important to consider SC as a dynamic feature rather than a fixed, inflexible barrier layer (see recent reviews and commentaries (Elias and Feingold 2006; Hoath 2001; Menon and Fartasch 2010; Menon 2003)).

Furthermore, the topic of the function and formation of the epidermal permeability barrier and the changes regarding its biophysical properties continues to be an important issue to understand regulation and development of the normal and abnormal epidermis (Fartasch 1997, 2004, 2005) and the perturbation of the epidermal permeability barrier, previously speculated to be just a symptom involved in skin diseases, is currently considered to be a primary pathophysiologic factor for many skin diseases.

A defective barrier function is characterized by an increased transepidermal water loss (TEWL), might be seen in disease entities with the disturbance of terminal differentiations (keratinisation disorders like different types of ichthyosis) and in inflammatory reactions of the epidermis, which influences epidermal proliferation and leads to incomplete cornification (like contact dermatitis, atopic dermatitis or psoriasis). In all cases the distribution, structure, and biochemistry of the intercellular lipid compartment of the SC, which are vital for the barrier function, are influenced leading to an impairment of the water diffusion barrier of the skin and probably facilitate penetration of various substances. Changes in epidermal differentiation of the corneocytes and lipid composition lead to a disturbed skin barrier, which allows the entry of environmental allergens, immunological reaction, and inflammation in atopic dermatitis. A disturbed skin barrier is important for the pathogenesis of contact dermatitis, ichthyosis, psoriasis, and atopic eczema.

2 Barrier: Structure and Biochemistry

The SC consists of protein-enriched differentiated extremely flattened and enucleated keratinocytes (Warner et al. 1995) filled with keratin and bounded with cornified envelope and cytoskeletal elements, as well as corneodesmosomes and lipid-enriched lamellar-arranged intercellular domains surrounding the corneocytes (➋ *Fig. 1.1*). The cornified cell envelope, a protein/lipid polymer structure, resides below the cytoplasmic membrane on the exterior of the corneocytes. The nucleated parts of the epidermis (➋ *Fig. 1.1*) also contribute to the barrier through tight, gap, and adherens junctions, as well as through desmosomes and cytoskeletal elements (so-called tonofibrils and the keratohyalin).

During epidermal differentiation lipids are synthesized in the keratinocytes of the lower parts of the

T. Rustemeyer, P. Elsner, S.M. John & H.I. Maibach (eds.), *Kanerva's Occupational Dermatology*,
DOI 10.1007/978-3-642-02035-3_1,

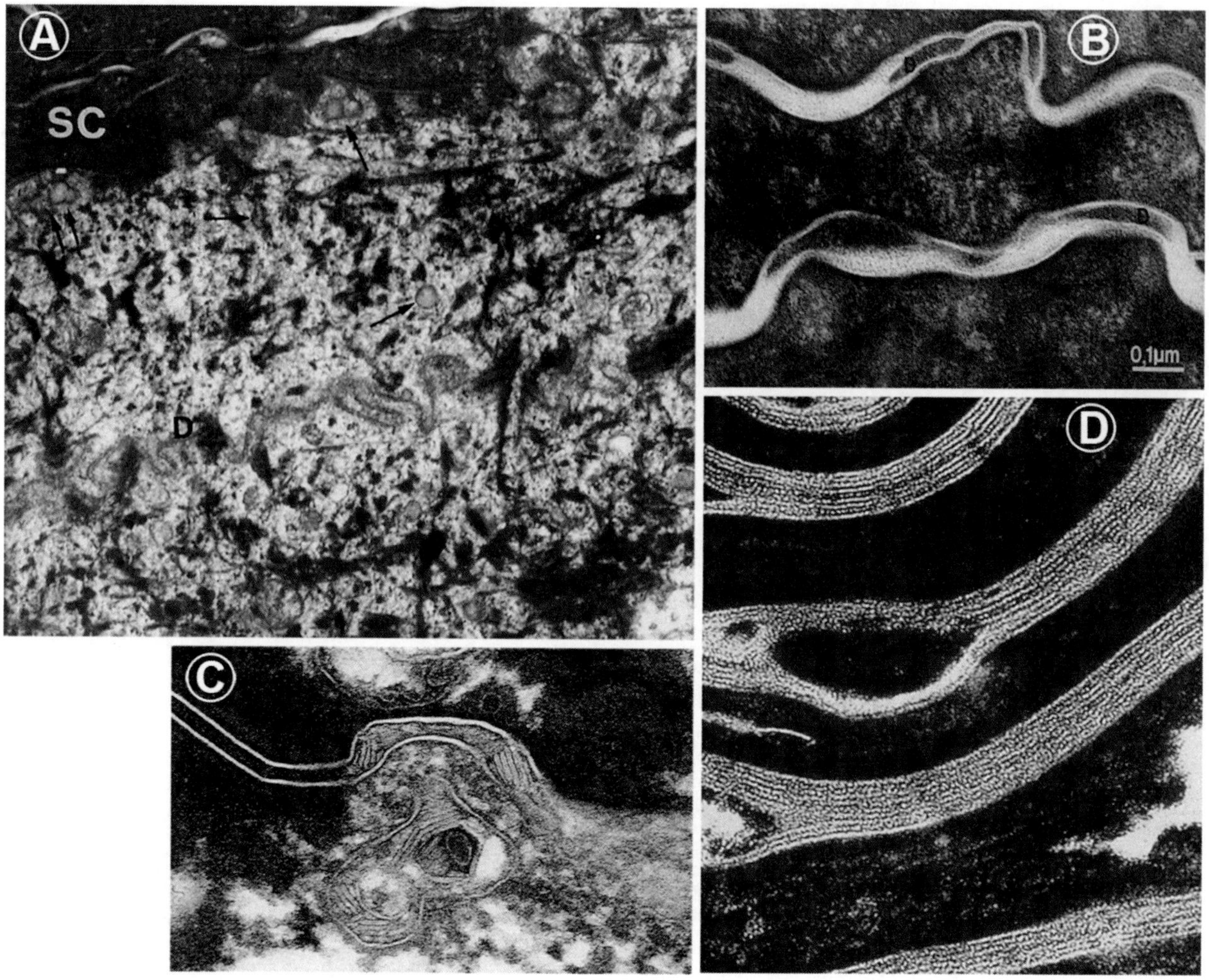

Fig.1.1
(a) Stratum corneum (*SC*)/Str. granulosum interface: The *upper layer* of stratum granulosum shows lamellar bodies (*arrow*) which are extruded in the intercellular spaces. (*D*) Desmosomes. (b) Stratum corneum shown by conventional OsO4 staining. (c) The lamellar bodies fuse with the upper membrane of the stratum granulosum cell and extrude their polar lipid content into the intercellular space. (d) After a transformation process the lipids are finally arranged into lipid bilayers. (b) and (d) RuO_4 staining

epidermal cells (stratum spinosum) and finally – in the upper parts of the epidermis (stratum granulosum/ stratum corneum interface) extruded into the extracellular domains via lamellar bodies (LB; Syn: keratinosomes, membrane-coating granules, and Odland bodies), where they form extracellular lipid-enriched layers. As most drugs and occupational substances applied onto the skin permeate in part along the lipid domains, the lipid organization is considered to be very important for the skin barrier function. Due to the exceptional stratum corneum lipid composition, with long chain ceramides, free fatty acids, and cholesterol as main lipid classes, the lipid organization is different from that of other biological membranes. In stratum corneum, two lamellar phases are present. Moreover, the lipids in the lamellar phases form predominantly crystalline lateral phases, but most probably a subpopulation of lipids forms a liquid phase (Bouwstra and Ponec 2006). The Ceramides A and B are covalently bound to cornified envelope proteins of the SC and form the backbone for the subsequent addition of free ceramides, free fatty acids, and cholesterol in the SC. Filaggrin – which forms the matrix of the corneocytes – is cross-linked to the cornified envelope and aggregates keratin filaments into macrofibrils. Formation and maintenance of barrier function is influenced by cytokines, 3', 5'-cyclic adenosine monophosphate and calcium.

3 The Role of the Epidermal Barrier Regarding Irritant and Allergic Contact Dermatitis

Contact dermatitis (Johansen et al. 1998), one of the most common skin diseases, has a great socioeconomic impact (Uter et al. 1998), especially as irritant contact dermatitis (ICD), is a frequent occupational disease, and represents a major health risk.

Irritation of the skin is accompanied by a complex array of epidermal and dermal metabolic responses. Previous studies have shown that structurally unrelated chemical irritants induce a different pattern of cellular damage to the viable parts of the epidermis when topically applied to human skin (Willis et al. 2001; Fartasch 1997). Further, the role of the epidermal barrier and its repair seems to be especially crucial for the epidermal responses since studies have shown that the epidermal keratinocyte actively participates in the modulation of inflammatory reactions induced by the injuring agent (Nickoloff and Naidu 1994; Tsai et al. 1994; von den Driesch et al. 1995; Wood et al. 1992). Additionally, there seems to be a precise relationship between barrier function (after barrier disruption) and cytokine expression (Nickoloff and Naidu 1994; Wilmer et al. 1994). The primary response to the irritation with the resulting barrier disruption should be the attempt to restore the protective barrier so that penetration of environmental hazards and further alteration of the keratinocytes are prevented.

The occurrence of allergic contact dermatitis (ACD) with previous or simultaneous irritation seems also to be common and this interaction has been investigated using human, animal, and in vitro skin models (Agner et al. 2002; Bonneville et al. 2007; Brasch et al. 1992; Grabbe et al. 1996; Jacobs et al. 2006; McLelland et al. 1991; Pedersen et al. 2004). Irritation and barrier alteration might facilitate the occurrence (induction) of allergic Type IV-contact dermatitis and Type I (immediate type reaction) reactions or aggravate allergic reaction (Bonneville et al. 2007). As mechanisms not only an enhanced penetration through skin barrier is discussed but also immunological effects (Agner et al. 2002; Basketter et al. 2007; Brasch et al. 1992; Grabbe et al. 1996; Jacobs et al. 2006; McLelland et al. 1991; Pedersen et al. 2004).

Combined effects of more allergens, more irritants, or allergens and irritants together are reported to produce an altered response compared to when applied separately (see Review (Pedersen et al. 2004)). Single versus repeated applications also elicits differential cytokine expressions in skin (de Jongh et al. 2007). The combined exposure of allergens and irritants may potentially influence irritant effects as well as allergenicity of the substances. Several types of interaction may exist: (1) an additive response, (2) a synergistic response, and (3) an antagonistic response (quenching), (Pedersen et al. 2004). In conclusion, the hapten-induced skin contact irritation conditions the development and the severity of ACD (Bonneville et al. 2007).

3.1 The Role of the Epidermal Barrier Regarding Type I (Immediate) and Type IV Sensitization of the Skin

3.1.1 Epidermal Barrier and Type I Reaction

Normally, aeroallergens do not make contact with antigen-presenting cells, such as Langerhans cells (LCs) in epidermis or other dendritic cells in subepithelial tissues, owing to the effectiveness of the cornified envelope, tight junctions between cells in the epidermis, and the barrier function of the basal lamina (details see also ➋ Chap. 14, "Mechanisms of Allergic Contact Dermatitis," by Rustemeyer).

But factors such as genetic, physical, chemical, and enzymatic activities of certain allergens like Der P 1 (de Jongh et al. 2008a, b), barrier alteration by mechanical or chemical trauma produced by house dust mites that affect one or more components of this multilayered barricade might increase the opportunities for allergens to penetrate into the epidermal layer and make contact with Langerhans cells which will initiate a T helper type II (Th II) response involving T cells, B cells, and immunoglobulin E (IgE) production, depending on the cytokine environment and/or other intrinsic properties of the host immune response. This has been supported by morphologic investigations using laser scanning method which have shown that the LHCs are also situated in the upper epidermis with their dendrocytes making contact with the lower regions of the SC (Bauer et al. 2001) and thus facilitating contact with foreign proteins which penetrate through small fissures in the barrier. Once initiated, this response is long lasting, with IgEs binding to mast cells in the skin, the lung, and other mucosae. Subsequent exposures of the host to allergens will activate mast cells, leading to allergic systemic symptoms such as conjunctivitis, rhinitis, asthma, urticaria, and angioedema (Incorvaia et al. 2008). Recent hypothesis (Callard and Harper 2007; Hudson 2006) also discuss an association between barrier dysfunction and IgE-mediated skin disorders (Type I reactions, immediate type) such as urticaria/angiodema which can be systemic in their expression and respiratory symptoms (with and without the combination with atopic dermatitis).

3.1.2 Epidermal Barrier and Type IV Reaction

Penetrating substances responsible for Type IV-contact dermatitis show certain physicochemical parameters and the ability for a certain chemical reactivity (Basketter et al. 2007; Kimber et al. 2003). Chemicals that possess the capacity to cause skin sensitization are reactive (electrophilic) or at least the precursors of an electrophile with a size less than 700 Da. The chemical species (haptens) covalently bound to skin protein then forms an antigen to which the immune system responds, and with sufficient exposure might lead to sensitization (Basketter et al. 2007). However, it is hypothesized that for this process to occur secondary stimuli (danger signals) are also necessary (Basketter et al. 2007; Bonneville et al. 2007; McLelland et al. 1991) and the sensitizing potency is linked to their ability to produce pro-inflammatory signal release which manifests clinically as ability for skin irritancy. They are capable to activate innate immunity causing irritant contact dermatitis and/or acquired specific immunity inducing allergic contact dermatitis (Saint-Mezard et al. 2004) and seem to stimulate Langerhans cells (LHC) – and induce their migration and maturation in antigen or non-antigen-dependent manner (Gallucci et al. 1999; Jacobs et al. 2006; McFadden and Basketter 2000).

Further, the presence and density of Langerhans cells play an important part in the induction of allergic type IV reactions. The constant ratio of epidermal Langerhans cells to other epidermal cells in healthy human skin (1 Langerhans cell keeps 53 epidermal cells under immune surveillance (Bauer et al. 2001)) is altered by experimental barrier disruption through acetone or sodium lauryl sulfate which increases the Langerhans cell density within the epidermis. Even standard patch testing using an occlusive patch test chamber, which leads to barrier disruption due to hyperhydration (Proksch and Brasch 1997) lead to altered LC ratios. Additionally, barrier disruption may in itself activate T-cells (Nishijima et al. 1997), indicating a link between the physical barrier and the immune barrier.

Studies using skin culture models have also shown that both skin irritation and contact allergens at nonirritating concentrations can accelerate LC migration (Jacobs et al. 2004) to the draining lymph nodes, indicating potential for initiating sensitization in vivo (see ➋ Chap. 104, "Identification of Skin Irritants and Allergens by In Vivo and In Vitro Methods").

3.1.3 Relationship Between Area of Barrier Exposure and Dose in Induction and Elicitation of Contact Hypersensitivity

One of the key questions is why do certain individuals develop allergic sensitization by vehicles whereas the larger majority of people tolerate contact with those substances without consequence (Friedmann 2006). Of course, some chemicals are more potent as sensitizers. A different exposure dose can be a factor; way of exposure, duration of exposure, and frequency of exposure are all factors that might influence the ability to induce a sensitization. Clearly studies with potent experimental sensitizers (2,4-dinitrochlorobenzne (DNCB), 2,4 dinitrofluornemzeme (DNFB)) have shown that an important factor seems to be the penetrating dose per unit area (Friedmann 2007) as key determinant of sensitization and with increasing concentration of allergen (e.g., DNCB v. 0.063%) a clear dose-response relationship (Friedmann et al. 1983; Friedmann 2007) is seen, whereas the total dose may vary over a wide range. Therefore crucial factors seem to be what is happening on the skin surface. A number of molecules of the antigen will diffuse into the stratum corneum, and in the case of ointments, drugs etc. the number being determined by the concentration in the vehicle and the partition coefficients and relative solubility of the substance in the vehicle and the SC.

3.2 Susceptibility of Individuals to Sensitization and Irritation

There are very strong interindividual variations in susceptibility to irritation which might be either explained by the differences in skin barrier properties as shown by analyzing SLS permeation rate through stratum corneum (de Jongh et al. 2006) but also due to the variations regarding the inflammatory response (Judge et al. 1996).

A combination between individual susceptibility to allergies (Type IV) and irritant reactions has been shown in persons who show cytokine gene polymorphism (IL1 genotypes, TNF-alpha genotypes) (Blomeke et al. 2008; de Jongh et al. 2008a, b; Westphal et al. 2003).

There is also clinical evidence that certain genetic disorders with barrier impairment show only an increase in type I reactions and not type IV. This is known for the barrier defect in Netherton's syndrome (NS), a rare autosomal recessive disorder characterized by a generalized inflammatory skin condition, a specific hair shaft abnormality (trichorrhexis invaginata) and invariably, atopic manifestations. NS shows loss of SC cohesion (desmoglein) due to defective LEKTI expression (loss of function mutations in SPINK5 chrom.5q31) (Chavanas et al. 2000) and probably secondarily induced altered lamellar body secretion and stratum corneum membrane structures (Fartasch et al. 1999). As a consequence, there is a loss of SC adhesion affecting skin barrier functions. NS shares several clinical features with atopic eczema (AE) and greater inflammatory reactivity.

AE, a common chronic inflammatory skin disease characterized by dry, scaly skin, increased TEWL, increased permeability to topical medications, and susceptibility to Type I allergy is the other disease where abnormality of barrier function and occurrence of Type I reaction is seen. Immunologically induced alterations in epidermal differentiation result in increased epidermopoises (Jensen et al. 2004; Proksch et al. 1990). Additionally, recent hypothesis discuss an association between barrier dysfunction, filaggrin mutation in subgroups of atopic eczema (associated with allergic asthma, rhinitis, Type-I-IgE sensitisation, early onset and persistence into adulthood of coexisting ichthyosis vulgaris (O'Reagan and Irvine 2008). There has always been ongoing discussion if the barrier in non-eczematous skin of atopics is disturbed and thus facilitates penetration. Recent studies have shown that penetration of SLS is increased in uninvolved skin of patients with atopic eczema (Jakasa et al. 2006). They also found that penetration coefficient of polyethylene glycols (PEGs) of varying molecular sizes through atopic skin was twice as high compared to normal skin. In some cases, the epidermis of nonaffected atopic skin shows signs of suppressed synthesis of keratohyalin (Profilaggrin) with a histologically perceptible reduction in thickness of granular layers (Fartasch et al. 1998; Jensen et al. 2004). Yet, recent molecular biological studies show a firm association between ichthyosis vulgaris and loss-of-function mutations in the filaggrin (FLG) gene as carried by 16.7–56% of all individuals with atopic dermatitis (Palmer et al. 2006). Additionally, recent studies have highlighted an association of FLG mutations in atopics with nickel sensitization (Type IV sensitization) and with reactions with jewelry but with lack of association with Type IV sensitizations to other common haptens (Novak et al. 2008). Since filaggrin is a precursors of natural moisturizing factors (NMF) inside of the corneocytes, the relation with penetration of small allergens is not clear (Kezic 2008).

References

Agner T, Johansen JD, Overgaard L et al (2002) Combined effects of irritants and allergens. Synergistic effects of nickel and sodium lauryl sulfate in nickel- sensitized individuals. Contact Dermatitis 47:21–26

Basketter DA, Kan-King-Yu D, Dierkes P et al (2007) Does irritation potency contribute to the skin sensitization potency of contact allergens? Cutan Ocul Toxicol 26:279–286

Bauer J, Bahmer FA, Worl J et al (2001) A strikingly constant ratio exists between Langerhans cells and other epidermal cells in human skin. A stereologic study using the optical disector method and the confocal laser scanning microscope. J Invest Dermatol 116:313–318

Blomeke B, Brans R, Dickel H et al (2008) Association between TNFA-308 G/A polymorphism and sensitization to para-phenylenediamine: a case-control study. Allergy 64(2):279–283

Bonneville M, Chavagnac C, Vocanson M et al (2007) Skin contact irritation conditions the development and severity of allergic contact dermatitis. J Invest Dermatol 127:1430–1435

Bouwstra JA, Ponec M (2006) The skin barrier in healthy and diseased state. Biochim Biophys Acta 1758:2080–2095

Brasch J, Burgard J, Sterry W (1992) Common pathogenetic pathways in allergic and irritant contact dermatitis. J Invest Dermatol 98:166–170

Callard RE, Harper JI (2007) The skin barrier, atopic dermatitis and allergy: a role for Langerhans cells? Trends Immunol 28:294–298

Chavanas S, Bodemer C, Rochat A et al (2000) Mutations in SPINK5, encoding a serine protease inhibitor, cause Netherton syndrome. Nat Genet 25:141–142

de Jongh CM, Jakasa I, Verberk MM et al (2006) Variation in barrier impairment and inflammation of human skin as determined by sodium lauryl sulphate penetration rate. Br J Dermatol 154:651–657

de Jongh CM, Lutter R, Verberk MM et al (2007) Differential cytokine expression in skin after single and repeated irritation by sodium lauryl sulphate. Exp Dermatol 16:1032–1040

de Jongh CM, John SM, Bruynzeel DP et al (2008a) Cytokine gene polymorphisms and susceptibility to chronic irritant contact dermatitis. Contact Dermatitis 58:269–277

de Jongh CM, Khrenova L, Kezic S et al (2008b) Polymorphisms in the interleukin-1 gene influence the stratum corneum interleukin-1 alpha concentration in uninvolved skin of patients with chronic irritant contact dermatitis. Contact Dermatitis 58:263–268

Elias PM, Feingold KR (2006) Permeability barrier homeostasis. In: Elias PM, Feingold KR (eds) Skin barrier. Taylor and Francis, New York \London

Fartasch M (1997) Epidermal barrier in disorders of the skin. Microsc Res Tech 38:361–372

Fartasch M (2004) The epidermal lamellar body: a fascinating secretory organelle. J Invest Dermatol 122:XI–XII

Fartasch M (2005) Atopic dermatitis and other skin diseases. In: Fluhr J, Elsner P, Berardesca E, Maibach F (eds) Bioengineering of the skin: water and stratum corneum, 2nd edn. CRC Press, Boca Raton, pp 160–169

Fartasch M, Schnetz E, Diepgen TL (1998) Characterization of detergent-induced barrier alterations – effect of barrier cream on irritation. J Investig Dermatol Symp Proc 3:121–127

Fartasch M, Williams ML, Elias PM (1999) Altered lamellar body secretion and stratum corneum membrane structure in Netherton syndrome: differentiation from other infantile erythrodermas and pathogenic implications. Arch Dermatol 135:823–832

Friedmann PS (2006) Contact sensitisation and allergic contact dermatitis: immunobiological mechanisms. Toxicol Lett 162:49–54

Friedmann PS (2007) The relationships between exposure dose and response in induction and elicitation of contact hypersensitivity in humans. Br J Dermatol 157:1093–1102

Friedmann PS, Moss C, Shuster S et al (1983) Quantitative relationships between sensitizing dose of DNCB and reactivity in normal subjects. Clin Exp Immunol 53:709–715

Gallucci S, Lolkema M, Matzinger P (1999) Natural adjuvants: endogenous activators of dendritic cells. Nat Med 5:1249–1255

Grabbe S, Steinert M, Mahnke K et al (1996) Dissection of antigenic and irritative effects of epicutaneously applied haptens in mice. Evidence that not the antigenic component but nonspecific proinflammatory effects of haptens determine the concentration-dependent elicitation of allergic contact dermatitis. J Clin Invest 98:1158–1164

Hoath S (2001) The skin as a neurodevelopmental interface. Neo Rev 2:269–281

Hudson TJ (2006) Skin barrier function and allergic risk. Nat Genet 38:399–400

Incorvaia C, Frati F, Verna N et al (2008) Allergy and the skin. Clin Exp Immunol 153(1):27–29

Jacobs JJ, Lehe CL, Cammans KD et al (2004) Assessment of contact allergens by dissociation of irritant and sensitizing properties. Toxicol In Vitro 18:681–690

Jacobs JJ, Lehe CL, Hasegawa H, Das PK et al (2006) Skin irritants and contact sensitizers induce Langerhans cell migration and maturation at irritant concentration. Exp Dermatol 15:432–440

Jakasa I, de Jongh CM, Verberk MM et al (2006) Percutaneous penetration of sodium lauryl sulphate is increased in uninvolved skin of patients with atopic dermatitis compared with control subjects. Br J Dermatol 155:104–109

Jensen JM, Folster-Holst R, Baranowsky A et al (2004) Impaired sphingomyelinase activity and epidermal differentiation in atopic dermatitis. J Invest Dermatol 122:1423–1431

Johansen JD, Skov L, Volund A et al (1998) Allergens in combination have a synergistic effect on the elicitation response: a study of fragrance-sensitized individuals. Br J Dermatol 139:264–270

Judge MR, Griffiths HA, Basketter DA et al (1996) Variation in response of human skin to irritant challenge. Contact Dermatitis 34:115–117

Kezic S (2008) Methods for measuring in-vivo percutaneous absorption in humans. Hum Exp Toxicol 27:289–295

Kimber I, Dearman RJ, Gerberick GF et al (2003) Designation of substances as skin sensitizing chemicals: a commentary. Hum Exp Toxicol 22:439–443

McFadden JP, Basketter DA (2000) Contact allergy, irritancy and "danger". Contact Dermatitis 42:123–127

McLelland J, Shuster S, Matthews JN (1991) "Irritants" increase the response to an allergen in allergic contact dermatitis. Arch Dermatol 127:1016–1019

Menon GK (2003) Caveolins in epidermal lamellar bodies: skin is an interactive interface, not an inflexible barrier. J Invest Dermatol 120:XV–XVI

Menon G, Fartasch M (2010) Structural and functional correlations of skin barrier in health and disease: models and evaluation. In: Monteiro-Riviere NA (ed) Toxicology of the skin: targets organ series. Informa Healthcare, New York

Nickoloff BJ, Naidu Y (1994) Perturbation of epidermal barrier function correlates with initiation of cytokine cascade in human skin. J Am Acad Dermatol 30:535–546

Nishijima T, Tokura Y, Imokawa G et al (1997) Altered permeability and disordered cutaneous immunoregulatory function in mice with acute barrier disruption. J Invest Dermatol 109:175–182

Novak N, Baurecht H, Schafer T et al (2008) Loss-of-function mutations in the filaggrin gene and allergic contact sensitization to nickel. J Invest Dermatol 128:1430–1435

O'Reagan GM, Irvine AD (2008) The role of filaggrin loss-of-function mutations in atopic dermatitis. Curr Opin Allergy Clin Immunol 8(5):406–410

Palmer CN, Irvine AD, Terron-Kwiatkowski A et al (2006) Common loss-of-function variants of the epidermal barrier protein filaggrin are a major predisposing factor for atopic dermatitis. Nat Genet 38:441–446

Pedersen LK, Johansen JD, Held E (2004) Augmentation of skin response by exposure to a combination of allergens and irritants – a review. Contact Dermatitis 50:265–273

Proksch E, Brasch J (1997) Influence of epidermal permeability barrier disruption and Langerhans' cell density on allergic contact dermatitis. Acta Derm Venereol 77:102–104

Proksch E, Elias PM, Feingold KR (1990) Regulation of 3-hydroxy-3-methylglutaryl-coenzyme A reductase activity in murine epidermis. Modulation of enzyme content and activation state by barrier requirements. J Clin Invest 85:874–882

Saint-Mezard P, Rosieres A, Krasteva M et al (2004) Allergic contact dermatitis. Eur J Dermatol 14:284–295

Tsai JC, Feingold KR, Crumrine D et al (1994) Permeability barrier disruption alters the localization and expression of TNF alpha/protein in the epidermis. Arch Dermatol Res 286:242–248

Uter W, Schnuch A, Geier J et al (1998) Epidemiology of contact dermatitis. The information network of departments of dermatology (IVDK) in Germany. Eur J Dermatol 8:36–40

von den Driesch P, Fartasch M, Huner A et al (1995) Expression of integrin receptors and ICAM-1 on keratinocytes in vivo and in an in vitro reconstructed epidermis: effect of sodium dodecyl sulphate. Arch Dermatol Res 287:249–253

Warner RR, Bush RD, Ruebusch NA (1995) Corneocytes undergo systematic changes in element concentrations across the human inner stratum corneum. J Invest Dermatol 104:530–536

Westphal GA, Schnuch A, Moessner R et al (2003) Cytokine gene polymorphisms in allergic contact dermatitis. Contact Dermatitis 48:93–98

Willis CM, Shaw S, De Lacharrière O et al (2001) Sensitive skin: an epidemiological study. Br J Dermatol 145(2):258–263

Wilmer JL, Burleson FG, Kayama F et al (1994) Cytokine induction in human epidermal-keratinocytes exposed to contact irritants and its relation to chemical-induced inflammation in mouse skin. J Invest Dermatol 102:915–922

Wood LC, Jackson SM, Elias PM et al (1992) Cutaneous barrier perturbation stimulates cytokine production in the epidermis of mice. J Clin Invest 90:482–487

2 Percutaneous Penetration

Aaron Wiener[1] · *Howard I. Maibach*[2]
[1]University of California (UCSF), Menlo Park, CA, USA
[2]Department of Dermatology, University of California (UCSF), San Francisco, CA, USA

Core Messages

- Percutaneous absorption is measured in vivo through different methods, including radioactivity measurements in blood and excreta, surface recovery, surface disappearance, biological and pharmacological responses, and the stripping method.
- In vitro methods include measuring absorption rates through excised skin into a receptacle designed to mimic actual dermatological conditions.
- Measuring the radioactivity in a subject's blood and excreta is commonly practiced, and involves administering a compound often radiolabeled, in order to measure the amount of the original dose that has penetrated the skin.
- Surface recovery and disappearance methods involve administering a compound on the skin and measuring the rate of recovery from the surface of the skin, or the rate of its disappearance.
- The stripping method deals with measuring the concentration of a chemical in the stratum corneum through successive tape applications and removals.
- The vehicle by which a compound is transferred to the skin has an effect on its absorption rate.

1 Introduction

Workplace chemical exposure especially when repetitive over weeks, months, and years has led to systemic (internal organ) toxicity such as bladder cancers and sterility. This chapter provides an introduction into the readily available techniques for quantification of some of the ten steps to percutaneous penetration. It is suspected that some idiopathic diseases will eventually be documented to be due to such occupational skin exposure. This summary will also provide an introduction to the methodology so that occupational health workers can most efficiently collaborate with laboratories performing such assays.

2 In Vivo Methods for Determining Absorption

2.1 Radioactivity in Excreta and Blood

Percutaneous absorption in vivo is commonly determined by chemical measurements (and/or radioactivity) taken in a subject's or animal's blood or excreta. Since levels of a compound are often found to be below the level required for detection after topical application, it may be necessary to use radiotracer methodology. The administered compound is usually labeled with ^{14}C or tritium, and is applied to the skin. Measurements of radioactivity are taken from blood, urine, or urine and feces combined. Radioactivity measurements include a mixture of both the applied compound and metabolites (Wester and Maibach 2002). Since the compound in question can be retained in the body, or exit through methods other than the measured excreta (sweating, breathing), the amount of radioactivity detected is corrected by measuring the amount of radioactivity excreted after parenteral administration.

The equation for determining percutaneous absorption is expressed as:

$$\frac{\text{Total Radioactivity After Topical Administration}}{\text{Total Radioactivity After Parenteral Administration}} \times 100 = \% \tag{2.1}$$

Measurements of radioactivity in the blood of a subject or animal have given similar results to those obtained through excreta (Wester and Maibach 2002). A limitation on using radioactivity as a means of measuring absorption is that metabolism by the skin is not accounted for.

2.2 Surface Recovery

This method of determining percutaneous absorption involves measuring the amount of compound that penetrates into the skin. It is assumed that the difference

T. Rustemeyer, P. Elsner, S.M. John & H.I. Maibach (eds.), *Kanerva's Occupational Dermatology*,
DOI 10.1007/978-3-642-02035-3_2,

between the applied dose and the residual dose collected after the trial period is the absorption. Finding accurate results with this approach is difficult, since materials are able to leave the surface of the skin without penetrating, thus full recovery of the residual compound is never assured. Properties of the radioisotope, penetrant and vehicle place limits on how useful this method can be (Wester and Maibach 2002).

2.3 Surface Disappearance

Using appropriate instrumentation, it is possible to measure the disappearance of a ^{14}C labeled compound from the surface of the skin. Disappearance of ^{14}C is due to both the movement of the compound into the skin, and the quenching effect of beta rays bouncing back into the measuring instrument, which places a limitation on this kind of measurement. Placing a sheet of stratum corneum over a quantity of radiolabeled chemical and then measuring the radioactivity with an external device will exhibit this effect (Wester and Maibach 2002).

2.4 Biological/Pharmacological Response

In this method of determining percutaneous absorption, a biological assay is substituted for a chemical assay. The great disadvantage of this method is that assays are limited to compounds that will elicit a response that can be easily and accurately measured. Results from this methodology are more qualitative than quantitative (Wester and Maibach 2002).

Another method to estimate in vivo percutaneous absorption in animals is whole body autoradiography. This procedure provides a picture of absorption followed by the involvement of other body tissues (Wester and Maibach 2002).

2.5 Stripping Method

The stripping method determines percutaneous absorption through measurements of the concentration of a chemical in the stratum corneum after a 30-min application period. Through linear extrapolation, the percutaneous absorption is predicted for application periods longer than 30 min. The chemical is applied to the skin of animals or humans, and after the application period, the stratum corneum is removed by successive tape application and removal (Rougier et al. 2002). A linear relationship between the stratum corneum's content of a tested chemical and the percutaneous absorption using standard radioactive excretion methods has been established. This method has considerable advantage over other methods in the fact that non-radiolabeled assays may be tested, and urinary and fecal excretions become unnecessary. This method requires more research to establish more accurate limitations (Wester and Maibach 2002).

3 In Vitro Methods for Determining Absorption

Skin removed from humans or animals can be used to measure percutaneous penetration of chemicals. The skin is stretched over the opening of a collecting receptacle, with the epidermal side facing up. The chemical in question is applied, and fluid in the receptacle is assayed at intervals to measure the penetration. The collecting fluid used is usually water or saline. Either the entire thickness of the skin or just the epidermis may be used for in vitro assays. Some variations on this method require that the excised skin be covered with fluid containing the chemical, but the preferred method is to expose one side of the skin to the air, while the underside is bathed in saline or other receptacle fluids. Since diffusion requires a concentration gradient, some receptacles have been designed to allow repeated replacement of the receptacle fluid. The fluid is usually continuously stirred and maintained at a temperature appropriate to the chemical in question (Maibach and Patrick 2001).

This method is advantageous to in vivo assays because it allows highly toxic chemicals to be tested, but just like any other method, it has limitations. Because skin must be stored before its use in an assay, it cannot be assumed that the skin will metabolize chemicals in the same manner as living skin. When using full thickness skin, the dermis can influence the absorptive process. This influence may be minimized by heat separating the dermis from the stratum corneum; however, the viability of the skin may be destroyed in the process. Often, the suitability of each specimen of skin is verified through a measurement of the penetration of titrated water through the tissue, prior to a chemical assay (Maibach and Patrick 2001).

4 Influence of Vehicle on Percutaneous Absorption

Substances added to a formula can influence the release, absorption, and action of an applied drug. Experiments have shown that doses administered through different vehicles will initially have differing absorption rates. As time passes, the influence of the vehicle decreases, and the absorption rate becomes constant for all vehicles. Vehicles have the ability to increase or decrease water levels in the stratum corneum, resulting in increased or decreased penetration. Additionally, it is hypothesized that a multiple-dose administration of a vehicle can "reactivate/solubilize" the original chemical preventing it from binding to the skin, as well as push the chemical into and through the skin (Wester and Maibach 2001).

5 Skin Cleansing and Decontamination

While it is largely assumed that washing with soap and water can decontaminate a chemical from the skin, the skin and the body are often subjected to enhanced penetration because the decontamination will increase absorption of the chemical. Soap and water washing is effective at removing visible dirt and odor, however, it may not be the best as a skin cleanser, especially in the case of fat-soluble materials (Maibach and Patrick 2001).

Taken together, utilization of techniques such as the above should aid the chemical and laboratory correlation of amounts of percutaneous penetration and biologic effect. Freeman documents examples of penetration leading to disease in man (Freeman and Maibach 1991), and the National Academy of Sciences implies that many human cancers may, in fact, be due to chemical exposure.

References

Freeman S, Maibach HI (1991) Systemic toxicity caused by absorption of drugs and chemicals through the skin. In: Marzulli FN, Maibach HI (eds) Dermatotoxicology, 4th edn. Hemisphere Publishing Corporation, New York, pp 851–875, Chap 35

Maibach H, Patrick E (2001) Dermatotoxicology. In: Hayes AW (ed) Principles and methods of toxicology. Taylor and Francis, Philadelphia, pp 1039–1084, Chap 22

Rougier A, Dupuis D, Lotte C, Maibach HI (2002) Stripping method for measuring percutaneous absorption in vivo. In: Bronaugh RL, Maibach HI (eds) Topical absorption of dermatological products. Marcel Dekker, New York, pp 241–245, Chap 16

Wester RC, Maibach HI (2001) Principles and practice of percutaneous absorption. In: Barel AO, Paye M, Maibach HI (eds) Handbook of cosmetic science and technology. Marcel Dekker, New York, pp 53–59, Part 3: Safety considerations, Chap 7

Wester RC, Maibach HI (2002) In vivo methods for percutaneous absorption measurement. In: Bronaugh RL, Maibach HI (eds) Topical absorption of dermatological products. Marcel Dekker, New York, pp 145–149, Chap 9

3 Quality of Life (QoL) in Relation to Occupational Skin Diseases

Tove Agner
Department of Dermatology, Bispebjerg Hospital, University of Copenhagen, Faculty of Health Science, Copenhagen, NV, Denmark

Core Messages

- Different instruments for assessment of QoL are compared and discussed. The influence of demographic and disease-related factors on HR-QoL is discused, and the importance of including HR-QoL instruments as outcomes in clinical trials is emphasized

1 Introduction

During the last decade, there has been an increased focus on research in health-related quality of life (HR-QoL). This concept generally refers to the perception of the effects of a disease and its impact on the patient's daily functioning, and incorporates the patient's personal perspective including the impact of disease on everyday life activities and life satisfaction. Research in QoL has rapidly become an important outcome variable in dermatology research, where today also other aspects such as the total burden of the disease are being taken into account. QoL instruments may be used in the clinical setting as part of severity assessment. Especially within the area of occupational (skin) diseases evaluation of QoL is important, since factors such as sick leave and job change or job loss may significantly influence the patient's perception of the severity of the disease. Different instruments for assessment of QoL will be discussed in this chapter.

Severity assessment of occupational hand eczema (OHE) is important in clinical settings as well as in research. Traditionally, severity of skin diseases is evaluated from the clinical appearance of the disease by the doctor. However, this evaluation may very well be misleading. The clinical picture reveals only the current situation, and not the frequency of eruptions, does not include the subjective perception of symptoms such as pain and itch, or psychosociological factors such as restraints on leisure activities, sick leave from work, impaired social contact, time-consuming treatments, and even embarrassment. The clinical symptoms may also bother different people to a very different degree: While some people as an example tend to live quite well with a mild or even moderate eczema, other people may find it extremely bothering, either due to limitation in handling of ordinary daily living activities or due to cosmetic reasons, and some may find it to cause a social handicap.

The relation between self-rated severity and severity assessment based on standardized medical certificates issued by dermatologists in a population of 758 patients with occupational hand eczema was recently compared. Major differences in the criteria for self-rated severity versus dermatologist-rated severity were found (Cvetkovski et al. 2005). While 40% of the patients responding to a questionnaire described themselves as having severe eczema, only 18% were judged as severe by the dermatologists. These data makes it clear that disease should be evaluated from more angles than just the classical medical angle, in research projects as well as in the daily clinical work.

Public health has been defined as "the science and art of promoting health," based on the understanding that health is a process engaging social, mental, spiritual, and physical well-being (Kickbusch 1989). Health-related quality of life (HR-QoL) generally refers to the perception of the effects of a disease and its impact on the patient´s daily functioning. HR-QoL is the perceived functioning in physical, psychological, and social dimensions and is therefore a more holistic assessment than the clinical examination.

During the last decade, there has been an increased focus on research in HR-QoL. This research incorporates the patient's personal perspective including the impact of disease on everyday life activities and life satisfaction. Since Finlay and Khan first introduced the Dermatology Life Quality Index (DLQI) as a practical clinical measure for disease severity (Finlay and Khan 1994), research in QoL has rapidly become an important outcome variable in dermatology research. Also other aspects such as the total burden of the disease, including the economical costs borne by the society, have increasingly been taken into account (Diepgen et al. 2007).

T. Rustemeyer, P. Elsner, S.M. John & H.I. Maibach (eds.), *Kanerva's Occupational Dermatology*,
DOI 10.1007/978-3-642-02035-3_3, © Springer-Verlag Berlin Heidelberg 2012

2 How Is QoL Assessed?

HR-QoL is usually assessed using patient questionnaires, either emailed or posted to patients or given to patient to fill in before, during, or after consultation. Three different instruments are used:

- *Generic questionnaires.* This type of questionnaire gives a global assessment of the impact on HR-QoL. These questionnaires are not specific for dermatological diseases, and incorporate information about influence of the general health status on QoL. Generic questionnaires can be used across different patient populations, enabling researchers to compare QoL in skin diseases with other medical conditions (Harlow et al. 2000; Moberg et al. 2009).
- *Dermatology-specific questionnaires.* These questionnaires are designed to assess the impact on QoL in different skin conditions and are therefore able to describe specific effects in dermatology. This type of questionnaire allows comparison between the impact on QoL between different skin diseases (Finlay and Khan 1994; Finlay 1998; Chren et al. 1996; Anderson and Rajagopalan 2001). This instrument has also been developed for children with skin diseases (Lewis-Jones and Finlay 1995).
- *Disease-specific questionnaires.* Disease-specific questionnaires focus on one particular skin condition, for example, acne (Mallon et al. 1999). At the moment a disease-specific questionnaire for hand eczema has not yet been developed.

2.1 Examples of Available Self-report Questionnaires

- Generic questionnaires:
  - SF36 (Short Form 36) (Harlow et al. 2000)

    The SF-36 is a multipurpose, short-form health survey with only 36 questions. It yields an 8-scale profile of functional health and well-being scores as well as psychometrically based physical and mental health summary measures.
  - EQ-5D (http://www.euroqol.org/, Moberg et al. 2009)

    The EQ-5D is a standardized instrument for use as a measure of health outcome. Applicable to a wide range of health conditions and treatments, it provides a simple descriptive profile and a single index value for health status. The EQ-5D is a generic instrument that has been developed and refined by an international group of researchers since 1987. Respondents complete the EQ-5D by choosing one of three severity levels on five questions covering five dimensions: mobility, self-care, usual activities, pain/discomfort, and anxiety/depression Responses on the five dimensions are used to create an index, a single value for each health profile.
- Dermatology-specific questionnaires
  - DLQI (Finlay and Khan 1994; Finlay 1998)

    The DLQI consists of 10 items (score range 0–30) covering six categories: symptoms and feelings, daily activities, leisure, work/school, personal relationships and treatment, and takes 3–5 min to complete. Score 0 means that QoL is totally unaffected by the disease, while a score of 30 is maximum. Scores above 10 are generally accepted as severe influence on QoL of the disease (Cvetkovski et al. 2006).
  - Skindex-29 (Chren et al. 1996)

    Skindex-29 consists of 29 items and one additional item concerning adverse effects of treatment. It consists of three separate subscales covering symptoms, functioning, and emotions. The response format is a five-point Likert scale. Completion time is estimated to be 5 min.
  - Dermatology-Specific Quality of Life (DSQL) (Anderson and Rajagopalan 2001)

    The DSQL consists of 52 items and is estimated to take 15 min to complete. The items cover seven different subscales: physical symptoms, activities of daily living, social functioning, work/school functioning, self-perception, general mental health, and vitality.
- Disease-specific questionnaires
  - Acne Quality of Life Questionnaire (Mallon et al. 1999)

    An example of a HR-QoL questionnaire aiming at assessing the effect of specific disease on QoL

For assessment of HR-QoL in dermatology, the best validated instruments/questionnaires are DLQI and Skindex-29 (Chren et al. 1997; De Korte et al. 2002; Zachariae et al. 2000). Components from the generic questionnaire, the SF-36, have been used to supplement a number of dermatology-specific questionnaires, and recently the use of EQ-5D has also been positively evaluated (Moberg et al. 2009).

3 QoL in Occupational Skin Disease

The most commonly notified and recognized occupational skin disease in Scandinavia as well as in most European countries is hand eczema, which comprises more than 90% of all occupational skin diseases. No major changes in the incidence of occupational hand eczema have taken place for the past few decades, despite preventive efforts and legislative regulations. In Scandinavia, the one-year prevalence of hand eczema is 9.5% (Meding and Jarvholm 2004), and it is estimated that 10% of all cases of hand eczema is due to occupational exposures (Lerbaek et al. 2008). The prognosis is generally poor (Shah et al. 1996; Wall and Gebauer 1991), and in a recent study, more than 70% of patients with occupational hand eczema reported activity in the eczema after 12 years (Meding et al. 2005). In some cases, hand eczema adversely affected patients' social lives. Hand eczema may constitute a considerable problem for the individual, since it may disturb sleep and hamper leisure activities and, as an occupational skin disease, it may lead to sick leave and eventually result in a change of occupation (Fowler 2008). Individuals with more severe, recurrent, or protracted hand eczema can endure serious psychosocial symptoms and a substantially impaired QoL.

It has also been investigated if people with hand eczema showed symptoms of depression. In a study comprising 758 individuals with work-related hand eczema, QoL and depression was investigated by questionnaires using the DLQI and the Hamilton score for depression, respectively. The mean DLQI total score was 5.5 for all patients and 7.8 for severe cases of occupational hand eczema. Twenty percent had low QoL defined as DLQI values above 10 (Cvetkovski et al. 2006). This means that patients with severe occupational hand eczema have equal impairment of QoL as patients with atopic dermatitis and psoriasis. The prevalence of moderate-to-severe depression was 9%, which is not far from the prevalence in the background population, and symptoms of depression could not directly be connected to hand eczema. An independent association was found between severe OHE and severely affected QoL. Also low socioeconomic status was independently associated with low QoL (Cvetkovski et al. 2006), and there was a trend showing that the negative effect on QoL was increasing with increasing age. A 12 months follow-up was performed, using the same questionnaires, and only minor changes in QoL and in depressive symptoms were found after 12 months of follow-up (➋ *Table 3.1*).

In a recent study, with participation of 10 different patch test clinics from different European countries, QoL was investigated in patients with hand eczema, using the DLQI instrument (Agner et al. 2008, 2009). A total of 416 (252 women and 164 men) were included, age 39 years, and 52% of all cases were reported as occupational hand eczema. DLQI was 8.0 for women and 7.0 for men, although the severity of hand eczema was assessed significantly higher for men than for women. High age and personal history of atopic eczema were independent risk factors for low QoL, and sick leave was also found to have a significantly negative influence on QoL. Severity of hand

◘ Table 3.1
Factors influencing QoL in patients with occupational hand eczema (OHE)

Factors influencing QoL	Influence on QoL	Reference
Severity	Severe OHE is associated with low QoL	Agner et al. 2008; Cvetkovski et al. 2006
Age	High age is related to low QoL	Agner et al. 2008; Cvetkovski et al. 2006
Gender	More impaired QoL for females than for males	Agner et al. 2008; Wallenhammar et al. 2004
Socioeconomic status	Low socioeconomic status is associated with low QoL	Cvetkovski et al. 2006
Atopy	Previous or current atopic eczema is associated with low QoL	Agner et al. 2008; Cvetkovski et al. 2006
Sick leave	Sick leave is associated with low QoL	Agner et al. 2008
Allergic contact dermatitis	The effect of allergic contact dermatitis is discussed	Kadyk et al. 2003; Diepgen et al. 2009
Early diagnosis	Early diagnosis has a positive influence on QoL.	Kadyk et al. 2003
Change of job	Associated with low QoL	Kadyk et al. 2003

eczema, as assessed by the HECSI scoring system (Held et al. 2005), was found significantly positively related to DLQI scores, while subgroups of hand eczema was not related to QoL (Diepgen et al. 2009).

The effect of allergic contact dermatitis on QoL was investigated (Kadyk et al. 2003). A total of 428 subjects with allergic contact dermatitis were, at varying times after diagnosis, mailed the Skindex-16 dermatology-specific questionnaire, modified to include an additional five items pertaining to occupational impact. The results showed that occupationally related allergic contact dermatitis was associated with worse QoL, and that hand involvement also had a significantly negative impact on QoL. Subjects that had changed jobs because of allergic contact dermatitis had more severe QoL impairment than any other group analyzed, with significantly worse scores on 17 of the 21 QoL items. Patients with allergic contact dermatitis of the face were significantly more bothered by the appearance of their skin. Early diagnosis was shown to have a positive influence of QoL. It was concluded that allergic contact dermatitis has an appreciable effect on QoL, especially when it affects the hands, the face, or is occupationally related. Of the four scales included in our study, the emotions scale suffered the greatest effect. Emotional impact is therefore an important measure of QoL in allergic contact dermatitis patients (Kadyk et al. 2003).

A comparison between a generic questionnaire (SF-36) and the dermatology-specific questionnaire (DLQI) for assessment of HR-QoL in patients with hand eczema was performed (Wallenhammar et al. 2004). The QoL was significantly negatively affected by hand eczema, measured with both SF-36 and DLQI. The SF-36 showed more impaired HR-QoL for females than for males, in the mental health dimension, whereas no gender-related differences were detected with the DLQI., and it was concluded that in this aspect the SF-36 was superior (Wallenhammar et al. 2004).

Another population-based study also used a generic questionnaire, the EQ-5D (Moberg et al. 2009). A questionnaire was sent to 57,009 randomly selected individuals aged 18–84 years. The questionnaire included a validated question concerning hand eczema ("have you ever had hand eczema"), as well as the EQ-5D. The study confirms that HR-QoL measured with the EQ-5D is negatively affected in individuals with hand eczema. The mean EQ-5D index was significantly lower for those with hand eczema than for those without, both in the group as a whole and within all age and gender subgroups. This indicates that hand eczema has an impact on HR-QoL for all those affected. The EQ-5D index was of the same size as those for psoriasis and asthma, all three common diseases with an impact on public health (Moberg et al. 2009).

4 QoL Score Used for Regulation of Therapies

In the last decade, new high-cost medical therapies have been marketed for a number of dermatological, with biologicals used for treatment of psoriasis as an example. Within the area of hand eczema, introduction of Alitretinoin is another example. To be able to control the costs for the society for these new medications regulation of when and to which patients the medicaments may be used has been introduced by the authorities. Severity assessment of the disease has become important within this discussion, and here also the impact of the disease on the quality of life of the patient has been looked upon (Smith et al. 2009; Ingram et al. 2009). Recently the NICE guidelines for use of Alitretinoin have used DLQI values for recommendation of treatment (DLQI above 15) (http://www.nice.org.uk/TA177, Rodgers et al. 2010).

Assessment of disease severity for work-related skin disease/occupational hand eczema is important when new treatment options become available and when multidisciplinary care for hand eczema is introduced (van Gils et al. 2009). HR-QoL has become an increasingly important aspect of this, but new instruments have become available which evaluates also the effect of treatment from the patient´s point of view. The "Patient Benefit Index" (PBI) is a validated instrument for the assessment of such benefits in patients with skin diseases, where patients rate the importance of specific treatment needs before treatment and benefits achieved after treatment (Augustin et al. 2009). This instrument has also been introduced for evaluation of treatment benefit in patients with hand eczema (Blome et al. 2009).

Counting the HR-QoL in the total assessment of severity of skin disease, including work-related skin diseases, has become an important part of outcome measures for epidemiological studies and RCT-studies, and is also used increasingly in the clinical setting, where treatment guidelines may sometimes demand that QoL should be assessed. To date, no specific instrument for chronic hand eczema (CHE) has been published. Dermatology-specific questionnaires, supplemented with some questions from generic questionnaires, seem today to be the most valid instruments.

References

Agner T, Andersen KE, Brandao FM, Bruynzeel DP, Bruze M, Frosch P, Gonçalo M, Goossens A, Le Coz CJ, Rustemeyer T, White IR, Diepgen T; EECDRG (2008) Hand eczema severity and quality of life: a cross-sectional, multicentre study of hand eczema patients. Contact Dermatitis 59:43–57

Agner T, Andersen KE, Brandao FM, Bruynzeel DP, Bruze M, Frosch P, Gonçalo M, Goossens A, Le Coz CJ, Rustemeyer T, White IR, Diepgen T; EECDRG (2009) Contact sensitisation in hand eczema patients-relation to subdiagnosis, severity and quality of life: a multicentre study. Contact Dermatitis 61(5):291–296

Anderson RT, Rajagopalan R (2001) Effects of allergic dermatosis on health-related quality of life. Curr Allergy Asthma Rep 1(4): 309–315

Augustin M, Radtke MA, Zschocke I, Blome C, Behechtnejad J, Schäfer I, Reusch M, Mielke V, Rustenbach SJ (2009) The patient benefit index: a novel approach in patient-defined outcomes measurement for skin diseases. Archives Dermatol Res 301(8):561–571

Blome C, Maares J, Diepgen T, Jeffrustenbach S, Augustin M (2009) Measurement of patient-relevant benefits in the treatment of chronic hand eczema–a novel approach. Contact Dermatitis 61(1):39–45

Chren MM, Lasek RJ, Quinn LM, Mostow EN, Zyzanski SJ (1996) SKINDEX: a quality of life measure for patients with skin disease. Reliability, validity and responsivness. J Invest Dermatol 107(5): 707–713

Chren MM, Lasek RJ, Quinn LM et al (1997) Convergent and discriminant validity of a generic and a disease-specific instrument to measure quality of life in patients with skin disease. J Invest Dermatol 108:103–107

Cvetkovski RS, Jensen H, Olsen J, Johansen JD, Agner T (2005) Relation between patients and physicians severity assessment of occupational hand eczema. Br J Dermatol 153(3):596–600

Cvetkovski RS, Zachariae R, Jensen H et al (2006) Quality of life and depression in a population of occupational hand eczema patients. Contact Dermatitis 54:106–111

De Korte J, Mombers FM, Sprangers MA et al (2002) The suitability of quality-of-life questionnaires for psoriasis research: a systematic literature review. Arch Dermatol 138:1221–1227

Diepgen TL, Agner T, Aberer W, Berth-Jones J, Cambazard F, Elsner P, McFadden J, Coenraads PJ (2007) Management of chronic hand eczema. Contact Dermatitis 57(4):203–210

Diepgen TL, Andersen KE, Brandao FM, Bruze M, Bruynzeel DP, Frosch P, Gonçalo M, Goossens A, Le Coz CJ, Rustemeyer T, White IR, Agner T; European Environmental and Contact Dermatitis Research Group (2009) Hand eczema classification: a cross-sectional, multicentre study of the aetiology and morphology of hand eczema. Br J Dermatol 160(2):353–358. Epub 2008 Oct 23

Finlay AY, Khan GK (1994) Dermatology life quality index (DLQI)–a simple practical measure for routine clinical use. Clin Exp Dermatol 19:210–216

Finlay AY (1998) Quality of life assessment in dermatology. Semin Cutan Med Surg 17(4):291–296

Fowler J (2008) Chronic hand eczema: a prevalent and challenging skin condition. Cutis 82(Suppl 4):4–8

Harlow D, Poyner T, Finlay AY et al (2000) Impaired quality of life of adults with skin disease in primary care. Br J Dermatol 143: 979–982

Held E, Skoet R, Johansen JD, Agner T (2005) The hand eczema severity index (HECSI): a scoring system for clinical assessment of hand eczema. A study of inter- and intraobserver reliability. Br J Dermatol 152(2):302–307

Ingram JR, Martin JA, Finlay AY (2009) Impact of topical calcineurin inhibitors on quality of life in patients with atopic dermatitis. Am J Clin Dermatol 10(4):229–237

Kadyk DL, McCarter K, Achen F et al (2003) Quality of life in patients with allergic contact dermatitis. J Am Acad Dermatol 49:1037–1048

Kickbusch I (1989) Approaches to an ecological base for public health. Health Promot 4:265–268

Lerbaek A, Kyvik KO, Ravn H, Menné T, Agner T (2008) Clinical characteristics and consequences of hand eczema – an 8-year follow-up study of a population-based twin cohort. Contact Dermatitis 58(4):210–216

Lewis-Jones MS, Finlay AY (1995) The children's dermatology life quality index (CDLQI): initial validation and practical use. Br J Dermatol 132(6):942–949

Mallon E, Newton JN, Klassen A, Stewart-Brown SL, Ryan TJ, Finlay AY (1999) The quality of life in acne: a comparison with general medical conditions using generic questionnaires. Br J Dermatol 140(4): 672–676

Meding B, Järvholm B (2004) Incidence of hand eczema-a population-based retrospective study. J Invest Dermatol 122(4):873–877

Meding B, Lantto R, Lindahl G, Wrangsjö K, Bengtsson B (2005) Occupational skin disease in Sweden–a 12-year follow-up. Contact Dermatitis 53(6):308–313

Moberg C, Alderling M, Meding B (2009) Hand eczema and quality of life: a population-based study. Br J Dermatol 161(2):397–403

Rodgers M, Griffin S, Paulden M, Slack R, Duffy S, Ingram JR, Woolacott N, Sculpher M (2010) Alitretinoin for severe chronic hand eczema: a NICE single technology appraisal. Pharmacoeconomics 28(5): 351–362

Shah M, Lewis FM, Gawkrodger DJ (1996) Prognosis of occupational hand dermatitis in metalworkers. Contact Dermatitis 34:27–30

Smith CH, Anstey AV, Barker JN, Burden AD, Chalmers RJ, Chandler DA, Finlay AY, Griffiths CE, Jackson K, McHugh NU, McKenna KE, Reynolds NJ, Ormerod AD; (Chair of Guideline Group). British association of dermatologists' guidelines for biologic interventions for psoriasis 2009. Br J Dermatol 161(5):987–1019

Van Gils RF, van der Valk PG, Bruynzeel D, Coenraads PJ, Boot CR, van Mechelen W, Anema JR (2009) Integrated, multidisciplinary care for hand eczema: design of a randomized controlled trial and cost-effectiveness study. BMC Public Health 9:438

Wall LM, Gebauer KA (1991) A follow-up study of occupational skin disease in Western Australia. Contact Dermatitis 24:241–243

Wallenhammar L-M, Nyfjäll M, Lindberg M et al (2004) Health-related quality of life and hand eczema – a comparison of two instruments, including factor analysis. J Invest Dermatol 122:1381–1389

Zachariae R, Zachariae C, Ibsen H et al (2000) Dermatology life quality index: data from Danish inpatients and outpatients. Acta Derm Venereol (Stockh) 80:272–276

4 Pharmacoeconomics of Occupational Diseases

Matthias Augustin
Institute for Health Services Research in Dermatology and Nursing (IVDP) and Hamburg Center for Health Economics (HCHE), University of Hamburg, Hamburg, Germany

Core messages

- From the economic point of view, occupational skin diseases are relevant to the payers, the patients, and society.
- Major cost drivers are treatment costs (direct costs), cost for losses of work productivity (indirect costs), and the patients' burden of disease (intangible costs).
- From the societal view, the great number of persons affected by occupational skin disease is crucial.
- Effective treatments for occupational skin diseases reduce the cost burden, and increase work productivity and the patients' quality of life.
- Preventive measures can be cost-effective if applied in time and provided to persons at defined risks.
- Cost–benefit evaluation of interventions for occupational skin diseases requires a long-term assessment period.

1 Introduction

Due to its increasing frequency and the wide-ranging consequences for the affected patients, occupational skin diseases are of great socioeconomic importance. In light of this, clinical and epidemiological research is devoted increasingly to the effect of the disease on quality of life and to costs. This chapter presents the status of research in these two areas.

In all studies published to date, there is a marked economic relevance of occupational skin diseases. Depending on the severity and the impact on work, the annual costs are in the same range or even exceed those for chronic inflammatory skin disease like psoriasis and atopic eczema. Moreover, significant limitations of quality of life are reported for patients with occupational skin diseases. The stress for these patients in many studies exceeds that of other skin diseases and also of other chronic diseases.

2 Basic Considerations on Economic Issues in Occupational Skin Diseases

Medical economy or health economy is an empirical and theoretical, interdisciplinary science that aims at recording the production and allocation of health services related to resource consumption and costs. The focus in this is a balanced use and distribution of goods, such as personnel, apparatus, medications, hospitals, and preventive and diagnostic measures, and the attendant efficiency, effectiveness, quality, and fairness in dealing with them.

Pharmacoeconomics is a subarea of health economics. It evaluates the costs and cost–benefit ratios of drugs and – in a larger sense – of therapeutic procedures. Medical interventions are economically sound if the costs are in an appropriate ratio to the benefits. "Benefit" is determined either in the form of medical parameters (such as skin scores), monetary units (such as costs of disease), or intangible values (such as quality of life, satisfaction).

It must be emphasized that from an economical point of view, there is no intervention which is per se "too expensive." The price is only to be viewed as in a favorable or unfavorable relationship to the achieved benefit. For this reason, a balance is needed between the costs accrued and the benefit achieved by an intervention.

2.1 Definition and Evaluation of Costs

According to international rules, costs in health economics are generally divided into three categories (➋ *Table 4.1*): direct costs, indirect costs, and intangible costs.

Direct costs are costs for the health service (public or private health insurance system, national health system) and costs for the patients (out-of-pocket expenses). They directly derive from diagnostic, therapeutic, and

T. Rustemeyer, P. Elsner, S.M. John & H.I. Maibach (eds.), *Kanerva's Occupational Dermatology*,
DOI 10.1007/978-3-642-02035-3_4,

Table 4.1
Forms of costs in pharmacoeconomic evaluations

Cost form	Perspective
Direct costs →	Costs in connection with treatment
	(a) Costs for the payers
	(b) Costs for the patient (out-of-pocket expenses)
Indirect costs →	Costs to the economy arising from illness
Intangible costs →	Non-monetary costs (e.g., quality of life impairment)

Table 4.2
Causes of relevant direct (1, 2) and indirect (3) costs in occupational skin diseases

1.Payer (Insurance/health service)	2. Patient	3. Economy
Drugs UV-therapy Outpatient Fees (consultations) Hospitalization Auxiliary materials Preventive measures (facultative)	Self-medication Care products Prescription fees Patient-paid transportation Extra dietary costs Extra costs for protective measures Informational material	Lost working days Loss of productivity at work Costs for changes of work place

preventive procedures. Indirect costs included the secondary impact of a disease due to losses of productivity and functional capacity. For this, they are accounted as costs for the national economy. Finally, "intangible costs" are raised to the patients for their burden of disease and losses of quality of life.

In discussing costs, it is thus necessary to cite the cost perspective. In many clinical studies, only the costs of the drugs, that is, only a part of the direct costs, are recorded. From the point of view of the health insurance system, the total treatment costs are relevant, but not the direct costs for the patient. From the perspective of the economy, the ability of the patient with occupational dermatitis to work and his productivity are of interest. This may raise a conflict of interest since payments from the health insurances for treatment of occupational diseases (raising direct costs for them) may lead to improved work ability (reducing indirect costs for the employers). For this, economists prefer to assess health economic parameters from a global societal perspective which includes all distinct perspectives.

In general, direct costs in health care derive from fees to doctors or hospitals and from costs for medication and other health devices (Spilker 1996). Moreover, transportation and other nonmedical costs can also be of importance. ➔ *Table 4.2* shows a summary of important cost-inducing factors in the direct costs.

International comparison shows that there are considerable differences in health systems and in the mechanisms of cost reimbursement for patients with occupational skin diseases. Direct and indirect costs and their perspectives strongly depend on the national health system, the health market, and the reimbursement system.

2.2 Definition and Evaluation of Quality of Life and Patient Benefits

The term "quality of life" (QoL) is a construct which cannot be directly measured. However, it is of crucial importance in outcomes measurement, being one of the major criteria for benefits from medical interventions. Parameters like QoL which need to be obtained directly from the patient are called "patient-reported outcomes" (PRO).

In its general sense, QoL includes all conditions necessary for the well-being of an individual in society. In a narrower sense, it reflects the well-being of a person in relation to his state of health. In such sense, QoL is termed "health-related quality of life" (HRQoL). Among the factors in health-related QoL are "physical health," "emotional health," "social life," and "functional capacity in everyday living" (Brock 1996; Schipper et al. 1996). The "health-related quality of life" can further be differentiated into "generic" quality of life, referring to general health conditions, and "disease-specific quality of life" which reflects the particular QoL situation in a given disease.

The patients' quality of life has been emphasized increasingly as a target criterion in almost every area of medicine over the past decade. In addition to the clinical course and effects of costs, quality of life is increasingly included as an outcomes parameter in economic studies (Spilker 1996).

Data on quality of life are needed not only in clinical studies, but also in everyday practice. It is self-explanatory that, in treating a patient with atopic dermatitis, we obtain an impression of whether that patient's quality of life is impaired and the extent to which the planned treatment measures will have an effect on this. The patient's quality of life has always been the focus of clinical treatment in this respect, even when it was not so explicitly stated in the past.

Moreover, quality of life is a decisional parameter in health economics and health politics in order to distribute the limited resources of the health system as fairly as possible where they are needed. It is an expressed health-political objective in all modern societies to apply the necessary financial resources to maintain or reinstate the quality of life in chronically ill patients. In order to do this, reliable data will be needed in the future on which to base these so-called cost allocations.

Assessing quality of life is based on the patient's subjective view. Thus, it can only be measured by interrogating the patient or his relatives ("proxies"). For methodological reasons, QoL is mostly assessed by standardized questionnaires instead of interviews. These questionnaires can be generic or diseases specific, the first permitting QoL assessment in a great range of diseases or even healthy persons, the latter being more adequate for the evaluation of problems specific to a certain disease. Hence, the choice of the right QoL questionnaire is strongly depending on the particular purpose and on the study design.

Numerous instruments have been published for the assessment of quality of life in dermatology and allergology, some being also feasible for occupational diseases. These include: Skindex-29, DLQI (Dermatology Life Quality Index; Chren et al. 1996), DSQL (Dermatology-specific Quality of Life; Anderson and Rajagopalan 1997), and DQOLS (Dermatology Quality of Life Scales; Morgan et al. 1997). The standards and methodology of assessing quality of life in skin diseases have been published by the German Dermatological Society (DDG) as guidelines (Augustin et al. 2004).

Another approach for assessing patient benefits in the care for patients with occupational diseases is the recording of patient-defined goals and their achievements by "goal attainment scaling." A particular method of such has been developed for use in dermatology (Augustin et al. 2009) and especially in chronic hand eczema (Blome et al. 2009). In this PRO technology, the patients rate their preferences for potential treatment goals before intervention. After the intervention, the grade of achievement of the single items is measured. A single, weighed index including all preferences and outcomes (patient benefit index, PBI) indicates the overall patient benefit.

2.3 Pharmacoeconomic Analyses

Economic evaluation is the comparison of two or more alternative courses of action in terms of both their costs and consequences (Drummond and McGuire 2001). It is obvious that the interpretation of the costs for a medical procedure is depending on the benefit that can be achieved. Thus, a validated comparison of the input (in monetary units) and the output (in monetary or other units) for any treatment or medication is necessary.

This input–output comparison can be performed on any level of the health system, e.g., the treatment of a single patient, the cost-effectiveness of a drug, the performance of a clinic, or the health system in total. Depending on the parameters to be compared, the analysis of costs versus outcome is called cost–benefit analysis (costs versus costs), cost–utility analysis (costs versus quality of life), or cost-effectiveness analysis (costs versus clinical parameters, like healing rate).

3 Special Pharmacoeconomic Aspects in Occupational Skin Diseases

3.1 Cost Factors in Occupational Skin Diseases

The number of scientific publications on the costs of occupational skin diseases (OSD) is small. In the United States, costs for OSD were estimated to be US$ 1.2 billion. In another study from Oregon, the average cost per claim of occupational skin diseases was $3,552, and the average disability time was 23.9 days (McCall et al. 2005).

Estimates or extrapolations indicate annual costs of disease of hundreds of million Euro each year in the EU. Most of these cost estimates take only into account the direct costs from the payers' perspective and indirect costs but not the out-of-pocket expenses and the intangible costs.

In recent studies, a few authors have published additional data on the costs-of-illness of occupational skin diseases in defined patient groups: In a single-center study, Diepgen et al. (2011) demonstrated a very high cost impact of about 9,000 € for patients of the German occupational health insurances.

In a German multicentre study on a representative random sample of patients with chronic hand eczema (CHE) insured by the statutory health insurances (SHI), the annual costs of disease amount to an average of 2,128 € for a patient with CHE; 1,512 € of these costs (71%) are direct costs for the statutory health insurances, 230 € (11%) costs for the patient, and 386 € (18%) indirect costs.

Important expenditure factors in CHE were: medication used (especially topical steroids and systemic therapy), frequent doctor's appointments, inpatient treatment days, own expenses for care products, sick days. Costs strongly correlated with the disease severity of the last 12 months (➋ *Fig. 4.1*).

Extrapolated for Germany, these data and data from other studies show total costs resulting from CHE of about 500 € Mio per year just for the SHI.

In another study section, these costs were compared with costs for patients being reimbursed by the occupational health insurances (Berufsgenossenschaften, BG). The results showed that annual costs for patients with chronic hand eczema being covered by the BG are strikingly higher than those for patients of the SHI (Diepgen et al. 2012). However, the subgroup of patients of the SHI associated with work impairments shows almost the same amount and pattern of costs as the BG patients (➋ *Fig. 4.2*): Direct costs for managing patients in the work-impaired group (GKV) and work-diseased group (BG) were 3,164 € and 3,309 € respectively, around double the costs for managing non-working and work-unaffected GKV patients.

3.2 Quality of Life and PRO in Occupational Skin Diseases

A variety of studies have shown that the quality of life (QoL) of patients with occupational skin diseases, in particular chronic hand eczema, is markedly reduced

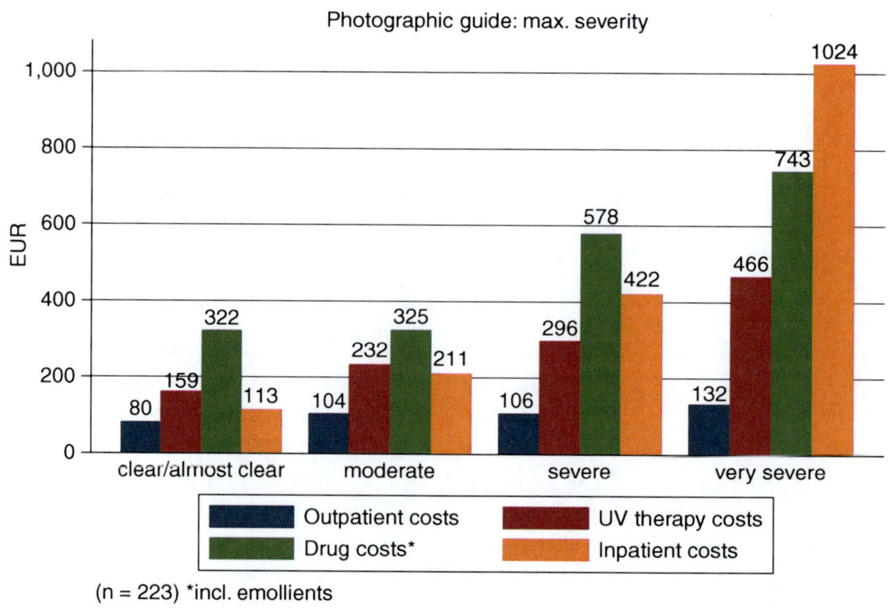

◘ Fig. 4.1
Costs-of-illness of patients with chronic hand eczema according to disease severity and cost groups (Augustin et al. 2011)

(Matterne et al. 2009; Rabin and Fraidlin 2007; Soder et al. 2007; Cvetkovski et al. 2006; Hutchings et al. 2001). In summary, it can be stated that significant limitations compared to healthy persons were found in most studies published on quality of life (Lau 2011). However, in a single publication on persons with occupational latex allergy, there were no relevant reductions of QoL (Nienhaus et al. 2008).

Conversely, there is at least some evidence that the QoL of patients with hand eczema and atopic eczema significantly improved in controlled clinical studies by means of various dermatological treatment procedures. Among these are: ciclosporin A (Harper et al. 2000; Salek et al. 1993), Tacrolimus (Drake et al. 2001), dermatological standard therapy with behavioral therapy (Lange et al. 1999), balneotherapy (Kubota et al. 1997), UV-therapy/photopheresis (Granlund et al. 2001; Mohla et al. 1999).

Also preventive interventions in occupational skin diseases induced improved QoL (Apfelbacher et al. 2009).

Regarding distinct patient-defined benefits, a noninterventional study on patients with chronic hand eczema, including occupational background, revealed a marked overall benefit from alitretinoin treatment, as measured with the PBI (Blome et al. 2009) (➋ *Fig. 4.3*).

In total, the following are the evidences on quality of life and patient benefits in occupational skin diseases:

- Clinically relevant losses of QoL due to the skin condition
- Marked improvements following guideline-compliant treatment
- Significant potential for improvements after the introduction of skin-preventive measures

3.3 Predictors of Costs in Occupational Diseases from the Societal Perspective

A major economic factor for the global costs of occupational skin diseases in a country is their epidemiology. Several publications indicate both the high prevalence and incidence in Western countries (Dickel et al. 2001; McDonald et al. 2006; Turner et al. 2007; Apfelbacher et al. 2008; Thyssen et al. 2010).

Moreover, the comorbidity and associated diseases must be taken into account, such as atopic risk factors (Nilsson et al. 1985; Coenraads and Diepgen 1998; Dickel et al. 2003). These additional conditions may aggravate the course of occupational disease and thus be an indicator of higher cost impact.

Given the chronic nature of occupational skin diseases, the long-term outcomes and the prevention of recurrences is also of relevance (Cherry et al. 2000; Mälkönen et al. 2009, 2010). Specific preventive programs – if effective and accepted by employers and employees – cannot just be clinically effective

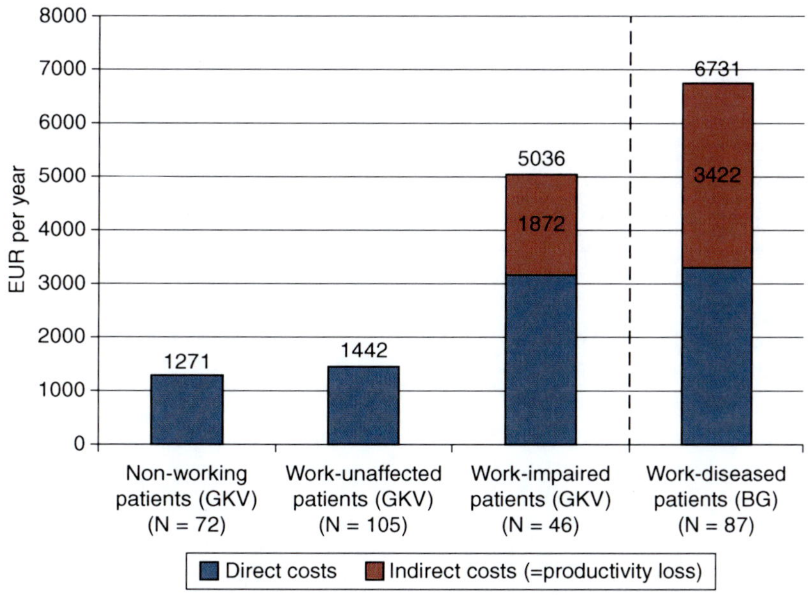

Fig. 4.2
Annual total, direct and indirect per patient costs for CHE treatment according to CHE impact on work (Diepgen et al. 2012)

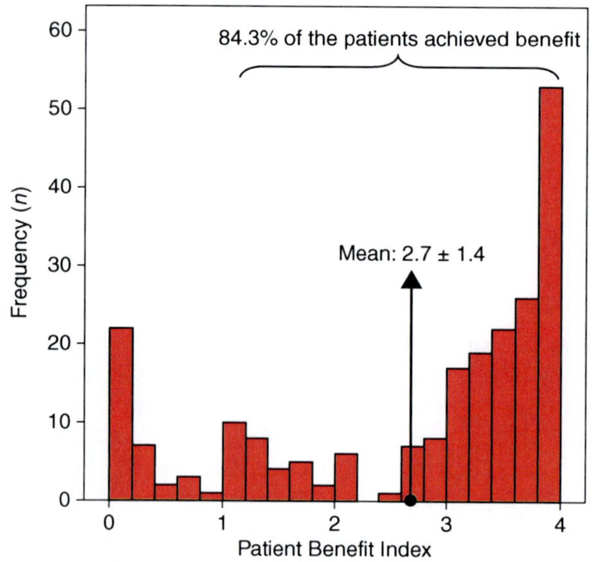

Fig. 4.3
Distribution of benefits achieved from treatment of chronic hand eczema with oral alitretinoin, as measured with the patient benefit index (PBI), n = 219

(Holness and Nethercott 1995; Dickel et al. 2002; Dulon et al. 2009; Held et al. 2002; Winker et al. 2009; Kütting et al. 2010) but also improve the economic prognosis of disease.

3.4 Cost-Effectiveness Data on Interventions in Occupational Skin Diseases

Most of the interventional studies on OSD have not been analyzed economically. Accordingly, in a recent systematic review, van Gils et al. have not found any publication on prevention programs in OSD which included cost assessments (van Gils et al. 2011).

However, some clinical drug studies have documented cost-effectiveness (C/E) of interventions for occupational skin diseases:

Blank et al. showed the C/E of oral alitretinoin in the treatment of chronic hand eczema in Switzerland (Blank et al. 2010). Annual costs of alitretinoin treatment were 2,212 €. Using a long-term Markov model, the incremental cost-effectiveness ratio resulted in 14,816 €/QALY gained, compared to standard care which is considered an acceptable ratio.

Findings of acceptable C/E ratios were also reported by Rodgers et al. appraising the C/E of alitretinoin for NICE (Rodgers et al. 2010 and Paulden et al. 2010).

3.5 Conclusions from the Economic Data on Occupational Skin Diseases

The following conclusions can be drawn:

- The great budget impact and the impairment of quality of life of patients with occupational skin diseases should be the impetus for qualified and inclusive disease management.
- The wide-ranging socioeconomic consequences of occupational skin diseases justify high investments in research, prevention, and therapy.
- A considerable proportion of costs could be saved by effective preventive measures. For the sake of better efficiency, they should be structured and provided by trained dermatologists.

References

Anderson RT, Rajagopalan R (1997) Development and validation of a quality of life instrument for cutaneous diseases. J Am Acad Dermatol 37(1):41–50

Apfelbacher CJ, Radulescu M, Diepgen TL, Funke U (2008) Occurrence and prognosis of hand eczema in the car industry: results from the PACO follow-up study. Contact Dermatitis 58:322–329

Apfelbacher CJ, Soder S, Diepgen TL, Weisshaar E (2009) The impact of measures for secondary individual prevention of work-related skin diseases in health care workers: 1-year follow-up study. Contact Dermatitis 60(3):144–149

Augustin M, Amon U, Braathen L, Bullinger M, Gieler U, Klein GF, Schultz-Amling W (2004) Erfassung von Lebensqualität in der Dermatologie (Leitlinie). J Dtsch Dermatol Ges 9:802–806

Augustin M, Radtke MA, Zschocke I, Blome C, Behechtnejad J, Schäfer I, Reusch M, Mielke V, Rustenbach SJ (2009) The patient benefit index: a novel approach in patient-defined outcomes measurement for skin diseases. Arch Dermatol Res 301(8):561–571

Augustin M, Kuessner D, Purwins S, Hieke K, Posthumus J, Diepgen TL (2011) Cost-of-illness of patients with chronic hand eczema in routine care: results from a multi-centre study in Germany. Br J Dermatol 165(4):845–851. doi:10.1111/j.1365-2133.2011.10427.x

Blanciforti LA (2010) Economic burden of dermatitis in US workers (corrected). J Occup Environ Med 52(11):1045–1054

Blank PR, Blank AA, Szucs TD (2010) Cost-effectiveness of oral alitretinoin in patients with severe chronic hand eczema – a long-term analysis from a Swiss perspective. BMC Dermatol 10:4

Blome C, Maares J, Diepgen T, Rustenbach SJ, Augustin M (2009) Measurement of patient-relevant benefits in the treatment of chronic hand eczema – a novel approach. Contact Dermatitis 61:39–45

Brock D (1996) Quality of life measures in health care and medical ethics. In: Spilker B (ed) Quality of life and pharmacoeconomics in clinical trials, 2nd edn. Lippincott-Raven, Philadelphia, pp 487–510 (Revised)

Bullinger M, Anderson R, Cella D, Aaronson N (1993) Developing and evaluating cross-cultural instruments from minimum requirements to optimal models. Qual Life Res 2(6):451–459

Cherry N, Meyer JD, Adisesh A, Brooke R, Owen-Smith V, Swales C, Beck MH (2000) Surveillance of occupational skin disease: EPIDERM and OPRA. Br J Dermatol 142:1128–1134

Chren MM, Lasek RJ, Quinn LM, Mostow EN, Zyzanski SJ (1996) Skindex, a quality-of-life measure for patients with skin disease: reliability, validity, and responsiveness. J Invest Dermatol 107(5):707–713

Coenraads PJ, Diepgen TL (1998) Risk for hand eczema in employees with past or present atopic dermatitis. Int Arch Occup Environ Health 71:7–13

Cvetkovski RS, Zachariae R, Jensen H, Olsen J, Johansen JD, Agner T (2006) Quality of life and depression in a population of occupational hand eczema patients. Contact Dermatitis 54(2):106–111

Dickel H, Kuss O, Blesius CR, Schmidt A, Diepgen TL (2001) Occupational skin diseases in Northern Bavaria between 1990 and 1999: a population based study. Br J Dermatol 145:453–462

Dickel H, Kuss O, Schmidt A, Diepgen TL (2002) Impact of preventive strategies on trend of occupational skin disease in hairdressers: population-based register study. Br Med J 324:1422–1423

Dickel H, Bruckner TM, Schmidt A, Diepgen TL (2003) Impact of atopic skin diathesis on occupational skin disease incidence in a working population. J Invest Dermatol 121:37–40

Diepgen TL, Scheidt R, Elke W, Hieke K (2011) Cost of illness of occupational hand eczema in Germany (Submitted)

Diepgen TL, Purwins S, John SM, Posthumus J, Kuessner D, Augustin M (2012) Cost of Illness of patients with chronic hand eczema in Germany: a comparison of patients in routine care from statutory and occupational health insurances (Submitted)

Drake L, Prendergast M, Maher R, Breneman D, Korman N, Satoi Y, Beusterien KM, Lawrence I (2001) The impact of tacrolimus ointment on health-related quality of life of adult and pediatric patients with atopic dermatitis. J Am Acad Dermatol 44:S65–S72

Drummond M, McGuire A (2001) Economic evaluation in health care. Oxford University Press, Oxford

Dulon M, Pohrt U, Skudlik C, Nienhaus A (2009) Prevention of occupational skin disease: a workplace intervention study in geriatric nurses. Br J Dermatol 161:337–344

Flyvholm MA, Mygind K, Sell L, Jensen A, Jepsen KF (2005) A randomised controlled intervention study on prevention of work related skin problems among gut cleaners in swine slaughterhouses. Occup Environ Med 62:642–649

Granlund H, Erkko P, Remitz A, Langeland T, Helsing P, Nuutinen M, Reitamo S (2001) Comparison of cyclosporin and UVAB phototherapy for intermittent one-year treatment of atopic dermatitis. Acta Derm Venereol 81:22–27

Harper JI, Ahmed I, Barclay G, Lacour M, Hoeger P, Cork MJ, Finlay AY, Wilson NJ, Graham-Brown RA, Sowden JM, Beard AL, Sumner MJ, Berth-Jones J (2000) Cyclosporin for severe childhood atopic dermatitis: short course versus continuous therapy. Br J Dermatol 142:52–58

Held E, Mygind K, Wolff C, Gyntelberg F, Agner T (2002) Prevention of work related skin problems: an intervention study in wet work employees. Occup Environ Med 59:556–561

Holness DL, Nethercott JR (1995) Work outcome in workers with occupational skin disease. Am J Ind Med 27:807–815

Hutchings CV, Shum KW, Gawkrodger DJ (2001) Occupational contact dermatitis has an appreciable impact on quality of life. Contact Dermatitis 45(1):17–20

Kubota K, Machida I, Tamura K, Take H, Kurabayashi H, Akiba T, Tamura J (1997) Treatment of refractory cases of atopic dermatitis with acidic hot- spring bathing. Acta Derm Venereol 77:452–454

Kütting B, Baumeister T, Weistenhöfer W, Pfahlberg A, Uter W, Drexler H (2010) Effectiveness of skin protection measures in prevention of occupational hand eczema: results of a prospective randomized controlled trial over a follow-up period of 1 year. Br J Dermatol 162:362–370

Lange S, Zschocke I, Langhardt S, Amon U, Augustin M (1999) Effects of combined dermatological and behavioural medicine therapy in hospitalized patients with psoriasis and atopic dermatitis. Hautarzt 50:791–7

Lau MY, Burgess JA, Nixon R, Dharmage SC, Matheson MC (2011a) A review of the impact of occupational contact dermatitis on quality of life. J Allergy (Cairo) 2011:964509, Epub 2011 Mar 16

Lau MY, Matheson MC, Burgess JA, Dharmage SC, Nixon R (2011b) Disease severity and quality of life in a follow-up study of patients with occupational contact dermatitis. Contact Dermatitis 65(3):138–145

Mälkönen T, Jolanki R, Alanko K, Luukonen R, Aalto-Korte K, Lauerma A, Susitaival P (2009) A 6-month follow-up study of 1048 patients diagnosed with an occupational skin disease. Contact Dermatitis 61:261–268

Mälkönen T, Alanko K, Jolanki R, Luukkonen R, Aalto-Korte K, Lauerma A, Susitaival P (2010) Long-term follow-up study of occupational hand eczema. Br J Dermatol 163:999–1006

Matterne U, Apfelbacher CJ, Soder S, Diepgen TL, Weisshaar E (2009) Health-related quality of life in health care workers with work-related skin diseases. Contact Dermatitis 61(3):145–151

McCall BP, Horwitz IB, Feldman SR, Balkrishnan R (2005) Incidence rates, costs, severity, and work-related factors of occupational dermatitis: a workers' compensation analysis of Oregon, 1990–1997. Arch Dermatol 141(6):713–718

McDonald JC, Beck MH, Chen Y, Cherry NM (2006) Incidence by occupation and industry of work-related skin diseases in the United Kingdom 1996–2001. Occup Med 56:398–405

Mohla G, Horvath N, Stevens S (1999) Quality of life improvement in a patient with severe atopic dermatitis treated with photopheresis. J Am Acad Dermatol 40:780–782

Morgan M, McCreedy R, Simpson J, Hay RJ (1997) Dermatology quality of life scales – a measure of the impact of skin diseases. Br J Dermatol 136(2):202–206

Nienhaus A, Kromark K, Raulf-Heimsoth M, van Kampen V, Merget R (2008) Outcome of occupational latex allergy – work ability and quality of life. PLoS One 3(10):e3459, Epub 2008 Oct 21

Nilsson GE, Mikaelsson B, Andersson S (1985) Atopy, occupation and domestic work as risk factors for hand eczema in hospital workers. Contact Dermatitis 13:216–223

Paulden M, Rodgers M, Griffin S, Slack R, Duffy S, Ingram JR, Woolacott N, Sculpher M (2010) Alitretinoin for the treatment of severe chronic hand eczema. Health Technol Assess 14(Suppl 1):39–46

Rabin B, Fraidlin N (2007) Patients with occupational contact dermatitis in Israel: quality of life and social implications. Soc Work Health Care 45(2):97–111

Rodgers M, Griffin S, Paulden M, Slack R, Duffy S, Ingram JR, Woolacott N, Sculpher M (2010) Alitretinoin for severe chronic hand eczema: a NICE single technology appraisal. Pharmacoeconomics 28(5): 351–362

Salek MS, Finlay AY, Luscombe DK, Allen BR, Berth-Jones J, Camp RD, Graham-Brown RA, Khan GK, Marks R, Motley RJ (1993) Cyclosporin greatly improves the quality of life of adults with severe atopic dermatitis. A randomized, double-blind, placebo-controlled trial. Br J Dermatol 129:422–430

Schipper H, Clinch JJ, Olweny CHLM (1996) Quality of life studies: definition and conceptual issues. In: Spilker B (ed) Quality of life and pharmacoeconomics in clinical trials. Lippincott-Raven, Philadelphia, pp 11–24

Soder S, Diepgen TL, Radulescu M, Apfelbacher CJ, Bruckner T, Weisshaar E (2007) Occupational skin diseases in cleaning and kitchen employees: course and quality of life after measures of secondary individual prevention. J Dtsch Dermatol Ges 5(8):670–676

Spilker B (ed) (1996) Quality of life and pharmacoeconomics in clinical trials. Lippincott-Raven, Philadelphia, pp 11–24

Thyssen JP, Johansen JD, Linneberg A, Menné T (2010) The epidemiology of hand eczema in the general population – prevalence and main findings. Contact Dermatitis 62(2):75–87

Turner S, Carder N, van Tongeren M, McNamee R, Lines S, Hussey L, Bolton A, Beck MH, Wilkinson M, Agius R (2007) The incidence of occupational skin disease as reported to The Health and Occupation Reporting (THOR) network between 2002 and 2005. Br J Dermatol 157:713–722

van Gils RF, Boot CR, van Gils PF, Bruynzeel D, Coenraads PJ, van Mechelen W, Riphagen II, Anema JR (2011) Effectiveness of prevention programmes for hand dermatitis: a systematic review of the literature. Contact Dermatitis 64(2):63–72

Winker R, Salameh B, Stolkovich S, Nikl M, Barth A, Ponocny E, Drexler H, Tappeiner G (2009) Effectiveness of skin protection creams in the prevention of occupational dermatitis: results of a randomized, controlled trial. Int Arch Occup Environ Health 82:653–662

5 Ethical Aspects

Nikolaus Knoepffler · Martin O'Malley
Department of Applied Ethics, Friedrich-Schiller-Universität, Jena, Germany

Core Messages

- Occupational dermatology is a professional field at the intersection of essentially four ethical realms: society, business, medical profession, and the individual.
- The fundamental ethical frameworks of most important occupational health ethical guidelines build upon the consensus principles of human dignity and human rights.
- Legal regimen and ethical guidelines are similar in that they build upon consensus social values, without which they are both illegitimate and ineffective.
- Ethical literature in the field is scant and focuses too narrowly upon dilemmas posed by the medical professional's conflicting loyalties to workers and employers.
- The "International Code of Ethics for Occupational Health Professionals" (ICOH Code) provides resources for a more adequate ethical approach to occupational dermatology.
- Among the key insights is the obligation to not just workers and employers, but also to society and the profession, i.e., to the social values and laws that share wide consensus, and to the principles and standards that have established the well-earned respect for medical care.
- Divided loyalties should be resolved *not* by reducing health surveillance or the flow of information between medical professionals and workers, but by establishing fully transparent guidelines: Medical officials should be able to attain the information they need to ensure the safest possible workplace and workers should be assured that their rights and privacy are not violated.
- Medical professionals have the duty to refrain from revealing information from employers when that revelation is a violation of workers' informed consent, or when such an action would endanger the trust in their integrity and impartiality.

1 Introduction

Occupational dermatology is a professional field at the intersection of essentially four ethical realms: society, business, health profession, and the individual. Each realm makes distinct ethical demands upon the health professional. *Society* makes demands in the form of social values and the explicit determinations of legal codes. *Business* forms a distinct ethical realm that deals with contractual obligations, market pressures, and professional standards. The *health profession* is a distinct realm even within the context of a business setting. Doctors, nurses, and other practitioners have a duty to uphold the integrity and reputation of medical practice. This is independent of their context of employment (business) and goes beyond what is merely required by the law (society). Finally, it is useful to consider the ethical demands of *individuals* as a realm distinct from that of society. All four realms are integrally related, but they are distinguished, as philosophers say, by their ends. That means that they each have distinct interests and goals. Ideally, these goals are in harmony, but experience teaches us that they often come into conflict. Ethics is the study of the nature and resolution of such conflicts according to established principles, practices, values, and procedures of resolution.

Rapid developments in science, medicine, and society necessitate legal regulations to establish the basic ethical framework for occupational dermatology. Laws are essential to deal with the hard cases that push established moral actions and principles into conflict. Laws set standards and stabilize expectations according to basic moral convictions within functioning societies. Laws prevent cases from being determined according to expediency or inflamed public opinions; laws insure that even the hard cases can be resolved according to processes that respect and reflect the moral convictions of a pluralistic society. Yet law is only one aspect of social ethics. Social ethics also involves the common moral values that transcend ideological differences – religious and secular. These values are distinct from the legal process, but they are integrally associated with the law. Both aspects of social ethics are relevant for occupational dermatology when resolving hard cases because the law may not sufficiently represent the full force of social values. How, for example, can a worker with a genetic disposition for certain dermatological diseases be protected in his working place when the law prohibits the employer from requiring genetic tests? How can a worker be protected in some countries where the law does not punish the use of dangerous substances?

Social ethics provide the general ethical context for occupational dermatology, or any other professional

T. Rustemeyer, P. Elsner, S.M. John & H.I. Maibach (eds.), *Kanerva's Occupational Dermatology*,
DOI 10.1007/978-3-642-02035-3_5, © Springer-Verlag Berlin Heidelberg 2012

person. Legal systems in modern democracies will not be perfect, but citizens must accept that they are governed by laws that represent their interests and values. They must also believe they share some participatory access to the continuing development of those regulations. This is a way of saying that the law has legitimacy. Legitimacy does not imply that the system of law represents a situation of perfect justice, especially in a pluralistic society with divergent notions of justice. The effectiveness of the law depends upon a people's conviction that the law reflects their fundamental moral convictions – or at least does not violate them. This applies to the specific ethics of health practitioners as well.

Business ethics deals with proper relationships and responsibilities within market-based enterprises. The end (or purpose) of society is human flourishing and business is oriented toward the creation of value in a competitive context. That created value is not exactly the same thing as the generation of profit for shareholders, but profit generation is necessary in business. Even if the workplace is not necessarily in a business context, but is in a not-for-profit or government organization, even that is a context where the organization's goals are limited by finite resources. Occupational dermatology has a responsibility to contribute toward the central objectives of the organization. That is an ethical demand for the health practitioner that must coexist with the ethical demands of professional medical codes. Doctors and nurses enjoy a respect in western society – and for good reason. People trust they act in the patients' best interests because the medical profession has zealously maintained standards of honorableness and competence over many decades. These standards impose an obligation on the practitioner that is distinct from both the social and business realms. Finally, the individual realm will be spelled out below, but is essentially comprised of the principles of human dignity and human rights – principles that are now universally recognized in such documents as the Universal Declaration of Human Rights (UDHR).

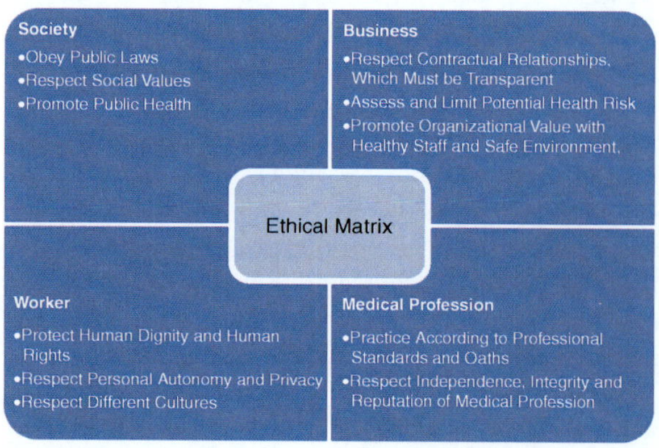

For the practitioner of occupational dermatology, the balance of these four ethical realms demands a core understanding of not only the realms themselves and the principles that govern them. It also requires an appreciation of that the achievement and maintenance of such an ethical balance parallels the process of achieving and maintaining a medical proficiency. As Aristotle famously taught, ethics is not merely the compliance with restrictive guidelines; it is the science of achieving the moral virtues necessary for living well.

The discussion below begins with a fundamental ethical framework and then argues that the existing codes in occupational health ethics represent an overlapping consensus that meets the demands of each of the four essential spheres outlined in the ethical matrix above. Next, specific questions relevant for occupational dermatology will be addressed, especially with respect to its relationship to the wider field of occupational medicine: What is the role of the physician in respect to patient (worker), employer, and other stakeholders? What are the responsibilities of worker and employer? What kind of therapies can be forced upon a worker? The discussion concludes with controversial questions regarding genetic screening of workers for specific dispositions for dermatological diseases. It considers whether some people should be excluded from some work in order to prevent them from getting diseases.

2 Fundamental Ethical Framework

Judgments in difficult bioethical cases are essentially dependent upon the ethical framework utilized. Thus it is important to be quite clear from the beginning that the ethical framework being proposed here is one built upon the principle of human dignity which has been established in international charters (UDHR) and national laws and which has achieved a distinct level of international consensus (see Knoepffler 2004, p. 7f, 2010, p. 65ff). The preamble of the UDHR recognizes "the inherent dignity and of the equal and inalienable rights of all members of the human family is the foundation of freedom, justice and peace in the world." This document was drafted in response to the cruel and inhuman beliefs of National Socialism, which rationalized the sacrifice of individual rights and personal dignity as necessary for the interests of the majority. The principle of human dignity stands as both a rejection of human debasement and a universal recognition of fundamental human worth. Every human being has value simply because they are human. Every human being shares a fundamental equality and fundamental human rights. No single philosophical or theological foundation was given to establish this ethical framework, even though it is certainly possible to do so (see Knoepffler 2004, pp. 33–49). Rather, the ethical framework was an historical achievement tied to the tragic experience of human degradation. This contingent context of the principle's creation does not imply that the principle itself is contingent. The context merely shows the background which lead to the formulation of an internationally recognized ethical principle. Hence, it is not a legalistic fallacy to consider that the principle of human dignity attained its status as a fundamental ethical "principle" precisely in the experience of human degradation during the period of National Socialism.

The fundamental principles of human dignity and human rights, once established by nearly unanimous international consent, lead to the recognition of the right of bodily integrity and welfare. Note the unambiguous formulation in the preamble of the World Health Organization:

- The enjoyment of the highest attainable standard of health is one of the fundamental rights of every human being without distinction of race, religion, political belief, economic or social condition.

Government organizations like the European Agency for Safety and Health at Work, National Institute for Occupational Safety and Health (USA) or the Work Safety & Health Council in Singapore, and the Information Center of Occupational Safety and Health in Israel all try to adopt what was stated by the Joint ILO/WHO Committee on Occupational Health at its first session in 1950 and revised at its twelfth session in 1995:

- Occupational health should aim at: the promotion and maintenance of the highest degree of physical, mental and social well-being of workers in all occupations; the prevention amongst workers of departures from health caused by their working conditions; the protection of workers in their employment from risks resulting from factors adverse to health; the placing and maintenance of the worker in an occupational environment adapted to his physiological and psychological capabilities; and, to summarize, the adaptation of work to man and of each man to his job.

In 2009, the Board of the German Society for Occupational Medicine and Environmental Medicine e.V. (DGAUM) and the Bureau of the Association of German Company and Factory Doctors e.V. (VDBW) formulated a code of ethics for occupational medicine. In article 2 they commit themselves explicitly to the UDHR and their respective principles: "Those doctors, scientists and medical ancillary staff entrusted with occupational medicine responsibilities agree to conform to internationally accepted ethical principles, as defined in the Universal Declaration of Human Rights and in German constitutional law, as well as to follow the specific ethical principles applicable to medicine in their professional behavior. The principle of each being treated equally always applies." The preamble consequently states "The goals of occupational medicine are to promote and maintain health and, in particular, to participate in the early detection of health impairments because of work and in the restoration of the health and employability of people in the workplace. This is facilitated, for example, through targeted medical and occupational toxicology, epidemiology and psycho-social research and, in practice, through comprehensive 'occupational health management' as is demanded of all participants and stakeholders in the promotion of health in the workplace."

These codes of ethics are very good at laying out the positive goals of occupational medicine that can be essentially boiled down to the maintenance of workers' good health through preventative and active measures. This is all fine and good, but as the recent literature shows, there is a perceived lack of concrete and useful ethical guidance (see Kuhn and Gensch 2009; London 2005; Brandt-Rauf 1989). This and other literature point to the dual loyalties posed by workers and employers as the essential problem. Workers have expectations of health service that include confidentiality and care. This might be understandable in light of the Brandt-Rauf's argument that ethical conflicts in occupational medicine are typically understood only according to traditional medical role models. Less emphasis is paid to the expectations of employers who have very different interests with respect to allowing sick leave and providing injury compensation, to name just two general examples. And even the expansion of consideration to dual loyalties neglects the ethical demands upon the occupational health professional (OHP) concerning the health profession and society in general.

There is a reciprocal relationship between the effectiveness and respect of the health professional. Thus even though the particular circumstances of occupational medicine may impose complex ethical responsibilities on the OHP, the field of the medicine poses a legitimate and independent set of responsibilities upon the practitioner. TL Guidotti (2008) rejects the disparagement of the profession posed in such accounts as Draper's "The Company Doctor: Risk, Responsibility, and Corporate Professionalism" (2003). Whether you follow Guidotti's positive history or Draper's more critical account of occupational medicine, the point stands that the reputation of the field is of critical importance for the integrity of the work of OHPs. No one is served by hazy ethical guidelines, violated boundaries, or an instrumentalized medical practice. This is more than just a guild mentality. It is an ethically responsible understanding of the great social good that the self-regulating health profession provides society.

We now turn to some practical examples of ethical dilemmas posed by occupational dermatology to explain the principles outlined above.

3 Some Hard Cases and the Role of the Physician

3.1 The Structural Problem

As we have seen, the principles of human dignity and human rights underlie the central importance of human life and bodily integrity, as well as the right to self-determination. There are essentially two aspects of human rights, the physical and the volitional, that frame a tension in the hard ethical cases of occupational dermatology.

A possible tension exists between the physical or "objective" claim to life and bodily integrity and the volitional or "subjective" claim to freedom that is associated with the right to self-determination, which the principle of human dignity also safeguards. The claim to freedom is subjective in the sense that the person has the freedom to choose his own good, at least to the degree that these choices do not infringe upon the self-determination of other people. The right to self-determination prioritizes the freedom of individuals over and against the structures of potentially over-reaching corporate and government structures. Protected freedoms can allow individuals to make bad or even tragic choices in selecting the place where they work. People can choose risky careers, for example. Nevertheless, modern liberal systems of law deem the restriction of freedom to be a greater evil.

Subjective rights protect the individual in a sphere of freedom, within which the individual may act according to her or his own desires, if those actions do not infringe upon the rights and freedoms of others. This is the classic definition of a right, subjectively understood. Ideally, we should not act in ways that are detrimental to our well-being. However, we do not have an ethical duty to protect our lives and bodies to the greatest possible degree according to some "objective" criteria. We have a right to life and bodily integrity. And we can freely choose a particular course of action such as working in a hazardous occupation that risks our lives and bodily integrity. Some (or even most) in society may judge this to be dumb or even morally problematic, but the greater social evil is posed by society's limit of our freedom to choose dumb things at least to a certain degree. Health professionals, employers and the social order all have obligations to uphold the rights protecting workers - despite the freedom that individuals have to take risks that potentially endanger themselves.

Just to mention some examples: Individuals may possess preconditions to disease or injury and nevertheless choose employment that poses distinct and peculiar risks to workers with such preconditions. Fair-skinned people with family histories of skin cancer may exercise their right to self-determination and choose a career that leaves them relentlessly exposed to the sun, for example. But even that is a situation where the preconditions and risks are blatantly manifest. Employers, however, have an interest in attaining the healthiest workers possible; for both the positive contribution and lack of risk they offer an organization. Thus, every employment situation poses a cost-benefit analysis that is dependent upon workers' health fitness and the risks posed by particular occupations. Piano moving presents risks very different from repetitive motion assembly lines or selling insurance. Ethical guidelines generally require a reasonable disclosure of fitness from prospective employment candidates and, from employers, a reasonable disclosure of an occupation's potential risks. The ICOH Code describes this level of reasonableness in terms of a general aim of contributing to the "establishment and maintenance of a safe and healthy working environment for all."

Problems potentially emerge when relevant information is excluded from the employment fitness analysis. Such a problem is posed by a worker with an undisclosed and infectious dermatological disease in an employment that includes close-range contact with other workers. The problems of scarce information or neglect of healthy working conditions are posed when the negative effects of limiting information are not associated with the perpetration of such actions. For example, there is a disassociation of actions and the negative effects of that action when a worker spreads an infection, but the cost of that infection are shouldered by the health insurer and the employer, but not the primary infector. The negative external effects go to other stakeholders like insurances (money of other insured people) or the state (taxpayer's money).

There is an inherent structural inefficiency posed by the fact that workers are protected by state laws in their withholding of certain medical conditions, and in their refusing to be submitted to certain health tests. Most western countries, for example, do not require workers to submit to genetic testing even if that testing could reveal genetic predispositions to diseases associated with elevated risks for environmental factors present in a desired place of employment. The person has a right "not to know." Even if the genetic predisposition is known to the person, there is a further protection such that such knowledge need not be handed over.

Using the example of genetic testing for certain dermatological hereditary predispositions: If the worker refuses to be tested, he is not obliged to do so. If a disease surfaces, the costs are then paid by the holder of the health-insurance policy. Whether the employer or the insurance agency foots the bill, there is a cost shift to the larger society when the resources from the common are dedicated to this treatment, rather than used for some other social good. Further, the employer has a high incentive to choose workers most fit for their work, i.e., they provide the greatest contribution and fewest risks. But if the costs of either providing increased health care and/or for replacing a worker are minimized through insurance leveraging or socialized medicine, there is a proportionate disincentive to actively attain healthy workers.

3.2 The Occupational Health Practitioner within the Fourfold Matrix of Ethical Responsibilities

Health practitioners may only reflect upon the ethics of their fields when they find themselves in situations of conflict. Then, they must go about resolving their particular dilemma according to some ethical-resolution strategy. Entering into such deliberation, it is important (following Westerholm 2007) to have a functional definition of health such as "the capacity and ability to achieve vital life goals." Next, one assembles all the information relevant to a case, whether medical, psychological, social, or other. Such a process may not lend itself simple to a process of evidence-based practice, but the skill set is analogous. After outlining the relevant values including dignity, rights, autonomy, competency, institutional well-being, etc., the practitioner can use the ethical matrix provided above to determine the specific spheres of loyalty that deserve attention. The OHP is responsible to (a) the worker as patient, (b) the employer/enterprise/or institutional structure involved (cf. London 2005), and to (c) maintaining the integrity of the profession. That is not all – though this consideration is neglected in most occupational medicine. A fourth party is involved, too, namely, the insurance industry and society as a whole that shoulders the financial and other burdens for the externalities caused by the information deficits present in the attaining of workers for risk-prone careers. Therefore, the OHP should understand the ethical responsibilities due society as well.

3.2.1 The OHPs Multiple Relationships of Accountability

As outlined in the chart above, the OHPs ethical matrix includes four essential realms of responsibility. The health provider is responsible to maintain the balance among all four while respecting human dignity and human rights and promoting the four values of beneficence, nonmaleficence, autonomy, and justice (or equality) (Westerholm 2007; Beauchamp and Childress 2001).

1. With respect to the worker as patient, there is the classical obligation of respecting the autonomy of the patient, following the values and principles included in the ethical medical codes that prioritize the health and well-being of the patient. As patient, the worker enjoys privileges of confidentiality and the respect of informed consent, which insures self-determination. These are all elements of the value of autonomy.
2. With respect to the employer, there is the classical obligation of respecting the norms and regulations of the corporation – as the health official is a loyal cooperator of the enterprise paying the health provider's salary. The value of justice, classically defined as "to each his own," insures the ethical consideration of the business and all those within and external to it who benefit from its productive functioning.
3. With respect to society/stakeholders, he or she has the classical has the classical obligation of a citizen in preventing the exploitation and contributing to public health.
4. Finally, there is the duty to uphold the reputation and standards of the health profession. Practitioners have a duty to promote good health, beneficence. Moreover, whether or not the OHP has taken an oath to do no harm, they are bound to this value of nonmaleficence.

3.2.2 The Potential for Loyalty Conflicts

The OHP should never enter into a strictly commercial relationship with an organization to act solely in its best interests. Such a one-sided loyalty compromises the OHPs responsibilities to the other three ethical realms. Most importantly, it jeopardizes the OHP's relationship with the worker and the commitment to the worker's best interests. Hence, there is no real relationship of health professional with a "patient." It may be necessary for an OHP to act overtly and prejudicially as a representative of the employer's interests, but such a position would necessarily be fully apparent to the worker. Such a role would arguably be only analogously a "health" role. Such a situation does call into question the situations where it is assumed that the occupational physician is bound by the medical code, and therefore acting both in the best interest of the patient and in the best interest of the organization.

Conflicts arise when these loyalties cannot be simultaneously preserved. Let us assume that a physician knows about the following risk: Predisposed workers have a high probability of incurring contact dermatitis from of a substance used by the firm. If it is in the (acknowledged) interest of the worker and employer to know about the predisposition, then there is no conflict. There is also no conflict when the rules or laws in a specific country allow the employer to demand a testing of the possible future worker concerning this specific predisposition. This is independent from the question whether the possible worker desperately needs the job or not.

A conflict arises, however, in the case where a worker with a genetic disposition for contact dermatitis is in grave financial need and testing for the specific predisposition is not obligatory or the test is legally prohibited, as is the case for genetic diagnosis in some regions. Germany's law on gene diagnosis, for example, prohibits employers from asking any questions regarding genetic predispositions. If the patient informs the physician about the predisposition under the reasonable presumption of confidentiality, the physician is bound by that confidentiality. A physician may only make use of persuasion to convince the patient not to apply for the position. In other countries where no such laws apply, the following conflict situations are possible:

Option 1: The physician does not break the confidentiality

The worker has a relatively high risk to get the disease and thus carries a high risk to bodily integrity. The employer, too, bears a high risk to be hurt economically. Depending upon the region's health-care structure, the long-term illness has to be paid by society or the participating members of the respective insurance. There is also another problem. Let us assume that after some years of work the worker attracts the disease he was predisposed for and then tells the employer that the physician was confidentially informed about his condition when he applied. The physician may fear that the employer will "punish" him for not telling him even though he was bound to maintain the confidentiality and the employer is not allowed to do so. Laws may protect OHPs, but there are indirect ways for businesses to apply punishment, e.g., denying career advancements and salary increases.

Option 2: The physician breaks the confidentiality

If the physician breaks the confidentiality, which is permissible in some countries, trust in the relationship and in the profession is damaged. The long-term result will be that no patient will reveal anything beyond the mere minimum required, and nothing will be revealed that could jeopardize job applications or security. The result will be that the distrusted physician is not able to try to convince someone not to apply for a position. This places the worker at a health risk because the OHP lacks necessary information. Further, the OHP and the business are placed in legal jeopardy because prospective applicants could seek legal remedies for broken patient confidentiality and damage done to future wage earnings.

Both options leave the physician in a dilemmatic situation. The solution consists in keeping confidentiality, because this is the foremost duty according to the ethical framework of human dignity and human rights. This solution respects the self-determination of the person, and is consistent with the framework of medical values worldwide, as well as the legal framework in most countries. Nevertheless, it is important that existing legal frameworks plainly address this problem to protect the physician, especially within national legal contexts that primarily categorize workers as a class of vulnerable persons (cf. Emanuel 2002). Instead, each party involved in the hiring process bears specific responsibilities, and these responsibilities should be as clearly delineated as possible. This protects the rights of the employer, the worker, and physician. Finally, advocating for fair rules and laws is the responsibility of each group, as citizens, and especially physicians and the medical community as specialists.

3.3 The Problem of a Duty of Complete Information

But what set of rules is adequate? On the one hand, it should be noted that OHPs are not primarily enmeshed in such conflictual situations, and that the great bulk of their work is applying technical and scientific knowledge to establish preventative safety and health policies and conditions, and that this is beneficial to all four ethical constituencies. Nevertheless, the potential for conflict means that the OHP ought to have responsibilities and loyalties clearly outlined for workers and management. The most conflict-ridden issue of divided loyalties should be resolved NOT by reducing health surveillance or the flow of information between medical professionals and workers. Rather, conflict resolution should be achieved by establishing clearly articulated boundaries: Medical officials should be able to attain the information they need to insure the safest possible workplace and workers should be assured that their rights and privacy are not violated. Where OHPs have obtained demonstrably relevant health information needed to make prudent medical decisions with respect to hazardous working conditions, the findings must be discretely relayed without revealing specific details of the examinations. (ICOH Code #10) Further, medical professionals have the duty to refrain from revealing information from employers when that revelation is a violation of workers' informed consent, or when such an action would endanger the trust in their integrity and impartiality. The ICOH Code is quite clear that to protect this independence, OHPs should insist that it be written into their contracts as standard practice (#19).

There are good reasons for applicants revealing all health information important for the position, and physicians should screen to exclude as much risk as possible. If this is the case, there is no inherent reason why genetic information must be dealt with differently if two conditions can be met: (1) that it can be reasonably demonstrated to predict predisposition to injury or disease; and (2) that injury or disease is reasonably grave and closely related to performing the occupational tasks. Genetic screening need not be prohibited if it is analogous with consisting regulations concerning nongenetic diseases and dispositions. A prohibition to reveal genetic information might appear to be ethically problematic for various reasons:

- Persons with diseases or predispositions for diseases considered conventional have to reveal a great deal of private information, some of them may not be currently understood. Therefore, they are not equally treated.
- Persons with genetic diseases or predispositions for diseases have the incentive mentioned above to exploit the system, if they are in desperate need of employment.

But if potentially valid and relevant monitoring and investigations are excluded for these two reasons, we face a situation of workers shielding medical information that places them and others at potential risk.

A more optimal solution (suggested by ICOH Code generally and especially #12) is the strict choosing of biological monitoring and investigations that have been proven valid and relevant "for the protection of the health of the worker concerned, with due regard to their sensitivity, their specificity, and their predictive value." This is not just a process of marginal cost-effectiveness analysis, although that analysis is certainly relevant. And there is room for flexibility among regions dependent upon their relative wealth. A good solution is for OHPs and the medical community as a whole to work together to establish the most high-risk predispositions or diseases for occupational populations. Employers should only be allowed to demand a screening for these agreed-upon respective predispositions and diseases. There is no inherent reason why genetic diseases and predispositions should be treated differently from conventional predispositions and diseases. Likewise, protections against discrimination should insure that genetic information is likewise not the cause of unfair exclusions from the job market for workers. If the fear or danger of discrimination is proven to be well founded, perhaps such genetic testing could be conducted by third-party health-care providers, who would maintain the genetic information independently from the place of employment.

4 Specific Ethical Case and Resolution for Occupational Dermatology

The discussion to this point has dealt with occupational health in general. This is a relevant discussion given that up to 50% of work-related illnesses are skin related (Peate 2002), but what follows focuses specifically upon occupational dermatology. According to Marks et al. (2002), the development of occupational skin disease is multifactorial in origin. It results from the interaction of predisposing risk factors in workers together with agents within the work environment such as chemicals, abrasions, plants, animals, sunlight, radiation, heat, cold, moisture, and others. The identity of such material causal agents suggests that occupational skin disease is an affliction that can be prevented with careful control of the work environment. Knowing that this condition is also one without a good prognosis makes it a reality especially open to ethical reflection. Only 25% of the people will be healed completely even though they change their occupation.

The following case presents a potential dilemma for the OHP and a pathway to an ethical treatment of the dilemma using the framework suggested above.

4.1 The Case: Chronic Allergic Contact Eczema Caused by the Chromate in Cement

Chronic allergic contact eczema, or concrete-induced dermatitis is a fairly common work-related disease and one that plagues the construction industry. In Germany, for example, between 1986 and 1996 there were approximately 300 cases diagnosed per year (Mettler 1999). The specific cause of the disease is a combination of factors that occur with the mixing of cement at construction sites. The concrete ingredients themselves are physically abrasive to the skin, causing scratches and the wearing down of the protective outer dermis. The cement mixture has a high alkaline content, causing chemical burns to the exposed, scratched, and degraded skin. That injured skin is especially sensitive to the chromium compounds found in the cement, and chromium is a common trigger for allergic reactions. Once sensitized, a person is a greater risk for repeat and serious allergic episodes. Indications can appear after weeks, but may take years. There is no known predisposition associated with greater risk for the disease. Preventative measures include reducing the chromate levels of cement (to less that 20 ppm), wearing protective clothing when handling the wet cement, reducing contact time with cement, avoiding extended time with wet hands, informing workers of the danger to increase probability that above conditions are enforced.

This ethical dilemma presented by this medical scenario is more structural than individual, as OHPs know the dangers, treatment and preventative measures relevant to the disease. Imagine, rather, a construction company operating in an economically deprived area employing workers from a large pool of available, but unskilled and nonunionized laborers, and operating with small profit margins in a not-so-rosy economic climate of escalated market competition. The OHP must outline an ethical approach to dealing with this scenario that appropriates the guidelines of the ICOH Code.

4.2 Start of a Solution

To deal with this problem in Germany, all the parties involved in the construction industry entered into a free-will commitment to reduce the chromium content in cement and cement products. This commitment remains in place but as free-will agreements tend to have little enforcement power, its goals were not achieved as of 2001. During that year, the LUBW (Baden-Württemberg's State Agency for the Environment, Measurement, and Environmental Protection) revealed that over two-thirds of construction sites were using cements with high chromium content. The revelation of noncompliance had a positive effect; within 1 year the chromium was reduced by 30%. But the experience demonstrates the inherently difficulties of goodwill agreements – and this is in a highly developed and prosperous nation.

4.3 Solution by the Framework of Rules

In January of 2005, the European Union set the standards for the construction industry. The rules stipulate that only cement with reduced chromium content may be used. This means that only cement with a soluble chromium (VI) content of <2 ppm. This rule was set not only for general-use cement, but also for products that contain cement such as mortar and tiling glue. The effects of this rule were substantial. Since the rule went into effect in 2005, the number of workers presenting concrete-induced dermatitis has been significantly reduced (Geier et al. 2011).

The example here shows that OHPs are very much dependent upon their industry's structure of rules, and that ethical considerations cannot be viewed independently from that structure. Individually, they are most aided by the competency standards set up for medical professionals. But the example of concrete-inducing dermatitis shows that the problems facing the OHP demand the support of the whole industry, medical community, and legal establishment. The factors leading to skin problems in workers are so complex, that individual approaches will tend to be ineffective. Issues such as market pressures in economically depressed regions make these issues more acutely felt, and there is room for regional variance, but the solution must nevertheless be a structural one. The example above with cement, for example, will have to be repeated in the near future for materials containing nanoparticles. The issues and health problems that are presented will be unique, but the solution will be analogous (also see ➋ Chap. 67, "Occupational Allergy to Natural Rubber Latex (NRL)").

References

Baur X, Letzel S, Nowak D (2009) Ethik in der Arbeitsmedizin. Orientierungshilfe in ethischen Spannungsfeldern. Ecomed, Landsberg

Beauchamp T, Childress J (2001) Principles of biomedical ethics, 5th edn. Oxford University Press, New York

Bercovitch L, Long TP (2007) Dermatoethics: a curriculum in bioethics and professionalism for dermatology residents at Brown Medical School. J Am Acad Dermatol 56:679–682

Board of the German Society for Occupational Medicine and Environmental Medicine e.V. (DGAUM) and the Bureau of the Association of German Company and Factory Doctors e.V. (VDBW) (2009) A code of ethics for occupational medicine. Ecomed, Landsberg

Brandt-Rauf PW (1989) Ethical conflict in the practice of occupational medicine. Br J Ind Med 46:63–66

Budnik LT, Baur X (2009) The assessment of environmental and occupational exposure to hazardous substances by biomonitoring. Dtsch Arztebl Int 106(6):91–97

Emanuel EJ (2002) Introduction to occupational medical ethics. Occup Med 17(4):549–558

Geier J, Krautheim A, Uter W, Lessmann H, Schnuch A (2011) Occupational contact allergy in the building trade in Germany: influence of preventive measures and changing exposure. Int Arch Occup Environ Health 84(4):403–411

Guidotti TL (2008) Occupational medicine and the construction of "difficult reputations". New Solut 18(3):285–298

International Commission on Occupational Health (2002) International Code of Ethics for Occupational Health Professionals. http://www.icohweb.org/core_docs.asp. Accessed 20 March 2010

Knoepffler N (2004) Menschenwürde in der Bioethik. Springer, Berlin

Knoepffler N (2010) Angewandte Ethik. Ein systematischer Leitfaden. Böhlau (UTB), Köln

Kuhn J, Gensch R (2009) Ethical aspects of workplace health management. Bundesgesundheitsblatt Gesundheitsforschung Gesundheitsschutz 52(5):535–552

London L (2005) Dual loyalties and the ethical and humans rights obligations of occupational health professionals. Am J Ind Med 47:322–332

Marks JG, Elsner P, DeLeo VA (2002) Etiology of occupational skin disease. In: Marks JG, Elsner P, DeLeo VA (eds) Contact and occupational dermatology, 3rd edn. Mosby, St. Louis, pp 303–313

Mettler H (1999) Problem Maurerkrätze: Es gibt eine Lösung. Trauma und Berufskrankheit 1:148–151

Peate WF (2002) Occupational skin disease. Am Fam Physician 66(6):1025–1032

Westerholm P (2007) Professional ethics in occupational health—Western European perspectives. Ind Health 45:19–25

Westerholm P, Nilstun T, Ovretveit J (2004) Practical ethics in occupational health. Radcliffe Medical Press, Oxford

World Health Organization (2006) Environmental health criteria 232. Static fields. World Health Organization, Geneva. http://www.who.int/peh-emf/publications/reports/ehcstatic/en/index.html. Accessed 11 Feb 2009

6 History of Occupational Dermatology

Jean-Marie Lachapelle
Unit of Occupational and Environmental Dermatology, Catholic University of Louvain, Montigny-le-Tilleul, Belgium

Core Messages

- Bernardino Ramazzini (1633–1714) is undoubtedly the father of modern occupational medicine.
- *De morbis artificum diatriba* is the first twenties dedicated to occupational medicine, but cases of occupational dermatology are poorly described.
- A major discovery in the eighteenth century was the cancer of the scrotum among chimney sweepers.
- The birth of dermatology during the nineteenth century had a limited impact on occupational dermatology.
- Josef Jadassohn is the father of Patch Testing (1895–1896).
- A breakthrough in occupational dermatology: Poul Bonnevie's pioneering work.
- Many books have been dedicated recently to occupational dermatology.

1 From the Ancient Times

1.1 Introduction

Michel Valentin wrote a detailed and very well documented history of occupational medicine (Valentin 1978) (➋ *Fig. 6.1*) and ergonomics, starting from the Egyptian period till the end of the seventeeth century. It is a goldmine of knowledge for historians, but, in all respects, it lacks of real interest for medical doctors. Indeed, the various stories collected in this book are too anecdotal and imprecise, and it seems difficult to adhere to the proposed conclusions.

Nevertheless, from the ancient Greek and Roman civilizations, the statements advanced by two Greats of that time have to be kept in memory:

- Hippocrates (circa 460–377 B.C.) considered environmental influences as possible causes of diseases (Cadwick and Mann 1950). His observations were prophetic but his conclusions somewhat tangential.
- Galen (A.D. 133–200) preceded the Environmental Protective Agency by 1900 years; he considered the noxious effect of air pollution in his work *De Temperamentis* (Siddiqui and Cormane 1976).

1.2 From Greece to Ramazzini

1.2.1 Bernardino Ramazzini, the Father of Occupational Medicine

Bernardino Ramazzini (1633–1714) is undoubtedly the father of modern occupational medicine. First of all, he appears to have been "one of the outstanding physicians of Italy of the time." He practised during all his life in Modena (Emilia) and was consulted by a vast number of patients; this was due to his scientific approach of the problems and his practical expertise. Obviously, he tried – as far as he could – to find out the presumable cause of the diseases encountered in daily life, but, of course, the general knowledge and the tools for appropriate diagnosis were very limited at that time!

When consulting his numerous writings, the reader is surprised by his encyclopedic medical erudition. Ramazzini was aware of the views and statements expressed by his Greek and Roman predecessors. He knew also very well the discoveries of the Arabic physicians, such as Rhazès or Avicenne (Ammar 1965). He fully agreed with some of them; but, sometimes, he argued strenuously against some precepts he considered nonsense.

Ramazzini was obviously an admirer of Hippocrates and seemed fascinated by his anamnestic approach, when Hippocrates was facing a new patient, sitting under the famous tree (still alive!) in Kos Island (Greece).

Nowadays, Hippocrates' questions, formulated two millennia ago, are still a part of the current propaedeutic heritage:

(a) What are your complaints?
(b) Have you any idea about the events that could have been responsible for their onset?
(c) When did the symptoms start?
 But Ramazzini had an additional question, very important for the real impact of occupational medicine in daily life:
(d) What is your current job?
 Which were your previous jobs?
 Can you tell me about the place you are living?
 Is there a particular environmental nuisance?

T. Rustemeyer, P. Elsner, S.M. John & H.I. Maibach (eds.), *Kanerva's Occupational Dermatology*,
DOI 10.1007/978-3-642-02035-3_6,

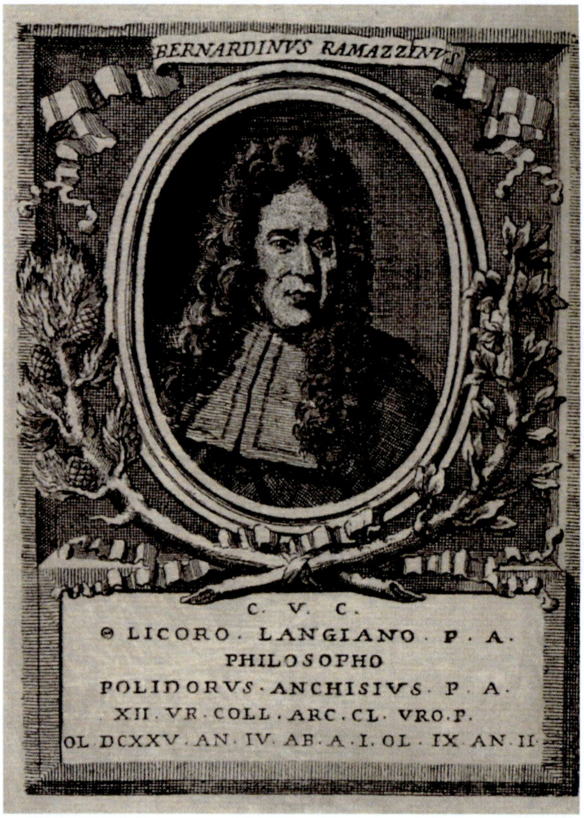

Fig. 6.1
Bernardino Ramazzini

This means that Ramazzini was very concerned by the occupational and social status of his patients and this led him to study occupational diseases in a roundabout way (Wright and Goldman 1979).

1.2.2 The First Treatise on Occupational Medicine: *De Morbis Artificum Diatriba*

Ramazzini began his lectures at the University of Modena on diseases of artisans in 1690. The first edition of his book: *De morbis artificum diatriba* ("About occupational diseases") was published at Modena in 1700 (Ramazzini 1700). The book was very innovative in its presentation and its contents (written in Latin).

It was divided into 40 chapters, each one being dedicated specifically to a well-defined occupation. Ramazzini emphasized the connection of many diseases with work conditions and urged that medical students study ways to protect workers. A second edition, expanded upon 52 chapters, was published in 1703 (*Fig. 6.2*).

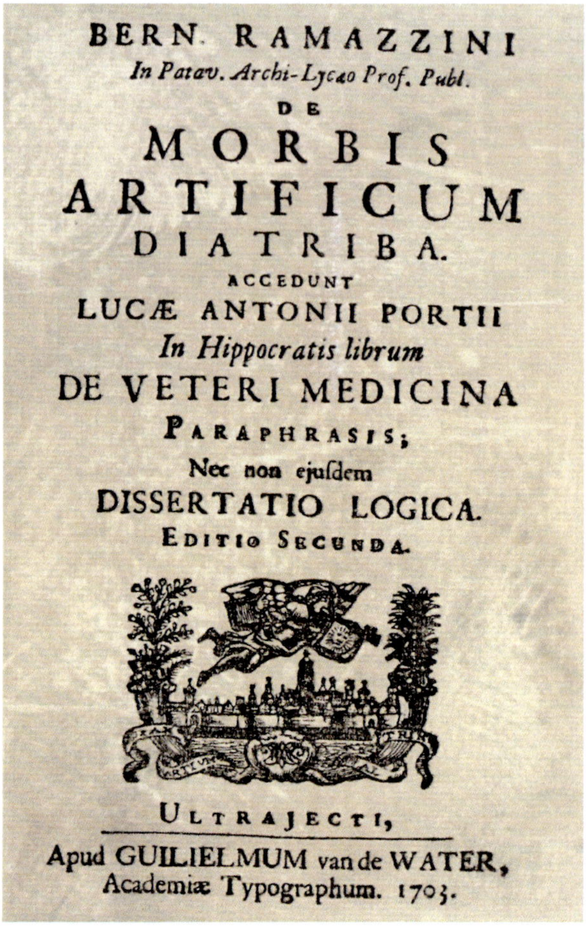
BERN. RAMAZZINI
In Patav. Archi-Lyceo Prof. Publ.
DE
MORBIS
ARTIFICUM
DIATRIBA.
ACCEDUNT
LUCÆ ANTONII PORTII
In Hippocratis librum
DE VETERI MEDICINA
PARAPHRASIS;
Nec non ejusdem
DISSERTATIO LOGICA.
EDITIO SECUNDA.

ULTRAJECTI,
Apud GUILIELMUM van de WATER,
Academiæ Typographum. 1703.

Fig. 6.2
Ramazzini's treatise: *De morbis artificum diatriba*

The success of the treatise was so important among the medical community throughout Europe that the French Royal Society asked a young brilliant doctor (circa 1780), Antoine de Fourcroy (1755–1809), to translate Ramazzini's opus into French. This translation was reedited in 1990 (de Fourcroy 1990), with a preface by Bernard Kouchner.

1.2.3 What About Occupational Dermatology in Ramazzini's Treatise?

Reading de Fourcroy's translation of Ramazzini's treatise, one is taken by surprise by the fact that skin diseases were so poorly described, as compared to other work-related diseases. However, one must remember that dermatology was not considered at that time a "speciality by itself." The

Table 6.1
Work-related skin diseases quoted in Ramazzini's treatise: *De morbis artificum diatriba* (1700)

Occupations	Skin diseases
Bakers and millers	Rheuma, i.e., seborrhoeic yellowish secretions around the eyes (from Meibomius' glands)
	Swollen and "painful hands"
Breastfeeding nurses	Impetigo of the breasts (with pustules)
	Scabies, etc.
Fishers (sea fishers and river fishers)	Wounds
	Leg ulcers
	Pustular reactions
Gilders	Mouth ulcers due to mercury vapors
Gold diggers	Chrysoderma
Horsemen	Hemorrhoids
	Anal clefts
Laundry women and soap workers	Irritant contact dermatitis of the hands and forearms attributed to repeated friction and direct contact with caustic substances
Midwives	Hand ulcers
	Syphilis (at risk). *Treponema pallidum* was not identified at that time, and the term "verola" was commonly used
Masons, bricklayers	Cement burns
Persons standing constantly at work	Varices
	Leg ulcers
Pharmacists	Lesions on the hands and forearms: pruritus, papules, scratch marks, etc. (these terms most probably prefigured "eczematous" lesions, either irritant or allergic)
Salt workers	Leg ulcers due to acids

work-related diseases were so dramatic, that skin lesions were considered ancillary. Most of the diseases described were life threatening, due to heavy poisoning by metals, for instance. Nevertheless, quoted in *Table 6.1* are some work-related skin diseases that were classically observed in the beginning of the eighteenth century.

It is clear that most skin conditions had not been identified as such in 1700 (i.e., eczemas, psoriasis, acne, various types of tumors, etc.). Therefore, the terms used in *Table 6.1* provide a flavor of popular medicine.

1.3 Some Reports of Occupational Dermatology During the Eighteenth Century

Some reports referring to occupational dermatology were published, somewhat isolated, during the eighteenth century (Wright and Goldman 1979). They were described as "dermatitis," mainly of the hands, forearms, and face. Some examples are quoted at random: cases of dermatitis due to lacquer varnish, laundry soaps, mercury, wax in shoe makers, etc.

In the United States, poison ivy dermatitis (unknown in European countries) was very frequent among foresters and agricultural workers. A. Rostenberg Jr., published a wonderful paper entitled *An Anecdotical Biographical History of Poison Ivy* (Rostenberg 1955). He explained at length how not only medical officers but also agricultural experts were implied in the problem-solving of the disease, which was a real disaster in some parts of the country. Experimental studies (including applications of various parts of the plant onto the skin) were conducted in many places, but all those efforts were forgotten for a long period of time.

1.4 A Major Discovery in the Eighteenth Century: The Cancer of the Scrotum Among Chimney Sweepers

During the eighteenth century, the most important discovery in occupational dermatology was the recognition of the occurence of cancers of the scrotum (defined later as squamous cell carcinomas) among chimney sweepers. This discovery was due to Sir Percival Pott (1775), in London. At that time, chimney sweepers were selected very young (even at the age of 5), in relation with their small size, and they worked for many years in the same job.

In his careful studies, Pott noticed that the tumors appeared at a late stage, when workers were aged 30–35 years. He considered that skin tumors were consecutive to a long exposure to soot, lack of protective clothing, and poor personal hygiene. In the next century, it was recognized that a number of coaltar products and certain forms of mineral oils in different industries could cause cutaneous cancers (Decoufle 1982).

Schwartz et al. (1957) believed that coaltar derivates were the most frequent causes of occupational cancer, with 35% caused by tar, 54% by pitch, and 5% by heavy tar oil. Nowadays, thanks to preventive measures, all these pathological events have almost completely disappeared.

2 The Birth of Dermatology in the Nineteenth Century

2.1 The Birth of Dermatology as a Separate Scientific Discipline During the Nineteenth Century: Its Impact on Occupational Dermatology

The knowledge of skin diseases and tumors blossomed in the beginning of the nineteenth century, almost simultaneously in many European countries. Attempts were made to classify adequately the elementary lesions that were observed on the skin of patients. Authors described carefully the morphological characteristics of each type of lesion; they also produced remarkable color drawings that they collected together in books of illustrations or in treatises. But there was still a pitfall: the etiology of most dermatoses was unknown, and, apart from the credit paid for the classification (like a stamp collection), no real progress could be reached.

Jean-Louis Alibert (1768–1837) is considered the father of French Dermatology. Alibert's tree of dermatoses is very famous but is of course obsolete nowadays (Alibert 1833). The tree of skin disorders is the testimony of Alibert's innovative work in picture form. As a result of the evolution of scientific knowledge over the past century, it has, of course, been superseded. Henceforth, it belongs to the historical patrimony of the Hôpital Saint-Louis to which the name of Alibert will be forever linked (Tilles 1989; Lachapelle et al. 1995).

The contribution of the English school at the same period was in retrospect more important for the future of occupational dermatology.

Thomas Bateman (1778–1821) worked in association with Robert Willan (1757–1812), the illustrious founder of the British Dermatology, at the Public Dispensary in London, an association which was to become far more than one of teacher and pupil, for Bateman became Willian's most trusted assistant, and the tremendous work of the latter interrupted by death (1811) was brought to its logical conclusion by Bateman in his masterful and most influential *A Practical Synopsis of Cutaneous Diseases*, (Bateman 1814). As with Socrates and Plato, it is difficult to determine where the work of one ends and the other's begins.

His description of eczema (he called it *eczema rubrum*) is very precise:

The disease is preceded by a sense of stiffness, burning, heat and itching, in the part where it commences. These sensations are soon followed by an appearance of redness, and the surface is somewhat rough to the touch. This, however, is not a simple erythema: for on examining it minutely between the light and the eye, or with a convex glass, the roughness is found to be occasioned by innumerable minute, red pellucid vesicles, which have been mistaken for papules. In two or three days, these vesicles, if they are not ruptured, obtain the size of a pin's head, and the included serum then becoming somewhat opaque and milky, the character of the eruption is obvious. When the vesicles begin to lose their transparency, they generally burst, and discharge from numerous points a thin acid fluid, which seems to irritate the surface. . . .

A detailed review of this fascinating story was edited by Shelley and Crissey (1953).

Von Hebra (1816–1880) marked the beginning of etiologic research by demonstrating that eczematous dermatitis could be induced by the application of croton oil on normal skin (Finnerud 1952). He utilized pathology to study a clinical dermatologic problem. Prior to his experiment, it was generally held that eczema was caused by morbid conditions of fluids of the body. While demonstrating that eczema could result from external substances, he realized that such a mechanism did not explain all skin diseases. He maintained that occupational exposure "per se" was not the cause of psoriasis.

2.2 Josef Jadassohn, the Father of Patch Testing

With the morphology and some pathophysiology established, some method of diagnostic confirmation was needed. Josef Jadassohn (1863–1936) developed the patch test, in 1895–1896 (Jadassohn 1896).

As recorded by Sulzberger in 1940 in his classic textbook, the key message of Jadassohn's paper was the fact that he recognized the process of delayed hypersensitivity to simple chemicals (Sulzberger 1940). He was the first to make a distinction between irritant and allergic reactions (the term "allergy" was not used at that time, since it was coined only in 1906 by von Pirquet).

3 The Life of Occupational Dermatology in the Twentieth Century

In fact, most cases of occupational dermatology observed during the twentieth century refer to contact dermatitis (either irritant or allergic) and more recently to contact urticaria and protein contact dermatitis (with or without an atopic background).

Therefore, there is a close connection between historical aspects of occupational dermatology, contact dermatitis, and patch testing. An extensive review of the evolution of patch testing has been made recently (Lachapelle 2009). The number of irritants and contact allergens has increased considerably, as it is fully explained in the different chapters.

It is out of the scope of this chapter to review the history of each individual allergen and/or irritant; it is more important to recall some general pathways which were applied in the field of occupational dermatology.

3.1 Occupational Dermatology in the First Half of the Twentieth Century

When reading many publications (dated 1900–1950) the overall impression was that occupational dermatology was not considered a specific entity: there was no real approach about it!

Most certainly, many papers were dealing with irritant and/or allergic contact dermatitis related to occupation, but during a long period of time no book was specially devoted to occupational dermatology. It was most probably due to the fact that no social structure did exist to help workers when they were facing skin problems.

3.2 Books Dedicated to Occupational Dermatology

Ronchese 1948 wrote a classical book entitled *Occupational Marks and Other Physical Signs. A Guide to Personal Identification.* His approach was interesting and quite original, but, of course, it had no practical implications. It is therefore not too surprising that it was rarely quoted in most textbooks of dermatology.

Gougerot and Carteaud 1952 published (in French) a book simply called *Occupational Dermatoses.* Its reading is intriguing for two reasons: (a) the section devoted to "eczemas" is limited to 22 pages; (b) on the other hand, 132 pages are dedicated to all other occupational dermatoses. They are listed in alphabetical order (*Table 6.2*). Some of these have completely disappeared in industrialized countries.

Table 6.2
List of occupational dermatoses quoted in Gougerot-Carteaud's book 1952

Achromias[a]
Acne (common)[a]
Actinic dermatitis
Anthrax[a]
Bullous dermatoses
Burns
Chloracne[a]
Chrome and/or nickel ulcer
Erysipeloid
Erythroderma
Frostbites
Glanders, farcy[a]
Hoffmann and Habermann's lichenoid melanoderma[a]
Keratoderma
Mycoses
Occupational cancers
Onychoses and perionyxis
Pruritus and prurigo
Purpura
Pyoderma
Radiodermatitis and radiumdermatitis[a]
Rhagades
Riehl's melanosis[a]
Syphilis[a]
Tattoos
Tuberculosis
Urticaria
Vaccinia[a]

[a]Dermatoses that have completely or almost completely disappeared in industrialized countries

3.3 A Breakthrough in Occupational Dermatology: Poul Bonnevie's Pioneering Work

The work initiated and developed by J. Jadassohn was pursued to a large extent by Bruno Bloch in Basel and in Zurich. Patch testing has become so important that some authors refer to the "Jadassohn-Bloch" technique. One of Bloch's trainees at the time was Poul Bonnevie from Copenhagen, who spent some time in Zurich. Bonnevie was also an occupational physician and he soon realized

Table 6.3
The standard series of patch tests proposed by Bonnevie 1939 and slightly modified by Marcussen 1962 (mainly in terms of nomenclature, and also with the addition of *Primula*)

1	Turpentine (50% olive oil)
2	Colophony resin (10% olive oil)
3	Balsams of Peru (25% lanolin)
4	Salicylic acid (5% lanolin)
5	Formalin (4% water)
6	Mercuric chloride (0.1% water)
7	Potassium dichromate (0.5% water)
8	Silver nitrate (2% water)
9	Nickel sulphate (5% water)
10	Resorcin (5% petrolatum)
11	*Primula obconica*
12	Sodium perborate powder (10% water)
13	Brown soap (as is)
14	Coal tar (pure)
15	Wood tars
16	Quinine HCl (1% water)
17	Iodine (0.5% ethanol)
18	Pyrogallol (5% petrolatum)
19	Paraphenylenediamine (2% petrolatum)
20	Paramidophenol, i.e., 4-amino-3 nitrophenol (2% petrolatum)
21	Adhesive plaster (as is)

how patch testing could be useful in the field of occupational dermatology. His book, edited simultaneously in German and in Danish in 1939, is a masterpiece of concision and knew a great success (Bonnevie 1939).

Bonnevie was the father of a "standard series" of patch tests, now called "baseline series" (➋ *Table 6.3*).

This "standard" or "baseline" series was used unchanged, and Marcussen 1962 an extensive statistical analysis of the results collected in Denmark.

The series was not dedicated in particular to occupational dermatology, but was a selection of the allergens, mainly encountered in the environment of that time. Nevertheless, it is obvious that some of them were primarily, but not exclusively, related to work activities, i.e., turpentine, formalin, potassium dichromate, nickel sulphate, brown soap, coal tar, wood tars, pyrogallol, paraphenylenediamine, and paramidophenol.

It is fascinating that about 30 years later, some allergens are still in the limelight (➋ *Table 6.4*).

Table 6.4
Bonnevie's series: allergens still present in the current standard series (Cadwick and Mann 1950)

1	Colophony
2	Balsams of Peru
3	Formaldehyde
4	Potassium dichromate
5	Nickel sulphate
6	Paraphenylenediamine
7	*Primula* (optional)
8	Adhesive plaster

Adhesive plaster as is; at that time, often allergenic (due to the presence of colophony). The material used today for patch testing is hypoallergenic

3.4 Later Events

The recent history of occupational dermatology is closely linked with the historical and scientific advances in the field of contact dermatitis. The creation of international groups of contact dermatitis, such as the ICDRG (International Contact Dermatitis Research Group), the NACDG (North American Contact Dermatitis Group), the ACDS (American Contact Dermatitis Society), the EECDRG (European Environmental and Contact Dermatitis Research Group), and the ECDS (European Contact Dermatitis Society), led to a blossom of knowledge in the field of contact dermatitis. The birth of national groups throughout the world boosted the discipline. Working parties on occupational dermatology were created, i.e., by the ECSD. Moreover, some departments, exclusively devoted to occupational dermatology, were opened in different countries.

3.5 Recent Books Related to Occupational Dermatology

Several books have been written in recent years about occupational dermatology. A French treatise on occupational and environmental dermatology has been published (Lachapelle et al. 1992) based on Gougerot and Carteaud's book (1952), it has been entirely actualized and adapted to modern life, including sports' activities and regulatory aspects, with a comparison between the French and the European legislation.

Robert Adams was a great specialist in occupational dermatology. His classical book was present in all librairies. The originality was that, for the first time, there were a lot of black-and-white photographs, illustrating various workplaces, thus allowing the reader to better understand skin problems encountered in different industrial sectors (Adams 1990).

Other condensed books appeared in the United States.

But the masterpiece in the field of occupational dermatology is Kanerva's book (Kanerva et al. 2000) that is a real encyclopedia, covering all aspects of occupational life.

A second edition was really needed!

References

Adams RM (1990) Occupational skin disease, 2nd edn. W.B. Saunders, Philadelphia, 706 pp

Alibert JL (1833) Clinique de l'Hôpital Saint-Louis, ou traité complet des maladies de la peau contenant la description de ces maladies et leurs meilleurs modes de traitement, orné de 63 planches, 1st edn. Cormon et Blanc, Paris, 390 pp

Ammar S (1965) En souvenir de la médecine arabe. Quelques uns de ses grands noms. Bascone et Touzat, Tunis, 209 pp

Bateman Th (1814) A practical synopsis of cutaneous diseases, 3rd edn. Longman, London, 344 pp

Bonnevie P (1939) Actiologic und Pathogenese der Ekzemkrankheiten. Klinische Studien über der Ursachen der Ekzeme unter besonderer Berücksichtigung des Diagnostischen Wertes der Ekzemproben. Busch, Copenhagen/Barth, Leipzig

Cadwick J, Mann WN (1950) The medical works of Hippocrates. Blackwell Scientific, London

de Fourcroy A (1990) Bernardino Ramazzini (1633–1714). Des maladies du travail (*De morbis artificum diatriba* – 1700) with a preface by Bernard Kouchner. Alexitère Editions, Paris, 340 pp

Decoufle P (1982) Occupation. In: Scottenfeld P, Fraumeni JF Jr (eds) Cancer epidemiology and prevention. W.B. Saunders, Philadelphia, pp 318–335

Finnerud CW (1952) Ferdinand von Hebra and the Vienna school of dermatology. Arch Dermatol Syphilol 66:223–232

Gougerot H, Carteaud A (1952) Dermatoses professionnelles. Maloine, Paris, 368 pp

Jadassohn J (1896) Zur Kenntnis der Medicamentösem Dermatosen. Verhandlungen der Deutschen Dermatologischen Gesellschaft, V Congress, 1895. Vienna, Austria; Braumüller, Vienna, pp 103–129

Kanerva L, Elsner P, Wahlberg JE, Maibach HI (2000) Handbook of occupational dermatology. Springer, Berlin, 1300 pp

Lachapelle JM (2009) Evolution of patch testing. Dermat 20:316–321

Lachapelle JM, Frimat P, Tennstedt D et al (1992) Précis de dermatologie professionnelle et de l'environnement. Masson, Paris, 400 pp

Lachapelle JM, Tennstedt D, Degreef H et al (1995) 2 centuries of dermatology. Jean-Louis Alibert (1768–1837). Glaxo Belgium, Brussels, 300 pp

Marcussen PV (1962) Variations in the incidence of contact hypersensitivities. Trans St Johns Hosp Dermatol Soc 48:40–49

Pott P (1775) Cancer scroti. In: Pott P (ed) Chirurgical observations. Hawes, Clarke and Collins, London, pp 63–68

Ramazzini B (1700) De morbis artificum diatriba. Impressoris Episcopalis, Modena

Ronchese F (1948) Occupational marks and other physical signs. A guide to personal identification. Grune and Stratton, New York, 176 pp

Rostenberg A Jr (1955) An anecdotal biographical history of poison Ivy. Arch Dermatol 72:438–455

Schwartz L, Tulipan L, Birmingham DJ (1957) Occupational diseases of the skin. Lea and Febiger, Philadelphia, pp 726–737

Siddiqui AH, Cormane RH (1976) Dermatologic origins and developments down to the early 20th century. J Invest Dermatol 66: 122–127

Sulzberger MD (1940) Dermatologic allergy. Thomas Springfield, Illinois, p 88

Tilles G (1989) La naissance de la dermatologie (1776–1880). Roger Dacosta, Paris, 320 pp

Valentin M (1978) Travail des hommes savants oubliés. Histoire de la médecine du travail, de la sécurité et de l'ergonomie. Docis, Paris, 329 pp

Wright RC, Goldman L (1979) Contact dermatitis: a historical perspective. Int J Dermatol 18:665–668

7 Classification of Occupations

Wolfgang Uter
Department of Medical Informatics, Biometry and Epidemiology, University of Erlangen/Nürnberg, Erlangen, Germany

Core Messages

- Occupational exposure can be represented either by the occupation (job title) or the industry a person is working in.
- Several international and even more national classification systems for both occupation and industry exist.
- As global classification of occupations, the "International Standard Classification of Occupations" (ISCO, presently ISCO-08) of the International Labor Organization is available.
- The "International Standard Industrial Classification of all Economic Activities" (ISIC), presently in its 4th revision, issued by the United Nations Statistics Division, is used to document industrial sectors.
- Depending on the circumstances, classification of occupation rather than industry may be preferable, or vice versa, or possibly use of both classification dimensions.
- Regarding all general classifications, medical use for representing relevant (skin) exposure has not been a major objective. Hence, additional categories may need to be added, while some original categories can be used on an aggregated level.

1 Introduction

The systematic surveillance of a population – from the world population to the members of a small or medium enterprise or community – is based on a number of classification systems. In the field of medical diagnoses, the International Classification of Diseases (ICD) by the WHO, presently in the 10th revision, is an accepted standard. While the classification of disease status concerns the outcome of epidemiological analyses, the classification of occupational exposure is needed to standardize a potential explanatory factor which can be linked to disease status. A certain occupation ("job title") can here be regarded as a more or less precise surrogate marker for a characteristic profile of medically relevant exposures, e.g., to carcinogens or allergens (Schnitzer et al. 1995). Beyond the simplest possible representation of occupational exposure by the job title itself, job titles can be expanded to standardized exposure profiles, termed job-exposure-matrix (JEM; Goldberg et al. 1993; Plato and Steineck 1993). JEM are used to link information on occupation with information on exposure to specific workplace hazards, e.g., for epidemiological risk analyses, if only data on occupation, but no individual data on exposure are available. The precision of JEM may vary, depending on whether they are designed for a company or an industrial sector and can therefore be based on a more detailed classification of occupations and better exposure information, or whether JEM are applied in population-based studies, where they necessarily have to be more general (Goldberg et al. 1993).

A competing concept of documenting medically (dermatologically) relevant descriptors, i.e., exposures and their duration and intensity, would be to classify not the individual occupation of the patient, but the type of industry he or she is working in. Examples of such classifications and some of their applications, e.g., by employers liability insurances or governmental labor statistics, are listed below. In many instances both types of classifications will achieve very similar results, for example, allowing either the classification of a patient as "hairdresser" ("ISCO-08" # 5141) or as a person working in "hairdressing and other beauty treatment" ("ISIC Rev. 4" # 9602), the latter being probably somewhat less specific. In other cases the classification according to industry may be more specific – at least comparing "ISCO-08" and "ISIC Rev. 4" – while "ISCO-08" aggregates "miners and quarriers" and "... laborers," respectively (# 8111, # 9311) irrespective of the minerals extracted, "ISIC Rev. 4" details already on the second hierarchical level the material extracted ("mining of coal ..." # 05, "mining of metal ores" # 07, etc.).

However, in other cases, particularly in large industrial plants, e.g., in the automobile industry ("manufacture of motor vehicles, trailers, and semi-trailers," ISIC Rev. 4 # 29), a whole range of different occupations (and very different exposures) is found in one industry, including, among others, cutting- and non-cutting metal workers ("ISCO-08" # 72: "Metal, machinery and related trades workers"), painters (# 7131 or # 8122), administrative personnel (# 1 – subgroups), cleaning (# 91 – subgroups), and kitchen (# 51 – subgroups) staff. Thus the

T. Rustemeyer, P. Elsner, S.M. John & H.I. Maibach (eds.), *Kanerva's Occupational Dermatology*,
DOI 10.1007/978-3-642-02035-3_7,

Table 7.1
"ISCO-08" occupational code numbers (different skill levels) and "ISIC Rev. 4" industrial code numbers, respectively, as appropriate, for selected occupations and industries, respectively. Code numbers selected on a hierarchical level as low as possible, i.e., as specific as possible. Exclusions in "job title" may not be applicable to the units identified by the number(s)

ISCO-08	Job title/Industrial sector	ISIC Rev.4
Various	Aircraft industry	3030
9312 (n.s.)	Air hammer operators	4210 (n.s.)
2230; 2269 (n.s.); 323	Aromatherapists	8690 (n.s)
8342 (n.s.); 9312 (n.s.)	Asphalt workers (Paving)	4210 (n.s)
7231	Automobile mechanics	4520
7512 (n.s.)	Bakers	1071; Part of 56 (n.s.)
5141	Barbers and hairdressers	9602 (n.s.)
5132	Bartenders	5630
5142 (n.s.)	Bath attendants	9311 (n.s.)
7318 (n.s.)	Batik manufacturing workers	1313 (n.s.)
7241 (n.s.)	Battery makers	2790 (n.s.)
6123	Beekeepers	0149 (n.s.)
751 (n.s.)	Biotechnical industry workers (food)	7210 (n.s.)
7115 (n.s.); 8142 (n.s.)	Boat builders	301
7231 (n.s.)	Brake-lining workers	2930 (n.s.)
7511 (n.s.); 8160 (n.s.)	Butchers and slaughterhouse workers	1010
7522	Cabinet makers	1623 (n.s.); 3100 (n.s.); 9524
8131 (n.s.)	Candle makers	3290 (n.s.)
7512 (n.c.)	Confectionery and candy makers	1073 (n.s.)
7115	Carpenters	4100 (n.s.)
Various	Car industry	29
8114	Cement workers	2394
7314; 8181 (n.s.)	Ceramic and pottery workers	2393
7513 (n.s.)	Cheese makers	1050 (n.s.)
3116; 3133; 8131	Chemists	20
5311	Child day-care workers	8510; 8790 (n.s.)
7516	Cigarette and cigar makers and tobacco workers	1200
Various	Construction workers	F (41–43)
5142 (n.s.)	Cosmetologists	9602 (n.s.)
2261; 3214; 3251; 5329	Dental personnel	8620 (n.s.)
5151; 7133; 911	Detergent workers (Cleaning staff)	812
7541	Divers	38 (n.s.)
3212	Electron microscopy workers	7420 (n.s.)
3114; 742; 8212	Electronic workers	26; 3313
8122 (n.s.)	Electroplaters	2592 (n.s.)
5163	Embalmers (including funeral service workers)	9603
7316 (n.s.)	Engravers	2592 (n.s.)
61; 631–3; 9211-3	Farmers and farm workers	011-017

Table 7.1 (Continued)

ISCO-08	Job title/Industrial sector	ISIC Rev.4
7122	Floor layers	4330 (n.s.)
5211 (n.s.); 522 (n.s.)	Florists	4773 (n.s.); 4789 (n.s.)
3143; 621; 9215	Forestry workers	2
3135	Foundry workers	1910
6129 (n.s.); 6224; 7531; 7532 (n.s.); 7535 (n.s.); 8155	Fur farmers and fur industry	014 (n.s.); 0170; 1420
7317; 752	Furniture manufacture	3100
2132; 6113; 9214	Gardeners	8130
7125; 7315; 8181 (n.s.)	Glass workers	2310; 2670 (n.s.); 3240 (n.s.)
7224	Grinders and brazers of hard-metal and stellite	Part of 25, 28, 29, and 30
322; 325 (excluding 3251); 532	Health care workers (except dental)	86 (n.s.)
9312 (n.s.)	Highway construction workers (except asphalt workers)	4210 (n.s.)
3212 (n.s.); 3219 (n.s.)	Histology technicians (except electron microscopy)	86 (n.s.)
5152; 9111	Domestic workers	
7124	Insulation workers	4329 (n.s.)
7313	Jewelers	321
3119; 3141; 321	Laboratory technicians	7120 (n.s.); 7500 (n.s.); 8690 (n.s.)
7318 (n.s.)	Leather industry	15
7222 (n.s.)	Locksmiths	4390 (n.s.)
7223	Machinists	Part of 25, 28, 29, and 30
2264 (n.s.); 3255	Masseurs	9609 (n.s.)
723	Mechanics	Part of 25, 28, 29, and 30
Various	Metal industry	24; 25; 26 and 27 (n.s.); 28; 29; 30 (n.s.); 33 (n.s.)
0	Military personnel	8422
1322; 3117; 3121; 7542; 8111; 9311	Mining (tunneling)	B (n.s.)
2652	Musicians	9000 (n.s.)
Various	Office workers	K; 68; 69; 70; 73; 82; P
8113	Oil rig workers	06 (n.s.); 0910 (n.s.)
2212; 2221	Operating room staff	86 (n.s.)
7131-2	Painters, lacquerers, and varnishers	2592 (n.s.); 4330 (n.s.); and others
8143; 8171	Paper industry, paper makers	17
3213	Pharmaceutical and cosmetic industry	21
3431; 8132	Photographers and photo lab workers	7420
6122	Poultry processors	0146; 1010 (n.s.)
9312 (n.s.)	Pitch workers	1910
7126	Plumbers and pipe fitters	4322
732	Printers and lithographers	1811
3421	Professional sports	93 (n.s.)
2144 (n.s.)	Railroad shop workers	3020
6121 (n.s.)	Reindeer herding	0149 (n.s.)

Table 7.1 (Continued)

ISCO-08	Job title/Industrial sector	ISIC Rev.4
7121	Roofers	4100 (n.s.)
7536; 8156	Shoe manufacturers and repairers	1520; 9523
7321	Silk-screen workers	1811 (n.s.)
7113	Stonemasons	2396; 4390 (n.s.)
7512 (n.s.)	Sugar artists	1073 (n.s.)
1431; 5419; 9129	Swimming pool workers	9311 (n.s.)
7131 (n.s.)	Tattoo artists	9609 (n.s.)
7318 (n.s.); 815 (excluding 8155–6)	Textile workers	13; 9601
324	Veterinary surgeons	7500
7212	Welders	2592 (n.s.)
6112; 7515; 8160	Wine makers	1102

n.s. non-specific
In case of multiple code numbers the original classifications should be consulted as to which number (entry) is most appropriate for the actual classification problem

documentation of occupation, and not of industry, appears preferable in this setting, as it mostly offers more precision (see also *Table 7.1*). A combination of both concepts may have advantages in some situations (Schnitzer et al. 1995).

Even a seemingly precise job title may hide quite varying exposure patterns, as illustrated by a comparison between a metal turner in a small workshop and a turner in a large, fully CNC equipped factory: the former will most likely heavily be exposed to cutting fluids, not being able to wear protective gloves because continually working with turning power tools, will probably use more aggressive hand cleansing because of greater soiling and will sometimes have no occupational safety or medical officers at hand. The latter turner may mostly feed crude workpieces into a completely encapsulated machine, check and pack finished workpieces, only occasionally setting or repairing the CNC lathe, being able to wear protective gloves at all times, and having easy access to safety and medical specialists.

Such differences may account for considerable variance of exposure, i.e., the need to employ more general (and imprecise) JEM the more heterogeneous the respective population is. As such characteristics may also vary a lot between countries – mostly depending on the degree of industrialization and labor division – a truly international meaning of one job title, particularly referring to a uniform exposure, can sometimes not be assumed.

These limitations have to be kept in mind considering any classification of occupations and, similarly, of industries. Despite this, the use of such a classification may be required by certain national regulations for selected purposes. In addition, and beyond legal requirements, the use of a set of well-defined entries of a catalog of occupations may facilitate standardized documentation for epidemiological analyses concerning occupational risk factors, e.g., patterns of sensitization (Uter et al. 2001), prevalence or incidence of dermatitis, etc. Therefore code numbers of the "ISCO-08," the current version, are given in *Table 7.1*, referring to occupations listed in the "Job Descriptions" section of this book. These numbers may also serve as an identifier or "common denominator" of job titles for different languages, as far as a national adaption of "ISCO-08" exists. Because some of the "Descriptions" refer to industries rather than occupations, and because most occupations can be related to one (or few) type(s) of industry(ies), "ISIC Rev. 4" code numbers have been supplemented additionally (*Table 7.1*).

2 International Standard Classification of Occupations (ISCO-08)

Regarding the classification of occupations (job titles), the International Labor Organization (ILO, www.ilo.org), Geneva, maintains the International Standard Classification of Occupations (ISCO). The ILO published the first edition of an international classification of occupations in 1952, comprising 1,727 occupations, based on national classifications of eight industrialized countries. Revisions followed in 1958, 1968, 1988, and 2007 (ISCO-08), the latter being the current version at the time this chapter is written. ISCO is a natural reference or starting point for occupational classifications developed and used in the context of occupational medicine. However, the ISCO is a truly universal classification also in the sense that it serves a variety of purposes unrelated to medicine, such as employment statistics, administrative uses, international trade and commerce, social sciences, etc. For the application in occupational dermatology, ISCO-08 partly has a degree of detail which is quite unnecessary, considering the special purpose of representing occupational skin exposure in a manageable and sensible format. For instance, many subtypes of "office workers" are listed. Conversely, in some other parts, even more detail than presented by the 4-digit level (see ➋ *Table 7.1*) appears desirable. This can be accommodated by expanding the respective 4-digit code number with a 5th (and, theoretically, further) digit with corresponding definitions, as long as (1) the hierarchical ordering is preserved and (2) mutual exclusiveness of the finest statistical units is maintained. Should a mapping to the original ISCO-08 catalog become necessary, e.g., for reporting purposes, the more detailed entries can simply be aggregated to the corresponding 4-digit level. Indeed, it has been suggested by the ILO to use the ISCO as a model for the development or adaption of national classifications, which may be extended to a finer structure. This refinement could be necessary to represent national characteristics of the labor market or more detailed occupational descriptions, which are "of particular interest . . . for vocational guidance and training, placement services, or analysis of occupation-specific morbidity and mortality" (ILO 2007). Thus, as judged by its authors, the 619 major groups, sub-major groups, minor groups, and unit groups contained in ISCO-08 may still be too gross – in parts – to serve some special demands, including occupational medicine (see also above). On an international level, ISCO-08 is used by the ILO, for statistical analyses published in the current "Yearbook of Labour Statistics."

ISCO is generally based both on the concept of "job," i.e., a certain kind of work performed by one person, which is the statistical unit of ISCO-08, and of "skill," i.e., the ability to carry out the tasks and duties of a given job, partly requiring some level of formal training. This division is useful not only from a social or economical point of view, but also from a medical, because exposure patterns may vary considerably between a chemical plant operator (# 8131), a chemical engineering technician (# 3116), a chemical processing plant controller (# 3133), a chemical engineer (# 2145) and a chemical scientist (# 2113), ordered by ascending level of skill, but all working, for instance, in the same plastic manufacturing plant. However, even within one of these units groups – which often encompass several actual occupations – marked differences in exposure may exist. As an example, in the group of hairdressers (# 5141) exposure to wet work is, at least in some countries, much heavier for apprentices – entailing a high risk of irritant hand dermatitis – than for skilled beauticians. Approaches to some specific problems in the classification of actual occupations are discussed within the "ISCO-08" (ILO 2007), which shall not be dealt with here in detail; the principles have been applied to the suggested code numbers (➋ *Table 7.1*).

3 International Standard Industrial Classification of All Economic Activities (ISIC Rev. 4)

The ISIC was first published in 1948 by the United Nations Statistics Division (UNSD); the last (fourth) revision was made in 2008. The ISIC provides a standard classification of economic activities arranged so that entities, such as persons, companies, or institutions, can be classified according to the activity they carry out. The categories of ISIC at the most detailed level (classes) are delineated according to what is in most countries the customary combination of activities described in statistical units. The groups and divisions, the successively broader levels of classification, combine the statistical units according to the character, technology, organization, and financing of production. The structure is hierarchical, consisting of 21 "Sections," 88 "Divisions," 238 "Groups," and 419 "Classes," the latter coded in 4-digit codes. This is a massive expansion since the 3rd revision, which comprised 292 "Classes." Wide use has been made of ISIC, both nationally and internationally, in classifying data according to kind of economic activity in the fields of population, production, employment, gross domestic product, and other economic activities. Other uses include demographic, social, and health analysis (e.g., ILO "Yearbook of Labour Statistics", see above).

4 Statistical Classification of Economic Activities (NACE Rev.2) of the EC

In 1970 a "General Industrial Classification of Economic Activities within the European Communities" was published by Eurostat, Luxembourg (French: "*Nomenclature statistique des activités économiques dans la*

Communauté européenne," hence the acronym NACE, corresponding to the Swiss "*Nomenclature Générale des Activités économiques* (NOGA)"). This was revised in 1990 and 2001 and made generally compatible with the ISIC, containing, however, some extensions as an adaption to European demands. On the finest, 4-digit level, NACE hosts 514 statistical units, corresponding to the ISIC classes. NACE is used as compulsory standard for Eurostat economic statistics from 1993 onward (Council Regulation EC No. 1893/2006) and regarded as part of the common statistical language being developed.

5 North American Industry Classification System (NAICS)

In January 1997, the North American Industry Classification System replaced the 1987 Standard Industrial Classification (SIC) system (Executive Office 1987) in the United States. The SIC had been used widely for national (US) statistics on occupational accidents and diseases, including occupational skin diseases (O'Malley et al. 1988; Mathias and Morrison 1988). The limitations of this system with respect to occupational dermatology have been commented on by Taylor (1988).

NAICS 2007, the latest revision at the time of writing, is an international system and has been developed in collaboration with Statistics Canada, Mexico's Instituto Nacional de Estadistica, Geografia e Information, and the US Office of Management and Budget, i.e., the NAFTA countries. NAICS 2007 is also organized in a hierarchical structure. The first two digits designate major Economic Sectors, such as Agriculture or Manufacturing. On this gross 2-digit level, it is relatively well compatible with the "ISIC Rev. 4." Readers from the three countries mentioned are referred to the US Census Bureau (http://www.census.gov/epcd/naics07/, last accessed 11-03-2010) for download, further information, and possible applications.

References

Council Regulation (EC) No. 1893/2006 establishing the statistical classification of economic activities NACE Revision 2 and amending Council Regulation (EEC) No 3037/90 OJ No L 393/1, 30 Dec 2006

Executive Office of the President, Office of Management and Budget (1987) Standard industrial classification manual, 2nd edn. N.T.I.S, Springfield

Goldberg M, Kromhout H, Guenel P et al (1993) Job exposure matrices in industry. Int J Epidemiol 22(suppl 2):S10–S15

ILO (2007) International Standard Classification of Occupations: ISCO-08. International Labour Office, Geneva. http://www.ilo.org/public/english/bureau/stat/isco/isco08/index.htm. Accessed 11 Mar 2010

Mathias CGT, Morrison JH (1988) Occupational skin diseases, United States: results from the bureau of labor statistics annual survey of occupational injuries and illnesses, 1973 through 1984. Arch Dermatol 124:1519–1524

O'Malley M, Thun M, Morrison J et al (1988) Surveillance of occupational skin disease using the supplementary data system. Am J Ind Med 13:291–299

Plato N, Steineck G (1993) Methodology and utility of a job-exposure matrix. Am J Ind Med 23:491–502

Schnitzer PG, Teschke K, Olshan AF (1995) A classification scheme for aggregating U.S. census occupation and industry codes. Am J Ind Med 28:185–191

Taylor JS (1988) Occupational disease statistics: in perspective. Arch Dermatol 124:1557–1558

United Nations (2008) International Standard Industrial Classification of all Economic Activities (ISIC – Rev. 4). http://unstats.un.org/unsd/cr/registry/isic-4.asp. Accessed 11 Mar 2010

Uter W, Schnuch A, Geier J et al (2001) Association between occupation and contact allergy to the fragrance mix: a multifactorial analysis of national surveillance data. Occup Environ Med 58:392–398

8 Occupational Contact Dermatitis

Thomas L. Diepgen[1] · *Pieter J. Coenraads*[2]
[1]Department of Clinical Social Medicine, Occupational and Environmental Dermatology, University of Heidelberg, Heidelberg, Germany
[2]Department of Dermatology, University Medical Centre Groningen, University Groningen, Groningen, The Netherlands

Core Messages

- Epidemiological studies play an important role in controlling outbreaks and disease trends, analyzing risk factors, and monitoring the efficacy of preventive measures.
- Occupational contact dermatitis constitutes up to 30% of notified occupational diseases. The average incidence rate of registered occupational contact dermatitis lies around 0.5–1.9 cases per 1,000 full-time workers per year.
- National registries and reporting systems are usually incomplete as a result of underdiagnosis and underreporting of occupational contact dermatitis, and it has been estimated that the incidence of occupational skin diseases is being grossly underestimated and mild cases are not included.
- The prognosis of occupational contact dermatitis is often poor. Changes in work practice or occupation favor the prognosis, but many patients continue to have skin problems, especially hand eczema.
- Wet work is the most important determinant of risk. Atopic skin diathesis is an important endogenous risk factor, or atopic eczema is activated by exposure.
- Primary and secondary prevention are essential fundamental components in the management of occupational contact dermatitis, and intervention studies are needed to demonstrate the efficacy of primary and secondary prevention measures.

1 Introduction

Epidemiological studies play an important role in controlling outbreaks and disease trends, analyzing risk factors, and monitoring the efficacy of preventive measures. Understanding the epidemiology of occupational contact dermatitis is essential, also for policy makers. Much knowledge about the epidemiology of occupational skin disease is derived from case-series, clinical studies of patients, compilations of patch-test clinics, official occupational disease notifications to labor agencies, or governmental health and employment departments. In addition, a number of cross-sectional studies and very few cohort studies have been performed in specific factories or branches of industry. All these data sources have their limitations, and need careful interpretation.

Occupational contact dermatitis often has consequences in daily life, and a person's nonoccupational contact dermatitis influences his/her work; typical examples are exposures to ubiquitous allergens such as nickel and chromate. Therefore, knowledge about the epidemiology of contact dermatitis is helpful; the reader can be referred to the relevant chapter in one of the major textbooks on this topic (Coenraads et al. 2011).

2 Incidence and Prevalence of Notified Occupational Contact Dermatitis

Occupational disease registries provide national incidence data based on the notification of occupational skin diseases and are available in many countries. Although the comparison of national data is hampered by differences across countries in reporting and definition of occupational diseases, the average incidence rate of registered occupational contact dermatitis in some countries lies around 0.5–1.9 cases per 1,000 full-time workers per year (Diepgen 2003).

Most of the national registers combine all types of skin disease, while no distinction is made with regard to eczema or contact dermatitis. Skin diseases constitute up to 30% of all notified occupational diseases, and it is estimated that eczema or contact dermatitis accounts for about 90–95% of all occupational skin diseases. Finland also keeps a register on occupational contact urticaria (Kanerva et al. 1996). Some of the occupational disease statistics give a breakdown by gender and occupation or branch of industry. Most national statistics do not provide information on the actual cause of contact dermatitis and predisposing factors.

National registries are usually incomplete as a result of underdiagnosis and underreporting of the disease. It has been estimated that the incidence of occupational skin diseases in the USA and Germany is being grossly

T. Rustemeyer, P. Elsner, S.M. John & H.I. Maibach (eds.), *Kanerva's Occupational Dermatology*,
DOI 10.1007/978-3-642-02035-3_8,

underestimated (Diepgen and Schmidt 2002), the milder cases of skin disease not being registered at all. The extent of underreporting is likely to differ between countries, because each country has its own system of notification and its own criteria for compensation. In the USA, occupational disease statistics are collected annually from private industries by the Bureau of Labor Statistics (BLS 2011). In the UK, the EPIDERM project in combination with OPRA (Occupational Physicians Reporting Activity) has evolved to THOR for recording occupational dermatoses: It requires dermatologists in a number of centers and occupational physicians to report confirmed or suspected cases of occupational skin disease, including the occupation of the patient concerned (McDonald et al. 2006; Turner et al. 2007). It is a voluntary system, and operates on the principle of simplicity, ensuring compliance. The epidemiological limitations are well recognized, but the system corrects the virtual absence of meaningful official statistics in the UK. A population-based study of occupational skin diseases in North Bavaria and the Saarland, Germany, is one of the few that can claim completeness in terms of new cases (numerator) and size of the occupational population as denominator (Bock et al. 2003; Dickel et al. 2002a).

In the UK (2002–2005), the average annual incidence rate of work-related contact dermatitis reported to THOR by dermatologists was 7/100,000, and by occupational physicians was 26/100,000 (Turner et al. 2007). Agents accounting for the highest number of allergic contact dermatitis cases were rubber, nickel, epoxy and other resins, aromatic amines, chromium, fragrances and cosmetics, and preservatives. Soaps, wet work, petroleum products, solvents, and cutting oils and coolants were the most frequently cited agents in cases of irritant dermatitis (Shum et al. 2003).

In 2009, occupational skin diseases were the most frequently recognized occupational diseases in Denmark, with an incidence of approximately 0.56/1,000 person-years (The official Web site of the National Board of Industrial Injuries in Denmark (Arbeidsskadestatitik 2009)). In 2009, health care workers accounted for 33% of the recognized occupational skin diseases in Denmark.

In Germany, occupational skin diseases excluding skin cancer are officially registered by the code "BK 5101," which is defined as "severe or recurrent skin diseases that force the discontinuation of any activity that causes or that could be causing the development, the worsening, or the recurrence of the skin disease." In the year 2009, the industrial nonprofit insurance institutions reported 17,238 such skin disease cases out of 61,341 notified occupational diseases. Occupational skin diseases without skin cancer constitute 28.1% of all occupational diseases in Germany. In Northern Bavaria, Germany, a detailed population-based prospective study was performed to classify all BK 5101 cases of occupational skin diseases (Dickel et al. 2001; Diepgen 2003). From 1990 to 1999, in total 5,285 cases were recorded. In cooperation with the State Institute of Labour and Occupation, the numbers of persons employed in different occupations during the same time period were collected. Since the number of employees in the different occupations was known, a population-based study was performed to investigate incidences and demographic characteristics in specific occupational groups. The estimated overall incidence was 0.67 cases per 1,000 workers per year. The highest incidence per 1,000 per year was in hairdressers (97), bakers (33), and florists (25). About 80% of all occupational skin diseases have been recorded in the following seven occupations: hairdressers, metalworkers, health care workers, food industry, cleaners, construction workers, and painters. The induction period was very short: about 2 years in hairdressers, 3 years in the food industry, and about 4 years in health service and in metalworkers. Females had a considerable higher risk to develop OCD than men. The incidence rate of contact dermatitis was highest between the age of 15 and 24 years. In about half of all cases, a delayed-type sensitization with occupational relevance was detected. In ➋ *Fig. 8.1*, the incidence rates of irritant contact dermatitis (ICD) and allergic contact dermatitis (ACD) of employees of the 12 groups with the highest risk for an occupational skin disease are presented. The population-based register in Northern Bavaria, Germany, could demonstrate a significant decline of the incidence of occupational skin disease among hairdressers between 1990 and 1999 (Dickel et al. 2002b). This supports a probable "intervention effect" by legislative and preventive measures that came into effect over the last decade for hairdressers. In the Scandinavian countries, the prevalence of potassium dichromate sensitization declined following the reduction of chromate levels, resulting from the addition of ferrous sulfate to cement.

In another German registry, all notified occupational skin diseases were assessed in the federal office for environmental and occupational protection in Saarbrücken, Germany (Apfelbacher et al. 2010). Data from 1,262 persons were available for analysis. Their average age was 37 years. The age distribution of the different occupational groups is shown in ➋ *Fig. 8.2*. The highest average age was observed in the cleaning sector and the lowest average age in the hairdressing trade. Irritant contact dermatitis was the most frequent diagnosis. Combinations of irritant contact dermatitis, allergic contact dermatitis, and atopic dermatitis occurred frequently (➋ *Fig. 8.3*).

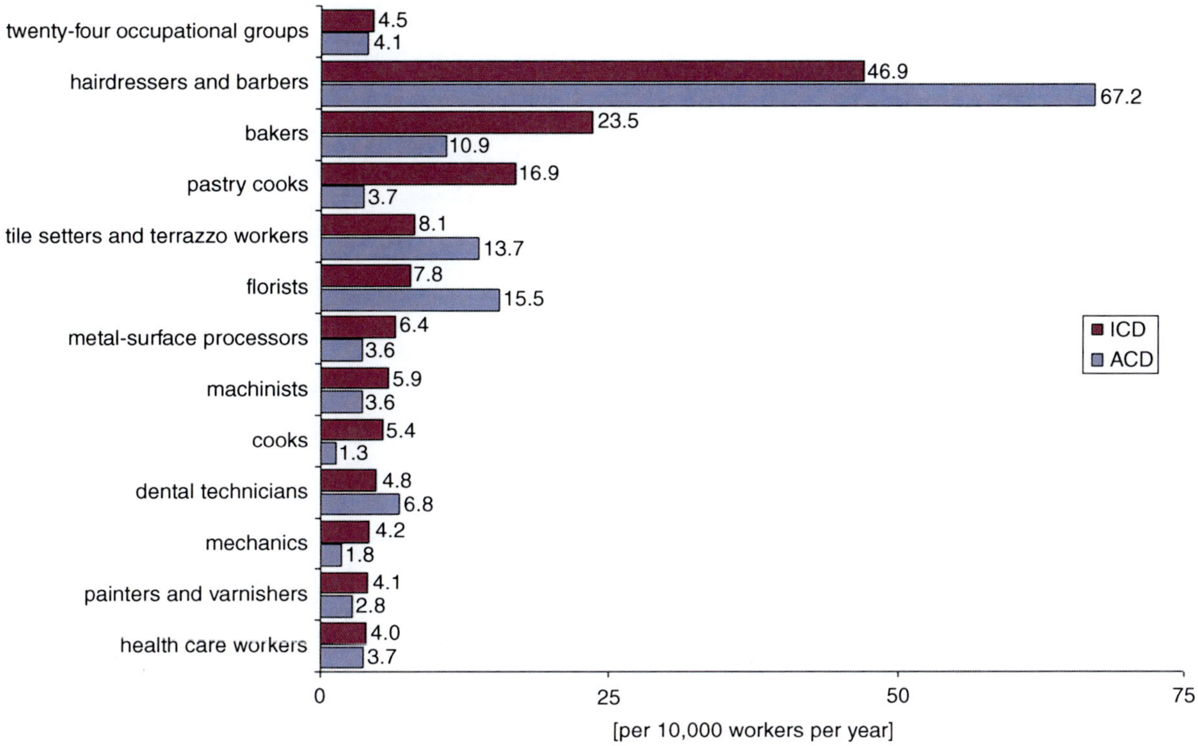

Fig. 8.1
Incidence rates (per 10,000 employees) of irritant contact dermatitis (ICD) and allergic contact dermatitis (ACD) in the 12 occupational groups with the highest risk for occupational skin diseases in North Bavaria (Dickel et al. 2001)

3 Prevalence and Incidence in Different Work Forces

During the past decades, several cross-sectional studies, mostly on hand eczema, have been performed among specific occupational groups. A major problem in such studies is the healthy worker effect and the fact that a clear relationship between skin disease and work is difficult to assess retrospectively.

A major issue is case definition based on ascertainment of the current (or past) presence of occupational contact dermatitis. In the published literature, ascertainment of cases varies from intensive efforts by a medical examination of all participants (Funke et al. 2001) to a relatively easy to apply self-administered questionnaire (Lind et al. 2007), or a combination of both. The validity of questionnaires has been investigated in several settings (Carstensen et al. 2006; de Joode et al. 2007). Based on a combination of consensus and validation, an extensive set of questions (NOSQ) has been developed for occupational skin diseases (Susitaival et al. 2003).

➋ *Table 8.1* summarizes the results of three prospective cohort studies in working populations. In the prospective Audi cohort study, 2,078 apprentices were examined at the start of their apprenticeship and systematically followed up over a 3-year period (Funke et al. 2001). The main outcome variable was the incidences of work-related hand eczema in different apprenticeships. The 1-year cumulative incidences of hand eczema were 9.2% in metalworkers, 8.8% in other blue-collar workers, and 4.6% in white-collar apprentices. The 3-year cumulative incidences of hand eczema were 15% in metalworkers, 14% in other blue-collar workers, and almost 7% in white-collar apprentices. The incidence was not uniformly distributed over the 3-year period: Within the first 6 months, a high rate of hand eczema occurred, which then declined and remained steady at a lower rate over the second and third years. Almost 10 years later, the same cohort was investigated again, showing a cumulative incidence of hand eczema of 29% (Apfelbacher et al. 2008).

In a prospective cohort study of 2,352 hairdressing apprentices, there were three examinations during their 3-year vocational training (Uter et al. 1998b). The point prevalence of (mostly slight) irritant skin changes of the hands increased from 35% in the initial examination to almost 48% in the intermediate examination and to 55%

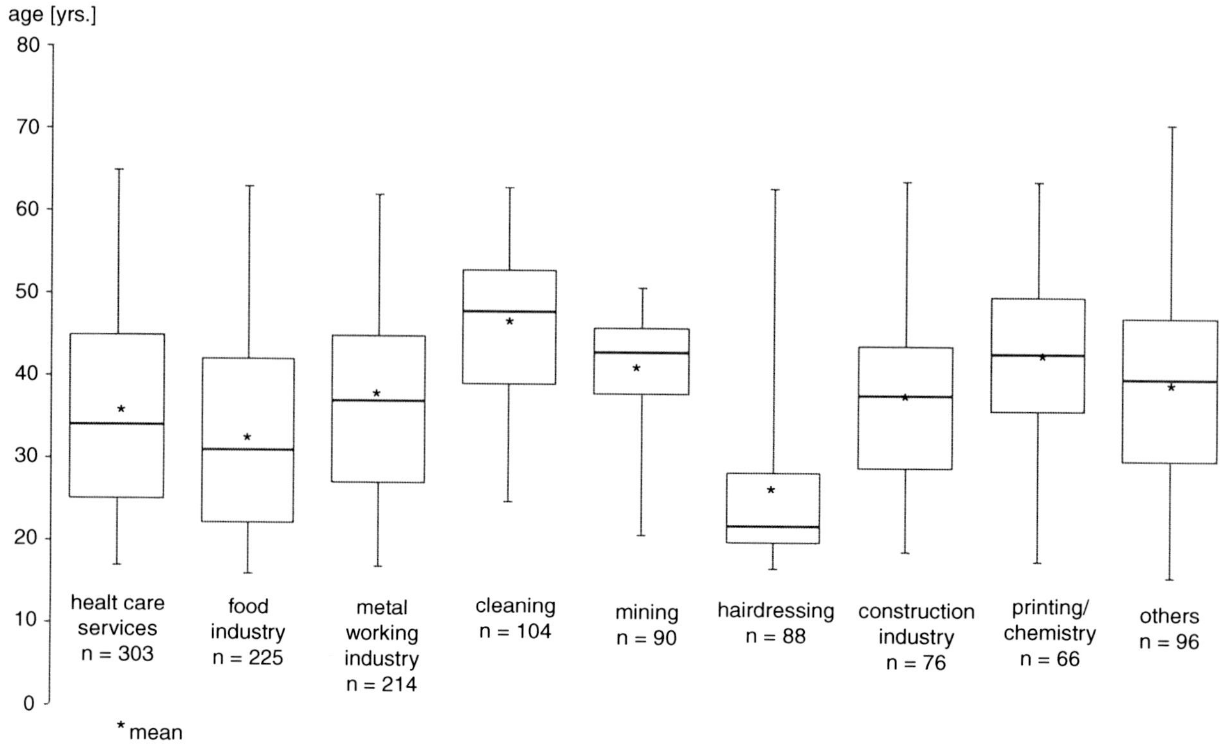

Fig. 8.2
Age distribution of 1,262 individuals with notified occupational skin diseases in different occupational groups in Saarland, Germany (According to Apfelbacher et al. 2010)

in the final examination. Given a more conservative definition of a case of "hand dermatitis," these estimates were almost 13%, 24%, and 24%, respectively. Altogether, about 34 and 15 cases of "skin changes (any degree)" and "hand dermatitis," respectively, per 100 person-years were observed during the study period. The incidence rate decreased in the course of the study. However, the proportion of dropouts until final follow-up was almost 52%. This study demonstrates that apprentices with skin problems leave the work force more often than healthy apprentices. A questionnaire-based retrospective cohort study among Swedish hairdressers found for hand eczema an incidence rate of 24/1,000 person-years, substantially higher than population-based controls, with most problems occurring at younger age (Lind et al. 2007).

4 Prognosis

A change of job does not necessarily lead to improvement of occupational contact dermatitis (Cvetkovski et al. 2006; Holness and Nethercott 1995; Mälkönen et al. 2009). Changes in work practice or occupation favor the prognosis, but many patients continue to have skin problems, especially hand eczema. The role of contact allergy is variable, and depends whether there is also exposure to the allergen outside the worker's occupation. An example is the role of nickel allergy (see Sect. 6 below). Poor prognosis has also been documented among workers with occupational contact dermatitis who are allergic to chromate, in spite of absence of occupational exposure (Mälkönen et al. 2009), but could not be confirmed in other reports (Cvetkovski et al. 2006). Nevertheless a recent study on nickel documented significant unnoticed exposure to nickel at the workplace (Jensen et al. 2011).

In a 1-year follow-up study on occupational hand eczema in Denmark, out of 564 patients with occupational hand eczema (response rate 91%) 25% had persistently severe or aggravated disease, 41% improved, and 34% had unchanged minimal or mild-to-moderate disease (Cvetkovski et al. 2006). Patients with atopic dermatitis fared poorly compared with other patients. Patients younger than 25 years fared clearly better than older groups. Furthermore, severe occupational hand eczema, age

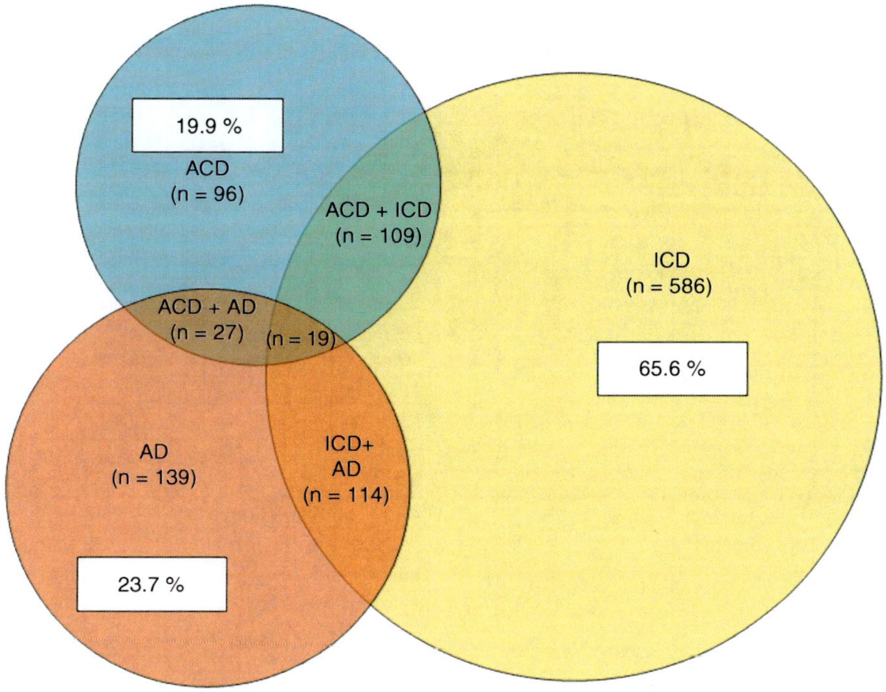

Fig. 8.3

Combinations of allergic contact dermatitis (ACD), irritant contact dermatitis (ICD), and atopic dermatitis (AD) in individuals with notified occupational skin diseases in Saarland, Germany (According to Apfelbacher et al. 2010)

40 years or greater, and severe impairment of quality of life at baseline appeared to be important predictors of prolonged sick leave and unemployment. Patients with lower socioeconomic status also had a high risk of prolonged sick leave, job change, and loss of job. Contact allergy was not found to be a risk factor for poor prognosis.

Long-term follow-up studies on the prognosis and consequences of occupational contact dermatitis (OCD) and the prognostic risk factors for persistent occupational contact dermatitis are sparse. In a recently published study from Finland, 605 patients diagnosed with occupational hand eczema completed a follow-up questionnaire 7–14 years after diagnosis (Mälkönen et al. 2010). The hand eczema had healed (no eczema during the last year) in 40% of patients with occupational hand eczema. The duration of hand eczema before diagnosis was strongly associated with the continuation of eczema. Age, sex, and diagnosis (allergic or irritant contact dermatitis) were not associated with the prognosis, but skin atopy and especially respiratory atopy were correlated with the continuation of hand eczema. Contact allergies in general were not risk factors for persistent occupational hand eczema, but the presence of a work-related chromate allergy was associated with poor healing. A total of 34% of patients had changed their occupation due to occupational hand eczema, and their long-term prognosis was better than those who had not. The hand eczema of patients originally in food-related occupations continued on an unfavorable course. In the logistic model, risk factors for the continuation of occupational hand eczema were a long duration of hand eczema before diagnosis, respiratory atopy, skin atopy, and continuation in the same occupation. Those who ended up changing occupation due to their occupational hand eczema had a better medical and economic prognosis.

5 Interventions

Well-designed intervention studies are difficult to perform in occupational contact dermatitis. Major problems are the time needed for follow-up and the difficulty of separating within the same plant the workers who participate in the intervention group versus those who are in the reference group (Coenraads and Diepgen 2003). However, prevention is an essential fundamental component in the management of occupational skin diseases and

Table 8.1

Prospective cohort studies on the incidence of work-related skin complaints (hand eczema (HE), contact sensitization, and contact dermatitis) in different professions

Author/year	Country	Target population	Method of case ascertainment	N	Outcome	Measures of incidence	Rate	Comment
Funke et al. (2001), Apfelbacher et al. (2008)	Germany	Apprentices in the car industry	Q, I, E	2,078	HE in metalworkers (apprentices)	1-year	9.2%	Prospective cohort study of high quality, follow-up rate 98.2%
						3-years	15.3%	
					HE in blue-collar apprentices	1-year	8.8%	
						3-years	14.1%	
					HE in white-collar apprentices	1-year	4.6%	
						3-years	6.9%	
Uter et al. (1998a)	Germany	Hairdressing apprentices	Q, I, E	2,352	HE at the first, second, and third examination during 3-year training	Point first year	12.9%	Prospective cohort study of high quality, high initial response rate (91.5%) but 51.8% dropouts until final follow-up
						Point second year	23.5%	
						Point third year	23.9%	
Lind et al. (2007)	Sweden	Hairdressing graduates from vocational schools	Q	4,061	HE	IR	24/ 1,000 PYE	Variable start of follow-up: from 1970 to 1995. Incidence rate compared to general population 2.5

Q questionnaire, *I* interview, *E* clinical examination, *PYE* person-years exposure

intervention studies are needed to demonstrate the efficacy of primary and secondary prevention. The aim of primary prevention is to help healthy individuals avoid disease (in this case, occupational contact dermatitis), that is, to decrease the incidence rate. Secondary prevention measures are indicated in patients who already have symptoms on the skin of the hands. The goal of secondary prevention is early detection of initial symptoms in order to initiate preventive measures as soon as possible.

An example is a workplace intervention study in geriatric nurses in Germany (Dulon et al. 2009). The objective was to determine whether a skin care program reduces skin disease on the hands of geriatric nurses and increases protective behavior and the provision of skin care products at the workplace. The intervention was based on a 2-h skin care training session and an occupational advisory service. The study design was a randomized intervention study with a control group; 388 geriatric nurses were included in the intervention group exposed to a skin care program (IG; n = 146) and in the control group (CG; n = 242). Both groups completed questionnaires on exposure and underwent clinical examinations of their hands at the beginning and after a 12-month period. At baseline, no difference between the intervention and the control group was found with respect to skin changes or work-related behavior. At follow-up, the frequency of skin disease was significantly reduced in the intervention group, from 26% at baseline to 17% at follow-up, whereas the frequency remained almost unchanged in the control group. Effects on behavior in the intervention group included significant increases in the use of moisturizers and hand disinfection instead of hand washing. The provision of cotton gloves and barrier cream products increased at intervention workplaces.

Other examples are publications about intervention studies in the meat industry (Flyvholm et al. 2005), in wet work employees in Denmark (Held et al. 2002), in the building and timber industry in Austria

(Winker et al. 2009), and the metal industry in Germany (Kütting et al. 2010). In the recent prospective four-arm intervention study with a 12-month follow-up, the effectiveness of skin care and skin protection measures were assessed in metal workers in Germany (Kütting et al. 2010). The largest and significant improvement was noted in the group following the skin protection program as it was generally recommended (skin care + protection) followed by skin protection alone as second best.

6 Risk Factors

Evidence has accumulated that past or present atopic dermatitis is a risk factor for irritant contact dermatitis (Coenraads and Diepgen 1998). Earlier studies indicated that atopy was almost three times as high among patients with hand eczema as in the general population or a healthy control group. Later it appeared that atopic dermatitis was particularly associated with irritant contact dermatitis, but not with contact allergy. The proportion of subjects with sporadic or continuous hand eczema was significantly greater in those with moderate and severe atopic dermatitis in childhood compared with those with respiratory allergy only, or a group without atopy. In a follow-up study of hospital workers, a history of atopic dermatitis increased the risk of developing hand eczema threefold (Nilsson et al. 1985). Population-based studies in the food industry calculated significantly greater risk of occupational contact dermatitis in employees with an atopic skin diathesis. The impact of atopic skin diathesis on occupational contact dermatitis could be analyzed by using attributable risk estimates; almost 22% of occupational skin disease cases may be ascribed to this endogenous risk factor (Tacke et al. 1995; Dickel et al. 2003).

Even if in epidemiological terms atopic dermatitis is an effect modifier, it can be argued that irritant contact dermatitis associated with atopy is primarily an exacerbation of underlying atopic dermatitis. Since atopic dermatitis is often associated with respiratory symptoms, respiratory atopy may appear as a risk factor. The same may apply to dry skin as an expression of atopic dermatitis.

The problem of contact dermatitis in a particular group of patients is easy to interpret when there is a straightforward cause-effect relationship: for example, hand eczema in a group of surgeons with a positive patch test to thiuram additives to their rubber gloves. However, the relevance of a positive patch test to very common allergens such as chromate or nickel may be difficult to assess in patients with an occupational (contact) dermatitis (Shum et al. 2003). As discussed above, there may be considerable (statistical) interaction between several exposure, or risk factors of interest. Elucidation of such interactions may have consequences for preventive or other public-health strategies. To illustrate this point, in ❯ *Table 8.2*, an example is created from the data (modified for this purpose) generated in two Scandinavian follow-up studies on hand eczema and exposure to irritants (Meding and Jarvholm 2002; Rystedt 1985).

Table 8.2
Relative risks (modified) of contact dermatitis of the hands according to the level of atopic skin diathesis and exposure to irritants (Coenraads and Diepgen 1998; Meding and Jarvholm 2002; Rystedt 1985)

	No irritant exposure	Exposure to irritants
No atopy	1	1,5
Mild atopic dermatitis	2	4
Severe atopic dermatitis	4	12

In ❯ *Table 8.2*, the relative risks of exposure to irritants on hand eczema are different according to the presence of a history of atopic dermatitis. There is an effect modification, meaning that the relative risks of exposure to irritants are not uniform (multiplicative) in the different levels of skin atopy: The risk of hand eczema in atopics is disproportionally increased by exposure to irritants.

The presence or absence of interactions between various factors operating on the risk of contact dermatitis (for example the role of chromate allergy in foot eczema) has not yet been investigated in detail. As mentioned above, there are indications that such phenomena operate on nickel allergy: In the absence of signs of atopic dermatitis, the relative risk of a positive nickel patch test on the risk of hand eczema was only 1.7 in hairdressers and only 1.1 in nurses (Smit et al. 1994). In a German study, nickel sensitivity was not associated with an elevated risk for hand eczema. Independent risk factors were: wet work, atopic skin, and exposure to permanent wave.

References

Apfelbacher CJ, Radulescu M, Diepgen TL, Funke U (2008) Occurrence and prognosis of hand eczema in the car industry: results from the PACO follow-up study. Contact Dermatitis 58:322–329

Apfelbacher CJ, Bernhard-Klimt C, Scheidt R, Diepgen TL (2010) Epidemiology of occupational skin disease in the Saarland, Germany. Exp Dermatol 19:220

Arbeidsskadestatitik (2009) www.ask.dk. Accessed Apr 2011

BLS (2011) Bureau of Labor Statistics. www.bls.gov/iif and www.bls.gov/iif/osh/case/ostb2045.txt. Accessed Apr 2011

Bock M, Schmidt A, Bruckner T, Diepgen TL (2003) Occupational skin disease in the construction industry. Br J Dermatol 149:1165–1171

Carstensen O, Rasmussen K, Ponten A, Gruvberger B, Isaksson M, Bruze M (2006) The validity of a questionnairebased epidemiological study of occupational dermatosis. Contact Dermatitis 55:295–300

Coenraads PJ, Diepgen TL (1998) Risk for hand eczema in employees with past or present atopic dermatitis. Int Arch Occup Environ Health 71:7–13

Coenraads PJ, Diepgen TL (2003) Problems with intervention studies on barrier creams and emollients at the workplace. Int Arch Occup Environ Health 76:362–366

Coenraads PJ, Uter W, Diepgen TL (2011) Epidemiology. In: Johansen JD et al (eds) Contact dermatitis, 5th edn. Springer, Heidelberg

Cvetkovski RS, Zachariae R, Jensen H, Olsen J, Johansen JD, Agner T (2006) Prognosis of occupational hand eczema: a follow-up. Arch Dermatol 142:305–311

de Joode BW, Vermeulen R, Heederik D, van Ginkel K, Kromhout H (2007) Evaluation of 2 self-administered questionnaires to ascertain dermatitis among metal workers and its relation with exposure to metalworking fluids. Contact Dermatitis 56:311–317

Dickel H, Kuss O, Blesius CR, Schmidt A, Diepgen TL (2001) Occupational skin diseases in Nothern Bavaria between 1990 and 1999: a population based study. Br J Dermatol 145:453–462

Dickel H, Bruckner T, Berhard-Klimt C, Koch T, Scheidt R, Diepgen TL (2002a) Surveillance scheme for occupational skin disease in the Saarland, FRG: first report from BKH-S. Contact Dermatitis 46:197–206

Dickel H, Kuss O, Schmidt A, Diepgen TL (2002b) Impact of preventive strategies on trend of occupational skin disease in hairdressers: population-based register study. Br Med J 324:1422–1423

Dickel H, Bruckner TM, Schmidt A, Diepgen TL (2003) Impact of atopic skin diathesis on occupational skin disease incidence in a working population. J Invest Dermatol 121:37–40

Diepgen TL (2003) Occupational skin-disease data in Europe. Int Arch Occup Environ Health 76:331–338

Diepgen TL, Schmidt A (2002) Werden Inzidenz und Prävalenz berufsbedingter Hauterkrankungen unterschätzt? Arbeitsmed Sozialmed Umweltmed 37:477–480

Dulon M, Pohrt U, Skudlik C, Nienhaus A (2009) Prevention of occupational skin disease: a workplace intervention study in geriatric nurses. Br J Dermatol 161:337–344

Flyvholm MA, Mygind K, Sell L, Jensen A, Jepsen KF (2005) A randomised controlled intervention study on prevention of work related skin problems among gut cleaners in swine slaughterhouses. Occup Environ Med 62:642–649

Funke U, Fartasch M, Diepgen TL (2001) Incidence of work-related hand eczema during apprenticeship: first results of a prospective cohort study in the car industry. Contact Dermatitis 44:166–172

Held E, Mygind K, Wolff C, Gyntelberg F, Agner T (2002) Prevention of work related skin problems: an intervention study in wet work employees. Occup Environ Med 59:556–561

Holness DL, Nethercott JR (1995) Work outcome in workers with occupational skin disease. Am J Ind Med 27:807–815

Jensen P, Thyssen JP, Johansen JD, Skare L, Menné T, Lidén C (2011) Occupational hand eczema caused by nickel and evaluated by quantitative exposure assessment. Contact Dermatitis 64:32–36

Kanerva L, Toikkanen J, Jolanki R, Estlander T (1996) Statistical data on occupational contact urticaria. Contact Dermatitis 35: 229–233

Kütting B, Baumeister T, Weistenhöfer W, Pfahlberg A, Uter W, Drexler H (2010) Effectiveness of skin protection measures in prevention of occupational hand eczema: results of a prospective randomized controlled trial over a follow-up period of 1 year. Br J Dermatol 162:362–370

Lind ML, Albin M, Brisman J, Kronholm Diab K, Lillienberg L, Mikoczy Z, Nielsen J, Rylander L, Torén K, Meding B (2007) Incidence of hand eczema in female Swedish hairdressers. Occup Environ Med 64:191–195

Mälkönen T, Jolanki R, Alanko K, Luukonen R, Aalto-Korte K, Lauerma A, Susitaival P (2009) A 6-month follow-up study of 1048 patients diagnosed with an occupational skin disease. Contact Dermatitis 61:261–268

Mälkönen T, Alanko K, Jolanki R, Luukkonen R, Aalto-Korte K, Lauerma A, Susitaival P (2010) Long-term follow-up study of occupational hand eczema. Br J Dermatol 163:999–1006

McDonald JC, Beck MH, Chen Y, Cherry NM (2006) Incidence by occupation and industry of work-related skin diseases in the United Kingdom 1996–2001. Occup Med 56:398–405

Meding B, Jarvholm B (2002) Hand eczema in Swedish adults – changes in prevalence between 1983 and 1996. J Invest Dermatol 118:719–723

Nilsson GE, Mikaelsson B, Andersson S (1985) Atopy, occupation and domestic work as risk factors for hand eczema in hospital workers. Contact Dermatitis 13:216–223

Rystedt I (1985) Hand eczema and long term prognosis in atopic dermatitis (thesis). Acta Derm Venereol (suppl) 117:1–59

Shum KW, Meyer JD, Chen Y, Cherry N, Gawkrodger DJ (2003) Occupational contact dermatitis to nickel: experience of the British dermatologists (EPIDERM) and occupational physicians (OPRA) surveillance schemes. Occup Environ Med 60:954–957

Smit HA, van Rijssen A, Vandenbroucke J, Coenraads PJ (1994) Individual susceptibility and the incidence of hand dermatitis in a cohort of apprentice hairdressers and nurses. Scand J Work Environ Health 20:113–121

Susitaival P, Flyvholm MA, Meding B, Kanerva L, Lindberg M, Svensson A, Olafsson JH (2003) Nordic occupational skin questionnaire (NOSQ-2002): a new tool for surveying occupational skin diseases and exposure. Contact Dermatitis 49:70–76

Tacke J, Schmidt A, Fartasch M, Diepgen TL (1995) Occupational contact dermatitis in bakers, confectioners and cooks. A population based study. Contact Dermatitis 33:112–118

Turner S, Carder N, van Tongeren M, McNamee R, Lines S, Hussey L, Bolton A, Beck MH, Wilkinson M, Agius R (2007) The incidence of occupational skin disease as reported to The Health and Occupation Reporting (THOR) network between 2002 and 2005. Br J Dermatol 157:713–722

Uter W, Pfahlberg A, Gefeller O, Schwanitz HJ (1998a) Hand eczema in a prospectively followed cohort of office workers. Contact Dermatitis 38:83–89

Uter W, Pfahlberg A, Gefeller O, Schwanitz HJ (1998b) Prevalence and incidence of hand dermatitis in hairdressing apprentices: results of the POSH study. Prevention of occupational skin disease in hairdressers. Int Arch Occup Environ Health 71:487–492

Winker R, Salameh B, Stolkovich S, Nikl M, Barth A, Ponocny E, Drexler H, Tappeiner G (2009) Effectiveness of skin protection creams in the prevention of occupational dermatitis: results of a randomized, controlled trial. Int Arch Occup Environ Health 82:653–662

9 Surveillance in Occupational Contact Dermatitis

Wolfgang Uter
Department of Medical Informatics, Biometry and Epidemiology, University of Erlangen/Nürnberg, Erlangen, Germany

Core Messages

- Surveillance is the continuous analysis, interpretation, and feedback of systematically collected data either on an (inter)national level or on the level of industrial plants.
- Occupational contact dermatitis does not separately appear in the general (national) statistics on occupational diseases and injuries; however, the proportion of occupational contact dermatitis among all occupational skin diseases is consistently estimated to be around 80%.
- Special registries, or special analyses of "routine" documentation systems generically including this data, enable the assessment of the spectrum of (occupational) contact allergens in different occupations.
- Clinical data on the frequency of irritant or allergic contact dermatitis, or on the prevalence of specific contact sensitization, cannot directly be interpreted as estimates of morbidity on the population level. Nevertheless, sufficiently standardized patient data are a valid basis of surveillance, addressing time trends (in subgroups) and risk factor assessment.

1 Introduction

Surveillance has been defined as "continuous analysis, interpretation, and feedback of systematically collected data, generally using methods distinguished by their practicality, uniformity, and rapidity rather than by accuracy or completeness. By observing trends in time, place, and persons, changes can be observed or anticipated and appropriate action, including investigative or control measures, can be taken" (Last 1995). Surveillance is used in several fields of public health. The most well-known application is probably infectious disease surveillance and cancer surveillance. Moreover, health surveillance is implemented in industrial production plants, if analysis of occupational risks by the employer or legal requirements indicates this is necessary (Anonymus 2004).

As a prerequisite for valid results, data acquisition procedures have (1) to follow a standardized protocol and (2) to ascertain sampling of representative data, if complete, population-wide registration is not feasible. Moreover, the sampling frame has to be large enough to render estimates of prevalence, incidence, trends, or comparisons between subgroups sufficiently precise and statistical tests adequately powerful. Regarding occupational contact dermatitis (OCD) as the most important occupational skin disease (OSD), a number of pertinent approaches are outlined in the following sections. Emphasis is on a systematic presentation of methods, and not on covering completely the results of the surveillance instruments.

2 Occupational Skin Disease as Part of General Occupational Statistics

In Germany, as in many other countries, record is kept by the employers liability insurance of all occupational diseases. Results are reported every few years ("BK-DOK"(1)). Notification of suspected cases of OSD has been declining since 1990, although to a lesser extent than all occupational diseases taken together (Haupt et al. 2005). This regular report provides insight into the distribution of suspected as well as confirmed cases of OSD across industrial sectors. However, to arrive at an estimation of the risk of specific occupations based on this morbidity statistic, additional statistics on the number of employed persons must be considered (for Germany: http://www.destatis.de/jetspeed/portal/cms/Sites/destatis/Internet/DE/Navigation/Statistiken/Arbeitsmarkt/Sozialversicherungspflichtige/Sozialversicherungspflichtige.psml, last accessed 2011-10-06).

In contrast, the US Bureau of Labor Statistics (www.bls.gov) provides not only absolute numbers of "skin diseases or disorders," as BK-DOK above, but also incidence rates calculated per standard full-time working hours as denominator, and grossly aggregated for

T. Rustemeyer, P. Elsner, S.M. John & H.I. Maibach (eds.), *Kanerva's Occupational Dermatology*,
DOI 10.1007/978-3-642-02035-3_9, © Springer-Verlag Berlin Heidelberg 2012

Table 9.1
Incidence rates (number of cases/10,000 working years) of occupational contact sensitization to three important metal allergens according to the Finnish registry of occupational (skin) diseases, 1991–1997 (Kanerva et al. 2000)

Nickel	Chromium	Cobalt
Footwear workers: 2.6	Tanners, fellmongers, and pelt dressers: 12.2	Printers: 0.80
Machine and metal products assemblers: 2.4	Cast concrete product workers: 6.9	Turners, machinists, and toolmakers: 0.36
Electrical and teletechnical equipment assemblers: 2.0	Leather goods workers: 4.7	Machine and engine mechanics: 0.17
Precision instrument mechanics: 1.7	Metal plating and coating workers: 3.7	
Postal officials: 1.5	Bricklayers: 3.4	

industrial sectors (http://www.bls.gov/iif/oshwc/osh/os/osh06_t6.pdf, last accessed 2011-10-06).

Similarly, the Finnish Institute of Occupational Health (www.ttl.fi, last accessed 2011-10-06) provides figures on OSD subdivided for:

- Diagnoses (e.g., in 2002, n = 330 cases of allergic contact dermatitis, n = 313 cases of irritant contact dermatitis, n = 115 cases of protein contact dermatitis and a number of other diagnoses among the 965 notified cases)
- Incidence of OSD aggregated by industries (e.g., in 2002, 16/10,000 cases in food and beverages manufacturing work, 14 cases/10,000 in manufacturing work not elsewhere classified and 12 cases/10,000 in agriculture, forestry, and fishing) (Riihimäki et al. 2002).

However, the information regarding OSD which can be provided by routine reporting from general statistics as those mentioned above is very general. Hence, occasional special analyses with a greater degree of detail, although still limited by the scope of data and classification detail inherent in the respective registration system, have been reported (e.g., Kanerva et al. 2000; O'Malley et al. 1988; Schnuch and Butz 1993).

Regarding the important aspect of occupational contact sensitization, a special analysis of the Finnish Institute of Occupational Health focused on the incidence rates of occupational allergic contact dermatitis caused by metals (Kanerva et al. 2000). Relating the numerator of notified cases of allergic contact dermatitis (n = 2,543; 1991–1997) with proven contact sensitization to nickel, chromium, or cobalt to the denominator of workers employed in the respective occupations, the incidence rates shown in Table 9.1 are calculated.

3 Specific Registration of Occupational Skin Disease

In some countries, specialized registration schemes for occupational skin diseases (OSD) have been implemented. In the United Kingdom, two voluntary surveillance systems exist which have been merged for analyses: EPIDERM for consultant dermatologists since 1993, and OPRA for occupational physicians since 1996 (Cherry et al. 2000; Turner et al. 2007). This system does not aim at a complete registration of all cases, but rather uses a representative sampling method and strives for completeness within this framework. According to this scheme, contact dermatitis is the most common OSD, with 79% of all registered cases, followed by neoplasia (12.8% of cases). The global annual incidence of occupational contact dermatitis (OCD) has been estimated as 12.9 cases/100,000 workers in the first reporting period (Cherry et al. 2000), and 6.8 cases reported by dermatologists and 26.0/100,000 by occupational physicians in a subsequent period (Turner et al. 2007). Interestingly, the "high risk" occupational areas, coded according to the UK Office of National Statistics, also varied by specialty:

- Dermatologists, via EPIDERM, identified printers (71/100,000 workers employed per year), machine tool operatives (56/100,000), and chemical, gas, and petroleum plant operatives (45/100,000) as most riskful occupations in men, and hairdressers and barbers (120/100,000), assemblers and line workers for vehicles and other metal goods (35/100,000), and routine laboratory testers (34/100,000) as high risk occupations in women.
- Occupational physicians, via OPRA, identified gas and petroleum plant operatives (182/100,000), assemblers and line workers for vehicles and other metal goods (109/100,000), and machine tool operatives (69/100,000 workers employed) in men, and biological scientists and biochemists (75/100,000), routine laboratory testers (52/100,000), and assemblers and line

workers (34/100,000) in women as occupations with a particularly high risk of OCD (Cherry et al. 2000).

The above differences between dermatologists and occupational physicians seem to illustrate the impact of the structure of occupational health care in a country, where, in this case, workers in the manufacturing industries are covered by occupational physicians, whereas workers in small-scale production or service units such as hairdressing salons are more likely to consult a dermatologist, be it after referral. This may have some impact on the results of surveillance based on either specialty, as illustrated above.

In Germany, a different approach has been followed in terms of temporarily implementing a regional, but presumably complete, registration of suspected cases of OSD (again mostly OCD) notified to the occupational liability insurance, first in Northern Bavaria (Dickel et al. 2001a) and later in Saarland (Dickel et al. 2002). A total of 5,285 cases, registered between 1990 and 1999, were assessed in Northern Bavaria. Combining morbidity data with regionally matched employment data, incidence rates in 24 different occupational groups were estimated. Among 3,097 cases of OSD (median age 25 years) in the main 24 occupational groups, a significant decline in overall incidence of OSD with 10.7 cases per 10,000 workers/year at the beginning and 4.9 cases per 10,000 workers/year at the end of the study period was noted. Hairdressing was associated with the greatest risk of OSD (97/10,000 workers per year), followed by bakers (33/10,000), florists (24/10,000) and pastry cooks (21/10,000). The largest number of notifications concerned hairdressers (n = 997), health care workers (n = 607), and household and restaurant service workers (n = 288) (Dickel et al. 2001a).

Evidently, incidence estimates for a trade which may be regarded as fairly comparable between nations in the "developed" countries, namely, hairdressing, vary greatly, if above statistics are compared. This may partly be due to variation of (1) actual risk of OCD, modified by the effectiveness of occupational safety regulations, (2) case definitions used, and (3) the sensitivity and specificity of the surveillance scheme used toward that case definition.

The degree of detail in most of the above-mentioned surveillance schemes, for instance, regarding the role of contact allergens or irritants, is mostly limited. The BKH-S and -N project included documentation and analysis of contact allergens in different occupations. However, as only a limited period was covered, and a relatively limited number of cases were included, no time trends and subgroup analyses, respectively, were feasible. This shortcoming can be overcome by utilizing routine clinical data collected by a contact allergy surveillance network, as described in the next section. Interestingly, within the scope covered by both systems, results in terms of the significance of single contact allergens in certain occupations were quite comparable (Dickel et al. 2001b).

4 Clinical Contact Allergy Data

An increasing number of national or multinational contact dermatitis research groups have established networks

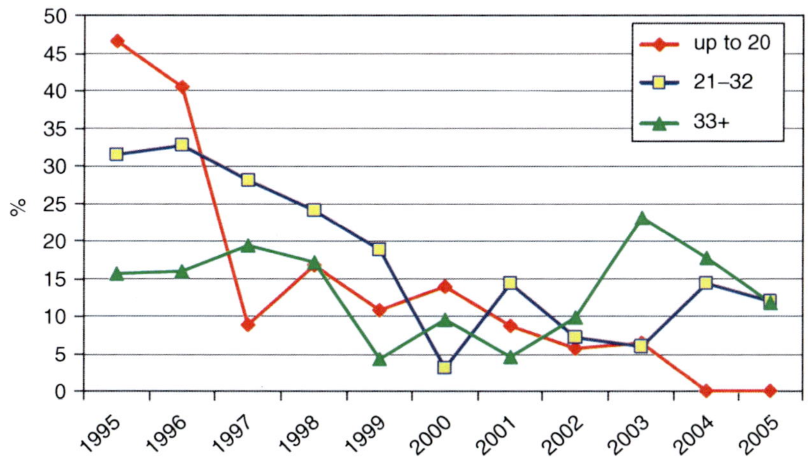

Fig. 9.1

Time course of the prevalence of sensitization to glyceryl monothioglycolate among hairdressers with occupational contact dermatitis, subdivided into three age strata (Reproduced with kind permission from Uter et al. (2006))

for the collection and continual analysis of patch test data, along with core information from the patients' history (Uter et al. 2011). In virtually all networks, data on occupational causation of dermatitis (often categorized as "certain," "probable," and "not likely," respectively, or as "exclusive," "partial," or "none," respectively) is collected. Additionally, the current occupation(s), and sometimes previous occupations, if relevant, are documented. Based on such data, the frequency of certain specific contact allergies in different occupations can be examined. If confounding of the association between occupation and target sensitization by factors such as age or gender is suspected, age and sex standardization, an adjusted, multifactorial analysis (e.g., Uter et al. 2001, 2004a), or other suitable methods for the control of confounding should be employed (Uter et al. 2004b).

Moreover, the analysis of time trends enables the identification of emerging problems (in certain occupational subgroups) which could target further in-depth investigation, or increased preventive efforts, as appropriate. Conversely, the success of preventive action aiming at the reduction or elimination of allergen exposure can be evaluated by examining the time trend after such action. For example, the withdrawal and subsequent regulation of glyceryl monothioglycolate, a component previously used in so-called acid perming solutions, has led to a sharp decline of overall sensitization frequency in hairdressers. In a more detailed age-stratified analysis, sensitization prevalence in the youngest subgroup of hairdressers, who entered working life only after withdrawal of GMTG, even arrived at 0% (Uter et al. 2006) (see ❯ *Fig. 9.1*). However, in other instances, if a compound is not completely and effectively withdrawn, a certain residual exposure and sensitization risk may remain. At any rate, the prevalence in those who became exposed only recently is the best possible approximation of incidence, based on such routine clinical data, and thus preferable to evaluate the effects of exposure changes.

In other cases, clinical surveillance data may point to a persisting or even increasing problem. This has been illustrated by a recent analysis of contact sensitization to thiuram mix in different occupational subgroups

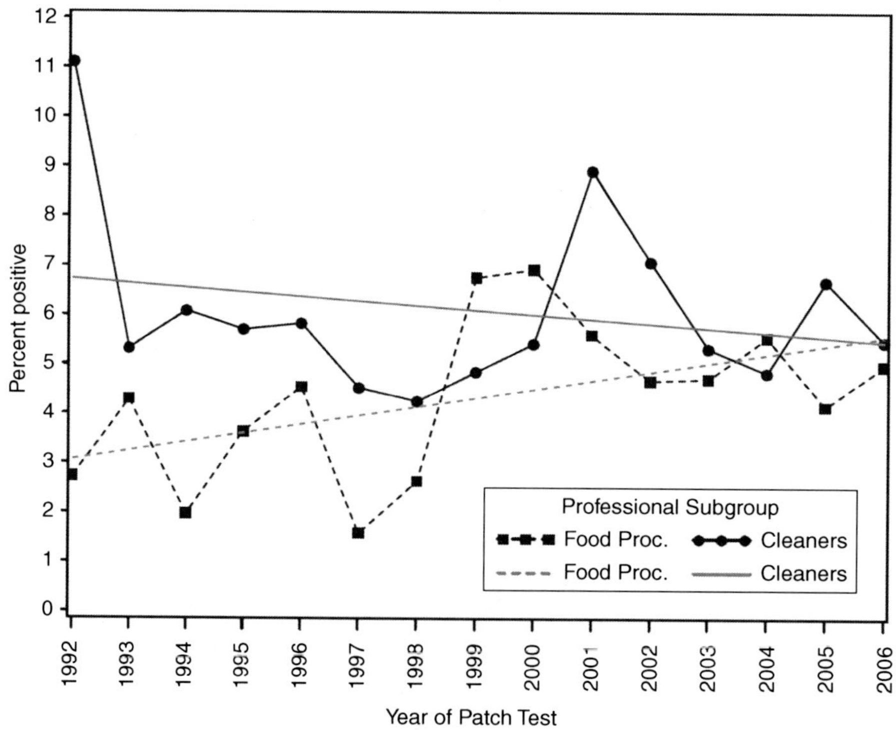

Fig. 9.2
Time trend of sensitization to the thiuram mix in food handlers and cleaners, respectively. Sensitization prevalence is directly age standardized. *Straight gray lines* represent fitted regression lines to represent a linear subgroup-specific trend (Reproduced with kind permission from Uter et al. (2010))

(Uter et al. 2010). While in health care workers, coinciding with the advent of improved quality gloves and possibly also due to the use of different vulcanizing agents in this sector, a significant decline of contact sensitization to thiurams was observed, the sensitization frequency in cleaners was largely stable and even slightly increasing in food handlers, see *Fig. 9.2.*

As patients consulting a dermatologist for suspected allergic contact dermatitis, to be patch tested, are a selected clinical sample, estimates of prevalence based on such clinical data cannot directly be regarded as representative of the prevalence (or incidence) in the population. Presumably, the clinical estimates overestimate prevalence on the population level. However, the main objective of "clinical surveillance of contact allergy" is not to arrive at estimates of morbidity and its changes or differences on the population level. Rather, within a given clinical sampling frame, which is regarded as largely stable, continual evaluation of this data can provide valid information on time trends and clustering in subgroups without direct reference to the population. Obviously, possible bias induced by selection effects must be carefully considered when relying on routine clinical data.

References

Anonymus (2004) Medical aspects of occupational skin disease, Guidance Note MS 24. Health and Safety Executive, Norwich

Cherry N, Meyer JD, Adisesh A et al (2000) Surveillance of occupational skin disease: EPIDERM and OPRA. Br J Dermatol 142:1128–1134

Dickel H, Kuss O, Blesius CR et al (2001a) Occupational skin diseases in Northern Bavaria between 1990 and 1999: a population-based study. Br J Dermatol 145:453–462

Dickel H, Uter W, Schmidt A et al (2001b) Auswertung von Datenbanken bzw. Registern von Hauttestergebnissen zur Relevanz arbeitsbedingter Faktoren (Schriftenreihe der Bundesanstalt für Arbeitsschutz und Arbeitsmedizin: Forschungsbericht, Fb 939), Wirtschaftsverlag NW Verlag für neue Wissenschaft GmbH, Bremerhaven

Dickel H, Bruckner T, Bernhard-Klimt C et al (2002) Surveillance scheme for occupational skin disease in the Saarland, FRG. First report from BKH-S. Contact Dermatitis 46:197–206

Haupt B, Drechsel-Schlund C, Guldner K-H et al (2005) Dokumentation des Berufskrankheiten-Geschehens in Deutschland – BK-DOK 2005. DGUV, St. Augustin

Kanerva L, Jolanki R, Estlander T et al (2000) Incidence rates of occupational allergic contact dermatitis caused by metals. Am J Contact Dermat 11:155–160

Last JM (1995) A dictionary of epidemiology. Oxford University Press, New York/Oxford/Toronto

O'Malley M, Thun M, Morrison J et al (1988) Surveillance of occupational skin disease using the supplementary data system. Am J Ind Med 13:291–299

Riihimäki H, Kurppa K, Karjalainen A et al (2002) Occupational diseases in Finland in 2002. New cases of occupational diseases reported to the Finnish Register of Occupational Diseases. Finnish Institute of Occupational Health, Helsinki

Schnuch A, Butz M (1993) Kosten berufsbedingter Hauterkrankungen für die Berufsgenossenschaften. Derm Beruf Umwelt 41:10–19

Turner S, Carder M, van Tongeren M et al (2007) The incidence of occupational skin disease as reported to The Health and Occupation Reporting (THOR) network between 2002 and 2005. Br J Dermatol 157:713–722

Uter W, Schnuch A, Geier J et al (2001) Association between occupation and contact allergy to the fragrance mix: a multifactorial analysis of national surveillance data. Occup Environ Med 58:392–398

Uter W, Rühl R, Pfahlberg A et al (2004a) Contact allergy in construction workers: results of a multifactorial analysis. Ann Occup Hyg 48: 21–27

Uter W, Schnuch A, Gefeller O (2004b) Guidelines for the descriptive presentation and statistical analysis of contact allergy data. Contact Dermatitis 51:47–56

Uter W, Geier J, Lessmann H et al (2006) Is contact allergy to glyceryl monothioglycolate still a problem in Germany? Contact Dermatitis 55:54–56

Uter W, Hegewald J, Pfahlberg A et al (2010) Contact allergy to thiurams: multifactorial analysis of clinical surveillance data collected by the IVDK network. Int Arch Occup Environ Health 83(6):675–881 doi:10.1007/s00420-009-0503-9

Uter W, Schnuch A, Giménez-Arnau A et al (2011) Databases and networks. The benefit for research and quality assurance in patch testing. In: Johansen JD, Frosch PJ, Lepoittevin JP (eds) Contact dermatitis. Springer, Heidelberg, 5th edn., pp 1053–1064

10 Occupational Skin Cancer

Thomas L. Diepgen[1] · *Hans Drexler*[2]
[1]Department of Clinical Social Medicine, Occupational and Environmental Dermatology, University of Heidelberg, Heidelberg, Germany
[2]Institute and Outpatient Clinic of Occupational, Social and Environmental Medicine, Friedrich-Alexander-University, Erlangen, Germany

Core Messages

- Occupational skin cancer can be induced due to industrial exposure to chemical carcinogens, but nowadays more important due to occupational exposure to UV radiation (UVR).
- Occupational skin cancer is characterized by long induction periods (years or decades) and its first manifestation is often seen many years after the occupational exposure or even when the affected individuals are not more occupationally exposed.
- Important industrial chemicals are arsenic and inorganic arsenic compounds, polycyclic aromatic hydrocarbons (PAHs) with particularly high levels in brown coal tars (soft coal tars), coal tars (black coal tars), coal tar pitches, coal tar oils, and coke oven emissions and can cause basal cell carcinomas and squamous cell carcinomas.
- A recently published systematic appraisal of the epidemiologic literature and meta-analysis clearly indicates that occupational UV-light exposure is a substantial and robust risk factor for the development of cutaneous squamous cell carcinoma (SCC).
- The actually available evidence of the epidemiologic literature could also clearly show a significant risk increase for occupationally UV-exposed workers to develop basal cell carcinoma (BCC) compared to nonexposed workers.
- There is enough scientific evidence that outdoor workers have an increased risk to develop work-related occupational skin cancer due to natural UVR exposure and adequate prevention strategies have to be implemented.
- The three measures that are successful and of particular importance in the prevention of nonmelanoma skin cancer in outdoor workers are the following:
  1. Changes in behavior regarding awareness of health and disease resulting from exposure to natural UV radiation
  2. Protection from direct UV radiation by wearing suitable clothing
  3. Regular and correct use of appropriate sunscreens

1 Introduction

Occupational skin cancer is, especially in the historical sense due to industrial exposure to chemical carcinogens, important, but nowadays the relation of skin cancer to occupation is often confounded by concurrent sun exposure from leisure pursuits. The term "skin cancer" is nonspecific. Under such a heading come different clinicopathological entities with different etiologic factors, presentation, clinical course, and prognosis (Naldi and Diepgen 2007). A distinction is usually made between "cutaneous melanoma" and "nonmelanoma skin cancer." The term "nonmelanoma skin cancer" includes a large number of different disorders, especially basal cell carcinoma (BCC) and squamous cell carcinoma (SCC). Nonetheless, it is common practice to use it with reference to only two entities, which, by far, are the most frequent ones, namely, basal cell carcinoma and squamous cell carcinoma, also collectively labeled as "keratinocyte carcinomas" or "epidermal skin cancer." Besides the above-mentioned disorders, a large number of clinicopathological entities may be listed as representing "skin cancer" (➋ *Table 10.1*).

In contrast to most inflammatory occupational skin diseases, especially allergic and irritant contact dermatitis and contact urticaria, occupational skin cancer is characterized by long induction periods (years or decades) and its first manifestation is often seen many years after the occupational exposure or even when the affected individual is not more occupationally exposed.

An additional problem related to occupational skin cancer is the fact that skin cancer nowadays is a widespread disease, especially in Caucasians, and is comparable rarely induced by occupational carcinogens but by constitutional (skin type) and lifestyle factors (sun exposure).

This chapter introduces different types of occupational skin cancer and discusses its occupational hazards. In the last paragraph, measures for the prevention of occupational skin cancer are presented.

T. Rustemeyer, P. Elsner, S.M. John & H.I. Maibach (eds.), *Kanerva's Occupational Dermatology*,
DOI 10.1007/978-3-642-02035-3_10, © Springer-Verlag Berlin Heidelberg 2012

Table 10.1
Classification of skin cancer (According to Naldi and Diepgen 2007)

	Example
Epidermal skin tumors	Basal cell carcinoma
	Squamous cell carcinoma
	Paget's disease
	Keratoacanthoma
Tumors of skin appendages	
Hair-follicle tumors	Pilary complex carcinoma
Sebaceous glands	Sebaceous carcinoma
Apocrine gland tumors	Apocrine carcinoma
Eccrine gland tumors	Sweat gland carcinoma
	Microcystic adnexal carcinoma
	Eccrine epithelioma
	Mucinous eccrine epithelioma
	Adenoid cystic carcinoma
	Lymphoepithelioma-like carcinoma
Melanocytic tumors	Melanoma
	Malignant blue nevus
Langerhans cell tumors	Histiocytosis X
Mast cell tumors	Lymphadenopathic mastocytosis and eosinophilia
Subcutaneous tissue tumors	Liposarcoma
Fibrohistiocytic tumors	Dermatofibrosarcoma protuberans
	Atypical fibroxanthoma
	Malignant fibrous histiocytoma
Neoplasms of the vessel wall	Angiosarcoma
	Kaposi's sarcoma
Smooth muscle tumors	Superficial leiomyosarcoma
Neural and neuroendocrine tumors	Granular cell tumor
	Neuroendocrine and Merkel cell carcinoma
Cutaneous lymphoproliferative disease	
T cell	Mycosis fungoides
	Sézary syndrome
	Adult T-cell leukemia/lymphoma
	Primary cutaneous CD30+ lymphoproliferative disorders
B cell	Primary cutaneous marginal zone B-cell lymphoma
	Primary cutaneous diffuse large B-cell lymphoma, leg type
Precursor hematologic neoplasms	

2 Epidemiology of Melanoma and Nonmelanoma Skin Cancer

Melanoma and nonmelanoma (basal and squamous cell carcinomas) skin cancer (NMSC) are now the most common types of cancer in the white populations and the incidence of skin cancer has reached epidemic proportions (Diepgen and Mahler 2002; Madan et al. 2010). According to population-based studies from Australia, the incidence rate is over 2% for basal cell carcinoma in males and 1%

for squamous cell carcinoma, and there are over 50 new cases of melanoma per 100,000 (Buettner and Raasch 1998). Without doubt, skin cancer is by far the most common kind of cancer diagnosed in many western countries. The chance of developing a skin cancer in British Columbia, Canada is approximately 1 in 7, over lifetime (Demers et al. 2005). This corresponds to perhaps 1 in 3 for a white population in California (Rigel et al. 1996), and even higher for a white population in Queensland, Australia (Staples et al. 2006). The most common skin cancer is basal cell carcinoma, followed by squamous cell carcinoma and melanoma.

The chance of developing a malignant melanoma during a lifetime, in North America, is in the order of 1 in 100 (Merrill and Feuer 1996). This is a startling increase over the figures of, for instance, 1935, when the rate was 1 in 1,500. Predictions of future incidence of skin cancer in the Netherlands suggest that if the rates continue to increase and population growth and aging remain unabated, a rise in annual demand for care of more than 5% could occur by the year 2015, a heavy burden on the health system (de Vries et al. 2005).

3 Types of Occupational Skin Cancer

3.1 Nonmelanoma Skin Cancer

The term "nonmelanoma skin cancer" (NMSC) covers those cancers of the skin (epidermis) which are not malignant melanomas. The two commonest NMSCs are basal cell carcinoma and squamous cell carcinoma of the skin. Both of these types of malignant tumor arise from the epidermal tissues: squamous cell carcinomas from the epidermal keratinocytes and basal cell carcinomas from the basal cells of the epidermis. Basal cell carcinoma is the commonest malignant tumor in fair-skinned people: It is extremely locally invasive and destructive but only rarely metastasizes.

Different types of basal cell carcinoma can be distinguished clinically: nodular, cystic, pigmented, superficial (multicentric), morphoea-like, and ulcerative. The nodular and cystic variants are usually found on the face and are up to 10 mm or more in diameter. The morphoeic type shows scarring and a diffuse edge and is often found on the face too, whereas the multicentric superficial tumors, which can extend to several centimeters in diameter, typically occur on the trunk. Exposure to the sun, to ionizing radiation, and to chemical carcinogens including tar products can be involved in the causation of basal cell carcinoma.

Like squamous cell carcinoma, it is more commonly found in men than in women. Basal cell carcinoma occurs about four times more frequently than squamous cell carcinoma, which is the second most common form of skin cancer. Squamous cell carcinoma has a destructive pattern of growth and it metastasizes. It nearly always arises from characteristic precancerous lesions; actinic keratoses (AKs) are preinvasive squamous cell carcinomas and can therefore be regarded as carcinoma in situ. Basal cell carcinomas and squamous cell carcinomas exhibit both epidemiological and biological differences.

Squamous cell carcinomas and basal cell carcinomas are the commonest skin cancers in fair-skinned people all over the world (Wang and Diepgen 2006). In the USA, it has even been estimated that the incidence rate of NMSCs (basal cell and squamous cell carcinomas combined) is about as high as all other types of cancer put together (American Cancer Society: http://www.cancer.org, 2006). In the year 2002, some one million Americans were diagnosed with NMSC. Because of the high morbidity and associated treatment costs, NMSCs represent a heavy burden on the health-care system, even though they are not usually associated with very high mortality. NMSC has therefore been included in the top 10 health-care priorities in the USA for this decade, currently occupying place eight. Since the 1960s, the annual incidence of NMSC has increased by 3–8% (Glass and Hoover 1989; Green 1992).

Sex-related differences in exposure to the sun during occupational and leisure activities, in the use of sun protection, and scalp hair are probably reasons for the higher prevalence of nonmelanoma skin cancer in men (Oberyszyn 2008; Hall et al. 1997).

Basal cell and squamous cell carcinomas are usually considered together under the heading "nonmelanoma skin cancer" but they present rather different distribution and etiologic factors. The two tumors share the difficulties of obtaining reliable incidence data and the limited contribution of mortality to understand their distribution and burden. Incidence estimates for "cancer of the skin other than melanoma" based on registry data, range from around 0.5/100,000 in Hispanics, Blacks, and Asians to more than 100/100,000 in white people in Switzerland and Ireland (Parkin et al. 2005). However, few cancer registries provide reliable data on nonmelanoma skin cancer and ad hoc studies should be better conducted.

Within populations of European descent, the incidence of squamous cell carcinoma is lower in those with darker skins (Mediterranean skin type). In Australia and the USA, the incidence of squamous cell carcinoma increases with proximity to the equator. Squamous cell carcinoma of the skin shows clear associations with geographical latitude of the domicile and measured UVB radiation. Lifetime cumulative exposure is decisive for risk. In contrast to malignant melanomas and basal cell carcinomas, the incidence of squamous cell carcinoma shows an exposure-response curve without any plateau phase. Benign UV-light-induced skin changes (lentigo, telangiectasia, and elastosis) also show a strong association with the incidence of squamous cell carcinoma.

3.1.1 Risk Factors for NMSC

➋ *Table 10.2* shows the similarities and differences in the risk factors for basal cell carcinoma and squamous cell carcinoma. Whereas squamous cell carcinomas are clearly associated with chronic exposure to UV light, occur on areas of skin exposed to light and, in Caucasian populations, show clear associations with the geographical latitude of domicile and measured UVB radiation, important risk factors for basal cell carcinomas also include intermittent exposure to sunlight and a genetic predisposition. A decisive factor for the development of squamous cell carcinoma is the cumulative lifetime UV exposure. In contrast to malignant melanomas and basal cell carcinomas, the incidence of squamous cell carcinoma shows an exposure-response curve without a plateau phase.

Besides UV radiation, other influences such as ionizing radiation, exposure to tar and other carcinogens, smoking, DNA repair defects (such as xeroderma pigmentosum), and/or immunosuppression may induce nonmelanoma skin cancer. Smoking and other types of tobacco use are clearly associated with squamous cell carcinoma of the lip. Malignant tumors of the skin may form in scars. Burns and other firm scar tissue are predisposed to skin cancer. Most of them are squamous cell carcinomas or basal cell carcinomas, although the former are more common (Kowal-Verna and Criswell 2005). Simultaneous exposure to UV light and benzopyrenes considerably intensifies the development of cancer.

▫ Table 10.2
Risk factors for nonmelanoma skin cancer (NMSC): basal cell carcinomas and squamous cell carcinomas – similarities and differences

Risk factor	NMSC: squamous cell carcinomas and basal cell carcinomas
Age	Clear increase with age
Sex	More common in men
Genetics	Increased risk with a positive family history of basal cell carcinoma, but not of squamous cell carcinoma
Phototype	Higher incidence in fair-skin types – people who do not tan easily, have many freckles, and get sunburn easily, and who have red or blonde hair
Past history of skin cancer	36–52% probability of the occurrence of a new skin cancer within the next 5 years
Ethnic group	More common in people of Caucasian origin
Geographical location	The incidence increases in Caucasian people with proximity to the equator
Medical causes	Chronic ulceration, burn scars, xeroderma pigmentosum, immunosuppression (organ transplantation), and HPV[a] infections are associated with increased risk
Occupation	Higher incidence of squamous cell carcinoma, but also of basal cell carcinoma, in outdoor workers
Exposure to chemicals and other substances	Ionizing radiation, PUVA therapy, and exposure to tar increase the risk. Smoking is a risk factor for squamous cell carcinoma; arsenic exposure is a more important risk factor for basal cell carcinoma
Exposure to sunlight	
Cumulative	The highest individual risk factor for squamous cell carcinoma, less important (together with other risk factors) for basal cell carcinoma
Sporadic	Intensive, intermittent exposure with sunburn and blistering especially in childhood/adolescence is associated with an increased risk of basal cell carcinoma but not of squamous cell carcinoma

[a]Human papilloma virus

In white transplant recipients, risk of squamous cell carcinoma increases 65–250-fold and risk of basal cell carcinoma 10–16-fold compared with the nontransplanted population (Lindelof et al. 2000; Moloney et al. 2006). The risk of developing actinic keratosis (AK) is about 250 times greater in organ transplant recipients (Stockfleth et al. 2002; Stoff et al. 2010).The ratio of squamous cell to basal cell carcinoma also reverses in iatrogenic immunosuppression, because squamous cell carcinomas and actinic keratosis occur more frequently in transplant recipients than do basal cell carcinomas.

Although basal cell carcinomas usually occur in light-exposed areas, unlike squamous cell carcinomas, they may also occur in areas hardly exposed to sunlight at all and without any significant actinic damage, such as the trunk. UV light is also the most potent causative factor for basal cell carcinoma, but its effects are less evident than in squamous cell carcinoma.

A carcinogen typically associated with basal cell carcinomas is arsenic. An increased incidence of basal cell carcinomas has been reported with a hereditary syndrome of congenital defects (basal cell nevus syndrome). A sebaceous nevus may enhance the development of basal cell carcinomas. Apart from the genetic predisposition, intermittent intense exposure to UV light with sunburn is a key risk factor.

People who already have one squamous cell carcinoma of the skin have an approximately 50% risk of developing a second malignant skin lesion (nonmelanoma skin cancer) in the following 3–5 years (Hemminki and Dong 2000).

3.2 Malignant Melanoma

Malignant melanoma (MM) occurs among all adequately studied racial and ethnic groups. Its incidence is much lower compared to NMSCs but has been rising in fair-skinned populations throughout the world for several decades (Armstrong and Kricker 1994). The incidence of malignant melanoma varies over 100-fold around the world (Naldi and Diepgen 2007). According to data provided in Cancer Incidence in Five Continents, the lowest rates reported around 1993–1997 were 0.3–0.5/100,000 person-years, in parts of Asia, and in Asian and black people in the USA, while the highest were up to 50/100,000 in Queensland, Australia (Parkin et al. 2005). Incidence rates have risen significantly over the last 30–40 years and continue to increase in the USA, Canada, Australia, and Europe, being perceived as a major public health concern. Geographic variations with incidence of cutaneous melanoma appear to reflect the combined effect of constitutional characteristics and latitude. Epidemiological data from the USA and Australia show that melanoma incidence in white people increases the closer to the equator people live.

In contrast to nonmelanoma skin cancer, the greatest numbers of melanomas are found on the intermittently sun-exposed areas of the back and legs. Increases in incidence in populations of European origin have been most pronounced on the trunk and other intermittently exposed areas, particularly in men, while the incidence of melanoma of the face has remained reasonably stable over time (Bulliard and Cox 2000; Thorn et al. 1990). The anatomical distribution in black people and people of Asian origin is quite different with most melanomas occurring on the soles of the feet (Cress and Holly 1997).

There are important clinical and epidemiological differences in risk factors for the different subtypes of cutaneous malignant melanoma (superficial spreading melanoma, nodular melanoma, lentigo maligna melanoma, and acrolentigo melanoma). The following are the most important risk factors for malignant melanoma:

Skin type/ethnicity: Increased incidence in those with fair complexions; those who burn easily, tan poorly and freckle; those who have red, blonde or light brown hair; and those of Celtic ancestry.

Family history: Occurrence of melanoma in a first- or second-degree relative confers increased risk. Familial atypical molemelanoma syndrome (FAMMS) confers even higher risk.

Nevi: A large number of melanocytic nevi and giant pigmented congenital nevi confer increased risk. Melanocytic nevi are markers for risk, not precursor lesions.

Geographic location: Higher incidence in whites living near the equator.

Sun exposure: Cumulative sun exposure probably does not influence risk, but intense, intermittent exposure and blistering sunburns in childhood and adolescence are associated with increased risk. However, lentigo maligna melanoma occurs in sun-exposed sites, typically on the face, and is typically associated with prolonged exposure to sunlight, usually over a period of many years, in somebody employed in outdoor work.

Occupation: Higher incidence in indoor workers, as well as those with higher education and income.

Medical conditions: Xeroderma pigmentosum, immunosuppression, other malignancies, and previous nonmelanoma skin cancer all increase risk. Previous melanoma is associated with increased risk.

The single greatest predictor of risk for developing melanoma is the total number of nevi (Gandini et al. 2005b). Studies over the last decades have revealed a great deal about the way nevi develop and the relationship between nevi and melanoma. Interestingly, red-haired children have a reduced count of nevi as compared to other skin phenotypes, but a higher melanoma risk, suggesting different pathways to melanoma development.

Intermittent sun exposure and sunburn history were shown to play considerable roles as risk factors for melanoma, whereas a high occupational sun exposure seemed to be inversely associated to melanoma (Gandini et al. 2005a). Overall, high occupational exposure is inversely associated with melanoma and directly related to the risk of squamous cell carcinoma.

4 Other Occupational Skin Cancers

Actinic (solar) keratoses clinically are brownish or reddish scaly areas, sometimes with a popular component or with inflammation, a few millimeters in diameter and a rough surface. They are located on sun-exposed sites, typically the dorsal aspects of the hands, the forearms, the face, and the scalp. They may be associated with other stigmata of sun-damaged skin, such as telangiectasia, irregular pigmentation, solar elastosis, or skin atrophy. Actinic keratoses are nowadays considered as a squamous cell carcinoma in situ and belong therefore to NMSC (Röwert-Huber et al. 2007).

Tar keratoses are related to exposure to coal tar, pitch, shale oil, and products of the distillation of coal (Gawkrodger 2004). They may appear some years after the period of exposure. Clinically they are brown-colored, flat-topped, round, or oval small plaques a few millimeters in diameter, with a tendency to be clustered. Their surface may be smooth or warty. They tend to be seen on the dorsal aspects of the hands, the forearms, and around the face.

Arsenical keratoses are typically seen as punctate keratoses on the palms of the hands and soles of the feet in subjects exposed to arsenic and are not seen with any other condition. They are usually multiple and may progress to squamous cell carcinoma. Intraepidermal carcinoma or multiple basal cell carcinomas may be associated (Gawkrodger 2004).

Keratoacanthoma is a rapidly growing dome-shaped nodule up to 2 cm in diameter, with a central keratinous plug, that is usually found in sun-exposed areas such as the face, dorsa of hands, and the forearms (Gawkrodger 2004). Histologically, they resemble squamous cell carcinomas, but spontaneous resolution may occur. It is associated with sunlight and tar exposure (Letzel and Drexler 1998).

Intraepidermal carcinoma (Bowen's disease) is in situ squamous cell carcinoma. It occurs as scaly red plaques up to several centimeters in size, located on the sun-exposed sites of the lower legs, face, or arms (Gawkrodger 2004). Progression to invasive carcinoma may occur. It is typically associated with arsenic ingestion.

5 Occupational Hazards

5.1 Arsenic

Arsenic occurs naturally in ores together with zinc, lead, copper, and iron. In the past, it was used for paints, pesticides, and as a medicine. Today arsenic is only used in the semiconductor and microchip industry. Arsenic and inorganic arsenic compounds are mainly absorbed via inhalation and ingestion. Several studies show that the internal exposure to arsenic correlates well with the external exposure. Therefore, dermal absorption under workplace conditions does not seem to be relevant. Arsenic and inorganic arsenic compounds are distributed rapidly in all organs. Accumulation is observed particularly in the liver, kidneys, and lungs. Long-term exposure to arsenic in humans cause fever, sleep disorders, weight loss, swelling of the liver, dark discoloration of the skin, sensory and motor neuropathy, and encephalopathy with symptoms such as headaches, poor concentration, deficits in the learning of new information, difficulties in remembering, mental confusion, anxiety, and depression. Long-term exposure to arsenic can also cause peripheral vascular effects such as acrocyanosis, Raynaud's disease, and tissue necrosis on the extremities (blackfoot disease). Long-term exposure to dust containing arsenic causes irritation of the conjunctiva and mucous membranes of the nose and throat. The pustular or follicular skin reactions observed after contact with inorganic arsenic compounds are usually attributed to irritative effects and not to sensitizing effects of the arsenic compounds.

Arsenic and inorganic arsenic compounds are carcinogenic in humans. The target organs of the carcinogenic effects after inhalation are the lungs and after ingestion the bladder, kidneys, lungs, and skin (Greim 2005).

The premalignat skin tumors are punctuate keratoses on the palms of the hand and soles of the feet in subjects exposed to arsenic. They cannot be observed under other conditions and are therefore pathognomonic for chronic arsenic exposure. They are usually multiple and may progress to squamous cell carcinoma (Gawkrodger 2004). Besides the squamous cell carcinomas which can also occur on each position on the skin beside palms and soles, superficial basaliomas are often associated with a chronic arsenic exposure.

5.2 Polycyclic Aromatic Hydrocarbons (PAHs)

In 1773, Sir Percival Pott was the first to describe the occurrence of occupational causes of cancers. He observed the frequent occurrence of squamous cell carcinomas of the scrotum in young chimney sweeps and identified soot as the causal agent. Soot is a pyrolysis product of organic materials which contain, among numerous other substances, polycyclic aromatic hydrocarbons (PAHs). The extremely complex mixtures which have been examined to date contain, simultaneously and in widely differing proportions, carcinogenic components and substances which promote cancer development. Many of the PAHs, which occur regularly in pyrolysis products, are carcinogenic in animal studies. They exist at particularly high levels in brown coal tars (soft coal tars), coal tars (black coal tars), coal tar pitches, coal tar oils, and coke oven emissions (DFG 2010).

The carcinogenic effect after occupational exposure to these mixtures of aromatic compounds has been demonstrated in epidemiological studies. Therefore, they are classified into the category of the human cancerogens.

In the organism, PAHs are enzymatically converted into carcinogenic metabolites. The enzymes required for this activation are monooxygenases (CYP 1A1, 1A2, 1B1) and are found in the hair follicles of the skin. Therefore, the initial cancers ("tar warts") develop – in contrast to solar keratosis – in the deeper layers of the epidermis.

PAHs can cause basal cell carcinomas and squamous cell carcinomas. Direct skin contact seems to be a prerequisite. The latency of the initial exposure to PAHs to an onset of skin tumors may be relevant for years to decades. Skin cancer can occur even after termination of exposure. Often there are other signs of a so-called tar or pitch skin disease (e.g., folliculitis, acne, diffuse brownish pigmentation, and hyperkeratosis). The tumors can also occur without these signs. The skin tumors are localized, in particular, in the exposed areas including nose, periorbital region, ears, and on the backs of the hands and forearms. The location seems to deviate from that of the light-induced tumors (more often lower lip than upper lip, more often nasal vestibule than bridge) (Letzel and Drexler 1998).

5.3 Ionizing Radiation

Ionizing radiation consists of particles (alpha particles, beta particles, neutrons) or electromagnetic waves (gamma rays with wavelengths less than 0.01 nm, which is less than the diameter of an atom, and X-rays with wavelengths from 0.01 to 10 nm). Alpha particles are absorbed completely in the stratum corneum and do not cause a damage in the skin. Under high acute radiation exposure (1 Sv and above), the development of acute radiation dermatitis is expected with redness, itching, and infiltration of the skin. Higher doses may cause bleeding into the skin, blisters, and necrosis. The final stage can be a chronic dermatitis with radio atrophy of the skin, increasing sclerosis, keratinization disorders, pigmentary changes, and dryness developing due to loss of sebaceous glands, hair loss, and telangiectasia.

Ionizing radiation can cause malignant diseases of the skin, especially squamous cell and basal cell carcinomas and less often sarcomas. Actinic keratoses caused by X-rays are carcinomas in situ and were often observed in the past at the hands of surgeons and radiologists. Today, in compliance with the radiation limits, however, no higher incidence of radiation-induced diseases is observed in occupationally to ionizing radiation-exposed persons. The radiation exposure from accidents such as Chernobyl or Fukushima, in contrast, is much higher and suitable to cause both stochastic damages (cancer) and deterministic damages (inflammation to necrosis) on the skin.

5.4 UV Radiation

The spectrum of ultraviolet (UV) light comprises wavelengths of 100–400 nm and is therefore below the range of visible light (400–780 nm). Depending on its wavelength, UV radiation is divided into UVA (315–400 nm), UVB (280–315 nm), and UVC (100–280 nm), although on the Earth human beings are exposed only to UVA and UVB. Natural solar UV radiation on this planet consists of $>95\%$ UVA and $\leq 5\%$ UVB.

UV radiation is the most important cause of skin aging and skin cancer. It causes chronic cutaneous photodamage (Saladi and Persaud 2005). The carcinogenic effects of UV radiation on the skin and eyes are well documented both experimentally and epidemiologically (Saladi and Persaud 2005). UV radiation acts as a carcinogen both directly, by inducing cell damage (DNA mutations), and indirectly, by inducing immunosuppression (suppression of T lymphocytes).

There is good evidence that UVB radiation acts directly through specific changes in oncogenes and p53 tumor suppressor genes, which are responsible for the initiation and progression of skin cancer. UV radiation, and in particular UVB, leads to the formation of pyrimidine dimers in deoxyribonucleic acid (DNA) and ribonucleic acid (RNA). This gives rise to mutations in keratinocytes and hence to neoplastic transformation. Particularly significant mutations affect the telomerase gene and the p53 tumor suppressor gene. These mutations are important steps toward neoplastic transformation.

UVB radiation causes direct damage to DNA and RNA by inducing covalent bond formation between adjacent pyrimidines, leading to generation of mutagenic photoproducts such as cyclopyrimidine dimers (TT) and pyrimidine-pyrimidine (6-4) adducts (Rünger 2007). UVA is less mutagenic than is UVB, and causes indirect DNA damage via a photo-oxidative-stress-mediated mechanism, resulting in formation of reactive oxygen species, which interact with lipids, proteins, and DNA to generate intermediates that combine with DNA to form adducts (Ridley et al. 2009). Several complex DNA repair systems are needed to prevent the harmful effects of these premutagenic adducts (Lear et al. 2000).

UVA radiation, which penetrates deeper into the skin, reinforces the carcinogenic effects of UVB rays and causes aging and immunosuppression. In this way, both UVB and UVA are involved in the development of skin cancer.

The relationship between UV radiation and skin cancer has been well demonstrated at various levels by epidemiology, clinical distribution of the tumors, molecular biology, and plausible mechanisms. However, some aspects in the development of the disease and in the counter-regulatory mechanisms, the interaction of various photobiological processes, and the secondary biochemical effects after irradiation are still unclear.

Light skin complexion (especially light skin and blond-red hair), freckling, and tendency to burn, not tan, after sun exposure, are constitutional variables which affect the risk of skin cancer. People from Southern European ethnic origin are at a significantly lower risk than those from English, Celtic, and Scandinavian origin. Those who migrate early in their life from such regions to lower latitudes increase their exposure levels to sunlight and show a higher risk of developing skin cancer. It can be further stated that the timing and character of sun exposure may affect differently the risk of different skin cancers. Cutaneous melanoma and basal cell carcinoma are most significantly linked to early exposure to ultraviolet light. Intermittent sun exposure and sunburn history are more important than cumulative dose in predicting adult risk for these tumors. Basal cell carcinoma and melanoma tumors appear to have a rapidly accelerating relative risk with relatively low exposures, followed by a broad plateau. Among sensitive individuals, sun avoidance behavior in adulthood may not markedly reduce risk for these tumors. On the contrary, squamous cell carcinoma is associated with total lifetime sun exposure. It has also been demonstrated that intermittent and chronic sun exposure is a risk factor for basal cell carcinoma (Walther et al. 2004).

Outdoor workers such as farmers, welders, watermen, police officers, physical education teachers, pilots, and cabin attendants have an increased risk of skin cancer (Ramirez et al. 2005). There is scientific and epidemiological evidence to recognize squamous cell carcinoma induced by occupational UV-light exposure as an occupational disease since a doubling of risk due to occupational UV radiation can be demonstrated (Diepgen and Drexler 2004). Two recently published systematic reviews demonstrate the increased risk of nonmelanoma skin cancer in outdoor workers (Schmitt et al. 2011; Bauer et al. 2011).

Schmitt et al. 2011demonstrated in a systematic review and meta-analysis that occupational UV-light exposure increases the risk for the development of cutaneous squamous cell carcinoma. The authors performed a systematic electronic literature search in PubMed (until May 2010) supplemented by handsearch identified 18 relevant studies that were included in the review. Eighteen studies (6 cohort studies, 12 case-control studies) met the eligibility criteria and were included in the systematic review. Sixteen studies (89%) found an increased risk of SCC in individuals with occupational UV-light exposure compared to individuals without occupational UV-light exposure, reaching statistical significance in 12 studies. Two studies found no association between occupational UV-light exposure and SCC occurrence. The pooled OR (95%CI) was 1.77 (1.40–2.22) and did not differ significantly between cohort studies (OR; 95%CI: 1.68; 1.08–2.63) and case-control studies (OR; 95%CI: 1.77; 1.37–2.30). Meta-regression analyses suggested an increasing strength of the association between occupational UV-light exposure and SCC risk with decreasing latitude. In addition, the authors identified several reasons why the observed increase in the risk for cutaneous SCC among individuals with work-related UV-light exposure compared to indoor workers is an underestimation of the true association. This systematic appraisal of the epidemiologic literature and meta-analysis clearly indicates that occupational UV-light exposure is a substantial and robust risk factor for the development of cutaneous SCC. These findings are of significant public health impact as they highlight the need for preventive measures for individuals with high levels of work-related UV-light exposure.

It is reasonable to assume that outdoor workers with a long history of work-related UV exposure are at increased risk of developing BCC; however, it has not yet been demonstrated epidemiologically as clearly as for cutaneous SCC. Recently, Bauer et al. (2011) summarized the actually available evidence of the epidemiologic literature and could also clearly show a significant risk increase for occupationally UV-exposed workers to develop BCCs compared to nonexposed workers. In this systematic review and meta-analysis, 24 relevant epidemiologic studies (5 cohort studies, 19 case-control studies) were identified. Twenty-three studies reported sufficient data to be included in the meta-analysis. The pooled OR for the association between outdoor work and BCC risk was 1.43 (95% CI: 1.23–1.66; $p = 0.0001$). Studies adjusting for sex ($p < 0.0001$) and individual nonoccupational UV exposure ($p = 0.014$) showed a significant stronger association of occupational UV exposure and BCC risk. Taking into account that the majority of the studies published to date lack precision in the assignment of workers to indoor and outdoor tasks as well as concerning UV-exposure measurements and adjustment for major confounders, it is most likely that the real risk is largely underestimated. In addition, meta-regression revealed a significant inverse relationship between occupational UV-light exposure and BCC risk with latitude ($p = 0.015$). This systematic review indicates that outdoor workers are at significantly increased risk for BCC. This study is important to inform occupational safety representatives, stimulate the implementation of prevention strategies, and encourage further research in this important field.

It has been estimated by the IARC that outdoor workers had the two to three times higher UV-radiation dose than indoor workers (IARC 1992). In subjects older than 20 years, the UV radiation (UVR) exposure is not related to age but to occupation, outdoor sports activities, or being a sun worshipper (Thieden et al. 2004). Thieden et al. (2004) developed a personal electronic UVR dosimeter in a wristwatch and measured continuously time-related UVR doses in standard erythema dose (SED). They demonstrated that the median estimated yearly UVR dose was 132 SEDs for indoor workers but 224 SEDs for gardeners. Knuschke et al. (2007) also found significantly increased UVR doses in different outdoor workers compared to indoor workers. It was estimated that the average annual UVR exposure of the general population is 130 SED per year in Germany (Knuschke et al. 2008).

In conclusion, there is enough scientific evidence that outdoor workers have an increased risk to develop a work-related occupational nonmelanoma skin cancer due to natural UVR exposure during working hours. In contrast to natural UVR exposure, epidemiological studies are still missing to demonstrate an increased risk of occupational skin cancer due to occupational exposure to artificial UVR.

5.5 Malignant Skin Tumors in Scars

Malignant skin tumors can develop within scars. Thus they can be caused indirectly by an industrial accident. Only burn scars and other tight scars are premalignant conditions for squamous cell carcinomas and basal cell carcinomas. Squamous cell carcinomas occur more frequently. (Kowal-Verna and Criswell 2005; Dix 1960). In order to postulate a causal context between the tumor and accidental scar, according to Ewing (cited in Kowal-Verna and Criswell 2005) the following conditions must be met:

1. The presence of a scar.
2. The tumor has developed within the boundaries of the scar.
3. The absence of a preexisting tumor of the same type.
4. Any tumor cells must correspond to the cells of the primary tumor in the scar (this item is only relevant for metastasis).
5. An adequate time interval between the scar and the development of the neoplasm.

6 Prevention

6.1 Primary Prevention

Risk assessment is the systematic identification and evaluation of relevant risks of workers with the aim of necessary measures for safety and health at work. It is based on an assessment of the hazard. Hazardous substances are labeled by many organizations regarding their potential effects (carcinogen, absorbed through the skin, sensitizing, irritating, etc.). To remove differences in the existing international systems of classification and labeling, a Globally Harmonized System of Classification and Labeling of Chemicals (GHS) was developed. The exposure is important too, which makes an assessment of the activities associated with the inhalation (breathing), dermal uptake (through skin contact), and the physical-chemical hazards necessary. If occupational exposure limits (OELs) are available, it must be ensured that these values are not exceeded. In many situations (skin absorption, long half-life time of the hazards, etc.) the concentration of a hazardous substance in workplace air is less significant. A biological monitoring is more suitable to assess the individual risk of an exposed subject (Drexler et al. 2008).

6.2 Occupational Skin Cancer Prevention Strategies for Outdoor Workers

Experts believe that 90% of nonmelanoma skin cancer and two-thirds of melanomas may be attributed to excessive exposure to the sun. The aim of primary skin cancer prevention is therefore to limit UVR exposure. Campaigns to prevent skin cancer have incorporated numerous messages including the need to avoid sunburn and generally reduce exposure to ultraviolet radiation by staying out of the midday sun (between 11 a.m. and 3 p.m.), wearing protective clothing, seeking shade, and applying sunscreen. These campaigns are also needed for outdoor workers and subjects with an increased occupational UVR exposure.

There are three measures which are successful and of particular importance in the prevention of nonmelanoma skin cancer in outdoor workers:

1. Changes in behavior regarding awareness of health and disease resulting from exposure to natural UV radiation
2. Protection from direct UV radiation by wearing suitable clothing
3. Regular and correct use of appropriate sunscreens

In the first place, changes in behavior have to be aimed at avoiding direct exposure to natural UV light between 11 o'clock in the morning and 3 o'clock in the afternoon, wearing suitable clothing when outdoors, applying sunscreen regularly, and keeping in the shade (Fry and Verne 2003). This applies not only to exposure during leisure activities, at weekends, or on holiday, but also to occupational exposure to natural UV radiation.

Suitable clothing must cover the arms and legs and should not have low-cut backs or necklines. Broad-brimmed hats should not only cover the head and face but also protect the ears and back of the neck. Materials used should be sufficiently thick in weave and in dark colors; clothing should not be too tight-fitting. Materials that are to be worn in the sun for any length of time should have an UV protection factor (UPF) greater than 40 (Gambichler et al. 2006). The European Committee for Standardization (CEN) has developed a new standard on requirements for test methods and labeling of sun-protective garments. This document has now been completed and is published. The first part of the standard (EN 13758-1) deals with all details of test methods (e.g., spectrophotometric measurements) for textile materials and part 2 (EN 13758-2) covers classification and marking of apparel textiles. UV-protective cloths for which compliance with this standard is claimed must fulfill all stringent instructions of testing, classification, and marking, including a UV protection factor (UPF) larger than 40 (UPF 40+), average UVA transmission lower than 5%, and design requirements as specified in part 2 of the standard. A pictogram, which is marked with the number of the standard EN 13758-2 and the UPF of 40+, shall be attached to the garment if it is in compliance with the standard. Garment manufacturers and retailers may now follow these official guidelines for testing and labeling of UV-protective summer clothes, and the sun-aware consumer can easily recognize garments that definitely provide sufficient UV protection.

In the year 2001 a study carried out by Gambichler et al. (2001) had demonstrated that one-third of European textiles are unsuitable and have a UPF of less than 15. Wet or damp clothing reduces the protective effects by one-third.

The regular use of appropriate photoprotective agents has been shown to protect against the development of UV-induced skin cancers in experimental, clinical, and epidemiological studies. Using a broad-spectrum sunscreen with a high sun protection factor (SPF) has been clearly shown to protect against UV-induced immunosuppression (Roberts et al. 1995).

Several randomized clinical trials carried out in Australia have shown that consistent use of sunscreens not only reduces the occurrence of new actinic keratoses (AKs) but also causes existing lesions to regress (Thompson et al. 1993; Darlington et al. 2003). Also in Texas, USA, a prospective 2-year study showed a reduction in actinic keratosis by the regular use of sun protection agents (Naylor et al. 2004). Likewise, over an observation period of 4.5 years, a prospective epidemiological study in Queensland showed that the incidence of squamous cell carcinoma is significantly reduced by the daily use of sunscreens (Green et al. 1999).

Regular use of a sunscreen is therefore part of the treatment of chronically photodamaged skin. Particularly in high-risk patients, the regular use of an appropriate sunscreen of SPF 50+ has to be strongly recommended. In an open interventional study published recently, it was shown that daily use of a liposomal sunscreen with photostable broad-spectrum filters (Daylong actinica) significantly reduced the occurrence of new actinic keratoses and squamous cell carcinomas in organ recipients over a follow-up period of 24 months (Ulrich et al. 2009). While nine invasive squamous cell carcinomas were diagnosed in the control group of 60 transplant patients using freely selected sunscreens, not a single new squamous cell carcinoma appeared in the interventional group using a sunscreen of SPF 50+ every day. During the 24-month study, 42 of the 120 patients developed 82 new actinic keratoses (all in the control group). In the sunscreen group, 102 actinic keratoses healed spontaneously.

It is also important to use a photoprotective agent with a high SPF, as sunscreens are often applied too thinly. This means that the actual protective effect is very much lower than that stated on the packaging. The SPF is based on the application of 2 mg sunscreen per cm^2 skin. In fact, on average, only 0.5 mg/cm^2 (range: 0.39–0.79 mg/cm^2) is applied (Neale et al. 2002; Autier et al. 2001). The sun protection factor does not show a linear correlation with the insufficient amount of sunscreen applied, but rather an exponential one, so that a sunscreen of SPF 16 is reduced to SPF 2 if only 0.5 mg/cm^2 is applied (Wulf et al. 1997). This has also been demonstrated recently for sunscreens with high SPFs (Kim et al. 2010).

A change in health awareness regarding exposure to UV radiation, knowledge of the previously mentioned preventative measures, and observing and regularly applying them, are all important for the high-risk group in particular. Appropriate preventative health-care concepts need to be developed. Halpern and Kopp (2005) found significant differences in awareness of skin cancer and sun protection habits between normal people in Australia, the USA, and Europe. In Australia, where the incidence of skin cancer is very high, more than 80% of survey responders expressed concerns about the dangers of sun exposure and skin cancer, while the figures were only 30% in Germany and 34% in France.

Another important public health message is that patients should promptly seek medical (dermatological) attention when they notice a suspicious or changing skin lesion. The detection of skin cancer at an early stage when it is most likely to be cured by simple outpatient excision is classified as secondary prevention. UVR-induced skin cancerogenesis is a multistep process that provides an excellent chance for effective prevention strategies to reduce the incidence, morbidity, and mortality of skin cancer and its precursor lesions. Therefore, outdoor workers should be screened for skin cancer regularly.

In Australia, where skin cancer is of epidemic proportions, aggressive public health campaigns have been underway since the 1980s. In addition to identifying tumors at an early stage, Australia managed an exciting educational program on photodamage prevention and sets standards for a wide variety of sun-protective products to include sunscreens, photoprotective apparel, sunglasses, and occupational standards for sun exposure. There, attitudes have already shifted positively toward avoiding exposure to the sun and away from desire for a tan.

The mainstay of sun protection is through avoidance of deliberate sun tanning; use of adequate protection measures such as wearing wide-brimmed hats, sunglasses, and protective clothing; and avoidance of peak hours for UV light. Sunscreens cannot be a substitute for other protective means. However, sunscreen use is the most popular form of sun protection and can significantly reduce the risk of developing skin cancer (Green et al. 1999). However, the results of a study from the UK, France, Italy, Germany, and Spain showed that both the general public and the majority of outdoor workers do not regularly apply sunscreens (MacKie 2004). Concern has also been raised that they may directly or indirectly increase the risk of malignancy, primarily because of poor application and increased exposure to the sun. The thickness of application has been shown to be less than half that officially tested and key exposed sites are often missed completely (Johnson et al. 2001).

For future public health policy, it is important to increase skin cancer awareness among outdoor workers, together with safe sun practices, such as application of sunscreen, wearing protective clothing, and avoiding the sun during times of peak solar intensity.

References

American Cancer Society (2006) http://www.cancer.org

Armstrong BK, Kricker A (1994) Cutaneous melanoma. Cancer Surv 19:219–239

Autier P, Boniol M, Severi G, Doré JF (2001) Quantity of sunscreen used by European students. Br J Dermatol 144:288–291

Bauer A, Diepgen TL, Schmitt J (2011) Is occupational solar UV-irradiation a relevant risk factor for basal cell carcinoma? A systematic review and meta-analysis of the epidemiologic literature. Br J Dermatol 165:612–625 [Epub ahead of print]

Buettner PG, Raasch BA (1998) Incidence rates of skin cancer in Townsville, Australia. Int J Cancer 78(5):587–593

Bulliard JL, Cox B (2000) Cutaneous malignant melanoma in New Zealand: trends by anatomical site, 1969–1993. Int J Epidemiol 29:416–423

Cress RD, Holly EA (1997) Incidence of cutaneous melanoma among non- Hispanic whites, Hispanics, Asians, and blacks: an analysis of California cancer registry data, 1988–93. Cancer Causes Control 8:246–252

Darlington S, Williams G, Neale R et al (2003) A randomized controlled trial to assess sunscreen application and beta carotene supplementation in the prevention of solar keratoses. Arch Dermatol 139:451–455

de Vries E, van de Poll-Franse LV, Louwman WJ, de Gruijl FR, Coebergh JW (2005) Predictions of skin cancer incidence in the Netherlands up to 2015. Br J Dermatol 152:481–488

Demers AA, Nugent Z, Mihalcioiu C, Wiseman MC, Kliewer EV (2005) Trends of nonmelanoma skin cancer from 1960 through 2000 in a Canadian population. J Am Acad Dermatol 53:320–328

DFG (Deutsche Forschungsgemeinschaft) (2010) List of MAK and BAT values 2010. Commission for the Investigation of Health Hazards of chemical compounds in the work area, Report No. 45. Wiley-VCH, Weinheim

Diepgen TL, Drexler H (2004) Skin cancer and occupational disease. Hautarzt 55:22–27

Diepgen TL, Mahler V (2002) The epidemiology of skin cancer. Br J Dermatol 146(Suppl 61):1–6

Drexler H, Göen Th, Schaller KH (2008) Biological tolerance values: change in a paradigm concept from assessment of a single value to use of an average. Int Arch Occup Environ Health 82:139–142

Fry A, Verne J (2003) Preventing skin cancer. BMJ 326:114–115

Gambichler T, Rotterdam S, Altmeyer P, Hoffmann K (2001) Protection against ultraviolet radiation by commercial summer clothing: need for standardised testing and labelling. BMC Dermatol 1:6

Gambichler T, Laperre J, Hoffmann K (2006) The European standard for sun-protective clothing: EN 13758. J Eur Acad Dermatol Venereol 20:125–130

Gandini S, Sera F, Cattaruzza MS, Pasquini P, Picconi O, Boyle P, Melchi CF (2005a) Meta-analysis of risk factors for cutaneous melanoma: II. Sun exposure. Eur J Cancer 41:45–60

Gandini S, Sera F, Cattaruzza MS, Pasquini P, Abeni D, Boyle P, Melchi CF (2005b) Meta-analysis of risk factors for cutaneous melanoma: I. Common and atypical naevi. Eur J Cancer 41:28–44

Gawkrodger DJ (2004) Occupational skin cancers. Occup Med 54:458–463

Glass AG, Hoover RN (1989) The emerging epidemic of melanoma and squamous cell skin cancer. JAMA 262:2097–2100

Green A (1992) Changing patterns in incidence of non-melanoma skin cancer. Epithelial Cell Biol 1:47–51

Green A, Williams G, Neale R et al (1999) Daily sunscreen application and betacarotene supplementation in prevention of basal-cell and squamous-cell carcinomas of the skin: a randomised controlled trial. Lancet 354(9180):723–729

Greim H (ed) (2005) Arsenic and its inorganic compounds. The MAK-collection Part I: MAK value documentations, vol 21. DFG, Deutsche Forschungsgemeinschaft. Wiley-VCH, Weinheim

Halpern AC, Kopp LJ (2005) Awareness, knowledge and attitudes to non-melanoma skin cancer and actinic keratosis among the general public. Int J Dermatol 44:107–111

Hemminki K, Dong C (2000) Subsequent cancers after in situ and invasive squamous cell carcinoma of the skin. Arch Dermatol 136:647–651

IARC, Cancer IAfRo (1992) Solar and ultraviolet radiation, vol 55. International Agency for Research on Cancer, Lyon

Johnson K, Davy L, Boyett T, Weathers L, Roetzheim RG (2001) Sun protection practices for children: knowledge, attitudes, and parent behaviors. Arch Pediatr Adolesc Med 155(8):891–896

Kim SM, Oh BH, Lee YW, Choe YB, Ahn KJ (2010) The relation between the amount of sunscreen applied and the sun protection factor in Asian skin. J Am Acad Dermatol 62:218–222

Knuschke P, Unverricht I, Ott G, Janssen M (2007) Personenbezogene Messung der UV-Exposition von Arbeitnehmern im Freien. Schriftenreihe der Bundesanstalt für Arbeitsschutz und Arbeitsmedizin, Forschung, F 1777. Dortmund/Berlin/Dresden. ISBN 978-3-88261-060-4

Knuschke P, Janßen M, Ott G (2008) Referenzbasis solarer UV-Expositionen zur Bewertung der Expositionslevel in der Bevölkerung und an Arbeitsplätzen im Freien. In: Kaase H, Serick F (Hrg) Licht und Gesundheit. Berlin, pp 24–29. ISBN 3-9807635-0-3

Kowal-Verna A, Criswell BK (2005) Burn scar neoplasms: a literature review and statistical analysis. Burns 31:403–413

Laperre J, Gambichler T (2001) Determination of the ultraviolet protection factor of textile materials: measurement precision. Photodermatol Photoimmunol Photomed 17(5):223–229

Lear JT, Smith AG, Strange RC, Fryer AA (2000) Detoxifying enzyme genotypes and susceptibility to cutaneous malignancy. Br J Dermatol 142:8–15

Letzel S, Drexler H (1998) Occupationally related tumors in tar refinery workers. J Am Acad Dermatol 39:712–720

Lindelof B, Sigurgeirsson B, Gabel H et al (2000) Incidence of skin cancer in 5356 patients following organ transplantation. Br J Dermatol 143:513–519

MacKie RM (2004) Awareness, knowledge and attitudes to basal cell carcinoma and actinic keratoses among the general public within Europe. J Eur Acad Dermatol Venereol 18:552–555

Madan V, Lear JT, Szeimies RM (2010) Non-melanoma skin cancer. Lancet 375:673–685

Merrill RM, Feuer EJ (1996) Risk-adjusted cancer-incidence rates (United States). Cancer Causes Control 7:544–552

Moloney FJ, Comber H, Conlon PJ et al (2006) The role of immunosuppression in the pathogenesis of basal cell carcinoma. Br J Dermatol 154:790–791

Naldi L, Diepgen TL (2007) The epidemiology of skin cancer. In: Lim HW, Hönigsmann H, Hawk JLM (eds) Photodermatology. Informa Healthcare, New York

Naylor MF, Boyd A, Smith DW, Cameron GS, Hubbard D, Neldner KH (2004) High sun protection factor sunscreens in the suppression of actinic neoplasia. Arch Dermatol 131:170–175

Neale R, Williams G, Green A (2002) Application patterns among participants randomized to daily sunscreen use in a skin cancer prevention trial. Arch Dermatol 138:1319–1325

Oberyszyn TM (2008) Non-melanoma skin cancer: importance of gender, immunosuppressive status and vitamin D. Cancer Lett 261(2):127–136

Parkin DM, Whelan SL, Ferlay J, Storm H (2005) Cancer incidence in five continents, vol I–VIII, IARC Cancer Base No. 7. IARC, Lyon

Ramirez CC, Federman DG, Kirsner RS (2005) Skin cancer as an occupational disease: the effect of ultraviolet and other forms of radiation. Int J Dermatol 44:95–100

Ridley AJ, Whiteside JR, McMillan TJ, Allinson SL (2009) Cellular and sub-cellular responses to UVA in relation to carcinogenesis. Int J Radiat Biol 85:177–195

Rigel DS, Friedman RJ, Kopf AW (1996) Lifetime risk for development of skin cancer in the U.S. population: current estimate is now 1 in 5. J Am Acad Dermatol 35:1012–3

Röwert-Huber J, Patel MJ, Forschner T, Ulrich C, Eberle J, Kerl H, Sterry W, Stockfleth E (2007) Actinic keratosis is an early in situ squamous cell carcinoma: a proposal for reclassification. Br J Dermatol 156(Suppl 3):8–12

Rünger TM (2007) How different wavelengths of the ultraviolet spectrum contribute to skin carcinogenesis: the role of cellular damage responses. J Invest Dermatol 127:2103–2105

Saladi RN, Persaud AN (2005) The causes of skin cancer: a comprehensive review. Drugs Today (Barc) 41:37–53

Schmitt J, Seidler A, Diepgen TL, Bauer A (2011) Occupational UV-light exposure increases the risk for the development of cutaneous squamous cell carcinoma: a systematic review and meta-analysis. Br J Dermatol 164:291–307

Staples MP, Elwood M, Burton RC, Williams JL, Marks R, Giles GG (2006) Non-melanoma skin cancer in Australia: the 2002 national survey and trends since 1985. Med J Aust 184:6–10

Stockfleth E, Ulrich C, Meyer T, Christophers E (2002) Epithelial malignancies in organ transplant patients: clinical presentation and new methods of treatment. Recent Results Cancer Res 160:251–258

Stoff B, Salisbury C, Parker D, O'Reilly Zwald F (2010) Dermatopathology of skin cancer in solid organ transplant recipients. Transplant Rev 24:172–189

Thieden E, Philipsen PA, Heydenreich J, Wulf HC (2004) UV radiation exposure related to age, sex, occupation, and sun behavior based on time-stamped personal dosimeter readings. Arch Dermatol 140:197–203

Thompson SC, Jolley D, Marks R (1993) Reduction of solar keratoses by regular sunscreen use. N Engl J Med 329:1147–1151

Thorn M, Bergstrom R, Adami HO, Ringborg U (1990) Trends in the incidence of malignant melanoma in Sweden, by anatomic site, 1960–1984. Am J Epidemiol 132:1066–1077

Ulrich C, Jurgensen JS, Degen A et al (2009) Prevention of non-melanoma skin cancer in organ transplant patients by regular use of a sunscreen: a 24 months, prospective, case-control study. Br J Dermatol 161(Suppl 3):78–84

Walther U, Kron M, Sander S, Sebastian G, Sander R, Peter RU, Meurer M, Krähn G, Kaskel P (2004) Risk and protective factors for sporadic basal cell carcinoma: results of a two-centre case-control study in southern Germany. Clinical actinic elastosis may be a protective factor. Br J Dermatol 151:170–178

Wang H, Diepgen TL (2006) The epidemiology of basal cell and squamous cell carcinoma. In: Reichrath J (ed) Molecular mechanisms of basal cell and squamous cell carcinomas. Springer, New York, pp S.1–S.9

Wulf HC, Stender IM, Lock-Andersen J (1997) Sunscreens used at the beach do not protect against erythema: a new definition of SPF is proposed. Photodermatol Photoimmunol Photomed 13:129–132

11 Other Occupational Skin Diseases

Elke Weisshaar · Thomas L. Diepgen
Department of Clinical Social Medicine, Occupational and Environmental Dermatology, University of Heidelberg, Heidelberg, Germany

Core Messages

- Erysipeloid is an acute infection due to *Erysipelothrix rhusiopathiae*, a gram-positive bacillus. It may present as a localized cutaneous form, a generalized cutaneous form with widespread erythematous-edematous lesions and symptoms such as, e.g., fever, lymphadenitis, and arthralgia. Healing normally occurs spontaneously in 2 weeks with desquamation or suppuration. Diagnosis is mainly clinical. Recommended treatment centers on antibiotics with, e.g., penicillins. Prevention includes, e.g., good sanitation, reduction of trauma, systematic slaughtering of infected animals, and wearing of protective gloves.
- Query (Q) fever is a worldwide zoonosis caused by *Coxiella burnetii*, a gram-negative bacterium. Farm animals and pets are the main reservoir of human infections. Epidemiological studies indicate Q fever as a public health problem in many countries. Therapy centers on doxycycline. Query fever infections resolve in most cases. Prevention includes protection measures such as, e.g., protective clothing, tick control strategies, good hygiene practice, and systematic slaughtering of infected animals.
- Tinea pedis is caused by dermatophytes and usually leads to an infection of the feet or toes. Living in an institution, especially when washing facilities are shared, is likely to increase the chances of infection. All professions demanding shoes that may occlude the skin are more frequently affected by tinea pedis. Diagnosis is made clinically and by fungal culture. Mild interdigital tinea pedis can be treated topically with broad-spectrum antifungal. Prevention includes treatment of onychomycosis if present, treatment of associated diseases such as vesicular eczema and hyperhidrosis and adequate hygiene of the feet.
- Vitiligo-like skin lesions may occur in the rubber industry when thiols and quinones are used as additives. Treatment comprises identifying the underlying etiology and prevention of skin contact with the causing agent.
- Psoriasis of the hands may present as keratotic patches on the palms, usually not displaying the classical features of psoriatic lesions elsewhere on the body. In the work environment, skin trauma and mechanical irritation of the hands are aggravating factors of psoriasis. No specific occupation predominates. It is estimated that occupational contact psoriasis probably accounts for 1.2% of all occupational dermatoses.
- Borreliosis is the most common tick-transmitted disease in the Northern hemisphere caused by spirochaetes of the *Borrelia burgdorferi* species. Diagnosis is made by the clinical findings, a history of tick bites (up to 50% of patients do not remember the tick bite), and laboratory test. Prevention of tick bites and borreliosis comprises a combination of primary prevention, early diagnosis, and treatment.

1 Erysipeloid

Erysipeloid is an acute infection due to *Erysipelothrix rhusiopathiae*, a gram-positive, nonsporulating, nonmotile bacillus. Infections are worldwide in distribution (Reboli and Farrar 1989). It also named in the past Rosenbach's disease and pseudoerysipelas (Veraldi et al. 2009). *E rhusiopathiae* colonizes a wide variety of animals worldwide, including mammals, birds, foal, fish, and shellfish. Human infection is contracted by direct contact from an animal or environmental source, most commonly from carcasses. This is the reason why the occupations mainly affected by the disease are slaughtermen, butchers, abattoir workers, meat-processing workers, cooks, fishermen, farmers, veterinarians, leather workers, and housewives (Brooke and Riley 1999; Reboli and Farrar 1989; Wang et al. 2010). Scratches or pricks are the usual mode of incubation. Although *E rhusiopathiae* is killed by moist heat at 55°C for 15 min, it is resistant to environmental influences such as salting, pickling, and smoking (Reboli and Farrar 1989) and can survive for long periods such as several months (Brooke and Riley 1999; Veraldi et al. 2009).

Reporting to health authorities of infection due to *E rhusiopathiae* is not required, so it is difficult to report incidence and prevalence of erysipeloid. The risk of human infection with *E rhusiopathiae* is closely related to the opportunity for exposure to the organism (Reboli and Farrar 1989). Most human cases are related to occupational exposure (Brooke and Riley 1999; Reboli and Farrar 1989).

T. Rustemeyer, P. Elsner, S.M. John & H.I. Maibach (eds.), *Kanerva's Occupational Dermatology*,
DOI 10.1007/978-3-642-02035-3_11,

Technological changes in industries that use animal products have probably resulted in reduced contact between *E rhusiopathiae* and humans (Reboli and Farrar 1989). Human-to-human infection has not been documented. Older studies showed that an average of 20–40% of healthy swine, and in some herds up to 98%, harbor *E rhusiopathiae* in the lymphoid tissue of the alimentary tract, particularly in the tonsils (Brooke and Riley 1999). Infections in man and animals appear to have a seasonal incidence with most cases occurring in the summer months (Brooke and Riley 1999). It is not clear if this is related to the biological activity of the temperature or to increased contact between people and sources of infections during these months.

Erysipeloid may present as a localized cutaneous form, a generalized cutaneous form with widespread erythematous-edematous lesions, fever, lymphadenitis, arthralgia and myalgia, and a rare septicemic form (Veraldi et al. 2009; Wang et al. 2010). Generalized skin infection and septicemia are seen sometimes in severe cases, e.g., immunosuppressed persons (Veraldi et al. 2009). Complications are encephalitis, meningitis, endocarditis, peritonitis, renal failure, and sepsis. Clinical symptoms are usually obvious about 2 days after inoculation. A hot, violaceous and tender erythema develops around the inoculation site and extends centrifugally but irregularly with a sharp and sometimes great border. This may also be vesicular. Erysipeloid is a true cellulitis. The lesions are most frequently located on the fingers, hands, and forearms (Veraldi et al. 2009; Wang et al. 2010). Fever and mild generous symptoms such as arthralgia are present in 10% of cases. Healing normally occurs spontaneously in 2 weeks with desquamation or suppuration. Diagnosis is mainly clinical. Isolation of *E rhusiopathiae* is difficult. Two PCR assays have been described for swine erysipelas, one of which can be used in cases of human erysipeloid (Veraldi et al. 2009; Wang et al. 2010).

Recommended treatment centers on antibiotics with, e.g., penicillins, cephalosporins, tetracyclines, and erythromycin. Prevention includes several measures such as sound husbandry, good sanitation, reduction of trauma, systematic slaughtering of infected animals, and wearing of protective gloves.

2 Query Fever

Query fever is a worldwide zoonosis caused by *Coxiella burnetii*, an obligate intracellular gram-negative bacterium (Angelakis and Raoult 2010). The time of incubation is 2–4 weeks. Farm animals and pets are the main reservoir of human infections. Query fever can be transmitted to humans by ticks, rodents, sheep, cattle, goats, and other wildlife animals. Persons at risk are farmers, veterinarians, abattoir workers, persons working with dairy products, and laboratory personnel. Infection occurs aerogenic by contaminated dust or by direct contact with animals including their excretions. Person-to-person transmission is rare, sexual transmission of Q fever in animals has been demonstrated (Angelakis and Raoult 2010). There are several studies in which young age seems to be protective against *Coxiella burnetii* (Angelakis and Raoult 2010). The prevalence of clinical cases increases with age. Men are symptomatic more often than women despite comparable exposure and seroprevalence (Angelakis and Raoult 2010).

Epidemiological studies indicate Q fever as a public health problem in many countries like, e.g., the United Kingdom, the Netherlands, Germany, France, and Canada (Angelakis and Raoult 2010; van der Hoek et al. 2010; Wallensten et al. 2010).

Query fever presents with high fever, headache, loss of weight, atypical pneumonia, and endocarditis. Granulomatous hepatitis, cardiac involvement, skin rash, and neurologic manifestation such as disorientation, encephalitis, meningoencephalitis, and peripheral neuropathy may occur as a complication. Up to 50% of infections are asymptomatic. Chronic Q fever infection may develop months to years after initial infection manifesting as bacterial culture-negative endocarditis (Angelakis and Raoult 2010). The diagnosis is made based on a significant increase in serum antibody titers.

Differential diagnosis includes all other causes of pneumonia. Therapy centers on antibiotics: doxycycline 100 mg twice daily for 2–3 weeks. In cases of endocarditis, doxycycline is combined with chinolon or rifampicin plus ciprofloxacin for up to several years (Angelakis and Raoult 2010). Query fever infections resolve in most cases. Lethality is 1–2%. Prevention includes protection measures such as dust masks, protective clothing, tick control strategies, good hygiene practice, and systematic slaughtering of infected animals.

3 Tinea Pedis

Tinea pedis is caused by dermatophytes and usually leads to an infection of the feet or toes. Three anthropophilic species, *Trichophyton rubrum*, *Trichophyton mentagrophytes*, and *Epidermophyton floccosum*, are responsible for the vast majority of cases. Tinea pedis is the most common form of dermatophytosis in most countries. It is estimated that about 10% of the total population are infected. The German "Foot Check Study" showed that the prevalence of tinea pedis and/or onychomycosis was 31.6% (Seebacher et al. 2008). Many patients are asymptomatic. Living in an institution, especially when washing facilities are shared, is likely to increase the chances of infection. Prevalences as high as 18% have been reported in some factories or sport institutes. However, tinea pedis may be equally well transmitted within the family bathroom. Reinfection from the environment is usual, with the same or another species or with combined species. Maceration of the toe clefts plays an important role. In adolescents and children, swimming pools are the major source of infection. Tinea pedis may more frequently occur in professions with wet environment and wearing of rubber boots. All professions demanding shoes that may occlude the skin are more frequently affected by tinea pedis. Occupational groups such as miners, soldiers, employees of meat and dairy product factories, fishermen, employees of chemistry works, forestry workers, farmers, zookeepers in aquariums, people working in swimming pools, and athletes are exposed to particularly high infection risk. The frequency of tinea pedis in these professions ranges from 13% to 73% (Seebacher at al. 2008).

The most common form of tinea pedis is located in the toe webs. The fourth interdigital web is preferentially infected, but the other webs can also be infected on one or both feet. The clinical symptoms are characterized by whitish, diffuse maceration in the cleft marginated by a collarette of continuous desquamation. In some cases, there is a small painful fissure running along the line of the cleft. The entire area is ulcerative and macerated from microbial superinfection. Itching is usually present. A squamous hyperkeratotic variety may occur in *Trichophyton rubrum* infections. This may occur chronically and partially resistant to treatment. Tinea pedis may also affect the soles, heels, and sides of the feet ("moccasin foot"). Associated onychomycosis is common. Tinea pedis is sometimes associated with plantar hyperhidrosis, plantar pompholyx, and vesicular eczema.

Diagnosis is made clinically and by fungal culture. Mild interdigital tinea pedis can be treated topically with broad-spectrum antifungals. Severe or refractory tinea pedis can be treated with oral antifungal, e.g., terbinafine 250 mg twice daily for 2 weeks, itraconazole 200 mg twice daily for 1 week. Prevention includes treatment of onychomycosis if present, treatment of associated diseases such as vesicular eczema and hyperhidrosis, adequate hygiene of the feet, and use of socks and shoes permeable to air.

4 Vitiligo-like Skin Diseases

Vitiligo-like skin lesions may occur in the rubber industry when thiols and quinones are used as additives. Chemical substances such as phenols and hydrochinon may also lead to vitiligo-like skin changes. Phenols in disinfectants may also cause pseudovitiligo or vitiligo-like skin lesions because they are more intensely released when used occlusively, e.g., by wearing protective gloves. Differential diagnosis includes vitiligo, hypopigmentation by systemic medications, e.g., chloroquine and leukoderma caused by skin diseases, e.g., psoriasis, eczema, and autoimmune disease such as systemic sclerosis.

There are no epidemiological data about the frequency of vitiligo-like skin lesions. This may be caused by the fact that affected persons have single skin lesions only and besides cosmetic impairment, they are usually not presented to a physician.

Vitiligo-like skin lesions often appear clinically different compared to vitiligo. They are frequently located symmetrically, e.g., on the underarms when caused by increased release of phenols by gloves' occlusion. Vitiligo-like skin lesions are usually not located in the typical body sites like the genital and anal area, face, and back of hands. They are usually located where skin contact to the releasing substance occurred.

Treatment comprises identifying the underlying etiology and prevention of skin contact with the causing agent. Repigmentation may occur spontaneously, local PUVA or other forms of UV phototherapy may help to repigmentate the affected skin site.

5 Psoriasis

Psoriasis is a chronic proliferative inflammatory skin disease. The severity of this disease ranges from mild focal enrollment to generalized forms. The clinical cause is unpredictable.

Psoriasis of the hands may present as keratotic patches on the palms, usually not displaying the classical features of psoriatic lesions elsewhere on the body. The presence of psoriatic lesions elsewhere, e.g., at elbows, knees, and scalp, often helps to establish the diagnosis. If these skin locations are not affected, diagnosis may be difficult. The most frequent differential diagnosis is hand eczema. It is often difficult to differentiate palmar psoriasis from chronic eczema. Skin biopsies often show nonspecific changes of eczema rather than that of psoriasis, and the histological findings often do not help to confirm a diagnosis.

In the work environment, skin trauma and mechanical affections of the hands are aggravating factors of psoriasis. No specific occupation predominates. Manufacturer and craftsmen are mainly affected. Pressure of hands in metal workers, bus drivers with the pressure of the steering wheel, health-care workers, and other professions with a high degree of mechanical trauma and pressure of the hands are some examples. Unilateral palmar lesions are usually located on the dominant hand. Patients with palmar lesions involved in regular manual work tend to show lesions restricted to areas exposed to pressure (Kumar et al. 2002).

It is estimated that occupational contact psoriasis probably accounts for 1.2% of all occupational dermatoses (Moroni et al. 1988). Other epidemiological data are not available. Palmar psoriasis is only noted as part of larger studies on psoriasis or palmoplantar psoriasis (Kumar et al. 2002).

Diagnosis can be obtained by clinically demonstrable psoriasis localized on the hands, mainly palms without significant involvement elsewhere, or psoriasis affecting other sites of the body except the hands with further development of lesions on the hands after engaging in a particular job.

Therapy of psoriasis of the hands can be a challenge. Local PUVA therapy is very helpful as well as topical antipsoriatics such as calcipotriol. Depending on the clinical picture, keratolytic topicals such as salicylic acid may be necessary. Prevention comprises mainly the identification of individuals with a propensity to develop occupational contact psoriasis during the cause of work. This can be reached by preemployment evaluation including psoriasis and clinical examination of the skin with specific emphasis on scalp, elbows, knees, pitting of the nails, hyperkeratoses of the palms in winter time, hyperkeratoses with persistent fissures on heel and dry perionychium and eponychium with rhagades.

6 Borreliosis

Borreliosis is the most common tick-transmitted disease in the Northern hemisphere caused by spirochaetes of the *Borrelia burgdorferi* species (Stanek and Strle 2003). The skin is the most frequently affected organ, mostly as erythema migrans and also as borrelial lymphocytoma, both occurring days to weeks after the infectious tick bite and acrodermatitis chronica atrophicans occurring months to years later. Influenza-like or unspecific symptoms such as, for instance, malaise, fatigue, fever, headache, myalgia, and arthralgia may occur.

A Swedish study found that there is a 4% risk of being tick-bitten per 10 h spent outdoors and the risk of contracting borreliosis was 1/221 tick bites (Stjernberg and Berglund 2002). In Germany, the state of Baden-Wuerttemberg was tested for antibodies against *Borrelia burgdorferi sensu lato* revealing human seroprevalence rates in forestry workers ranging from 18% to 52% depending on the county of the state (Oehme et al. 2002). Own data showed that children in forest kindergarten have a 2.8 higher risk for getting at least one tick bite and 4.6 higher risk for coming down with borreliosis compared to children in conventional kindergarten. Attending and working in a forest kindergarten is a risk factor for acquiring tick bites and for suffering from borreliosis (Weisshaar et al. 2006). Professions at risk are outdoor workers like, e.g., forest workers, gardeners, farmers, and nursery nurses working in so-called forest kindergartens (Weisshaar et al. 2006).

Diagnosis is made by the clinical findings, a history of tick bites (up to 50% of patients do not remember the tick bite), and laboratory test (ELISA and Western immunoblot assay for IGM and IgG). Doxycycline is generally considered as first-line therapy using 200 mg daily for 14–21 days. Advanced disease needs intravenous ceftriaxone 2 g daily for 3–4 weeks. Prevention is very important including behavioral prevention such as wearing appropriate clothes (long-sleeved, white or light color), use of insect repellents, and careful (self) skin inspection for ticks (Hayes and Piesman 2003). Educational prevention comprises disseminating information via different media such as TV, newspapers, and magazines, providing advice, changing attitudes and behavior including practical approaches, e.g., prompt removal of the tick in case of tick bites. A population-based, randomized study showed that an educational intervention can increase the proportion of people who check themselves and use repellents (Malouin et al. 2003). Prevention of tick bites and borreliosis comprises a combination of primary prevention, early diagnosis, and treatment.

References

Angelakis E, Raoult D (2010) Q fever. Vet Microbiol 140:297–309

Brooke CJ, Riley TV (1999) Erysipelothrix rhusiopathiae: bacteriology, epdidemiology and clinical manifestation of an occupational pathogen. J Med Microbiol 48:789–799

Hayes EB, Piesman J (2003) How can we prevent lyme disease? N Engl J Med 348:2424–2430

Kumar B, Saraswat A, Kaur I (2002) Palmoplantar lesions in psoriasis: a study of 3065 patients. Acta Derm Venereol 82:192–195

Malouin R, Winch P, Leontsini E, Glass G, Simon D, Hayses EB, Schwartz BS (2003) Longitudinal evaluation of an educational intervention for preventing tick bites in an area with endemic lyme disease in Baltimore County, Maryland. Am J Epidemiol 157:1039–1051

Moroni P, Cazzaniga R, Pierini F, Panella V, Zerboni R (1988) Occupational contact psoriasis. Dermatosen 36:163–164

Oehme R, Hartelt K, Backe H, Brockmann S, Kimmig P (2002) Foci of tick-borne disease in Southwest Germany. Int J Med Microbiol 291(suppl 33):22–29

Reboli AC, Farrar WE (1989) Erysipelothrix rhusiopathiae: an occupational pathogen. Clin Microbiol Rev 2:354–359

Seebacher C, Bouchara JP, Mignon B (2008) Updates on the epidemiology of dermatophyte infections. Mycopathologica 166:335–352

Stanek G, Strle F (2003) Lyme borreliosis. Lancet 362:1639–1647

Stjernberg L, Berglund J (2002) Risk of acquiring tick bites in Southeastern Sweden. Scand J Infect Dis 34:840–844

van der Hoek W, Dijkstra F, Schimmer B, Schneeberger PM, Vellema P, Wijkmans C, Scheggert R, Hackert V, van Duynhoven Y (2010) Q fever in the Netherlands: an update on the epidemiology and control measures. Euro Surveill 15(12):pii = 19520

Veraldi S, Girgenti V, Dassoni F, Gianotti R (2009) Erysipeloid. A review. Clin Experimental Dermatol 34:859–62

Wallensten A, Morre P, Webster H, Johnsons C, van der Burgt G, Pritchard G, Oliver I (2010) Q fever outbreak in Cheltenham, United Kingdom, in 2007 and the use of dispersion modelling to investigate the possibility of airborne spread. Euro Surveill 15(12):pii = 19521

Wang Q, Chang BJ, Riley TV (2010) Erysipelothrix rhusiopathiae. Veterinary Microbiology 140:405–17

Weisshaar E, Schäfer A, Scheidt RW, Bruckner T, Apfelbacher CJ, Diepgen TL (2006) Epidemiology of tick bites abd borreliosis in children attending kindergarten or so-called "forest kindergarten" in Southwest Germany. J Invest Dermatol 126:584–590

Section 2

Occupational Skin Diseases: Clinical

12 Contact Dermatitis Due to Irritation

Dimitar Antonov · Sibylle Schliemann · Peter Elsner
Department of Dermatology, University Hospital Jena, Jena, Germany

Core Messages

- Irritant contact dermatitis (ICD) denotes inflammation of the skin which results from a contact with external agent and does not require prior sensitization of the immune system.
- Irritant contact dermatitis is the most frequent cause for occupational contact dermatitis.
- The clinical features are quite diverse and there are ten clinical types described: acute; acute delayed; irritant reaction; cumulative; traumiterative; exsiccation eczematid; traumatic; pustular and acneiform; nonerythematous; subjective.
- Distinction from allergic contact dermatitis (ACD) usually relies on time course (quicker onset in irritation), subjective symptoms (itch in ACD vs burning or pain in ICD), and morphology (spread outside the contact area, more infiltration and vesiculation in ACD). However, distinction may be clinically very difficult or impossible; histology, pathogenesis, and therapy are also very similar.
- Atopic skin predisposition is the best established risk factor for irritant contact dermatitis; respiratory manifestations of atopy are less predictive than skin manifestations.
- Prevention, early recognition, and therapy are decisive in averting chronic and persistent forms.

1 Introduction

Irritant contact dermatitis (ICD), defined as inflammation of the skin resulting from exposure to an exogenous agent (Chew and Maibach 2006) which does not require prior sensitization of the immune system, is a leading cause of occupational disease in dermatology and causes economic damage to workers, companies, and social security systems worldwide. The perception of ICD as more trivial than the more intellectually appealing problem of allergic sensitization has changed dramatically. In Germany, skin diseases are the second most frequent occupational disease following musculoskeletal disorders. Occupational skin disease is usually among the top five occupational diseases in many countries (Keegel et al. 2009). Most occupational dermatoses are cases of contact dermatitis. Of the two varieties of contact dermatitis, irritant and allergic, a higher prevalence of ICD is predominantly reported; only in few sources a higher frequency of ACD is to be found (Keegel et al. 2009). Epidemiologic studies on hand eczema from various countries show that irritation is the most frequent cause and in many further cases is a contributing factor to allergy or atopy (Lofgren and Warshaw 2006; Thyssen et al. 2010a).

In contrast to ACD, ICD is defined as being the result of a primarily unspecific damage to the skin, i.e., it does not require prior sensitization of the immune system. ICD is not a clinical entity, but rather a spectrum of diseases. The clinical aspect of ICD is determined by the dose–effect relationship (Patil and Maibach 1994). The morphology of acute ICD shows erythema; edema; vesicles that may coalesce, bullae, and ooze (➋ *Figs. 12.1, 12.2*). Necrosis and ulceration are seen with corrosive materials (➋ *Fig. 12.3*). The clinical features of chronic ICD include redness, lichenification, excoriations, scaling, and hyperkeratosis (➋ *Figs. 12.4, 12.5*). Any skin site may be affected. However, most frequently affected by ICD are the hands, as they are the human "tools" that interact with the environment most and have intensive contact to irritants. Spilling of fluids may irritate the forearms or other body sites, especially when fluids soak through work clothes.

2 Clinical Types of Irritant Contact Dermatitis

Irritants produce a wide range of clinical features. Cutaneous responses depend on the type of irritant (detergent, acid, alkali, oil, organic solvent, oxidant, reducing agent, water – ➋ *Table 12.1*), the concentration at which the irritant comes into contact with the skin, the type of exposure, and the individual response. Clinical manifestations of the ICD syndromes are also modified by external factors such as environmental factors (mechanical pressure, temperature, and humidity (Fluhr et al. 2005)) and predisposing characteristics of the individual (age, sex, ethnic origin, preexisting skin disease, atopic skin diathesis, and anatomic region exposed) (Pinnagoda et al. 1989; Wilkinson and Willis 1998).

T. Rustemeyer, P. Elsner, S.M. John & H.I. Maibach (eds.), *Kanerva's Occupational Dermatology*,
DOI 10.1007/978-3-642-02035-3_12,

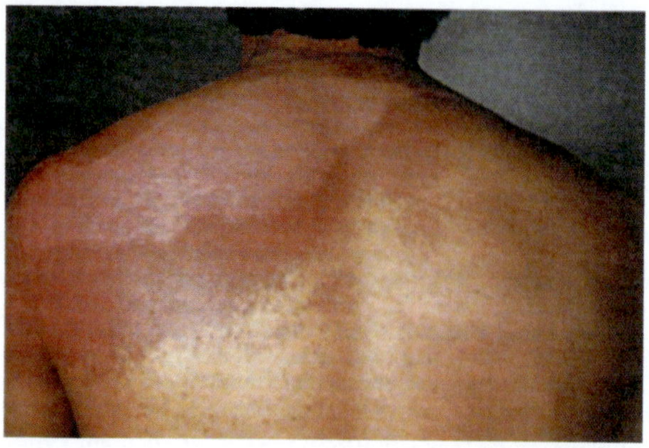

■ **Fig. 12.1**
Chemical burn caused by tear gas in a policeman

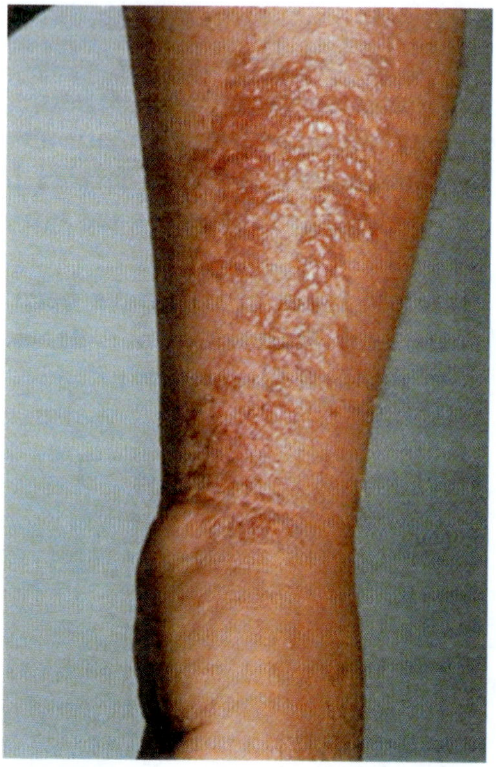

■ **Fig. 12.2**
Jellyfish reaction in a lifeguard

For example, elderly people are not only affected more often by contact dermatitis because of their reduced epidermal barrier, they also show more severe symptoms (Patil and Maibach 1994; Ghadially et al. 1995). Environmental influences, such as cold and low ambient humidity, are important factors decreasing the water content of the stratum corneum (Mozzanica 1992). Cold alone can also reduce the plasticity of the horny layer and lead to cracking. Occlusion increases the water content of the stratum corneum with consequent enhanced percutaneous absorption of water soluble substances. A list of the factors which influence the irritant potential of the irritants is presented in ❯ *Table 12.2.*

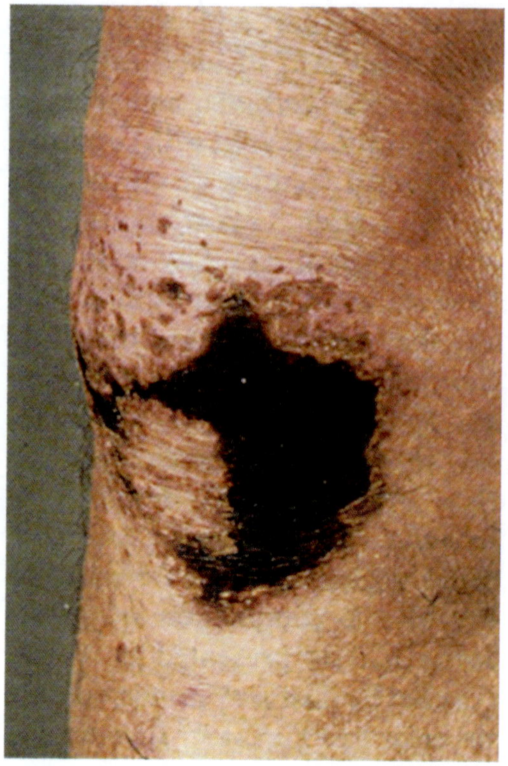

■ **Fig. 12.3**
Caustic reaction caused by cement

Several different types of ICD have been described (❯ *Table 12.3*).

2.1 Acute ICD

Acute ICD develops when the skin is exposed to a strong irritant or caustic chemical. Usually this happens as an accident at work or in special emergency situations. The irritant reaction reaches its peak quickly, and then starts to heal; this is called the decrescendo phenomenon. Because the lag time is short (usually minutes to hours after exposure) and the association between exposure and skin symptoms is usually clear, the diagnosis is easy in most cases. It may become difficult when the patient was

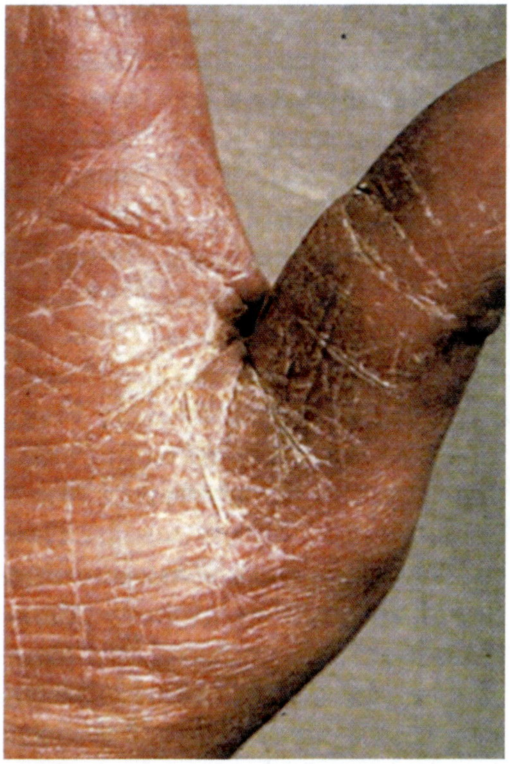

Fig. 12.4
Housewives'eczema due to chronic wet work

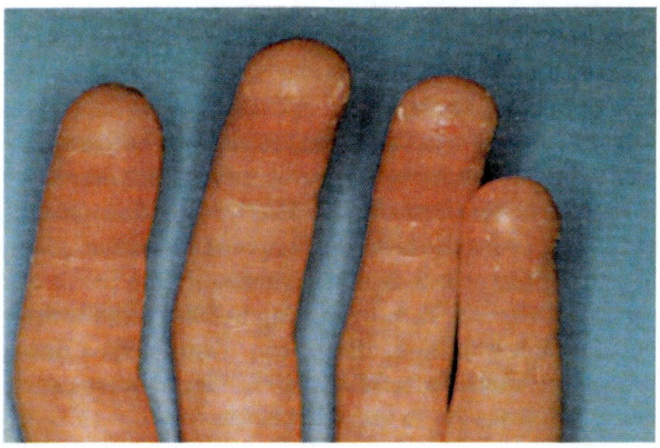

Fig. 12.5
Fingertip eczema due to physical trauma in a cellist

unaware of an exposure. Acute ACD has to be considered as differential diagnosis, which is caused by a delayed sensitization reaction, and requires 24–48 h after allergen contact for symptoms to appear; this type of contact dermatitis is characterized by the crescendo phenomenon (i.e., a transient increase of signs and symptoms despite removal of the allergen). The clinical appearance of acute ICD is highly variable, and it may even be indistinguishable from the allergic type. There are numerous reports in the literature of even experienced dermatologists being misled into an initial assumption of ACD which later, after a careful workup, turned out to be "only irritation" (Frosch and John 2011). Furthermore, the combination of allergic and irritant dermatitis is frequent, e.g., "black-spot poison ivy dermatitis" (Hurwitz et al. 1984), as an acute ICD superimposed upon an ACD.

Table 12.1
Common irritants and their modes of action (Elsner 1994)

Substances	Mechanisms of toxicity
Detergents	Solubilization and/or disorganization of the barrier lipids and the natural moisturizing factor in the stratum corneum (SC); protein denaturation; membrane toxicity
Acids	Protein denaturation, cytotoxicity
Alkali	Barrier-lipid denaturation, cytotoxicity through cell swelling
Oils	Disorganization of barrier lipids
Organic solvents	Solubilization of barrier lipids; membrane toxicity; retrograde inflammation through release of mediators from the dermis
Oxidants	Cytotoxicity
Reducing agents	Keratolysis
Water	If barrier is disrupted, cytotoxicity through swelling of viable epidermal cells

Symptoms of acute irritant dermatitis are burning, stinging, and soreness of the skin. Signs are erythema, edema, bullae, and possibly necrosis. These lesions are restricted to the area where the irritant or toxicant damaged the tissue. Borders are mostly sharply demarcated, and the asymmetrical pattern of the lesions hints at an exogenous cause (*Figs. 12.1*, *12.2*, *12.3*). The prognosis of this type is good (Elsner 1994). The most frequent potent irritants leading to acute ICD are acids and alkaline solutions (Eichmann and Amgwerd 1992). A typical accident situation is chemical burning in construction workers (Skogstad and Levy 1994) when alkaline concrete fluid soaks through garments or spills into work boots.

Chemical burns by fluoric acid are the most dangerous of all injuries caused by acids, and need special treatment. But even substances thought to be less toxic, such as N-methyl-2-pyrrolidone, may cause acute ICD (Malten et al. 1979).

Table 12.2
Factors influencing the irritancy potential (Wilkinson and Willis 1998)

Exogenous	Endogenous	Cofactors
Chemical characteristics Molecular structure pH pKa Hydrophobicity (log of the partition coefficient) Inherent toxicity Concentration/dose Penetration characteristics Vehicle Solubility Duration of contact Type of contact	Individual susceptibility Atopy Race/skin color/phototype Age Hormonal Barrier function Repair capacity Eczema elsewhere Other skin disease Other unknown Cite of exposure	Mechanical Thermal Climatic

Table 12.3
Subtypes of ICD and their prognosis (based on Chew and Maibach 2006; Frosch and John 2006)

Types of ICD	Prognosis
Acute	Good
Acute delayed	Good
Irritant reaction	Good
Cumulative	Variable
Traumiterative	Variable
Exsiccation eczematid	Variable
Traumatic	Variable
Pustular and acneiform	Variable
Nonerythematous	Variable
Subjective	Excellent

2.2 Acute Delayed ICD

Acute delayed ICD is characteristic for certain irritants, such as benzalkonium chloride, anthralin, calcipotriol, tretinoin, and others (Table 12.4) that elicit a retarded inflammatory response. Delayed irritation may be more common than generally thought. Clinically, acute delayed ICD resembles acute ICD. The visible inflammation is not seen until 8–24 h or more after

Table 12.4
Chemicals inducing delayed acute irritation (Lammintausta and Maibach 1990)

Anthralin
Calcipotriol
Benzalkonium chloride
Tretinoin
Bis(2-chloroethyl)sulfide
Hexanediol and butanediol diacrylates
Dichloro(2-chlorovynil)arsene
Epichlorhydrin
Ethylene oxide
Hydrofluoric acid
Hydroxypropylacrylate
Podophylline
Propane sulfone

exposure (Malten et al. 1979). Irritant patch-test reactions to benzalkonium chloride may be papular and increase in intensity with time, thus imitating ACD and the crescendo phenomenon. On the normal skin surrounding psoriatic plaques, dithranol causes redness and edema, which may become very severe on the legs because of venous stasis. Irritation due to tretinoin develops after a few days, and is characterized by mild to fiery redness followed by desquamation or large flakes of stratum corneum. The symptoms are burning rather than itching which is a helpful indicator to distinguish from ACD. The skin becomes sensitive to touch and to water (Frosch and John 2006). Patch testing helps differentiate acute delayed ICD from ACD (Chew and Maibach 2006).

2.3 Irritant Reaction ICD

Irritant reaction ICD is a type of subclinical irritant dermatitis in individuals exposed to wet work, such as hairdressers or metal workers, in their first months of training. This diagnosis is made if the clinical picture is monomorphic rather than polymorphic, and characterized by the predominance of one of the following signs: scaling, redness, vesicles, pustules, and erosions (Frosch and John 2011).

On the hands it often begins under rings and then may spread over the fingers to the hands and the forearms. It usually affects the dorsum of the hands and fingers, but irritants can also cause eczema of the palmar sides of the fingers and the hands.

This distribution occurs in caters and, described as dyshidrotic eczema, it has been reported in metal workers with an ICD from cooling lubricants (Cronin 1995). Frequently, this condition heals spontaneously, resulting in hardening of the skin; sometimes it progresses to cumulative irritant dermatitis.

2.4 Cumulative (Chronic) ICD

According to Malten (➋ *Fig. 12.6*) cumulative ICD is a consequence of multiple subthreshold damages to the skin if the time between the insults is too short for complete restoration of skin barrier function (Malten 1981). It may be the result of too frequent repetition of one impairing factor (see ➋ traumiterative ICD), but is more commonly the result of a variety of stimuli, each beginning to be active before recovery from the foregoing stimuli has been completed. Clinical symptoms will develop only when the damage exceeds a certain "manifestation threshold," which is individually determined. The development of visible changes in irritant dermatitis has also been compared to being only the "tip of the iceberg" of functional derangement (Freeman and Maibach 1988). Persons with sensitive skin are characterized by a decreased threshold or an increased restoration time leading to earlier development of clinical irritant dermatitis. The "manifestation threshold" is not a fixed value for an individual, but it may decrease with the disease. This explains why in patients with cumulative ICD even a limited irritant exposure may perpetuate the condition. Cumulative ICD is linked to exposure to weak irritants, rather than potent irritants. It develops slowly, after repeated subthreshold irritations over a period ranging from days to weeks or even years (Chew and Maibach 2006). Very often, this exposure occurs not only at work but also in private life. Because the link between exposure and disease is often not obvious to the patient, diagnosis may be delayed considerably. This is one of the reasons for the rather doubtful prognosis of this disease (Belsito 2005).

Cumulative and chronic ICD are synonymous, because the same phenomenon is deemed to take place in chronic ICD, i.e., new insults occur before the restoration of the skin is completed. Such insults may occur not only through the exposure to irritants which can cause acute ICD by themselves. Repeated exposure to many weak irritants, which would otherwise be well tolerated by a healthy skin, could prolong the condition into chronic ICD. For the diagnosis of chronic ICD to be made, the disease duration should exceed the proposed arbitrary limit of 6 weeks (Chew and Maibach 2006). Symptoms of chronic irritant dermatitis are itching and pain due to cracking of the hyperkeratotic skin. Signs include dryness, erythema, and vesicles, but mainly lichenification, hyperkeratosis, and chapping. In contrast to acute irritant dermatitis, the lesions are less sharply demarcated. Xerotic dermatitis is the most frequent type of cumulative toxic dermatitis (Eichmann and Amgwerd 1992).

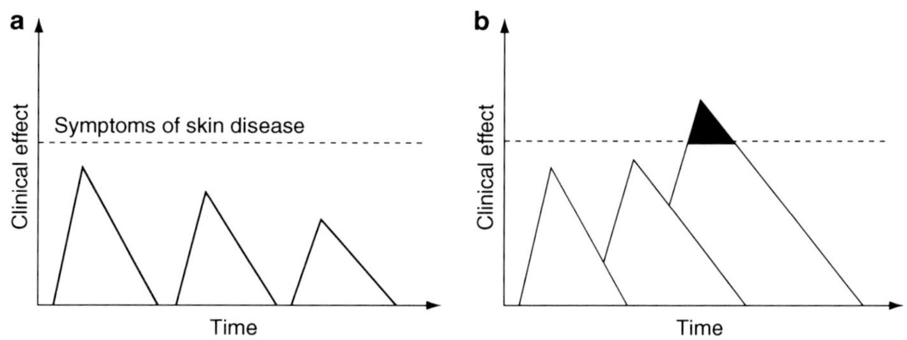

Fig. 12.6
Model of the pathogenesis of chronic irritant contact dermatitis, according to Malten. (a) subliminal irritants do not lead to clinical irritant dermatitis if exposures are far enough apart for restoration of skin barrier function. (b) When the same irritants follow each other closely or when the manifestation threshold is reduced, irritant dermatitis develops (based on Malten 1981)

2.5 Traumiterative ICD

In contrast to cumulative ICD resulting from a too early repetition of exposures differing in type, traumiterative ICD is a result of too early repetition of just one type of load (Malten and den Arend 1985). Nevertheless, these two types are very similar clinically and are often combined in one group.

2.6 Exsiccation Eczematid

Other terms frequently used for this condition are asteatotic eczema and eczema cracquelé (Chew and Maibach 2006; Thong and Maibach 2008). Exsiccation eczematid is a special variant of ICD that is seen mainly in elderly individuals with a history of frequent showering and bathing without remoisturizing their skin. Patients suffer from intensive itching and sensation of "skin tightness," and their skin appears dry, cracked, and with ichthyosiform scaling. Mostly the legs, the backs of the hands, and the arms are affected. The condition mainly occurs during the winter months, when humidity is low.

2.7 Traumatic ICD

Traumatic ICD may develop after acute skin trauma, such as burns, lacerations, and acute ICD. Patients should also be asked whether they have cleansed the skin with strong soaps or detergents. The syndrome is characterized by delayed healing and eczematous lesions, such as erythema, papules, vesicles, and scaling (Chew and Maibach 2006). This eczematous condition persists for a considerable time period, with a minimum of 6 weeks (Frosch 1995). In the later stages it may resemble nummular dermatitis (Chew and Maibach 2006).

The most common location is the hands. In a fully developed case, redness, infiltration, and scaling with fissuring are seen all over the affected areas.

2.8 Pustular and Acneiform ICD

Pustular and acneiform ICD is a result of exposure to certain irritants, such as croton oil, mineral oils, tars, greases, naphthalenes, chlorinated aromatic hydrocarbons ("chlor acne"), fluorinated compounds (Steciuk et al. 1997), and others. This syndrome must always be considered in conditions in which acneiform lesions develop outside the typical acne age. Those most affected are patients with seborrhoea, macroporous skin conditions, and prior acne vulgaris, as well as atopics. The pustules are sterile and transient, however, subcorneal pustular eruption may also be a manifestation of allergy (ACD). An example is the allergy to trichlorethylene, which has to be considered as a differential diagnosis in patients with appropriate history (Goh 1995).

Pustular and vesicular reactions are typical for the acute irritant dermatitis caused by the contact with the hemolymph of crushed bodies or sometimes with the whole bodies of certain bugs. While in Paederus dermatitis, the subtype caused by the bugs from the Paederus family, the lesions are inflamed, linear "whiplash-" or burn-shaped, the lesions induced by the vesiculant from other insects, cantheridin, are vesicles and bullae on uninflamed skin (Zargari et al. 2003). Outbreaks in factories or deployed military personnel are reported (Dursteler and Nyquist 2004; Huang et al. 2009).

2.9 Nonerythematous ICD

Nonerythematous ICD may be defined as a subclinical form of ICD with early stages of skin irritation characterized only by changes in the stratum corneum barrier function (detectable by bioengineering methods) without a clinical correlate, i.e., not exceeding the "manifestation threshold" or not reaching the "tip of the iceberg," as discussed in the ➋ Cummulative ICD section (van der Valk et al. 1985; Berardesca and Maibach 1988; Lammintausta et al. 1988).

2.10 Subjective ICD

Subjective or sensory ICD is characterized by the lack of clinical signs, but individuals complain of a subjective sensation of stinging, burning, smarting, or even pain after contact with certain chemicals, such as lactic acid, which is also a model irritant for this type of invisible cutaneous irritation. This reaction may be reliably reproduced in a double-blinded exposure test. The property of the chemical agents to elicit such sensations depends on their concentration and vehicle. Neural pathways are considered to be responsible (Lee et al. 2009). Frosch (Frosch and John 2011) distinguishes between immediate-type stinging, caused by chemicals such as chloroform and methanol (1:1) or 95% ethanol, and delayed-type stinging. The delayed type is mostly caused by sunscreen agents, insect repellants and several dermatological therapeutic agents and vehicles that are used in cosmetics and topical medicaments (Frosch and John 2011; Frosch and Kligman 1977). With some irritants, for example, chloroform and methanol (1:1) or some caustic chemicals, the sensations of burning, stinging, etc., can be viewed as an early warning signal and an initial phase of irritation, because the continued exposure would invariably produce damaging effects (Frosch and John 2011). Substances which produce non-immunologic contact urticaria, like cinnamic aldehyde, also produce only sensorial irritation, when applied at concentrations too low to induce a detectable reaction. The sensory irritant properties do not correspond with the actual corrosive or irritant characteristics. For example, undiluted kerosene and others may induce severe irritation without any accompanying sensation (Frosch and John 2011).

2.11 Other Forms of ICD

Airborne ICD is not separated as a distinct type, because it develops through similar mechanisms as the other types listed above. What sets it apart is the fact that the irritants are dispersed and carried by the air before they come into contact with uncovered skin (Chew and Maibach 2006). Mainly sensitive exposed skin is affected, such as the face and especially the periorbital region (Dooms-Goossens et al. 1986; Patiwael et al. 2005; Lachapelle 2006). Which areas are affected and the morphology of the lesions are related to the physical form of the irritant: dust or fibers, where a mechanical friction is important, or sprays, vapors and gases (Lachapelle 2006). Most reports concern occupational exposure (Santos and Goossens 2007). Airborne ICD caused by industrial dust adhered to the clothing may mimic textile dermatitis, with lesions most prominent in sites with close skin–garment contact, such as the axilla, the gluteal region, or the thighs (Hafner et al. 1995). More detailed information is given in ➋ Chap. 17, "Airborne Contact Dermatitis" of this book.

The aspects of pigmented contact dermatitis are reviewed in ➋ Chap. 27, "Pigment Disorders". Pigmentary changes may arise on the sites of irritation dermatitis as a postinflammatory hyperpigmentation. Melanodermatitis toxica is viewed to be a phototoxic dermatitis due to tars, pitch, or oil products. The phototoxic reactions are reviewed in ➋ Chap. 15, "Phototoxic Dermatitis". Other less common related conditions, in the sense that they are caused by contact with external substances and irritants, but have a morphology other than eczema/dermatitis, are also the subject of separate chapters in this book – granulomatous reactions (➋ Chap. 28, "Noneczematous Occupational Contact Reactions") and non-immunologic contact urticaria (➋ Chap. 21, "Frictional Trauma/ Mechanic Skin Diseases").

3 Irritation or Allergy?

The distinction between irritant and allergic contact dermatitis has become increasingly blurred. Despite their different pathogenesis, ACD and ICD, especially of the chronic type, show a remarkable similarity with respect to clinical appearance, histology, and immunohistology. It is apparent that some of the same inflammatory immune mechanisms are important both in ACD and ICD (Brasch et al. 1992; Dika et al. 2004). The epidermal and dermal cell activity that produces the cascade of inflammation appears to be similar and applicable to both irritants and allergens. However, although inflammatory and immunological mediators may be activated, in contrast to ACD no memory T-cell function is involved. Many comparative studies suggest these two entities are more alike than they are not (Dika et al. 2004). Histologically, irritant contact dermatitis reactions show much greater pleomorphism than those elicited by allergens. Various alterations of epidermal cells can be observed according to the nature and concentration of the irritant applied, the type and duration of exposure, and the individual reactivity of the skin. Frequently, even therapy is similar. Additionally, the concept that irritants are thought to cause symptoms and signs within minutes to hours whereas allergens take days has been disqualified for one of the most widely studied irritants. Occlusion of sodium lauryl sulfate (SLS) for 24 h resulted in clearly more signs of inflammation at 48 h, a time course more characteristic of allergic reactions (Rietschel 1997; Dika et al. 2004).

4 Pathogenesis

The various irritants may cause damage through different mechanisms, which depend on the nature and the dose of the irritant (Elsner 1994; Fluhr et al. 2008). Some may, for example, disrupt the organization of the lipids in SC, swell or denaturate proteins, cause damage to the keratinocytes or penetrate and reach the dermis and release inflammatory mediators there (➋ *Table 12.1*). Whatever their exact mechanisms may be, they elicit irritation either by disrupting the epidermal barrier, by causing an epidermal cellular damage, or a combination of both (Berardesca and Distante 1994; Welss et al. 2004). Inflammatory response follows through the secretion of cytokines and chemokines by the keratinocytes. There are identical stages in this process among various irritants and allergens (Hoefakker et al. 1995; Dika et al. 2004; Spiekstra et al. 2005).

The cytokine IL-1α is available as a preformed pool in the keratinocytes and is quickly secreted upon keratinocyte damage or activation (Kupper 1990; Wood et al. 1996). The release of IL-1α has been called the "main switch" in the activation of the inflammatory cascade in the skin (Welss et al. 2004), but there is evidence that it is not the only primary inflammatory mediator (Corsini and Galli 2000). TNFα is another early cytokine, which is not shown to be readily stored in the keratinocytes, but is secreted by them upon activation. IL-1α, IL-1β, and TNFα are considered "primary" cytokines, as they can trigger inflammation independently, without additional stimuli (Kupper 1990; Welss et al. 2004). The release of IL1α and TNFα can be viewed as a primary general "alarm signal" which is a common phase in the response to various stimuli, including irritants and allergens (Spiekstra et al. 2005). The secretion of other cytokines follows, such as IL-6, IL-8, GM-SCF, and other cyto- and chemokines which recruit inflammatory cells to the injured skin (Corsini and Galli 2000). Such cytokines are considered "secondary," because although they modulate the inflammation, they could not trigger it alone (Kupper 1990; Corsini and Galli 2000). Other pathways are also shown to be activated, for example, the arachidonic acid cascade in experimental models with surfactants (Welss et al. 2004) and other irritants (Thong and Maibach 2008).

The irritation causes the keratinocytes to secrete anti-inflammatory and modulatory cytokines as well, like IL-1 receptor antagonist (ILRA) and IL-10 (de Jongh et al. 2006, 2007). The main function of the ILRA is to balance the inflammatory properties of IL-1 (Arend and Guthridge 2000). The ILRA to IL-1α ratio is what directs the inflammatory response (de Jongh et al. 2007). This ratio is decreased after a single irritation with sodium lauryl sulfate (SLS) and is increased after repeated SLS applications which model the cumulative ICD (de Jongh et al. 2006, 2007). The studies on cutaneous cytokines show dissimilar cytokine levels in the acute versus cumulative irritation with SLS, implying different pathogenesis of the acute and cumulative ICD (de Jongh et al. 2006, 2007). These studies also reveal great interpersonal variability in the cytokine responses to the standardized single and repetitive irritation with SLS, as well as variability in the baseline cytokine levels (de Jongh et al. 2006). It has been suggested that the uneven personal susceptibility to acute and chronic irritation might be due to different levels of certain cytokines in the skin (de Jongh et al. 2006). Correlation between higher baseline ILRA and IL-8 levels and stronger irritation responses to SLS has been reported (de Jongh et al. 2006). An association is reported between genetic polymorphisms in the TNFα and IL-1α genes and the susceptibility to chronic hand eczema (de Jongh et al. 2008a). These findings may have implications for identifying individuals with a higher risk of developing chronic dermatitis (de Jongh et al. 2008a).

The differences in the irritation responses, evoked by the diverse irritants, are thought to be due to the varying properties of these irritants to activate inflammatory and cytokine pathways (Corsini and Galli 2000). For example, benzalkonium chloride does not induce a detectable production of TNFα at a concentration which induces skin irritation, unlike other irritants (Holliday et al. 1997; Corsini and Galli 2000; Thong and Maibach 2008). Another example is the difference in the epidermal cytokines, induced in the initial steps of irritation with SLS compared to nonanoic acid (NAA) (Grangsjo et al. 1996). When these model irritants were applied at concentrations which cause a similar cellular injury at 24 h, NAA provoked a more consistent expression of IL-6 mRNA, while only SLS led to a GM-CSF mRNA expression (Grangsjo et al. 1996). The same irritants were also compared in a recent study using gene expression analysis with microarray chips at early and late time-points (Clemmensen et al. 2010). This technology allowed the comparison of the expression of 47,000 transcripts between the two irritants and to discern the common and the distinct pathways activated at early (acute irritation) and late stages and after cumulative irritation. A complex picture was revealed where most of the early activated genes are quickly turned off. The two irritants exhibited very different expression profiles while at the same time commonly expressed transcripts were identified which could be potential biomarkers for cumulative skin irritation (Clemmensen et al. 2010). Besides elucidating the pathways involved in the pathogenesis of the irritation, this technology may have diagnostic uses. Discrimination between irritant or allergic dermatitis and even the identification of the causative irritants could be possible, if their specific transcription profiles are known (Wong et al. 2004). RNA could be sampled for this purpose with minimally invasive tape-stripping procedures (Wong et al. 2004). The expression patterns after irritation with other irritants have also been investigated on various models, such as on rats, cultured human keratinocytes, human skin equivalents, and human volunteers (Fletcher et al. 2001; Rogers et al. 2003; Borlon et al. 2007; McDougal et al. 2007; Clemmensen et al. 2010).

The cytokines secreted during irritation not only orchestrate the inflammation response, they also trigger the keratinocyte proliferation and the lipid synthesis and secretion, needed for the epidermal barrier restoration (Feingold et al. 2007). Such function is demonstrated for IL-1, TNFα, and IL-6 in mice experiments (Proksch et al. 2008). It is therefore considered that the chronic increase in these cytokines could be responsible for the hyperproliferation of the epidermis seen in chronic dermatitis (Proksch et al. 2008). Additional mechanisms, activated when the stratum corneum barrier is disrupted and/or the epidermis is damaged, include the changes in the gradients of the calcium and other ions, the change in the pH gradient, the serine protease/proteinase-activated receptor-2 (PAR-2) pathway and the nitric oxide (NO) pathway (Feingold et al. 2007). While some of these accelerate the barrier repair, like the cytokines and the ion gradients, others downregulate it (PAR-2 and NO pathways). The function of the interrelated positive and negative signals is considered to finely tune the barrier homeostasis (Feingold et al. 2007).

5 Epidemiology

While population-based epidemiological studies on the frequency of ICD are rare, there is agreement that irritant dermatitis is more frequent than ACD, although ACD tends to have more severe consequences for the patient. Coenraads and Smit reviewed international prevalence studies for eczema due to all causes conducted with general populations in five countries (England, The Netherlands, Norway, Sweden, United States). They showed point prevalence rates of 1.7–6.3%, and 1- to 3-year-period prevalence rates of 6.2–10.6% (Coenraads and Smit 1995).

Contact Dermatitis (all types) represents 90–95% of all cases with occupational skin disease in the Western countries (Keegel et al. 2009). The hands are usually involved (Dickel et al. 2001), but in studies on hand eczema which are population-based, the effects of the occupation may be diluted within the other types of eczema and therefore, less evident (Thyssen et al. 2010a). A recent review found that the rates of ICD are higher than ACD in most studies on occupational contact dermatitis (OCD) (Keegel et al. 2009). The reviewed epidemiology data were strongly influenced by the method of information gathering in each country, reporting systems, definitions and degrees of industrialization (Keegel et al. 2009). The general opinion is that many cases of OCD remain undetected, undiagnosed, or unreported. The incidence of reported OCD is similar in countries with a compulsory reporting systems and comparable rates of industrialization, such as Germany, Denmark, and Finland and is in the range of 5–8 cases per 10,000 workers per year (Keegel et al. 2009). The voluntary systems of reporting, like the EPIDERM in the UK and a similar one in the Netherlands, rely on the voluntary submission of data from various physicians – dermatologist, general practitioners, and occupational physicians. Their estimated incidence rates per 10,000 workers are more variable – 15 in the Netherlands, 1.3 in the UK, and 2.2 in Australia. Studies based on self-reporting (mailed questionnaires or interviews) have the highest rates of OCD (Keegel et al. 2009). The National Health Interview Survey in the USA which included randomly selected households, estimated a 1-year-period prevalence of 170 cases per 10,000 workers of occupational skin disease in 1988 (Lushniak 2003). An interesting fact is the statistically significant decrease in the incidence of OCD, reported in Bavaria for the period 1990–1999 (Dickel et al. 2001). This decrease seems to be a consequence of preventive public health initiatives and legislative measures for the occupational groups at highest risk (Dickel et al. 2001).

The perception that irritant dermatitis is more frequent than ACD in the occupational setting is supported by data from Singapore. Of 557 patients with occupational dermatoses, 55.7% (310) had ICD, 38.6% (215) had ACD, and 5.7% (32) had noncontact dermatitis (Goh 1987). However, the incidence rates of ICD and ACD in a population-based study in North Bavaria showed different predominance of ICD or ACD in the different occupational groups (Diepgen and Coenraads 1995). Since cases of irritant dermatitis tend to be less severe and chronic than those of ACD, the latter may outnumber the former in specialized occupational dermatology clinics (Kanerva et al. 1988). More information on the epidemiology of ICD and OCD are given in ➋ Chap. 8, "Occupational Contact Dermatitis".

6 Risk Factors

A number of individual factors for irritant dermatitis have been identified. Although occupational irritant hand dermatitis is more frequent in women (Meding 2000), no sex difference of irritant reactivity could be established experimentally (Hogan et al. 1990; Thyssen et al. 2010a). It is suspected that the increased exposure to irritants at home accounts for the higher prevalence in women (Meding 2000). This is supported by the observation that caring for children under the age of 4 years and the lack of dish washing machine significantly increased the risk of contracting hand eczema in a population of female hospital workers (Nilsson 1986). Irritant reactivity declines with increasing age. This is true not only for acute but also for cumulative irritant dermatitis (Suter-Widmer and Elsner 1996). In population studies on hand eczema, there was a trend of declining frequency with age (Thyssen et al. 2010a). The self-reported rates of hand eczema were highest for women in their twenties. The prevalence among men was less age-dependent, but there was also a declining trend with age (Thyssen et al. 2010a). Atopy is probably the best established risk factor for irritant hand dermatitis (Meding and Swanbeck 1990; Diepgen 2003). It has to be stressed, however, that respiratory manifestations of atopy seem to be less predictive of irritant reactivity compared with a skin manifestation. In a study with metal worker trainees, it was the personal history of flexural eczema in the past, rather than the total atopic score, which indicated an increased risk of occupational contact dermatitis (Berndt et al. 2000). On the level of the individual, there remains considerable uncertainty in the prediction of irritant reactivity. As was shown in a Swedish study, about 25% of the atopics in extreme risk occupations, such as ladies' hairdressers and nursing assistants, did not develop hand eczema (Rystedt 1985).

Genetic factors other than atopy may contribute to the susceptibility to hand eczema (all types), according to twin studies (Bryld et al. 2003; Lerbaek et al. 2007). Patch testing of twins with three model irritants in the past suggests that for some irritants there might be a genetic predisposition for the higher susceptibility (Holst and Moller 1975).

Filaggrin mutations could be additional genetic factors. The insufficient or absent function of filaggrin leads to xerosis and impairment of the stratum corneum barrier function and is a known predisposing factor for atopic dermatitis (de Jongh et al. 2008b). Filaggrin loss-of-function mutations were linked to an increased risk of occupational chronic irritant contact dermatitis, but it is still unclear if it is a risk factor independent from atopy (de Jongh et al. 2008b). Another study found an association between filaggrin mutations and a particular type of chronic hand eczema, a combined form of allergic and irritant contact dermatitis (Molin et al. 2009). More on the genetic predictors is given in ➋ Chap. 107, "Genetic Identification of Individuals with Increased Risk of Developing Occupational Skin Diseases".

Prediction of the individual susceptibility to irritation by means of bioengineering testing with model irritants, such as DMSO (dimethyl sulfoxide) and sodium hydroxide has been attempted, but the correlations were weak and no single test was found to be sufficient by itself (Bangha et al. 1996). A combination of tests showed better results (Berndt et al. 1999). It is generally considered that, with a few exceptions, the higher sensitivity to a given irritant does not predict sensitivity to other irritants (Marriott et al. 2005), perhaps due to the high interpersonal variability in the sensitivity to irritants (Robinson 2001). Further details are provided in ➋ Chap. 103, "Prediction of Skin Irritation by Noninvasive Bioengineering Methods".

The influence of lifestyle factors has been investigated in hand eczema in the general population (Thyssen et al. 2010a). No association with alcohol consumption was consistently found, while for smoking there are controversies and some studies have reported such an association (Thyssen et al. 2010b).

The incidence of ICD correlates with irritant exposure of the workers in a given profession (Goldner 1994). Some high-risk occupations are caterers (Wood and Greig 1997), construction workers (Avnstorp 1996), hospital workers, nurses (Kassis et al. 1984), cleaners, kitchen workers, hairdressers (Diepgen and Coenraads 1999; Dickel et al. 2001), and metal workers (Elsner et al. 1995; Wigger-Alberti et al. 1997). Recently, apart from chemical irritants, additional important risk factors for the development of occupational hand dermatitis in metal worker trainees have been examined: atopic disposition, mechanical irritation, and insufficient amount of skin regeneration time (Berndt et al. 2000). Generally, occupations involving "wet work" are especially prone to irritant dermatitis. The various occupational groups were classified into "exceedingly high risk" and "high risk" according to the yearly incidence of occupational skin disease (all types), reported to the compulsory system in Germany (Dickel et al. 2001). Some occupations in the exceedingly high group were hairdressers and barbers, bakers, florists, health-care workers, machinists, metal-surface processors, and others. The high-risk group included cooks, painters, metal processors, mechanics, housekeepers and cleaners and others (Dickel et al. 2001). More detailed lists of specific occupational hazards are given in the chapters with job descriptions.

7 Diagnosis

ICD has to be diagnosed by excluding other causes of contact and endogenous dermatitis. While this is more easily done on the basis of signs and symptoms for acute ICD, it is usually more difficult for cumulative irritant dermatitis. ACD, which tends to show spreading papules and vesicles, is the most important diagnosis to be excluded. It is hard to differentiate in the chronic state. Irritant dermatitis may be diagnosed if patch tests remain negative, if there is an exposure to irritants, and if the disease develops and heals, depending on the frequency and intensity of the irritant exposure. However, many allergens are also good irritants and may confuse the interpretation of patch testing (Moshell 1997). The interplay of ICD with ACD and atopy to produce the clinical picture of hand eczema was demonstrated in a study which gathered data from ten European patch-test clinics and proposed a relevant classification of the subdiagnoses of hand eczema (Diepgen et al. 2009b). ICD was the subdiagnosis of 21.5% of patients, ICD+ACD in 15.2%, and ICD+atopic hand eczema in 7.8% (Diepgen et al. 2009b).

Since cumulative ICD may become chronic in a later stage, the relation between exposure and disease tends to weaken. Histologic examination of a biopsy cannot differentiate between chronic irritant and allergic or atopic dermatitis. However, chronic ICD differs morphologically from acute ICD (Willis 1996). Immunohistologic staining has not shown any significant differences in the inflammatory infiltrate of chronic irritant and allergic dermatitis (Brasch et al. 1992). Whereas a biopsy may be helpful to exclude palmar psoriasis, psoriasis can usually be excluded or confirmed on clinical grounds that consider sharply demarcated hyperkeratotic or pustular lesions in contrast to the fuzzy borders of eczema while searching for other features such as nail and scalp involvement.

Visual evaluation of skin erythema and surface changes is still widely used to assess irritant reactions. However, various non-invasive techniques have been developed that permit objective evaluation of skin changes compared to a visual assessment (Fluhr et al. 2001). The bioengineering techniques such as measuring transepidermal water loss as an indicator of epidermal barrier function are well suited to detect minute epidermal barrier impairment earlier than clinical examinations and to assess the grade of dermatitis quantitatively. However, they are not useful in making a safe differential diagnosis between ACD and ICD. They rather offer the possibility to evaluate inflammation parameters such as redness, scaling and infiltration objectively and to quantify these reactions. More on the diagnosis of occupational contact dermatitis can be found in ➋ Chaps. 79–88.

8 Treatment and Prognosis

Avoiding the irritant(s) remains the basis of treating occupational ICD. This is achieved through technical measures (exchange of working substances, encapsulation of irritating fluids), individual skin protection (gloves, protective suits, protective creams), and, if necessary, sick leave until the epidermal barrier has completely regenerated. The epidermal barrier recovery may be a lengthy process, especially in cumulative irritant dermatitis. For example, a study on tertiary individual prevention foresees a period of 6 weeks (3 weeks inpatient treatment, followed by additional 3 weeks off-work) for patients with chronic occupational contact dermatitis in order to promote recovery (Skudlik et al. 2009).

The use of topical corticosteroids in the successful treatment of ACD has been questioned in irritant dermatitis (van der Valk and Maibach 1989). They may be effective in chronic, hyperkeratotic irritant dermatitis, but their prolonged use may lead to epidermal atrophy and consequently increased irritant sensitivity (see also ➋ Chap. 92, "Topical and Systemic Corticosteroids"). Other therapeutic options recommended by the published guidelines include topical tars, calcineurine inhibitors, phototherapy (UVB or PUVA), and retinoids (Diepgen et al. 2009a; English et al. 2009) (see also ➋ Chaps. 89–98). In difficult cases of chronic irritant hand dermatitis, radiation therapy may be indicated but it is ever less frequently used or even obsolete in some countries due to the need for licensed equipment and personnel, the safety concerns, and the availability of newer therapies (Warner and Cruz 2008). Bacterial superinfection may be a complication of contact dermatitis; it is treated with topical or systemic antibiotics. Potential irritants not only in the workplace but also in the home environment, such as irritant cleansing products, must be identified and whenever possible eliminated (Diepgen et al. 2009a).

The treatment modalities for contact dermatitis influence the barrier function repair. While both topical and systemic corticosteroids and retinoids such as alitretinoin have negative effects, the topical calcineurine inhibitors allow normal recovery, and UV-phototherapy up-regulates the barrier function of the skin. A key component of the therapy of ICD is the basic topical therapy with emollients (see ➋ Chap. 94, "Emollients: Effects, Evidence, and Side Effects"). It has been shown to promote the healing of dermatitis and the restoration of the skin barrier.

Prognosis for acute ICD is good if irritant contact is avoided. Cumulative irritant dermatitis, however, has a doubtful prognosis. The prognoses of occupational and nonoccupational contact dermatitis, ICD, and ACD are often compared in review-articles. The conflicting conclusions may be due to the improved response to therapy over time (Belsito 2005) or to the fact that the various subtypes of ICD have different prognoses, for example, cumulative ICD has a worse prognosis than ACD or acute ICD (Belsito 2005). According to Cahill et al. the prognosis is more likely to be poor for occupational ACD than for ICD in general (Cahill et al. 2004), although other opinions are also published. The prognoses of ICD and ACD were reported to be similar by Hogan et al. (1990). According to Goh, most studies appear to indicate that patients with ICD have a poorer prognosis than those with ACD (Goh 1997). A reason could be that in allergic dermatitis a specific causative allergen can be identified and avoided and the specific cause of ICD is often unknown.

A well-known factor that causes a poor prognosis of ICD is the existence of atopic dermatitis (Hogan et al. 1990). It contributes to the poor prognosis through a higher susceptibility to irritation and probably a slower healing (Chew and Maibach 2003). It is considered that atopic workers more frequently continue to suffer from persistent hand dermatitis even after changing the job (Belsito 2005). The term "persistent post-occupational dermatitis (PPOD)," with pertinent criteria, has been proposed for the cases where the dermatitis has the tendency to persist, even when all conceivable triggering causes have been removed (Wall and Gebauer 1991; Sajjachareonpong et al. 2004). For example, metal workers with cutting fluid dermatitis took up to several years to recover despite job change and avoidance of irritants (Elsner et al. 1995). This stresses the importance of early intervention in irritant dermatitis before it reaches the chronic stage.

The influence of job change on the prognosis of occupational contact dermatitis (all types) has been assessed in various studies over decades (Hogan et al. 1990; Cahill et al. 2004; Belsito 2005). These studies revealed that a job change did not affect the course of the disease; the workers with OCD who change jobs often have reasons other than dermatitis and that the social prognosis without a job change might be better despite ongoing OCD (Hogan et al. 1990; Cahill et al. 2004; Belsito 2005). More information on the prognosis of ICD is given in ➋ Chap. 100, "Prognosis of Irritant Contact Dermatitis".

9 Prevention

Considering the high incidence of ICD at the workplace, preventive measures play an important role. In order to increase the awareness of this health risk and to achieve an optimal compliance with the protective measures, employees should be adequately instructed already at the start of their training. It was shown in a study on the risk behavior that metal working apprentices were very poorly informed about skin diseases, the potential risk of hand eczema at the workplace and the benefit of skin care (Itschner et al. 1996). Considering this finding, it seems urgent to intensify health and safety education in high-risk workplaces.

The general scheme of prevention in public health divides it into primary, secondary, and tertiary prevention, and this classification is transferred to OCD as well. Primary prevention tries to prevent the development of disease in the healthy individual. Secondary prevention is targeted at the diseased individual trying to inhibit a relapse of contact dermatitis. In tertiary prevention (rehabilitation), a chronically diseased patient is treated and reintegrated into the working environment (Wigger-Alberti and Elsner 1997). Prevention of ICD requires an integrated approach that considers both the exposure and the exposed individual. The responsibility for primary prevention rests mainly with manufacturers and producers of chemicals and products, government agencies, consumer organizations, industrial physicians and nurses, and safety engineers. A multidimensional approach with eight basic elements of prevention planning has been proposed by Mathias (1990): recognition of potential cutaneous irritants and allergens, engineering controls or chemical substitution to prevent skin exposure, personal protection with appropriate clothing or protective creams, personal and environmental hygiene, regulation of potential allergens and irritants within the workplace, educational efforts to promote awareness of potential allergens and irritants, motivational techniques to promote safe work conditions and practices, and preemployment and periodic health screening.

In the prevention of exposure, the main elements are technical measures, i.e., avoidance of the irritant through its removal from the workplace or through technical shielding by the use of potent irritants in closed systems or automation, irritant replacement or removal (Lachapelle 1995), and personal protection of the workers (Wigger-Alberti and Elsner 1998). On the individual's side, screening for predisposition to irritant dermatitis and counseling of sensitive individuals may be appropriate preventive measures. More on the prevention of occupational dermatoses is given in the dedicated section in this book (➋ Chaps. 103–115).

References

Arend WP, Guthridge CJ (2000) Biological role of interleukin 1 receptor antagonist isoforms. Ann Rheum Dis 59(Suppl 1):i60–i64

Avnstorp C (1996) Irritant contact eczema. In: van der Valk PG, Maibach H (eds) The irritant contact dermatitis syndrome. CRC Press, Boca Raton, pp 111–119

Bangha E, Hinnen U et al (1996) Irritancy testing in occupational dermatology: comparison between two quick tests and the acute irritation induced by sodium lauryl sulphate. Acta Derm Venereol 76(6):450–452

Belsito DV (2005) Occupational contact dermatitis: etiology, prevalence, and resultant impairment/disability. J Am Acad Dermatol 53(2): 303–313

Berardesca E, Distante F (1994) The modulation of skin irritation. Contact Dermatitis 31(5):281–287

Berardesca E, Maibach HI (1988) Racial differences in sodium lauryl sulphate induced cutaneous irritation: black and white. Contact Dermatitis 18(2):65–70

Berndt U, Hinnen U et al (1999) Is occupational irritant contact dermatitis predictable by cutaneous bioengineering methods? Results of the Swiss metalworkers' eczema study (PROMETES). Dermatology 198(4):351–354

Berndt U, Hinnen U et al (2000) Hand eczema in metalworker trainees–an analysis of risk factors. Contact Dermatitis 43(6):327–332

Borlon C, Godard P et al (2007) The usefulness of toxicogenomics for predicting acute skin irritation on in vitro reconstructed human epidermis. Toxicology 241(3):157–166

Brasch J, Burgard J et al (1992) Common pathogenetic pathways in allergic and irritant contact dermatitis. J Invest Dermatol 98(2): 166–170

Bryld LE, Hindsberger C et al (2003) Risk factors influencing the development of hand eczema in a population-based twin sample. Br J Dermatol 149(6):1214–1220

Cahill J, Keegel T et al (2004) The prognosis of occupational contact dermatitis in 2004. Contact Dermatitis 51(5–6):219–226

Chew AL, Maibach HI (2003) Occupational issues of irritant contact dermatitis. Int Arch Occup Environ Health 76(5):339–346

Chew A-L, Maibach HI (2006) Ten genotypes of irritant contact dermatitis. In: Chew A-L, Maibach HI (eds) Irritant dermatitis. Springer, Berlin, pp 5–9

Clemmensen A, Andersen KE et al (2010) Genome-wide expression analysis of human in vivo irritated epidermis: differential profiles induced by sodium lauryl sulfate and nonanoic acid. J Invest Dermatol 130(9):2201–2210

Coenraads PJ, Smit J (1995) Epidemiology. In: Rycroft RJG, Menne T, Frosch PJ (eds) Textbook of contact dermatitis. Springer, Berlin, pp 133–150

Corsini E, Galli CL (2000) Epidermal cytokines in experimental contact dermatitis. Toxicology 142(3):203–211

Cronin E (1995) Hand eczema. In: Rycroft RJG, Menne T, Frosch PJ (eds) Textbook of contact dermatitis. Springer, Berlin, pp 207–218

de Jongh CM, Verberk MM et al (2006) Stratum corneum cytokines and skin irritation response to sodium lauryl sulfate. Contact Dermatitis 54(6):325–333

de Jongh CM, Lutter R et al (2007) Differential cytokine expression in skin after single and repeated irritation by sodium lauryl sulphate. Exp Dermatol 16(12):1032–1040

de Jongh CM, John SM et al (2008a) Cytokine gene polymorphisms and susceptibility to chronic irritant contact dermatitis. Contact Dermatitis 58(5):269–277

de Jongh CM, Khrenova L et al (2008b) Loss-of-function polymorphisms in the filaggrin gene are associated with an increased susceptibility to chronic irritant contact dermatitis: a case-control study. Br J Dermatol 159(3):621–627

Dickel H, Kuss O et al (2001) Occupational skin diseases in Northern Bavaria between 1990 and 1999: a population-based study. Br J Dermatol 145(3):453–462

Diepgen TL (2003) Occupational skin-disease data in Europe. Int Arch Occup Environ Health 76(5):331–338

Diepgen TL, Coenraads PJ (1999) The epidemiology of occupational contact dermatitis. Int Arch Occup Environ Health 72(8):496–506

Diepgen T, Coenraads PJ, Diepgen T, Coenraads PJ (1995) What can we learn from epidemiological studies on irritant contact dermatitis? In: Elsner P, Maibach H (eds) Irritant dermatitis: new clinical and experimental aspects. Karger, Basel, pp 18–27

Diepgen T, Elsner P et al (2009a) Management von Handekzemen Leitlinie ICD-10-Ziffer: L20. L23. L24. L25. L30. J Dtsch Dermatol Ges 7(s3):s1–s16

Diepgen TL, Andersen KE et al (2009b) Hand eczema classification: a cross-sectional, multicentre study of the aetiology and morphology of hand eczema. Br J Dermatol 160(2):353–358

Dika E, Branco N et al (2004) Immunologic patterns in allergic and irritant contact dermatitis: similarities. Exog Dermatol 3:113–120

Dooms-Goossens AE, Debusschere KM et al (1986) Contact dermatitis caused by airborne agents. A review and case reports. J Am Acad Dermatol 15(1):1–10

Dursteler BB, Nyquist RA (2004) Outbreak of rove beetle (Staphylinid) pustular contact dermatitis in Pakistan among deployed U.S. personnel. Mil Med 169(1):57–60

Eichmann A, Amgwerd D (1992) Toxic contact dermatitis. Schweiz Rundsch Med Prax 81(19):615–617

Elsner P (1994) Irritant dermatitis in the workplace. Dermatol Clin 12(3):461–467

Elsner P, Baxmann F et al (1995) Metal working fluid dermatitis: a comparative follow-up study in patients with irritant and nonirritant hand dermatitis. In: Elsner P, Maibach H (eds) Irritant dermatitis: new clinical and experimental aspects. Karger, Basel, pp 77–88

English J, Aldridge R et al (2009) Consensus statement on the management of chronic hand eczema. Clin Exp Dermatol 34(7):761–769

Feingold KR, Schmuth M et al (2007) The regulation of permeability barrier homeostasis. J Invest Dermatol 127(7):1574–1576

Fletcher ST, Baker VA et al (2001) Gene expression analysis of EpiDerm following exposure to SLS using cDNA microarrays. Toxicol In Vitro 15(4–5):393–398

Fluhr JW, Kuss O et al (2001) Testing for irritation with a multifactorial approach: comparison of eight non-invasive measuring techniques on five different irritation types. Br J Dermatol 145(5):696–703

Fluhr JW, Akengin A et al (2005) Additive impairment of the barrier function by mechanical irritation, occlusion and sodium lauryl sulphate in vivo. Br J Dermatol 153(1):125–131

Fluhr JW, Darlenski R et al (2008) Skin irritation and sensitization: mechanisms and new approaches for risk assessment. 1. Skin irritation. Skin Pharmacol Physiol 21(3):124–135

Freeman S, Maibach H (1988) Study of irritant contact dermatitis produced by repeat patch test with sodium lauryl sulfate and assessed by visual methods, transepidermal water loss, and laser Doppler velocimetry. J Am Acad Dermatol 19(3):496–502

Frosch PJ (1995) Cutaneous irritation. In: Rycroft RJG, Menne T, Frosch PJ (eds) Textbook of contact dermatitis. Springer, Berlin, pp 28–61

Frosch PJ, John SM (2006) Clinical aspects of irritant contact dermatitis. In: Frosch PJ, Menné T, Lepoittevin JP (eds) Contact dermatitis. Springer, Berlin, pp 255–294

Frosch PJ, John SM (2011) Clinical aspects of irritant contact dermatitis. In: Johansen JD, Frosch PJ, Lepoittevin JP (eds) Contact dermatitis. Springer, Berlin, pp 305–345

Frosch PJ, Kligman AM (1977) A method for appraising the stinging capacity of topically applied substances. J Soc Cosmet Chem 28:197–209

Ghadially R, Brown BE et al (1995) The aged epidermal permeability barrier. Structural, functional, and lipid biochemical abnormalities in humans and a senescent murine model. J Clin Invest 95(5): 2281–2290

Goh CL (1987) Occupational skin disease in Singapore: epidemiology & causative agents. Ann Acad Med Singapore 16(2):303–305

Goh CL (1995) Noneczematous contact reactions. In: Rycroft RJG, Menne T, Frosch PJ (eds) Textbook of contact dermatitis. Springer, Berlin, pp 221–236

Goh CL (1997) Prognosis of contact and occupational dermatitis. Clin Dermatol 15(4):655–659

Goldner R (1994) Work-related irritant contact dermatitis. Occup Med 9(1):37–44

Grangsjo A, Leijon-Kuligowski A et al (1996) Different pathways in irritant contact eczema? Early differences in the epidermal elemental content and expression of cytokines after application of 2 different irritants. Contact Dermatitis 35(6):355–360

Hafner J, Ruegger M et al (1995) Airborne irritant contact dermatitis from metal dust adhering to semisynthetic working suits. Contact Dermatitis 32(5):285–288

Hoefakker S, Caubo M et al (1995) In vivo cytokine profiles in allergic and irritant contact dermatitis. Contact Dermatitis 33(4):258–266

Hogan DJ, Dannaker CJ et al (1990) The prognosis of contact dermatitis. J Am Acad Dermatol 23(2 Pt 1):300–307

Holliday MR, Corsini E et al (1997) Differential induction of cutaneous TNF-alpha and IL-6 by topically applied chemicals. Am J Contact Dermat 8(3):158–164

Holst R, Moller H (1975) One hundred twin pairs patch tested with primary irritants. Br J Dermatol 93(2):145–149

Huang C, Liu Y et al (2009) An outbreak of 268 cases of Paederus dermatitis in a toy-building factory in central China. Int J Dermatol 48(2):128–131

Hurwitz RM, Rivera HP et al (1984) Black-spot poison ivy dermatitis. An acute irritant contact dermatitis superimposed upon an allergic contact dermatitis. Am J Dermatopathol 6(4):319–322

Itschner L, Hinnen U et al (1996) Prevention of hand eczema in the metal-working industry: risk awareness and behaviour of metal worker apprentices. Dermatology 193(3):226–229

Kanerva L, Estlander T et al (1988) Occupational skin disease in Finland. An analysis of 10 years of statistics from an occupational dermatology clinic. Int Arch Occup Environ Health 60(2):89–94

Kassis V, Vedel P et al (1984) Contact dermatitis to methyl methacrylate. Contact Dermatitis 11(1):26–28

Keegel T, Moyle M et al (2009) The epidemiology of occupational contact dermatitis (1990–2007): a systematic review. Int J Dermatol 48(6): 571–578

Kupper TS (1990) Immune and inflammatory processes in cutaneous tissues. Mechanisms and speculations. J Clin Invest 86(6):1783–1789

Lachapelle JM (1995) Principles of prevention and protection in contact dermatitis (with special reference to occupational dermatology). In: Rycroft RJG, Menne T, Frosch PJ (eds) Textbook of contact dermatitis. Springer, Berlin, pp 695–702

Lachapelle JM (2006) Airborne irritant dermatitis. In: Chew AL, Maibach H (eds) Irritant dermatitis. Springer, Berlin, pp 71–79

Lammintausta K, Maibach HI (1990) Contact dermatitis due to irritation: general principles, etiology, and histology. In: Adams RM (ed) Occupational skin disease. W.B. Saunders, Philadelphia, pp 1–15

Lammintausta K, Maibach HI et al (1988) Mechanisms of subjective (sensory) irritation. Propensity to non-immunologic contact urticaria and objective irritation in stingers. Derm Beruf Umwelt 36(2):45–49

Lee E, An S et al (2009) Development of a novel method for quantitative evaluation of sensory skin irritation inhibitors. Skin Res Technol 15(4):464–469

Lerbaek A, Kyvik KO et al (2007) Heritability of hand eczema is not explained by comorbidity with atopic dermatitis. J Invest Dermatol 127(7):1632–1640

Lofgren SM, Warshaw EM (2006) Dyshidrosis: epidemiology, clinical characteristics, and therapy. Dermatitis 17(4):165–181

Lushniak BD (2003) The importance of occupational skin diseases in the United States. Int Arch Occup Environ Health 76(5):325–330

Malten KE (1981) Thoughts on irritant contact dermatitis. Contact Dermatitis 7(5):238–247

Malten KE, den Arend JA (1985) Irritant contact dermatitis. Traumiterative and cumulative impairment by cosmetics, climate, and other daily loads. Derm Beruf Umwelt 33(4):125–132

Malten KE, den Arend JA et al (1979) Delayed irritation: hexanediol diacrylate and butanediol diacrylate. Contact Dermatitis 5(3): 178–184

Marriott M, Holmes J et al (2005) The complex problem of sensitive skin. Contact Dermatitis 53(2):93–99

Mathias CG (1990) Prevention of occupational contact dermatitis. J Am Acad Dermatol 23(4 Pt 1):742–748

McDougal JN, Garrett CM et al (2007) Effects of brief cutaneous JP-8 jet fuel exposures on time course of gene expression in the epidermis. Toxicol Sci 95(2):495–510

Meding B (2000) Differences between the sexes with regard to work-related skin disease. Contact Dermatitis 43(2):65–71

Meding B, Swanbeck G (1990) Occupational hand eczema in an industrial city. Contact Dermatitis 22(1):13–23

Molin S, Vollmer S et al (2009) Filaggrin mutations may confer susceptibility to chronic hand eczema characterized by combined allergic and irritant contact dermatitis. Br J Dermatol 161(4):801–807

Moshell AN (1997) Workshop on irritant contact dermatitis. Am J Contact Dermat 8(2):79–105

Mozzanica N (1992) Pathogenetic aspects of allergic and irritant contact dermatitis. Clin Dermatol 10(2):115–121

Nilsson E (1986) Individual and environmental risk factors for hand eczema in hospital workers. Acta Derm Venereol Suppl (Stockh) 128:1–63

Patil S, Maibach HI (1994) Effect of age and sex on the elicitation of irritant contact dermatitis. Contact Dermatitis 30(5):257–264

Patiwael JA, Wintzen M et al (2005) Airborne irritant contact dermatitis due to synthetic fibres from an air-conditioning filter. Contact Dermatitis 52(3):126–129

Pinnagoda J, Tupker RA et al (1989) The intra- and inter-individual variability and reliability of transepidermal water loss measurements. Contact Dermatitis 21(4):255–259

Proksch E, Brandner JM et al (2008) The skin: an indispensable barrier. Exp Dermatol 17(12):1063–1072

Rietschel RL (1997) Comparison of allergic and irritant dermatitis. Immunol Allergy Clin North Am 17:359–364

Robinson MK (2001) Intra-individual variations in acute and cumulative skin irritation responses. Contact Dermatitis 45(2):75–83

Rogers JV, Garrett CM et al (2003) Gene expression in rat skin induced by irritating chemicals. J Biochem Mol Toxicol 17(3):123–137

Rystedt I (1985) Work-related hand eczema in atopics. Contact Dermatitis 12(3):164–171

Sajjachareonpong P, Cahill J et al (2004) Persistent post-occupational dermatitis. Contact Dermatitis 51(5–6):278–283

Santos R, Goossens A (2007) An update on airborne contact dermatitis: 2001–2006. Contact Dermatitis 57(6):353–360

Skogstad M, Levy F (1994) Occupational irritant contact dermatitis and fungal infection in construction workers. Contact Dermatitis 31(1): 28–30

Skudlik C, Weisshaar E et al (2009) Multicenter study "medical-occupational rehabilitation procedure skin - optimizing and quality assurance of inpatient-management (ROQ)". J Dtsch Dermatol Ges 7(2):122–126

Spiekstra SW, Toebak MJ et al (2005) Induction of cytokine (interleukin-1alpha and tumor necrosis factor-alpha) and chemokine (CCL20, CCL27, and CXCL8) alarm signals after allergen and irritant exposure. Exp Dermatol 14(2):109–116

Steciuk A, Dompmartin A et al (1997) Pustular contact dermatitis from fluorine in an antirust solution. Contact Dermatitis 36(5):276–277

Suter-Widmer J, Elsner P (1996) Age and irritation. In: van der Valk PG, Maibach H (eds) The irritant contact dermatitis syndrome. CRC Press, Boca Raton, pp 257–261

Thong H-Y, Maibach HI (2008) Irritant dermatitis as a model of inflammation. Drug Discovery Today: Disease Mechanisms 5(2): e221–e228

Thyssen JP, Johansen JD et al (2010a) The epidemiology of hand eczema in the general population–prevalence and main findings. Contact Dermatitis 62(2):75–87

Thyssen JP, Linneberg A et al (2010b) The effect of tobacco smoking and alcohol consumption on the prevalence of self-reported hand eczema: a cross-sectional population-based study. Br J Dermatol 162(3):619–626

van der Valk PG, Maibach HI (1989) Do topical corticosteroids modulate skin irritation in human beings? Assessment by transepidermal water loss and visual scoring. J Am Acad Dermatol 21(3 Pt 1):519–522

van der Valk PG, Nater JP et al (1985) Vulnerability of the skin to surfactants in different groups of eczema patients and controls as measured by water vapour loss. Clin Exp Dermatol 10(2):98–103

Wall LM, Gebauer KA (1991) A follow-up study of occupational skin disease in Western Australia. Contact Dermatitis 24(4):241–243

Warner JA, Cruz PD Jr (2008) Grenz ray therapy in the new millennium: still a valid treatment option? Dermatitis 19(2):73–80

Welss T, Basketter DA et al (2004) In vitro skin irritation: facts and future. State of the art review of mechanisms and models. Toxicol In Vitro 18(3):231–243

Wigger-Alberti W, Elsner P (1997) Preventive measures in contact dermatitis. Clin Dermatol 15(4):661–665

Wigger-Alberti W, Elsner P (1998) Do barrier creams and gloves prevent or provoke contact dermatitis? Am J Contact Dermat 9(2):100–106

Wigger-Alberti W, Hinnen U et al (1997) Predictive testing of metalworking fluids: a comparison of 2 cumulative human irritation models and correlation with epidemiological data. Contact Dermatitis 36(1):14–20

Wilkinson JD, Willis CM (1998) Contact dermatitis: irritant. In: Champion RH, Burton JL, Burns DA, Breathnach SM (eds) Textbook of dermatology. Blackwell, London, pp 709–731

Willis CM (1996) The histopathology of irritant contact dermatitis. In: van der Valk PGM, Maibach HI (eds) The irritant contact dermatitis syndrome. CRC Press, Boca Raton, pp 291–303

Wong R, Tran V et al (2004) Use of RT-PCR and DNA microarrays to characterize RNA recovered by non-invasive tape harvesting of normal and inflamed skin. J Invest Dermatol 123(1):159–167

Wood BP, Greig DE (1997) Occupational dermatitis–what's new? Catering industry. Clin Dermatol 15(4):567–571

Wood LC, Elias PM et al (1996) Barrier disruption stimulates interleukin-1 alpha expression and release from a pre-formed pool in murine epidermis. J Invest Dermatol 106(3):397–403

Zargari O, Kimyai-Asadi A et al (2003) Paederus dermatitis in northern Iran: a report of 156 cases. Int J Dermatol 42(8):608–612

13 Chemical Skin Burns

Audris Chiang[1] · *Magnus Bruze*[1,2] · *Sigfrid Fregert*[2] · *Birgitta Gruvberger*[2]
[1]University of California Medical School, San Francisco, CA, USA
[2]Department of Occupational and Environmental Dermatology, Skåne University Hospital Malmö, Lund University, Malmö, Sweden

Core Messages

- Chemical skin burns are common in industry, but can also occur in non-work-related environments.
- Chemical burns from household products may not be noticeable, but oftentimes the cause of a burn is obvious and medical treatment is not sought.
- Usually chemical burn damage is minimal, but some chemical burns have risk of complications and long-term disabilities.
- The severity of a burn can be diminished if treated properly and promptly.
- It is important for physicians to understand corrosive chemicals as well as chemical burns in regards to their clinical manifestations, mechanism, medical treatment, and preventive measures.

1 Introduction

Chemical skin burns are particularly common in industry, but they also occur in non-work-related environments. Occupationally induced chemical burns are frequently noticed when visiting and examining workers at their work sites. Corrosive chemicals used in hobbies are an increasing cause of skin burns. Disinfectants and cleansers are examples of household products which can cause chemical burns. However, in most cases, the cause of a chemical burn is obvious to the affected persons and damage is minimal and heals without medical care, so medical attention is not sought. Sometimes the chemical burns are severe and extensive, with the risk of complications and long-term disability. In the acute stage, there is a varying risk of systemic effects, including a fatal outcome, depending on exposure conditions and the incriminating agent. For these reasons it is important for the physician to have knowledge of corrosive chemicals as well as of chemical burns with regard to their clinical manifestations, specific medical treatments, and preventive measures.

2 Definition

A caustic burn (chemical burn) is an acute, severe irritant reaction by which the cells have been damaged to a point where there is no return to viability; in other words, a necrosis develops (Stewart 1985; Sykes et al. 1986; Cartotto et al. 1996). One single skin exposure to certain chemicals can result in a chemical burn. These chemicals react with intra- and intercellular components in the skin. However, the action of toxic (irritant) chemicals varies, causing partly different irritant reactions morphologically. They can damage the horny layer, cell membranes, lysosomes, mast cells, leukocytes, DNA synthesis, blood vessels, enzyme systems, and metabolism. The corrosive action of chemicals depends on their chemical properties, concentration, pH, alkalinity, acidity, temperature, lipid/water solubility, interaction with other substances, and duration and type (e.g., occlusion) of skin contact. It also depends on the body region, previous skin damage, and possibly on individual resistance capacity.

Many substances cause chemical burns only when they are applied under occlusion from, for example, gloves, boots, shoes, clothes, caps, face masks, adhesive plasters, and rings. Skin folds may be formed and act occlusively in certain body regions, e.g., under breasts and in the axillae. Many products, which under ordinary skin exposure conditions cause weak irritant reactions or irritant contact dermatitis, can under occlusion cause chemical burns, e.g., detergents, emulsifiers, solvents, plants, woods, topical medicaments, toiletries, insecticides, pesticides, preservatives, cleansers, polishes, plastic monomers, and portland cement. Wet cement can usually be handled without causing a chemical burn, but when present under occluding clothes for some hours, it can cause severe skin damage, e.g., on knees. White spirit causes only slight dryness at open application, but causes blisters under occlusion.

T. Rustemeyer, P. Elsner, S.M. John & H.I. Maibach (eds.), *Kanerva's Occupational Dermatology*,
DOI 10.1007/978-3-642-02035-3_13,

There are different mechanisms for reactions between skin components and agents causing chemical and thermal burns. Chemical agents cause progressive damage until either no more chemical remains unreacted in the tissue or the agent is inactivated by treatment, while thermal damaging effects cease shortly after removal of the heat source.

The most commonly reported chemicals that can cause chemical burns are listed in ❯ *Table 13.1.* Acids and alkalis have been grouped separately, as the corrosive effect within the respective group is exerted through the same mechanism. These groups contain both strong and weak acids and alkalis, respectively. The other compounds are listed together although their corrosive effects are mediated through different mechanisms. Most of these compounds are neutral. However, some are weak acids or alkalis but are considered to be corrosive due to properties other than acidity or alkalinity, respectively.

3 Mechanism

A chemical burn occurs when two chemical entities, one acting as the donor and the other as the acceptor, interact with each other. The strength of the aggressor affects the weakness of its biochemical target until it consumes it completely, then the aggressor continues to attack species of subsequently higher energy levels until exhausting its own concentration.

Chemical agents can have corrosive effects on tissues by damaging cytoplasmic membranes, by denaturing or coagulating proteins, or by chelating trace elements essential to cellular function.

Six types of elementary reactions delineate the possible mechanisms of a chemical burn: acid-base reaction, redox reaction, chelation, addition, substitution, and solvation. Depending on the type of elementary reaction, different types of entities are exchanged: electrons for redox reactions, ions for acid-base and chelating reactions, and atoms or molecules for additions and substitutions.

Acid-base and redox reactions modify the balances of chemical reactivity.

For acid-base reactions, protons are exchanged until reaching an equilibrium pH. Given the concentration and pK of a substance, it is possible to predict the resulting degree of irritability. Above a certain threshold concentration and pK lower than 4 or above 10, a burn will develop from the aggressor substance. Levels of cellular structures are successively destroyed from the surface downward until exhaustion of the aggressor molecules. An acid with a given energy level pK consumes all bases of weaker energy level (with a bigger pK) beginning with the weakest base. The transfer of H^+ ions modifies the H^+/OH^- balance of the chemical environment, thus changing the acidity/basicity of the environment, possibly resulting in irritation or corrosion.

For redox reactions, the oxidizing agent oxidizes reducing agents with weaker potentials than its own, accepting electrons to complete its orbitals and thus become stable. For example, chlorine bleaches can cause skin burns. This is because they contain the strong oxidizer hypochlorite and the by-products of the oxidation reaction are corrosive. Redox reactions, similar to acid-base reactions, can generate lesions to tissues.

Addition and substitution reactions modify biological molecules, for example, by disintegrating the 3D configuration of proteins or by coagulation of proteins.

Chelation and solvation cause the disappearance of an active entity. For example, the F^- ion from hydrofluoric acid chelates calcium and magnesium ions, changing physiological balance by disrupting biochemical metabolisms until cell death and, consequently, tissue necrosis occurs.

Burgher provides significant detail for eye burns (Burgher et al. 2011); the principles delineated above probably relate equally to the skin.

4 Diagnosis

It is usually easy to arrive at a diagnosis of chemical skin burn, as the symptoms are easily recognized and the exposure to a corrosive agent obvious. However, sometimes the exposure is concealed, at least initially. For example, hospital personnel may be exposed to ethylene oxide, which may remain in gowns and straps after sterilization (Biro et al. 1974), and cleaners may occasionally be exposed to a corrosive agent contaminating nonhazardous objects in a laboratory. Corrosive substances under occlusion may also, at least initially, confuse and delay the diagnosis. Occasionally, a chemical burn can mimic other dermatoses, e.g., ethylene oxide can mimic bullous impetigo.

5 Clinical Features

Not only the skin but also the eyes, lips, mouth, esophagus, nose septum, glottis, and lungs can be directly affected. As a result of resorption, toxic chemicals can damage the blood, bone marrow, liver, kidneys, nerves, brain, and other organs. The most common locations of chemical burns on the skin are the hands and face/neck, but the whole body can be affected. The exposure usually

Table 13.1

Agents causing chemical burns. The chemicals listed are the most common reported to cause chemical burns in industries, hobbies, and households. The list features strong corrosive substances and also less irritating compounds that require special conditions, for example, occlusion, to cause chemical burns

Acids	Alkalis	Miscellaneous
Acetic acid	Amines	Acetyl chloride
Acrylic acid	Ammonia	Acrolein
Benzoic acid	Barium hydroxide	Acrylonitrile
Boric acid	Calcium carbonate	Alkali ethoxides
Bromoacetic acid	Calcium hydroxide	Alkali methoxides
Chloroacetic acids	Calcium oxide	Allyl diiodine
Chlorosulfuric acid	Hydrazine	Aluminum bromide
Fluorophosphoric acid	Lithium hydroxide	Aluminum chloride
Fluorosilicic acid	Potassium hydroxide	Aluminum trichloride
Fluorosulfonic acid	Sodium carbonate	Ammonium difluoride
Formic acid	Sodium hydroxide	Ammonium persulfate
Fumaric acid	Sodium metasilicate	Ammonium sulfide
Hydrobromic acid		Antimony trioxide
Hydrochloric acid		Aromatic hydrocarbons
Hydrofluoric acid		Arsenic oxides
Lactic acid		Benzene
Nitric acid		Benzoyl chloride
Perchloric acid		Benzoyl chlorodimethylhydantoin
Peroxyacetic acid		Benzoyl chloroformate
Phosphonic acids		Borax
Phosphoric acids		Boron tribromide
Phthalic acids		Bromine
Picric acid		Bromotrifluoride
Propionic acid		Calcium carbide
Salicylic acid		Cantharides
Sulfonic acids		Carbon disulfide
Sulfuric acid		Carbon tetrachloride
Tartaric acid		Chlorobenzene
Toluenesulfonic acid		Chlorinated acetophenones (tear gas)
		Chlorinated solvents
		Chloroform
		Chlorocresols
		Chlorophenols
		Chromates
		Chromium oxychloride
		Chromium trioxide
		Cresote
		Cresolic compounds
		Croton aldehyde
		Dichloroacetyl chloride
		Dichromates
		Dimethyl acetamide
		Dimethyl formamide
		Dimethyl sulfoxide (DMSO)
		Dioxane
		Dipentene
		Dithranol
		Epichlorohydrine

Table 13.1 (Continued)

Acids	Alkalis	Miscellaneous
		Epoxy reactive diluents
		Ethylene oxide
		Ferric chloride hexahydrate
		Fluorides
		Fluorine
		Fluorosilicate
		Formaldehyde
		Gasoline
		Gentian violet
		Glutaraldehyde
		Halogenated solvents
		Hexylresorcinol
		Iodine
		Isocyanates
		Kerosene fuel
		Limonene
		Lithium
		Lithium chloride
		Mercury compounds
		Methylchloroisothiazolinone
		Methylenedichloride
		Methylisothiazolinone
		Morpholine
		Perchloroethylene
		Peroxides
		Benzoyl
		Cumene
		Cyclohexanone
		Hydrogen
		Methylethylketone
		Potassium
		Phenolic compounds
		Phosphorus
		Phosphorus bromides
		Phosphorus chlorides
		Phosphorus oxychloride
		Phosphorus oxides
		Piperazine
		Potassium
		Potassium cyanide
		Potassium difluoride
		Potassium hypochlorite
		Potassium permanganate
		Povidone iodine
		Propionic oxide
		Propylene oxide
		Quarternary ammonium compounds
		Reactive diluents
		Sodium
		Sodium borohydride
		Sodium difluoride
		Sodium hypochlorite

Table 13.1 (Continued)

Acids	Alkalis	Miscellaneous
		Sodium sulfite Sodium thiosulfate Styrene Sulfur dichloride Sulfur dioxide Sulfur mustard Thioglycollates Thionyl chloride Tributyltin oxide Trichloroethylene Turpentine Vinyl pyridine White spirit Zinc chloride

occurs by accident. However, occasionally, a chemical burn is the result of malingering. The major symptoms are burning and smarting. Morphologically, chemical burns are characterized by erythema, blisters, erosions, ulcers, and necrosis with surrounding erythema. Usually, the symptoms develop immediately or in close connection to exposure, but certain chemicals, such as phenols, weak hydrofluoric acid, and sulfur mustard gas, can give delayed reactions which first appear several hours, or even a day, after the exposure.

Strong acids coagulate skin proteins, and further penetration is decreased by the barrier formed. Some common toxic chemicals affect the skin in a special way (Kuniyuki and Oonishi 1997). Principally, all strong acids give the same symptoms and major features, including erythema, blisters, and necrosis. Some acids discolor the skin, e.g., producing a yellow color from nitric acid. Sulfuric acid, as an example, dehydrates the skin by creating excessive heat in the tissue, producing coagulation necrotic eschars with thrombus formation in the lesion's microvasculature (Flammiger and Maibach 2006). The action of hydrofluoric acid in the skin differs from other strong acids (Vance 1990; Kirkpatrick et al. 1995). It causes liquefaction necrosis, and the penetration may continue for days. When an area above 1% of the total body surface is affected, systemic effects can arise. In the skin, this acid causes much stronger pains than other acids. Diluted hydrofluoric acid can cause pain starting several hours or even a day after the exposure. For example, when bricklayers use this acid at a concentration of 10–30% for rinsing brick walls, it may penetrate into their nail beds and, thereby, cause severe pain after several hours. The strong pain is due to the capacity of fluorine ions to bind calcium in the tissue, which affects the nervous system. Hydrofluoric acid can penetrate to the bone and cause decalcification there. Also, fluorides and fluorosilicic acid can give the same types of symptoms.

Alkalis often cause more severe damage than acids, except hydrofluoric acid (Gelmetti and Cecca 1992; Winemaker et al. 1992; Beausang and Herbert 1994). The necrotic skin first appears dark brown, then changes to black. Later, skin becomes hard, dry, and cracked. Generally, no blisters appear in the skin. Alkalis split proteins and lipids, and there is a saponification of the released fatty acids. The emulsifying effect of the soap formed facilitates further penetration of the alkali into deeper layer of the skin. Chemical burns from alkaline chemicals are more painful than from acids, except from hydrofluoric acid. Because of its alkalinity, cement mixed with water can cause acute ulcerative damage (Stoermer and Wolz 1983; McGeown 1984; Lane and Hogan 1985; Fisher 1986; Onuba and Essiet 1986; Tosti et al. 1989; Adams 1990; Morley et al. 1996). Severe skin damage has involved the lower limbs, often after kneeling on wet concrete or when it gets inside boots or shoes. Sometimes, necrotic skin appears 8–12 h after exposure. Rarely, hands can also be affected, particularly when the insides of gloves have been contaminated. The alkalinity can also vary considerably between batches from the same cement factory.

Phenolic compounds such as phenol, cresol, chlorocresol, and unhardened phenolic resins penetrate the skin easily and can damage peripheral nerves, resulting in insensibility. Sometimes, peripheral nerves can be affected without visible damage to the skin. After exposure to phenolic compounds, the local blood vessels become constricted, which can contribute to the development of the necrosis. Shock and renal damage can appear after absorption of phenolic compounds (Lin and Yang 1992; Horch et al. 1994; Shibata et al. 1994).

Sulfur mustard, 2,2′-dichlorodiethyl sulfide, is a chemical warfare agent (Newman-Taylor and Morris 1991; Smith and Dunn 1991; Ruhl et al. 1994). It has been dumped into the sea, and fishermen have been injured when leaking containers get in their nets. The chemical is a viscous liquid below and a gas above 14°C. On the skin, the liquid causes blisters and necrosis 10–12 h after skin exposure. The gas attacks mainly the eyes and the respiratory organs. Sometimes the skin is also affected by direct contact with the gas, and the chemical burn then clinically appears 3–6 h after exposure; initial redness is followed by blisters and ulcers. Tear gas can give a bullous dermatitis (Zekri et al. 1995).

Ethylene oxide gas used for sterilization of surgical instruments, textile, and plastic material can remain in these objects for several days if not ventilated well enough (Biro et al. 1974; Fisher 1990). Thus, when hospital personnel handle such objects, there is possible exposure to ethylene oxide, which is not obvious, and the symptoms, including erythema, edema, and large bullae, may therefore be misdiagnosed as another skin disease. Accidental skin exposure to chemicals under high pressure, for example hydraulic oil, can result in deep penetration into the skin, where a chemical burn with necrosis can develop.

6 Treatment

Repair cannot proceed until the responsible agent is inactivated by chemical reaction with tissues, neutralized, or removed. As long as the chemical is present, tissue destruction will continue, so skin decontamination is important (Flammiger and Maibach 2006). Rinsing with water is the first-aid treatment; preferably, tepid running tap water should be used. Irrigation should not be done at high pressure, as the corrosive agent may be splashed onto other parts of the body or on the persons treating the burn. It is important that the treatment starts immediately after exposure and that copious volumes of water be supplied, sometimes for hours. Occasionally, chemical burns are caused by corrosive substances insoluble in water; therefore, a solution of water and soap should frequently be used instead. However, sometimes specific antidotes for certain types of chemical burns are required. Clothes, watches, rings, shoes, etc. can be contaminated with the corrosive agent, so they should be removed.

Theoretically, neutralizing solutions should be an alternative treatment to water after exposure to acids and alkalis (Dunn et al. 1992; Yano et al. 1994; Erdmann et al. 1996). However, neutralization of the corrosive agent with weak acids/bases is not recommended for two reasons: (1) irrigation should not be delayed while waiting for a specific antidote – immediate irrigation provides the best removal of the agent, and (2) neutralization of the corrosive agent may produce an exothermic reaction, and the heat can cause further damage (Sawhney and Kaushish 1989).

Heat is generated when strong sulfuric and phosphoric acids are exposed to water; hence, a thermal burn can add to the chemical burn. Even so, an experimental study by Davidson found less skin injury when the agent, sulfuric acid, was removed by dilution with water when compared to treatment with neutralizers (Davidson 1927). Thus to prevent a burn, it is important that copious volumes of running water be applied. However, water is contraindicated in extinguishing burning metal fragments of sodium, potassium, and lithium, because a chemical burn can be caused by hydroxides formed when water is added to hot metals. These metals spontaneously ignite when exposed to water. To extinguish the burning metal, sand can be used. The burn should then be covered with cooking or mineral oil to isolate the metal from water. Metal pieces should be mechanically removed. Embedded pieces should be removed surgically. First, though, the area should be irrigated with water to prevent an alkali burn from the hydroxides already formed from the metal and water naturally present in the skin.

Skin exposed to hydrofluoric acid should be carefully irrigated with copious volumes of running tap water as soon as possible. The results of a study by Bromberg et al. on the effect of an 1 h water irrigation on hydrochloric acid burns in mice showed that less severe burns were noted when treatment began immediately, and severity of burns worsened with greater delay in treatment, even with 5 s intervals (Bromberg et al. 1965). After water irrigation, the target site then should be treated with calcium gluconate gel (2.5%) by massaging into the burned skin for at least 30 min ("K-Y Jelly," Johnson and Johnson Products, Inc., New Brunswick, NJ, USA) (Anderson and Anderson 1988; Chick and Borah 1990; Seyb et al. 1995; Dunn et al. 1996). The calcium gluconate gel can also be made by mixing 3.5 g calcium gluconate with 150 g of a water-soluble lubricant. A variation of this treatment is suggested – ten 10-g tablets of calcium carbonate (648 mg) crushed to a fine powder. The powder is mixed with 20 ml of a water-soluble lubricant to create a slurry. This calcium preparation is applied repeatedly to the skin until the pain has disappeared. Necrotic tissue should be excised, blisters debrided, and the underlying tissue treated with the calcium preparation. Nails should be removed if the acid penetrates to the nail bed and matrix and causes severe pain there. If there is no effect of the topical treatment within 2 h, 10% calcium gluconate (0.5 ml/cm^2) should be injected into and under the lesions. No anesthetics should be given, since the disappearance of pain is a sign of successful treatment. Without treatment, the burn can increase in depth for several weeks.

Superficial chemical burns from chromic acid with an area greater than 1% of the total body surface imply a high risk of systemic damage to many organs, including erythrocytes (Terrill and Gowar 1990). Therefore, immediate irrigation of the burn with copious volumes of water is necessary. Thereafter, and within 2 h after the exposure, all burnt tissue must be excised. To remove circulating chromium, peritoneal dialysis has to be carried out during the first 24 h. Solid particles of lime, cement, and phosphorus, for example, tend to fix to the skin and should be mechanically removed before or during irrigation.

Phosphorus, above all white phosphorus, is oxidized by air and can ignite spontaneously, thus causing thermal burns (Kaufman et al. 1988; Eldad and Simon 1991; Eldad et al. 1992; Eldad et al. 1995). In water, oxidized phosphorus is transformed into phosphoric acid, which can cause a chemical burn; therefore, it is important to remove particles mechanically before washing with soap and water. The skin is then washed with 1% copper(II) sulfate in water, which reacts with phosphorus to form black copper phosphite, which makes any remaining phosphorous visible and thus easily removable. Wet dressings of copper sulfate should never be applied to wounds because of the risk of systemic copper poisoning. To minimize the copper absorption, a water solution of 5% sodium bicarbonate and 3% copper sulfate suspended in 1% hydroxyethyl cellulose can be used for irrigation instead of the 1% copper sulfate solution. However, it should be stressed that copper is a potentially toxic substance, which can cause systemic effects. Copper sulfate must therefore be used only for a few minutes in order to visualize phosphorous and, after mechanical removal of the phosphide, it is important to irrigate the skin with water.

Skin contaminated with bromine or iodine should be washed frequently with soap and water and treated with 5% sodium thiosulfate, which reacts with bromine and iodine, forming ions less hazardous to the skin (White and Joseet 1990; Corazza et al. 1997).

Skin contaminated with phenolic compounds can initially be washed with soap and water, and treated as early as possible with undiluted polyethylene glycol 300 or 400, or with 10% ethanol, which all dissolve phenolic compounds (Lin and Yang 1992; Horch et al. 1994; Shibata et al. 1994). Tissues with deep damage from phenolic compounds should be excised immediately, as the compounds easily penetrate further with subsequent damage of, for example, nerves.

Skin contaminated with sulfur mustard liquid should be treated with a mixture of 75% calcium hypochlorite and 25% magnesium sulfate for some minutes before washing with soap and water. Contaminated objects should also be treated with this mixture (Newman-Taylor and Morris 1991; Smith and Dunn 1991; Ruhl et al. 1994).

Hot tar, pitch, and asphalt cause burns mainly due to the heat. They stick to the skin and should not be removed mechanically, as the skin can be further damaged and thus increase the risk of secondary infection. The material falls off spontaneously in due time.

Generally, an antibacterial cream should be given to chemical skin burns to protect the surface and to prevent secondary infection. If there is a significant element of inflammation in non-necrotic areas, a mild topical corticosteroid preparation can be used. Frequent examinations of primarily superficial and limited burns are also advisable, as they can become deeper in a few days.

Surgical treatments, such as excision, debridation of blisters, transplantation, and removal of nails can be of great value. When a limb is affected circumferentially, there is a risk of blood-vessel compression. The best method for treating the black, adherent necrotic tissue caused by cement and other toxic compounds is excision. For example, the healing time of cement burns on knees can be diminished from 8–10 weeks to 3 weeks if the necrotic tissue is excised.

Several chemicals can also produce systemic effects without severe skin injury, e.g., phenolic compounds, hydrofluoric acid, chromic acid, sulfur mustard, and gasoline (Andersen 1990; Chan et al. 1995). When the chemical burn is not minimal, there is risk of systemic damage, and an analysis including hematological screening and liver and kidney function should be made both at the first examination and then later in the course of treatment, depending on the intensity and extension of the chemical burn as well as on the results of the laboratory investigations. These analyses are performed mainly to enable precautions and measures necessary to prevent and diminish damage to internal organs, in addition to legal reasons.

Patients with severe and extensive skin damage and/or with systemic symptoms after exposure to corrosive agents should be treated in intensive care units. It should be noted that hydrofluoric acid or chromic acid exposure affecting even 1% of the total body surface of a person means risk of severe systemic effects. Hospitalization is also recommended for persons who have concurrent illnesses, implying that they are high-risk patients, as well as for persons with chemical burns on the hands, feet, and perineum (Andersen 1990; Chan et al. 1995).

7 Complications

Chemical skin burns can cause hyper- or hypopigmentation. Chemical burns involving deeper parts of the skin heal with scarring. Tumors of both malignant and benign types may rarely develop in scars. In the acute stage of chemical burns from, for example, phenolic compounds and hydrofluoric acid/fluorides, the sensory nerve system is frequently affected.

Many contact sensitizers also have irritant properties. Patch testing with such sensitizers at high concentrations can cause an irritant reaction or a chemical burn, which seems to facilitate active sensitization. However, only a few sensitizers can cause chemical burns without occlusion, e.g., formaldehyde, chromic acid, amines, chloroacetophenone, some plastic monomers, and methylisothiazolinones. Even one single contact with these chemicals can both cause a chemical burn and induce sensitization, with subsequent possible development of allergic contact dermatitis (Bruze et al. 1990; Kanerva et al. 1994). Therefore, when a potential sensitizer has caused a chemical burn, the patient should be patch tested with the sensitizer after healing of the burn, independent of any subsequent development of eczema.

Another type of eczematous dermatitis that can follow after a chemical burn is "post-traumatic eczema" (Mathias 1988). It can present as discoid eczema and is a poorly understood complication of skin injuries (Wilkinson 1979). It can appear after either physical or chemical skin injuries, including chemical burns, and is always unrelated to infection and topical treatment.

8 Prevention

Employees should be informed of the risks of exposure to corrosive agents and be well trained to handle the chemicals as well as to act when they have been exposed. Showers for rapid irrigation with water should be easily accessible. A 1% copper sulfate solution, polyethylene glycol 300 or 400, 5% sodium thiosulfate solution, and a proper calcium preparation should be present in the first-aid kit. A calcium preparation for topical treatment should also be present near employees' work site where hydrofluoric acid or fluorides are used. Workers at risk should wear proper protective equipment, which may include eye glasses, face masks, gloves, boots, and safety dresses.

In industries in which corrosive chemicals are handled, certain procedures frequently lead to accidents, resulting in exposure to the chemicals. Such procedures include the repairing as well as charging and discharging of procedure vessels, during which chemicals can be spilt and splashed. Accidents can be caused by breakage of hoses or connections with snap couplings. A non-accidental but unintended exposure may occur due to material sterilized with ethylene oxide; thus, the material should be well ventilated and not used until a week after the sterilization procedure. For these reasons, it is important to prevent chemical burns via careful planning and supervision of the working environment.

9 Summary

Thousands of chemicals and products can cause chemical skin burns, some only under special circumstances, for example, occlusion. Most chemical burns are due to accidents and the majority are occupationally induced, but chemical burns also frequently occur in households and while engaged in hobbies. Clinically, a chemical burn is characterized by erythema, blisters, and necrotic skin. Some corrosive chemicals, such as phenolic compounds, sulfur mustard, chromic acid, hydrofluoric acid, and gasoline, may cause systemic effects that require hospitalization. Other chemical burns, particularly those affecting hands, feet, and perineum, may also require hospitalization. To prevent and diminish the damage after exposure to corrosive agents, it is important to administer immediate treatment. Irrigation with copious volumes of water is a universal remedy, except for treatment of burning metal fragments of sodium, potassium, and lithium. First-aid treatment after exposure to water-insoluble corrosive agents consists of washing with soap and water. Sometimes specific antidotes are needed, as for chemical burns from hydrofluoric acid, phenolic compounds, phosphorous, iodine, bromine, and sulfur mustard (➋ *Table 13.2*). Surgical intervention may be required for certain chemical burns. A few corrosive compounds are potential sensitizers, and one single exposure to such a compound may cause both a chemical burn and induce sensitization

Table 13.2
Treatment for chemical skin burns caused by some specific chemicals

Chemical	Treatment
Hydrofluoric acid	Calcium gluconate gel (2.5%)
Phosphorous	Copper (II) sulfate in water (1%)
Bromine, iodine	Sodium thiosulfate in water (5%)
Phenolic compounds	Polyethylene glycol 300 or 400; ethanol in water (10%)
Sulfur mustard liquid	Mixture of 75% calcium hypochlorite and 25% magnesium sulfate

with subsequent allergic contact dermatitis. To prevent chemical burns, it is important to use as few corrosive agents as possible and, when unavoidable, to use the weakest ones possible, particularly in households and while engaged in hobbies. In the working environment, well-informed workers, access to first-aid treatment, careful planning, and supervision are required to prevent chemical burns.

References

Adams RM (1990) Cement burns. In: Adams RM (ed) Occupational skin disease, 2nd edn. Saunders, Philadelphia, pp 15–16

Andersen KE (1990) Systemic toxicity from percutaneous absorption of industrial chemicals. In: Adams RM (ed) Occupational skin disease, 2nd edn. Saunders, Philadelphia, pp 73–88

Anderson WJ, Anderson JR (1988) Hydrofluoric acid burns of the hand: mechanism of injury and treatment. J Hand Surg [Am] 13:52–57

Beausang E, Herbert K (1994) Burns from a dust explosion. Burns 20:551–552

Biro L, Fisher AA, Price E (1974) Ethylene oxide burns. Arch Dermatol 110:924–925

Bromberg BE, Song IC, Walden RH (1965) Hydrotherapy of chemical burns. Plast Reconstr Surg 35(1):85–95

Bruze M, Dahlquist I, Gruvberger B (1990) Chemical burns and allergic contact dermatitis due to Kathon WT. Am J Contact Dermat 1:91–93

Burgher F, Mathieu L, Blomet J (2011) The chemical agents and the involved chemical reactions. In: Schrage N, Burgher F, Blomet J, Bodson L, Gerard M, Hall A, Josset P, Mathieu L, Merle H (eds) Chemical ocular burns. Springer, Berlin/Heidelberg/New York, pp 17–48

Cartotto RC, Peters WJ, Neligan PC et al (1996) Chemical burns. Can J Surg 39:205–211

Chan TC, Williams SR, Clark RF (1995) Formic acid skin burns resulting in systemic toxicity. Ann Emerg Med 26:383–386

Chick LR, Borah G (1990) Calcium carbonate gel therapy for hydrofluoric acid burns of the hand. Plast Reconstr Surg 86:935–940

Corazza M, Bulciolu G, Spisani L et al (1997) Chemical burns following irritant contact with povidone-iodine. Contact Dermatitis 36:115–116

Davidson EC (1927) The treatment of acid and alkali burns. Ann Surg 85(4):481–489

Dunn BJ, MacKinnon MA, Knowlden NF et al (1992) Hydrofluoric acid dermal burns. An assessment of treatment efficacy using an experimental pig model. J Occup Environ Med 34:902–909

Dunn BJ, MacKinnon MA, Knowlden NF et al (1996) Topical treatment for hydrofluoric acid dermal burns. Further assessment of efficacy using an experimental pig model. J Occup Environ Med 38:507–514

Eldad A, Chaouat M, Weinberg A et al (1992) Phosphorous pentachloride chemical burn – a slowly healing injury. Burns 18:340–341

Eldad A, Simon GA (1991) The phosphorous burn – a preliminary comparative experimental study of various forms of treatment. Burns 17:198–200

Eldad A, Wisoki M, Cohen H et al (1995) Phosphorous burns: evaluation of various modalities for primary treatment. J Burn Care Rehabil 16:49–55

Erdmann D, Hussmann J, Kucan JO (1996) Treatment of a severe alkali burn. Burns 22:41–146

Fisher AA (1986) Chromate dermatitis and cement burns. In: Fisher AA (ed) Contact dermatitis, 3rd edn. Lea and Febiger, Philadelphia, pp 762–772

Fisher AA (1990) Ethylene oxide (EO) burns. In: Adams RM (ed) Occupational skin disease, 2nd edn. Saunders, Philadelphia, pp 17–18

Flammiger A, Maibach H (2006) Sulfuric acid burns (corrosion and acute irritation): evidence-based overview to management. Cutan Ocul Toxicol 25(1):55–61

Gelmetti C, Cecca E (1992) Caustic ulcers caused by calcium hydroxide in 2 adolescent football players. Contact Dermatitis 27:265–266

Horch R, Spilker G, Stark GB (1994) Phenol burns and intoxications. Burns 20:45–50

Kanerva L, Tarvainen K, Pinola A et al (1994) A single accidental exposure may result in a chemical burn, primary sensitization and allergic contact dermatitis. Contact Dermatitis 31:229–235

Kaufman T, Ullmann Y, Har-Shai Y (1988) Phosphorus burns: a practical approach to local treatment. J Burn Care Rehabil 9:474–475

Kirkpatrick JJ, Enion DS, Burd DA (1995) Hydrofluoric acid burns: a review. Burns 21:483–493

Kuniyuki S, Oonishi H (1997) Chemical burn from acetic acid with deep ulceration. Contact Dermatitis 36:169–170

Lane PR, Hogan DJ (1985) Chronic pain and scarring from cement burns. Arch Dermatol 121:368–369

Lin CH, Yang JY (1992) Chemical burn with cresol intoxication and multiple organ failure. Burns 18:162–166

Mathias CGT (1988) Post-traumatic eczema. Dermatol Clin 6:35–42

McGeown G (1984) Cement burns of the hands. Contact Dermatitis 10:246

Morley SE, Humzah D, McGregor JC et al (1996) Cement-related burns. Burns 22:646–647

Newman-Taylor AJ, Morris AJR (1991) Experience with mustard gas casualties. Lancet 337:242

Onuba O, Essiet A (1986) Cement burns of the heels. Contact Dermatitis 14:325–326

Ruhl CM, Park SJ, Danisa O et al (1994) A serious skin sulfur mustard burn from an artillery shell. J Emerg Med 12:159–166

Sawhney CP, Kaushish R (1989) Acid and alkali burns: considerations in management. Burns 15:132–134

Seyb ST, Noordhoek L, Botens S et al (1995) A study to determine the efficacy of treatments for hydrofluoric acid burns. J Burn Care Rehabil 16:253–257

Shibata K, Yoshita Y, Matsumoto H (1994) Extensive chemical burns from toluene. Am J Emerg Med 12:353–355

Smith WJ, Dunn MA (1991) Medical defense against blistering chemical warfare agents. Arch Dermatol 127:1207–1213

Stewart CE (1985) Chemical skin burns. Am Fam Physician 31:149–157

Stoermer D, Wolz G (1983) Cement burns. Contact Dermatitis 9:421–422

Sykes RA, Mani MM, Hiebert JM (1986) Chemical burns: retrospective review. J Burn Care Rehabil 7:343–347

Terrill PJ, Gowar JP (1990) Chromic acid burns; beware, be aggressive, be watchful. Br J Plast Surg 43:699–701

Tosti A, Peluso AM, Varotti C (1989) Skin burns due to transit-mixed Portland cement. Contact Dermatitis 21:58

Vance MV (1990) Hydrofluoric acid (HF) burns. In: Adams RM (ed) Occupational skin disease, 2nd edn. Saunders, Philadelphia, pp 18–21

White A, Joseet M (1990) Burns from iodine. Anaesthesia 45:75

Wilkinson DS (1979) Discoid eczema as a consequence of contact with irritants. Contact Dermatitis 5:118–199

Winemaker M, Douglas L, Peters W (1992) Combination alkali/thermal burns caused by "black liquor" in the pulp and paper industry. Burns 18:68–70

Yano K, Hata Y, Matsuka K et al (1994) Effects of washing with a neutralizing agent on alkaline skin injuries in an experimental model. Burns 20:36–39

Zekri AMB, King WWK, Yeung R et al (1995) Acute mass burns caused by o-chlorobenzylidene malononitrile (CS) tear gas. Burns 21:586–589

14 Mechanisms of Allergic Contact Dermatitis

Thomas Rustemeyer[1] · *Ingrid M. W. van Hoogstraten*[2] · *B. Mary E. von Blomberg*[2] · *Rik J. Scheper*[2]
[1]Department Dermatology/Allergology, VU University Medical Center, Amsterdam, The Netherlands
[2]Department Pathology, VU University Medical Center, Amsterdam, The Netherlands

Core Messages

- Allergenicity depends on several factors determined by the very physicochemical nature of the molecules themselves, i.e., their capacity to penetrate the horny layer, lipophilicity, and chemical reactivity. The sensitizing property of the majority of contact allergens could be predicted from these characteristics (Patlewicz et al. 2004; Gerberick et al. 2008). Two other factors, however, further contribute to the allergenicity of chemicals, viz. their pro-inflammatory activity and capacity to induce maturation of LC. These issues will be dealt with in more detail in the following sections.
- Along with their migration and settling within the draining lymph nodes, haptenized LC further mature, as characterized by their increased expression of costimulatory and antigen-presentation molecules (Cumberbatch et al. 1997; Heufler et al. 1988). In addition, they adopt a strongly veiled, interdigitating appearance, thus maximizing the chances of productive encounters with naive T lymphocytes and recognition of altered self (Steinman et al. 1995; Furue et al. 1996; Schuler and Steinman 1985).
- The intricate structure of lymph node paracortical areas, the differential expression of chemokines and their receptors, the characteristic membrane ruffling of IDC, and the predominant circulation of naïve T lymphocytes through these lymph node areas provide optimal conditions for T-cell-receptor binding, i.e., the first signal for induction of T-cell activation (Banchereau and Steinman 1998). Intimate DC–T-cell contacts are further strengthened by secondary signals, provided by sets of cellular adhesion molecules, and growth-promoting cytokines (reviewed in Hommel (2004), Cella et al. (1997)).
- In healthy individuals, primary skin contacts with contact allergens lead to differentiation and expansion of allergen-specific effector T cells displaying Th1, Th2, and/or Th17 cytokine profiles. The same allergens, if encountered along mucosal surfaces, favor the development of allergen-specific Th2 and Th17 effector cells, and/or Th3 and Tr1 allergen-specific regulatory T cells. Whereas the first two subsets may assist or replace Th1 cells in pro-inflammatory effector functions, the latter two subsets are mainly known for downregulating immune responsiveness. For most, if not all allergens, along with prolonged allergenic contacts, the role of Th2 cells as effector cells gradually increases given reduced longevity of Th1 responses.
- The respective contributions of similar subsets of allergen-specific $CD8^+$ T cells are still unknown, but distinct effector roles of allergen-specific Tc1 and Tc2 have been postulated.
- Priming via the skin results in CLA positive T cells, which upon inflammatory stimuli preferentially enter the skin; on the other hand, gut homing T cells have been primed and generated along mucosal surfaces. Upon priming, T cells loose much of their capacity to recirculate via the lymph nodes, but gain the capacity to enter the tissues. In particular recently activated T cells will enter skin inflammatory sites. ACD reactions are primarily infiltrated by CD4 and/or CD8 pro-inflammatory cells, later reactions may be dominated by Th2 cells and regulatory T cells. Skin infiltation by T cells is fine-tuned by sets of adhesion molecules and chemokine receptors, whose expression is not rigid, but can be modulated by micro-environmental factors.
- After antigenic activation the progeny of primed T cells is released via the efferent lymphatics into the bloodstream. Circulating allergen-specific cells can be challenged in vitro to provide diagnostic parameters for contact hypersensitivity. At least for water-soluble allergens, like metal salts, the degree of allergen-specific proliferation and cytokine production, in particular type-2 cytokines, correlate with clinical allergy. For routine application of a broad spectrum of allergens, culture conditions still need to be improved. For mechanistic in vitro studies in ACD, however, with selected sets of relatively nontoxic allergens, peripheral blood provides an excellent source of lymphocytes and antigen-presenting cells.

T. Rustemeyer, P. Elsner, S.M. John & H.I. Maibach (eds.), *Kanerva's Occupational Dermatology*,
DOI 10.1007/978-3-642-02035-3_14,

- ACD reactions can be mediated by classical effector cells, i.e., allergen-specific $CD4^+$ type-1 T cells which, upon triggering by allergen-presenting cells, produce IFN-γ to activate nonspecific inflammatory cells like macrophages. However, $CD8^+$ T cells, and other cytokines, including IL-4, IL-17, and IL-22 can also play major roles in ACD. The conspicuous difference with DTH reactions induced by intradermal administration of protein antigens, i.e., the epidermal infiltrate, can largely be attributed to hapten-induced chemokine release by keratinocytes.

1 Introduction

During the past few decades, the understanding of why, where, and when allergic contact dermatitis (ACD) might develop has rapidly increased. Critical discoveries include the identification of T cells as mediators of cell-mediated immunity, their thymic origin and recirculation patterns, and the molecular basis of their specificity to just one or few allergens out of the thousands of allergens known (Janeway 2008). Progress has also resulted from the identification of genes that determine T-cell function, and the development of monoclonal antibodies that recognize their products. Moreover, the production of large amounts of recombinant products, e.g., cytokines and chemokines, and the breeding of mice with disruptions in distinct genes (knockout mice) or provided with additional genes of interest (transgenic mice), have allowed in-depth analysis of skin-inflammatory processes, such as those taking place in ACD.

Although humoral antibody-mediated reactions can be a factor, ACD depends primarily on the activation of allergen-specific T cells (Bergstresser 1989), and is regarded as a prototype of delayed hypersensitivity, as classified by Turk (1975) and Gell and Coombs (type IV hypersensitivity) (Gell et al. 1975). Evolutionarily, cell-mediated immunity has developed in vertebrates to facilitate eradication of microorganisms and toxins. Elicitation of ACD by usually nontoxic doses of small molecular weight allergens indicates that the T-cell repertoire is often slightly broader than one might wish. Thus, ACD can be considered to reflect an untoward side effect of a well-functioning immune system.

Subtle differences can be noted in macroscopic appearance, time course, and histopathology of allergic contact reactions in various vertebrates, including rodents and man (Mestas and Hughes 2004). Nevertheless, essentially all basic features are shared. Since both mouse and guinea pig models, next to clinical studies, have greatly contributed to our present knowledge of ACD, both data sets provide the basis for this chapter.

In ACD, a distinction should be made between induction (also known as sensitization or primary) and effector (also known as elicitation or secondary) phases (Saint-Mezard et al. 2003) (➋ *Fig. 14.1*). The induction phase includes the events following a first contact with the allergen and is complete when the individual is sensitized and capable of giving a positive ACD reaction. The effector phase begins upon elicitation (challenge) and results in clinical manifestation of ACD. The entire process of the induction phase requires at least 4 days to several weeks, whereas the effector phase reaction is fully developed within 1–4 days. Main episodes in the induction phase (steps 1–5) and effector phase (step 6) are:

1. *Binding of allergen to skin components.* The allergen penetrating the skin readily associates with all kinds of skin components, including major histocompatibility complex (MHC) proteins. These molecules, in humans encoded for by histocompatibility antigen (HLA) genes, are abundantly present on epidermal antigen-presenting cells, called Langerhans cells (LC) (Lepoittevin 2006; Gerberick et al. 2008; Divkovic et al. 2005).
2. *Hapten-induced activation of allergen-presenting cells.* Allergen-carrying LC become activated, mature, and travel via the afferent lymphatics to the regional lymph nodes, where they settle as so-called interdigitating cells (IDC) in the paracortical T-cell areas.
3. *Recognition of allergen-modified LC by specific T cells.* In nonsensitized individuals the frequency of T cells with certain specificities is usually far below 1 per million. Within the paracortical areas, conditions are optimal for allergen-carrying IDC to encounter naive T cells that specifically recognize the allergen–MHC molecule complexes. The dendritic morphology of these allergen-presenting cells strongly facilitates multiple cell contacts, leading to binding and activation of allergen-specific T cells.
4. *Proliferation of specific T cells in draining lymph nodes.* Supported by interleukin (IL)-1, released by the allergen-presenting cells, activated T cells start producing several growth factors, including IL-2 (Hoyer et al. 2008). A partly autocrine cascade follows since at the same time receptors for IL-2 are upregulated in these cells, resulting in vigorous blast formation and proliferation within a few days.
5. *Systemic propagation of the specific T-cell progeny.* The expanded progeny is subsequently released via the efferent lymphatics into the blood flow and begins to recirculate. Thus, the frequency of specific

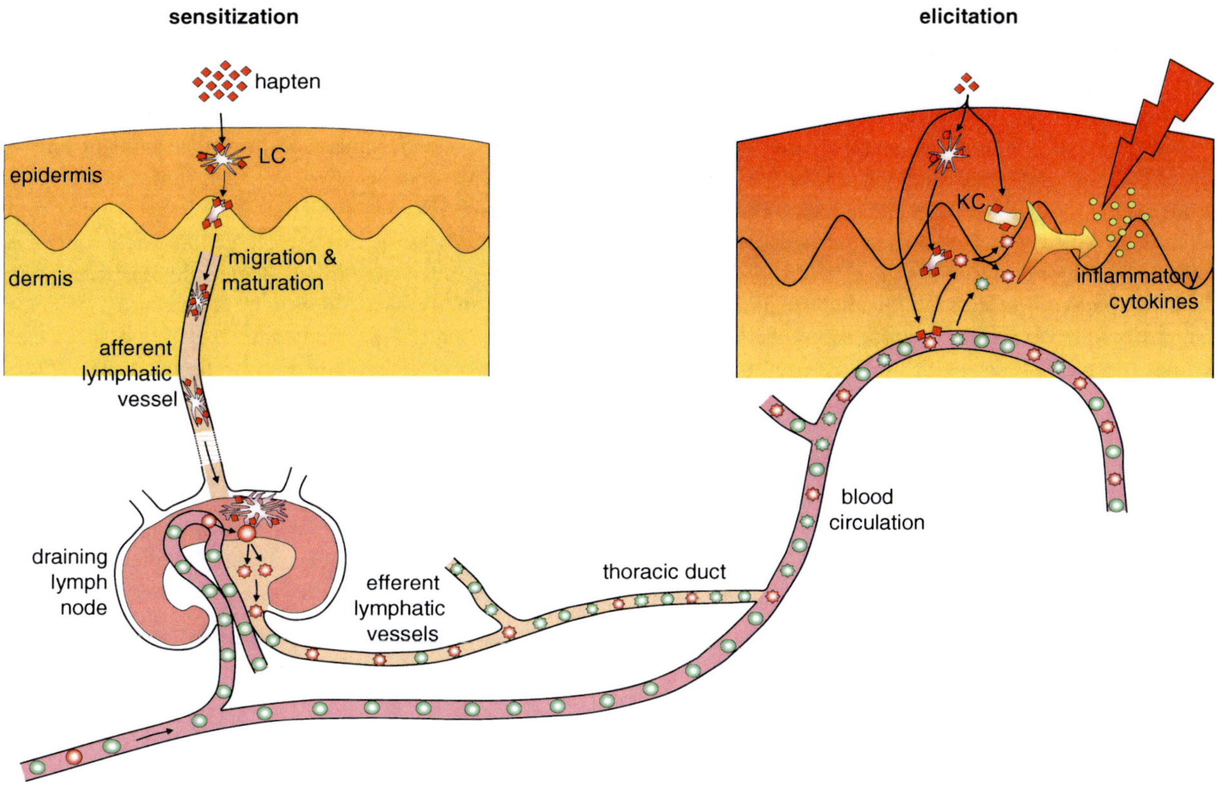

Fig. 14.1

Immunological events in allergic contact dermatitis (ACD). During the induction phase (*left*), skin contact with a hapten triggers migration of epidermal Langerhans cells (*LC*) via the afferent lymphatic vessels to the skin-draining lymph nodes. Haptenized LC home into the T cell-rich paracortical areas. Here, conditions are optimal for encountering naïve T cells that specifically recognize allergen–MHC molecule complexes. Hapten-specific T cells now expand abundantly and generate effector and memory cells, which are released via the efferent lymphatics into the circulation. With their newly acquired homing receptors, these cells can easily extravasate peripheral tissues. Renewed allergen contact sparks off the effector phase (*right*). Due to their lowered activation threshold, hapten-specific effector T cells are triggered by various haptenized cells, including *LC* and keratinocytes (*KC*), to produce proinflammatory cytokines and chemokines. Thereby, more inflammatory cells are recruited further amplifying local inflammatory mediator release. This leads to a gradually developing eczematous reaction, reaching a maximum within 18–48 h, after which reactivity successively declines

effector-memory T cells in the blood may rise to as high as one in a thousand, whereas most of these cells display receptor molecules facilitating their migration into peripheral tissues. In the absence of further allergen contacts, their frequency gradually decreases in subsequent weeks or months, but does not return to the low levels found in naive individuals.

6. *Effector phase.* By renewed allergen contact, the effector phase is initiated, which depends not only on the increased frequency of specific T cells, and their altered migratory capacities, but also on their low activation threshold. Thus, within the skin, allergen-presenting cells and specific T cells can meet, and lead to plentiful local cytokine and chemokine release. The release of these mediators, many of which have a pro-inflammatory action, causes the arrival of more inflammatory cells, thus further amplifying local mediator release. This leads to a gradually developing eczematous reaction that reaches its maximum after 18–72 h and then declines.

The following sections discuss these six main episodes of the ACD reaction in more detail. Furthermore, the chapter will discuss local hyperreactivity, such as flare-up and retest reactivity, and hyporeactivity, i.e., upon desensitization or tolerance induction.

2 Binding of Contact Allergens to Skin Components

Chemical Nature of Contact Allergens. Most contact allergens are small, chemically reactive molecules with a molecular weight less than 500 Da (Bos and Meinardi 2000) (➋ *Fig. 14.2*). Since these molecules are too small to be antigenic themselves, contact sensitizers are generally referred to as haptens.

Upon penetration through the epidermal horny layer, haptens readily conjugate to endogenous epidermal and dermal molecules. Sensitizing organic compounds may covalently bind to protein nucleophilic groups, such as thiol, amino, and hydroxyl groups, as is the case with poison oak/ivy allergens (reviewed in Roberts and Lepoittevin 1998). Examples of contact allergens containing electrophilic components include aldehydes, ketones, amides, or polarized bonds. Metal ions, e.g., nickel cations, instead form stable metal–protein chelate complexes by coordination bonds (Budinger and Hertl 2000). The most reactive nucleophilic side chains are those found in the amino acids lysine, cysteine, and histidine (Gerberick et al. 2008). Of note, their degree of ionization and hence nucleophilicity is dependent on the pH of the microenvironment which is influenced by surrounding amino acids as well as protein location within the epithelium (Divkovic et al. 2005). Predicting the chemicals that can function as haptens in allergic contact dermatitis as well as identifying cutaneous proteins involved in hapten–protein complexes is the subject of current intense investigations (Gerberick et al. 2008; Mutschler et al. 2009; Lepoittevin 2006).

Hapten Presentation by Langerhans cells (LC). Sensitization is critically dependent on direct association of haptens with epidermal LC-bound MHC molecules, or peptides present in the groove of these molecules. Both MHC class I and class II molecules may be altered this way, and thus give rise to allergen-specific $CD8^+$ and $CD4^+$

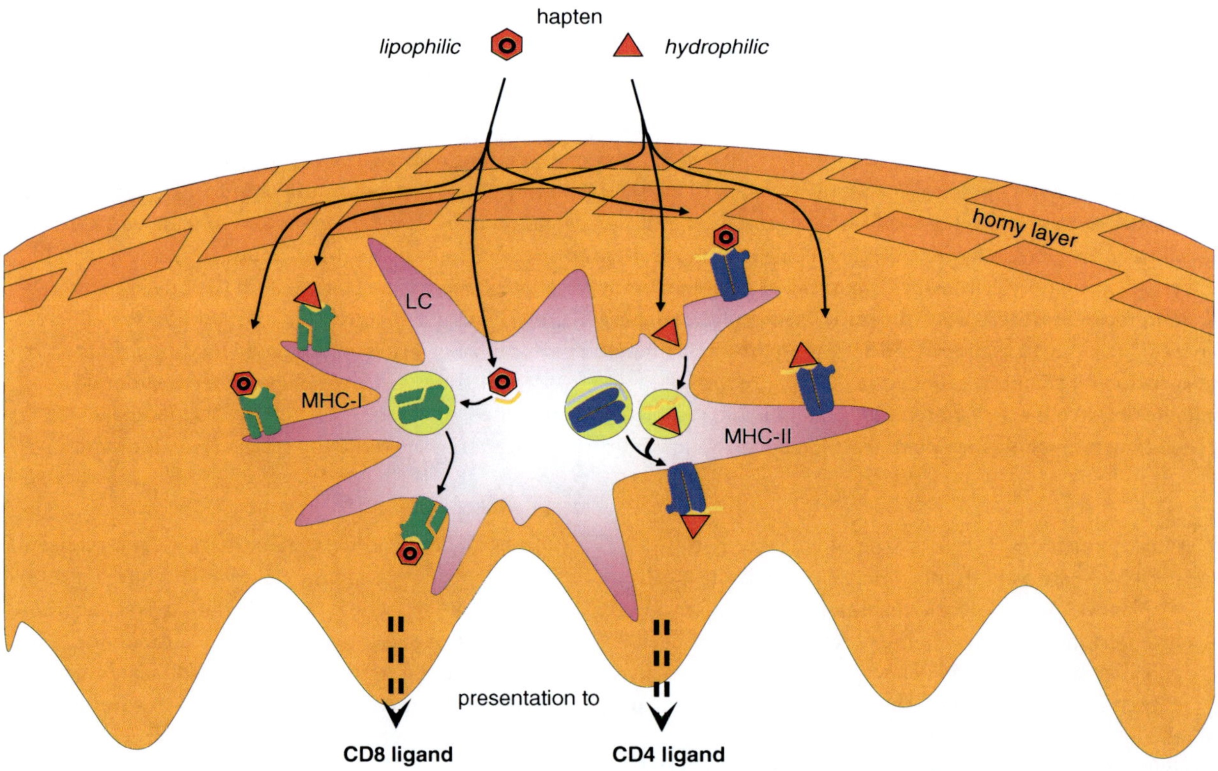

Fig. 14.2
Hapten presentation by epidermal Langerhans cells. Allergen penetrating into the epidermis readily associates with all kinds of skin components, including major histocompatibility complex (*MHC*) proteins, abundantly present on epidermal Langerhans cells (*LC*). Both MHC class I and class II molecules may be altered directly or via intracellular hapten processing and, subsequently, be recognized by allergen-specific $CD8^+$ and $CD4^+$ T cells

T cells, respectively. Distinct differences between allergens can, however, arise from differences in chemical reactivity and lipophilicity (➋ *Fig. 14.2*), since association with MHC molecules may also result from internalization of the haptens, followed by their intracellular processing as free hapten molecules or hapten–carrier complexes. Lipophilic haptens can directly penetrate into LC, conjugate with cytoplasmic proteins and be processed along the "endogenous" processing route, thus favoring association with MHC class I molecules (Blauvelt et al. 2003). In contrast, hydrophilic allergens such as nickel ions may, after conjugation with skin proteins, be processed along the "exogenous" route of antigen processing and thus favor the generation of altered MHC class II molecules. Thus, the chemical nature of the haptens can determine to what extent allergen-specific $CD8^+$ and/or $CD4^+$ T cells will be activated (Kimber et al. 2002; Liberato et al. 1981; Kalish et al. 1994; Toebak et al. 2006).

Pre- and Prohaptens. Whereas most contact allergens can form hapten–carrier complexes spontaneously, some need activation first. Contact allergens requiring activation outside the body, e.g., by UV-light or oxygen, are called prehaptens (Naisbitt 2004; Lepoittevin 2006). The typical photoallergen tetrachlorosalicylanilide is a prototype of this. Tetrachlorosalicylanilide, which undergoes photochemical dechlorination with UV irradiation, ultimately provides photoadducts with skin proteins (Epling et al. 1988). Contact allergens dependent on activation inside the body, e.g., by enzyme-induced metabolic conversion, are referred to as prohaptens. A classical prohapten is *p*-phenylenediamine, which needs to be oxidized by *N*-acetyltransferases to a reactive metabolite which can form a trimer, known as Bandrowski's base (Krasteva et al. 1993; Merk et al. 2004). Reduced enzyme activity in certain individuals, related to genetic enzyme polymorphisms, explains the reduced risk of sensitization to prohaptens that need enzymatic activation (Schnuch et al. 1998; Karlberg et al. 2008; Blömeke et al. 2009).

3 Hapten-Induced Activation of Allergen-Presenting Cells

Physiology of Langerhans Cells. Although originally thought to be neurons based on their staining properties and cellular morphology (Langerhans 1868), LC subsequently were surmised to function as "professional" antigen-presenting cells (Wilson and Villadangos 2004). They form a contiguous network within the epidermis and represent 2–5% of the total epidermal cell population (Hoath and Leahy 2003). Their principal functions are internalization, processing, transport, and presentation of skin-encountered antigens (Breathnach 1988; Romani et al. 2003). As such, LC play a pivotal role in the induction of cutaneous immune responses to infectious agents as well as to contact sensitizers (Kimber and Dearman 2003; Inaba et al. 1986; Kimber and Cumberbatch 1992). Recent studies of LC indicate that this cell type has direct epidermal innervations and can respond to a number of neurotransmitters (among them are calcitonin gene-related peptide, α-melanocyte stimulating hormone and substance P) (Luger 2002). Most of the experimental evidence to date indicates a suppressive effect of the neurohormones and neuropeptides on Langerhans cell function and cutaneous inflammation, but it has become evident lately that the timing of exposure to a stimulus is critical to the outcome of the immune response (Romagnani 2006). Thus, administration of a stress hormone or exposure to a stressor before the LC encounters an allergen may diminish the immune response toward that substance, while a stressor may enhance immune function when acting on a maturing LC or before reexposure to the allergen (Seiffert et al. 2006). LC originate from $CD34^+$ bone marrow progenitors, entering the epidermis via the blood stream (Dieu et al. 1998). Their continuous presence in the epidermis is also assured by local proliferation (Stingl et al. 1978; Czernielewski and Demarchez 1987). They reside as relatively immature DC, characterized by a high capacity to gather antigens by macropinocytosis, whereas their capacity to stimulate naïve T cells is still underdeveloped at this stage (Streilein and Grammer 1989). Their prominent dendritic morphology and the presence of distinctive Birbeck granules were observed long ago (Langerhans 1868; Birbeck 1961; Braathen 1980). In the last decade, their pivotal function in the induction of skin immune responses was explained by high expression of molecules mediating antigen presentation (e.g., MHC class I and II, CD1), as well as of cellular adhesion and costimulatory molecules (e.g., CD54, CD80, CD86, and cutaneous lymphocyte antigen [CLA]) (Kimber et al. 1998, 2002; Park et al. 1998).

Hapten-Induced LC Activation. Upon topical exposure to contact sensitizers, or other appropriate stimuli (e.g., trauma, irradiation), up to 40% of the local LC become activated (Weinlich et al. 1998; Richters et al. 1994), leave the epidermis, and migrate, via afferent lymphatic vessels, to the draining lymph nodes (Jakob et al. 2001) (➋ *Fig. 14.3*). This process of LC migration results from several factors, including contact allergen-induced production of cytokines favoring LC survival (Ozawa et al. 1996; Wong et al. 1997; Aiba and Tagami 1999) and

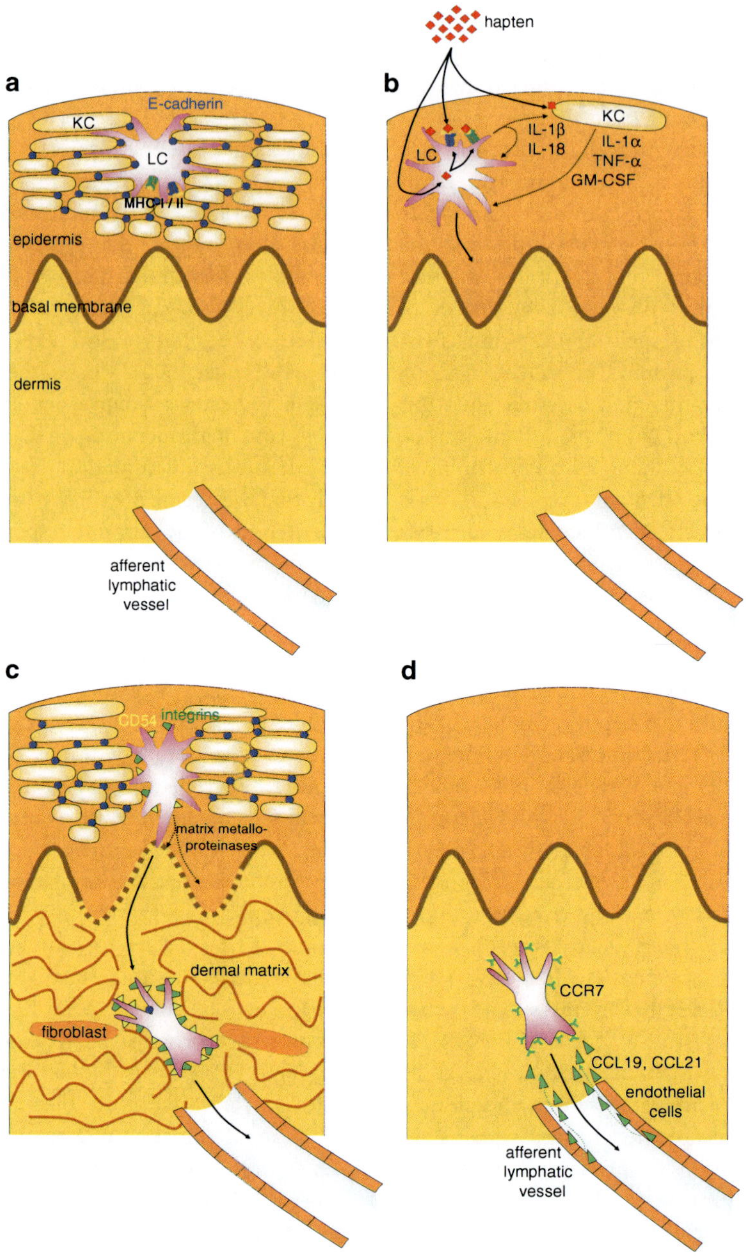

Fig. 14.3

(a–d) Hapten-induced migration of Langerhans cells. (a) In a resting state, epidermal Langerhans cells (*LC*) reside in suprabasal cell layers, tightly bound to surrounding keratinocytes (*KC*), e.g., by E-cadherin. (b) Early after epidermal hapten exposure, LC produce IL-1β and IL-18, which induces the release of IL-1α, TNF-α and GM-CSF from keratinocytes. Together, these three cytokines facilitate migration of LC from the epidermis toward the lymph nodes. (c) Emigration of LC starts with cytokine-induced disentanglement from surrounding keratinocytes (e.g., by downregulation of E-cadherin) and production of factors facilitating penetration of the basal membrane (e.g., matrix metalloproteinases) and interactions with extracellular matrix and dermal cells (e.g., integrins and integrin ligands). (d) Once in the dermis, LC migration is directed toward the draining afferent lymphatic vessels, guided by local production of chemokines (e.g., CCL19 and CCL21) acting on newly expressed chemokine receptors, such as CCR7, on activated LC. Along their journey, haptenized LC further mature as characterized by their increased dendritic morphology and expression of costimulatory and antigen-presentation molecules

loosening from surrounding keratinocytes (Inaba et al. 1993; Jakob and Udey 1998; Schwarzenberger and Udey 1996). Thus, within 15 min after exposure to a contact sensitizer, production of IL-1β mRNA is induced (Enk 1992; Enk et al. 1993). Along with this, caspase-1, formerly known as interleukin-1-converting enzyme, is activated and cleaves the active IL1 β cytokine from the translated precursor-IL1β protein. Caspase-1 activates also IL-18 from its precursor form. These inflammatory processes are now viewed at as making up the "inflammasome" (Iversen and Johansen 2008). IL-1β in concert with IL-18 stimulates release of tumor necrosis factor (TNF)-α and granulocyte-macrophage colony-stimulating factor (GM-CSF) from keratinocytes (Iversen and Johansen 2008). Together, these three cytokines facilitate migration of LC from the epidermis toward the lymph nodes (Wang et al. 2003; Steinman et al. 1995). IL-1β and TNF-α downregulate membrane-bound E-cadherin expression and thus cause disentanglement of LC from surrounding keratinocytes (➋ *Fig. 14.3*) (Schwarzenberger and Udey 1996; Tang et al. 1993; Jakob and Udey 1998). Simultaneously, adhesion molecules are upregulated promoting LC migration by mediating interactions with the extracellular matrix and dermal cells, such as CD54, α_6 integrin, and CD44 variants (Ma et al. 1994; Rambukhana et al. 1995; Price et al. 1997; Weiss et al. 1997; Brand et al. 1999). Also, production of the epidermal basement membrane degrading enzyme metalloproteinase-9 is upregulated in activated LC (Kobayashi 1997).

Next, LC migration is directed by hapten-induced alterations in chemokine receptor levels (Randolph 2001). Upon maturation, LC downregulate expression of receptors for inflammatory chemokines (e.g., CCR1, 2, 5, and 6), whereas others (including CCR4, 7, and CXCR4) are upregulated (➋ *Fig. 14.3*) (reviewed by Sallusto (1998a), Zlotnik et al. (1999), Caux et al. (2000), Sallusto et al. (1999)). Notably, CCR7 may guide maturing LC into the draining lymphatics and the lymph node paracortical areas, since two of its ligands (CCL19 and 21) are produced by both lymphatic and high endothelial cells (Saeki et al. 1999; Gunn et al. 1998). Importantly, the same receptor-ligand interactions cause naive T cells, which also express CCR7, to accumulate within the paracortical areas (Kim and Broxmeyer 1999). Migratory responsiveness of both cell types to CCR7 ligands is promoted by leukotriene C4, released from these cells via the transmembrane transporter molecule Abcc1 (previously called MRP1) (Randolph 2001; Robbiani et al. 2000; Honig et al. 2003; van de Ven et al. 2009). Interestingly, Abcc1 belongs to the same superfamily as the transporter associated with antigen-processing TAP, known to mediate intracellular peptide transport in the "endogenous route" which favors peptide association with MHC Class I molecules. Final positioning of the LC within the paracortical T-cell areas may be due to another CCR7 ligand, EBI1-ligand chemokine (ELC, CCL19), produced by resident mature DC (Sallusto 1998).

4 Recognition of Allergen-Modified Langerhans' Cells by Specific T Cells

Homing of Naive T Cells into Lymph Nodes. More than 90% of naive lymphocytes present within the paracortical T-cell areas have entered the lymph nodes by high endothelial venules (HEV) (Haig et al. 1999). These cells are characterized not only by CCR7 but also by the presence of a high molecular weight isoform of CD45 (CD45RA) (Haig et al. 1999; Altin and Sloan 1997). Entering the lymph nodes via HEV is established by the lymphocyte adhesion molecule L-selectin (CD62L), which allows rolling interaction along the vessel walls by binding to peripheral node addressins (PNAd), such as GlyCAM-1 or CD34 (Schon et al. 2003; von Andrian and Mrini 1998; Vestweber and Blanks 1999). Next, firm adhesion is mediated by the interaction of CD11a/CD18 with endothelial CD54, resulting in subsequent endothelial transmigration. Extravasation and migration of naïve T cells to the paracortical T-cell areas is supported by chemokines such as CCL18, 19, and 21 produced locally by HEV and by hapten-loaded and resident DC (Robbiani et al. 2000; Adema et al. 1997; Ngo et al. 1998; Nagira et al. 1997). In non-sensitized individuals, frequencies of contact-allergen-specific T cells are very low, and estimates vary from 1 per 109 to maximally 1 per 106 (Haig et al. 1999; Rustemeyer et al. 1999). Nevertheless, the preferential homing of naive T cells into the lymph node paracortical areas, and the large surface area of interdigitating cells, make allergen-specific T-cell activation likely with only few dendritic cells exposing adequate densities of haptenized MHC molecules (Crivellato et al. 2004; Itano and Jenkins 2003).

Activation of Hapten-Specific T Cells. As outlined in "Binding of Contact Allergens to Skin Components," the chemical nature of the hapten determines its eventual cytoplasmic routing in antigen-presenting cells (APC), and thus whether presentation will be predominantly in context of MHC class I or II molecules (➋ *Fig. 14.2*). T cells, expressing CD8 or CD4 molecules can recognize hapten-MHC class I or II complexes showing stabilized MHC membrane expression (Griem et al. 1998; Moulon et al. 1995).

Chances of productive interactions with T cells are high since each MHC-allergen complex can trigger a high number of T-cell receptor (TCR) molecules ("serial triggering") (Li et al. 2004). Moreover, after contacting specific $CD4^+$ T cells, hapten-presenting DC may reach a stable super-activated state, allowing for efficient activation of subsequently encountered specific $CD8^+$ T cells (Schoenberger et al. 1998). The actual T-cell activation is executed by TCRξ-chain mediated signal transduction, followed by an intracellular cascade of biochemical events, including protein phosphorylation, inositol phospholipid hydrolysis, increase in cytosolic Ca^{2+} (Gascoigne and Zal 2004; Cantrell 1996), and activation of transcription factors, ultimately leading to gene activation (➲ *Fig. 14.4*) (Kuo and Leiden 1999).

For activation and proliferation, TCR triggering ("signal 1") is insufficient, but hapten-presenting APC also provide the required costimulation (➲ *"signal 2"; Fig. 14.5*) (Davis and van der Merwe 2003; Trautmann and Randriamampita 2003). The costimulatory signals may involve secreted molecules, such as cytokines (IL-1), or sets of cellular adhesion molecules (CAMs) and their counter-structures present on the outer cellular membranes of APC and T cells. Expression levels of most of these CAMs vary with their activational status, and thus can provide positive stimulatory feedback loops. For example, as mentioned above, after specific TCR binding and ligation of CD40L (CD154) on T cells with CD40 molecules, APC reach a superactivated state, characterized by overexpression of several CAMs, including CD80 and CD86 (➲ *Fig. 14.4*) (Acuto and Michel 2003; Quezada et al. 2004). In turn, these molecules bind to and increase expression of CD28 on T cells. This interaction stabilizes CD154 expression, causing amplified CD154–CD40 signaling (Dong et al. 2003).

The activational cascade is, as illustrated above, characterized by mutual activation of both hapten-presenting APC and hapten-reactive T cells. Whereas this activation protects the APC from apoptotic death and prolongs their life to increase the chance of activating their cognate T cells, only the latter capitalize on these interactions by giving rise to progeny. As discussed below, to promote T-cell growth, cellular adhesion stimuli need to be complimented by a broth of cytokines, many of which are released by the same APC. Together, elevated expression levels of (co-)stimulatory molecules on APC and local abundance of cytokines overcome the relatively high activation threshold of naive T cells (Viola and Lanzavecchia 1996).

5 Proliferation and Differentiation of Specific T Cells

T-Cell Proliferation. Upon their activation, naive allergen-specific T cells start producing several cytokines, including IL-2, the classical T-cell growth factor (Crispin 2009; Malek 2009). In particular, ligation of T cell-bound CD28 receptors unleashes full-scale IL-2 production in T cells by increasing IL-2 transcription and mRNA stabilization (Pei 2008). T-cell IL-2 production peaks within 24 h and declines subsequently (Villarino 2007). Concomitant upregulation of the IL-2 receptor α-chain facilitates the assembly of high-affinity IL-2 receptor complexes which augment autocrine T-cell responsiveness, thus providing a positive feedback loop leading to T-cell clonal expansions up to 1,000 fold (Lan 2008). The process of proliferation can be visible as an impressive, sometimes painful lymph node swelling.

T-Cell Differentiation. Whereas allergen specificity remains strictly conserved along with their proliferation, within few days T cells show distinct expression of transcription factors associated with varying cytokine production profiles and surface marker expression (Zhu and Paul 2008; Sallusto 2009; Dong 2008; Oboki 2008). Thus, the recent offspring of allergen-specific $CD4^+$ T cells can show at least five distinct cytokine profiles, generally associated with helper/effector or regulatory/suppressive functions (➲ *Fig. 14.5*). Type-1 Th cells are characterized by a predominant release of IFN-γ, IL-2, and TNF-β, all known as prototypical pro-inflammatory and cytotoxic cytokines. Type-2 Th cells secrete IL-4, IL-5, IL-13, which have distinct pro-inflammatory activities but are most prominent in promoting humoral antibody production, e.g., along mucosal surfaces where IgA contributes to exclusion of microbial entry (Dabbagh and Lewis 2003; Faria and Weiner 2006). Next, the Th3 subset is distinguished by its release of transforming growth factor (TGF)-β, which displays anti-inflammatory activities (Allan et al. 2008; Faria and Weiner 2006). Recently, Th-17 cells have been recognized as a separate lineage of pro-inflammatory T cells, characterized by production of IL-17A and IL-17E, as well as IL-22, all of which play pivotal roles in auto-immune diseases, e.g., by recruiting neutrophils and macrophages (Korn et al. 2009; Louten 2009). Finally, still another subset of $CD4^+$ T cells is recognized for its strong regulatory role in controlling inflammatory reactivities, i.e., the Tr1 cells or "inducible Tregs," characterized by the secretion of IL-10 (Zhu and Paul 2008; Allan et al. 2008; Sallusto 2009). This $CD4^+$ T-cell population is phenotypically remarkably heterogeneous, with part of the cells expressing high amounts of the high affinity IL-2 receptor ("$CD25^{high}$"), either or not

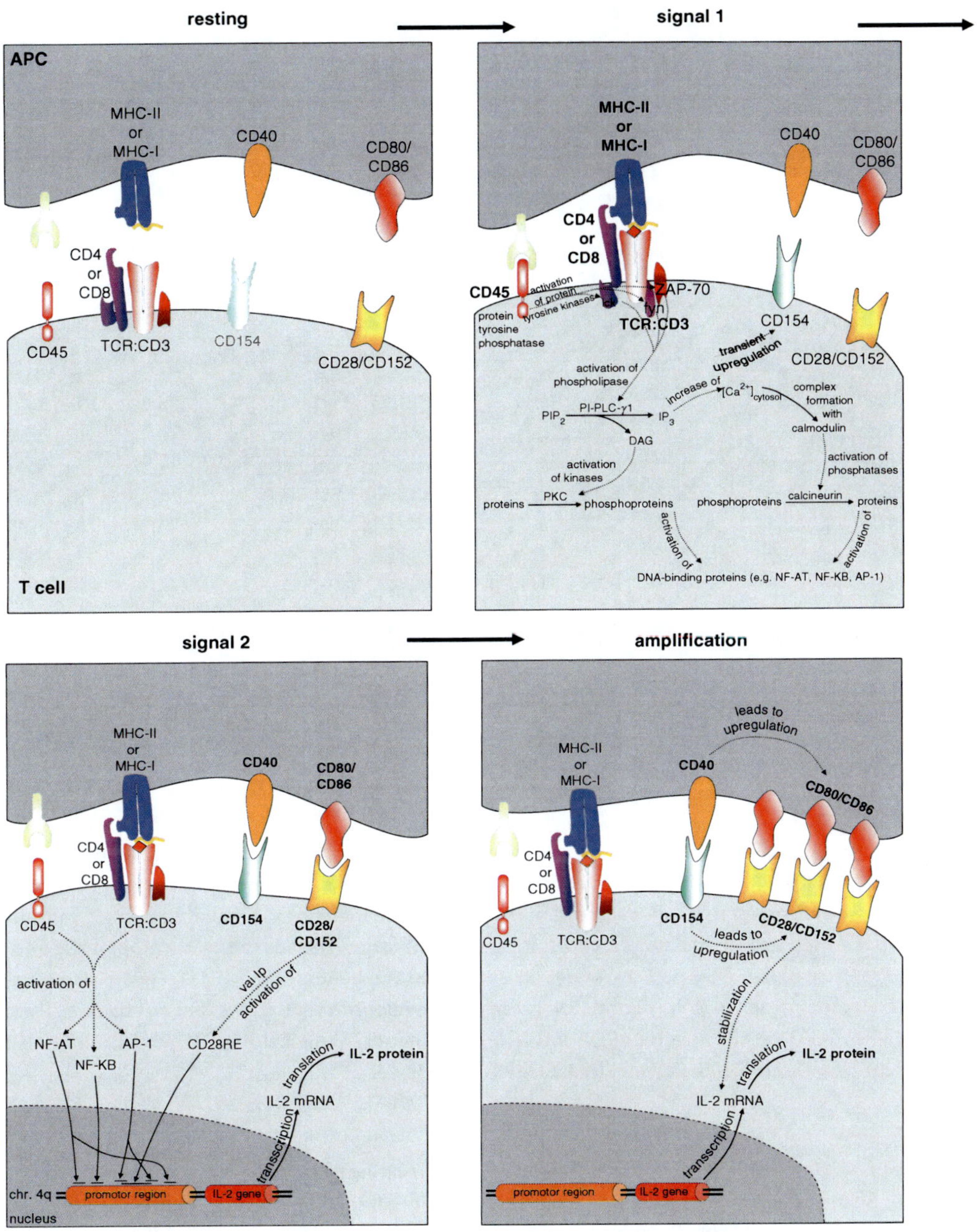

■ **Fig. 14.4**

Activation of hapten-specific T cells. T-cell receptor (TCR) triggering by hapten–major histocompatibility complex (*MHC*) complexes ("signal 1") is insufficient for T-cell activation. But "professional" antigen-presenting cells (*APC*), such as Langerhans cells, can provide the required costimulation ("signal 2"), involving secreted molecules, such as cytokines, or sets of cellular adhesion molecules present on the outer cellular membranes of APC and T cells. T cells, stimulated in this way, activate nuclear responder elements (e.g., CD28RE). Together with nuclear transcription factors (*NF*), produced upon TCR triggering, these nuclear responder elements enable transcription of T-cell growth factors, e.g., IL-2. APC–T cell interaction gives rise to mutual activation ("amplification"): on APC, ligation of CD40 with CD154 molecules on T cells induces overexpression of several costimulatory molecules, including CD80 and CD86. In turn, these molecules bind to and increase expression of CD28 on T cells. This interaction stabilizes CD154 expression, causing amplified CD154–CD40 signaling, and preserves strong IL-2 production, finally resulting in abundant T-cell expansion

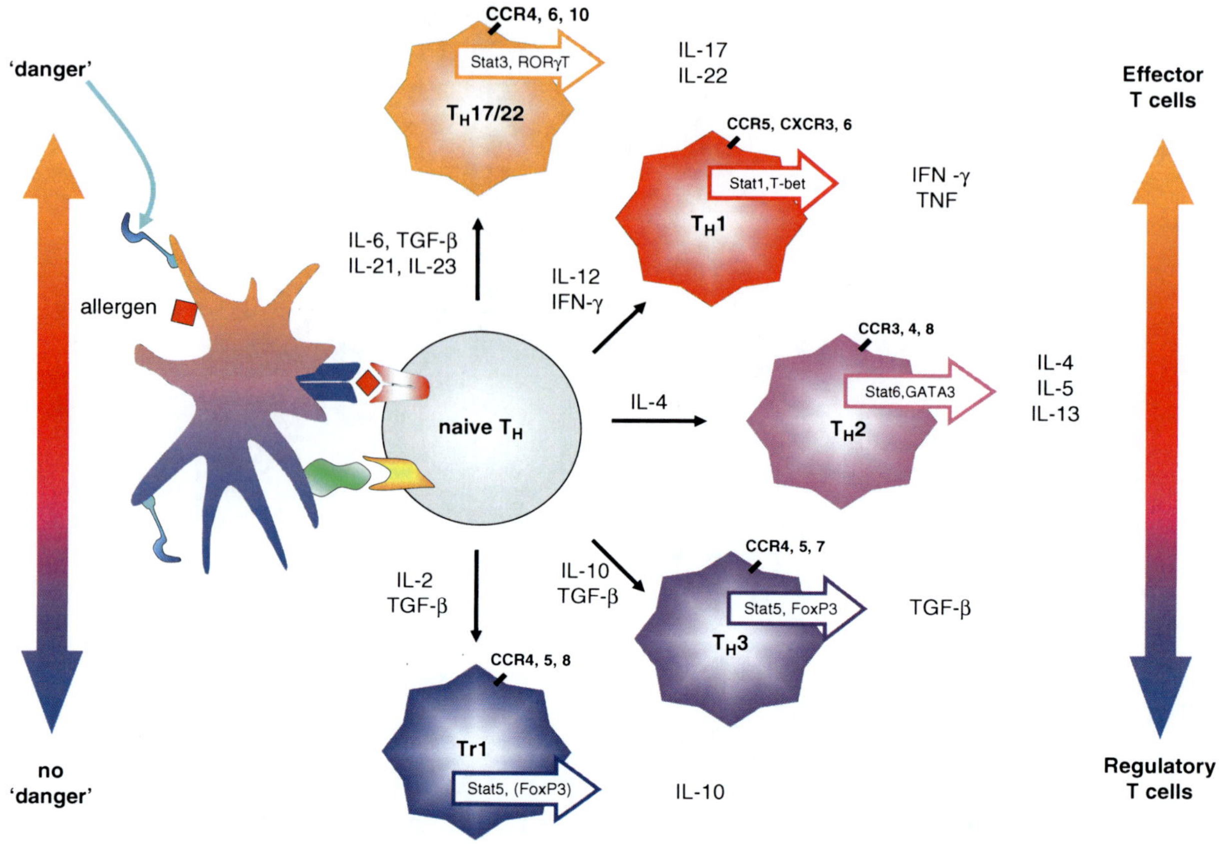

Fig. 14.5

Spectrum of allergen driven CD4$^+$ T cell differentiation: current schematic view. Depending on the immunological microenvironment (amount of allergen, danger signals, and other soluble mediators), activated naïve T cells are skewed into distinct phenotypes. The presence of allergen and sufficient danger signals leads to the development of effector T cell phenotypes of ACD. Presence of IL-6, TGF-β, IL-21, and IL-23 stimulates the generation of TH17/Th23 cells. Development of TH1 cells is stimulated by the presence of IL-12 and IFN-γ, and the development of TH2 is favored by IL-4. The absence of sufficient danger signals stimulates the development of tolerogenic phenotypes, including TH3 and Tr1 (Larsen 2009; Dong 2008; Zhu 2008; Duhen 2009; Ward 2009; Cavani 2008; Sallusto 2009)

accompanied by expression of the transcription factor FoxP3 (Romagnani 2006; Feuerer 2009; Cavani 2008) (➋ *Fig. 14.5*). Tr1 cells have essential roles in maintenance of immune homeostasis, regulating effector T-cell responses and preventing their potentially pathogenic effects by various indirect ways, e.g., by suppressing macrophage functions (Wu et al. 2007; Shevach 2009). Each of these five cytokine profiles is under control of distinct sets of transcription factors which are shown in ➋ *Fig. 14.5*, but discussed further elsewhere (e.g., Zhu and Paul 2008; Wilson 2009; Zhou and Littman 2009; Basso et al. 2009; Dong 2008).

To some extent the same distinct cytokine profiles may develop in CD8$^+$ T cells, where at least type 1 and 2 cytokine-releasing CD8$^+$ cells are known to contribute to allergic contact dermatitis (Kimber and Dearman 2002; Coulter et al. 2010).

Several factors are thought to contribute to the above-described polarized cytokine production profiles in allergen-specific T cells, including (1) the site and cytokine environment of first allergenic contact, (2) the molecular nature and concentrations of the allergen, and (3) the neuroendocrine factors.

Cytokine Environment. In the skin-draining lymph nodes, allergen-activated LC and dermal dendritic cells rapidly produce large amounts of IL-12, switching off IL-4 cytokine production, thus promoting the differentiation of Th1 cells (Nakamura et al. 1997b; Kang et al. 1996;

Pulendran 2004). Of note, since Th1 cells retain, next to IL12R, high IL-4R expression they remain sensitive to IL-4 as a growth factor (Kubo et al. 1997). Thus, they also retain the capacity to shift cytokine production toward the type-2 profile. In contrast, type-2 T cells, e.g., developing in mucosa-draining lymph nodes, rapidly lose the genes encoding the IL-12-R β2 chain and thus, type-2 differentiation is irreversible (Rogge et al. 1997; Zhou and Chong 2009).

Early differentiation of type-1 T cells is promoted by microbial danger-signal-induced IL-12 and IL-18, leading to IFN-γ release by nonspecific "bystander" cells, e.g., DC and NK cells, within the lymph nodes (Nakamura et al. 1997; Orange and Biron 1996). IFN-γ interferes with skewing toward other cytokine profiles. Since Th1 cells rapidly lose functional IFN-γR expression, these cells, in contrast to e.g., Th2, Th3 and Th17 cells, become refractory to the growth-inhibitory effects of IFN-γ (Groux et al. 1997; Gajewski and Fitch 1988; Takatori et al. 2008). Interestingly, T-cell skewing may also be facilitated by primary contact-mediated signals, e.g., Th1 skewing by CD154 ligation through APC-bound CD40 [124], or Th2 skewing by ligation of CD134 (OX40) through APC-bound CD252 (Ohshima et al. 1997; Croft et al. 2009).

In the process of T-cell skewing toward the other major cytokine profiles, TGF-β plays a central role. TGF-β can be produced by various cell types, including Th3 cells themselves, but is most prominently produced by mucosal epithelial cells (Zhu and Paul 2008; Takatori et al. 2008; Iliev et al. 2009). Apparently, in conjunction with IL-10 production, e.g., produced by mucosal B cells, allergen-stimulated T cells rapidly initiate endogenous TGF-β production thus revealing the Th3 phenotype (Izcue et al. 2009). These cells may stimulate IgA production along the mucosae, but elsewhere immunosuppressive activities prevail. Interestingly, in conjunction with abundant local IL-2 production, such as induced by strong antigenic stimulation involving most effective CD28 triggering, TGF-β favors skewing toward IL-10 production, thus providing an effective immunoregulatory feedback loop (Hoyer et al. 2008; Letourneau 2009). Still, in the presence of strong and persistant microbial molecule-induced danger/growth signals, e.g., IL-6, IL-21, and IL-23, TGF-β induces the development of Th17 and/or Th22 cells, which both have been postulated to contribute to various allergic and autoimmune disorders (Larsen 2009; Oboki 2008; Louten 2009; Oukka 2009; Takatori et al. 2008) (➋ *Fig. 14.5*).

Thus, ACD may be caused by any combination of at least three distinct types of effector T cells, releasing type-1, -2, and -17/22 cytokines, respectively. Considering that contact allergens will mainly enter via the skin, type-1 pro-inflammatory T cells are thought to represent the primary effector cells in ACD (Edele et al. 2007; Fyhrquist-Vanni et al. 2007). Nevertheless, in sensitized individuals, type-2 T cells also play a role, as shown by both IL-4 production and allergen-specific type-2 T cells in the blood and at ACD reaction sites (see ➋ Sect. 7) (Werfel et al. 1997; Probst et al. 1995; Grewe et al. 1998). Their role may increase along with the longevity of sensitization, since several factors contribute to shifting type-1 to type-2 responses, including reversibility of the former and not of the latter T cells, as mentioned above (Perez et al. 1995; Ulrich et al. 2001). Still, other sets of cytokines, including IL-17 and/or IL-22, are important in immune defense mechanisms, and thus Th17 and or Th22 cells have also been found to mediate allergic and autoimmune disorders (van Beelen et al. 2007). Given rapid local release of both IL-4 and TGF-β within mucosal tissues, mucosal allergen contacts, if accompanied by strong danger signals, may lead in particular to Th2 and Th17 effector cells. Without these signals, rather immunoregulatory subsets (Th3, Tr1) would develop, as is observed in the induction of "oral tolerance" (see below) (Mucida and Salek-Ardakani 2009).

Nature of the Allergen. A second factor in determining T-cell cytokine-production profiles, although still poorly understood, is the molecular character of the contact allergen itself, and the resulting extent of TCR triggering (Constant and Bottomly 1997; Constant et al. 1995). For both protein and peptide antigens, high doses of antigen might favor type-2 responses, whereas intermediate/low doses would induce type-1 T-cell responses (Constant and Bottomly 1997; Bretscher et al. 1997). Strong antigenic stimulation was also shown to upregulate CD40L expression on T cells and, in combination with microbial-induced IL-6, to promote, Th17 differentiation (Lezzi 2009). To what extent this translates to contact allergens is still unclear. Certainly, endogenous capacities of contact allergens to provide danger signals and activate the "inflammasome," in combination with their capacity to induce differentiation-skewing cytokines (in particular IL-4, IL-6, IL-12, and IL-23), will affect the outcome (Toebak and Moed 2006; Watanabe 2008). In this respect, some contact allergens are notorious for inducing type-2 responses, even if their primary contact is by the skin route, e.g., trimellitic acid, which is also known as a respiratory sensitizer (Kanerva et al. 1997).

Neuroendocrine Factors. Diverse neuroendocrine factors co-determine T-cell differentiation (Geenen and Brilot 2003; Luger and Lotti 1998, 2002). An important link has been established between nutritional deprivation and decreased T-cell-mediated allergic contact reactions (Lord et al. 1998). Apparently, adipocyte-derived leptin, a hormone released by adequately nourished and functioning fat cells, is required for type-1 T-cell differentiation. Administration of leptin to mice restored ACD reactivity in mice during starvation (Lord et al. 1998). Also, androgen hormones and adrenal cortex-derived steroid hormones, e.g., dehydroepiandrosterone (DHEA), promote type-1 T-cell and ACD reactivity. DHEA, like testosterone, may favor differentiation of type-1 T cells by promoting IFN-γ and suppressing IL-4 release (Morfin et al. 2000; Cutolo et al. 2002). In contrast, the female sex hormone progesterone furthers the development of type-2 $CD4^+$ T cells and even induces, at least transient, IL-4 production and CD30 expression in established type-1 T cells (Kidd 2003; Piccinni 1995). Type-2 T-cell polarization is also facilitated by adrenocorticotrophic hormone (ACTH) and glucocorticosteroids (Vieira et al. 1998), and by prostaglandin $(PG)E_2$ (Calder et al. 1992). PGE_2, released from mononuclear phagocytes, augments intracellular cAMP levels, resulting in inhibition of pro-inflammatory cytokine production, like IFN-γ and TNF-α (Uotila 1996; Demeure et al. 1997; Abe et al. 1997; Kalinski et al. 1997), and thus can influence the development of effector T cells in ACD.

6 Systemic Propagation of the Specific T-Cell Progeny

T-Cell Recirculation. Upon sensitization via the skin, the progeny of primed T cells is released via the efferent lymphatic vessels of the skin draining lymph nodes and the thoracic duct into the blood (➋ *Fig. 14.6*). If the first encounter with allergen occurs via the intestinal route (e.g., along with induction of oral tolerance), priming will take place in the Peyer's patches and mesenteric lymph nodes, and primed T cells will be released from there to the circulation. The subsequent recirculation and homing pattern of primed T cells is guided by adhesion molecules and chemokine receptors which they express on the cell membrane (➋ *Table 14.1*). As outlined below, expression of these molecules is determined by the site of priming, as well as by the activational state of the T cells. In addition, there is a distinct relationship between the sets of chemokine and homing receptors expressed by T cells and their type of differentiation.

First, primed T cells have different homing receptors depending on the site of priming, a process called "imprinting" (Woodland 2009; Edele 2008). During priming of allergen-specific T cells in the skin draining lymph nodes, both $CD4^+$ and $CD8^+$ T cells are stimulated to express cutaneous lymphocyte antigen (CLA; Fuhlbrigge et al. 1997) and the chemokine receptors CCR4 and CCR10, a phenotype that predisposes for eventual migration to the skin. In the mesenteric lymph nodes, on the other hand, T cells are stimulated to express the integrin α4:β7 and the chemokine receptor CCR9, a phenotype which predisposes for gut homing. An instructive role of the peripheral tissues in this imprinting process was demonstrated in a mouse model on T cell priming by dendritic cells, where either dermal or intestinal cells were added to the cultures, resulting in T cells expressing mouse "CLA" or α4:β7 integrin, respectively (Edele 2008). Whereas for the imprint of gut homing retinoic acid was identified as a crucial factor, for the imprint of skin homing, the active metabolite of vitamin D3 was shown to be essential, because it induces CCR10 expression in T cells (Sigmundsdottir 2008). Still, for induction of CLA and thus for establishing the full skin homing profile, cell-cell contact and/or other mediators like IL-12 seem to be required (Edele 2008).

After priming and imprinting, circulating gut homing memory T lymphocytes, bearing the α4:β7 integrin, can attach to intestinal endothelial cells by binding to the mucosal vascular addressin MAdCAM-1. Further infiltration in the mucosa is guided by chemokines, such as CCL25, produced by small intestinal epithelial cells (Miles 2008). Thus, along the gut, T lymphocyte progeny is attracted that has been generated in other mucosal tissues. Likewise, in the skin, CLA-positive cells are attracted that have been generated in skin draining lymph nodes. CLA binds to E-selectin (CD62E) on dermal endothelial cells, while CCR4 and CCR10 expression allow the lymphocytes to migrate in the skin toward CCL17 and CCL27 produced by keratinocytes in the epidermis.

At least as important for the recirculation and homing characteristics of T cells is the activational state of the cells. In this respect, primed T cells can be divided into two main subsets: the central memory T cells (T_{CM}) and the effector memory T cells (T_{EM}). Like their naive precursors, T_{CM} can still enter the peripheral lymphoid tissues, due to the fact that they continue to express CD62L and CCR7, allowing for binding to high endothelial venules in the lymph nodes and migration into the paracortical areas. T_{EM}, on the other hand, have lost these molecules and migrate, due to simultaneous upregulation of several other adhesion molecules, preferentially to peripheral inflamed tissues. T_{EM} are characterized by rapid effector function upon antigenic stimulation, but, in the absence of antigenic stimuli, T_{EM} eventually convert to T_{CM} by

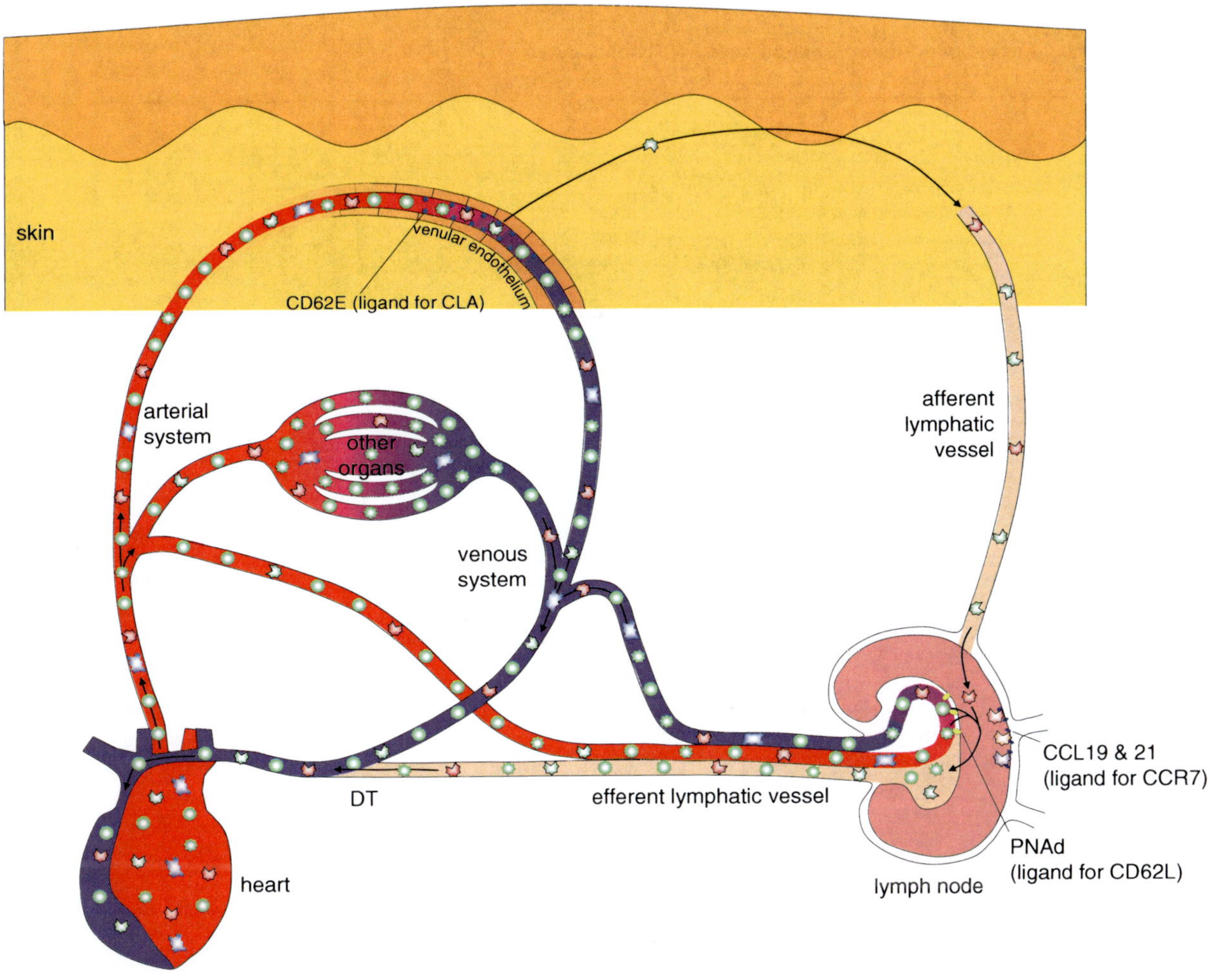

Fig. 14.6

Systemic propagation of hapten-specific T cells. From the skin-draining lymphoid tissue, the progeny of primed T cells is released via the efferent lymphatic vessels and the thoracic duct (*DT*) into the blood and becomes part of the circulation. Like their naïve precursors, these CCR7$^+$ effector/memory T cells can still enter lymphoid tissues and settle in paracorticale areas by binding to its ligands CCL19 and CCL21. But increased expression of skin-homing molecules, e.g., cutaneous lymphocyte antigen (*CLA*), facilitates their spontaneous migration in the skin

reacquiring CCR7 and CD62L. In turn, T_{CM} may convert to T_{EM} upon antigenic restimulation (Sallusto et al. 1999, 2004; Woodland 2009; Sallusto 2009).

Peripheral endothelial binding and extravasation of T cells to inflamed tissues requires the expression of both selectins and integrins on the T cell membrane, such as LFA-1, VLA-4, and PSGL-1. The vascular expression of their respective ligands (➋ *Table 14.1*) is strongly increased by cytokines released at inflammatory sites. The density of adhesion molecules on the T cell membrane is generally upregulated upon activation, in particular in T_{EM}. Since their expression is highest only for short periods after activation, only recently activated T cells show a unique propensity to enter skin sites and exert effector functions.

Third, the differentiation of T cells (Th1, Th2, etc.) is clearly associated with distinct homing chracteristics. T cells biased toward a pro-inflammatory phenotype show a higher propensity to enter skin sites, as compared to mucosal tissues (Austrup et al. 1997; Fuhlbrigge et al. 1997; Larsen 2009; Duhen 2009). In mice, the early influx of type-1 T cells into delayed-type hypersensitivity (DTH) reactions was found to be more efficient than that of type-2 T cells, although both cell types expressed CLA. Here, CD162, highly expressed by type-1 T cells, was

◘ Table 14.1
Molecules involved in the migration of hapten-specific T lymphocytes

Receptor/ Ligand	T Cell	Ligand / Receptor	Cell	Tissue	References
CD62L (L-selectin)	T_{naive} T_{CM}	CD34, GlyCAM-1 (PNAd)	HEV	lymph node	Janeway 2008, Sallusto 2004
CCR7		CCL19,CCL21	Stromal cells, DC		Sallusto 2004
CD11a/CD18 (αL:β2-integrin, LFA-1)	T_{EM}; increased upon activation	CD54, CD102 (ICAM-1, ICAM-2)	Endothelial cells	skin	Janeway 2008
CD49d (α4:β1-integrin, VLA-4)	increased upon activation	CD106, fibronectin (VCAM-1)	Endothelial cells		Janeway 2008
CD162 (P-selectin ligand, PSGL-1)	increased upon activation	CD62P (P-selectin)	Endothelial cells		Woodland 2009
CLA	skin homing	CD62E (E-selectin)	Cutaneous endothelial cells		Woodland 200
CCR4	Th2	CCL17 (TARC)	Keratinocytes		Woodland 2009
CCR5	Th1	CCL2 (MCP-1)? CCL3 (MIP-1α)	Keratinocytes (a.o.)		Meller 2007, Gaga 2008
CCR6	Th17	CCL20 (MIP-3α / LARC)	Langerhans cells Endothelial cells		Larsen 2009 Meller 2007
CCR10	Th22, CLA+	CCL27 (CTACK)	Keratinocytes Langerhans cells		Duhe 2009, Homey 2002, Kagami 2008, Woodland 2009
CXCR3	Th1	CXCL9 and CXCL10 (Mig and IP-10)	Keratinocytes		Moed 2004 Meller 2007
α4:β7-integrin	T cells; gut homing	MAdCAM-1	Endothelial cells	gut	Janeway 2008
CCR9	T cells	CCL25 (TECK)	Epithelial cells		Grimm 2008; Miles 2008

found to be important for this preferential homing (Borges et al. 1997). Also the pattern of chemokine receptors differs between the Th subsets (➋ *Table 14.1*). Some receptors, such as CXCR3, are preferentially expressed on Th1 cells, whereas others like CCR4 and CCR8 are in particular expressed by Th2 cells (Ward 2009; Cavani 2008; Hudak 2002; Sallusto 2009). The latter chemokine receptors are not only overexpressed on type-2 cytokine-producing T cells, but also on basophils and eosinophils. Together, these cells strongly contribute to local immediate allergic hyperresponsiveness. The more recently described Th17 and Th22 lymphocyte subsets expressing CCR4, CCR6, and CCR10 (Ward 2009; Duhen 2009) are attracted to the skin by epidermal CCL17, CCL20, and CCL27, respectively (➋ *Table 14.1*, ➋ *Fig. 14.5*). Overall, results obtained thus far favor the view that the pro-inflammatory subsets (Th1 and Th17/22) will be the first to enter skin sites upon local inflammatory stimuli, their primary function being an early control of antigenic pressure, e.g., through amplification of macrophage effector functions. The ACD reaction is, however, a dynamic process, in which the first influx of cells influences the local chemokine environment and determines the type of subsequent infiltrating cells. Thus, upon repeated exposure to contact allergens gradually Th2 cells and regulatory cells may dominate (Kitagaki 1997). Interestingly, also at the T-cell level modulation of the cytokine and chemokine receptor profiles may occur, thereby maintaining plasticity of the immune response (Wilson 2009; Sallusto 2009). Of note, the actual composition of the T-cell infiltrate in ACD skin lesions does not only depend on the influx of lymphocytes, but should rather be regarded as the resultant of infiltration, apoptosis, and retention of lymphocytes, next to their emigration to the lymphatics.

Finally, the antigen specificity of T cells contributes to their migration pattern. Allergens penetrated via the epidermis and displayed at the dermal endothelial surface may be recognized by allergen-specific T cells, thus resulting in activation, immobilization, and transendothelial migration of these cells at sites of allergen exposure (Ward 2009).

Allergen-Specific T-Cell Recirculation: Options for In Vitro Testing. The dissemination and recirculation of primed, allergen-specific T cells in the body suggests that peropheral blood offers a most useful and accessible source for T cell based in vitro assays for ACD (➋ *Fig. 14.6*). A major advantage of in vitro testing would be the noninterference with the patient's immune system, thus eliminating any potential risk of primary sensitization and boosting by in vivo skin testing. Although such tests have found several applications in fundamental research, e.g., on recognition of restriction elements, cross-reactivities and cytokine-profile analyses, their use for routine diagnostic purposes is still limited. Even in highly sensitized individuals, frequencies of contact allergen-specific memory/effector cells may still be below 1 per 10^4 (Cavani et al. 1998; Lindemann 2008; Kalish 1990). Given the relatively small samples of blood obtainable by venepuncture (at only one or a few time points), numbers of specific T cells in any culture well used for subsequent in vitro testing would typically be below 100 cells/well. For comparison, in vivo skin test reactions recruit at least 1,000 times more specific T cells from circulating lymphocytes passing by for the period of testing, i.e., at least 24 h (von Blomberg et al. 1991).

Therefore, the sensitivity of in vitro assays, e.g., allergen-induced proliferation or cytokine production may not always be sufficient to pick up weak sensitization. Intermediate or strong sensitization is, however, readily detected in vitro by both proliferation and cytokine production assays (Lindemann 2008; Bordignon 2008; Minang 2005; Moed 2005). With respect to the latter, both the "Elispot" assay, where allergen induced cytokine production is evaluated at the single cell level, and the cytokine evaluation in allergen-stimulated culture supernatants provide adequate information (Rustemeyer et al. 2004; Spiewak 2007; Minang 2005). Notably with respect to cytokine production, type-2 cytokines appear to provide most specific parameters for contact sensitization in these assays (Rustemeyer et al. 2004; Minang 2008), although generally both Th1 and Th2 cytokines are being produced in vitro by allergic individuals upon allergen exposure (Moed 2005; Minang 2006).

Importantly, most of the above-mentioned, successful in vitro studies evaluated hydrophilic allergens, like nickel, chromium, and palladium salts. Reports on successful in vitro assays with other hydrophobic and more toxic allergens are scarce (Moed 2005; Wahlkvist 2007; Skazik 2008). Appropriate allergen presentation is a major hurdle in in vitro studies, because of the broad range of requirements for different allergens with unique solubilities, toxicities, and reactivity profiles. Moreover, in the absence of LC, monocytes are the major source of APC, and their numbers in peripheral blood vary substantially within and between donors. Of note, optimal APC function is particularly critical for in vitro activation of resting memory T cells, since, in the absence of repeated allergenic contacts, activated effector memory T cells (T_{EM}) may finally revert to a more naïve phenotype, with a higher threshold for triggering (Sallusto et al. 2004; Boyman 2009). Supplementing in vitro test cultures with appropriate mixtures of cytokines may, however, compensate for suboptimal APC function (Rustemeyer et al. 1999, 2004; Moed 2005).

7 The Effector Phase of Allergic Contact Dermatitis

Elicitation of ACD. Once sensitized, individuals can develop ACD upon reexposure to the contact allergen. Positive patch test reactions mimic this process of allergen-specific skin hyperreactivity. Thus, skin contacts induce an inflammatory reaction that, in general, is maximal within 2–3 days and, without further allergen supply, declines thereafter (➋ *Fig. 14.7*). Looked at superficially, the mechanism of this type of skin hyperreactivity is straightforward: allergen elicitation or challenge leads to the (epi)dermal accumulation of contact allergen-specific memory/effector T lymphocytes which, upon encountering allergen-presenting cells, are reactivated to release pro-inflammatory cytokines. These, in turn, spark the inflammatory process, resulting in macroscopically detectable erythema and induration. As compared to immediate allergic reactions, developing within a few minutes after mast-cell degranulation, ACD reactions show a delayed

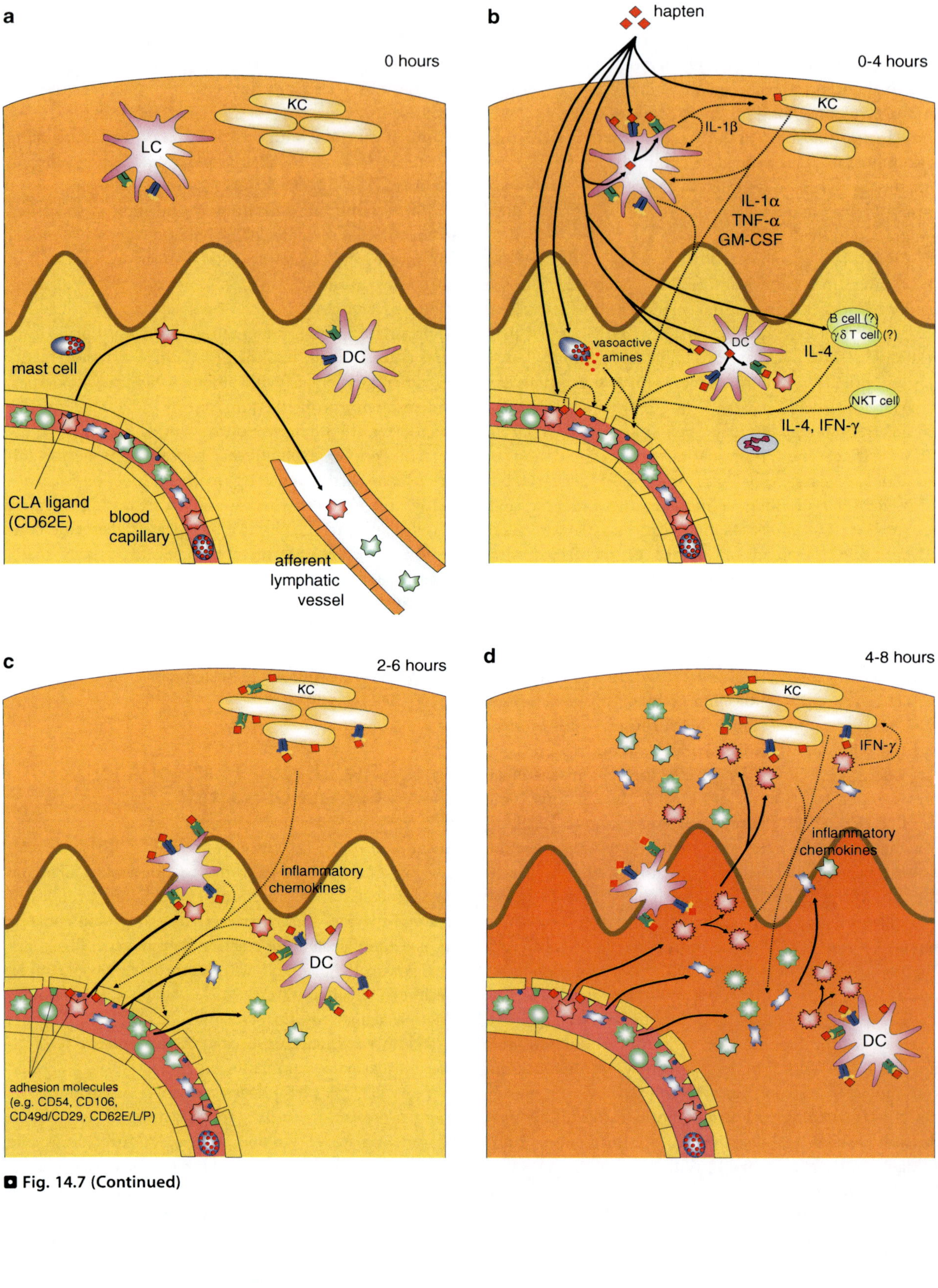

Fig. 14.7 (Continued)

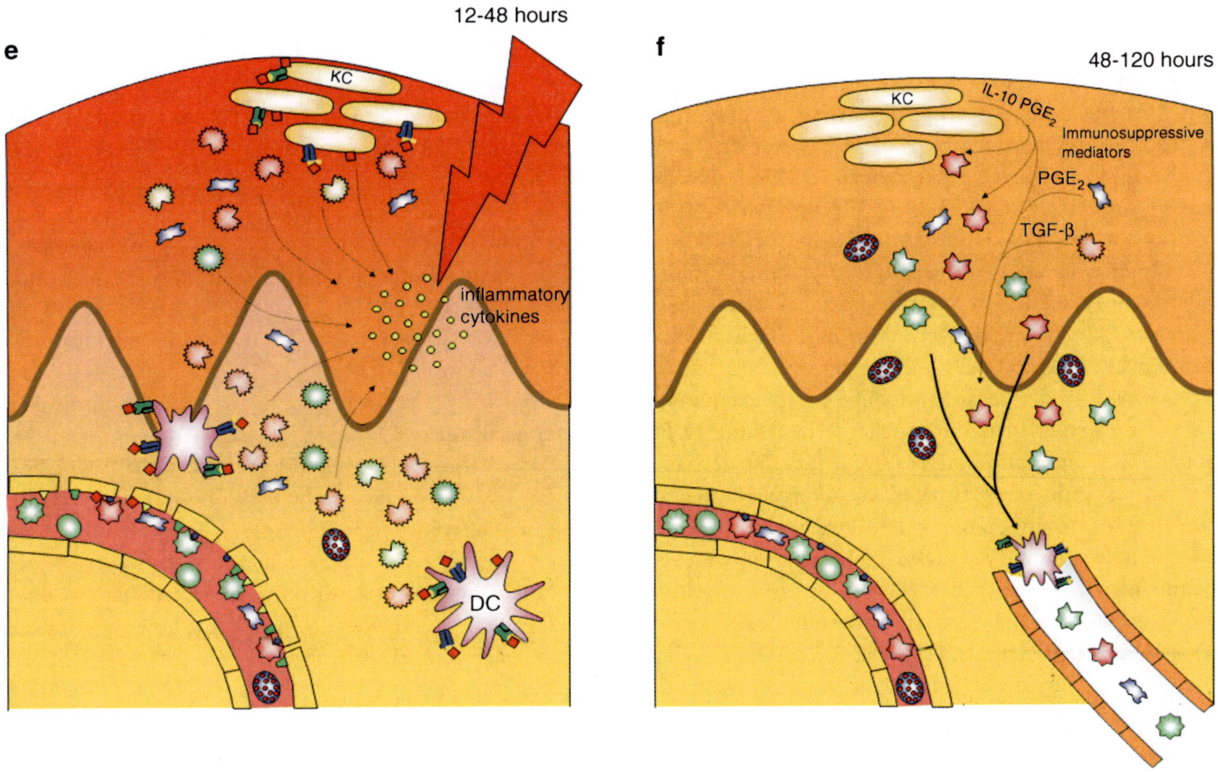

Fig. 14.7

The effector phase of allergic contact dermatitis. (a) 0 h: In resting skin relatively few randomly patrolling, skin-homing CLA$^+$ T cells are present. (b) 0–4 h: Reexposure of the contact allergen, binding to (epi)dermal molecules and cells, induces release of proinflammatory cytokines. (c) 2–6 h: Influenced by inflammatory mediators, activated epidermal Langerhans cells (*LC*) start migrating toward the basal membrane and endothelial cells express increased numbers of adhesion molecules. Endothelial cell-bound hapten causes preferential extravasation of hapten-specific T cells, which are further guided by inflammatory chemokines. (d) 4–8 h: Hapten-activated T cells release increasing amounts of inflammatory mediators, amplifying further cellular infiltration. (e) 12–48 h: The inflammatory reaction reaching its maximum, characterized by (epi) dermal infiltrates, oedema, and spongiosis. (f) 48–120 h: Gradually, downregulatory mechanisms take over, leading to decreased inflammation and disappearance of the cellular infiltrate. Finally, primordial conditions are reconstituted except for a few residual hapten-specific T cells causing the local skin memory. *KC* keratinocyte, *DC* dendritic cell

time course, since both the migration of allergen-specific T cells from the dermal vessels and local cytokine production need several hours to become fully effective. Still, the picture of the rise and fall of ACD reactions is far from clear. Some persistent issues are discussed below, notably: (1) irritant properties of allergens, (2) role of early-phase reactivity, (3) T-cell patrol and specificity, (4) effector T-cell phenotypes, and (5) down regulatory processes.

Irritant Properties of Allergens. Within a few hours after allergenic skin contact, immunohistopathological changes can be observed, including vasodilatation, upregulation of endothelial adhesion molecules (Goebeler et al. 1993, 1995), mast-cell degranulation (Walsh et al. 1990; Waldorf et al. 1991), keratinocyte cytokine and chemokine production (Spiekstra 2005; Meller 2007), influx of leucocytes (Bangert et al. 2003; Houck et al. 2004), and LC migration toward the dermis (Rambukhana et al. 1995; Silberberg-Sinakin et al. 1976; Hill et al. 1990; Toebak 2009). These pro-inflammatory phenomena, which are also observed in non-sensitized individuals (Sterry et al. 1991) and in T-cell-deficient nude mice (Herzog et al. 1989), strongly contribute to allergenicity (Saint-Mezard et al. 2003). Clearly most, if not all, of these effects can also be caused by irritants and, therefore, do not unambiguously discriminate between irritants and contact allergens (Willis et al. 1986; Hoefakker et al. 1995; Brasch et al. 1992;

Spiekstra 2005). Apparently, true differences between these types of compounds depend on whether or not allergen-specific T cells become involved. Thus, only after specific T-cell triggering distinctive features might be observed, e.g., local release of certain chemokines, such as the Th1 associated chemokines CXCL9, CXCL10 (IP-10), and CXCL11 (I-TAC/IP-9) ([206], Meller 2007) or the Th2-related chemokines CCL11, CCL17, and CCL22 (Flier et al. 1999; Meller 2007). Certainly, pro-inflammatory effects of contact allergens increase, in many ways, the chance of allergen-specific T cells meeting their targets. The first cells affected by skin contact, i.e., keratinocytes and LC, are thought to represent major sources of pivotal mediators such as IL-1β and TNF-α (Enk 1992; Kondo and Sauder 1995). First, as described in "Hapten-Induced Activation of Allergen-Presenting Cells," these cytokines cause hapten-bearing LC to mature and migrate toward the dermis (Kimber et al. 1998; Steinman et al. 1995; Toebak 2009). But, these cytokines also cause (over)expression of adhesion molecules on dermal postcapillary endothelial cells and loosen intercellular junctions. Thereby, extravasation of leucocytes, including allergen-specific T cells, is strongly promoted (Wardorf et al. 1991; Pober et al. 1986; Shimizu et al. 1991; Ward 2009). Moreover, haptens can stimulate nitric oxide (NO) production of the inducible NO-synthase (iNOS) of LC and keratinocytes, which contributes to local edema, vasodilatation, and cell extravasation (Ross et al. 1998; Rowe et al. 1997; Virag et al. 2002). In addition to these pathomechanisms that contribute to inflammatory responses, toll-like receptors (TLR) can be involved in triggering sensitization. Recent studies have indicated that at least the contact allergen nickel can specifically trigger human TLR-4, which adds to the release of unspecific danger signals (Rothenberg 2010; Schmidt et al. 2010).

Histopathological analyses support the view that the major causative events take place in the papillary dermis, close to the site of entry of allergen-specific T cells, for instance at hair follicles, where haptens easily penetrate and blood capillaries are nearby (Szepietowski et al. 1997). Here, perivascular mononuclear cell infiltrates develop, giving the highest chance of encounters between allergen-presenting cells and specific T cells. Once triggered, extravasated T cells will readily enter the lower epidermal layers, in which haptenized keratinocytes produce lymphocyte-attracting chemokines, like CXCL9/10, CCL17, CCL20, and CCL27 (Flier et al. 1999; Larsen 2009; Meller 2007; Woodland 2009, ➋ *Table 14.1*). Subsequently, since effector memory T cells can also be triggered by "non-professional" APC, including KC, fibroblasts, and infiltrating mononuclear cells, ACD reactivity is amplified in the epidermis (Hommel 2004; Viola and Lanzavecchia 1996). Together, these events result in the characteristic epidermal damage seen in ACD, such as spongiosis and hyperplasia. Notably, in ongoing ACD reactions, the production of chemokines attracting lymphocytes and monocytes/macrophages, in addition to the production of cytokines, adds to the nonspecific recruitment and activation of leucocytes (Yu et al. 1994; Buchanan and Murphy 1997). Thus, like the very early events in the effector phase reaction, the final response to a contact allergen is antigen-non-specific. It is therefore not surprising that allergic and irritant reactions are histologically alike.

Early Phase Reactivity. In the elicitation phase allergen-specific T cells are triggered by MHC-bound allergen, just like in the afferent phase. The role of Langerhans cells in allergen presentation upon elicitation is, however, less prominent, and also other cells, like mast cells, macrophages and keratinocytes may now contribute, since effector T cells are easily triggered and do not require professional antigen presentation. The role of keratinocytes in the onset of the ACD reaction is important, because of the cytokines and chemokines they produce upon hapten application (Meller 2007; Spiekstra 2005), thereby facilitating the influx of effector T cells. In addition, a variety of other cells and mediators may contribute to the initiation of the ACD reaction, as summarized below.

The role of neutrophils in the onset of ACD reactions has not been well established, though recent studies in mice demonstrate that skin reactivity to haptens largely depends on CXCL1, released from endothelial cells when the first hapten-specific CD8 T cells encounter the allergen and produce IL-17. CXCL1 may then attract neutrophils to the elicitation site, thus facilitating further influx of allergen-specific T cells (Kish 2009). In the human system, neutrophil infiltration was also observed in skin biopsies from nickel patch tests, presumably as a result of IL-17/IL-22-mediated inflammation (Larsen 2009). Moreover, it has been shown that IL-8/CXCL8, a potent neutrophil chemoattractant, is readily produced by human antigen presenting cells upon hapten exposure (Toebak et al. 2006); this could also contribute to an early influx of neutrophils in ACD reactions.

The role of an antibody-mediated early phase reaction in the development of ACD is still unclear in man, although Askenase and his colleagues have generated robust data to support this view in murine models (Askenase 2000): Hapten-specific IgM, produced upon sensitization by distant hapten-activated B-1 cells, can bind antigen early after challenge and activate complement. The resulting C5a causes the release of serotonin and TNF-α from local mast cells and platelets, leading to vascular dilatation and permeabilization, detectable as an early ear swelling peaking at 2 h (Van Loweren et al. 1983). Furthermore, C5a and TNF-α induce the upregulation of adhesion molecules on local endothelial cells (Foreman et al. 1994; Groves et al. 1995), thereby contributing to the recruitment of T cells in hapten challenge sites (Groves et al. 1995; Tsuji et al. 1997). In addition, human T cells were found to express the C5a receptor and are chemoattracted to endothelium-bound C5a (Nataf et al. 1999). However, against most contact allergens, including nickel, no antibodies have been detected in man, arguing against humoral mechanisms playing more than a minor role in clinical ACD (Wilkinson et al. 1994; Shirakawa et al. 1992). Interestingly in mice, immunoglobulin light chains, which have long been considered as the meaningless remnants of a spillover in the regular immunoglobulin production of B cells, were discovered to mediate very early hypersensitivity reactions by mast cell activation (Redegeld and Nijkamp 2003; vd Heyden 2006).

In addition to an auxiliary role of B cells and antibodies, natural killer (NK) cells have been reported to play a role in the onset of ACD reactions. Mice lacking both T- and B-cells (RAG2−/−) could still be sensitized to contact allergens and $Thy1^+$ NK cells were identified here as effector cells with a prominent role for the activating NK receptor NKG2D (O'Leary 2006). Interestingly, another NK-like cell, the invariant NKT cell, that recognizes CD1d bound glycolipids resulting in rapid IL-4 and IFN-γ release, was also found to play a role in the elicitation of contact sensitivity in mice: Blocking of CD1d prevented both sensitization and elicitation by contact allergens (Nieuwenhuis 2005). Notably, in human ACD reactions relatively high frequencies of invariant NKT cells have been observed, ranging from 1.7% to 33% of total infiltrating T cells, which is 10–100 fold higher than the frequency found in the circulation (Gober 2008). Also other T cells with relatively restricted TCR repertoire such as Tγδ cells have been reported to contribute in a non-antigen-specific, probably non-MHC-restricted manner, to (early) elicitation responses (Dieli et al. 1998).

To conclude, using various mouse models, different types of early allergen specific reactivity have been claimed to play initiating roles in ACD, but clinical evidence for such mechanisms is still lacking.

T-Cell Patrol and Specificity of T-Cell Infiltrates. Whereas early nonspecific skin reactivity to contact allergens is pivotal for both sensitization and elicitation, full-scale development of ACD, of course, depends on allergen-specific T cells within the (epi)dermal infiltrates. In healthy skin there is a constant flow of memory T cells ending up in the draining lymph nodes: about 200 T cells/h/cm^2 skin (Brand et al. 1999, ➲ *Fig. 14.6*). Since one single antigen-specific T cell can already trigger visible skin inflammation (Milon et al. 1981; Marchal et al. 1982), randomly skin-patrolling memory/effector T cells might account for the initiation of the allergen-specific effector phase. However, since frequencies of hapten-specific T cells in sensitized individuals may still remain below 1 in 10,000, this does not seem to be a realistic scenario. Thus, augmented random and/or specific T-cell infiltration accompanies the development of ACD. Apparently, local chemokine release upon allergen contact is pivotal in this respect (see *T-Cell recirculation*; Meller 2007). Chemokine gene expression evaluated 48 h after NiSO4 application was increased for both Th1-related cytokines (CXCL9, CXCL10, and CXCL11) and Th2-related cytokines (CCL11, CCL17, and CCL22). CCL27, on the other hand, which attracts preferentially CCR10 bearing Th17/22 cells is constitutively produced in resting skin, but is rapidly released upon allergen contact to accumulate in the draining lymph nodes (Huang 2008).

The question concerning the specificity of ACD T-cell infiltrates has so far received little attention. In a guinea pig model, preferential entry of dinitrochlorobenzene (DNCB)-specific T cells was observed within 18 h after elicitation of skin tests with DNCB, as compared to non-related compounds (Scheper et al. 1985). Probably, extravasation of hapten-specific T cells benefits from T cell receptor-mediated interactions with endothelial MHC molecules, presenting hapten penetrated from the skin (Ward 2009). Within minutes after epicutaneous application, hapten can indeed be found in dermal tissues and on endothelial cells (Goebeler et al. 1993; Macatonia et al. 1987; Lappin et al. 1996). Indeed, the frequency of allergen-specific cells in positive patch tests to urushiol was found to be 10- to 100-fold higher than in the blood (Kalish 1990). Interestingly, whereas preferential entry may already contribute to relatively high frequencies of allergen-specific T cells (within 48 h up to 10%) (Probst et al. 1995; Milon et al. 1981), at later stages, when the ACD reaction fades away, the local frequency of allergen-specific T cells may increase even further, due to allergen-induced proliferation and rescue from apoptosis. Thus, at former skin reaction sites these cells can generate "local skin memory" (see ➲ Sect. 8).

Effector T-Cell Phenotypes. The debate on phenotypes of effector T cells in ACD is still ongoing and the number of T cell subsets potentially involved is growing every year (➲ *Fig. 14.7*). Consensus exists, however, on the phenotype of the skin homing T cell, i.e., CLA postive. This molecule enables binding to cutaneous endothelial cells via E-selectin (CD62E) and thus migration into the dermis.

Since cutaneous infiltrates show a clear preponderance of $CD4^+$ T cells, it is not surprising that these cells have most often been held responsible for mediating ACD. In nickel allergic individuals, indeed, allergen-responding cells were found to be $CD4^+CLA^+$ memory T cells (Moed 2004a, b). Other studies, however, revealed $CD8^+CLA^+$ nickel reactive T cells as most discriminating for allergic individuals, since $CD4^+$ nickel-reactive T cells were also found in healthy controls (Cavani et al. 1998). While the effector mechanism of $CD4^+$ T cells is mainly based on cytokine production, $CD8^+$ T cells may mediate skin inflammation also through killing of hapten-bearing target cells. In mice, generally $CD8^+$ T cells are found to cause contact sensitivity reactions, certainly to strong allergens, like DNFB (Kish 2009; Gober 2008). In mice $CD4^+$ T cells are rather found to be regulatory, as shown by the fact that contact sensitization to weak allergens succeeded only after depletion of the $CD4^+$ T cells (Vocanson 2006). Of note, most model allergens studied in mice are hydrophobic molecules like DNFB and oxazolone, whereas in human studies very often water soluble metal salts, such as $NiSO_4$ are used as model allergen. This could, at least partly explain the different T-cell subsets involved (➋ *Figs. 14.2* and ➋ *14.5* MHCI/II presentation). So, taken together, it has become clear that both $CD4^+$ and $CD8^+$ T cells can act as effector cells in DTH and ACD reactions. Likewise, neither of these subsets can be regarded simply as regulatory or suppressor cells, although both of these subsets may, depending on the allergen models and read-out assays, play such roles (Kimber et al. 2002; Abe et al. 1996).

An essentially similar conclusion holds true for T-cell subsets (whether $CD4^+$ or $CD8^+$), releasing type-1, type-2, or type-17 cytokines or combinations thereof. Whereas type-1 cytokines, in particular IFN-γ, display well-established pro-inflammatory effects by increasing MHC and ICAM-1 expression (Saulnier 1995; Kish 2009) thereby contributing to improved allergen presentation and infiltration, IL-4, a hallmark type-2 cytokine, can cause erythema and induration, when released in the skin (Rowe and Bunker 1998; Asherson et al. 1996). Indeed, blockage of IL-4 can interfere with ACD (Asherson et al. 1996). IL-17 plays a role in recruitment and activation of neutrophils. It was shown to be produced both by $CD8^+$ T cells (in mouse models with DNFB; Kish 2009) and by $CD4^+$ T cells (in human nickel patch tests; Larsen 2009). The latter study shows, interestingly, that within a few hours after challenge CCL20 expression is upregulated in the skin, attracting CCR6 positive cells. Since all Th17 cells do express this receptor, an early preferential influx of Th17, and as a consequence IL-17 and IL-22 production, could be an essential early event in the development of the ACD reaction.

Thus, a picture emerges in which ACD reactions can be caused both by allergen-specific type-1, type-2, and type-17 T cells (Cavani et al. 1998; Rustemeyer et al. 2004; Moed 2004; Larsen 2009; Gober 2008; Oboki 2008). In retrospect, the down regulatory effects of IL-4 on ACD reactions observed earlier in some mouse models (Asada et al. 1997) might be ascribed to accelerated allergen-clearance rather than to blunt suppression. Still, both with time and repeated allergen-pressure, type-2 responsiveness may rapidly take over (Kitagaki et al. 1995; Kitagaki 1997). Allergen-specific T cells isolated from skin test sites of sensitized individuals, as compared to blood, showed a strong bias toward type-2 cytokine profiles (Werfel et al. 1997). Additional local IFN-γ release seems, however, indispensable, since for a broad panel of contact allergens, clinical ACD reactions were characterized by increased expression of mRNA encoding IFN-γ-inducible chemokines (Flier et al. 1999). In addition, transgenic mice expressing IFN-γ in the epidermis showed strongly increased ACD reactivity (Carroll et al. 1997).

Downregulatory Processes. Resolution of ACD reactions and risk factors for the development of chronicity are not yet fully understood. Of course, if the allergen source is limited, as with skin testing, local concentrations of allergen usually rapidly decrease, thus taking away the critical trigger of the ACD reaction cascade. Since even ACD reactions due to chronic exposure to allergen seldom result in permanent tissue destruction and scarification, immunoregulatory factors most likely contribute to prevention of excessive cytotoxicity and fatal destruction of the basal membrane. Both IL-1 and heparinase, secreted from activated keratinocytes and T cells, protect keratinocytes from TNF-α-induced apoptosis (Lider et al. 1995; Kothny-Wilkes et al. 1998). Moreover, activated effector T cells can undergo activation-induced cell death (AICD) during the resolution phase (Orteu et al. 1998). Notably, pro-inflammatory type 1 T cells, expressing high levels of Fas-ligand (CD95L) and low amounts of apoptosis-protecting FAP-1 protein, are more susceptible to AICD than type-2 cells (Zhang et al. 1997). This may partly explain the shift toward type-2 reactivity that is observed upon prolonged allergen exposure (Kitagaki et al. 1995). Moreover, during the late phase of ACD, keratinocytes, infiltrated macrophages and T cells start producing IL-10 (Enk 1992; Schwarz et al. 1994; Berg et al. 1995), which has many anti-inflammatory activities, including suppression of antigen-presenting cell and macrophage functions ([110], Lalani et al. 1997; Morel and Oriss 1998). In addition, the release of factors, such as PGE_2 and TGF-β, derived from activated keratinocytes and infiltrated leucocytes, e.g., type-3 T cells, contribute to dampening of the immune response (Epstein et al. 1991; Lawrence et al. 1997). Release of PGE_2, on the one hand, inhibits production of pro-inflammatory cytokines (Kalinski et al. 1997; Walker et al. 1983) and, on the other hand, activates basophils (Weston and Peachell 1998). These may constitute up to 5–15% of infiltrating cells in late phase ACD reactions (Dvorak et al. 1976) and are also believed to contribute to down regulation of the inflammatory response (Marone et al. 1994; Lundeberg et al. 1999). TGF-β silences activated T cells and inhibits further infiltration by down regulating the expression of adhesion molecules on both endothelial and skin cells (Sallusto et al. 2004). Regulatory cells producing these suppressive mediators might even predominate in skin sites, frequently exposed to the same allergen, and known to show local (allergen-specific) hypo-responsiveness [283]. It is of interest in this context that $CD4^+$ memory T cells expanded from late DTH reactions could be educated to become $CD4^+CD25^{++}$ regulatory T cells expressing Foxp3 (Vukmanovic 2008).

8 Flare-up and Retest Reactivity

Local allergen-retention. Flare-up reactivity of former ACD and patch test reaction sites is sometimes observed (Jensen et al. 2003; Hindsen et al. 2001; Larsson et al. 1997). From the basic mechanisms of ACD, it can be inferred that allergen-specific flare-up reactions depend either on local allergen or T-cell retention at these skin sites. Upon short-lasting, low-dose contacts, e.g., by skin testing, local allergen retention usually does not exceed a 2-week period, which is actually long enough to exceed the time required for active sensitization. In experimental guinea-pig studies we observed that skin tests with DNCB, chromium or penicillin could become positive even if primary sensitization was postponed to 1 week after skin testing. Apparently effector T cells released into the circulation at that late time still detected sufficient residual allergen at the former skin test sites to cause flare-up reactivity (Scheper et al. unpublished results). Maximum allergen-persistence for around 14 days was also reported by Saint-Mezard et al. (2003), using the hapten fluorescein-isothiocyanate in a mouse model for flare-up reactivity. Also in humans flare-up reactions due to locally persisting allergen can be observed, when from about 4–6 days after primary sensitization, peripheral effector T-cell frequency increases (Skog 1976). Clinically, this phenomenon can explain anomalous results from patch testing with multiple contact allergens. When a patient suspected for penicillin allergy was patch tested with cross-reactive penicillin derivatives, a regular 24–72 h reaction was only observed to one of the penicillins, but all others also became positive from about 8–9 days after skin testing. The first penicillin derivative turned out to release formaldehyde to which the patient was found to be allergic. Positive reactivity to formaldehyde apparently had potentiated primary sensitization to penicillin, causing the other, previously negative reaction sites to flare up (Neering, personal communication). Thus, skin test sites may occasionally flare-up if the testing dose itself led to the release or activation of sufficiently high numbers of effector T cells in the circulation.

Local T-cell retention. In contrast, allergen-specific T cells may persist for at least several months in the skin causing "local skin memory"(➋ *Fig. 14.8*) (Scheper et al. 1983; Moed 2004). Thus, locally increased allergen-specific hyperreactivity, detectable through either accelerated "retest" reactivity (after repeated allergenic contact at the same skin site) or flare-up reactivity (after allergen entry from the circulation, e.g., derived from food ingestion), may be observed for long periods of time at former skin reaction sites (Christensen et al. 1985; Hindsen and Christensen 1992). Typically, the erythematous reactions peak between 2 and 6 h after contact with the allergen. Histological examination of such previously positive skin reaction sites shows that the majority of remaining T cells is $CD4^+$ $CCR10^+$ (Moed 2004). The remarkable flare-up reactivity at such sites can be understood by considering that just one specific effector T cell can be sufficient to generate macroscopic reactivity (Marchal et al. 1982). Moreover, a very high frequency of the residual T cells may be specific for the allergen, as discussed above in "The Effector Phase of Allergic Contact Dermatitis." Apparently, local specific T-cell retention is highly advantageous in combating microbial infections, since memory T cells localized in peripheral tissues contribute to robust protection e.g., to viral infections (Woodland 2009). Only in highly sensitized individuals unrelated skin test sites may also show flare-up reactions (Scheper et al. 1983) and even generalized erythematous macular eruptions can be observed with higher allergen doses (Polak 1968). The latter reactivities probably relate to the fact that recently activated T cells show strong expression of adhesion and homing molecules, e.g., CLA and chemokine receptors,

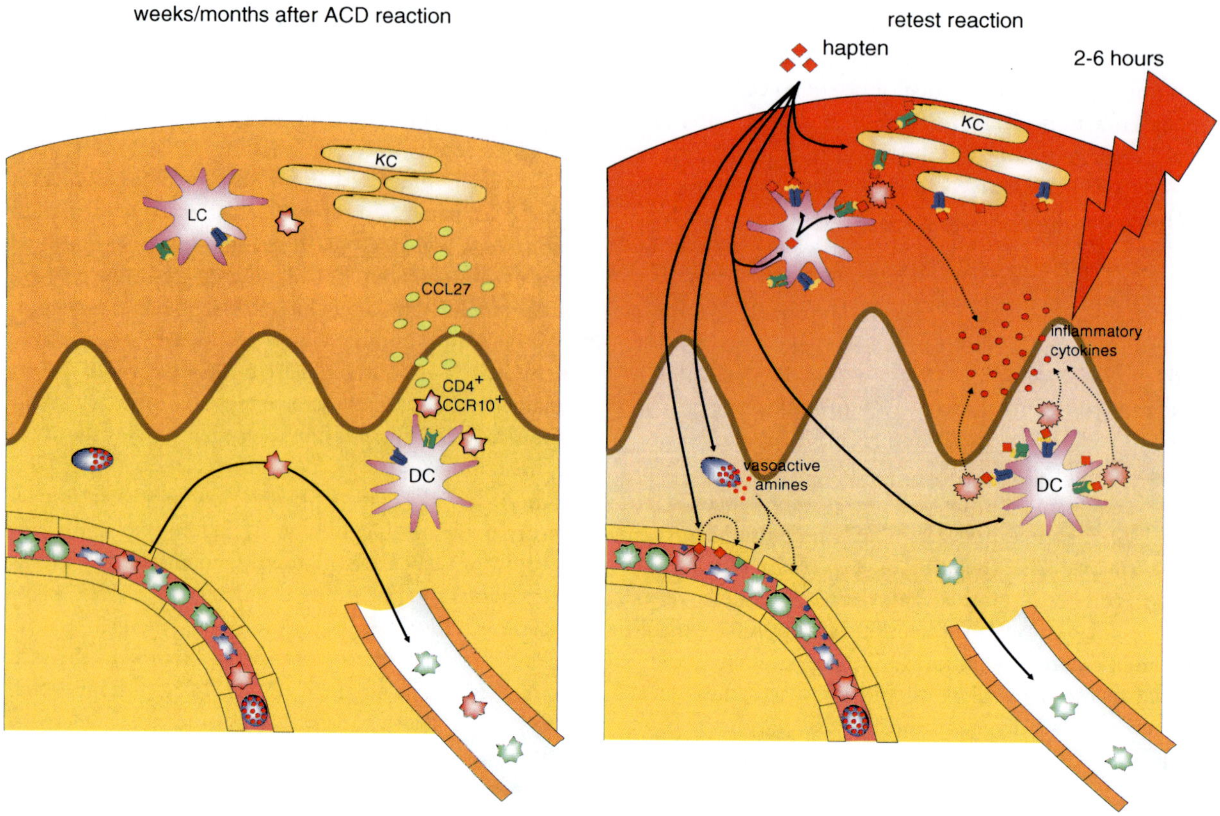

◘ Fig. 14.8

Local skin memory. In former allergic contact dermatitis sites a few hapten-specific T cells can remain, mainly close to dermal dendritic cells (*DC*). Retest reaction: renewed hapten contact can induce a rapid onset of an erythematous reaction, sparked off by the residual hapten-specific T cells. *KC* keratinocyte, *LC* Langerhans cell

such as CCR5, facilitating random migration into peripheral tissues and thus allergen-specific T-cell patrol in the skin (Moser et al. 1998; Woodland 2009). Upon subsequent allergen entry from the circulation, these allergen-specific T cells could mediate generalized erythematous reactions (Hindsen et al. 2001).

Interestingly, local allergen-specific T-cell retention/"local skin memory" can be clinically exploited to discriminate between simultaneous sensitization to different sensitizers ("concomitant sensitization") and cross-reactivity between different sensitizers (Rustemeyer et al. 2002; Matura 1998; Inerot and Moller 2000). Using several different combinations of contact allergens in a guinea pig model, we retested guinea pigs previously sensitized to DNCB and methyl methacrylate (MMA), with the same allergens and some other methacrylate congeners. Accelerated retest reactivities were observed with the latter congeners on the former MMA, but not DNCB, patch test sites (Rustemeyer et al. 2002). Thus, with preferential local retention of MMA-specific T cells at the MMA skin test site, no accelerated retest reactivity could be elicited with DNCB, but to varying degrees with all four MMA-related compounds. In clinical practice using this approach, Matura et al. (1998) confirmed positive cross-retest reactions for cloprednol and tixocortol pivalate, both belonging to group A, and budesonide, amcinonide, and triamcinolone, all belonging to group B corticosteroids (see also Isaksson and Bruze 2003).

9 Hyporeactivity: Tolerance and Desensitization

Of course, uncontrolled development and expression of T-cell-mediated immune function would be detrimental to the host. During evolution, several mechanisms developed to curtail lymph node hyperplasia or to prevent excessive skin damage upon persisting antigen exposure.

Regulation of Immune Responses. First, allergen contacts, e.g., by oral or intravenous administration, may lead to large-scale presentation of allergen by cells other than skin DC (➋ *Fig. 14.9*). In the absence of appropriate costimulatory signals (as described above in "Recognition of Allergen-Modified Langerhans' Cells") allergen presented by e.g., immature Langerhans' cells may anergize naive T cells, i.e., cause receptor-downregulation associated with an unresponsive state, eventually leading to their death by apoptosis (➋ *Fig. 14.10*) (Zinkernagel 2004; Piccirillo and Thornton 2004; Benson and Whitacre 1997). With increasing densities of MHC-antigen complexes on the surface of professional APC, at least three different levels of T-cell tolerance may be induced, characterized by active suppression, anergy or deletion (Ferber et al. 1994; Morgan et al. 1999). Unresponsiveness of T cells, induced by allergenic contacts at skin sites where LC/DC functions have been damaged, e.g., by UV irradiation, or are naturally absent, e.g., in the tail skin of mice, may be ascribed to T-cell anergy, frequently associated with TCR/CD4 or CD8 down regulation, and apoptosis/deletion (Shreedhar et al. 1998; Semma and Sagami 1981). Whereas anergy and deletion reflect "passive" unresponsiveness, tolerance by active suppression may also be induced under similar circumstances (Taams et al. 1999). Actually, with increasing dose and exposure times, even regular epicutaneous allergenic contacts not only induce T effector cells but also lymphocytes controlling T-cell proliferation (afferently acting regulatory cells) and/or causing decreased skin reactivity (regulatory cells of effector phase). Thus, allergic contact hypersensitivity is the resultant of a delicate balance between effector and regulatory mechanisms (Boerrigter and Scheper 1987; Girolomoni et al. 2004).

Cellular Basis of Active Tolerance. Upon preferential stimulation of regulatory cells, e.g., by feeding non-primed, naïve individuals with contact allergens, strong and stable allergen-specific, active tolerance may develop (Mayer et al. 2001; Weiner 1997; Wang 2008). The concept of active regulatory ("suppressor") cells controlling ACD is based on the fact that, in experimental animal models, such allergen-specific tolerance can be transferred by lymphoid cells from tolerant to naive animals (Dieli et al. 1998; Rustemeyer et al. 2001). Active suppression, as revealed by these adoptive cell transfers, is a critical event in regulating T-cell responses to contact sensitizers, and to all possible peptide/protein antigens, including bacterial, autoimmune, and graft rejection antigens (Miller et al. 1977; Polak 1980; Weiner 1997).

Like effector T cells in ACD, regulatory cells are not a single subpopulation of cells. As outlined above,

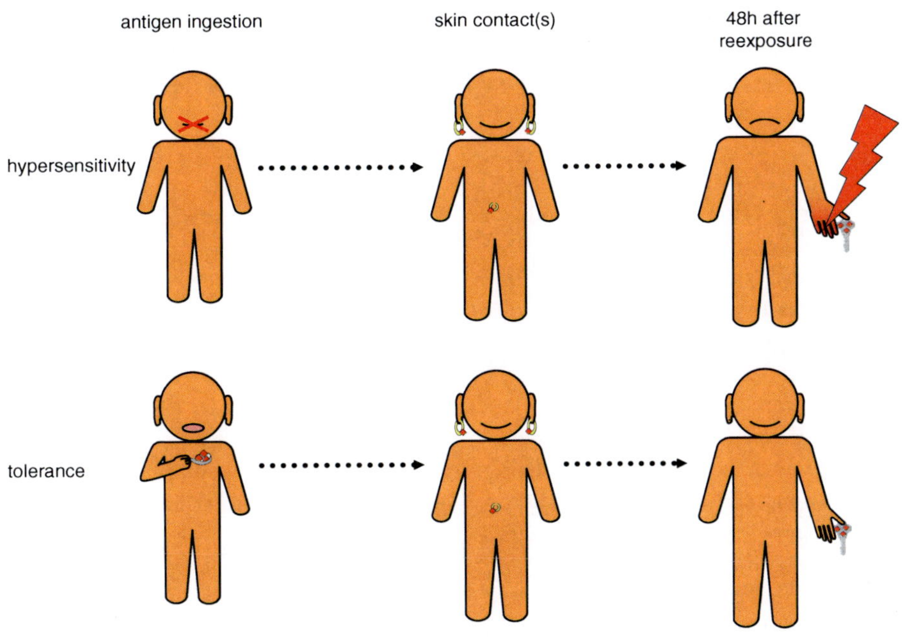

Fig. 14.9

Induction of oral tolerance. Hapten ingestion, prior to potential sensitizing skin contact(s), can induce hapten-specific tolerance

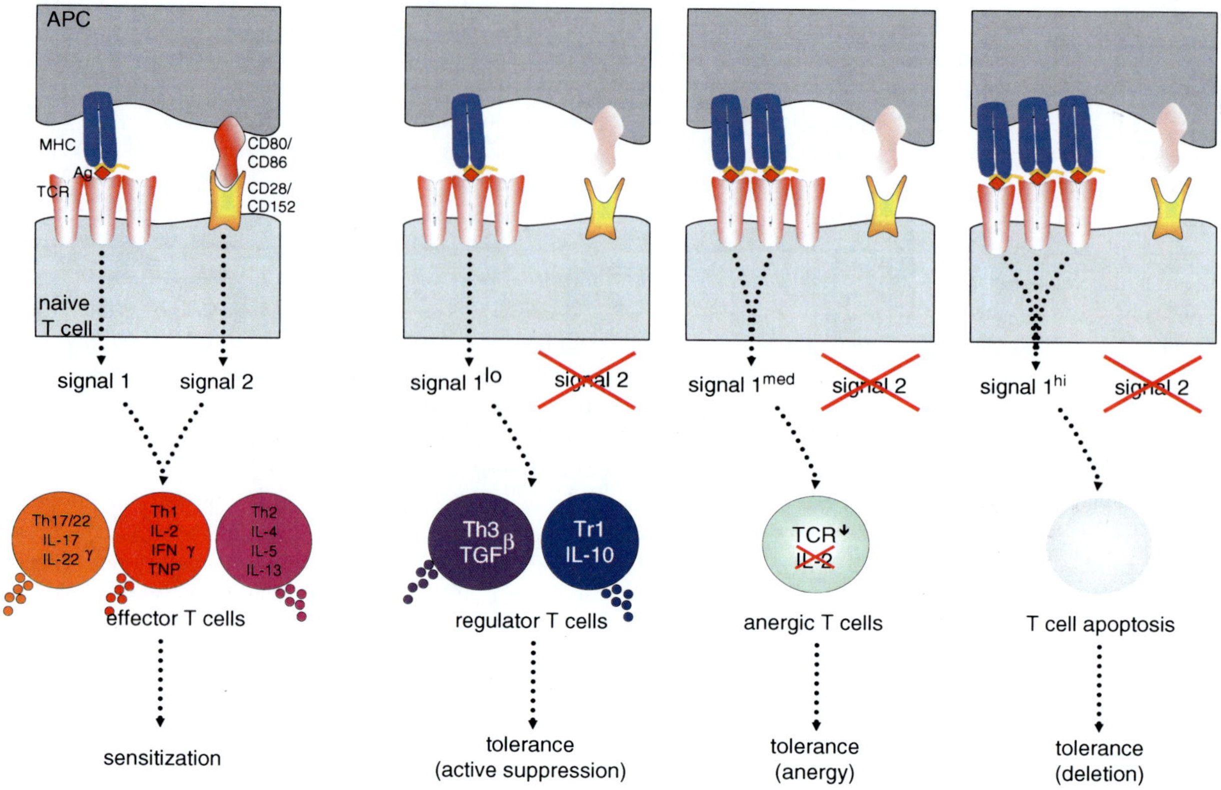

Fig. 14.10

The character of the APC–T-cell interaction determines the immunological outcome. Sensitization: Naïve T cells, activated by antigen-presenting cells (*APC*) providing both hapten-specific ("signal 1") and appropriate costimulatory ("signal 2") signals, develop into effector T cells, characterized by Th-17/22, -1, and -2 cytokine secretion profiles. Tolerance: In the absence of appropriate costimulatory signals, immunological tolerance may develop. With increasing density of MHC-hapten complexes on the surface of APC, activating "signal 1" T-cell pathways, multiple levels of T-cell tolerance might be induced

depending on e.g., the nature of the allergen and route of exposure, ACD can be mediated by both $CD4^+$ and $CD8^+$ T cells, either or both releasing Th1, Th2, Th3, Th17/22 cytokines. With distinct effector phenotypes for particular allergens, each of the other phenotypes can act as regulatory cells (Weigle and Romball 1997; Arnaboldi 2009). Notwithstanding, type-2 cytokine producing cells are prominent in regulating ACD, with allergic contact hypersensitivity enhanced and tolerance reversed by interfering with type-2 T-cell functions (Zembala and Ashershon 1973; Boerrigter and Scheper 1984; Mokyr et al. 1998). Also, interferons and IL-12, both impairing Th2 and Th17/22 cells, were shown to inhibit regulatory cells and to stimulate effector-cell functions in mouse models (Knop et al. 1982; Zhang and Michael 1990; Claessen et al. 1996). In particular after mucosal allergen contact stimulation, T cells producing IL-10 and/or TGF-β (type-3 cytokine profile), many of which co-expressing CD4, CD25 and the transcription factor Foxp3 (Treg), may act as regulatory cells (Bridoux et al. 1997; Cavani et al. 2003; Feuerer 2009). These T cells promote anti-inflammatory immunity, e.g., by switching antibody production to IgA, which mediates secretory immunity and thus contributes to antigen exclusion in the lumen, e.g., of the gastrointestinal tract (Hafler et al. 1997). Of note, TGF-β strongly suppresses development of both type-1 and -2 effector T cells, and can silence T cells in a semi-naïve state (O'Garra 1998).

Regulatory Mechanisms of the Effector Phase. A critical feature of the regulatory principles involving mutual regulation of T-cell subpopulations by Th1, Th2, Th3 and Th17/22 cytokines, is that regulatory functions are most effective during initiation of immune responses (➋ *Fig. 14.5*). Thus, once established, effector T cell and cytokine profiles show remarkable stability and refractoriness to regulatory forces. Down-regulation of allergic skin reactions may, therefore, take considerable time. Of course, the preliminary factor facilitating decreased allergic skin reactivity is removal of hapten by exudate and innate immune cells of the inflammatory infiltrate. But, at chronically exposed sites also specific regulatory mechanisms can be involved, such as $CD8^+$ T cells, acting either as regulator/suppressor ($CD28^-CD11b^+$) or cytotoxic ($CD28^+CD11b^-$) T cells (Lonati et al. 1998; De panfilis 1998), which may downregulate skin reactivity by targeting allergen-presenting DC [331]. Multiplicity and reduncancy of regulatory mechanisms have thus far hampered development of robust clinical treatments exploiting regulatory T-cell functions to provide for allergen-specific downregulation of the effector phase of ACD. The development of potential therapeutic applications of regulatory cells in various disorders, such as allergic contact dermatitis and autoimmune diseases, therefore, needs much more time than envisioned earlier (Ilan 2009).

Redundancy of Tolerance Mechanisms. Besides regulatory T cells, producing different cytokines, or exerting distinct cytotoxicities, other mechanisms may also contribute to immune regulation and tolerance. Clearly, the risk of excessive immune reactivity should be very low. These mechanisms involve allergen-specific T cells shedding truncated T-cell receptors, acting as antagonists and blocking allergen presentation (Kuchroo 1998), and high-dose allergen-induced anergic T cells (Morgan et al. 1999). Possibly, the latter cells, by actively suppressing DC functions, can function as "active" suppressor cells (Taams et al. 1998, 2000). Interestingly, DC, becoming suppressive by this mechanism (Taams et al. 1998) or by suppressive cytokines like IL-10 and PGE_2 (Kumar and Sercarz 1998; Kalinski et al. 1998), can, in turn, act themselves as suppressor cells by conferring antigen-specific anergy to subsequently encountered T cells (Steinbrink et al. 1999; Taams et al. 2000). Although, at present, consensus has been reached about a critical role of regulatory/suppressor cells in the development and expression of ACD, the relative contributions of each of the various mechanisms are still far from clear.

Induction of Lasting Tolerance Only in Naive Individuals. Both clinical and experimental findings indicate that full and persistent tolerance can only be induced prior to any sensitizing allergen contacts (Van Hoogstraten et al. 1989; Strobel and Mowat 1998; Wang 2008). Upon primary allergenic contacts, naive T cells differentiate to produce polarized cytokine profiles (➋ *Figs. 14.5* and ➋ *14.9*). Once polarized, however, T-cell profiles are irreversible, due to loss of cytokine (receptor) genes, or at least very stable, due to the mutually suppressive activities of T-cell cytokines. An important corollary of the latter concept of active suppression is the bystander effect, in which the response to any antigen can be downregulated by immunosuppressive cytokines acting in a local tolerogenic microenvironment (von Herrath 1997). The latter was observed for both protein antigens (Fowler and Weiner 1997) and methacrylate contact allergens (Rustemeyer et al. 2001). Stable polarization/skewing may also explain why even low, non-sensitizing doses of nickel applied to the skin prevented subsequent tolerance induction by feeding the metal allergen (Van Hoogstraten et al. 1994). Apparently, the progeny of naïve allergen-specific cells, once "on the stage," have been triggered to a "subclinical" degree toward effector cell differentiation and become refractory to regulatory cell action (➋ *Fig. 14.10*). This may also have contributed to incomplete tolerance induction in earlier clinical studies when feeding with poison ivy-/oak-derived allergens (Epstein 1987). Indeed, to our knowledge, permanent reversal of existing ACD in healthy individuals has, as yet, never been achieved. Nevertheless, as described above, effector cells still seem susceptible, though transiently, to the downregulation of allergen reactivity, as was observed in desensitization procedures (Van Hoogstraten et al. 1994; Morris 1998).

Transient Desensitization in Primed Individuals. For dermatologists, methods by which patients might be desensitized for existing ACD would be a welcome addition to the currently prevailing symptomatic therapies, and investigators have made a wide variety of attempts to achieve this goal. Unfortunately, as mentioned above, therapeutic protocols involving ingestion of poison ivy allergen, penicillin, or nickel sulfate were of only transient benefit to the patients (Epstein 1987; Wendel et al. 1985; Panzani et al. 1995; Tammaro et al. 2009). Similarly in animal models, only a limited and transient degree of hyposensitization was obtained by Chase (1946) when feeding DNCB-contact-sensitized guinea pigs with the allergen, whereas, for achieving persistent chromium-unresponsiveness in presensitized animals, Polak and Turk (1968a, b) needed a rigorous protocol involving up to lethal doses of the allergen. As outlined above, mechanisms underlying specific desensitization in ACD probably depend on direct interference of allergen with effector T-cell function, by blocking or downregulating T-cell receptors, leading to anergy and apoptosis (Polak and Rinck 1978). As the onset of desensitization is immediate, no suppressor mechanisms may initially be involved. Apparently in the absence of LC, MHC class II-positive keratinocytes can serve as APC and are very effective in rendering allergen-specific effector cells anergic (Gaspari et al. 1988). Moreover, at later stages active suppression may come into play resulting from secondary inactivation of DC function by anergized T cells (Shreedhar et al. 1998). Nevertheless, major problems with in vivo desensitization procedures relate to the refractoriness of effector T cells to regulatory cell functions, and the rapid replacement of anergized effector cells by naïve T cells from relatively protected peripheral lymphoid tissues provides a source of new effector cells upon sensitizing allergen contacts. The same conclusions can be drawn from attempts to achieve local desensitization. It was found that local desensitization by repeatedly applying allergen at the same skin site did not result from local skin hardening or LC inactivation, as local reactivity to an unrelated allergen at the site was unimpaired (Boerrigter and Scheper 1987). Persistence of cellular infiltrates, in the absence of erythematous reactivity, at a desensitized skin site could reflect local anergy, but also locally active regulatory cells. Upon discontinuation of allergen exposure, however, local unresponsiveness was rapidly (within 1 week) lost. Collectively, this data illustrates the problems encountered in attempting to eradicate established effector-T-cell function, not only in ACD but also in autoimmune diseases (Weiner 1997; Wang 2008).

10 Summary and Conclusions

Extensive research has led to a better understanding of the mechanisms of ICD and ACD. The primary role of innate immune cells in coping with exogenous potential harmful threats is rapidly being uncovered. Also, the basic immunology of ACD is now well-defined, including T-cell migratory patterns, recognition of distinct allergens, interactions with other inflammatory cells to generate inflammation, and cytokine profiles. But new complexities have emerged. For instance, in contrast to earlier belief, many of the currently known T-cell subpopulations can act either or both as effector and regulatory cells, depending on the nature of the allergen, the route of entry, frequency of exposure, and many other, still ill-defined factors. In particular, the poor understanding of regulatory mechanisms in ACD still hampers further therapeutic progress. So far, no methods of permanent desensitization have been devised.

Nevertheless, next to the established anti-inflammatory drugs, recently defined cellular interaction molecules and mediators provide promising targets for new generations of anti-inflammatory drugs, some of which have already entered clinical trials. Clearly, drugs found to be effective in preventing severe T-cell-mediated conditions, e.g., rejection of a vital organ graft, should be very safe before their use in ACD would seem appropriate. To date, prudence favors alternative measures to prevent ICD and ACD, be it through legal action to outlaw the use of certain materials or through avoiding personal contact with these materials. In the meantime, for difficult-to-avoid allergens, further studies on the potential value of tolerogenic treatments prior to possible sensitization seem warranted.

References

Abe M, Kondo T, Xu H, Fairchild RL (1996) Interferon-gamma inducible protein (IP-10) expression is mediated by CD8+ T cells and is regulated by CD4+ T cells during the elicitation of contact hypersensitivity. J Invest Dermatol 107:360–366

Abe N, Katamura K, Shintaku N, Fukui T, Kiyomasu T, Lio J, Ueno H, Tai G, Mayumi M, Furusho K (1997) Prostaglandin E2 and IL-4 provide naïve CD4+ T cells with distinct inhibitory signals for the priming of IFN-gamma production. Cell Immunol 181:86–92

Acuto O, Michel F (2003) CD28-mediated co-stimulation: a quantitative support for TCR signalling. Nat Rev Immunol 3:939–951

Adema GJ, Hartgers F, Verstraten R, de Vries E, Marland G, Menon S, Foster J, Xu Y, Nooyen P, McClanahan T, Bacon KB, Figdor CG (1997) A dendritic-cell-derived C–C chemokine that preferentially attracts naïve T cells. Nature 387:713–717

Aiba S, Tagami H (1999) Dendritic cell activation induced by various stimuli, e.g. exposure to microorganisms, their products, cytokines, and simple chemicals as well as adhesion to extracellular matrix. J Dermatol Sci 20:1–13

Allan SE, Broady R, Gregori S, Himmel ME, Locke N, Roncarolo MG, Bacchetta R, Levings MK (2008) CD4+ T-regulatory cells: toward therapy for human diseases. Immunol Rev 223:391–421

Altin JG, Sloan EK (1997) The role of CD45 and CD45-associated molecules in T cell activation. Immunol Cell Biol 75:430–445

Asada H, Linton J, Katz SI (1997) Cytokine gene expression during the elicitation phase of contact sensitivity – regulation by endogenous IL-4. J Invest Dermatol 108:406–411

Asherson GL, Dieli F, Sireci G, Salerno A (1996) Role of IL-4 in delayed type hypersensitivity. Clin Exp Immunol 103:1–4

Austrup F, Vestweber D, Borges E, Lohning M, Brauer R, Herz U, Renz H, Hallmann R, Scheffold A, Radbruch A, Hamann A (1997) P- and E selectin mediate recruitment of T-helper-1 but not T-helper-2 cells into inflamed tissues. Nature 385:81–83

Banchereau J, Steinman RM (1998) Dendritic cells and the control of immunity. Nature 392:245–252

Bangert C, Friedl J, Stary G, Stingl G, Kopp T (2003) Immunopathologic features of allergic contact dermatitis in humans: participation of plasmacytoid dendritic cells in the pathogenesis of the disease? J Invest Dermatol 121:1409–1418

Basso AS, Cheroutre H, Mucida D (2009) More stories on Th17 cells. Cell Res 19(4):399–411

Benson JM, Whitacre CC (1997) The role of clonal deletion and anergy in oral tolerance. Res Immunol 148:533–541

Berg DJ, Leach MW, Kuhn R, Rajewsky K, Muller W, Davidson NJ, Rennick D (1995) Interleukin 10 but not interleukin 4 is a natural suppressant of cutaneous inflammatory responses. J Exp Med 182:99–108

Bergstresser PR (1989) Sensitization and elicitation of inflammation in contact dermatitis. In: Norris DA (ed) Immune mechanisms in cutaneous disease. Dekker, New York, pp 219–246

Birbeck M (1961) An electron microscope study of basal melanocytes and high level clear cells (Langerhans cells) in vitiligo. J Invest Dermatol 37:51–56

Blauvelt A, Hwang ST, Udey MC (2003) Allergic and immunologic diseases of the skin. J Allergy Clin Immunol 111:S560–S570

Blömeke B, Brans R, Coenraads PJ, Dickel H, Bruckner T, Hein DW, Heesen M, Merk HF, Kawakubo Y (2009) Para-phenylenediamine and allergic sensitization: risk modification by *N*-acetyltransferase 1 and 2 genotypes. Br J Dermatol 161(5):1130–1135

Boerrigter GH, Scheper RJ (1984) Local administration of the cytostatic drug 4-hydroperoxy-cyclophosphamde (4-HPCY) facilitates cell mediated immune reactions. Clin Exp Immunol 58:161–166

Boerrigter GH, Scheper RJ (1987) Local and systemic desensitization induced by repeated epicutaneous hapten application. J Invest Dermatol 88:3–7

Boerrigter GH, de Groot J, Scheper RJ (1986) Intradermal administration of 4-hydoperoxy-cyclophosphamde during contact sensitization potentiates effector T cell responsiveness in draining lymph nodes. Immunopharmacology 1:13–20

Borges E, Tietz W, Steegmaier M, Moll T, Hallmann R, Hamann A, Vestweber D (1997) P-selectin glycoprotein ligand-1 (PSGL-1) on T helper 1 but not on T helper 2 cells binds to P-selectin and supports migration into inflamed skin. J Exp Med 185:573–578

Bos JD, Meinardi MMHM (2000) The 500 Dalton rule for the skin penetration of chemical compounds and drugs. Exp Dermatol 9:165–169

Braathen LR (1980) Studies on human epidermal Langerhans cells. III. Induction of T lymphocyte response to nickel sulphate in sensitized individuals. Br J Dermatol 103:517–526

Brand CU, Hunger RE, Yawalkar N, Gerber HA, Schaffner T, Braathen LR (1999) Characterization of human skin-derived CD1a-positive lymph cells. Arch Dermatol Res 291:65–72

Brasch J, Burgard J, Sterry W (1992) Common pathways in allergic and irritant contact dermatitis. J Invest Dermatol 98:166–170

Breathnach SM (1988) The Langerhans cell. Centenary review. Br J Dermatol 119:463–469

Bretscher PA, Ogunremi O, Menon JN (1997) Distinct immunological states in murine cutaneous leishmaniasis by immunizing with different amounts of antigen: the generation of beneficial, potentially harmful, harmful and potentially extremely harmful states. Behring Inst Mitt 98:153–159

Bridoux F, Badou A, Saoudi A, Bernard L, Druet E, Pasquier R, Druet P, Pelletier L (1997) Transforming growth factor beta (TGF-beta)-dependent inhibition of T helper cell 2 (Th2)-induced autoimmunity by self-major histocompatibility complex (MHC) class II-specific, regulatory CD4+ T cell lines. J Exp Med 185:1769–1775

Buchanan KL, Murphy JW (1997) Kinetics of cellular infiltration and cytokine production during the efferent phase of a delayed-type hypersensitivity reaction. Immunology 90:189–197

Budinger L, Hertl M (2000) Immunologic mechanisms in hypersensitivity reactions to metal ions: an overview. Allergy 55:108–115

Calder PC, Bevan SJ, Newsholme EA (1992) The inhibition of T-lymphocyte proliferation by fatty acids is via an eicosanoid-independent mechanism. Immunology 75:108–115

Cantrell D (1996) T cell receptor signal transduction pathways. Annu Rev Immunol 14:259–274

Carroll JM, Crompton T, Seery JP, Watt FM (1997) Transgenic mice expressing IFN-gamma in the epidermis have eczema, hair hypopigmentation, and hair loss. J Invest Dermatol 108:412–422

Caux C, Ait-Yahia S, Chemin K, de Bouteiller O, Dieu-Nosjean MC, Homey B, Massacrier C, Vanbervliet B, Zlotnik A, Vicari A (2000) Dendritic cell biology and regulation of dendritic cell trafficking by chemokines. Springer Semin Immunopathol 22:345–369

Cavani A, Mei D, Guerra E, Corinti S, Giani M, Pirrotta L, Puddu P, Girolomoni G (1998) Patients with allergic contact dermatitis to nickel and nonallergic individuals display different nickel-specific T cell responses. Evidence for the presence of effector CD8+ and regulatory CD4+ T cells. J Invest Dermatol 111:621–628

Cavani A, Nasorri F, Ottaviani C, Sebastiani S, De Pita O, Girolomoni G (2003) Human CD25+ regulatory T cells maintain immune tolerance to nickel in healthy, nonallergic individuals. J Immunol 171:5760–5768

Cella M, Sallusto F, Lanzavecchia A (1997) Origin, maturation and antigen presenting function of dendritic cells. Curr Opin Immunol 9:10–16

Chase MW (1946) Inhibition of experimental drug allergy by prior feeding of the sensitizing agent. Proc Soc Exp Biol Med 61:257–259

Christensen OB, Beckstead JH, Daniels TE, Maibach HI (1985) Pathogenesis of orally induced flare-up reactions at old patch sites in nickel allergy. Acta Derm Venereol 65:298–304

Claessen AME, von Blomberg BME, de Groot J, Wolvers DAE, Kraal G, Scheper RJ (1996) Reversal of mucosal tolerance by subcutaneous administration of interleukin-12 at the site of attempted sensitization. Immunology 88:363–367

Constant SL, Bottomly K (1997) Induction of Th1 and Th2 CD4+ T cell responses: the alternate approaches. Annu Rev Immunol 15: 297–322

Constant SL, Pfeiffer C, Woodard A, Pasqualini T, Bottomly K (1995) Extent of T cell receptor ligation can determine the functional differentiation of naïve CD4+ T cells. J Exp Med 5:1591–1596

Coulter EM, Jenkinson C, Farrell J, Lavergne SN, Pease C, White A, Aleksic M, Basketter D, Williams DP, King C, Pirmohamed M, Park BK, Naisbitt DJ (2010) Measurement of CD4+ and CD8+ T-lymphocyte cytokine secretion and gene expression changes in *p*-phenylenediamine allergic patients and tolerant individuals. J Invest Dermatol 130:161–174

Crivellato E, Vacca A, Ribatti D (2004) Setting the stage: an anatomist's view of the immune system. Trends Immunol 25:210–217

Croft M, So T, Duan W, Soroosh P (2009) The significance of OX40 and OX40L to T-cell biology and immune disease. Immunol Rev 229(1):173–191

Cumberbatch M, Dearman RJ, Kimber I (1997) Interleukin 1-beta and the stimulation of Langerhans cell migration – comparisons with tumour necrosis factor alpha. Arch Dermatol Res 289:277–284

Cutolo M, Seriolo B, Villaggio B, Pizzorni C, Craviotto C, Sulli A (2002) Androgens and estrogens modulate the immune and inflammatory responses in rheumatoid arthritis. Ann N Y Acad Sci 966:131–142

Czernielewski SM, Demarchez M (1987) Further evidence for the self-reproducing capacity of Langerhans cells in human skin. J Invest Dermatol 88:17–20

Dabbagh K, Lewis DB (2003) Toll-like receptors and T-helper-1/T-helper-2 responses. Curr Opin Infect Dis 16:199–204

Davis SJ, van der Merwe PA (2003) TCR triggering: co-receptor-dependent or -independent? Trends Immunol 24:624–626

De Panfilis G (1998) CD8+ cytolytic T lymphocytes and the skin. Exp Dermatol 7:121–131

Demeure CE, Yang LP, Desjardins C, Raynauld P, Delespesse G (1997) Prostaglandin E-2 primes naïve T cells for the production of anti-inflammatory cytokines. Eur J Immunol 27:3526–3531

Dieli F, Ptak W, Sireci G, Romano GC, Potestio M, Salerno A, Asherson GL (1998) Cross-talk between V-beta-8(+) and gamma-delta(+) T lymphocytes in contact sensitivity. Immunology 93:469–477

Dieu M-C, Vanbervliet B, Vicari A, Bridon J-M, Oldham E, Ait-Yahia S, Brière F, Zlotnik A, Lebecque S, Caux C (1998) Selective recruitment of immature and mature dendritic cells by distinct chemokines expressed in different anatomic sites. J Exp Med 188:373–386

Divkovic M, Pease CK, Gerberick GF, Basketter DA (2005) Hapten-protein binding: from theory to practical application in the in vitro prediction of skin sensitization. Contact Dermatitis 53(4):189–200

Dong C (2008) TH17 cells in development: an updated view of their molecular identity and genetic programming. Nat Rev Immunol 8(5):337–348

Dong C, Nurieva RI, Prasad DV (2003) Immune regulation by novel costimulatory molecules. Immunol Res 28:39–48

Dvorak HF, Mihm MC Jr, Dvorak AM (1976) Morphology of delayed-type hypersensitivity reactions in man. J Invest Dermatol 64: 391–401

Edele F, Esser PR, Lass C, Laszczyk MN, Oswald E, Strüh CM, Rensing-Ehl A, Martin SF (2007) Innate and adaptive immune responses in allergic contact dermatitis and autoimmune skin diseases. Inflamm Allergy Drug Targets 6(4):236–244

Eliasson E, Kenna JG (1996) Cytochrome P450 2E1 is a cell surface autoantigen in halothane hepatitis. Mol Pharmacol 50:573–582

Enk AH, Katz SI (1992a) Early molecular events in the induction phase of contact sensitivity. Proc Natl Acad Sci USA 89:1398–1402

Enk AH, Katz SI (1992b) Identification and induction of keratinocyte-derived IL-10. J Immunol 149:92–95

Enk AH, Angeloni VL, Udey MC, Katz SI (1993) An essential role for Langerhans cell-derived IL-1b in the initiation of primary immune responses in skin. J Immunol 150:3698–3704

Epling GA, Wells JL, Yoon UC (1988) Photochemical transformations in salicylanilide photoallergy. Photochem Photobiol 47:167–171

Epstein WL (1987) The poison ivy picker of Pennypack Park: the continuing saga of poison ivy. J Invest Dermatol 88:7–9

Epstein SP, Baer RL, Thorbecke GJ, Belsito DV (1991) Immunosuppressive effects of transforming growth factor beta: inhibition of the induction of Ia antigen on Langerhans cells by cytokines and of the contact hypersensitivity response. J Invest Dermatol 96:832–837

Faria AM, Weiner HL (2006) Oral tolerance and TGF-beta-producing cells. Inflamm Allergy Drug Targets 5(3):179–190

Ferber I, Schönrich G, Schenkel J, Mellor AL, Hämmerling GJ, Arnold B (1994) Levels of peripheral T cell tolerance induced by different doses of tolerogen. Science 263:674–676

Flier J, Boorsma DM, Bruynzeel DP, van Beek PJ, Stoof TJ, Scheper RJ, Willemze R, Tensen CP (1999) The CXCR3 activating chemokines IP-10, MIG and IP-9 are expressed in allergic but not in irritant patch test reactions. J Invest Dermatol 113:574–578

Foreman KE, Vaporciyan AA, Bonish BK, Jones ML, Johnson KJ, Glovsky MM, Eddy SM, Ward PA (1994) C5a-induced expression of P-selectin in endothelial cells. J Clin Invest 94:1147–1155

Fowler E, Weiner HL (1997) Oral tolerance: elucidation of mechanisms and application to treatment of autoimmune diseases. Biopolymers 43:323–335

Fuhlbrigge RC, Kieffer JD, Armerding D, Kupper TS (1997) Cutaneous lymphocyte antigen is a specialized form of PSGL-1 expressed on skin-homing T cells. Nature 389:978–981

Furue M, Chang CH, Tamaki K (1996) Interleukin-1 but not tumor necrosis factor a synergistically upregulates the granulocyte-macrophage colony-stimulating factor-induced B7–1 expression of murine Langerhans cells. Br J Dermatol 135:194–198

Fyhrquist-Vanni N, Alenius H, Lauerma A (2007) Contact dermatitis. Dermatol Clin 25(4):613–623

Gajewski TF, Fitch FW (1988) Antiproliferative effect of IFN-gamma in immune regulation. I. IFN-gamma inhibits the proliferation of Th2 but not Th1 murine helper T lymphocyte clones. J Immunol 140:4245–4252

Gascoigne NR, Zal T (2004) Molecular interactions at the T cell-antigen-presenting cell interface. Curr Opin Immunol 16:114–119

Gaspari AA, Jenkins MK, Katz SI (1988) Class II MCH-bearing keratinocytes induce antigen-specific unresponsiveness in hapten-specific TH1 clones. J Immunol 141:2216–2220

Geenen V, Brilot F (2003) Role of the thymus in the development of tolerance and autoimmunity towards the neuroendocrine system. Ann N Y Acad Sci 992:186–195

Gell PDH, Coombs RRA, Lachman R (1975) Clinical aspects of immunology, 3rd edn. Blackwell, London

Gerberick F, Aleksic M, Basketter D, Casati S, Karlberg AT, Kern P, Kimber I, Lepoittevin JP, Natsch A, Ovigne JM, Rovida C, Sakaguchi H, Schultz T (2008) Chemical reactivity measurement and the predicitve identification of skin sensitisers. The report and recommendations of ECVAM Workshop 64. Altern Lab Anim 36(2):215–242

Girolomoni G, Gisondi P, Ottaviani C, Cavani A (2004) Immunoregulation of allergic contact dermatitis. J Dermatol 31:264–270

Goebeler M, Meinardus-Hager G, Roth J, Goerdt S, Sorg C (1993) Nickel chloride and cobalt chloride, two common contact sensitizers, directly induce expression of intercellular adhesion molecule-1 (ICAM-1), vascular cell adhesion molecule-1 (VCAM-1), and endothelial leukocyte adhesion molecule (ELAM-1) by endothelial cells. J Invest Dermatol 100:759–765

Goebeler M, Roth J, Brocker EB, Sorg C, Schulze-Osthoff K (1995) Activation of nuclear factor-kappa B and gene expression in human endothelial cells by the common haptens nickel and cobalt. J Immunol 155:2459–2467

Grewe M, Bruijnzeel-Koomen CA, Schöpf E, Thepen T, Langeveld-Wildschut AG, Ruzicka T, Krutmann J (1998) A role for Th1 and Th2 cells in the immunopathogenesis of atopic dermatitis. Immunol Today 19(8):359–361

Griem P, Wulferink M, Sachs B, Gonzales JB, Gleichmann E (1998) Allergic and autoimmune reactions to xenobiotics: how do they arise? Immunol Today 19:133–141

Groux H, Sornasse T, Cottrez F, de Vries JE, Coffman RL, Roncarolo MG, Yssel H (1997) Induction of human T helper cell type-1 differentiation results in loss of IFN-g receptor b-chain expression. J Immunol 158:5627–5631

Groves RW, Allen MH, Ross EL, Barker JN, MacDonald DM (1995) Tumor necrosis factor alpha is pro-inflammatory in normal human skin and modulates cutaneous adhesion molecule expression. Br J Dermatol 132:345–352

Gunn MD, Tangemann K, Tam C, Cyster JG, Rosen SD, Williams LT (1998) A chemokine expressed in lymphoid high endothelial venules promotes the adhesion and chemotaxis of naïve T lymphocytes. Proc Natl Acad Sci USA 95:258–263

Hafler DA, Kent SC, Pietrusewicz MJ, Khoury SJ, Weiner HL, Fukaura H (1997) Oral administration of myelin induces antigen-specific

TGF-beta 1 secreting T cells in patients with multiple sclerosis. Ann N Y Acad Sci 835:120–131

Haig DM, Hopkins J, Miller HRP (1999) Local immune responses in afferent and efferent lymph. Immunology 96:155–163

Herzog WR, Meade R, Pettinicchi A, Ptak W, Askenase PW (1989) Nude mice produce a T cell-derived antigen-binding factor that mediates the early component of delayed-type hypersensitivity. J Immunol 142:1803–1812

Heufler C, Koch F, Schuler G (1988) Granulocyte/macrophage colony-stimulating factor and interleukin 1 mediate the maturation of epidermal Langerhans cells into potent immunostimulatory dendritic cells. J Exp Med 167:700–705

Hill S, Edwards AJ, Kimber I, Knight SC (1990) Systemic migration of dendritic cells during contact sensitization. Immunology 71:277–281

Hindsen M, Christensen OB (1992) Delayed hypersensitivity reactions following allergic and irritant inflammation. Acta Derm Venereol 72:220–221

Hindsen M, Bruze M, Christensen OB (2001) Flare-up reactions after oral challenge with nickel in relation to challenge dose and intensity and time of previous patch test reactions. J Am Acad Dermatol 44:616–623

Hoath SB, Leahy DG (2003) The organization of human epidermis: functional epidermal units and phi proportionality. J Invest Dermatol 121:1440–1446

Hoefakker S, Caubo M, van Herve EHM, Roggeveen MJ, Boersma WJA, Van't Joost Th, Notten WRF, Claassen E (1995) In vivo cytokine profiles in allergic and irritant contact dermatitis. Contact Dermatitis 33:258–266

Hommel M (2004) On the dynamics of T-cell activation in lymph nodes. Immunol Cell Biol 82:62–66

Honig SM, Fu S, Mao X, Yopp A, Gunn MD, Randolph GJ, Bromberg JS (2003) FTY720 stimulates multidrug transporter- and cysteinyl leukotriene-dependent T cell chemotaxis to lymph nodes. J Clin Invest 111:627–637

Houck G, Saeed S, Stevens GL, Morgan MB (2004) Eczema and the spongiotic dermatoses: a histologic and pathogenic update. Semin Cutan Med Surg 23:39–45

Hoyer KK, Dooms H, Barron L, Abbas AK (2008) Interleukin-2 in the development and control of inflammatory disease. Immunol Rev 226:19–28

Iliev ID, Mileti E, Matteoli G, Chieppa M, Rescigno M (2009) Intestinal epithelial cells promote colitis-protective regulatory T-cell differentiation through dendritic cell conditioning. Mucosal Immunol 2(4):340–350

Inaba K, Schuler G, Witmer MD, Valinsky J, Atassi B, Steinman RM (1986) Immunologic properties of purified epidermal Langerhans cells. Distinct requirements for stimulation of unprimed and sensitized T lymphocytes. J Exp Med 164:605–613

Inaba K, Schuler G, Steinman RM (1993) GM-CSF – a granulocyte/macrophage/dendritic cell stimulating factor. In: Van Furth R (ed) Hemopoietic growth factors and mononuclear phagocytes. Karger, Basel, pp 187–196

Inerot A, Moller H (2000) Symptoms and signs reported during patch testing. Am J Contact Dermatol 11:49–52

Isaksson M, Bruze M (2003) Late patch-test reactions to budesonide need not be a sign of sensitization induced by the test procedure. Am J Contact Dermatol 14:154–156

Itano AA, Jenkins MK (2003) Antigen presentation to naive CD4 T cells in the lymph node. Nat Immunol 4:733–739

Iversen L, Johansen C (2008) Inflammasomes and inflammatory caspases in skin inflammation. Expert Rev Mol Diagn 8(6):697–705

Izcue A, Coombes JL, Powrie F (2009) Regulatory lymphocytes and intestinal inflammation. Annu Rev Immunol 27:313–338

Jakob T, Udey MC (1998) Regulation of E-cadherin mediated adhesion in Langerhans cell-like dendritic cells by inflammatory mediators that mobilize Langerhans cells in vivo. J Immunol 160:4067–4073

Jakob T, Ring J, Udey MC (2001) Multistep navigation of Langerhans/dendritic cells in and out of the skin. J Allergy Clin Immunol 108:688–696

Jensen CS, Menne T, Lisby S, Kristiansen J, Veien NK (2003) Experimental systemic contact dermatitis from nickel: a dose–response study. Contact Dermatitis 49:124–132

Kalinski P, Hilkens CMU, Snijders A, Snijdewint FGM, Kapsenberg ML (1997) IL-12 deficient dendritic cells, generated in the presence of prostaglandin E2, promote type-2 cytokine production in maturing human naïve T helper cells. J Immunol 159:28–35

Kalinski P, Schuitemaker JH, Hilkens CM, Kapsenberg ML (1998) Prostaglandin E2 induces the final maturation of IL-12 deficient CD1a + CD83+ dendritic cells. J Immunol 161:2804–2809

Kalish RS, Wood JA, LaPorte A (1994) Processing of urushiol (poison ivy) hapten by both endogenous and exogenous pathways for presentation to T cells in vitro. J Clin Invest 93:2039–2047

Kanerva L, Hyry H, Jolanki R, Hytonen M, Estlander T (1997) Delayed and immediate allergy caused by methylhexahydrophthalic anhydride. Contact Dermatitis 36:34–38

Kang KF, Kubin M, Cooper KD, Lessin SR, Trinchieri G, Rook AH (1996) IL-12 synthesis by human Langerhans cells. J Immunol 156:1402–1407

Karlberg AT, Bergström MA, Börje A, Luthman K, Nilsson JL (2008) Allergic contact dermatitis–formation, structural requirements, and reactivity of skin sensitizers. Chem Res Toxicol 21(1):53–69

Kidd P (2003) Th1/Th2 balance: the hypothesis, its limitations, and implications for health and disease. Altern Med Rev 8:223–246

Kim CH, Broxmeyer HE (1999) Chemokines: signal lamps for trafficking of T and B cells for development and effector function. J Leukoc Biol 65:6–15

Kimber I, Cumberbatch M (1992) Dendritic cells and cutaneous immune responses to chemical allergens. Toxicol Appl Pharmacol 117: 137–146

Kimber I, Dearman RJ (2002) Allergic contact dermatitis: the cellular effectors. Contact Dermatitis 46:1–5

Kimber I, Dearman RJ (2003) What makes a chemical an allergen? Ann Allergy Asthma Immunol 90:28–31

Kimber I, Dearman RJ, Cumberbatch M, Huby RJ (1998) Langerhans cells and chemical allergy. Curr Opin Immunol 10:614–619

Kimber I, Basketter DA, Gerberick GF, Dearman RJ (2002) Allergic contact dermatitis. Int Immunopharmacol 2:201–211

Kitagaki H, Fujisawa S, Watanabe K, Hayakawa K, Shiohara T (1995) Immediate-type hypersensitivity response followed by late reaction is induced by repeated epicutaneous application of contact sensitizing agents in mice. J Invest Dermatol 105:749–755

Knop J, Stremmer R, Neumann C, Dc Maeyer D, Macher E (1982) Interferon inhibits the suppressor T cell response of delayed-type hypersensitivity. Nature 296:775–776

Kobayashi Y (1997) Langerhans cells produce type IV collagenase (MMP-9) following epicutaneous stimulation with haptens. Immunology 90:496–501

Kondo S, Sauder DN (1995) Epidermal cytokines in allergic contact dermatitis. J Am Acad Dermatol 33:786–800

Korn T, Bettelli E, Oukka M, Kuchroo VK (2009) IL-17 and Th17 cells (review). Annu Rev Immunol 27:485–517, PubMed PMID: 19132915

Kothny-Wilkes G, Kulms D, Poppelmann B, Luger TA, Kubin M, Schwarz T (1998) Interleukin-1 protects transformed keratinocytes from tumor necrosis factor-related apoptosis-inducing ligand. J Biol Chem 273:29247–29253

Krasteva M, Nicolas JF, Chabeau G, Garrigue JL, Bour H, Thivolet J, Schmitt D (1993) Dissociation of allergenic and immunogenic functions in contact sensitivity to para-phenylenediamine. Int Arch Allergy Immunol 102:200–204

Kubo M, Ransom J, Webb D, Hashimoto Y, Tada T, Nakayama T (1997) T-cell subset-specific expression of the *IL-4* gene is regulated by a silencer element and STAT6. EMBO J 16(13):4007–4020

Kuchroo VK, Byrne MC, Atsumi Y, Greenfeld E, Connol JH, Whitters MJ, O'Hara RM, Collins M, Dorf ME (1991) T cell receptor alpha chain plays a critical role in antigen-specific suppressor cell function. Proc Natl Acad Sci USA 88:8700–8704

Kumar V, Sercarz E (1998) Induction or protection from experimental autoimmune encephalomyelitis depends on the cytokine secretion profile of TCR peptide-specific regulatory CD4 T cells. J Immunol 161:6585–6591

Kuo CT, Leiden JM (1999) Transcriptional regulation of T lymphocyte development and function. Annu Rev Immunol 17:149–187

Lalani I, Bhol K, Ahmed AR (1997) Interleukin-10 biology, role in inflammation and autoimmunity. Ann Allergy Asthma Immunol 79:469–484

Langerhans P (1868) Über die nerven der menschlichen haut. Virchows Arch Pathol Anat 44:325–337

Lappin MB, Kimber I, Norval M (1996) The role of dendritic cells in cutaneous immunity. Arch Dermatol Res 288:109–121

Larsson A, Moller H, Björkner B, Bruze M (1997) Morphology of endogenous flare-up reactions in contact allergy to gold. Acta Derm Venereol 77:474–479

Lawrence JN, Dickson FM, Benford DJ (1997) Skin irritant-induced cytotoxicity and prostaglandin E-2 release in human skin keratinocyte cultures. Toxicol Vitro 11:627–631

Lepoittevin JP (2006) Metabolism versus chemical transformation or pro-versus prehaptens? Contact Dermatitis 54(2):73–74

Li QJ, Dinner AR, Qi S, Irvine DJ, Huppa JB, Davis MM, Chakraborty AK (2004) CD4 enhances T cell sensitivity to antigen by coordinating Lck accumulation at the immunological synapse. Nat Immunol 5:791–799

Liberato DJ, Byers VS, Ennick RG, Castagnoli N (1981) Region specific attack of nitrogen and sulfur nucleophiles on quinones from poison oak/ivy catechols (urushiols) and analogues as models for urushiol-protein conjugate formation. J Med Chem 24:28–33

Lider O, Cahalon L, Gilat D, Hershkoviz R, Siegel D, Margalit R, Shoseyov O, Cohen IR (1995) A disaccharide that inhibits tumor necrosis factor alpha is formed from the extracellular matrix by the enzyme heparinase. Proc Natl Acad Sci USA 92:5037–5041

Lonati A, Licenziati S, Marcelli M, Canaris D, Pasolini G, Caruso A, de Panfilis G (1998) Quantitative analysis "at the single cell level" of the novel CD28-CD11b- subpopulation of CD8+ T lymphocytes. ESDR meeting, Cologne

Lord GM, Matarese G, Howard LK, Baker RJ, Bloom SR, Lechler RI (1998) Leptin modulates the T-cell immune response and reverses starvation-induced immunosuppression. Nature 394:897–901

Luger TA (2002) Neuromediators–a crucial component of the skin immune system. J Dermatol Sci 30(2):87–93

Luger TA, Lotti T (1998) Neuropeptides: role in inflammatory skin diseases. J Eur Acad Dermatol Venereol 10:207–211

Lundeberg L, Mutt V, Nordlind K (1999) Inhibitory effect of vasoactive intestinal peptide on the challenge phase of allergic contact dermatitis in humans. Acta Derm Venereol 79:178–182

Ma J, Wing J-H, Guo Y-J, Sy M-S, Bigby M (1994) In vivo treatment with anti-ICAM-1 and antiLFA-1 antibodies inhibits contact sensitization-induced migration of epidermal Langerhans cells to regional lymph nodes. Cell Immunol 158:389–399

Macatonia SE, Knight SC, Edwards AJ, Griffiths S, Fryer P (1987) Localization of antigen on lymph node dendritic cells after exposure to the contact sensitizer fluorescein isothiocyanate. Functional and morphological studies. J Exp Med 166:1654–1667

Marchal G, Seman M, Milon G, Truffa-Bachi P, Zilberfarb V (1982) Local adoptive transfer of skin delayed-type hypersensitivity initiated by a single T lymphocyte. J Immunol 129:954–958

Marone G, Spadaro G, Patella V, Genovese A (1994) The clinical relevance of basophil releasability. J Allergy Clin Immunol 94:1293–1303

Matura M (1998) Contact allergy to locally applied corticosteroids. Thesis, Leuven

Mayer L, Sperber K, Chan L, Child J, Toy L (2001) Oral tolerance to protein antigens. Allergy 56:12–15

Merk HF, Abel J, Baron JM, Krutmann J (2004) Molecular pathways in dermatotoxicology. Toxicol Appl Pharmacol 195:267–277

Mestas J, Hughes CC (2004) Of mice and not men: differences between mouse and human immunology. J Immunol 172:2731–2738

Miller SD, Sy M-S, Claman HN (1977) The induction of hapten-specific T cell tolerance using hapten-modified lymphoid membranes. II. Relative roles of suppressor T cells and clone inhibition in the tolerant state. Eur J Immunol 7:165–170

Milon G, Marchal G, Seman M, Truffa-Bachi P (1981) A delayed-type hypersensitivity reaction initiated by a single T lymphocyte. Agents Actions 11:612–614

Moed H, Boorsma DM, Stoof TJ, von Blomberg BM, Bruynzeel DP, Scheper RJ, Gibbs S, Rustemeyer T (2004a) Nickel-responding T cells are CD4+ CLA+ CD45RO+ and express chemokine receptors CXCR3, CCR4 and CCR10. Br J Dermatol 151:32–41

Moed H, Boorsma DM, Tensen CP, Flier J, Jonker MJ, Stoof TJ, Von Blomberg BM, Bruynzeel DP, Scheper RJ, Rustemeyer T, Gibbs S (2004b) Increased CCL27-CCR10 expression in allergic contact dermatitis: implications for local skin memory. J Pathol 204:39–46

Mokyr MB, Kalinichenko T, Gorelik L, Bluestone JA (1998) Realization of the therapeutic potential of CTLA-4 blockade in low-dose chemotherapy-treated tumor-bearing mice. Cancer Res 58:5301–5304

Morel PA, Oriss TB (1998) Crossregulation between Th1 and Th2 cells. Crit Rev Immunol 18:275–303

Morfin R, Lafaye P, Cotillon AC, Nato F, Chmielewski V, Pompon D (2000) 7 alpha-hydroxy-dehydroepiandrosterone and immune response. Ann N Y Acad Sci 917:971–982

Morgan DJ, Kreuwel HTC, Sherman LA (1999) Antigen concentration and precursor frequency determine the rate of CD8(+) T cell tolerance to peripherally expressed antigens. J Immunol 163:723–727

Morris DL (1998) Intradermal testing and sublingual in desensitization for nickel. Cutis 61:129–132

Moser B, Loetscher M, Piali L, Loetscher P (1998) Lymphocyte responses to chemokines. Int Rev Immunol 16:323–3244

Moser K, Kriwet K, Naik A, Kalia YN, Guy RH (2001) Passive skin penetration enhancement and its quantification in vitro. Eur J Pharm Biopharm 52:103–112

Moulon C, Vollmer J, Weltzien H-U (1995) Characterization of processing requirements and metal crossreactivities in T cell clones from patients with allergic contact dermatitis to nickel. Eur J Immunol 25:3308–3315

Mucida D, Salek-Ardakani S (2009) Regulation of TH17 cells in the mucosal surfaces. J Allergy Clin Immunol 123(5):997–1003

Murphy K, Travers P, Walport M (eds) (2008) Janeway's immunobiology, 7th edn. Garland Science/Taylor & Francis Group, New York/Oxford

Mutschler J, Giménez-Arnau E, Foertsch L, Gerberick GF, Lepoittevin JP (2009) Mechanistic assessment of peptide reactivity assay to predict skin allergens with Kathon CG isothiazolinones. Toxicol In Vitro 23(3):439–446

Nagira M, Imai T, Hieshima K, Kusuda J, Ridanpaa M, Takagi S, Nishimura M, Kakizaki M, Nomiyama H, Yoshie O (1997) Molecular cloning of a novel human CC chemokine secondary lymphoid-tissue chemokine that is a potent chemoattractant for lymphocytes and mapped to chromosome 9p13. J Biol Chem 272:19518–19524

Naisbitt DJ (2004) Drug hypersensitivity reactions in skin: understanding mechanisms and the development of diagnostic and predictive tests. Toxicology 194:179–196

Nakamura T, Kamogawa Y, Bottomly K, Flavell RA (1997a) Polarization of IL-4- and IFN-gamma-producing CD4(+) T cells following activation of naive CD4(+) T cells. J Immunol 158:1085–1094

Nakamura T, Lee RK, Nam SY, Podack ER, Bottomly K, Flavell RA (1997b) Roles of IL-4 and IFN-g in stabilizing the T helper cell type-1 and 2 phenotype. J Immunol 158:2648–2653

Nataf S, Davoust N, Ames RS, Barnum SR (1999) Human T cells express the C5a receptor and are chemoattracted to C5a. J Immunol 162:4018–4023

Ngo VN, Tang LH, Cyster JG (1998) Epstein-Barr virus-induced molecule 1 ligand chemokine is expressed by dendritic cells in lymphoid tissues and strongly attracts naïve T cells and activated B cells. J Exp Med 188:181–191

O'Garra A (1998) Cytokines induce the development of functionally heterogeneous T helper cell subsets. Immunity 8:275–283

Ohshima Y, Tanaka Y, Tozawa H, Takahashi Y, Maliszewski C, Delespesse C (1997) Expression and function of OX40 ligand on human dendritic cells. J Immunol 159:3838–3848

Orange JS, Biron CA (1996) An absolute and restricted requirement for IL-12 in natural killer cell IFN-g production and antiviral defense. J Immunol 156:1138–1142

Orteu CH, Poulter LW, Rustin MHA, Sabin CA, Salmon M, Akbar AN (1998) The role of apoptosis in the resolution of T cell-mediated cutaneous inflammation. J Immunol 161:1619–1629

Oukka M (2008) Th17 cells in immunity and autoimmunity. Ann Rheum Dis 67(Suppl 3):iii26–iii29

Ozawa H, Nakagawa S, Tagami H, Aiba S (1996) Interleukin-1b and granulocyte-macrophage colony stimulating factor mediate Langerhans cell maturation differently. J Invest Dermatol 106:441–445

Panzani RC, Schiavino D, Nucera E, Pellegrino S, Fais G, Schinco G, Patriarca G (1995) Oral hyposensitization to nickel allergy: preliminary clinical results. Int Arch Allergy Immunol 107:251–254

Park SH, Chiu YH, Jayawardena J, Roark J, Kavita U, Bendelac A (1998) Innate and adaptive functions of the CD1 pathway of antigen presentation. Semin Immunol 10:391–398

Patlewicz GY, Basketter DA, Pease CK, Wilson K, Wright ZM, Roberts DW, Bernard G, Arnau EG, Lepoittevin JP (2004) Further evaluation of quantitative structure–activity relationship models for the prediction of the skin sensitization potency of selected fragrance allergens. Contact Dermatitis 50:91–97

Perez VL, Lederer JA, Lichtman AH, Abbas AK (1995) Stability of Th1 and Th2 populations. Int Immunol 7:869–875

Piccirillo CA, Thornton AM (2004) Cornerstone of peripheral tolerance: naturally occurring CD4+ CD25+ regulatory T cells. Trends Immunol 25:374–380

Pober JS, Bevilacqua MP, Mendrick DL, Lapierre LA, Fiers W, Gimbrone MA Jr (1986) Two distinct monokines, interleukin 1 and tumor necrosis factor, each independently induce biosynthesis and transient expression of the same antigen on the surface of cultured human vascular endothelial cells. J Immunol 136:1680–1687

Polak L (1980) Immunological aspects of contact sensitivity. An experimental study. Monogr Allergy 15:4–60

Polak L, Rinck C (1978) Mechanism of desensitization in DNCH-contact sensitive guinea pigs. J Invest Dermatol 70:98–104

Polak L, Turk JL (1968a) Studies on the effect of systemic administration of sensitizers in guinea-pigs with contact sensitivity to inorganic metal compounds. II. The flare-up of previous test sites of contact sensitivity and the development of a generalized rash. Clin Exp Immunol 3:253–262

Polak L, Turk SL (1968b) Studies on the effect of systemic administration of sensitizers in guinea pigs with contact sensitivity to inorganic metal compounds. I. The induction of immunological unresponsiveness in already sensitized animals. Clin Exp Immunol 3:245–251

Price AA, Cumberbatch M, Kimber I (1997) α6 integrins are required for Langerhans cell migration from the epidermis. J Exp Med 186:1725–1735

Probst P, Küntzlin D, Fleischer B (1995) TH2-type infiltrating T cells in nickel-induced contact dermatitis. Cell Immunol 165:134–140

Pulendran B (2004) Modulating TH1/TH2 responses with microbes, dendritic cells, and pathogen recognition receptors. Immunol Res 29:187–196

Quezada SA, Jarvinen LZ, Lind EF, Noelle RJ (2004) CD40/CD154 interactions at the interface of tolerance and immunity. Annu Rev Immunol 22:307–328

Rambukhana A, Bos JD, Irik D, Menko WJ, Kapsenberg ML, Das PK (1995) In situ behaviour of human Langerhans cells in skin organ culture. Lab Invest 73:521–531

Randolph GJ (2001) Dendritic cell migration to lymph nodes: cytokines, chemokines, and lipid mediators. Semin Immunol 13:267–274

Redegeld FA, Nijkamp FP (2003) Immunoglobulin free light chains and mast cells: pivotal role in T-cell-mediated immune reactions? Trends Immunol 24:181–185

Richters CD, Hoekstra MJ, van Baare J, Du Pont JS, Hoefsmit EC, Kamperdijk EW (1994) Isolation and characterization of migratory human skin dendritic cells. Clin Exp Immunol 98:330–336

Robbiani DF, Finch RA, Jager D, Muller WA, Sartorelli AC, Randolph GJ (2000) The leukotriene C(4) transporter MRP1 regulates CCL19 (MIP-3beta, ELC)-dependent mobilization of dendritic cells to lymph nodes. Cell 103:757–768

Roberts DW, Lepoittevin J-P (1998) Allergic contact dermatitis: the molecular basis. In: Lepoittevin J-P, Basketter DA, Goossens A, Karlberg A-T (eds) Springer, Berlin/Heidelberg/New York, pp 81–1118

Rogge L, Barberis-Maino L, Biffi M, Passini N, Presky DH, Gubler U, Sinigaglia F (1997) Selective expression of an interleukin-12 receptor component by human T helper 1 cells. J Exp Med 185:825–831

Romagnani S (2006) Regulation of the T cell response. Clin Exp Allergy 36(11):1357–1366

Romani N, Holzmann S, Tripp CH, Koch F, Stoitzner P (2003) Langerhans cells – dendritic cells of the epidermis. Acta Pathol Microbiol Immunol Scand 111:725–740

Ross R, Gilitzer C, Kleinz R, Schwing J, Kleinert H, Forstermann U, Reske-Kunz AB (1998) Involvement of NO in contact hypersensitivity. Int Immunol 10:61–69

Rothenberg ME (2010) Innate sensing of nickel. Nat Immunol 11(9):781–782

Rowe A, Bunker CB (1998) Interleukin-4 and the interleukin-4 receptor in allergic contact dermatitis. Contact Dermatitis 38:36–39

Rowe A, Farrell AM, Bunker CB (1997) Constitutive endothelial and inducible nitric oxide synthase in inflammatory dermatoses. Br J Dermatol 136:18–23

Rustemeyer T, von Blomberg BME, de Ligter S, Frosch PJ, Scheper RJ (1999) Human T lymphocyte priming in vitro by haptenated autologous dendritic cells. Clin Exp Immunol 117:209–216

Rustemeyer T, de Groot J, von Blomberg BME, Frosch PJ, Scheper RJ (2001) Induction of tolerance and cross-tolerance to methacrylate contact sensitizers. Toxicol Appl Pharmacol 176:195–202

Rustemeyer T, de Groot J, von Blomberg BME, Frosch PJ, Scheper RJ (2002) Assessment of contact allergen cross-reactivity by retesting. Exp Dermatol 11:257–265

Rustemeyer T, von Blomberg BME, van Hoogstraten IMW, Bruynzeel DP, Scheper RJ (2004) Analysis of effector and regulatory immune-reactivity to nickel. Clin Exp Allergy 34(9):1458–1466

Saeki H, Moore AM, Brown MJ, Hwan ST (1999) Secondary lymphoid-tissue chemokine (SLC) and CC chemokine receptor 7 (CCR7) participate in the emigration pathway of mature dendritic cells from the skin to regional lymph nodes. J Immunol 162:2472–2475

Saint-Mezard P, Krasteva M, Chavagnac C, Bosset S, Akiba H, Kehren J, Kanitakis J, Kaiserlian D, Nicolas JF, Berard F (2003) Afferent and efferent phases of allergic contact dermatitis (ACD) can be induced after a single skin contact with haptens: evidence using a mouse model of primary ACD. J Invest Dermatol 120:641–647

Sallusto F, Lanzavecchia A, Mackay CR (1998a) Chemokines and chemokine receptors in T-cell priming and Th1/Th2-mediated responses. Immunol Today 19:568–574

Sallusto F, Schaerli P, Loetscher P, Schaniel C, Lenig D, Mackay CR, Qin S, Lanzavecchia A (1998b) Rapid and coordinated switch in chemokine receptor expression during dendritic cell maturation. Eur J Immunol 28:2760–2769

Sallusto F, Palermo B, Lenig D, Miettinen M, Matikainen S, Julkunen I, Forster R, Burgstahler R, Lipp M, Lanzavecchia A (1999) Distinct patterns and kinetics of chemokine production regulate dendritic cell function. Eur J Immunol 29:1617–1625

Sallusto F, Geginat J, Lanzavecchia A (2004) Central memory and effector memory T cell subsets: function, generation, and maintenance. Annu Rev Immunol 22:745–763

Scheper RJ, von Blomberg BME, Boerrigter GH, Bruynzeel D, van Dinther A, Vos A (1983) Induction of local memory in the skin. Role of local T cell retention. Clin Exp Immunol 51:141–148

Scheper RJ, van Dinther-Janssen AC, Polak L (1985) Specific accumulation of hapten-reactive T cells in contact sensitivity reaction sites. J Immunol 134:1333–1336

Schmidt M, Raghavan B, Müller V, Vogl T, Fejer G, Tchaptchet S, Keck S, Kalis C, Nielsen PJ, Galanos C, Roth J, Skerra A, Martin SF, Freudenberg MA, Goebeler M (2010) Crucial role for human Toll-like receptor 4 in the development of contact allergy to nickel. Nat Immunol 11(9):814–819

Schnuch A, Westphal GA, Muller MM, Schulz TG, Geier J, Brasch J, Merk HF, Kawakubo Y, Richter G, Koch P, Fuchs T, Gutgesell T, Reich K, Gebhardt M, Becker D, Grabbe J, Szliska C, Aberer W, Hallier E (1998) Genotype and phenotype of *N*-acetyltransferase 2 (NAT2) polymorphism in patients with contact allergy. Contact Dermatitis 38:209–211

Schoenberger SP, Toes REM, Vandervoort EIH, Offringa R, Melief CJM (1998) T-cell help for cytotoxic T lymphocytes is mediated by CD40-CD40L interactions. Nature 393:480–483

Schon MP, Zollner TM, Boehncke WH (2003) The molecular basis of lymphocyte recruitment to the skin: clues for pathogenesis and selective therapies of inflammatory disorders. J Invest Dermatol 121:951–962

Schuler G, Steinman RM (1985) Murine epidermal Langerhans cells mature into potent immune-stimulatory dendritic cells in vitro. J Exp Med 161:526–546

Schwarz A, Grabbe S, Riemann H, Aragane Y, Simon M, Manon S, Andrade S, Luger TA, Zlotnik A, Schwarz T (1994) In vivo effects of interleukin-10 on contact hypersensitivity and delayed-type hypersensitivity reactions. J Invest Dermatol 103:211–216

Schwarzenberger K, Udey MC (1996) Contact allergens and epidermal proinflammatory cytokines modulate Langerhans cell E-cadherin expression in situ. J Invest Dermatol 106:553–558

Seiffert K, Granstein RD (2006) Neuroendocrine regulation of skin dendritic cells. Ann N Y Acad Sci 1088(1):195–206

Semma M, Sagami S (1981) Induction of suppressor T cells to DNFB contact sensitivity by application of sensitizer through Langerhans cell-deficient skin. Arch Dermatol Res 271:361–364

Shimizu Y, Newman W, Gopal TV, Horgan KJ, Graber N, Beall LD, van Seventer GA, Shaw S (1991) Four molecular pathways of T cell adhesion to endothelial cells: roles of LFA-1, VCAM-1, and ELAM-1 and changes in pathway hierarchy under different activation conditions. J Cell Biol 113:1203–1212

Shirakawa T, Kusaka Y, Morimoto K (1992) Specific IgE antibodies to nickel in workers with known reactivity to cobalt. Clin Exp Allergy 22:213–218

Shreedhar V, Giese T, Sung VW, Ullrich SE (1998) A cytokine cascade including prostaglandin E2, IL-4, and IL-10 is responsible for UV-induced systemic immune suppression. J Immunol 160:3783–3789

Silberberg-Sinakin I, Thorbecke GJ, Baer RL, Rosenthal SA, Berezowsky V (1976) Antigen-bearing Langerhans cells in skin, dermal lymphatics, and in lymph nodes. Cell Immunol 25:137–151

Skog E (1976) Spontaneous flare-up reactions induced by different amounts of 1,3-dinitro-4-chlorobenzene. Acta Derm Venereol 46:386–395

Steinbrink K, Jonuleit H, Muller G, Schuler G, Knop J, Enk AH (1999) Interleukin-10-treated human dendritic cells induce a melanoma-antigen-specific anergy in CD8(+) T cells resulting in a failure to lyse tumor cells. Blood 93:1634–1642

Steinman RM, Hoffman L, Pope M (1995) Maturation and migration of cutaneous dendritic cells. J Invest Dermatol 105:2S–7S

Sterry W, Künne N, Weber-Matthiesen K, Brasch J, Mielke V (1991) Cell trafficking in positive and negative patch test reactions: demonstration of a stereotypic migration pathway. J Invest Dermatol 96:459–462

Stingl G, Katz SI, Clement L, Green I, Shevach EM (1978) Immunological functions of Ia-bearing epidermal Langerhans cells. J Immunol 121:2005–2013

Streilein JW, Grammer SF (1989) In vitro evidence that Langerhans cells can adopt two functionally distinct forms capable of antigen presentation to T lymphocytes. J Immunol 143:3925–3933

Strobel S, Mowat AM (1998) Immune responses to dietary antigens: oral tolerance. Immunol Today 19:173–181

Szepietowski JC, McKenzie RC, Keohane SG, Walker C, Aldridge RD, Hunter JA (1997) Leukaemia inhibitory factor: induction in the early phase of allergic contact dermatitis. Contact Dermatitis 36:21–25

Taams LS, van Rensen AJML, Poelen MC, van Els CACM, Besseling AC, Wagenaar JPA, van Eden W, Wauben MHM (1998) Anergic T cells actively suppress T cell responses via the antigen presenting cell. Eur J Immunol 28:2902–2912

Taams LS, van Eden W, Wauben MHM (1999) Dose-dependent induction of distinct anergic phenotypes: multiple levels of T cell anergy. J Immunol 162:1974–1981

Taams LS, Boot EPJ, van Eden W, Wauben MHM (2000) 'Anergic' T cells modulate the T-cell activating capacity of antigen-presenting cells. J Autoimmun 14:335–341

Takatori H, Kanno Y, Chen Z, O'Shea JJ (2008) New complexities in helper T cell fate determination and the implications for autoimmune diseases. Mod Rheumatol 18(6):533–541

Tammaro A, De Marco G, Persechino S, Narcisi A, Camplone G (2009) Allergy to nickel: first results on patients administered with an oral hyposensitization therapy. Int J Immunopathol Pharmacol 22(3):837–840

Tang A, Amagai M, Granger LG, Stanley JR, Udey MC (1993) Adhesion of epidermal Langerhans cells to keratinocytes mediated by E-cadherin. Nature 361:82–85

Toebak MJ, Moed H, von Blomberg MB, Bruynzeel DP, Gibbs S, Scheper RJ, Rustemeyer T (2006) Intrinsic characteristics of contact and respiratory allergens influence production of polarizing cytokines by dendritic cells. Contact Dermatitis 55(4):238–245

Trautmann A, Randriamampita C (2003) Initiation of TCR signalling revisited. Trends Immunol 24:425–428

Tsuji RF, Geba GP, Wang Y, Kawamoto K, Matis LA, Askenase PW (1997) Required early complement activation in contact sensitivity with generation of local C5-dependent chemotactic activity, and late T cell interferon g: a possible initiating role of B cells. J Exp Med 186:1015–1026

Turk JL (1975) Delayed hypersensitivity, 2nd edn. North-Holland, Amsterdam

Ulrich P, Grenet O, Bluemel J, Vohr HW, Wiemann C, Grundler O, Suter W (2001) Cytokine expression profiles during murine contact allergy: T helper 2 cytokines are expressed irrespective of the type of contact allergen. Arch Toxicol 75(8):470–479

Uotila P (1996) The role of cyclic AMP and oxygen intermediates in the inhibition of cellular immunity in cancer. Cancer Immunol Immunother 43:1–9

van Beelen AJ, Teunissen MB, Kapsenberg ML, de Jong EC (2007) Interleukin-17 in inflammatory skin disorders. Curr Opin Allergy Clin Immunol 7(5):374–381

van de Ven R, Scheffer GL, Scheper RJ, de Gruijl TD (2009) The ABC of dendritic cell development and function. Trends Immunol 30(9):421–429

Van Hoogstraten IMW, Andersen JE, von Blomberg BME, Boden D, Bruynzeel DP, Burrows D, Camarasa JMG, Dooms-Goossens A, Lahti A, Menné T, Rycroft R, Todd D, Vreeburg KJJ, Wilkinson JD, Scheper RJ (1989) Preliminary results of a multicenter study on the incidence of nickel allergy in relationship to previous oral and cutaneous contacts. In: Frosch PJ, Dooms-Goossens A, Lachapelle JM, Rycroft RJG, Scheper RJ (eds) Current topics in contact dermatitis. Springer, Berlin/Heidelberg/New York, pp 178–184

Van Hoogstraten IMW, von Blomberg BME, Boden D, Kraal G, Scheper RJ (1994) Non-sensitizing epicutaneous skin tests prevent subsequent induction of immune tolerance. J Invest Dermatol 102:80–83

Van Loweren H, Meade R, Askenase PW (1983) An early component of delayed type hypersensitivity mediated by T cells and mast cells. J Exp Med 157:1604–1617

Vestweber D, Blanks JE (1999) Mechanisms that regulate the function of the selectins and their ligands. Physiol Rev 79:181–213

Vieira PL, Kalinski P, Wierenga EA, Kapsenberg ML, Dejong EC (1998) Glucocorticoids inhibit bioactive IL-12P70 production by in vitro-generated human dendritic cells without affecting their T cell stimulatory potential. J Immunol 161:5245–5251

Viola A, Lanzavecchia A (1996) T cell activation determined by T cell receptor number and tunable thresholds. Science 273:104–106

Virag L, Szabo E, Bakondi E, Bai P, Gergely P, Hunyadi J, Szabo C (2002) Nitric oxide-peroxynitrite-poly(ADP-ribose) polymerase pathway in the skin. Exp Dermatol 11:189–202

Von Andrian UH, Mrini C (1998) In situ analysis of lymphocyte migration to lymph nodes. Cell Adhes Commun 6:85–96

von Blomberg BME, Bruynzeel DP, Scheper RJ (1991) Advances in mechanisms ofallergic contact dermatitis: in vitro and in vivo research. In: Marzulli FN, Maibach HI (eds) Dermatotoxicology, 4th edn. Hemisphere Publishing Corporation, New York, pp 255–362

von Herrath MG (1997) Bystander suppression induced by oral tolerance. Res Immunol 148:541–554

Waldorf HA, Walsh LJ, Schechter NM, Murphy GF (1991) Early molecular events in evolving cutaneous delayed hypersensitivity in humans. Am J Pathol 138:477–486

Walker C, Kristensen F, Bettens F, deWeck AL (1983) Lymphokine regulation of activated (G1) lymphocytes. I. Prostaglandin E2-induced inhibition of interleukin 2 production. J Immunol 130:1770–1773

Walsh LJ, Lavker RM, Murphy GF (1990) Determinants of immune cell trafficking in the skin. Lab Invest 63:592–600

Wang B, Esche C, Mamelak A, Freed I, Watanabe H, Sauder DN (2003) Cytokine knockouts in contact hypersensitivity research. Cytokine Growth Factor Rev 14:381–389

Wardorf HA, Walsh LJ, Schechter NM (1991) Early cellular events in evolving cutaneous delayed hypersensitivity in humans. Am J Pathol 138:477–486

Weigle WO, Romball CG (1997) CD4+ T-cell subsets and cytokines involved in peripheral tolerance. Immunol Today 18:533–538

Weiner HL (1997) Oral tolerance: immune mechanisms and treatment of autoimmune diseases. Immunol Today 18:335–343

Weiner HL, Gonnella PA, Slavin A, Maron R (1997) Oral tolerance: cytokine milieu in the gut and modulation of tolerance by cytokines. Res Immunol 148:528–533

Weinlich G, Heine M, Stössel H, Zanella M, Stoitzner P, Ortner U, Smolle J, Koch F, Sepp NT, Schuler G, Romani N (1998) Entry into afferent lymphatics and maturation in situ of migrating murine cutaneous dendritic cells. J Invest Dermatol 110:441–448

Weiss JM, Sleeman J, Renkl AC, Dittmar H, Termeer CC, Taxis S, Howells N, Hofmann M, Kohler G, Schöpf E, Ponta H, Herrlich P, Simon JC (1997) An essential role for CD44 variant isoforms in epidermal Langerhans cell and blood dendritic cell function. J Cell Biol 137:1137–1147

Wendel GD, Stark BJ, Jamison RB, Molina RD, Sullivan TJ (1985) Penicillin allergy and desensitization in serious infections during pregnancy. N Engl J Med 312:1229–1232

Werfel T, Hentschel M, Kapp A, Renz H (1997) Dichotomy of blood- and skin-derived IL-4-producing allergen-specific T cells and restricted V beta repertoire in nickel-mediated contact dermatitis. J Immunol 158:2500–2505

Weston MC, Peachell PT (1998) Regulation of human mast cell and basophil function by cAMP. Gen Pharmacol 31:715–719

Wilkinson SM, Mattey DL, Beck MH (1994) IgG antibodies and early intradermal reactions to hydrocortisone in patients with cutaneous delayed-type hypersensitivity to hydrocortisone. Br J Dermatol 131:495–498

Willis CM, Young E, Brandon DR, Wilkinson JD (1986) Immunopathological and ultrastructural findings in human allergic and irritant contact dermatitis. Br J Dermatol 115:305–316

Wilson NS, Villadangos JA (2004) Lymphoid organ dendritic cells: beyond the Langerhans cells paradigm. Immunol Cell Biol 82:91–98

Wong BR, Josien R, Lee SY, Sauter B, Li HL, Steinman RM, Choi YW (1997) TRANCE (Tumor necrosis factor [TNF]-related activation-induced cytokine), a new TNF family member predominantly expressed in T cells, is a dendritic cell-specific survival factor. J Exp Med 186:2075–2080

Wu K, Bi Y, Sun K, Wang C (2007) IL-10-producing type 1 regulatory T cells and allergy. Cell Mol Immunol 4(4):269–275

Yu X, Barnhill RL, Graves DT (1994) Expression of monocyte chemoattractant protein-1 in delayed type hypersensitivity reactions in the skin. Lab Invest 71:226–235

Zembala M, Ashershon GL (1973) Depression of T cell phenomenon of contact sensitivity by T cells from unresponsive mice. Nature 244:227–228

Zhang ZY, Michael JG (1990) Orally inducible immune unresponsiveness is abrogated by IFN-gamma treatment. J Immunol 144:4163–4165

Zhang X, Brunner T, Carter L, Dutton RW, Rogers P, Bradley L, Sato T, Reed JC, Green D, Swain SL (1997) Unequal death in T helper cell (Th)1 and Th2 effectors: Th1, but not Th2, effectors undergo rapid Fas/FasL-mediated apoptosis. J Exp Med 185:1837–1849

Zhou L, Littman DR (2009) Transcriptional regulatory networks in Th17 cell differentiation (review). Curr Opin Immunol 21(2): 146–152

Zhou L, Chong MM, Littman DR (2009) Plasticity of CD4+ T cell lineage differentiation (review). Immunity 30(5):646–655, PubMed PMID: 19464987

Zinkernagel RM (2004) On 'reactivity' versus 'tolerance'. Immunol Cell Biol 82:343–352

Zlotnik A, Morales J, Hedrick JA (1999) Recent advances in chemokines and chemokine receptors. Crit Rev Immunol 19:1–47

15 Phototoxic Dermatitis

Margarida Gonçalo
Clinic of Dermatology, Unit of Skin Allergy, University Hospital and Faculty of Medicine, University of Coimbra, Coimbra, Portugal

Core Messages

- Phototoxic dermatitis from exogenous chemicals can be polymorphic.
- It is not always easy to distinguish phototoxicity from photoallergy.
- Phytophotodermatitis from plants containing furocoumarins is one of the main causes of phototoxic contact dermatitis.
- Topical and systemic drugs are a frequent cause of photosensitivity, often with phototoxic aspects.
- The main clinical pattern of acute phototoxicity is an exaggerated sunburn.
- Subacute phototoxicity from systemic drugs can present as pseudoporphyria, photoonycholysis, and dyschromia.
- Exposure to phototoxic drugs can enhance skin carcinogenesis.

1 Introduction

Photosensitivity represents an abnormal inflammatory skin reaction to the sun, presenting under a wide spectrum of clinical reaction patterns. It is usually due to the abnormal presence, in the skin, of an endogenous or exogenous substance that is selectively activated by solar radiation – a chromophore. Apart from exogenous photoactive chemicals, there are several causes for photosensitivity: congenital or acquired errors may hinder DNA repair after ultraviolet (UV) aggression (xeroderma pigmentosum, Bloom's syndrome) and reduce the natural UV protection (albinism and vitiligo) or the antioxidative response to UV light (pellagra due to reduced levels of niacin in diet or from alcohol consumption); accumulation of endogenous photoactive chemicals, like in porphyria; idiopathic photodermatosis, inflammatory or immune-mediated reactions whose antigen has not been well characterized, like solar urticaria, polymorphos light eruption, "lucite estvial benigne," actinic prurigo, and chronic actinic dermatitis (Hawk 1999).

Considering only photosensitivity from exogenous agents, both chemicals applied topically or those that reach the skin by the systemic route, there is still a wide spectrum of skin reactions. Some involve predominantly a specific T-cell-dependent response, including photoallergy, both photoallergic contact dermatitis and systemic photoallergy, and autoimmunity with photosensitivity, as in drug-induced photosensitive lupus erythematosus in Ro-positive patients taking terbinafine, thiazide diuretics, calcium channels blockers, or taxanes (Farhi et al. 2006; Sontheimer et al. 2008; Cohen 2009). Phototoxic dermatitis, on the other hand, does not involve specific immune hypersensitivity reactions.

Although these mechanisms are well characterized, their participation in each case of photosensitivity can be more complex. For instance, in chronic actinic dermatitis, the extreme photosensitivity to UV light may be initially triggered by a photosensitive reaction or by contact allergy to perfumes, sesquiterpene lactones, or colophony, but in its evolution, individuals become extremely photosensitive even with no further exposure to the exogenous chromophore or allergen: An autoantigen may be formed during the acute reaction (DNA or RNA modified by plant products) and/or, in the absence of the expected UV-induced immunosuppression, sensitization to a new epidermal autoantigen may occur (Hawk 2004; Béani 2009).

When considering only phototoxic and photoallergic dermatitis there is also an overlap between these two reaction patterns. Except for a few chemicals, as piroxicam and olaquindox, which do not have an intrinsic phototoxic potential and induce only photoallergic reactions (Figueiredo 1994), most substances can induce both photoallergic and phototoxic reactions. For instance, potent phototoxic agents like psoralens can induce photoallergy in some individuals. There is also some overlap between phototoxicity and photoallergy in the clinical characteristics of the reaction and their time course. Most phototoxic reactions are well recognized, are not severe, and do not call medical attention. Others may be severe and are often misdiagnosed, as their relation to sun exposure is not so obvious, namely, the recently described UV-induced skin cancers in patients on voriconazole (McCarthy et al. 2007; Cowen et al. 2010).

Photoallergy from exogenous agents is now considered rare (Darvay et al. 2001; Bryden et al. 2006), but it may be underreported or underdiagnosed (Zeeli et al. 2006). Many photosensitizers have been recognized and

T. Rustemeyer, P. Elsner, S.M. John & H.I. Maibach (eds.), *Kanerva's Occupational Dermatology*,
DOI 10.1007/978-3-642-02035-3_15,

removed from the market (salicylanilides, PABA) or sun avoidance is recommended when they are used (lomefloxacin). Also, there is an increasing concern on premarketing studies on the photosensitizing potential of chemicals for human use. Nevertheless, photosensitivity is still a field on intense research. New photosensitizers are discovered, either causing skin disease (Chang et al. 2009) or for therapeutic purposes. Also, new mechanisms underlying the photosensitizing potential of chemicals and new aspects of clinical presentation of photosensitivity are recognized, which may be important to understand diseases that course with photosensitivity, as HIV infection (Béani 2009).

2 General Mechanisms of Phototoxicity from Exogenous Chemicals

Normal skin is prepared to live with sunlight and takes benefit from it. Skin chromophores are activated upon sun exposure and undergo chemical reactions which are important for survival under the sun and necessary for human life: 7-dehydrocholesterol is activated by UVB to form pro-vitamin D3 and Vitamin D.

Photosensitivity develops when an abnormal chromophore is present in the skin or when a normal chromophore in present in exaggerated amounts. When excited by a photon these molecules receiving the energy suffer changes within the molecule itself, often also within neighboring molecules, in a cascade of events that result in skin damage and inflammation. The energy received by the molecule excites the electrons in the outer orbits; the molecule becomes reactive and can undergo several types of modifications within itself (isomerization, breaking of double bounds, oxidation) or react with neighboring molecules, eventually forming free radicals or reactive oxygen species (ROS). These ROS and other free radicals damage cellular organelles by modifying unsaturated lipids of cell membranes, aromatic amino acids of proteins, and pyrimidine bases of DNA or RNA. If the repair mechanisms do not act immediately, there is damage of these cellular structures and suffering or death of skin cells. In this process, inflammatory mediators are generated (prostaglandins, leukotrienes, IL-1, 6, 8, other cytokines and chemokines) with consequent visible skin lesions – this is briefly the mechanism of phototoxicity (Hawk 1999; Ferguson 1999). In photoallergy, the energy of the photon transforms the chromophore into a photoproduct or enhances its reaction with an endogenous peptide forming a hapten or an allergen that is specifically recognized by the immune system.

Several phototoxic substances, like psoralens, chlorpromazine, and fluorquinolones, apart from the capacity to generate free radicals and cell death responsible for acute phototoxicity, also enhance chromosomal damage in the presence of UVR, both in vitro and in vivo (Seto et al. 2010). Therefore, they are photogenotoxic and photomutagenic, which is usually associated with photoimmunosupression, and have consequent implications in animal photocarcinogenesis (Klecak et al. 1997; Marrot et al. 2003; Lhiaubet-Vallet et al. 2009; Müller et al. 1998). Epidemiological studies and recent reports also show enhancement of photocarcinogenesis in humans exposed to photoactive chemicals (Cowen et al. 2010; Placzek et al. 1999; Miller et al. 2010).

From the solar spectrum that reaches the earth, UV radiation, and particularly UVA (320–400 nm), is responsible for most cases of photosensitivity. Even though some chromophores absorb in the UVB (290–320 nm) and UVB is more energetic, UVA penetrates the skin more deeply and, particularly for systemic chromophores, this is certainly the most important spectrum for inducing photodermatosis (Hawk 1999). Only exceptional cases have a well-documented exogenous photosensitivity exclusively from UVB (Fujimoto et al. 2009).

2.1 Phototoxicity Versus Phototoallergy

In theory, it is easy to differentiate photoallergy from phototoxicity, but there are many overlapping aspects, as presented below.

Classically, photoallergy develops only in a limited number in individuals, needs previous sensitization but occurs also with cross-reactive chemicals, is not dose-dependent, develops on low UV dose, appears as eczema that can spread to nonexposed sites and, on skin biopsy, there is mainly T-cell infiltration, spongiosis, and vesicles. Phototoxicity is more frequent, develops in every individual, as long as enough photosensitizer and sun exposure are present, occurs on a first and single contact, with no flare-ups or cross-reactions, appears mainly as well-demarcated erythema exclusively on sun exposed areas (mimicking sunburn), resolves with hyperpigmentation and, on histology, apoptotic keratinocytes (sunburn cells) are abundant (➲ *Table 15.1*).

These are the two polar aspects of photosensitivity, but, as referred previously, some molecules may induce both phototoxic and photoallergic reactions and, in the

◘ Table 15.1
Distinction between phototoxicity and photoallergy

	Phototoxicity	Photoallergy
Frequency	High	Low
Latency period/ sensitization	No	Yes
Doses of UV/ photosensitizer	High	Low
Cross-reactions	No	Yes
Morphology of lesions	Sunburn, polymorphic	Eczema, erythema multiforme
Sharp limits	Yes	No
Covered areas	Not involved	Possibly involved
Resolution	Quick	May recur, persistent reactors
Residual hyperpigmentation	Yes	No
Histology	Sunburn cells	Eczema
Pathomechanism	DNA/cell damage ROS/ inflammation	Type IV hypersensitivity Photoproduct

same patient, aspects that resemble phototoxicity may coexist with others that suggest photoallergy.

After contact with plant furocoumarins (*Ruta graveolens, Ficus carica, Umbelliferae*) or during photochemotherapy, some individuals can become reactive to very low concentrations of psoralens (Karimian-Teherani et al. 2008) and with phototoxic drugs like promethazine and lomefloxacin, patients may develop photoallergy, reacting to very low doses of the drug or sun exposure (Gonçalo 1998; Oliveira et al. 1996; Kurumajin and Shono 1992). Very probably, as for contact allergens that have an inherent "irritant" potential to awaken the innate immune system promoting sensitization (Neves et al. 2008), photoallergens are photoactive molecules with some inherent phototoxicity. This innate inflammatory reaction can work as the "danger signal" necessary to initiate the sensitizing process.

Although phototoxicity can occur on a first contact and photoallergy needs previous sensitization, individuals previously sensitized by contact or photocontact to a similar molecule can react on a first exposure. This occurs in individuals with contact allergy to thimerosal and its moiety thiosalicylic acid who develop photoallergy to piroxicam on the first drug intake and patients allergic to perfumes (cinnamic alcohol) who may have photoallergic contact dermatitis from ketoprofen on a first exposure (Foti et al. 2008). Upon UVA irradiation, piroxicam is photodecomposed into a molecule very similar antigenically and structurally to thiosalicylic acid (Gonçalo et al. 1992; Hariva et al. 1993) and there are conformational similarities between cinnamate derivatives and ketoprofen photoproducts (Foti et al. 2008; Pigatto et al. 1996)

Phototoxicity is considered to occur in every patient as long as enough chromophore and sun are present at the same time, but even in drug phototoxicity and phytophotodermatitis there is some individual susceptibility, even though the parameters that characterize this susceptibility are not precisely known.

3 Clinical Patterns of Photosensitivity from Exegenous Chemicals

As referred, clinical and evolutive aspects suggesting of a phototoxic dermatitis from exogenous chemicals can coexist with signs of photoallergy or other photo-immune reactions; therefore, in most instances it is best to call photosensitivity. Nevertheless, in this chapter, clinical patterns that are more suggestive of phototoxicity will be described.

The clinical patterns of phototosensitivity from exogenous chemicals vary from urticaria through eczema or subacute lupus erythematosus up to vitiligo-like lesions or squamous cell carcinomas (Gonçalo 1998; Ferguson 1999; McCarthy et al. 2007). They can be very typical, like phytophotodermatitis or acute exaggerated sunburn from a phototoxic drug, but sometimes, the diagnosis or even the suspicion of photosensitivity is not so obvious. It is the example of cases involving nonexposed areas, which occurs mainly in photoallergy, or when there is no immediate or evident relation with exposure to the sun and exogenous chemicals, as in actinic keratosis and skin cancer in patients chronically exposed to photoactive drugs (➋ *Table 15.2*).

Skin reactions can occur immediately after sun exposure, as in photocontact urticaria, but the appearance of skin lesions may be delayed 1 or 2 days, as in most phototoxic or photoallergic contact dermatitis or systemic photoallergy, several days or weeks, as in pseudoporphyria or subacute lupus erythematosus, or even years, in photocarcinogenesis enhanced by a long exposure to the sun and the photoactive chemicals.

Table 15.2
Clinical patterns of photosensitivity

Predominant in phototoxicity	In photoallergy
Exaggerated "sunburn"	Urticaria in sun-exposed area
Pseudoporphyria	Acute or subacute eczema
Photoonycholysis	Cheilitis
Hyperpigmentation	Erythema multiform-like
Hypopigmentation (vitiligo-like lesions)	Lichenoid reactions
Telangiectasia Purpura	Subacte or chronic lupus erythematosus
Pellagra-like reactions	
Actinic keratosis and squamous cell carcinoma	

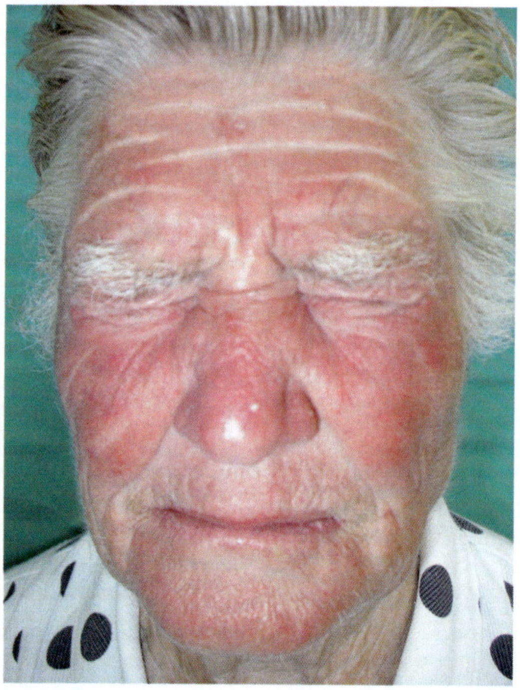

Fig. 15.1
Acute phototoxicity from amiodarone, mimicking sunburn and sparing the deep wrinkles

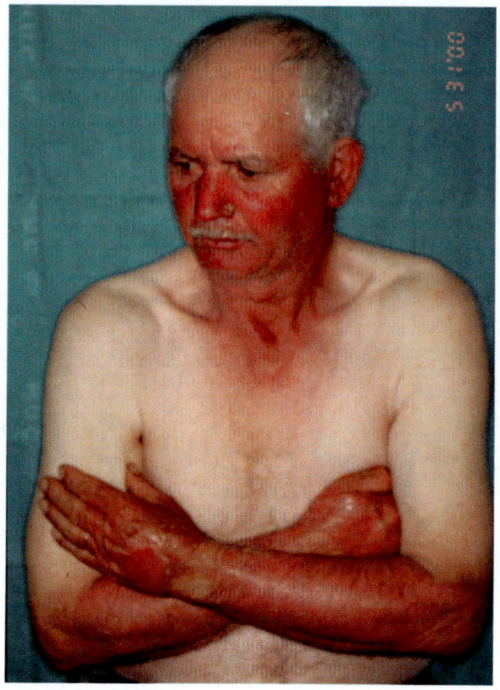

Fig. 15.2
Photosensitivity from systemic lomefloxacin, sparing the sunshaded areas and the wrist protected from the watch

Localization of the lesions depends on whether the photoactive chemical is applied on the skin (photocontact dermatitis) or the photosensitizer is a systemic drug. In photocontact dermatitis from a topical agent, dermatitis draws the area of application and concomitant sun exposure, but distant lesions can occur in areas of accidental contact, as in a contralateral limb (kissing faces of the legs) or in areas of inadvertent spread by the hands or contaminated objects (Hindsén et al. 2004). Some topical drugs, as nonsteroidal anti-inflammatory drugs (NSAIDs), are considerably absorbed through the skin and lesional distribution can be similar to systemic photosensitivity.

In systemic photosensitivity the reaction usually involves, in a symmetric distribution, all exposed areas of the face, the V-shaped area of the neck and upper chest, dorsum of the hands and forearms, while shaded areas are spared. This corresponds, in the face, to the upper eyelids, upper lip, deep wrinkles (➋ *Fig. 15.1*), retroauricular areas, submandibular area, and areas covered by the beard or hair. Large body folds, like the axillae, groins, finger webs, and areas covered by clothing or other accessories (watch strip, shoes) (➋ *Fig. 15.2*) are also usually spared. Involvement of these shaded areas suggests dermatitis from an airborne allergen or irritant.

In exceptional cases where sun exposure is asymmetric, this pattern can be different, as in car drivers who only expose the left arm. Sometimes, in systemic photosensitivity, the lower lip is mainly or almost exclusively involved, because of its higher exposure and, very probably, because of the thinner corneal layer more prone to phototoxic reactions (Auffret et al. 2006; Cardoso et al. 2009).

3.1 Acute Patterns of Phototoxicity

3.1.1 Immediate Reactions

Apart from idiopathic solar urticaria, for which a chromophore is not identified, immune or nonimmune urticaria as a manifestation of photosensitivity from an exogenous substance has been rarely described with 5-aminolevulinic acid, used in photodynamic therapy (Kerr et al. 2007), with oxybenzone in sunscreens (Collins and Ferguson 1994) and chlorpromazine (Lovell et al. 1986). Nevertheless for some drugs, like amiodarone and benoxaprofen (already removed from the market), immediate prickling and burning with transient erythema may occur as a manifestation of photosensitivity (Ferguson 1999).

3.1.2 Acute Phototoxic Dermatitis, Mimicking Sunburn

The main clinical pattern of acute phototoxicity, mimicking exaggerated sunburn develops within 12–24 h of sun exposure. It consists on a well-demarcated erythema with prickling and burning, eventually with skin pain but typically without pruritus. Erythema can progress to vesicles and bullae, but eczematous lesions with small vesicles or multiforme-like lesions involving also covered areas is not usual in phototoxicity and recalls mainly photoallergy.

Like in exaggerated sunburn, acute phototoxicity progresses to large sheets of epidermal detachment within the next days and resolves with residual hyperpigmentation. In this pattern of phototoxicity, there is typically a very sharp limit between affected and nonaffected shaded area (➋ *Fig. 15.2*).

3.2 Subacute Patterns of Phototoxicity

Some clinical patterns of photosensitivity develop within days or weeks after exposure to the photosensitizer and the sun. These patterns that evoke mainly a phototoxic reaction are pseudoporphyria, photoonycholsys, hyper or hypopigmentation, telangiectasia, and purpura.

3.2.1 Pseudoporphyria

Pseudoporphyria presents as chronic skin fragility with flaccid bullae on non-inflamed exposed skin, occasionally with later milia formation, that resembles porphyria cutanea tarda both clinically and on histopathology (bullae formation below the lamina densa). It occurs in individuals with no inborn error in porphyrin metabolism and no increase of endogenous porphyrins.

It was observed in individuals regularly exposed to solarium (Kochs et al. 2009) or to some systemic drugs. Nalidixic acid, furosemide, and naproxen predominantly in children (Ferguson 1999; Figueiredo 1994) were initially described as causing pseudoporphyria but, more recently, many others drugs are associated with this phototoxic reaction: ciprofloxacin (Schmutz et al. 2008), celecoxib (Cummins et al. 2000; Schmutz et al. 2006), voriconazole (Auffret et al. 2006), torasemide (Pérez-Bustillo et al. 2008), and imatinib (Timmer-de Mik et al. 2009). This represents a typical phototoxic reaction where the drug, as the uroporphyrin in the hereditary disease, probably induces phototoxicity through singlet oxygen (Ferguson 1999; Figueiredo 1994).

3.2.2 Photoonycholysis

Photoonycholysis, with a half-moon distal onycholysis of one or several nails, is a typical pattern of phototoxicity, occurring most often as the single manifestation of phototoxicity (➋ *Fig. 15.3*). It appears late (2–3 weeks after drug intake and sun exposure), sometimes preceded by pain in the nail apparatus. It occurs mainly with tetracyclines (demethylchlortetracycline or doxycycline)

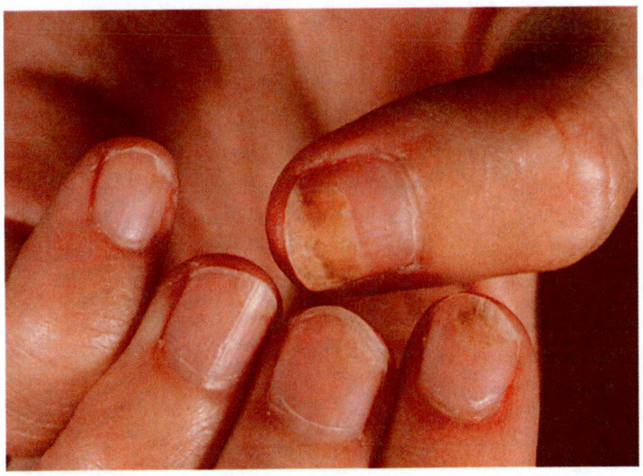

Fig. 15.3
Photoonycolysis from chlortetracycline

(Passier et al. 2004), psoralens, and fluorquinolones (Baran and Juhlin 2002). There is no definite explanation for the single involvement of the nail: The nail bed is relatively unprotected from sunlight, it contains less melanin, the nail plate may work as a lens, and the inflammatory reaction induces detachment of the nail plate from the nail bed (Passier et al. 2004; Baran and Juhlin 2002; Gregoriou et al. 2008).

3.2.3 Dyschromia

Hyperpigmentation that follows mainly an acute phototoxic reaction is frequently due to the residual melanocytic hyperpigmentation, and is very typical in phytophotodermatitis (➋ *Fig. 15.3*).

In rare occasions, like in flutamide-induced photosensitivity, vitiliginous lesions with sharp limits occur after the acute reaction (Gonçalo et al. 1999; Vilaplana et al. 1990).

Dyschromia from the accumulation of the photoactive drug or its metabolites in the dermis occurs in a smaller percentage of patients after acute phototoxicity from amiodarone, minocycline, or phenothiazines (Ammoury et al. 2008; Vassileva et al. 1998). Some patients with lower phototypes also develop a golden-brown, slate gray, or bluish color on sun-exposed areas, that persists much longer than residual melanocytic hyperpigmentation (Ferguson 1999; Ammoury et al. 2008).

3.2.4 Other Clinical Patterns

Telangiectasia as a manifestation of photosensitivity has been reported with calcium channel blockers (Ferguson 1999) and the telangiectatic pattern of photoaging with lesions mainly in the lateral folds of the neck, sparing the shaded skin under the chin, is frequently observed in patients chronically exposed to the sun or to photoactive drugs. In rare cases, petechial purpura with sharp limits on the transition to the shaded areas was described with ciprofloxacin (Urbina et al. 2006).

Pellagra is associated with the prolonged use of isoniazid, that consumes niacin for its metabolization, and pellagroid reactions were reported with the anticancer agents, like 6-mercaptopurine and 5-fluorouracil.

3.3 Delayed and Late Effects of Phototoxicity

Patients that are chronically exposed to photoactive drugs may develop other patterns of skin lesions, like chronic actinic dermatitis and lupus erythematosus where autoimmune reactions are predominantly involved, or accelerated photoaging and skin cancers, that are explained by the photogenotoxic effect of some phototoxic molecules.

There is a consensual agreement on the increased risk of skin cancers after longtime therapeutic exposure to PUVA phototherapy (Ferguson 1999) but, apart from psoralens, other drugs like naproxen, chlorpromazine, and the fluorquinolones, particularly lomefloxacin, also augment in vitro UV-induced DNA aggression and increase epidermal neoplasia in animals (Klecak et al. 1997). Recent reports and epidemiological data also correlate chronic human exposure to photoactive drugs with an increased risk of developing actinic keratoses, nonmelanoma skin cancer and, even, malignant melanoma (Placzek et al. 1999; McCarthy et al. 2007; Jensen et al. 2008). In 1999, the group of Przybilla showed an association between actinic keratosis and the use of potentially photosensitizing chemicals (Placzek et al. 1999). More recent studies tend to confirm an increased risk for skin cancer in patients chronically exposed to psoralens, fluoroquinolones, and diuretics (Jensen et al. 2008) and voriconazole (McCarthy et al. 2007; Cowen et al. 2010; Miller et al. 2010). Also, patients with severe chronic photosensitivity may develop skin cancers in the photoexposed areas, like squamous cell carcinoma with ciprofloxacin (personal experience) and both squamous cell carcinoma and melanoma with voriconazole (Cowen et al. 2010; Miller et al. 2010).

Also the photoaging process may be enhanced by the exposure to topical or systemic photosensitizers.

4 Main Sources of UV Exposure

The sun is the main source of UV exposure even in the occupational setting. Farmers, gardeners, construction workers, fishermen, sailors, policemen, ski instructors, oil-field workers, and road workers are occupations where sun exposure can be heavy, prolonged, and begin at an early age.

Artificial sources of UV exposure are present in several occupational settings and, even though protective measures and instructions for UV avoidance are active, UV exposure can be relevant in some of them. Some examples are the rooms for solarium and phototherapy, plants for UV curing of printing inks, lacquers, dental acrilates, or nail modeling acrilates, indoor working places artificially illuminated with UVA light sources with no plastic/glass cover, and areas of food cooking where insect traps have UVA emission to attract the insects.

The highest artificial UV exposure in occupational setting occurs in welders, particularly in electric arc welding. These individuals may suffer UV-induced erythema, burns, and keratitis (welder's flash) during inadvertent exposure during the arc welding process (Hawk 1999).

Exposure to the more energetic UVC rays (260–265 nm) can also occur during sterilization or disinfection of water for drinking, for cosmetic or pharmaceutical industries or for swimming pools, during sterilization of the air in cabinets, research laboratories, and operating theaters and during the treatment of sewage effluents (Hawk 1999).

5 Main Topical and Systemic Photosensitizers

There is a large and increasing list of photoactive molecules to which we can be exposed to in our daily life and that can induce photosensitivity (Table 15.3). But there has been a higher concern on the evaluation of the phototoxic potential of cosmetics and consumer products before marketing and many photosensitizers have been removed or highly reduced in our ambience.

These "historical" photosensitizers include some predominantly photoallergic others mainly phototoxic: musk ambrette and natural bergamot oil were removed by the perfume industry, the sunscreen isopropyl–dibenzoylmethane was withdrawn in 1994, the sunscreen PABA (para-aminobenzoic acid) which sensitized about 4% of the American population in the 1950s is no longer used (Lowe 2006), the antibiotic olaquindox, a swine feed additive, was banned in 1998 by the European Commission (Emmert et al. 2007), and the halogenated salicylanylides were removed from disinfectants and hygiene products in most countries, since 1976. Nevertheless, even though some products are not available in Europe, they can be "imported" from other countries and induce photosensitivity (Emmert et al. 2007; Waters et al. 2009).

In most reports from Europe and the USA, the main topical photosensitizers are the UV filters (Darvay et al. 2001; Sheuer and Warshaw 2006) which represent 5.6–80% of the cases diagnosed by photopatch testing (Darvay et al. 2001; Cardoso et al. 2009; Bakkum and Heule 2002; Leonard et al. 2005), but they represent photoallergic reactions in the vast majority of cases. Furocoumarin-rich plants are an important source of phototoxicity, mainly in more sunny countries, and

Table 15.3
Main agents causing exogenous photosensitivity

1. Sunscreens[c]	
2. Plants[b]	**Umbelliferae** *Ammi majus* *Apium graveolens* (celery) *Pastinaca sativa* (parsnip) *Petroselinum crispum* (parsley) *Heracleum mantegazzianum* (giant hogweed)
	Rutacea Citrus spp, *Citrus aurantica v. bergamia* (bergamot) *Citrus aurantifolia* (lime) *Citrus limon* (lemon) *Ruta graveolans* (common rue) *Dictamus albus* (burning bush)
	Moracea *Ficus carica* (fig)
3. Drugs	**Antimicrobials**
	Tetracyclines[b] (doxycycline, minocycline)
	Sulphonamides (sulfametoxazole)
	Fluorquinolones (lomefloxacin[b], ciprofloxacin[b])
	Voriconazole[b], griseofulvin[b], efavirenz
	Nonsteroidal anti-inflammatory drugs (NSAIDs)
	Arylpropionic acids: Ketoprofen[a], tiaprofenic acid[b], suprofen, naproxen, ibuprofen, ibuproxam, carprofen Piroxicam[a], benzydamine, etofenamate[a] azapropazone, diclofenac, fenilbutazone, indometacine
	Phenotiazines
	Chlorpromazine, thioridazine Promethazine[a], Chorproethazine[a]
	Antidepressants
	clomipramine, imipramine, sertraline
	Cardiovascular drugs
	Amiodarone[b], quinidine, Furosemide and thiazide diuretics
	Anticancer agents
	Paclitaxel, 5-fluoruracil, Dacarbazine, methotrexate
	Miscellaneous
	Flutamide, sulfonylureas, fenofibrate, simvastatin

Table 15.3 (Continued)

4. "Historical" photosensitizers	**Perfumes:** musk ambrette and bergamot oil[b]
	Halogenated salicylanilides: tetrachlorsaliiynilide trichlorocarbanilide tribromsalicylanide
	Sunscreens: isopropyldibenzoylmethane, PABA
	Antibiotics: Olaquindox[a]

[a]Mainly photoallergic
[b]Mainly phototoxic
[c]Sunscreens are not detailed as they are responsible mainly for photoallergy

drugs, both phototoxic and photoallergic are, by far, the most frequent photosensitizers in Southern Europe (Cardoso et al. 2009; La Cuadra-Oyanguren et al. 2007; Leonard et al. 2005; Pigatto et al. 2008)

5.1 UV Filters

Due to the increased awareness of the sun-damaging effects, sunscreens are widely used, and UV filters are also included in moisturizing and facial creams, lipstick, nail varnish, shampoos, and other hair products, but adverse skin reactions from UV filters are not reported proportionally (Darvay et al. 2001). Also, as referred, most represent allergic, photoallergic, or photoaggravated allergic contact dermatitis, not phototoxicity (Bryden et al. 2006; Berne and Ros 1998; Pigatto et al. 2008; Leonard et al. 2005; La Cuadra-Oyanguren et al. 2007; Cardoso et al. 2009).

The newer UV filters – Mexoryl SX (terephtalydene dicamphor sulfonic acid), Tinosorb M (methylene-bis-benzotriazolyl tetramethylbutylphenol or bisoctrizole), and Tinosorb S (bis-ethylhexyloxyphenol methoxyphenyl triazine) – are photostable molecules and, in mixtures of several sunscreens, are able to photostabilize older photolabile UV filters, like butyl-methoxydibenzoylmethane and cinnamates. Therefore, they seem to be more efficient in protecting from the harmful effects of UVR (Lowe 2006) and, eventually, in reducing photosensitivity from the other UV filters.

5.2 Plants Causing Phytophotodermatitis

Photoactive furocoumarins, e.g., bergapten (5- methoxypsoralen), 8-methoxypsoralen, 5,6 dimethoxyisopsoralen, sphondin (6-methoxyisopsoralen), and isobergapten (5-methoxyisopsoralen) run in the sap of several plants, in variable amounts. They are beneficial for the plant which uses them as a protection against fungus and insects.

Since the antiquity, these substances have been used in folk medicine in the treatment of vitiligo and, more recently, in photochemotherapy (PUVA), but their acute and chronic phototoxic potential is well known and measures are regularly considered to avoid these adverse effects: A low UV dose is used in the beginning of therapy and in patients with lower phototypes, children under 16 are not usually admitted on PUVA therapy, and a cumulative dose below 1,000–1,500 J/cm^2 of UVA is advised for patients on photochemotherapy to reduce the potential risk of photocarcinogenesis and photoaging.

Aromatic oils rich in furocoumarins were used by the cosmetic industry in tanning oils, but their use has been considerably reduced as this accelerated tanning is harmful – the photosensitizer in the oil enhances UV-induced DNA aggression.

The natural bergamot oil, extracted from the rind of *Citrus bergamia,* previously included in oils and perfumes, was responsible for a very particular type of phototoxic dermatitis, "breloque dermatitis," or berlock dermatitis. It presented as erythema followed by hyperpigmentation, in a very particular shape of a pendant-like figure simulating a breloque, beginning in the face or neck and descending down to the collar. It corresponded to the place where the first drop of perfume is applied and the adjacent and dependent draining area. The natural oil of bergamot is no more used in perfumes and breloque dermatitis is an image of the past, but citrus oils containing psoralens can still induce phototoxicity when used in aromatic oils in sauna or in massages (Lovell 2000).

Nowadays, phototoxic dermatitis from psoralens occurs mainly from inadvertent contact with plants, either during recreation or in occupational settings. Main occupational exposures occur in rural workers or gardeners who harvest fruits or vegetables (parsnip, figs) or cut bushes and weeds (common rue – *Ruta graveolens*, burning bush – *Dictamnus albus*, or fig trees – *Ficus carica*) (Gonçalo et al. 1989; Lovell 2000) and in barmen who squeeze and peal the lime (*Citrus aurantifolia*) and other citrus fruits to prepare cocktails in the sunny weather (Wagner et al. 2002; Gonçalo 2004; Lovell 2000) (*Fig. 15.4*).

The most typical pattern of phytophotodermatitis was described by Oppenheim in 1934 – *dermatosis bullosa striata pratensis.* Corresponding to the contact with the damaged leaves of the plant, prickling linear erythematous

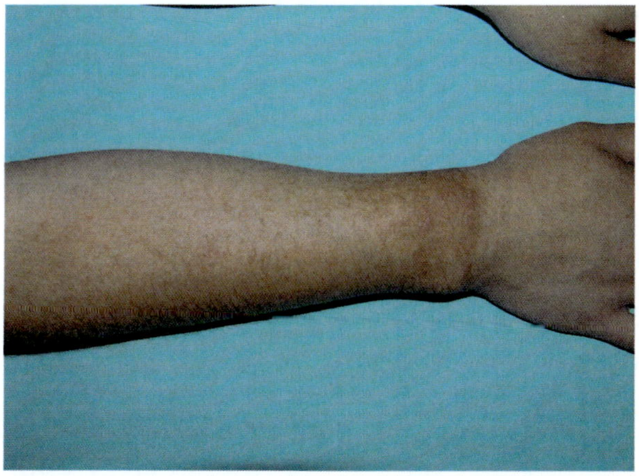

Fig. 15.4
Residual pigmentation in the forearms in a barman who squeezed limes and lemons for cocktails, during an outdoor summer festival (note limit due to glove protection)

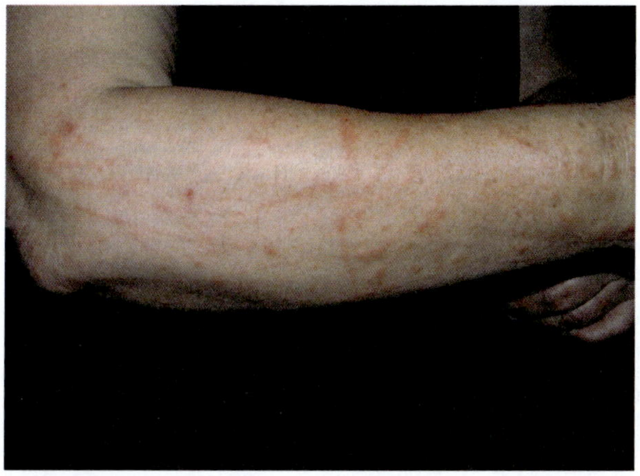

Fig. 15.5
Phytophotodermatitis with linear streaks of erythema and hyperpigmentation in a patient who contacted Ruta graveolens from her garden

skin streaks develop within 24–48 h followed by painful vesicles and bullae (*Figs. 15.5* and *15.6*). This gradually gives rise to long-lasting typical browny linear hyperpigmentation which, sometimes, allows a retrospective diagnosis (Gonçalo 2004).

Other patterns of phytophotodermatitis are the "strimmer dermatitis," a more diffuse involvement as the sap of the plant is sprayed all over the body by the string trimmer (Lovell 2000), a leg dermatitis in walkers who develop lesions only above the socks, and skin lesions in children who make trumpets or pea shooters from the

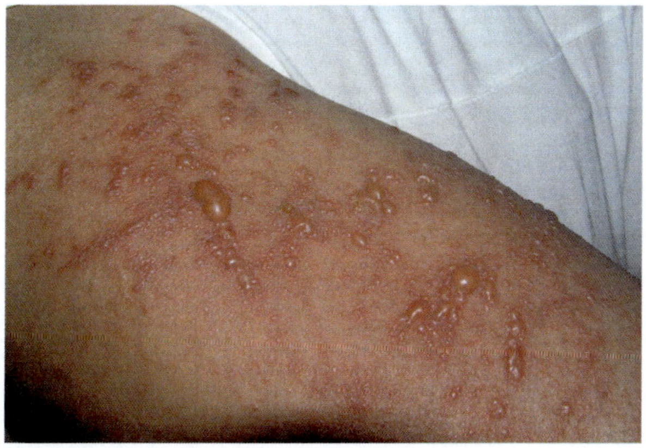

Fig. 15.6
Phytophotodermatitis with linear bullous lesions in the arms, after cutting a fig tree during a sunny day

hollow stems of the giant hogweed (*Heracleum mantegazzianum*) and developed blisters around their mouth (Lovell 2000).

Very occasionally, the ingestion of these plants can induce a systemic photosensitivity as in the cases of celery, parsnip or infusions of St. John's wort (*Hypericum perforatum L.*) used to treat depression (Lovell 2000). Also, they are occasionally used topic drug as a "folk medicine" with impressive adverse effects, as in a recent report where an infusion of *Ruta graveolens* was applied topically to relieve pain in fibromyalgia (Arias-Santiago et al. 2009).

Plants rich in furocoumarins causing phytophotodermatitis occur all over the globe and belong mainly to the families of Umbelliferae, Rutacea, and Moracea (*Table 15.3*)

5.3 Photosensitive Drugs

Drugs used systemically or applied topically are the main cause of exogenous photosensitivity, particularly in Southern European countries (Cardoso et al. 2009; La Cuadra-Oyanguren et al. 2007; Leonard et al. 2005; Pigatto et al. 2008).

Drugs manipulated in an occupational setting can induce photosensitivity: carprofen, a NSAID no more used in humans, induced photoallergic contact dermatitis in workers who manufacture the drug for animals (Kerr et al. 2008a; Walker et al. 2006), and photosensitivity has been reported in nurses and family members who smashed the tablets of chlorpromazine to give to their patients/relatives (Cardoso et al. 2009).

The main systemic drugs inducing photosensitivity are antimicrobials, particularly tetracyclines, fluorquinolones, sulfonamides, and some antifungals, NSAIDs, phenothiazines, and cardiovascular drugs. After topical application, NSAIDs are by far the most frequent cause (Cardoso et al. 2009; La Cuadra-Oyanguren et al. 2007; Leonard et al. 2005; Pigatto et al. 2008).

5.3.1 Antimicrobials

Systemic tetracyclines, particularly doxycycline and minocycline, are highly phototoxic, induce photoonycholysis and pseudoporphyria and, the latter, can also induce a bluish persistent pigmentation (Vassileva et al. 1998; Ferguson 1999).

The fluorquinolones induce phototoxic reactions, in some cases presenting as pseudoporphyria (Schmutz et al. 2008), as initially described for the first quinolone antibiotic, nalidixic acid (Vassileva et al. 1998). Ciprofloxacin was also responsible for purpura in photo-exposed areas (Urbina et al. 2006). Phototoxicity is particularly important and frequent (4–15% of treated patients) with fleroxacin, lomefloxacin, sparfloxacin, pefloxacin, and less frequent with ciprofloxacin, norfloxacin, ofloxacin, and enoxacin (Ferguson 1999). The recommendation to take the drug by the end of the day, therefore reducing drug concentrations in the circulation and in the skin during midday, can reduce this phototoxic reaction.

Although in vitro and in vivo tests prove the high phototoxic potential of fluorquinolones, photoallergy has also been reported with lomefloxacin (Oliveira et al. 1996; Kurumajin and Shono 1992) and enoxacin (Vassileva et al. 1998), sometimes with cross-reaction to other fluorquinolones (ciprofloxacin and flerofloxacin) (Kimura and Kawada 1998; Correia et al. 1994), positive lymphocyte stimulation tests, and drug-specific Th1 cells that recognize skin cells combined with UV irradiated fluorquinolone (Tokura et al. 2001). Moreover, the fluorquinolones also photosensitize DNA and may be photomutagenic and photocarcinogenic (Klecak et al. 1997). A patient on long-term ciprofloxacin therapy for multiresistant tuberculosis developed photosensitivity and highly aggressive squamous cell carcinomas of the face (personal experience).

Sulfonamide antibacterials, as well as sulfa-drug analogs (thiazide diuretics, hypoglycemic sulfonylureas, and celecoxib) and dapsone (diaminodiphenylsulfone) have been reported to cause photosensitivity within the spectrum both of UVB and UVA (Vassileva et al. 1998; Yazici et al. 2004) but this side effect is not so frequent with cotrimoxazole (trimethoprim/sulfamethoxazole) (Vassileva et al. 1998; Ferguson 1999).

Grisefulvin is a known phototoxic drug and can aggravate lupus erythematosus, as the more recent antifungal, terbinafine, which also induced subacute lupus erythematosus in patients with anti-Ro antibodies (Farhi et al. 2006). Another antifungal from a different chemical group, voriconazole, has recently been reported to cause severe photosensitivity (Béani 2009; Frick et al. 2010) and was considered responsible for skin cancer, including malignant melanoma (Auffret et al. 2006; McCarthy et al. 2007; Cowen et al. 2010; Miller et al. 2010).

5.3.2 Nonsteroidal Anti-inflammatory Drugs

Benoxaprofen marketed between 1980 and 1982 called the attention to photosensitivity from this class of drugs. Thereafter, photosensitivity was reported with all the other arylpropionic derivatives (carprofen, naproxen, suprofen, tiaprofenic acid, ketoprofen, and ibuprofen) and NSAIDs from other groups (azapropazone, diclofenac, piroxicam, fenilbutazone, celecoxib, benzydamine, and etofenamate) (Figueiredo 1994). The in vitro and in vivo phototoxic potential has been documented particularly for tiaprofenic acid (Figueiredo 1994). In humans, photopatch testing showed typically phototoxic reactions in more than half patients tested with tiaprofenic acid (5% pet) and 5 J/cm^2 of UVA (Gonçalo and Figueiredo 1992; Neumann et al. 1994, 2000), but in other studies tiaprofenic acid was typically photoallergic (Pigatto et al. 1996; LeCoz et al. 1998; Foti et al. 2008), therefore calling the attention to the concomitancy of both patterns of photosensitivity with the same drug.

Most topically applied NSAIDs are absorbed through the skin and cause distant lesions, resembling systemic photosensitivity. Benzydamine, widely used in the oral or genital mucosa, causes photosensitivity at distant sites (Elgezua et al. 2004), eventually after systemic absorption (Cardoso et al. 2009; La Cuadra-Oyanguren et al. 2007) and, when used in the mouth, can induce cheilitis and chin dermatitis as a manifestation of photoallergy (Cardoso et al. 2009).

Although ketoprofen and piroxicam are not the most sold NSAIDs, they cause most cases of photosensitivity (Cardoso et al. 2009; La Cuadra-Oyanguren et al. 2007; Leonard et al. 2005), particularly photoallergy and with a peculiar pattern of cross-reactions (Imai et al. 2005) (Béani 2009; Cardoso et al. 2009): cinnamic alcohol and aldehyde, oxybenzone, octocrylene, and fenofibrate for ketoprofene (Pigatto et al. 1996; LeCoz et al. 1998; Devleeschouwer et al. 2008; Foti et al. 2008), and thimerosal and thiosalicylic acid for piroxicam (Gonçalo et al. 1992; Hariva et al. 1993).

5.3.3 Other Drugs as Photosensitizers

Phenothiazines used systemically (chlorpromazine and thioridazine) can induce photosensitivity, often with a lichenoid pattern and with residual pigmentation (Ferguson 1999). They are typically phototoxic, both in vitro and in vivo, but some cases of photoallergy also occur (Cardoso et al. 2009). Promethazine is a highly phototoxic drug that is still used as a topical antipruritic, at least in Portugal and Greece. In this setting, it induces many cases of photosensitivity, many of them photoallergic (Cardoso et al. 2009; Katsarou et al. 2008). Its analogue, chlorproethazine, marketed in France as Neuriplege® cream for muscle pain (Genevrier, Antibes, France), is also a frequent cause of photoallergic contact dermatitis (Barbaud et al. 2001a; Kerr et al. 2008b).

The antiarrhythmic amiodarone is a well-known photosensitizer that is still widely used. Apart from erythema in sun-exposed areas, it induces a bluish-gray hyperpigmentation in sun-exposed areas due to the accumulation of drug metabolites in the dermis (Ammoury et al. 2008).

The list of drugs causing photosensitivity is very large and always increasing, with the recent inclusion of biologics, namely, vandetanib, an orally effective VEGF-inhibitor used in oncology (Chang et al. 2009). Therefore, whenever a patient has a photosensitive eruption a systematic inquiry for drugs should be carefully conducted.

6 Diagnostic Procedures in Photosensitivity

Sometimes the lesions are so typical for a dermatologist, as in phytophotodermatitis or in exaggerated sunburn after the use of a systemic phototoxic drug, that no further diagnostic procedures are needed. A simple questionnaire can find the responsible agent. Also, in typical phototoxic reactions, both photopatch and photoprovocation tests are positive in the great majority of tested individuals. Therefore, they are not particularly useful for confirming the etiology of a phototoxic reaction, but they can disclose a hidden photoallergy.

Photopatch testing should be performed according to a standardized procedure (Bruynzeel et al. 2004), using a photoallergen series adapted to the geographic area (Cardoso et al. 2009; Gonçalo 2011) with additions according to patient exposure. Irradiation of one set of allergens at day 1 or day 2 with 5 J/cm2 of UVA is advised and readings should be performed immediately after irradiation and also 48 and/or 72 h thereafter (Bruynzeel et al. 2004).

Photopatch tests results have to be carefully interpreted. A reaction only in the irradiated side mainly with erythema and edema, without pruritus, exclusively limited to the test chamber area, with very sharp limits that begins shortly after irradiation, has its highest intensity by 24 h and regress by 48/72 h (decrescendo reaction) with hyperpigmentation, suggests a phototoxic reaction. A similar reaction may be observed in many individuals tested in the same conditions and, if histology is performed, there are many sunburn cells in the epidermis. On the other hand, a pruritic erythema with vesicles, diffuse limits extending beyond the chamber limit, that increases in intensity until 48–72 h after UV irradiation (crescendo reaction), suggests photoallergy (Neumann et al. 1994). But sometimes the photopatch test pattern is not so typical and the difficulties previously referred in the interpretation of clinical cases also occur in the interpretation of the photopatch tests.

The main indication for photopatch testing is the diagnosis of photallergic contact dermatitis, but photopatch testing can also be useful in the study of systemic drug photosensitivity (Gonçalo 1998, 2010; Barbaud et al. 2001b).

7 Conclusions

Phototoxic, photoallergic, and overlapping photosensitive reactions are still a frequent problem. They have a highly polymorphic clinical presentation, with different time courses and variations in the responsible agents depending on geographic areas and over times. Therefore, the dermatologist must be highly alert to search for a possible involvement of an exogenous chromophore in a photosensitive patient and try to confirm its contribution to photosensitivity. A correct questionnaire should be conducted and, although not so important in typical phototoxic cases, complementary tests including photopatch and photoprovocation tests may contribute to the final etiologic diagnosis and, consequently, allow an adequate patient advice concerning further eviction of the photosensitizer and related chemicals.

References

Ammoury A, Michaud S, Paul C, Prost-Squarcioni C, Alvarez F, Lamani L, Launay F et al (2008) Photodistribution of blue-gray hyperpigmentation after amiodarone treatment. Molecular characterization of amiodarone in the skin. Arch Dermatol 144:92–96

Arias-Santiago S, Fernandéz-Pugnaire M, Anamzán-Fernandéz F, Serrano-Franco C, Serrano-Ortega S (2009) Phytophotodermatitis due to Ruta graveolens prescribed for fibromyalgia. Rheumatol 48(11):1401

Auffret N, Janssen F, Chevalier P, Guillemain R, Amrein C, Le Beller C (2006) Photosensibilisation au voriconazole. Ann Dermatol Venereol 133:330–332

Bakkum R, Heule F (2002) Results of photopatch testing in Rotterdam during a 10-year period. Br J Dermatol 146:275–279

Baran R, Juhlin L (2002) Photoonycholysis. Photodermatol Photoimmunol Photomed 18:202–207

Barbaud A, Collet E, Martin S, Granel F, Tréchot P, Lambert D, Schmutz J (2001a) Contact sensitization to chlorproéthazine can induce persistent light reaction and cross photoreactions to other phenothiazines. Contact Dermatitis 44:373

Barbaud A, Gonçalo M, Bircher A, Bruynzeel D (2001b) Guidelines for performing skin tests with drugs in the investigation of cutaneous adverse drug reactions. Contact Dermatitis 45:321–328

Béani J (2009) Les photosensibilisations graves. Ann Dermatol Venereol 136:76–83

Berne B, Ros A (1998) 7 years experience of photopatch testing with sunscreen allergens in Sweden. Contact Dermatitis 38:61–64

Bruynzeel D, Ferguson J, Andersen K, Gonçalo M, English J, Goossens A, Holzle E et al (2004) Photopatch testing: a consensus methodology for Europe. J Eur Acad Dermatol Venereol 18:679–682

Bryden A, Moseley H, Ibbotson S, Chowdhury M, Beck M, Bourke J, English J et al (2006) Photopatch testing of 1115 patients: results of the U.K. multicentre photopatch study group. Br J Dermatol 155:737–747

Cardoso J, Canelas M, Gonçalo M, Figueiredo A (2009) Photopatch testing with an extended series of photoallergens. A 5-year study. Contact Dermatitis 60:314–319

Chang C, Chang J, Hui C, Yang C (2009) Severe photosensitivity reaction to Vandetanib. J Clin Oncol 27(27):114–115

Cohen P (2009) Photodistributed erythema multiforme:paclitaxel-related, photosensitive conditions in patients with cancer. J Drugs Dermatol 8:61–64

Collins P, Ferguson J (1994) Photoallergic contact dermatitis to oxybenzone. Br J Dermatol 131:124–129

Correia O, Delgado L, Barros M (1994) Bullous photodermatosis after lomefloxacin. Arch Dermatol 130(6):808–809

Cowen E, Nguyen J, Miller D, Mcshane D, Arron S, Prose N, Turner M et al (2010) Chronic phototoxicity and aggressive squamous cell carcinoma of the skin in children and adults during treatment with voriconazole. J Am Acad Dermatol 62:31–37

Cummins R, Wagner-Weiner L, Paller A (2000) Pseudoporphyria induced by celecoxib in a patient with juvenile rheumatoid arthritis. J Rheumatol 27:2938–2940

Darvay A, White I, Rycroft R, Jones A, Hawk J, McFadden J (2001) Photoallergic contact dermatitis is uncommon. Br J Dermatol 145:597–601

Devleeschouwer V, Roelandts R, Garmyn M, Goossens A (2008) Allergic and photoallergic contact dermatitis from ketoprofen: results of (photo) patch testing and follow-up of 42 patients. Contact Dermatitis 58:159–166

Emmert B, Schauder S, Palm H, Haliier E, Emmert S (2007) Disabling work-related persistent photosensitivity following photoallergic contact dermatitis from chlorpromazine and olaquindox in a pig breeder. Ann Agric Environ Med 14:329

Farhi D, Viguier M, Cosnes A, Reygagne P, Dubertret L, Revuz J, Roujeau J (2006) Terbinafine-induced subacute cutaneous lupus erythematosus. Dermatology 212:59–65

Ferguson J (1999) Drug and chemical photosensitivity. In: Hawk's photodermatology, 1st edn. Oxford University Press, New York, pp 155–169

Figueiredo A (1994) Fotossensibilidade aos anti-inflamatórios não esteróides. Estudo fisiopatológico (Thesis). Coimbra, Portugal

Foti C, Bonamonte D, Conserva A, Stingeni L, Lisi P, Lionetti N, Rigano L et al (2008) Allergic and photoallergic contact dermatitis from ketoprofen: evaluation of cross-reactivities by a combination of photopatch testing and computerized conformational analysis. Curr Pharm Des 14(27):2833–2839

Frick M, Soler-Palacin P, Nalda A, Guarmer M, Nadal C (2010) Photosensitivity in immunocompromised patients receiving long-term therapy with oral voriconazole. Pediatr Infect Dis J 29(5): 480–481

Fujimoto N, Danno K, Wakabayashi M, Uenishi T, Tanaka T (2009) Photosensitivity with eosinophilia due to ambroxol and UVB. Contact Dermatitis 60:110–113

Gonçalo M (1998) Explorations dans les photo-allergies médicamenteuses. Em *GERDA.Progrès en Dermato-Allergologie.* Nancy/John Libbey Eurotext, pp 67–74

Gonçalo M (2004) Dermatitis por plantas y maderas. In: Em Conde-Salazar Gómez L, Ancona-Alayón A (eds) Dermatologia profesional. Aula Médica Ediciones, Madrid, pp 193–210

Gonçalo M (2011) Photopatch testing. In: Johanssen JD, Frosch P, Leppoitevin J-P (eds) Textbook of contact dermatitis, 5th edn. Springer, Berlin/Heidelberg, pp 519–531

Gonçalo M, Figueiredo A (1992) Photopatch testing with nonsteroidal anti-inflammatory drugs. Em Proceedings of the 1st european symposium of contact dermatitis, Brussels, pp 25

Gonçalo S, Correia C, Couto J, Gonçalo M (1989) Contact and photocontact dermatitis from *Ruta chalepensis.* Contact Dermatitis 21(3):200–201

Gonçalo M, Figueiredo A, Tavares P, Ribeiro C, Teixeira F, Baptista A (1992) Photosensitivity to piroxicam: absence of cross-reaction with tenoxicam. Contact Dermatitis 27(5):287–290

Gonçalo M, Domingues J, Correia O, Figueiredo A (1999) Fotossensibilidad a flutamida. Boletim Informativo del GEIDC 29:45–48

Gregoriou S, Karagiorga T, Stratigos A, Volonakis K, Kontochristopoulos G, Rigopoulos D (2008) Photo-onycholysis caused by olanzapine and aripiprazole. J Clin Psychopharmacol 28:219–220

Hariva T, Kitamura K, Osawa J, Ikezawa Z (1993) A cross-reaction between piroxicam-photosensitivity and thiosalicylate hypersensitivity in lymphocyte proliferation test. J Dermatol Sci 5(3):165–174

Hawk J (1999) Photodermatology, 1st edn. Oxford University Press, New York

Hawk J (2004) Chronic actinic dermatitis. Photodermatol Photoimmunol Photomed 20:312–314

Hindsén M, Isaksson M, Persson L, Zimersson E, Bruze M (2004) Photoallergic contact dermatitis from ketoprofen induced by drug-contaminated personal objects. J Am Acad Dermatol 50:215–219

Imai S, Atarashi K, Ikesue K, Akiyama K, Tokura Y (2005) Establishment of murine model of allergic photocontact deermatitis to ketoprofen and characterization of pathogenic T cells. J Dermatol Sci 41:127–136

Jensen A, Thomsen H, Engebjerg M, Olesen A, Sorensen H, Karagas M (2008) Use of photosensitising diuretics and risk of skin cancer: a population based case-control study. Br J Cancer 99:1522–1528

Karimian-Teherani D, Kinaciyan T, Tanew A (2008) Photoallergic contact dermatitis from Heracleum giganteum. Photodermatol Photoimmunol Photomed 24:99–101

Katsarou A, Makris M, Zarafonitis G, Lagogianni E, Gregoriou S, Kalogeromitros D (2008) Photoallergic contact dermatitis: the 15-year experience of a tertiary reference center in a sunny Mediterranean city. Int J Immunopathol Pharmacol 21:725–727

Kerr A, Ferguson J, Ibbotson S (2007) Acute phototoxicity with urticarial features during topical 5-aminolaevulinic acid photodynamic therapy. Clin Exp Dermatol 32:201–202

Kerr A, Muller F, Ferguson J, Dawe R (2008a) Occupational carprofen photoallergic contact dermatitis. Br J Dermatol 159:1303–1308

Kerr A, Woods J, Ferguson J (2008b) Photocontact allergic and phototoxic studies of chlorproethazine. Photodermatol Photoimmunol Photomed 24:11–15

Kimura M, Kawada A (1998) Photosensitivity induced by lomefloxacin with cross-photosensitivity to ciprofloxacin and fleroxacin. Contact Dermatitis 38:130

Klecak G, Urbach F, Urwyler H (1997) Fluoroquinolone antibacterials enhance UVA-induced skin tumors. J Photochem Photobiol B 37:174–181

Kochs C, Mühlenstädt E, Neumann N, Hanneken S (2009) Solarium-induced pseudoporphyria and variegate porphyria as rare differential diagnoses of porphyria cutanea tarda. Hautarzt 60:790–793

Kurumajin Y, Shono M (1992) Scarified photopatch testing in lomefloxacin photosensitivity. Contact Dermatitis 26:5–10

La Cuadra-Oyanguren J, Pérez-Ferriols A, Lecha-Carralero M, Giménez-Arnau A, Fernández-Redondo V, Ortiz de Frutos F, Silvestre-Salvador J et al (2007) Resultdos y evaluación del fotoparche en España: hacia una nueva batería estánder de fotoalergenos. Actas Dermosifiliogr 98:96–101

Lasa Elgezua O, Gorrotxategi P, Gardeazabal Gracia J, Ratón Nieto J, Pérez J (2004) Photoallergic hand eczema due to benzydamine. Eur J Dermatol 14(1):69–70

LeCoz C, Bottlaender A, Scrivener J, Santinelli F, Cribier B, Heidei E, Grosshans E (1998) Photocontact dermatitis from ketoprofen and tiaprofenic acid: cross-reactivity study in 12 consecutive patients. Contact Dermatitis 38:245–252

Leonard F, Adamski H, Bonnevalle A, Bottlaender A, Bourrain J, Goujon-Henry G, Leroy D et al (2005) Étude prospective multicentrique 1991–2001 de la batterie standard des photopatch-tests de la Société Française de Photodermatologie. Ann Dermatol Venereol 132:313–320

Lhiaubet-Vallet V, Bosca F, Miranda M (2009) Photosensitized DNA damage: the case of fluoroquinolones. Photochem Photobiol 85:861–868

Lovell C (2000) Phytophotodermatitis. In: Avalos J, Maibach HI (eds) Dermatological botany. CRC Press, Boca Raton, pp 51–65

Lovell C, Cronin E, Rhodes E (1986) Photocontact urticaria from chlorpromazine. Contact Dermatitis 14:290–291

Lowe N (2006) An overview of ultraviolet radiation, sunscreens and photo-induced dermatosis. Dermatol Clin 24:9–17

Marrot L, Belaïdi J, Jones C, Perez P, Riou L, Sarasin A, Meunier J (2003) Molecular responses to photogenotoxic stress induced by the antibiotic lomefloxacin in human skin cells: from DNA damage to apoptosis. J Invest Dermatol 121:596–606

McCarthy K, Playforf E, Looke D, Whitby M (2007) Severe photosensitivity causing multifocal squamous cell carcinomas secondary to prolonged voriconazole therapy. Clin Infect Dis 44:e55–e56

Miller D, Cowen E, Nguyen J, McCalmont T, Fox L (2010) Melanoma associated with long-term voriconazole therapy: a new manifestation of chronic photosensitivity. Arch Dermatol 146(3):300–304

Müller L, Kasper P, Kersten B, Zhang J (1998) Photochemical genotoxicity and photochemical carcinogenesis – two sides of a coin? Toxicol Lett 102–103:383–387

Neumann N, Holzle E, Lehmann P, Benedikter S, Tapernoux B, Plewig G (1994) Patterns analysis of photopatch test reactions. Photodermatol Photoimmunol Photomed 16:65–73

Neumann N, Holzle E, Plewig G, Schwatz T, Pannizzon R, Breit R, Ruzicka T et al (2000) Photopatchtesting: the 12-year experience of the german, Austrian and swiss photopatch test group. J Am Acad Dermatol 42:183–192

Neves B, Cruz M, Francisco V, Gonçalo M, Figueiredo A, Duarte C, Lopes M (2008) Differential modulation of CXCR4 and CD40 protein levels by skin sensitizers and irritants in the FSCD cell line. Toxicol Lett 177:74–82

Oliveira H, Gonçalo M, Figueiredo A (1996) Photosensitivity from lomefloxacine. A clinical and photobiological study. Photodermatol Photoimmunol Photomed 16:116–120

Passier A, Smits-van Herwaarden A, van Puijenbroek E (2004) Photo-onycholysis associated with the use of doxycycline. BMJ 329:265

Pérez-Bustillo A, Sánchez-Sambucety P, Suárez-Amor O, Rodríiguez-Prieto M (2008) Torasemide-induced pseudoporphyria. Arch Dermatol 144(6):812–813

Pigatto P, Bigardi A, Legori A, Valsecchi R, Picardo M (1996) Cross reactions in patch testing and photopatch testing with ketoprofen, tiaprofenic acid and cinnamic aldehyde. Am J Contact Dermat 7:220–223

Pigatto P, Guzzi G, Schena D, Guarrera M, Foti C, Francalanci S, Cristaudo A et al (2008) Photopatch tests: an Italian multicentre study from 2004 to 2006. Contact Dermatitis 59(2):103–108

Placzek M, Eberlein-könig B, Przybilla B (1999) Association between actinic keratoses and potentially photosensitizing drugs. N Engl J Med 341:1474–1475

Schmutz J, Barbaud A, Tréchot P (2006) Pseudoporphyria and coxib. Ann Dermatol Venereol 133:213

Schmutz J, Barbaud A, Tréchot P (2008) Ciprofloxacin and pseudoporphyria. Ann Dermatol Venereol 135(11):804

Seto Y, Ochi M, Onoue S, Yamada S (2010) High-throughput screening strategy for photogenotoxic potential of pharmaceutical substances using fluorescent intercalating dye. J Pharm Biomed Anal 52(5):781–786

Sheuer E, Warshaw E (2006) Sunscreen allergy: a review of epidemiology, clinical characteristics, and responsible allergens. Dermatitis 17:3–11

Sontheimer R, Henderson C, Grau R (2008) Drug-induced subacute cutaneous lupus erythematosus: a paradigm for bedside-to-bench patient-oriented translational clinical investigation. Arch Dermatol Res 301(1):65–70

Timmer-de Mik L, Kardaun S, Krammer M, Hayes D, Bousema M (2009) Imatinib-induced pseudoporphyria. Clin Exp Dermatol 34(6):705–707

Tokura Y, Seo N, Fujie M, Takigawa M (2001) Quinolone-photoconjugated major histocompatibility complex class II-binding peptides with lysine are antigenic for T cells mediating murine quinolone photoallergy. J Invest Dermatol 117(5):1206–1211

Urbina F, Barrios M, Sudy E (2006) Photolocalized purpura during ciprofloxacin therapy. Photodermatol Photoimmunol Photomed 22:111–112

Vassileva S, Matev G, Parish L (1998) Antimicrobial photosensitive reactions. Arch Intern Med 158:1993–2000

Vilaplana J, Romaguera C, Azón A, Lecha M (1990) Flutamide photosensitivity-residual vitiliginous lesions. Contact Dermatitis 38:68–70

Wagner A, Wu J, Hansen R, Nigg H, Beiere R (2002) Bullous phytophotodermatitis associated with high natural concentrations of furanocoumarins in limes. Am J Contact Dermat 13(1):10–14

Walker S, Ead R, Beck M (2006) Occupational photoallergic contact dermatitis in a pharmaceutical worker manufacturing carprofen, a canine nonsteroidal anti-inflammatory drug. Br J Dermatol 154:551–577

Waters A, Sandhu D, Lowe G, Ferguson J (2009) Photocontact allergy to PABA: the need for continous vigilance. Contact Dermatitis 60(3):172–173

Yazici A, Baz K, Ikizoglu G, Kokturk A, Uzumlu H, Tataroglu C (2004) Celecoxib-induced photoallergic drug eruption. Int J Dermatol 43(6):459–461

Zeeli T, David M, Trattner A (2006) Photopatch tests: any news under the sun? Contact Dermatitis 55:305–307

16 Photoallergic Contact Dermatitis

James Ferguson · Alastair C. Kerr
Photobiology Unit, Ninewells Hospital and Medical School, Dundee, Scotland, UK

Core Messages

- Topical photoallergic contact dermatitis (PACD) is thought to represent a delayed-type hypersensitivity reaction when an exogenous agent combines with some component of the skin in the presence of ultraviolet (UV) and/or visible light.
- Although PACD is relatively rare, it is also underdiagnosed as a cause of sunlight-exposed site dermatitis.
- Photopatch testing is the investigation of choice for topical PACD and a European consensus methodology for photopatch testing should allow greater comparison between centers.
- Currently, organic UV sunscreen filters and topical nonsteroidal anti-inflammatory drugs (NSAIDs) are the commonest photohaptens encountered by patients.
- Clinicians should be aware of potential new photohaptens in the environment and have a low threshold for photopatch testing such agents.

1 Introduction

Photoallergic contact dermatitis (PACD) describes the reaction seen in the skin when an exogenous agent comes into contact with the skin topically in the presence of ultraviolet (UV) or visible light. Therefore, it presents as a dermatitis which predominantly affects sunlight-exposed skin.

2 Differential Diagnoses

Phototoxicity – Whether this is due to systemic exposure to a drug or topical exposure to a drug or chemical, it does cause diagnostic difficulties. Phototoxicity (which does not involve an immune mechanism) will arise in any individual, providing there is enough chemical and subsequent light exposure of appropriate wavelength within the skin. The clinical history is of key importance to determine the temporal relationship between commencement of medication and onset of the eruption. Although in many cases this may be weeks, it can also be many months or years. Phototoxicity is more common than PACD and often presents as a sunburn-like confluent erythema or lichenoid eruption. Well-described groups include phytophotodermatitis (usually due to psoralen exposure) or tar pitch phototoxicity, and on some occasions phototoxic dyestuffs, such as benzanthrone.

Allergic contact dermatitis – Certain contact allergens, such as airborne allergens, fragrances, or sunscreens, can cause dermatitis with a predominantly exposed site distribution.

Chronic actinic dermatitis (CAD) – CAD is a syndrome which has severe photosensitivity and usually multiple contact allergies. It may arise on a background of chronic dermatitis (atopic or contact) and can present as either a sunlight-exposed site dermatitis or may be entered into via a contact dermatitis presentation. Monochromator or solar simulator phototesting will show objective evidence of photosensitivity with skin biopsy of phototest responses revealing a dermatitis histopathology, rather than a sunburn reaction as seen in a phototoxic reaction (➋ *Fig. 16.1*).

Polymorphic light eruption (PLE) – PLE more commonly presents as a pruritic, papular or papulovesicular rash of sunlight-exposed skin (➋ *Fig. 16.2*). However, atypical forms may have a scaling or dermatitic appearance during resolution. Actinic prurigo may also cause diagnostic problems (➋ *Fig. 16.3a, b*).

Cutaneous lupus – Cutaneous manifestations of systemic lupus erythematosus (SLE) as well as subacute cutaneous lupus (SCLE) can present as an erythematous and scaling eruption affecting sunlight-exposed skin (➋ *Fig. 16.4*). In such cases, there may be other systemic manifestations of lupus. Skin biopsy with direct immunofluorescence and peripheral blood autoimmune tests should aid diagnosis.

Porphyria – Porphyria cutanea tarda (PCT) and other cutaneous porphyrias can lead to a sunlight-exposed skin eruption. Skin fragility, bullae, and milia may be present and a peripheral blood porphyria plasma scan should aid diagnosis. Pseudoporphyria due to drug phototoxicity with or without renal failure may present in a similar fashion, although the porphyrin assay is usually within the normal range.

T. Rustemeyer, P. Elsner, S.M. John & H.I. Maibach (eds.), *Kanerva's Occupational Dermatology*,
DOI 10.1007/978-3-642-02035-3_16, © Springer-Verlag Berlin Heidelberg 2012

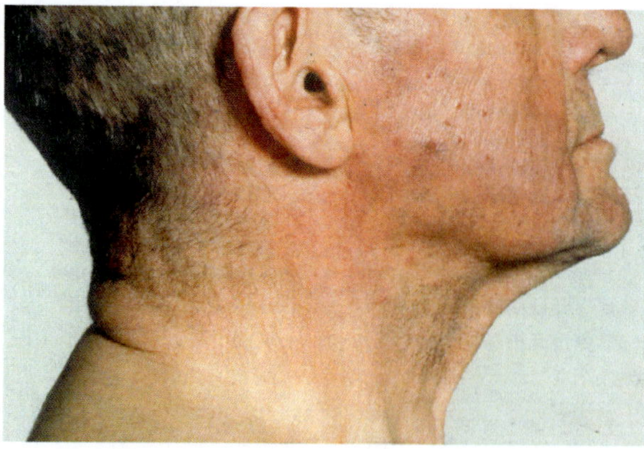

Fig. 16.1
Chronic actinic dermatitis (CAD) showing a photoexposed site dermatitis, with sparing in the photoprotected area behind the ear and under the chin

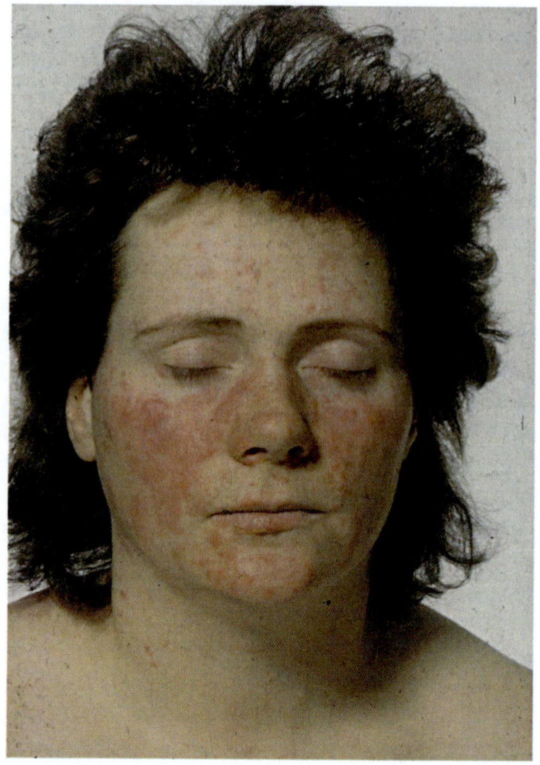

Fig. 16.2
Polymorphic light eruption (PLE) showing an erythematous papulovesicular rash on the photoexposed skin of the face with relative sparing of the forehead due to the fringe

3 Mechanism of PACD

The exact molecular basis of topical PACD has not been fully elucidated. However, experimental evidence suggests that in most cases, an exogenous low molecular weight compound (photohapten) binds to an endogenous substance in the skin or circulation, most likely a protein. The resulting protein–hapten conjugate is then recognized as antigenic by antigen presenting cells within the body and leads to a delayed-type hypersensitivity reaction. Crucially, the conjugation of protein and hapten will only occur in the presence of UV and/or visible light.

4 Incidence

PACD is relatively uncommon. Among patients that have been referred to tertiary referral centers with a photoexposed site dermatosis, a frequency between 2% and 10% has been reported (Bell and Rhodes 2000; Darvay et al. 2001; Bryden et al. 2006). The true incidence in the general population is not known, but will be significantly lower than this.

5 Historical Photosensitizers

Historically, many diverse compounds have been recognized as responsible for PACD. Epstein was among the first to use the term "photoallergy," when investigating skin problems due to topical sulfanilamide in 1939 (Epstein 1939). However, it was not until an outbreak of PACD due to the halogenated salicylanilides in the 1960s that clinicians became generally aware of its importance. Salicylanilides were compounds added to soaps as germicidal agents and it was the use of these with subsequent sunlight exposure that led to many, sometimes severe cases of PACD (Wilkinson 1961). After their strong photoallergic potential was discovered, their usage was gradually reduced and the problem essentially cleared.

In the 1970s, musk ambrette, a synthetic compound added to men's fragrances, became a recognized photohapten (Raugi et al. 1979). As with halogenated salicylanilides, usage of these agents in Europe and the USA has all but ceased, although interestingly it remains available for purchase via the Internet.

In the 1970s, the veterinary food additive quindoxin was reported as a cause of PACD among pig farmers in Europe (Scott and Dawson 1974). Again, it was withdrawn from the marketplace and replaced with a derivative, olaquindox. Unfortunately, this compound also proved to be a photohapten and was itself removed from further usage (Schauder et al. 1996).

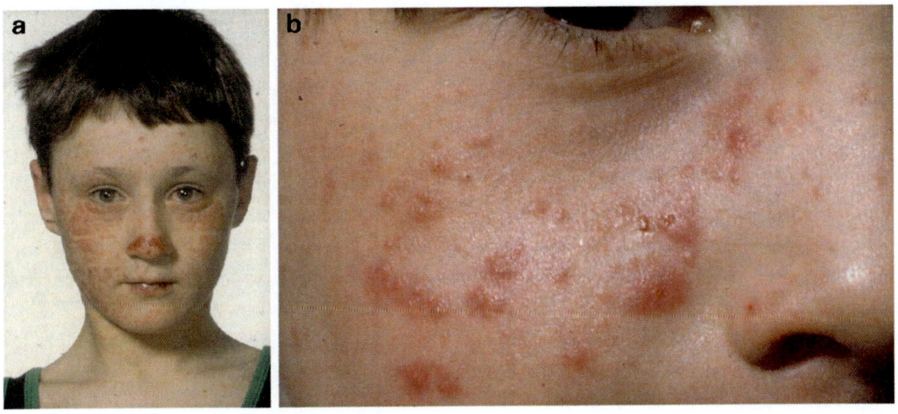

Fig. 16.3
(a, b) Actinic prurigo showing an excoriated papulo-nodular rash on the photoexposed skin of the face, with characteristic involvement of the tip of the nose

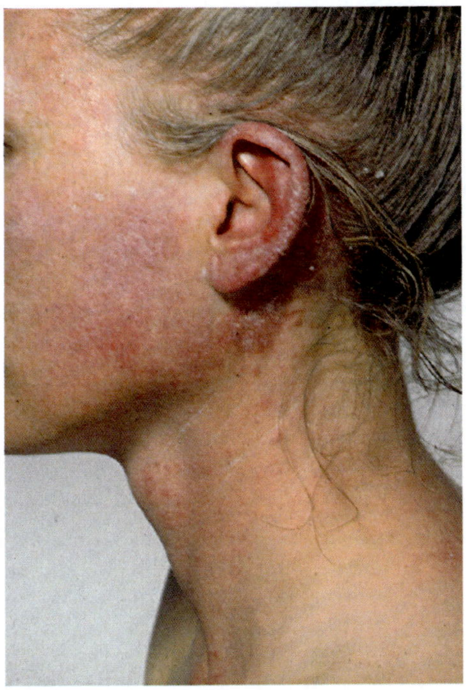

Fig. 16.4
Cutaneous lupus erythematosus (LE) showing an infiltrated and scaly eruption affecting photoexposed skin

The major tranquillizer, chlorpromazine, was also shown to elicit photoallergy as well as phototoxicity (Epstein 1968). PACD was often seen among carers of psychiatric patients who had to crush up tablets for those with swallowing difficulties but the subsequent introduction of a syrup formulation contributed to a reduction in this problem.

6 Current Photohaptens

6.1 Sunscreens

Sunscreens are currently the largest group of photohaptens that most people come into contact with regularly. They are freely available to consumers over the counter without prescription and are very widely used by all age groups of healthy individuals. They are found not only in products marketed primarily as sun protection products, but also in many other cosmetics, many of which are marketed with "antiaging" properties. Filters are also added to prolong the shelf life of products in translucent packaging by helping to slow photodegradation of other constituents.

When a consumer purchases a proprietary sunscreen, this can contain 30 or more individual ingredients, only 3–6 of which may be active organic UV filters. These filters work by absorbing those sunburn-causing, shorter UVB and UVA wavelengths, which raise the molecule to an excited state. As the molecule returns to the ground state, it releases the energy in the form of less harmful, longer UVA wavelengths. A sunscreen may also contain inorganic filters such as titanium dioxide or zinc oxide. These work as physical reflectants of incoming UV and seem to have little or no photoallergic potential.

When a patient presents with possible sunscreen-related photoallergy, it is important to attempt to ascertain which organic UV filters may be implicated. If the patient has brought the bottle which contained the sunscreen to the clinic, the ingredients may be listed. Unfortunately, over time, many of the individual filters have acquired many synonyms, due to the complex nature of their chemical structures and also due to use of commercial/proprietary names. Where possible, clinicians should use the International Nomenclature of Cosmetic Ingredients (INCI) name and if necessary, the Chemical Abstracts Service (CAS) number when ordering agents and performing patch and photopatch testing. ➲ *Table 16.1* lists some commonly used organic UV sunscreen filters with their CAS numbers and a list of synonyms. As can be seen from the table, if a positive contact allergic or photocontact allergic reaction is demonstrated in a patient, it would be advisable to provide the patient with all synonyms of the agent to aid future avoidance.

When photopatch testing to sunscreens, as with conventional patch testing, it is important to test the patient's own proprietary product "as is." It is possible that testing to individual filters that are within the product may be negative, while the "as is" product testing is positive. There may be several reasons for this including differing filter concentration, different filter vehicle and unknown effects of the many other excipients when tested under photopatch test conditions. Indeed, it is possible that other excipients within the product have been the cause of the contact or photocontact allergy. If there is no alternative product or if the patient wishes more in-depth investigation, the clinician must then attempt to obtain all the individual excipients of the product by contacting the manufacturer. Often the manufacturer may oblige and provide the various ingredients in a form suitable for photopatch testing.

Two situations the clinician should be aware of are the unsuspecting sunscreen user who is unaware that they are exposed to an organic UV filter in the form of an "antiaging" cream or a cosmetic product that contains a sun barrier with the purpose of extending its shelf life. Another problem is the incorrect assumption that the ingredients of a named commercial product remain constant. This is certainly not the case and all products should be checked by examination of the ingredient list on the box or product itself, which may be revealing.

When photopatch testing organic UV sunscreen filters, petrolatum is a suitable vehicle for most although occasionally other vehicles may be required (e.g., terephthalylidene dicamphor sulfonic acid, which needs to be tested in water). In the European Union, no organic filter can be used in cosmetic products at a concentration of greater than 15%. However, in some across the counter (ATC) products, there are agents which use much lower concentrations. This has the advantage of reducing the potential for induction of PACD. Although the optimum concentration to perform photopatch tests has not yet been fully elucidated, most filters can be photopatch tested at a concentration of 10%, without a significant risk of leading to false-positive irritant responses (Kerr et al. 2009). Most agents are, therefore, usually photopatch tested at 10% concentration.

While most organic UV filters have been reported as causing both contact and photocontact allergy, certain agents seem to have a greater photoallergic potency than others (Schauder and Ippen 1997). Over time, the accumulation of reports citing adverse cutaneous effects have led to the withdrawal of certain filters (e.g., PABA and isopropyl dibenzoylmethane). A high level of literature reports may not simply be due to the photoallergic contact potential of a particular agent. For example, the quantity and concentration of use may impact, with some ubiquitous sunscreens having a greater number of reports simply due to a greater exposure rather than greater photoallergic potency.

When a new drug or sunscreen is now developed, photosafety testing during product development is increasingly required. This is capable of picking up photoallergy as well as phototoxicity and can be studied first in the laboratory with the guinea pig maximization test before considering human volunteer testing. Within the European Union, sunscreens are classed as cosmetic ingredients and a "list of UV filters which cosmetic products may contain" is available under Annex VII of the CosIng section of the European Commission Web site (European Commission, Enterprise and Industry, Cosmetic Ingredients and Substances 2011). This annex contains information about the maximum concentration at which each filter can be used as well as links to existing safety data for each filter.

In order to create and update such regulation, the EU works closely with Colipa, the European cosmetics trade association which represents companies working in the cosmetics industry. Colipa continually collects, reviews, and presents data on usage of UV sunscreen filters. This data (plus other sources available) is then studied by a group of independent scientists (a scientific committee on consumer products – SCCP) and a report is published with their opinion of the safety of a substance. This information is circulated by the European commission to an Ad Hoc Working Party (AHWP), on the cosmetic directive not all of whom are scientifically trained, and decisions made about inclusion or updating of information in the annex (Mascotto 2005).

In the USA, the Food and Drug Administration (FDA) regulates products which contain a sunscreen active but make no claim for sunburn protection (e.g., products with a sunscreen added to protect color) as cosmetics. Those products which do claim sunburn protective qualities

Table 16.1
Commonly used organic UV filters with their CAS number, INCI name, USAN, and commercial synonyms

Chemical Abstracts Service (CAS) Number	International Nomenclature of Cosmetic Ingredients (INCI) name	Other names	United States adopted name (USAN)	Proprietary/trade names (all registered trademarks)
150-13-0	PABA	4-Aminobenzoic acid		
118-60-5	Ethylhexyl salicylate	Octyl salicylate	Octisalate	Escalol 587, Eusolex OS, Neo Heliopan OS
8045-71-4	Homosalate	Homomenthyl salicylate	Homosalate	Eusolex HMS, Neo Heliopan HMS
6197-30-4	Octocrylene	Octocrilene	Octocrylene	Escalol 597, Eusolex OCR, Neo Heliopan 303, Parsol 340, Uvinul 539T
5466-77-3	Ethylhexylmethoxycinnamate	Octyl methoxycinnamate	Octinoxate	Escalol 557, Eusolex 2292, NeoHeliopan AV, Parsol MCX, Tinosorb OMC, Uvinul MC 80
71617-10-2	Isoamyl-*p*-methoxycinnamate		Amiloxate	Neo Heliopan E1000
131-57-7	Benzophenone-3		Oxybenzone	Escalol 567, Eusolex 4360, Neo Heliopan BB, Tinosorb B3, Uvinul M40
4065-45-6	Benzophenone-4		Sulisobenzone	Escalol 577, Uvinul MS 40
70356-09-1	Butyl methoxydibenzoylmethane	4-*Tert*-butyl-4′-methoxydibenzoylmethane	Avobenzone	Escalol 517, Eusolex 9020, NeoHeliopan 357, Parsol 1789
36861-47-9	4-Methylbenzylidene camphor		Enzacamene	Eusolex 6300, Neo Heliopan MBC, Parsol 5000, Uvinul MBC 95
27503-81-7	Phenylbenzimidazole sulfonic acid		Ensulizole	Eusolex 232, Neo Heliopan Hydro
207574-74-1	Polysilicone-15			Parsol SLX
88122-99-0	Ethylhexyl triazone	Octyl triazone		Uvinul T150
154702-15-5	Diethylhexyl butamido triazone		Iscotrizinol	Uvasorb HEB
90457-82-2	Terephthalylidene dicamphor sulfonic acid		Ecamsule	Mexoryl SX
302776-68-7	Diethylamino hydroxybenzoyl hexyl benzoate			Uvinul A Plus
180898-37-7	Disodium Phenyl Dibenzimidazole Tetrasulfonate		Bisdisulizole disodium	Neo Heliopan AP
187393-00-6	Bis-Ethylhexyloxyphenol methoxyphenyl triazine		Bemotrizinol	Escalol S, Tinosorb S
103597-45-1	Methylene bis-benzotriazolyl tetramethylbutylphenol	MBBT	Bisoctrizole	Tinosorb M
155633-54-8	Drometrizole trisiloxane			Mexoryl XL, silatrizole

are regulated as over the counter (OTC) drugs. Nearly all such products are regulated under the Final Monograph for Sunscreen Drug products for over the counter (OTC) use, which was published on May 21, 1999, and can be accessed via the FDA Web site. The Time and Extent Application (TEA) is a regulatory process that may allow the inclusion of new agents, not yet included in the monograph, if sufficient data on long-term use from other countries exists (Holman and Shetty 2005; Murphy 2005; U.S. Food and Drug Administration 1999).

In order to keep up with consumer and industry demand for more UVA and broad-spectrum filters, new agents continue to be developed and it is likely that some of these may also cause photoallergy. Only by intermittently performing large multicenter photopatch studies which include existing and new filters will it be possible to reliably guide clinicians as to which agents should be included in test series. As above, all such data helps inform regulators and industry as to which agents to use at which concentration.

6.2 Topical NSAIDs

Nonsteroidal anti-inflammatory drugs (NSAIDs) are administered most commonly by systemic routes as analgesic and anti-inflammatory agents. However, over recent years there has been an increase in the number and usage of NSAIDs within topical preparations. These agents are usually made up as gels which are semisolid thickened aqueous solutions containing high molecular weight polymers. They dry after application, leaving a film of the active ingredient on the surface of the skin. Such preparations have the advantage of improving symptoms at the local site of application without any associated potential systemic adverse effects, a mechanism supported by some observations (Guy and Maibach 1983). However, because many NSAIDs are photohaptens, there have been consequent reports of PACD to such products (Ophaswongse and Maibach 1993). In some cases, NSAIDs are incorporated into adhesive dressings and the patient may not forward this information, possibly erroneously assuming the skin reaction to be due to some other constituent of the dressing.

As with organic sunscreen filters, NSAIDs seem to vary in their photoallergic potency (Diaz et al. 2006). Some molecules, notably ketoprofen and carprofen appear to be very potent, with exposure to even minute quantities capable of eliciting severe PACD (Hindsen et al. 2004; Kerr et al. 2008). When photopatch testing, cross-reactions between different members of the same class of NSAID are described. As one would expect, close chemical structural similarity appears to increase the likelihood of such reactions occurring. Within the arylpropionic acid derivatives, reactions are more common between ketoprofen and tiaprofenic acid than with either ibuprofen or naproxen (Le Coz et al. 1998). The benzophenone moiety of ketoprofen (and benzophenone-like ring in tiaprofenic acid) can also lead to cross-reactions with non-NSAID molecules, for example, benzophenone UV sunscreen filters and the lipid-lowering agent fenofibrate (Leroy et al. 1997; Le Coz et al. 1998; Hindsen et al. 2006) (➋ *Fig. 16.5*). Patients who develop photoallergy to ketoprofen may also cross react with and develop contact allergy to certain fragrance substances, notably the cinnamic derivatives (Girardin et al. 2006). As with sunscreens, anybody may potentially come into contact with topical NSAIDs through treating musculoskeletal injuries. However, an occupational history may reveal that an individual is an employee of a pharmaceutical company which is involved in the manufacture and packaging of NSAIDs. Alternatively, a careful social history may reveal the patient is a pet-owner who has been administering their pet the veterinary NSAID carprofen.

7 Photopatch Testing

Like patch testing, photopatch testing is based upon provocation of the eczematous reaction produced by an

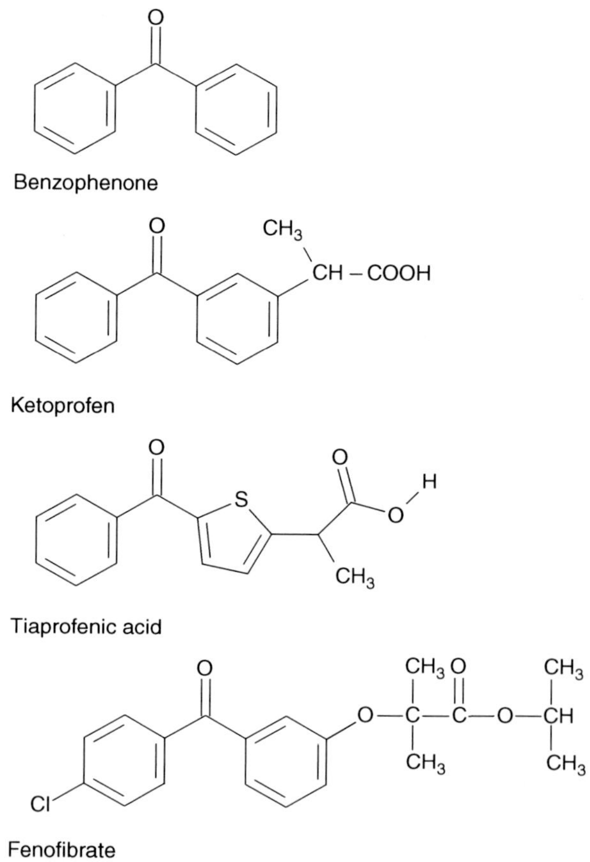

Fig. 16.5
Chemical structural similarity of benzophenone, ketoprofen, tiaprofenic acid, and fenofibrate

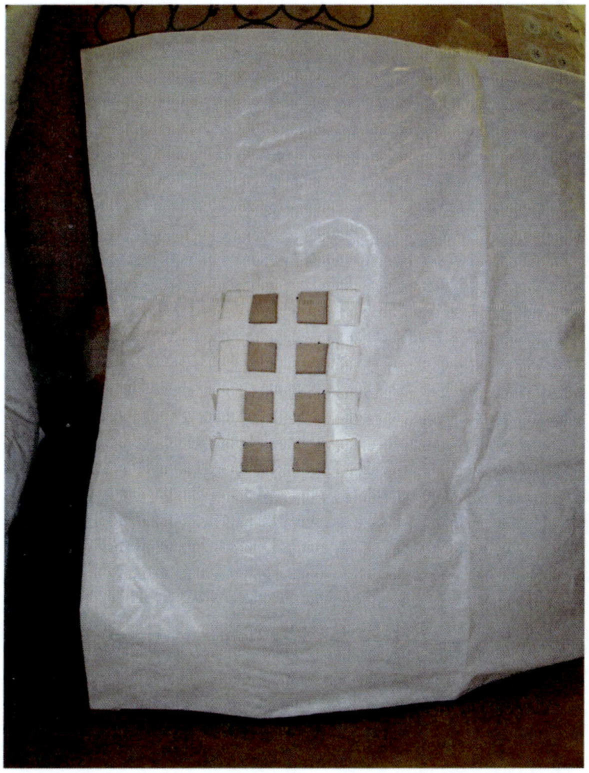

■ Fig. 16.6
The MED template is taped to the skin of the patient's back. It is composed of four layers of UV-opaque white polythene with eight square apertures of 15 mm^2 area, arranged in two columns of four at 10 mm intervals. Each aperture has its own door which can be closed and held shut with adhesive tape

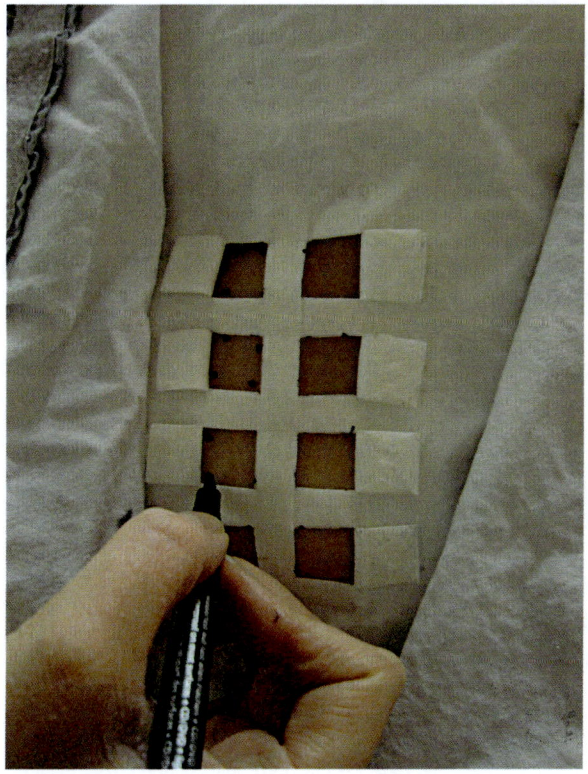

■ Fig. 16.7
Each corner of each aperture should be marked with a dot from a skin-safe marker to allow later identification of the MED test site

exogenous agent on the skin. However, it requires the additional step of irradiation of the skin with an external light source. The perceived added complexity of irradiation is one of the reasons that it is underused as an investigation by clinicians in comparison to patch testing. This has not been aided by historical discrepancies in methodology between different centers. However, a consensus methodology for Europe now exists and should allow easier comparison of results across different centers (Bruynzeel et al. 2004). Other factors that have contributed to the underuse of photopatch testing are the presence of obsolete agents in standard commercially available test series and an apparent lack of confidence in the use of the UVA irradiation source.

As with patch testing, the first step is to record a careful history to guide the selection of appropriate agents for testing. Most clinicians performing patch testing are familiar with the use of a "standard" set and further more specific sets of allergens to investigate different likely causative allergens (e.g., medicaments, oils, plants). Although such series may vary between centers and countries, they have generally been selected on the basis of experience and many years of discussion between experts. In contrast to this, the present situation is that no single multinational "standard" set of photopatch test allergens exists. One of the primary reasons for this is that the most widely used organic UV sunscreen filters change relatively frequently. This stems from the continual development of new agents by industry to keep pace with the demand for ever-better sunscreens. This means that such a "standard" series would become obsolete more quickly than many agents used in patch test series. For this reason there must continue to be intermittent large multicenter photopatch test studies which test these new agents and allow the informed updating of such series.

Despite such problems, many organic sunscreen filters and topical NSAIDs are available commercially through patch test agent suppliers for photopatch testing. As with patch testing, it is very important to consider photopatch

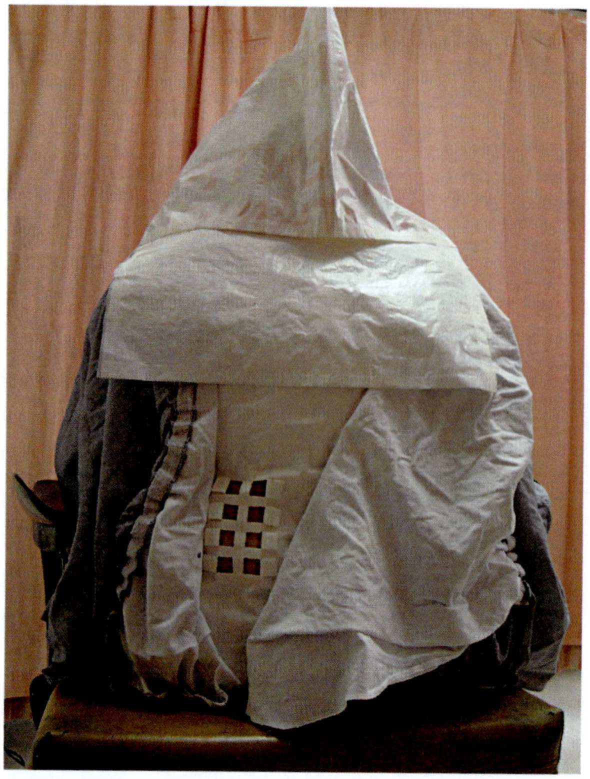

Fig. 16.8
The remainder of the patient is then covered with UV-opaque material

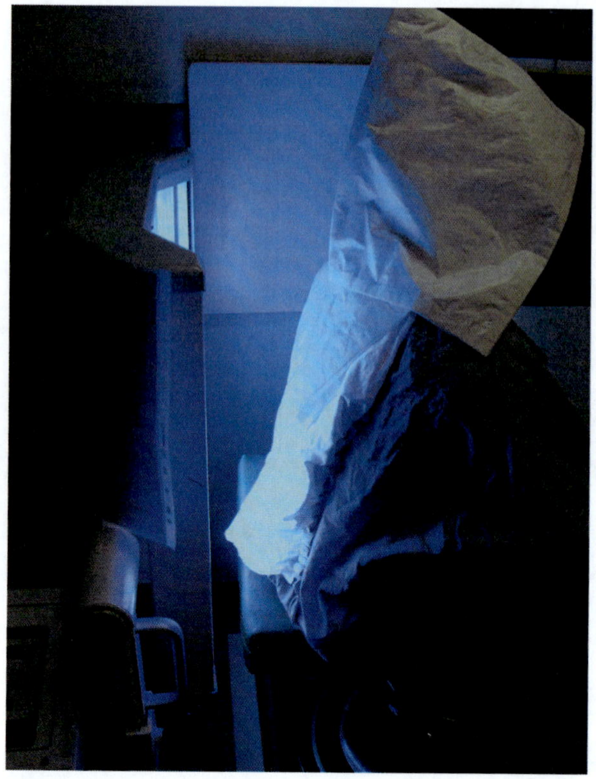

Fig. 16.9
The MED test site is then irradiated with the UVA source. This should be positioned parallel to the MED test site at a distance of 20 cm. During the period of irradiation, this distance should be episodically checked with a measuring rod, as the patient may move slightly

testing "as is" any of the patients' own agents that they have identified as a potential source of PACD, as long as safety data sheets are available and testing it would not be dangerous (i.e., irritant/corrosive/toxic). Reference to textbooks and scientific literature on such agents can aid choice of concentration and vehicles for such agents (de Groot 1994).

7.1 Irradiation Source

Historically, various types of light source have been used to irradiate photopatch tests. In the past, polychromatic sources (which contain UVB, UVA, and visible light) have been employed, as have UVB sources. However, these have largely fallen out of usage, as the doses of UVB required to elicit a delayed-type PACD reaction are often greater than that required to provoke a sunburn-like erythema, and so false positives can occur (Anonymous 1997). As a result, UVA sources are now the most widely employed when performing photopatch testing. Ideal characteristics of a UVA source include a continuous, broad, and stable emission with high irradiance over a uniform field. Fluorescent UVA lamps, such as those found in PUVA cabinets, are therefore suitable, although some metal halide or monochromators may also be suitable in some cases. The output of the source must be measured at regular intervals using a calibrated meter to ensure accurate doses are used. Once the UVA source has been decided upon, the first step of photopatch testing is to perform a UVA minimal erythemal dose (MED).

7.2 Performing a UVA MED

A UVA MED is usually performed on Day 0 (D0) on the skin of the back at a different area to the site of photopatch testing. It is performed in order to determine whether the patient has abnormal objective photosensitivity to the UVA source that is to be used for the subsequent irradiation of the photopatch test site. Possible causes

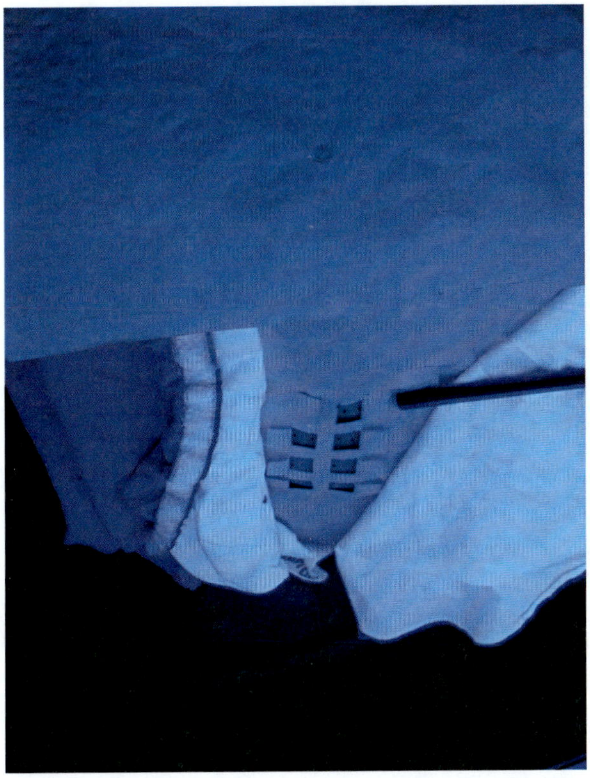

◘ Fig. 16.10
To deliver the eight doses required, each door is manually closed at the appropriate time. The person performing this should have their hand and arm protected by UV-opaque material and wear UV-protective eyewear. This view from above shows that the door of the first aperture has been closed using a handheld rod

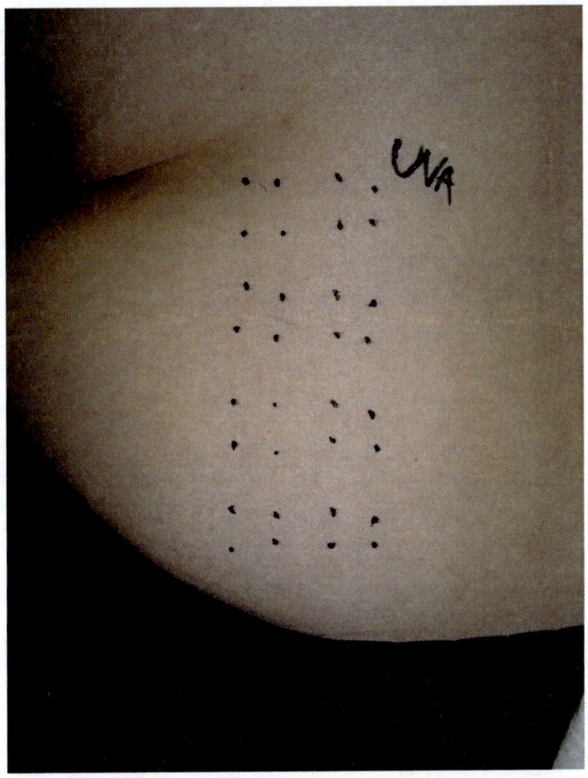

◘ Fig. 16.11
Twenty-four hours after irradiation, the UVA MED test site is visually inspected and the dose at which minimally perceptible erythema is seen is recorded as the MED. In this case no erythema is visible, indicating that the MED is greater than 4.7 Jcm^{-2} and a dose of 5 Jcm^{-2} can be used for irradiation of the photopatch test site

of such photosensitivity include systemic drug-induced phototoxicity, chronic actinic dermatitis, and cutaneous lupus. In conventional MED testing, eight incremental doses of UVA are used (e.g., 1.0, 1.5, 1.8, 2.2, 2.7, 3.3, 3.9, and 4.7 Jcm^{-2}). The doses from 1.8 Jcm^{-2} and above are approximately 20% increments from the previous dose. Such doses allow an even spread of values up to approximately 5 Jcm^{-2}.

A UVA MED can be performed using an automated device, or manually, where each incremental dose site is covered by hand sequentially with a "door" of UV-opaque material after the appropriate time corresponding to the dose of UVA has elapsed. The area of each dose of the MED test series (often a 15 × 15 mm^2) must be marked out on the skin to enable subsequent identification of any reactions after 24 h. In both cases, the remainder of the patients back, neck, and head must be covered with UV-opaque material to avoid unnecessary irradiation of these areas. The (previously warmed-up) UVA source is then positioned at a distance of 20 cm, parallel to the skin of the MED test site. The actual irradiation time for each dose will depend on the output of the UVA source used. After 24 h (D1), prior to irradiation of the photopatch test site, the MED test site is visually inspected and the dose at which minimally perceptible erythema can be discerned is recorded as the MED (➋ *Figs. 16.6–16.11*). If no erythema is seen at any dose, a dose of 5 Jcm^{-2} can be safely used to irradiate the photopatch test site. If erythema is seen, a dose of 50% of the MED has been suggested as a reasonable dose for irradiation of the photopatch tests, but even this may be too high (Anonymous 1997). If there is marked UVA sensitivity, it is advisable not to irradiate the photopatch tests with any UVA as a large area of confluent erythema at the photopatch test site may result.

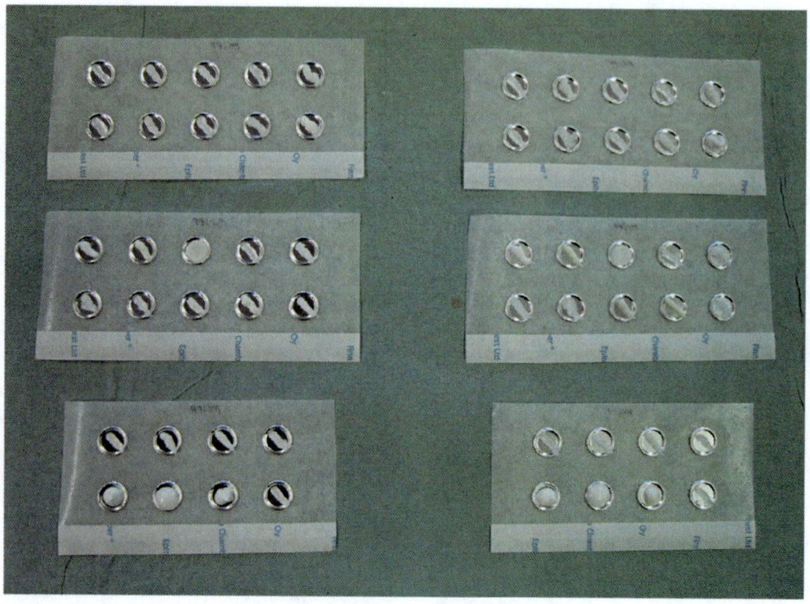

Fig. 16.12
The agents for photopatch testing are prepared in duplicate. One set to serve as a control and one set for irradiation

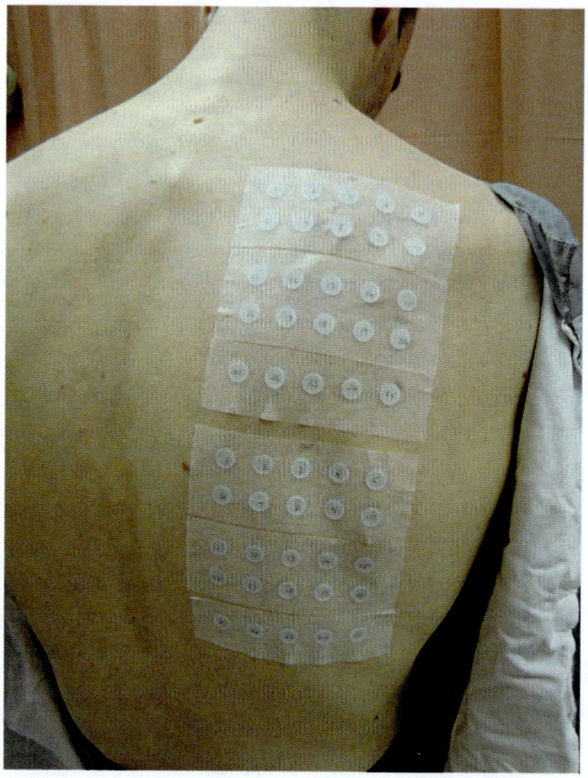

Fig. 16.13
The duplicate sets of agents are then applied on the skin of the back and left in place for 24 or 48 h

7.3 Photopatch Testing

Once the photopatch test agents have been selected for testing, two identical sets, one for irradiation and one as control, are prepared. They are applied under occlusion to the skin of the back as one would apply patch tests. The length of application of photopatch test agents is either 24 or 48 h. In many photobiology units, 24 h is used, but in many contact dermatitis units, 48 h is used. It may be that application for 48 h picks up more positive reactions (Batchelor and Wilkinson 2006), but clinicians should choose a duration of application that does not disrupt the provision of care and other investigations in their unit. After this time the agents are removed and the test site is visually inspected. Any reactions seen should be recorded using the International Contact Dermatitis Research Group (ICDRG) grading scale (Wahlberg 2001) and their relevance noted with a scale such as the COADEX system (Bourke et al. 2001).

The next step is to cover the control set of photopatch test agents with a UV-opaque material (such as a thick, flexible plastic-containing dressing sheet). As with UVA MED testing, all other areas of the back, neck, and head apart from the set of photopatch agents chosen for irradiation are then covered with a similar material, to reduce unnecessary exposure of the patient to UVA. As with UVA MED testing, the UVA source is then positioned parallel to the set of photopatches to be irradiated at a distance of

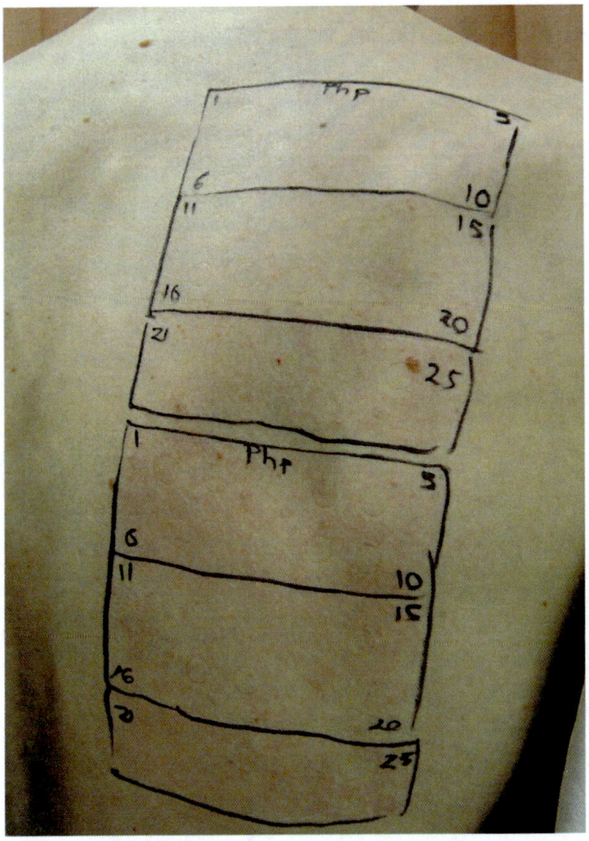

Fig. 16.14
Before removal, the area of patch application is marked with a skin-safe pen. The patches are then removed and the site visually inspected for any positive reactions

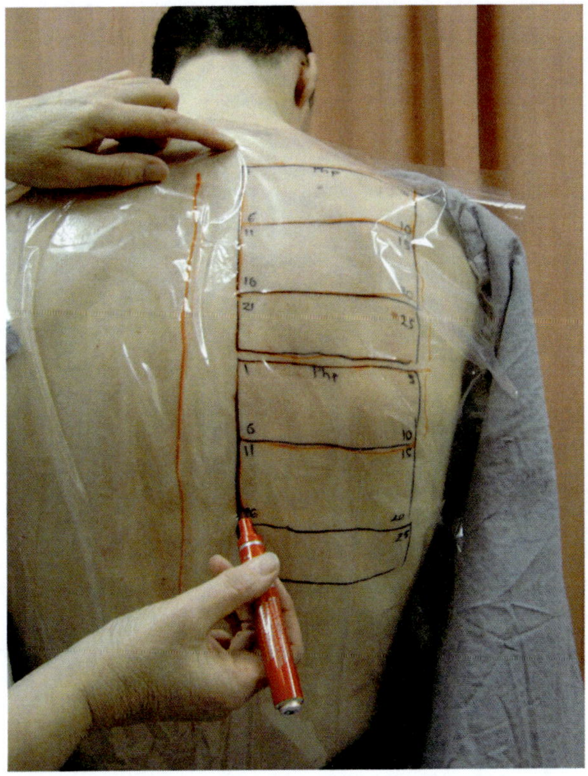

Fig. 16.15
A map of the photopatch application site is then made using a clear polythene sheet. Landmarks, including the spine and nevi are marked to aid future placement

20 cm and a dose of 5 Jcm^{-2} (or less if the UVA MED is reduced) is administered. Immediately following the removal of the UV-opaque material, the test site is again visually inspected and any reactions are graded and recorded. Readings of both sets of photopatch test agents are made at various time-points after irradiation, conventionally multiples of 24 h. The most important of these is 48 h, although 24, 72, 96, and 120 h readings can be performed depending on the logistics of the local unit and patient availability (*Fig. 16.12–16.18*).

7.4 Interpretation of Photopatch Test Results

As above, positive photopatch test results are graded and their intensity recorded, conventionally using the ICDRG scale. Because there are two identical sets of reagents, one irradiated and the other not, there are more potential combinations of reactions that need interpreted than in standard patch testing. The main four patterns of immunologically mediated reactions possible for a single agent are summarized below:

1. Photoallergic contact dermatitis – a positive reaction (of any ICDRG grade) is seen in the irradiated set only. The same site in the control set is negative.
2. Allergic contact dermatitis – a positive reaction (of any ICDRG grade) is seen in the irradiated set and a reaction of equal grade is seen at the same site in the control set.
3. Photoaugmentation of allergic contact dermatitis – a positive reaction is seen in the control set and a positive reaction which is at least one ICDRG grade higher is seen at the same site in the irradiated set. This pattern is uncommon.
4. Photoinhibition of allergic contact dermatitis – a positive reaction is seen in the control set and a positive reaction which is at least one ICDRG grade lower is seen at the same site in the irradiated set. This pattern is uncommon.

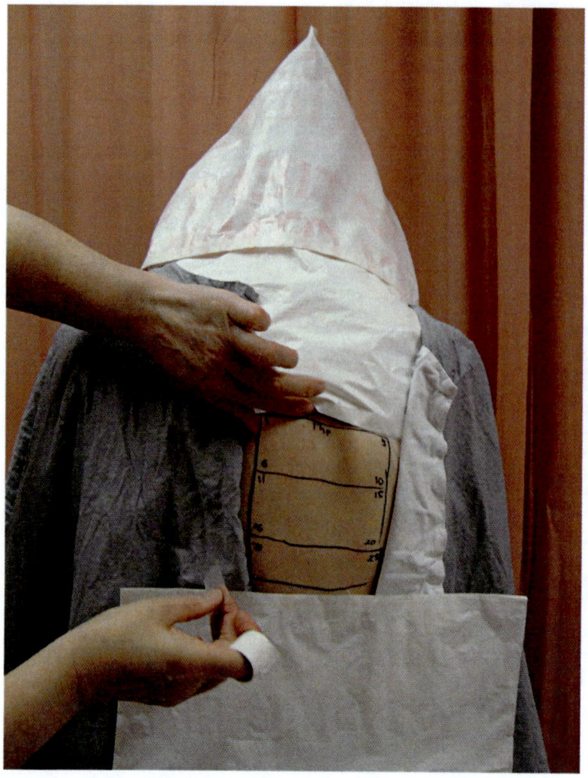

◘ Fig. 16.16
One set of photopatches is covered with UV-opaque material, leaving the other set exposed for irradiation

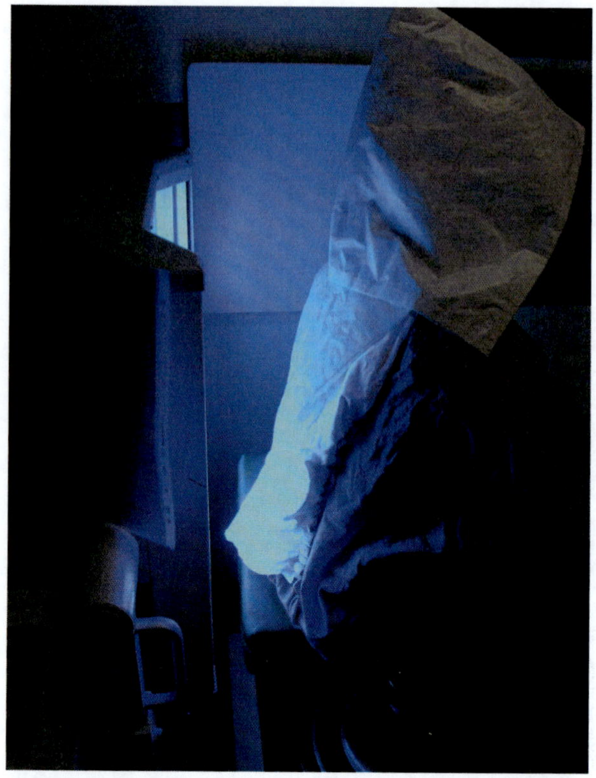

◘ Fig. 16.17
The set of exposed photopatch test agents is then irradiated using a dose of UVA determined by the UVA MED. As with UVA MED testing, the patient should be placed such that the irradiation site is 20 cm from the parallel UVA source

As in standard patch testing, irritant reactions can also occur, as well as non-immunological phototoxic reactions, which are classically flat, "decrescendo" reactions that do not extend out with the area of agent application.

8 Investigating Occupational PACD/ Factory Visits

As with cases of occupational contact dermatitis, cases of PACD can arise within the workplace environment. In such cases, it may be necessary to perform a factory visit, possibly in a legal/regulatory capacity. Such a visit is undertaken to ascertain objective evidence as to the possibility of one or more employees being exposed to potential photohaptens there. It is important to enter into open communication with the management of such a factory, often at an early stage as it may conceivably be months or even years before the actual visit goes ahead. Once communication is established, one should arrange a suitable time for the visit to take place. Ideally, this should be at a time when there is no restriction of access to any areas of the factory that may be relevant. Because ultraviolet and/or visible light may be involved in a PACD reaction, a portable spectroradiometer may be useful to measure the output of any sources in the factory. It may be advisable to take a colleague (e.g., a medical physicist) who is familiar with the correct method for operating such a device.

When in the factory, the exact nature of employee duties must be ascertained and recorded, if necessary by use of practical demonstration. In some cases, this should be with an employee present as well as management so that an accurate account can be corroborated by both sides. However, in certain cases, it may be necessary to get an account from the employee alone, as they may not feel able to disclose all accurate information in the presence of the employer, for fear of consequences for their job. By doing this, an idea can be obtained as to the instances during an employee's work practices when they

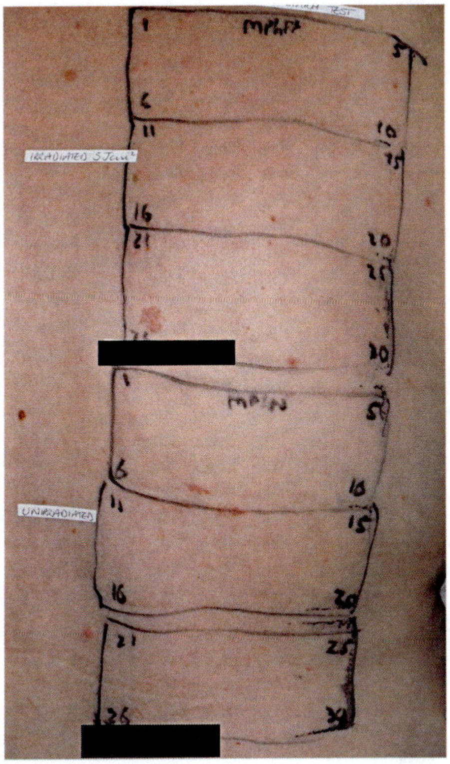

Fig. 16.18
At 24-h intervals after irradiation (i.e., 24, 48, 72 h) the photopatch test site is visually inspected and any positive reactions graded and recorded using the ICDRG scale. In this case, a positive result in the irradiated set only at position 26 has confirmed a diagnosis of PACD to a proprietary sunscreen preparation tested "as is"

may come into contact with potential photohaptens. A record should also be made of the number of employees over time that may have come into contact with potential photohaptens through a work practice. Note must be made of the protective equipment provided and level of usage by employees, the ventilation/extraction systems in operation, how many areas the potential photohapten is present in, and the potential for contamination of areas other than the main area of potential exposure. By performing a factory visit, it may be possible to confirm a diagnosis of occupational PACD, which may otherwise not have been made (Kerr et al. 2008).

Because of the additional possibility of UV and/or visible light contributing to the development of PACD, note must be made of such sources if any are present. For windows, this would include their position relative to employees, size, age, type, and number. Similar note must be made for artificial light sources, fluorescent, and others, along with and the presence or otherwise of protective diffusers. There may also be other less obvious sources, such as UV insect-killing devices. These observations must be made for the main work area but also for other areas, such as changing/washing areas. While potential photohaptens may be present in the main working area, perhaps as part of the main processes taking place within the factory, one should have a low threshold for suspecting other potential agents. To illustrate this, in the initial outbreak of salicylanilide PACD reported by Wilkinson in the 1960s, the factory was involved in metalworking but the source of the outbreak was a germicidal soap used by the workers (Wilkinson 1961).

As mentioned above it is preferable to test the employee (if safe to do so) with the potential photohapten "as is" and this may be supplied by the factory after written request. However, it is possible that an agent will not be released by the factory, and therefore the active part(s) of the potential photohapten may need to be ordered from chemical suppliers and photopatch testing performed using appropriate dilutions.

References

Anonymous (1997) Photopatch testing-methods and indications. British photodermatology group. Br J Dermatol 136:371–376

Batchelor RJ, Wilkinson SM (2006) Photopatch testing- a retrospective review using the 1 day and 2 day irradiation protocols. Contact Dermatitis 54:75–78

Bell HK, Rhodes LE (2000) Photopatch testing in photosensitive patients. Br J Dermatol 142:589–590

Bourke J, Coulson I et al (2001) British association of dermatologists. Guidelines for care of contact dermatitis. Br J Dermatol 145:877–885

Bruynzeel DP, Ferguson J et al (2004) Photopatch testing: a consensus methodology for Europe. J Eur Acad Dermatol Venereol 18:679–682

Bryden AM, Moseley H et al (2006) Photopatch testing of 1155 patients: results of the U.K. multicentre photopatch study group. Br J Dermatol 155:737–747

Darvay A, White IR et al (2001) Photoallergic contact dermatitis is uncommon. Br J Dermatol 145:597–601

de Groot AC (1994) Patch testing: test concentrations and vehicles for 3700 chemicals, 2nd edn. Elsevier, New York

Diaz RL, Gardeazabal J et al (2006) Greater allergenicity of topical ketoprofen in contact dermatitis confirmed by use. Contact Dermatitis 54:239–243

Epstein S (1939) Photoallergy and primary photosensitivity to sulfanilamide. J Invest Dermatol 2:43–51

Epstein S (1968) Chlorpromazine photosensitivity. Phototoxic and photoallergic reactions. Arch Dermatol 98:354–363

European Commission, Enterprise and Industry, Cosmetic Ingredients and Substances (2011) Annex VII, Part 1 – List of permitted UV filters which cosmetic products may contain. http://ec.europa.eu/enterprise/cosmetics/cosing/index.cfm?fuseaction=search.results&annex=VII&search. Accessed 18 Jan 2010

Girardin P, Vigan M et al (2006) Cross-reactions in patch testing with ketoprofen, fragrance mix and cinnamic derivatives. Contact Dermatitis 55:126–128

Guy RH, Maibach HI (1983) Drug delivery to local subcutaneous structures following topical administration. J Pharm Sci 72: 1375–1380

Hindsen M, Isaksson M et al (2004) Photoallergic contact dermatitis from ketoprofen induced by drug-contaminated personal objects. J Am Acad Dermatol 50:215–219

Hindsen M, Zimerson E et al (2006) Photoallergic contact dermatitis from ketoprofen in southern Sweden. Contact Dermatitis 54:150–157

Holman M, Shetty D (2005) The role of FDA in sunscreen regulation. In: Shaath NA (ed) Sunscreens. Regulations and commercial development, vol 28, 3rd edn, Cosmetic and technology series. Taylor & Francis, London

Kerr AC, Muller F et al (2008) Occupational carprofen photoallergic contact dermatitis. Br J Dermatol 159:1303–1308

Kerr AC, Niklasson B et al (2009) A double-blind, randomized assessment of the irritant potential of sunscreen chemical dilutions used in photopatch testing. Contact Dermatitis 60:203–209

Le Coz CJ, Bottlaender A et al (1998) Photocontact dermatitis from ketoprofen and tiaprofenic acid: cross-reactivity study in 12 consecutive patients. Contact Dermatitis 38:245–252

Leroy D, Dompmartin A et al (1997) Photodermatitis from ketoprofen with cross-reactivity to fenofibrate and benzophenones. Photodermatol Photoimmunol Photomed 13:93–97

Mascotto RE (2005) Regulatory aspects of sunscreens in Europe. In: Shaath NA (ed) Sunscreens. Regulations and commercial development, vol 28, 3rd edn, Cosmetic and technology series. Taylor & Francis, London

Murphy EG (2005) The final monograph. In: Shaath NA (ed) Sunscreens. Regulations and commercial development, vol 28, 3rd edn, Cosmetic and technology series. Taylor & Francis, London

Ophaswongse S, Maibach H (1993) Topical nonsteroidal antiinflammatory drugs: allergic and photoallergic contact dermatitis and phototoxicity. Contact Dermatitis 29:57–64

Raugi GJ, Storrs FJ et al (1979) Photoallergic contact dermatitis to men's perfumes. Contact Dermatitis 5:251–260

Schauder S, Ippen H (1997) Contact and photocontact sensitivity to sunscreens. Review of a 15-year experience and of the literature. Contact Dermatitis 37:221–232

Schauder S, Schroder W et al (1996) Olaquindox-induced airborne photoallergic contact dermatitis followed by transient or persistent light reactions in 15 pig breeders. Contact Dermatitis 35:344–354

Scott KW, Dawson TA (1974) Photo-contact dermatitis arising from the presence of quindoxin in animal feeding stuffs. Br J Dermatol 90:543–546

U.S. Food and Drug Administration (1999) Rulemaking history for OTC sunscreen drug products. http://www.fda.gov/Drugs/DevelopmentApprovalProcess/DevelopmentResources/Over-the-CounterOTCDrugs/StatusofOTCRulemakings/ucm072134.htm. Accessed 18 Jan 2010

Wahlberg JE (2001) Patchtesting. In: Rycroft R, Menne T, Frosch P, Lepoittevin J-P (eds) Textbook of contact dermatitis, 3rd edn. Springer, Berlin

Wilkinson DS (1961) Photodermatitis due to tetrachlorsalicylanilide. Br J Dermatol 73:213–219

17 Airborne Contact Dermatitis

Jean-Marie Lachapelle
Unit of Occupational and Environmental Dermatology, Catholic University of Louvain, Montigny-le-Tilleul, Belgium

Core Messages

- Occupational airborne irritant (frictional and/or chemical) contact dermatitis is due to fibers, dust particles, vapors, and/or gasses.
- Occupational airborne allergic contact dermatitis is a common problem, provoked by a large variety of allergens.
- Occupational airborne phototoxic and/or photoallergic contact dermatitis is a rare, but well documented event.
- Occupational airborne immunological contact urticaria can be caused by several chemicals and/or proteins. Allergy to latex proteins is the main problem.
- "Extrinsic" atopic dermatitis (face and neck dermatitis) is related to the penetration into the skin of aeroallergens, particularly dust mite.
- There is a vast range of procedures available to reach a proper etiological diagnosis of airborne contact dermatitis.
- Prevention and treatment of airborne contact dermatitis deserve special attention, and must be adapted to each individual situation.

1 Introduction

Most patients consulting in occupational dermatology are referred to as contact dermatitis cases; conceptually, the term "contact dermatitis" implies a direct contact of the skin with the offending (liquid and/or solid) agents. It is not surprising that in this respect, hand dermatitis is the major complaint; this is due to a direct manipulation – at work – of thousands of different products. It is clear that other skin sites can also be affected, either directly or indirectly (transfer of chemicals by hands; so-called by proxy contact dermatitis).

Apart from this "familiar landscape" the occurrence of occupational airborne dermatoses, that is, due to agents carried by or through the air, has been underestimated in the past. Pirilä (1950) was the first to promote the concept of airborne dermatoses on clinical and experimental grounds. In his extensive paper, the author called attention – almost exclusively – to allergic conditions, referring for instance to the cases of thiokol dermatitis he had observed in Finland after World War II. Later on, examples of occupational dermatoses closely related to airborne skin offenders were occasionally reported throughout the relevant literature (Pirilä et al. 1963).

In the 1980s, more attention was paid to the problem, after the publication of two review articles (Lachapelle 1986; Dooms-Goossens et al. 1986). In 2007, Santos and Goossens have updated in a review paper (2001–2006) a list of offending agents able to provoke airborne contact dermatitis. They consider that the figures are underestimated for two main reasons : (a) many original cases are never published and (b) in some papers, the term "airborne" does not appear in the key words and the publications are therefore omitted in general reviews.

Nowadays, each year brings a blossom of new observations, coming from various parts of the world. These publications reflect the diversity of problems encountered, in relation with new chemicals and/or modified technical procedures. A better knowledge of occupational airborne dermatoses has practical implications, in terms of diagnosis, treatment, and prevention. There is a clear distinction to be made between airborne dermatoses and the "sick building syndrome"; the latter refers to epidemics of subjective symptoms (itching or burning sensations) without any clinically visible signs, which occur in the work environment. This situation can be related for instance to a low relative humidity rate in the air, but may also represent a mass psychogenic illness.

Two papers are of particular interest for initiating a differential diagnosis between both conditions. One is referring to the skin disorders among construction workers following Hurricane Katrina and Hurricane Rita (Noe et al. 2007); the other deals with airborne occupational dermatoses experienced by aircrew (Legatt and Smith 2006).

2 Airborne Offending Agents

Airborne offending agents are present under various forms:

Fibers

Different types of fibers can be implied (Stam-Westerveld et al. 1994). The most classical example is fiberglass. Other examples include rockwool, carbon

T. Rustemeyer, P. Elsner, S.M. John & H.I. Maibach (eds.), *Kanerva's Occupational Dermatology*,
DOI 10.1007/978-3-642-02035-3_17,

fibers, plastic materials such as polypropylene fibers, etc. Fibers can be chemically inert, and provoke only mechanical trauma to the skin. Carbon fibers' dermatitis and most cases of fiberglass dermatitis are good examples of this condition. On the other hand, some fibers can produce allergic reactions, such as epoxy-coated fiberglass.

Dust particles

Dust is ubiquitous in the work environment. Dust particles are transported by air; they can accumulate on the surface of the skin, in a visible way or not. Like fibers, some dust particles are chemically inert but can provoke mechanical (frictional) injury to the skin, whereas others do contain chemicals which are dissolved by the sweat; according to their nature, these chemicals are responsible for several types of skin reactions (Lachapelle 1987).

Sprays

Water or other liquid-based products moving in a mass of dispersed droplets represent an important source of airborne offending agents. Any of numerous commercial products, including paints, cosmetics, and insecticides that are dispensed from containers in this manner, are good examples. Skin reactions are multifaceted: irritant, eczematous, urticarial, or combined.

Vapors and gasses

Vapor is defined as barely visible or cloudy diffused matter, such as mist, fumes, or smoke, suspended in the air. Gas has a more restricted meaning. Vapors and gasses may be like sprays, irritant, allergenic, or both.

3 Classification of Occupational Airborne Skin Diseases

Two categories of occupational airborne skin diseases have to be considered.

(a) "Systemic" occupational airborne skin diseases

Some skin conditions are as a result of the toxic effects of chemicals that have been absorbed by the body tissues either by inhalation or by transdermal penetration. We have coined the term "systemic" occupational airborne skin disease, by analogy with the term "systemic contact dermatitis" (Lachapelle 2009).

The most classical example is chloracne that, although rare, may serve as an extremely important indicator of internal poisoning and should be recognized by physicians treating occupational skin disease. Cloracneigenic substances such as polyhalogenated naphthalenes are well known (Coenraads et al. 1994); tetrachloro-2,3,7,8 dibenzo-p-dioxine was the agent incriminated in the Seveso catastrophe, which occurred in Northern Italy in 1976.

Another example of "systemic" occupational airborne skin disease is lepidopterism, a syndrome including all symptoms due to airborne contact with the barbed hairs of pine tree processionary caterpillars, that is, pruritic rash, conjunctival hyperemia, dyspnea, wheezing, and more exceptionally anaphylaxis. Foresters and agricultural workers are at risk. More generally, it is a growing public health problem: There is an increasing number of outbreaks. Children are also affected, and often more severely than adults (Gottschling et al. 2007; Shkalim et al. 2008).

(b) Occupational airborne contact dermatoses

This group refers to all skin symptoms directly related to airborne contact of the skin with the accountable agents. In fact, all varieties of contact dermatoses due to direct contactants can also be provoked by airborne contactants. Furthermore, in many cases, direct contact and airborne contact can occur simultaneously; contact urticaria to latex proteins (Lagier et al. 1990) or allergic contact dermatitis to epoxy resins (Le Coz et al. 1999) represent two good examples of such situations.

A classification of occupational airborne contact dermatoses has been proposed in *Table 17.1*. Although no specific criteria do exist to assess an airborne origin, some morphological and/or topographical aspects can help in the diagnostic procedure, as explained in the next paragraphs.

Table 17.1

Classification of occupational airborne contact dermatoses

1. Occupational airborne irritant (frictional and/or chemical) contact dermatitis
2. Occupational airborne allergic contact dermatitis
3. Occupational airborne phototoxic contact dermatitis
4. Occupational airborne photoallergic contact dermatitis
5. Occupational airborne (immunological and/or nonimmunological) contact urticaria
6. Exacerbation of "extrinsic" atopic dermatitis by aeroallergens

4 Occupational Airborne Irritant (Frictional and/or Chemical) Contact Dermatitis

4.1 Airborne Irritant Contact Dermatitis Due to Fibers

Subjective symptoms are always present. Itching, stinging, and burning sensations are the usual complaints of many patients, with or without objective signs. In particular, facial complaints are not often accompanied by detectable lesions; they correspond to the so-called subjective irritant dermatitis. The eyelids, cheeks, nasal folds, and neck are commonly involved.

Subjective symptoms may occur not only on covered parts of the body, mainly in the flexures (axillae, groins, cubital, and/or popliteal fossae), but also on the extensor aspects of the limbs or on the trunk.

Objective symptoms are usually present, but vary in severity from case to case. Scratch marks, tiny papules, or a maculopapular rash are the usual lesions (➋ *Fig. 17.1*). Severe cases could involve secondary infection (pustules) from scratching. The most typical example quoted in the literature is fiberglass dermatitis. Symptoms include itching and prickling in the skin areas coming into contact with fiberglass spicules present in the work environment. Scratch marks, papules, and pustules are sometimes present (Fisher 1982; Koh et al. 1992). To some extent, it may resemble scabies.

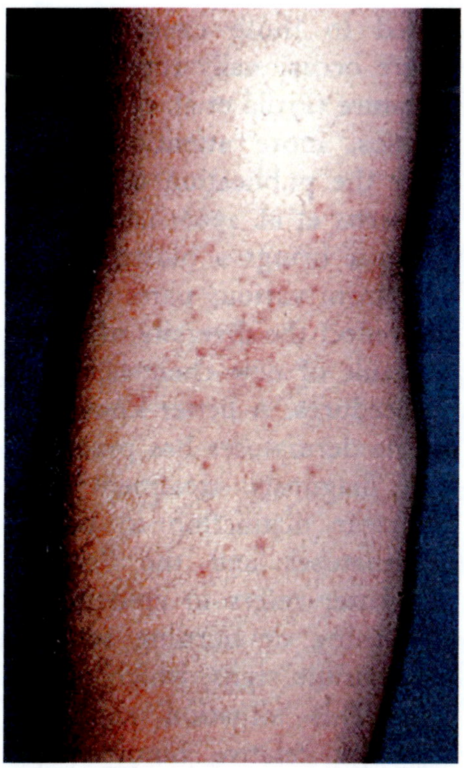

◘ Fig. 17.1
Fiberglass dermatitis: tiny papules and scratch marks

The presence of fibers encrusted in the horny layer of epidermis is clearly shown by the skin surface biopsy technique (Marks and Dawber 1971). The method consists of the following very simple steps: (a) a drop of cyanoacrylate glue is placed on the skin; (b) a clear glass slide is gently pressed on the drop for 30 s; (c) the slide is then removed. A slight modification consists of using polyester tape instead of glass as holder (Lachapelle et al. 1977). Foreign material present at the surface of the skin or encrusted in horny cells is removed with the adhesive which remains attached to the glass slide or the plastic sheet; it can be visualized under the microscope.

Fiberglass dermatitis is still a very important problem in occupational dermatology, as mentioned in recent papers (Cusano and Mariano 2007; Bordel-Gomez and Miranda-Romero 2008). A very interesting contribution has been made about the size and configuration of glass fibers by scanning electron microscopy (Hsieh et al. 2001).

Other examples of fibers' dermatitis include glasswool, rockwool, carbon fibers, ceramic fibers, polypropylene fibers, urea-formaldehyde insulating foam, etc. In all cases, the symptoms are similar to those observed in fiberglass dermatitis, but are usually milder. It is obvious that clinical manifestations are due to a mechanical effect, either frictional or consecutive to encrustment of fibers into the skin. The diameter of fibers seems crucial to explain the severity of skin symptoms (Lachapelle 1986; Stam-Westerveld 1997).

In our experience, the diameter of most fibers incriminated in airborne contact dermatitis was comprised between 6 mμ and 20 mμ. Atopics are undoubtedly more prone to develop severe symptoms than nonatopics (Björnberg et al. 1979). This can be clearly demonstrated when epidemics of fiberglass dermatitis do occur in factories. Björnberg was a visionary at that time; his work has been underestimated, but, nowadays, new developments in the comprehension of atopic dermatitis confirm his studies, based upon epidemiological investigations.

More recently, an outbreak of eight cases of occupational airborne irritant contact dermatitis has been reported in intensive care unit employees caused by synthetic (polypropylene and polyethylene) fibers from an air-conditioning filter (Patiwael et al. 2005). High filter pressure in the intensive care air-conditioning system, maintained to establish an outward airflow and prevent microorganisms from entering the ward, probably caused fibers from the filter to become airborne. Most patients recovered quickly after treatment with emollients and changing the filters.

And, finally, what about asbestos fibers? When asbestos was used extensively as an insulation procedure, very little was said about the potential irritant properties of asbestos. This is probably due to several factors: (a) asbestos is a mixture of dust and fibers; (b) most fibers have a diameter <1 mm; and (c) asbestos fibers can split longitudinally, which reduces even more the mean diameter of fibers.

An extensive program of removal of asbestos fibers is conducted in most industrialized countries, with their replacement by manmade vitreous fibers, such as glass or ceramic fibers. It occurs nowadays that some workers who remove asbestos fibers do complain of itching and prickling sensations, but this is certainly partly related to psychological factors, in relation with the propaganda fueled by the media on the toxicological properties of asbestos (Lachapelle 2006).

4.2 Airborne Irritant Contact Dermatitis Due to Dust Particles

Two different situations have to be taken into consideration:

(a) The dust particles are "chemically inert." Skin symptoms are related to the mechanical (frictional) properties of particles. It is not clear whether the shape of the particles (e.g., particles with sharp edges) plays an important role or not (➋ *Fig. 17.2*). Many other concomitant factors are most probably important, such as ambient heat, low humidity, sweating, and/or atopic state. The clinical symptoms are quite similar to those observed with fibers. Facial complaints are usually prominent: the eyelids, cheeks, nasal folds, retroauricular folds, and neck are commonly involved. Workers wearing ill-fitted masks sometimes complain of itching of the face, due to the accumulation of dust under the mask, particularly in the nasal folds. Subjective and objective complaints can also occur on covered parts of the body, due to the accumulation of dust particles under the garments. Indeed, solid particles can pass easily under protective clothes, most often between sleeves and gloves; dust particles can also accumulate on the skin of the feet even when workers wear safety shoes.

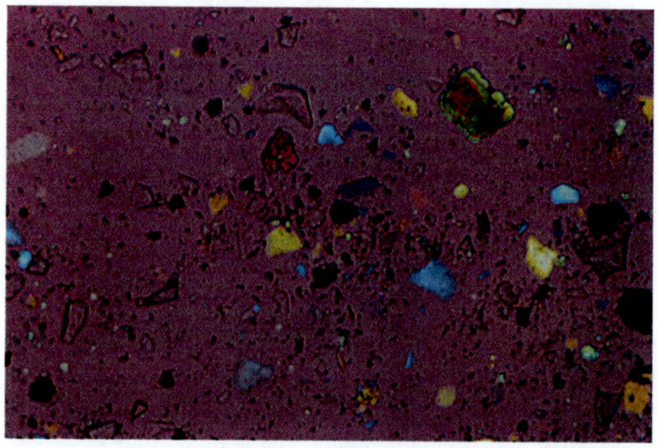

Fig. 17.2
Dust particles with sharp edges (Polarized light; x100)

(b) The dust particles are not chemically inert. They release irritant substances (acidic, alkaline, or neutral) that are responsible for true irritant (i.e., chemically-induced) contact dermatitis. When dust material is suspended in distilled water, the pH of the supernatant can be very alkaline, as mentioned in some reports (Lachapelle et al. 1984): anhydrite (pH: 11.2); sewage sludge (pH: 11); trona (pH: 10.5). Dried industrial dyes show a wide range of pH. In these various situations, clinical symptoms are unequivocally typical of irritant contact dermatitis. Eyelids are preferentially involved, due not only to the accumulation of particles, but also to the increased penetration of chemicals into the skin.

Periorbital dermatitis is a common problem encountered in occupational dermatology. Differential diagnosis of this entity is often difficult. Airborne irritant contact dermatitis to dust particles has to be taken into consideration as a potential etiological factor (Feser and Mahler 2009).

4.3 Airborne Irritant Contact Dermatitis due to Sprays, Vapors, and Gasses

On the contrary of fibers' and/or dust particles' dermatitis, that may affect covered as well as uncovered parts of the body, occupational airborne irritant contact dermatitis related to sprays, vapors, and/or gasses is almost exclusively limited to uncovered parts.

Face and neck are primarily involved: Clinical symptoms are typical of irritant contact dermatitis. Itching, stinging, and burning sensations are the usual complaints

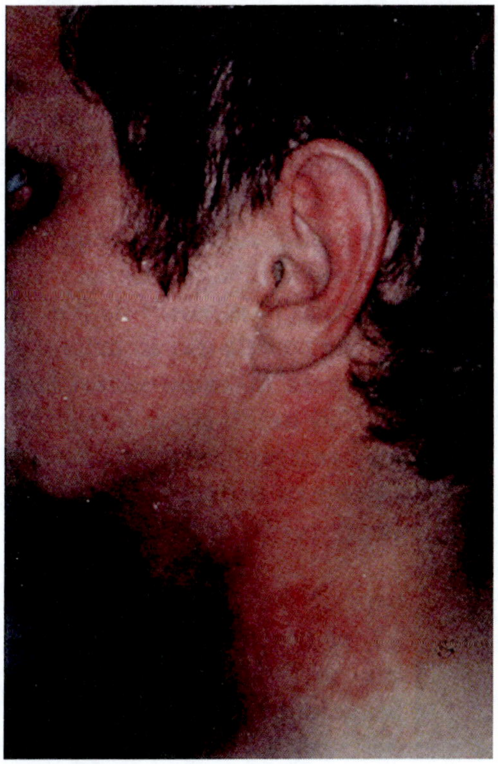

Fig. 17.3
Perchlorethylene fume irritant dermatitis after cleaning an unventilated tank. Extensive erythematous pruritic plaques on the lateral aspect of the neck

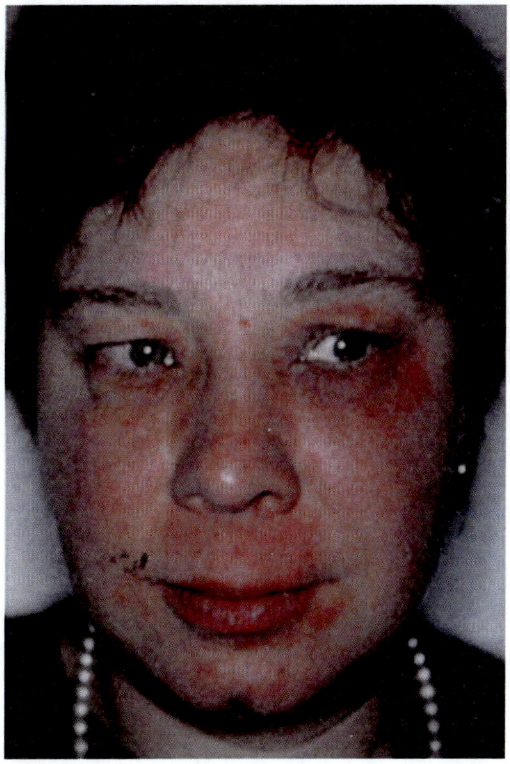

Fig. 17.4
Airborne allergic contact dermatitis to propacetamol (Pro-Dafalgan®) in a female nurse prior to injection into the infusion set. Erythematous intensely pruritic lesions of the face, with marked malar edema

that precede the occurrence of a maculopapular rash (*Fig. 17.3*). The lesions may be limited to the eyelids (periorbital dermatitis) or extend to the whole face and neck, sparing some partly protected areas, such as retroauricular folds or the margins of the scalp. Organic solvents, ammonia, and formaldehyde are often quoted as classical offending agents, but many others can be listed, such as acids and alkalis, domestic products (e.g., cleansing products), industrial solvents, carbonless copy paper, or phenol vapors (Dooms-Goossens et al. 1986).

5 Occupational Airborne Allergic Contact Dermatitis

Occupational airborne allergic contact dermatitis seems to be very frequent according to the recent literature.

Airborne "contact" allergens can be volatile (vapors and/or gasses), or transported under the form of sprays (mini-droplets), or present in dust particles: All physical forms are common in the work environment.

5.1 Clinical Symptoms

Clinical symptoms are typical of allergic contact dermatitis. There is no specific sign in relation with airborne contact. Eczematous lesions are symmetrical in most cases (*Fig. 17.4*); they are acute or chronic, depending on the environmental conditions: nature and/or concentration of the allergens, frequency of airborne contact, and so on. For instance, dermatitis from wood dust normally starts on the eyelids (*Fig. 17.5*) or the lower half of the face, often preceded by a period of itching. Swelling and redness spread to the neck, hands, and forearms. By the time the patient goes for treatment, a diffuse dermatitis might have developed, distinctly limited at the margins of the sleeves and collar. Because of the accumulation of dust and sweat, the elbow flexures and the skin under a tight collar are often lichenified. As already emphasized, airborne allergic contact dermatitis has no specific clinical features. Therefore, there is no magic clue that leads to an

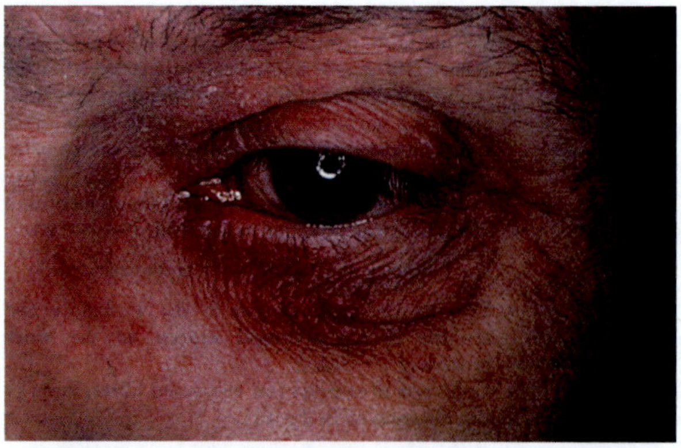

■ **Fig. 17.5**
Airborne allergic contact dermatitis to meranti (exotic wood) dust particles. Extensive eczematous lesions of the eyelids

unequivocal diagnosis. Anamnestic data, analysis of symptoms, and patch test results are needed to reach a correct conclusion.

In a recent observation, occupational conjunctivitis was the sole manifestation of airborne contact allergy to trimethylolpropane triacrylate (Mancuso and Berdondini 2008).

5.2 Differential Diagnosis

Differential diagnosis of facial airborne allergic contact dermatitis includes the following:

(a) "True" (or direct) contact allergic contact dermatitis. Asymmetry of facial lesions is a clinical sign in favor of "true" (or direct) allergic contact; this assertion has to be moderate, due to the fact that some airborne allergens can be sprayed on the face in an asymmetrical way at the workplace.
(b) Flare-up of the so-called id type, including eventually systemic contact dermatitis.
(c) Atopic dermatitis limited to the face. The distinction between both conditions is difficult to assess in many cases. The complexity of the problem has increased in recent years due to the current knowledge that facial signs of atopic dermatitis could be triggered, worsened, or even provoked by various allergens of high molecular weight (mainly proteins) present in house dust, pollens, molds, etc. This important current issue is discussed in detail in ➋ Sect. 8: Exacerbation of "Extrinsic" Atopic Dermatitis by Aero-allergens.
(d) Photoallergic contact dermatitis, bearing in mind that some photoallergic reactions can be airborne related.

■ **Table 17.2**
Selected allergens responsible for occupational airborne allergic contact dermatitis

Allergen
Animal feeds
Bryozoans: Dogger Bank itch
Budesonide
Chromate, i.e., from cement dust, or from welding fumes
Cinnamon
Cobalt, i.e., from cement dust
Colophony (in woodcutting and soldering)
Drugs (and/or chemicals used in the synthesis of drugs in the pharmaceutical industry)
Epoxy resin when heated, epoxy hardeners and epoxy reaction diluents
Formaldehyde
Isothiazolinones
Parthenium
Pesticides
Plastics such as acrylates, phenolformaldehyde resins, etc.
Sesquiterpene lactones, such as in Compositae or Frullania
Woods (wood dust from exotic or indigenous woods)

In contrast to allergic airborne contact dermatitis, some parts of the face are partly or completely spared in non-airborne photoallergic reactions: eyelids, submental region, retroauricular folds. In most cases, lesions of allergic airborne contact dermatitis are symmetrical.
(e) Seborrhoeic dermatitis, sometimes worsened by work conditions: irritant fumes or dusts, high temperature involving increased sweating, and so on.
(f) "Sebopsoriasis" is not uncommon and has also to be taken into account in the differential diagnosis. It can be triggered by work conditions, including contact with irritant fumes and dusts. Abundant sweating due to a high-temperature environment is a major cause of worsening of skin symptoms.

5.3 Main Allergens

The list of allergens responsible for occupational and/or environmental airborne allergic contact dermatitis is countless, as emphasized in the general review by Santos and Goossens 2007.

Referring to that review and to more recent reports, the most important groups of allergens are listed in ➋ *Table 17.2.*

Some problems of current interest deserve special attention:

- Occupational airborne allergic contact dermatitis to budesonide, even at very low concentrations, affecting nurses working in the hospital (Pontén 2006; Corazza et al. 2008; Baeck and Goossens 2009).
- Plastic resin systems have an increasing diverse array of applications, which induce health hazards, in particular occupational airborne allergic contact dermatitis. These resin systems include epoxies, (meth)acrylics, polyurethanes, phenol-formaldehydes, polyesters, amino resins (melamine-formaldehydes, urea-formaldehydes, etc.). Some papers summarize the risks encountered (Cao et al. 2009; Geraut et al. 2009).
- Parthenium dermatitis (*Parthenium hysterophorus*; parthenium weed) is a very common problem of occupational airborne allergic contact dermatitis in India, and was extensively studied in recent years. Dermatitis occurs in farmers, with exacerbations during summer. It is sometimes photoaggravated and rare cases of chronic actinic dermatitis have been recorded. Patch tests to Parthenium are positive (Sharma and Sethuraman 2007; Agarwal and D'Souza 2009).

6 Occupational Airborne Phototoxic and Photoallergic Contact Dermatitis

Phototoxic and/or photoallergic chemicals can be airborne. Practically, there is no clinical sign that allows a clear-cut distinction between direct contact and airborne contact.

Both produce a similar type of eruption. On theoretical grounds, phototoxic reactions are more sharply demarcated, whereas photoallergic reactions display ill-defined margins, but there are many exceptions to the general rule. On the other hand, it can be claimed that in non-airborne phototoxic or photoallergic reactions, some parts of the face are relatively or completely spared whereas in airborne ones, no part is spared. Once again, the rule has many exceptions. Diagnosis is therefore based on carefully completed anamnestic data, analysis of symptoms and signs, and patch test and photopatch test results (Lachapelle et al. 1992).

Occupational airborne phototoxic agents are rarely involved: coal tar and derivates, for example, anthracene, acridine, phenanthrene, pyrene; dyes; and furocoumarins are quoted in most textbooks. Photoallergenic molecules include fragrance ingredients (in the cosmetic industry), coal tar derivates, olaquindox, and several drugs (in the pharmaceutical industry).

Combined airborne and photoaggravated contact allergy, as seen with Compositae and lichens, presents difficulties in diagnosis (Thune 1977).

Parthenium dermatitis (mentioned above) is a good example of such difficult problems.

7 Occupational Airborne (Immunological and/or Nonimmunological) Contact Urticaria

Occupational airborne contact urticaria has been underestimated in the past. In most cases, it is the clinical expression of an immunological reaction, of the immediate type, mediated by IgE. Allergy to natural rubber latex has now become a major health-care issue. Direct contact urticaria due to latex gloves affects both hands, but natural rubber latex proteins are absorbed onto the maize starch powder of gloves; these are released into the air when the packets are opened or gloves are pulled out of multipack boxes. The particles contaminate the air, and in operating theaters with recirculated air systems, the allergens can be spread to the whole theater suite and cause different clinical problems: urticarial plaques on the face (➋ *Fig. 17.6*), conjunctivitis, rhinitis, and even asthma (Handfield-Jones 1998). The problem is more or less under control nowadays, due to the conjunction of three preventive measures: (a) the use of non-powdered latex gloves; (b) the improvement in the quality of latex gloves, in terms of allergenicity (removal of immunogenic proteins); and (c) the increasing use of non-latex surgical gloves (Kean and Mc Nally 2009). Other offending agents responsible for occupational airborne immunological contact urticaria are cosmetics, fruit, vegetables, animals' hair, ammonium persulfate, or anhydrides.

Nonimmunological airborne urticarial reactions are less frequent in occupational life.

8 Exacerbation of "Extrinsic" Atopic Dermatitis by Aeroallergens

It is convincingly proven that patients suffering from atopic dermatitis of exposed sites (the so-called face and neck dermatitis) are worsened by airborne contact with aeroallergens, especially house dust mite (Samochocki 2007). A recent study (Hallai and Gawkrodger 2009) has shown that 77% of patients presented with a positive

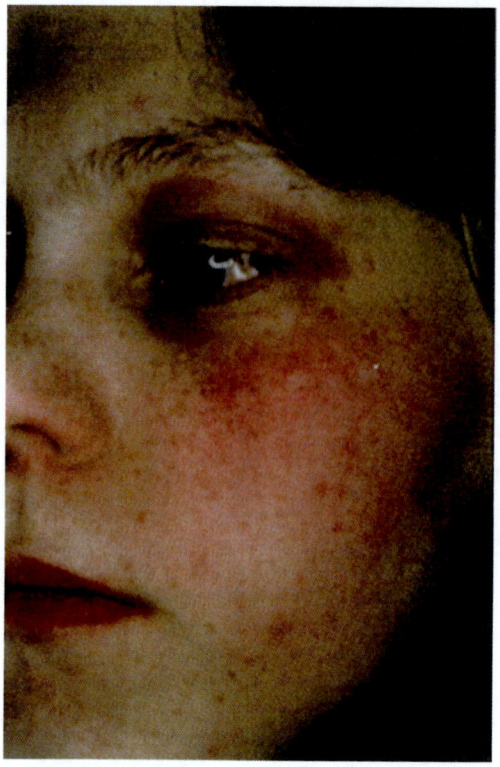

Fig. 17.6
Airborne immune contact urticaria of the face caused by the dispersion of cornstarch particles with a high latex protein content in a female operating theater nurse presensitized by latex gloves

atopy patch test reaction to human dust mite (20% in pet; Chemotechnique®) at day 4, as well as an elevated allergen-specific IgE level. This emphasizes the new concept of "extrinsic" atopic dermatitis, related to filaggrin haploinsufficiency in the stratum corneum; this allows an increased penetration of high-molecular-weight allergens into the skin. The impact of these studies has to be further evaluated in occupational dermatology.

9 Diagnostic Procedures

The diagnosis of occupational airborne contact dermatitis may be extremely difficult.

The approach of each individual case requires various steps that can be discussed in an algorithmic way. The major issue is to determine whether the clinical symptoms evocate or not such a diagnosis. The classical tools available for diagnosing occupational contact dermatitis in general can be applied to occupational airborne contact dermatitis. These include: anamnestic data, clinical symptoms, exacerbation (or not) of symptoms during work activities, determination of the occurrence of all offending agents at the workplace, knowledge of the chemical nature of these agents, etc.

When an airborne contact is reasonably suspected, the following strategy is recommended:

(a) Patch testing and/or photopatch testing

Patch tests and/or photopatch tests are performed in the usual way. There are no specific techniques that are recommended for airborne dermatitis. The methodology also includes additional procedures, such as open tests, semi-open tests, ROAT's, and eventually use tests.

(b) Prick testing

Prick tests are needed when airborne contact urticaria or protein contact dermatitis (i.e., to latex or pollen proteins) is suspected.

(c) Procedures useful in the diagnosis of occupational irritant airborne contact dermatitis

Some procedures are available that permit to evaluate the potential accountability of some offending agents for provoking airborne irritancy of the skin. This approach cannot be achieved without the collaboration of occupational physicians and/or safety officers. It also requires laboratory equipment and dermatological expertise in the field.

The following steps are usually recommended:

- Visit of the dermatologist at the workplace and analysis of the technical aspects of the work procedure.
- Collection of samples (i.e., suspected fibers, dusts, or liquids sprayed in the air).
- Analysis of samples, including pH, physical and chemical properties of chemicals, etc.
- Determination of the presence of particles (and eventually of chemicals) in the skin (i.e., using skin surface biopsy).
- Evaluation of the irritant potential of collected materials on the skin of workers or volunteers, by means of noninvasive techniques (such as transepidermal water loss, erythrometry, laser-Doppler flowmetry, and others).
- Evaluation of the relative rate of humidity in the air.
- Use of an exposure chamber designed for experiments with controlled exposure to airborne particles, mainly skin and respiratory allergens and irritants. The aims are to study skin effects and to develop methods for the measurement of deposition of particles on the skin (Lidén et al. 1998).

- Review of the relevant literature.
- Using such techniques does not lead – in many instances – to a final conclusion, but it allows recommendations in terms of preventive measures that will be applied and evaluated by occupational physicians.

10 Prevention and Treatment

Preventive measures are of course of prime importance to eradicate occupational airborne irritant and allergic contact dermatitis. They have been explained in detail in this chapter.

When dermatitis does occur, treatment strategies are multifaceted: topical treatments on the first line, that is, emollients, corticosteroids, and calcineurin inhibitors.

Tacrolimus ointment is the treatment of choice for periorbital dermatitis.

Systemic treatments are sometimes required; for example, in severe cases of parthenium dermatitis, azathioprine is very useful and superior to betamethasone (Verma et al. 2008).

References

Agarwal KK, D'Souza M (2009) Airborne contact dermatitis induced by parthenium: a study of 50 cases in South India. Clin Exp Dermatol 34:4–6

Baeck M, Goossens A (2009) Patients with airborne sensitization/contact dermatitis from budesonide-containing aerosols "by proxy". Contact Dermatitis 61:1–8

Björnberg A, Lowhagen G, Tengberg JE (1979) Relationship between intensities of skin test reactions to glass fibers and chemical irritants. Contact Dermatitis 5:171–174

Bordel-Gomez MT, Miranda-Romero A (2008) Fibreglass dermatitis: a report of 2 cases. Contact Dermatitis 59:120–122

Cao LY, Sood A, Taylor JS (2009) Hand/face/neck localized pattern: sticky problems-resins. Dermatol Clin 27:227–249

Coenraads PJ, Brouwer A, Olie K et al (1994) Chloracne. Some recent issues. Dermatol Clin 12:569–576

Corazza M, Baldo F, Osti F et al (2008) Airborne allergic contact dermatitis due to budesonide from professional exposure. Contact Dermatitis 58:318–319

Cusano F, Mariano M (2007) Fiberglass dermatitis: microepidemic in a primary school. Contact Dermatitis 57:351–352

Dooms-Goossens A, Debusschere KM, Gevers DM et al (1986) Contact dermatitis caused by airborne agents. J Am Acad Dermatol 15:1–10

Feser A, Mahler V (2009) Periorbital dermatitis: causes, differential diagnosis and therapy. J Dtsch Dermatol Ges 8:159–166

Fisher AA (1982) Fiberglass vs. mineral wool (rockwool) dermatitis. Cutis 29:415–416

Geraut C, Tripodi D, Brunet-Courtois B et al (2009) Occupational dermatitis to epoxydic and phenolic resins. Eur J Dermatol 19: 205–213

Gottschling S, Meyer S, Dill-Mueller D et al (2007) Outbreak report of airborne caterpillar dermatitis in a kindergarten. Dermatology 215:5–9

Hallai N, Gawkrodger DJ (2009) Patch testing to aeroallergens, especially house dust mite, is often positive in atopics with eczema of the face and hands. J Eur Acad Dermatol Venereol 23:728–729

Handfield-Jones SE (1998) Latex allergy in health-care workers in a English district general hospital. Br J Dermatol 138:273–276

Hsieh MY, Guo YL, Shiao JS et al (2001) Morphology of glass fibers in electronics workers with fiberglass dermatitis – a scanning electron microscopy study. Int J Dermatol 40:258–261

Kean T, Mc Nally M (2009) Latex hypersensitivity: a closer look at considerations for dentistry. J Can Dent Assoc 75:279–282

Koh D, Aw TC, Foulds IS (1992) Fibreglass dermatitis from printed circuit boards. Am J Ind Med 21:193–198

Lachapelle JM (1986) Industrial airborne irritant or allergic contact dermatitis. Contact Dermatitis 14:137–145

Lachapelle JM (1987) Industrial airborne irritant contact dermatitis due to dust particles. Boll Dermatol Allerg Profes 2:83–89

Lachapelle JM (2006) Airborne Irritant Dermatitis. In: Chew AL, Maibach HI (eds) Irritant dermatitis. Springer, Berlin

Lachapelle JM (2009) Eczémas "systémiques". In: Saurat JH, Lachapelle JM, Lipsker D, Thomas L (eds) Dermatologie et infections sexuellement transmissibles. Masson, Paris, pp 65–66

Lachapelle JM, Gouverneur JC, Boulet M et al (1977) A modified technique (using polyester tape) of skin surface biopsy. Br J Dermatol 97:49–52

Lachapelle JM, Mahmoud G, Van Herle R (1984) Anhydrite dermatitis in coal mines: an airborne irritant reaction assessed by laser Doppler flowmetry. Contact Dermatitis 11:188–189

Lachapelle JM, Frimat P, Tennstedt D et al (1992) Précis de Dermatologie Professionnelle et de l'Environnement. Masson, Paris, pp 107–111

Lagier F, Badier M, Martigny J et al (1990) Latex as aeroallergen. Lancet 336:516–517

Le Coz CJ, Coninx D, Van Rengen A et al (1999) An epidemic of occupational contact dermatitis from an immersion oil for microscopy in laboratory personnel. Contact Dermatitis 40:77–83

Legatt PA, Smith DR (2006) Dermatitis and aircrew. Contact Dermatitis 54:1–4

Lidén C, Lundgren L, Skare L et al (1998) A new whole-body exposure chamber for human skin and lung challenge experiments – the generation of wheat flour aerosols. Ann Occup Hyg 42:541–547

Mancuso G, Berdondini RM (2008) Occupational conjunctivitis as the sole manifestation of airborne contact allergy to trimethylolpropane triacrylate contained in a UV-cured paint. Contact Dermatitis 59:372–373

Marks R, Dawber RPR (1971) Skin surface biopsy: an improved technique for the examination of the horny layer. Br J Dermatol 84:117–123

Noe R, Cohen AL, Lederman E et al (2007) Skin disorders among construction workers following Hurricane Katrina and Hurricane Rita: an outbreak investigation in New Orleans, Louisiana. Arch Dermatol 143:1393–1398

Patiwael JA, Wintzen M, Rustemeyer T et al (2005) Airborne irritant contact dermatitis due to synthetic fibres from an air-conditioning filter. Contact Dermatitis 52:126–129

Pirilä V (1950) Thiokol as a frequent cause of dermatitis. Acta Allerg 3:319–328

Pirilä V, Noro L, Laamen A (1963) Air pollution and allergy. Acta Allerg 18:113–130

Pontén A (2006) Airborne occupational contact dermatitis caused by extremely low concentrations of budesonide. Contact Dermatitis 55:121–124

Samochocki Z (2007) Hypersensitivity to aeroallergens in adult patients with atopic dermatitis develops due to different immunological mechanisms. Eur J Dermatol 17:520–524

Santos R, Goossens A (2007) An update on airborne contact dermatitis: 2001–2006. Contact Dermatitis 57:353–360

Sharma VK, Sethuraman G (2007) Parthenium dermatitis. Dermatitis 18:183–190

Shkalim V, Herskovici Z, Amir J et al (2008) Systemic allergic reaction to tree processionary caterpillar in children. Pediatr Emerg Care 24:233–235

Stam-Westerveld EB (1997) Man-made mineral fibres: glasvezel- en steenwoldermatitis. Ned Tijdschr Dermatol Venereol 7:196–198

Stam-Westerveld EB, Coenraads PJ, van der Valk PJ et al (1994) Rubbing test responses of the skin to man-made mineral fibres of different diameters. Contact Dermatitis 31:1–4

Thune P (1977) Contact allergy due to lichens in patients with a history of photosensitivity. Contact Dermatitis 3:267–272

Verma KK, Mahesh R, Strivastava P et al (2008) Azathioprine versus betamethasone for the treatment of parthenium dermatitis: a randomized controlled study. Indian J Dermatol Venereol Leprol 74:453–457

18 Acute and Recurrent Vesicular Hand Dermatitis

Jacob P. Thyssen · Torkil Menné
Department of Dermato-Allergology, National Allergy Research Centre, Gentofte Hospital, Hellerup, Denmark

Core Messages

- Acute and recurrent vesicular hand dermatitis is a subtype of hand eczema.
- This term covers dyshidrotic hand dermatitis (eczema) and pompholyx, terms that should be abandoned.
- The disease is characterized by eruptive, vesicular dermatitis reactions that affect the palms, the palmar and lateral aspects of the fingers, and the periungual area.
- The vesicles or bullous lesions are often large and deep-seated.
- Causes and aggravating factors include emotional stress, hyperhidrosis, weather changes, atopy, mycosis, irritants, contact allergens, and systemic exposure to metals, drugs, and food. However, the cause is often unknown.
- Treatment includes primarily removal of causative exposures as well as topical corticosteroids, phototherapy, and in some cases systemic treatment.

1 Introduction

Acute and recurrent vesicular hand dermatitis is a term used to describe eruptive vesicular dermatitis reactions that affect the palms, the palmar and lateral aspects of the fingers, and the periungual area (Veien and Menné 2000; Veien 2009). Itch and burning sensitization often precede the development of lesions by 12–24 h. The vesicles or bullous lesions are deep-seated and are rarely observed outside the above-defined areas, e.g., the back of the hands or the forearms (Menné and Hjorth 1983; Veien 2009). However, similar vesicular lesions may also be observed on the soles and toes. Guillet et al., recently showed that among 120 patients with pompholyx, 70% had palmar lesions, 10% had plantar lesions, and 20% had lesions in both places (Guillet et al. 2007). Similar findings were reported by Castelain (1987) whereas Benedek (1974)found that among 1,835 military cases with acute and recurrent vesicular palmar or plantar dermatitis, 51% had foot involvement only. The palmar or plantar skin is usually not inflamed but inflammatory skin changes may be observed following repeated eruptions (Veien 2009). Scales tend to appear when the skin undergoes healing and returns to its normal appearance, typically after 2–3 weeks (Menné and Hjorth 1983; Veien 2009). Many patients have frequent attacks, 6–12 times per year (Menné and Hjorth 1983). As the skin may not clear between recurrent episodes, the patient will present a chronic dermatitis with desquamation, vesicles, and fissures (Menné and Hjorth 1983). The nail matrices may in some recurrent cases be damaged which will result in transverse ridging of the nailplates or even discoloration (Menné and Hjorth 1983). Each transverse ridge indicates an attack of recurrent vesicular hand dermatitis (Menné and Hjorth 1983). Also, in rare cases, lymphedema may develop due to failure of small initial lymphatics of the hand to absorb and drain lymph to regional nodes (Pearce and Mortimer 2009). Dermatologists may benefit from the use of a magnifying glass when searching for vesicles in the diagnostic workup of their patients (Veien 2009). This is of relevance as vesicular hand dermatitis at causal glance incorrectly may be diagnosed as chronic hand dermatitis (Veien 2009). The dyshidrotic eczema area and severity index (DASI) is a commonly used tool that quantifies clinical signs and symptoms of acute and recurrent vesicular hand dermatitis based on the number of vesicles, desquamation, erythema, itch, and extension (Vocks et al. 1999).

2 Nomenclature

Over time, acute and recurrent vesicular hand dermatitis has also been known as dyshidrotic eczema, dyshidrosis, pompholyx, and cheiropompholyx (pompholyx of the hands). Dyshidrosis and pompholyx come from Greek and mean "bad sweating" and "bubble," respectively. The term dyshidrosis was initially used since vesicular hand dermatitis was thought to be associated with occlusion of the sweat glands and ducts leading to sweat retention, and as clinical worsening was often observed during a swift to higher temperatures and during the warmer summer

T. Rustemeyer, P. Elsner, S.M. John & H.I. Maibach (eds.), *Kanerva's Occupational Dermatology*,
DOI 10.1007/978-3-642-02035-3_18,

months (Castelain 1987; Lodi et al. 1992). However, studies have rejected an association as histopathological examinations have revealed spongiotic dermatitis with intraepidermal vesicles and as the intraepidermal portion of the eccrine sweat duct (acrosyringium) is unaltered by the spongiosis (Christensen et al. 1981; Kutzner et al. 1986). Thus, sweat ducts are mostly pushed aside by vesicles or pass between them (Menné and Hjorth 1983). Recently, a case report described bile-colored vesicles in a patient with jaundice and the authors speculated whether secondary pathological damage to the ducts was driven by inflammatory spongiosis (Lee et al. 2009). Some authors distinguish between dyshidrotic hand eczema and pompholyx as they claim these subtypes have different clinical expression patterns (Löfgren and Warshaw 2006). Thus, dyshidrotic hand eczema is characterized by chronic and recurrent eruptions of small (1–2 mm) vesicles whereas a severe and explosive onset of larger bullae is observed in pompholyx (Löfgren and Warshaw 2006). The above-mentioned terms cover the same disease entity and they should all be addressed as (acute and) recurrent vesicular hand dermatitis to avoid confusion.

3 Epidemiology

The epidemiology of acute and recurrent vesicular hand dermatitis has been reviewed on several occasions (Veien and Menné 2000; Löfgren and Warshaw 2006; Veien 2009). So far, few studies have investigated the prevalence of vesicular hand dermatitis in the general population. Agrup questioned 107,206 subjects about skin changes on the hands (Agrup 1969): 2,499 (2.3%) gave an affirmative answer and 1,659 underwent clinical examination (Agrup 1969). In the latter group, 827 had hand dermatitis and 51 (6.1%) had dermatitis of recurrent vesicular morphology (Agrup 1969). In a large epidemiological study, Meding and Swanbeck also found that 6% of 1,032 subjects with hand dermatitis had vesicular morphology and that the female to male ratio was 1:0 (Meding and Swanbeck 1989). Thus, the overall estimated prevalence of vesicular hand dermatitis in the general population in Sweden was 0.2% in 1964–1965 and 0.3% in 1983–1984 (Meding and Swanbeck 1989). Slightly higher prevalences were identified by Latinga et al. 1984, as they showed that the prevalence of vesicular hand dermatitis was 0.9% in 1979 and 2.8% in 1982 among 1,992 adults from the Netherlands. More females than males were affected (Lantinga et al. 1984). More recently, Bryld et al. found that 300 (5.3%) of 5,673 Danish twins reported vesicles on the hands without other symptoms (Bryld et al. 2000) and Lerbaek et al. found that among 77 twins with hand dermatitis, 20% had vesicular morphology (Lerbaek et al. 2008).

Several reports have estimated the prevalence of vesicular hand dermatitis in clinical patients. Among 425 Swedish patch-tested dermatitis patients, 38% had vesicular hand dermatitis (Edman 1988). Among 714 Portuguese patients with hand dermatitis, 20.3% had vesicular hand dermatitis (Magina et al. 2003). Recently, Veien et al. found that 50% of 347 Danish female patients and 31% of 175 Danish male patients seen in private practice had vesicular hand dermatitis (Veien et al. 2008). In contrast to these high estimates, an older Swedish study estimated that vesicular hand dermatitis accounted for 1% of all hand dermatitis patients (Thelin and Agrup 1985). Furthermore, a recent European multicenter study found that vesicular hand dermatitis occurred in 9.3% of 319 patients with hand dermatitis (Diepgen et al. 2009). The authors found a predominance among men (Diepgen et al. 2009). Lodi et al. 1992 found that among 104 patients with vesicular hand dermatitis, 56% were men. Like other subtypes of hand dermatitis, vesicular hand dermatitis is associated with young age (Guillet et al. 2007). From the above, it can be appreciated that vesicular hand dermatitis is generally a minor subtype of hand dermatitis.

4 Causes and Aggravating Factors

Several etiological and aggravating factors of acute and recurrent vesicular hand dermatitis have been suggested (➋ *Table 18.1*). As vesicular hand dermatitis is infrequent in the general population, evidence is mainly derived from clinical studies which are known to be more biased. Furthermore, it should be remembered that hand dermatitis is a complex disorder with many causative factors and that these may interact differently in different individuals. The accumulation of evidence from the studies discussed below show that recurrent and vesicular hand dermatitis can be triggered by many different causes but the clinical expression and morphology is often similar. Thus, vesicular hand dermatitis is likely to be a nonspecific reaction pattern in predisposed individuals as previously suggested (Lodi et al. 1992). In a review, Menné and Hjorth (1983) found that vesicular hand dermatitis was not associated with genetic predisposition. However, one case report described a gene associated with a rare autosomal dominant form of pompholyx to chromosome 18q22-18q22.3 (Chen et al. 2006). Future genetic studies may help to further subdivide this disorder into etiological subtypes which will increase our understanding markedly.

Table 18.1
Possible causes and aggravating factors of acute and recurrent vesicular hand eczema

Causes and aggravating factors	Comments
External factors	
Fungal (id-reactions)	*Trichophyton* species. Convincing association
Irritants	E.g., water, detergents and solvents
Allergens	E.g., metals, fragrances and preservatives
Systemic allergic dermatitis reaction	E.g., foods, metals, implants and drugs
Hyperhidrosis	Patients may have a higher perspiration volume
Weather and temperature changes	Worsening during a shift to warmer or colder temperatures
Sunlight	UVA exposure
Parasites	Rare cause
HIV infection	One case
Smoking	Limited evidence
Internal factors	
Atopy	Doubtful association among Caucasians
Emotional or general stress	Evidence of improvement following biofeedback therapy
Hormones	Worsening during the pre-menstrual period

4.1 Atopy

Atopy has repeatedly been discussed as a risk factor for acute and recurrent vesicular hand dermatitis. Lodi et al. (1992) found a significantly higher prevalence of atopy among 104 subjects with vesicular hand dermatitis when they were compared with 208 controls (50% versus 11.5%). Pitché et al. (2006) found a strong association with atopy in a multivariate analysis performed in a recent prospective case–control study performed in Togo, Africa. In a comparison between 59 workers with vesicular hand dermatitis and 160 workers with other subtypes of hand dermatitis, no significant difference in the prevalence of atopy was found (42.4% versus 30.6%) (Lehucher-Michel et al. 2000). Also, the authors found no association with contact allergy of occupational relevance (Lehucher-Michel et al. 2000). De Boer et al. 1988, found that only 1 (4.7%) of 21 patients with occupational vesicular hand dermatitis had atopy. Edman et al. investigated 425 patients with hand dermatitis of which 92 had vesicular hand dermatitis and found no association with atopy (Edman 1988). Thelin and Agrup (1985) did not find a higher prevalence of atopy among 68 patients with vesicular hand dermatitis when they were compared to the expected prevalence in the Swedish general population. Finally, Bryld et al. (2003) rejected an association among 398 Danish twins. Taken together, atopy may only be weakly associated with vesicular hand dermatitis among European patients whereas a stronger association possibly exists for Africans.

4.2 Cutaneous Contact with Irritants and Allergens

The possible association between vesicular hand dermatitis on one hand and contact allergy and irritant reactions on the other hand, respectively, has been investigated on several occasions. However, these data are mainly observational and not generated from exposure studies. De Boer et al. (1988) showed that among 21 metal workers with vesicular hand dermatitis, only 3 had positive patch test reactions, suggesting that irritancy was associated with vesicular hand dermatitis. In contrast, Meneghini et al. found a high prevalence of contact allergy among 364 patients with vesicular hand dermatitis (Meneghini and Angelini 1979). Also, Jain et al. (2004) found a high prevalence of contact allergy among 50 patients with vesicular hand dermatitis. Of note, most investigators have found the strongest association between vesicular hand dermatitis and metal allergy (Menné and Hjorth 1983; Veien and Menné 2000; Veien 2009). Crosti and Lodi (1993) speculated that the higher prevalence of metal allergy among patients with vesicular hand dermatitis could be explained by the high frequency of hyperhidrosis as metal ions are readily released from metallic items upon contact with sweat. However, Guillet et al. (2007) found that cosmetics and personal hygiene products were more often associated with vesicular hand dermatitis when compared to metals. Finally, Bryld et al. (2003) rejected an association between vesicular hand dermatitis and nickel allergy among 398 Danish twins from the general population. Cutaneous skin contact with irritants as well as contact allergens may elicit vesicular hand dermatitis although study results are diverging and not very convincing. It may be difficult to adequately study this association by using epidemiological tools since vesicular hand dermatitis is relatively uncommon and as many other factors may play a role. Exposure studies such as those previously performed for other subtypes of hand dermatitis seems to be required (Nielsen et al. 1999).

4.3 Systemic Exposure to Allergens

Reports have described the development or aggravation of vesicular hand dermatitis following insertion of metallic implants such as orthodontic wires and dental plates, infusion needles, clips, pacemakers, and orthopedic plates and screws (Veien and Menné 2000; Veien 2009). On a large scale, such reactions are uncommon as shown by a Danish questionnaire study performed among 1,085 girls in active orthodontic treatment or retention (Staerkjaer and Menné 1990). Furthermore, there is substantial evidence that oral ingestion of food, metals, and drugs can result in vesicular hand dermatitis (Menné and Hjorth 1983; Veien and Menné 2000; Löfgren and Warshaw 2006; Thyssen and Maibach 2008; Veien 2009). However, the contribution of systemic reactivation in the pathogenesis of vesicular hand dermatitis was recently questioned as Guillet et al. found that only 6.7% of 120 patients had an internal reactivation of their hand dermatitis from food, drugs, or metals (Guillet et al. 2007). Oral provocation has repeatedly been shown to result in vesicular hand dermatitis since the pioneering work performed by Flood and Perry (Flood and Perry 1946; Veien 2009). In a double-blind, placebo-controlled study with 17 patients sensitized to balsam of Peru and 5 patients sensitized to spices, per oral challenge with balsam of Peru and spices resulted in an increased number of palmar vesicles (30–280%) (but not with placebo) in 8 patients and an increased number of vesicles in three patients using both the placebo and the active ingredients (Niinimaki 1995). Veien et al. found that 28 (60.9%) of 46 patients treated with long-term dietary restriction of balsams in food had improvement in their dermatitis (Veien et al. 1996).

Besides foods, there is substantial evidence that the ingestion of metals may elicit vesicular hand dermatitis in predisposed individuals (Veien et al. 1983; Veien and Menné 2000; Veien 2009). It is interesting that vesicular hand dermatitis is observed in both metal sensitized and nonsensitized individuals (Veien and Kaaber 1979; Veien et al. 1987). Whether this is explained by false-negative patch test reactions (Veien 2009), a "placebo" effect, or by direct activation of immunological reactions caused by metal ingestion is currently unknown (Thyssen and Maibach 2008). A study on systemic nickel allergy found a dose–response relationship between nickel ingestion and dermatitis flare-up. Thus, 0.3, 1, and 4 mg pure nickel as a sulfate hexahydrate gave dermatitis in 40%, 40%, and 70% of nickel allergic subjects (Jensen et al. 2003). From this study, it can be concluded that a single dose of 4 mg nickel will result in widespread dermatitis in most nickel-allergic patients. However, normal daily dietary nickel intake has been found to vary from 0.02 to 0.48 mg (Jensen et al. 2006). An open study found an effect of a 6-week low-nickel diet in 9 of 17 nickel-allergic patients that previously had reacted to 2.5 mg nickel exposure (Kaaber et al. 1978). Despite disulfiram, therapy may reduce the frequency of flares in nickel allergic-patients with vesicular dermatitis (Kaaber et al. 1983), the risk of severe side effects has prevented their routine use. Cobalt-allergic patients may experience worsening of their vesicular hand dermatitis upon oral exposure to 1 mg cobalt (Veien and Kaaber 1979; Veien et al. 1995). A point-based guide was recently published that reduced cobalt intake to <12 μg per day (Stuckert and Nedorost 2008). Finally, most chromate allergic patients reacted to an oral challenge with 2.5 mg chromium in a placebo-controlled study (Veien et al. 1994). Of note, the chromium content in food is much lower (Veien et al. 1994). Taken together, the association between high metal intake and elicitation of vesicular hand dermatitis is indisputable but it remains unclear why nonallergic subjects also may react to peroral challenge. The association may have been stronger in the middle of the twentieth century than today as cutaneous skin contact with higher metal concentrations occurred more frequently at that time. The difficulty of conducting randomized double-blinded placebo-controlled diet studies should be taken into account when one interprets data. Clearly, there is a need for further research to clarify the exact role of diets in the treatment of vesicular hand dermatitis.

The role of systemic drug exposure in the development of vesicular hand dermatitis was recently reviewed (Thyssen and Maibach 2008). Briefly, many drugs may be causative and they should always be suspected (Ekelund and Möller 1969). Of interest, case reports have described vesicular hand dermatitis following treatment with intravenous immunoglobulin in patients (Iannaccone et al. 1999).

4.4 Tinea Pedis

Tinea pedis is known to result in vesicular eruptions on the hands. In temperate climates, they are most often observed during the summer months (Veien and Menné 2000). Most cases are caused by *Trichophyton mentagrophytes* and *Trichophyton rubrum* (Veien and Menné 2000; Pitche et al. 2006). The classic example of "id" reaction is a dermatophytid, a symmetrical vesicular eruption on the hands caused by tinea pedis (Veien and Menné 2000). Veien refers to an early description by Sulzberger and Baer's which among other things requires that the onset of eruption on the hands must follow activation or irritation of the primary focus and that the eruption should disappear or subside within a reasonable time after the fungal infection has cleared (Veien and Menné 2000). In a Danish twin study, the point prevalence of vesicles on the hands was three times elevated among those with tinea pedis (Bryld et al. 2003). In a recent prospective study performed in Togo, Africa, a very strong association was found in a multivariate analysis (Pitche et al. 2006). Also, Guillet et al. found that 10% of 120 patients with vesicular hand dermatitis had mycosis (Guillet et al. 2007).

4.5 Tobacco Smoking

So far, two studies have investigated the association between tobacco smoking and vesicular hand dermatitis. A positive association was found in both studies but these results should be carefully interpreted as the studies were not designed optimally to address this question (Edman 1988; Guillet et al. 2007). In addition, other studies have investigated the association between smoking and hand dermatitis in general (any subtype) and found diverging results (Montnemery et al. 2005; Lerbaek et al. 2007; Meding et al. 2009). However, there is indirect evidence of an effect from tobacco smoking on the pathogenesis of vesicular hand dermatitis as smoking may negatively influence the effect of psoralen UVA (PUVA) therapy (Douwes et al. 2000). A possible positive association between smoking and vesicular hand dermatitis may be explained by the fact that nickel is found in tobacco plants as a result of absorption from soil, fertilizing products, or pesticides. Furthermore, the nickel content in cigarettes and tobacco is high regardless of its kind and origin (Stojanovic et al. 2004). One study examined the nickel concentration in 123 blood samples and 147 urine samples from smokers and nonsmokers. It revealed a significantly higher concentration of nickel in the urine but not in the blood of smokers in comparison to nonsmokers (Stojanovic et al. 2004). Further research is warranted.

4.6 Other Causes

Acute and recurrent vesicular hand dermatitis has also been associated with psychological stress or nervousness (Kellum 1973; Hansen et al. 1981). Biofeedback training appeared to have a positive effect in two different patient series (Miller and Coger 1979; Kodlys and Meyer 1979). Little research has been conducted in this field in recent years. Furthermore, seasonal variation can influence the development of vesicular hand dermatitis and can lead to aggravation. Lodi et al. found that 43 (41%) and 38 (37%) of 104 patients with vesicular hand dermatitis reported seasonal variation and worsening due to sweating, respectively (Lodi et al. 1992). However, Thelin and Agrup rejected an association with hyperhidrosis (Thelin and Agrup 1985). In an interesting study, Yokozeki et al. found that patients with vesicular hand dermatitis had a 2.5 higher perspiration volume than age- and sex-matched controls indicating an association between vesicular hand dermatitis and hyperhidrosis (Yokozeki et al. 1992). Also, iontophoresis has proved successful in the treatment of vesicular hand dermatitis in 20 patients (Odia et al. 1996). Recently, it was suggested that UVA exposure could play a role in the pathogenesis of vesicular hand dermatitis as Man et al. showed that UVA provocation on previously affected sites induced vesicular dermatitis in five patients (Man et al. 2004).

5 Differential Diagnoses

Several differential diagnoses to vesicular hand dermatitis should be considered (➋ *Table 18.2*). In the acute phase, vesicular and bullous disorders (e.g., pustulosis palmoplantaris, vesicular tinea manus) may mimic vesicular hand dermatitis, whereas in the chronic phase, it is rather the scaly and hyperkeratotic disorders that should be

◘ Table 18.2
Differential diagnoses of acute and recurrent vesicular hand eczema (Veien and Menné 2000; Löfgren and Warshaw 2006; Wollina 2008; Veien 2009)

Pustulosis palmo-plantaris
Superficial peeling (dyshidrosis lamellosa sicca)
Infantile acropustolosis
Protein contact dermatitis
Bullous pemphigoid
Pustular bactericid
Acrodermatitis continua
Hyperkeratotic hand eczema
Palmar psoriasis
Vesicular tinea manus and pedis
Scabies
Herpes simplex
Epidermolysis bullosa hereditaria
Herpes gestationes
Friction blisters

Table 18.3

Treatment options for acute and recurrent vesicular hand eczema

Treatment	Comments
Frequently used:	
Emollients	A mainstay in all therapy regimens but may in some cases cause irritancy
Cool compresses	Typically applied for a few days to dry up blisters
Topical corticosteroids (Veien et al. 1999; Veien 2009)	First line; these should often be potent
Oral corticosteroids (Veien 2009)	Only short-term treatment advised
Non-ionizing radiotherapy (Grattan et al. 1991; Schempp et al. 1997; Behrens et al. 1999; Petering et al. 2004; Schiener et al. 2005)	UVB/UVA-1/topical and oral PUVA therapy
Antibiotics	Bacteria should be suspected upon deterioration or when the skin is broken
Rarely used:	
Ionizing radiotherapy (King and Chalmers 1984; Fairris et al. 1984; Fairris et al. 1985; Stambaugh et al. 2000)	Should be used with caution due to harmful side effects
Aluminum chloride	Typically applied during night time for prevention of hyperhidrosis
Iontophoresis (Odia et al. 1996)	Rarely used but efficient in some patients
Botulinum toxin (Swartling et al. 2002; Wollina and Karamfilov 2002)	Two trials; some effect
Calcineurin inhibitors (Schnopp et al. 2002; Belsito et al. 2004)	Two trials; tacrolimus seem to be effective whereas pimecrolimus may only have a weak effect
Cromoglycate (Cox 1971)	One single-blind trial; significant effect
Mychophenolate mofetil (Pickenacker et al. 1998)	One case report
Methotrexat (Egan et al. 1999)	One case series
Azathioprine (Scerri 1999)	One case series
Cyclosporine (Petersen and Menné 1992)	One case report
Etanercept (Ogden et al. 2006)	One case report
Future option:	
Alitretinoin (Bollag and Ott 1999; Ruzicka et al. 2004; Ruzicka et al. 2008)	Promising effect in three trials

excluded (e.g., hyperkeratotic palmar hand eczema, superficial peeling, and psoriasis). Of note, vesicular hand dermatitis may be observed in the initial phase or concomitantly with other disorders, e.g., bullous pemphogoid, linear IgA disease, cutaneous T-cell lymphoma, and lichen planus (Veien and Menné 2000).

6 Treatment

Treatment modalities for acute and recurrent vesicular hand dermatitis were recently reviewed (➋ *Table 18.3*) (Löfgren and Warshaw 2006; Wollina 2008). Firstly, causative and aggravating exposures should be identified and removed. Low-diet treatment may be necessary in selected cases as described previously. Secondly, the use of emollients remains a cornerstone of all treatment protocols and should be applied liberally. In some cases, supplementary use of cool compresses to dry up blisters and to treat pruritus may be beneficial. In the rare case of lymphedema, prophylactic antibiotics together with aggressive treatment has proven to be efficient (Pearce and Mortimer 2009).

6.1 Corticosteroid Treatment

First-line therapy of vesicular hand dermatitis includes topical application of corticosteroids (Veien et al. 1999; Veien 2009), sometimes applied under occlusion (Volden 1992). Intermittent control is necessary to prevent atrophy. It is generally perceived that ointments are more efficient than creams. Short-term oral corticosteroid treatment is often effective (e.g., 30 mg/day for 1 week) (Veien 2009). Others have recommended higher treatment doses (Löfgren and Warshaw 2006; Wollina 2008). Long-term treatment with oral corticosteroids should be avoided due to the risk of systemic side effects.

6.2 Topical Calcineurin Inhibitors

Topical calcineurin inhibitor treatment may be effective for the treatment of vesicular hand dermatitis. In a randomized, single-blind study, 16 patients were treated twice daily for 4 weeks with either topical tacrolimus or momethasone furoate 0.1% ointment (Schnopp et al. 2002). The two therapies were equally efficient (both reduced the DASI score with 50%) and the authors suggested that the treatment could be used rotationally to prevent excessive corticosteroid use (Schnopp et al. 2002). Topical pimecrolimus therapy was used twice daily in a 3 week double-blind, randomized, placebo-controlled study of 294 patients with chronic hand dermatitis of which some had vesicular hand dermatitis (Belsito et al. 2004). A nonsignificant effect was observed in the pimecrolimus group when compared to the vehicle group (p = 0.068). Perhaps occlusive treatment with pimecrolimus may have a better effect as suggested by a case report (Schurmeyer-Horst et al. 2007). The exact role of tacrolimus in the treatment of vesicular hand dermatitis remained to be defined.

6.3 Botulinum Toxin-A Therapy

The efficacy of botulinum toxin-A was assessed among eight adult patients with vesicular hand dermatitis in an 8-week prospective, side-by-side controlled study using topical corticosteroid treatment on both hands in combination with intracutaneous injections of botulinum toxin-A on the more severely affected hand (Wollina and Karamfilov 2002). A significant improvement was observed over an 8-week period (Wollina and Karamfilov 2002). Furthermore, among 10 patients with vesicular hand dermatitis, botulinum toxin-A therapy resulted in improved self-assessment of hand dermatitis in the hand treated with injections in comparison to the untreated hand (Swartling et al. 2002). Double-blind studies are warranted but it is unlikely that injection treatment will become routine.

6.4 Iontophoresis

Iontophoresis is traditionally used for the treatment of hyperhidrosis. However, a significant effect was demonstrated in a single-blind right-left study performed in 20 patients with vesicular hand dermatitis (Odia et al. 1996). Treatment was performed for a total of 20 sessions (15 min each) on one hand for 3 weeks. Seventeen patients had a significant improvement.

6.5 Alitretinoin

Alitretinoin may be a novel treatment option for vesicular hand dermatitis. In a Swiss pilot study, 34 (89%) of 38 patients with chronic refractory hand dermatitis (of which 7 were diagnosed as having vesicular hand dermatitis) showed a good or very good response to systemic alitretinoin treatment (20 mg or 40 mg) lasting 1–5 months (Bollag and Ott 1999). "Good" and "very good" were defined as 61–80% and 81–100% reduction of lesions, respectively. All subtypes of hand dermatitis responded in a similar way. Only mild side effects such as cheilitis, transient headache, and transient flush to the head were recorded. The duration of remission after discontinuation of successful therapy was 1 month to more than 1 year (Bollag and Ott 1999). The initial findings were only supported to some degree in a double-blind, randomized, placebo-controlled multicenter study where treatment with oral alitretinoin was performed in 319 patients, of which 70 had vesicular hand dermatitis (Ruzicka et al. 2004). Treatment with either placebo (n = 78), alitretinoin 10 mg (n = 80), 20 mg (n = 80), or 40 mg (n = 81) was conducted over a 12-week period. Fifty-three percent of patients who were treated with 40 mg alitretinoin per day and 27% of those who received placebo therapy reported complete or nearly complete disappearance of disease signs and symptoms. Physician's global assessment showed that 12% of patients who received placebo and 43% of patients who received 40 mg alitretinoin per day had clearance of their hand dermatitis. However, the response rate was not significantly different among patients with vesicular hand dermatitis. In a recent randomized, double-blind, placebo-controlled multicentre trial, 1,032 patients with hand dermatitis (27% with vesicular hand dermatitis) were enrolled and randomized to treatment with 10 mg (n = 418) or 30 mg (n = 409) alitretinoin or placebo therapy (n = 205) for up to 24 weeks (Ruzicka et al. 2008). This study also found a dose-dependent effect of alitretinoin therapy as clear or almost clear hands was observed in 17% of those who received placebo and in up to 48% of those who received alitretinoin. Recurrence of 75% of symptoms was observed after typically 6 months (Ruzicka et al. 2008).

Taken together, alitretinoin may be a promising new treatment modality for vesicular hand eczema but the results from three trials have not yet convincingly determined its role.

6.6 Methotrexate

Methotrexate is rarely used for the treatment of vesicular hand eczema but seemed efficient in an open study with five patients treated with 12.5–20 mg per week for up to 20 weeks (Egan et al. 1999).

6.7 Azathioprine

The efficacy of azathioprine therapy was retrospectively evaluated in six patients with vesicular hand dermatitis (Scerri 1999). An oral dose of 50–100 mg/day was given for a mean duration of 33.5 months and resulted in excellent response (n = 3), good response (n = 1), and fair response (n = 2) (Scerri 1999).

6.8 Mycophenolate Mofetil

One case report showed that treatment with mycophenolate mofetil was efficient in a patient who had tried corticosteroids, iontophoresis, PUVA therapy, cyclosporine, dapsone, and topical tar (Pickenacker et al. 1998). Treatment with 1.5 g mycophenolate mofetil twice a day resulted in complete recovery after 4 weeks (Pickenacker et al. 1998). Of note, mycophenolate mofetil treatment following lever transplantation resulted in vesicular hand dermatitis in one patient (Semhoun-Ducloux et al. 2000).

6.9 Cyclosporine

Cyclosporine therapy may be efficient for vesicular hand dermatitis (Petersen and Menné 1992). However, no studies have so far been directed at evaluating the effect on vesicular hand dermatitis alone but this subtype has probably been a part of larger patient series (Löfgren and Warshaw 2006). Granlund et al. found that 3 mg cyclosporine per kilogram per day had a similar efficacy as topical betamethasone therapy in a randomized double-blind study with 41 patients suffering from chronic hand dermatitis (Granlund et al. 1996).

6.10 Cromoglycate

Cromoglycate therapy was significantly more efficient at reducing vesicular hand dermatitis than a low-nickel diet when used in a randomized, single-blind study including 24 patients with vesicular hand dermatitis (Cox 1971).

6.11 Etanercept

A patient with atopic dermatitis suffered from chronic vesicular hand dermatitis and was treated with 25 mg etanercept twice weekly (Ogden et al. 2006). Symptoms cleared at 6 week follow-up but the patient experienced flare-up after 4 months. When therapy was repeated (in double dose), no effect was observed.

6.12 Radiotherapy

Ionizing radiation techniques include the use of superficial x-rays, grenz rays, and megavoltage therapy. In some patient series, no information is given about hand dermatitis morphology and these articles have been discussed elsewhere (Löfgren and Warshaw 2006). Superficial radiotherapy given at 1-week intervals resulted in a significant better response than simulated therapy (placebo) after 1 month, whereas the difference was not apparent after 3 and 6 months (King and Chalmers 1984). In a double-blind trial of 24 patients with vesicular hand dermatitis, superficial x-ray therapy was given on one hand (and simulated therapy on the other) at intervals of 21 days and in combination with topical corticosteroids (Fairris et al. 1984). A significantly better result was obtained on hands that received superficial x-ray therapy when compared to hands that received placebo (Fairris et al. 1984). Among 25 patients with vesicular hand dermatitis that participated in a double-blind trial, superficial x-ray therapy resulted in a significantly better skin condition than Grenz ray therapy (given in three doses at 21 day intervals) at follow-up after 3, 6, 12, and 18 weeks (Fairris et al. 1985). Stambaugh et al. reported complete remission of severe vesicular hand dermatitis following low-dose external beam megavoltage therapy 1 month after therapy was initiated (Stambaugh et al. 2000).

Nonionizing radiotherapy includes the use of UVB, UVA-1, and topical or oral psoralen in combination with UVA irradiation (PUVA). In a clinical study of seven patients with vesicular hand dermatitis, oral PUVA therapy was given three times weekly and resulted in remission on the maintenance schedule for 2–6 months (LeVine et al. 1981). Promising results have also been found for topical PUVA therapy in small open patient series (Schempp et al. 1997; Davis et al. 1998; Behrens et al. 1999). There seems to be no difference in the efficacy of PUVA-gel versus PUVA-bath therapy (Schiener et al. 2005). Treatment with UVB irradiation was inferior to oral PUVA therapy when applied in 35 patients with chronic hand dermatitis (only one had acute and recurrent vesicular hand dermatitis) (Rosen et al. 1987). However, a recent prospective, comparative study found that local narrowband UVB therapy was as effective as paint-PUVA therapy in 15 patients (Sezer and Etikan 2007). In a double-blind controlled study including 28 patients with vesicular hand dermatitis, UVA-1 versus simulated irradiation given five times weekly for 3 weeks resulted in significant improvement after 2–3 weeks in the active treatment group (Polderman et al. 2003). Studies have suggested that UVA-1 therapy is equally efficient with topical and oral PUVA therapy (Grattan et al. 1991; Petering et al. 2004).

References

Agrup G (1969) Hand eczema and other hand dermatosis in South Sweden. Acta Derm Venereol 49:1–91

Behrens S, von Kobyletzki G, Gruss C, Reuther T, Altmeyer P, Kerscher M (1999) PUVA-bath photochemotherapy (PUVA-soak therapy) of recalcitrant dermatoses of the palms and soles. Photodermatol Photoimmunol Photomed 15:47–51

Belsito DV, Fowler JF Jr, Marks JG Jr, Pariser DM, Hanifin J, Duarte IA, Pires MC, Cruz PD Jr, Langley RG, Patel P, Bush C, Thurston M, Graeber M, Cherill R (2004) Pimecrolimus cream 1%: a potential new treatment for chronic hand dermatitis. Cutis 73:31–38

Benedek T (1974) Pompholyx of the hands and feet. Its etiology, pathogenesis and specific vaccine therapy. (Formerly: 'epidermophytosis' of hands and feet). Mycopathol Mycol Appl 53:25–44

Bollag W, Ott F (1999) Successful treatment of chronic hand eczema with oral 9-cis-retinoic acid. Dermatology 199:308–312

Bryld LE, Agner T, Kyvik KO, Brondsted L, Hindsberger C, Menné T (2000) Hand eczema in twins: a questionnaire investigation. Br J Dermatol 142:298–305

Bryld LE, Agner T, Menné T (2003) Relation between vesicular eruptions on the hands and tinea pedis, atopic dermatitis and nickel allergy. Acta Derm Venereol 83:186–188

Castelain PY (1987) Dysidrosis. Ann Dermatol Venereol 114:579–585

Chen JJ, Liang YH, Zhou FS, Yang S, Wang J, Wang PG, Du WH, Xu SJ, Huang W, Zhang XJ (2006) The gene for a rare autosomal dominant form of pompholyx maps to chromosome 18q22.1-18q22.3. J Invest Dermatol 126:300–304

Christensen OB, Lindstrom C, Löfberg H, Möller H (1981) Micromorphology and specificity of orally induced flare-up reactions in nickel-sensitive patients. Acta Derm Venereol 61:505–510

Cox JS (1971) Disodium cromoglycate. Mode of action and its possible relevance to the clinical use of the drug. Br J Dis Chest 65:189–204

Crosti C, Lodi A (1993) Pompholyx: a still unresolved kind of eczema. Dermatology 186:241–242

Davis MD, McEvoy MT, el-Azhary RA (1998) Topical psoralen-ultraviolet A therapy for palmoplantar dermatoses: experience with 35 consecutive patients. Mayo Clin Proc 73:407–411

de Boer EM, Bruynzeel DP, van Ketel WG (1988) Dyshidrotic eczema as an occupational dermatitis in metal workers. Contact Dermatitis 19:184–188

Diepgen TL, Andersen KE, Brandao FM, Bruze M, Bruynzeel DP, Frosch P, Goncalo M, Goossens A, Le Coz CJ, Rustemeyer T, White IR, Agner T (2009) Hand eczema classification: a cross-sectional, multicentre study of the aetiology and morphology of hand eczema. Br J Dermatol 160:353–358

Douwes KE, Karrer S, Abels C, Landthaler M, Szeimies RM (2000) Does smoking influence the efficacy of bath-PUVA therapy in chronic palmoplantar eczema? Photodermatol Photoimmunol Photomed 16:25–29

Edman B (1988) Palmar eczema: a pathogenetic role for acetylsalicylic acid, contraceptives and smoking? Acta Derm Venereol 68:402–407

Egan CA, Rallis TM, Meadows KP, Krueger GG (1999) Low-dose oral methotrexate treatment for recalcitrant palmoplantar pompholyx. J Am Acad Dermatol 40:612–614

Ekelund AG, Möller H (1969) Oral provocation in eczematous contact allergy to neomycin and hydroxy-quinolines. Acta Derm Venereol 49:422–426

Fairris GM, Jones DH, Mack DP, Rowell NR (1985) Conventional superficial X-ray versus Grenz ray therapy in the treatment of constitutional eczema of the hands. Br J Dermatol 112:339–341

Fairris GM, Mack DP, Rowell NR (1984) Superficial X-ray therapy in the treatment of constitutional eczema of the hands. Br J Dermatol 111:445–449

Flood JM, Perry DJ (1946) Recurrent vesicular eruption of the hands due to food allergy. J Invest Dermatol 7:309–327

Granlund H, Erkko P, Eriksson E, Reitamo S (1996) Comparison of cyclosporine and topical betamethasone-17,21-dipropionate in the treatment of severe chronic hand eczema. Acta Derm Venereol 76:371–376

Grattan CE, Carmichael AJ, Shuttleworth GJ, Foulds IS (1991) Comparison of topical PUVA with UVA for chronic vesicular hand eczema. Acta Derm Venereol 71:118–122

Guillet MH, Wierzbicka E, Guillet S, Dagregorio G, Guillet G (2007) A 3-year causative study of pompholyx in 120 patients. Arch Dermatol 143:1504–1508

Hansen O, Kuchler T, Lotz GR, Richter R (1981) Wilckens A [My fingers itch, but my hands are bound. An exploratory psychosomatic study of patients with dyshidrosis of the hands (cheiropompholyx)]. Z Psychosom Med Psychoanal 27:275–290

Iannaccone S, Sferrazza B, Quattrini A, Smirne S, Ferini-Strambi L (1999) Pompholyx (vesicular eczema) after i.v. immunoglobulin therapy for neurologic disease. Neurology 53:1154–1155

Jain VK, Aggarwal K, Passi S, Gupta S (2004) Role of contact allergens in pompholyx. J Dermatol 31:188–193

Jensen CS, Menné T, Johansen JD (2006) Systemic contact dermatitis after oral exposure to nickel: a review with a modified meta-analysis. Contact Dermatitis 54:79–86

Jensen CS, Menné T, Lisby S, Kristiansen J, Veien NK (2003) Experimental systemic contact dermatitis from nickel: a dose-response study. Contact Dermatitis 49:124–132

Kaaber K, Menné T, Veien N, Hougaard P (1983) Treatment of nickel dermatitis with Antabuse; a double blind study. Contact Dermatitis 9:297–299

Kaaber K, Veien NK, Tjell JC (1978) Low nickel diet in the treatment of patients with chronic nickel dermatitis. Br J Dermatol 98:197–201

Kellum RE (1973) Dyshidrotic hand eczema: a psychotherapeutic approach. Cutis 16:875–878

King CM, Chalmers RJ (1984) A double-blind study of superficial radiotherapy in chronic palmar eczema. Br J Dermatol 111:451–454

Kodlys KW, Meyer RP (1979) Biofeedback training in the therapy of dyshidrosis. Cutis 24:219–221

Kutzner H, Wurzel RM, Wolff HH (1986) Are acrosyringia involved in the pathogenesis of "dyshidrosis"? Am J Dermatopathol 8:109–116

Lantinga H, Nater JP, Coenraads PJ (1984) Prevalence, incidence and course of eczema on the hands and forearms in a sample of the general population. Contact Dermatitis 10:135–139

Lee WJ, Lee DW, Kim CH, Won CH, Chang SE, Lee MW, Choi JH, Moon KC (2009) Pompholyx with bile-coloured vesicles in a patient with jaundice: are sweat ducts involved in the development of pompholyx? J Eur Acad Dermatol Venereol 24(2):235–236

Lehucher-Michel MP, Koeppel MC, Lanteaume A, Sayag J (2000) Dyshidrotic eczema and occupation: a descriptive study. Contact Dermatitis 43:200–205

Lerbaek A, Kyvik KO, Ravn H, Menné T, Agner T (2007) Incidence of hand eczema in a population-based twin cohort: genetic and environmental risk factors. Br J Dermatol 157:552–557

Lerbaek A, Kyvik KO, Ravn H, Menné T, Agner T (2008) Clinical characteristics and consequences of hand eczema – an 8-year follow-up study of a population-based twin cohort. Contact Dermatitis 58:210–216

LeVine MJ, Parrish JA, Fitzpatrick TB (1981) Oral methoxsalen photochemotherapy (PUVA) of dyshidrotic eczema. Acta Derm Venereol 61:570–571

Lodi A, Betti R, Chiarelli G, Urbani CE, Crosti C (1992) Epidemiological, clinical and allergological observations on pompholyx. Contact Dermatitis 26:17–21

Löfgren SM, Warshaw EM (2006) Dyshidrosis: epidemiology, clinical characteristics, and therapy. Dermatitis 17:165–181

Magina S, Barros MA, Ferreira JA, Mesquita-Guimaraes J (2003) Atopy, nickel sensitivity, occupation, and clinical patterns in different types of hand dermatitis. Am J Contact Dermat 14:63–68

Man I, Ibbotson SH, Ferguson J (2004) Photoinduced pompholyx: a report of 5 cases. J Am Acad Dermatol 50:55–60

Meding B, Alderling M, Albin M, Brisman J, Wrangsjö K (2009) Does tobacco smoking influence the occurrence of hand eczema? Br J Dermatol 160:514–518

Meding B, Swanbeck G (1989) Epidemiology of different types of hand eczema in an industrial city. Acta Derm Venereol 69:227–233

Meneghini CL, Angelini G (1979) Contact and microbial allergy in pompholyx. Contact Dermatitis 5:46–50

Menné T, Hjorth N (1983) Pompholyx-dyshidrotic eczema. Semin Dermatol 2:75–80

Miller RM, Coger RW (1979) Skin conductance conditioning with dyshidrotic eczema patients. Br J Dermatol 101:435–440

Montnemery P, Nihlen U, Lofdahl CG, Nyberg P, Svensson A (2005) Prevalence of hand eczema in an adult Swedish population and the relationship to risk occupation and smoking. Acta Derm Venereol 85:429–432

Nielsen NH, Menné T, Kristiansen J, Christensen JM, Borg L, Poulsen LK (1999) Effects of repeated skin exposure to low nickel concentrations: a model for allergic contact dermatitis to nickel on the hands. Br J Dermatol 141:676–682

Niinimaki A (1995) Double-blind placebo-controlled peroral challenges in patients with delayed-type allergy to balsam of Peru. Contact Dermatitis 33:78–83

Odia S, Vocks E, Rakoski J, Ring J (1996) Successful treatment of dyshidrotic hand eczema using tap water iontophoresis with pulsed direct current. Acta Derm Venereol 76:472–474

Ogden S, Clayton TH, Goodfield MJ (2006) Recalcitrant hand pompholyx: variable response to etanercept. Clin Exp Dermatol 31:145–146

Pearce VJ, Mortimer PS (2009) Hand dermatitis and lymphoedema. Br J Dermatol 161:177–180

Petering H, Breuer C, Herbst R, Kapp A, Werfel T (2004) Comparison of localized high-dose UVA1 irradiation versus topical cream psoralen-UVA for treatment of chronic vesicular dyshidrotic eczema. J Am Acad Dermatol 50:68–72

Petersen CS, Menné T (1992) Cyclosporin A responsive chronic severe vesicular hand eczema. Acta Derm Venereol 72:436–437

Pickenacker A, Luger TA, Schwarz T (1998) Dyshidrotic eczema treated with mycophenolate mofetil. Arch Dermatol 134:378–379

Pitche P, Boukari M, Tchangai-Walla K (2006) Factors associated with palmoplantar or plantar pompholyx: a case-control study. Ann Dermatol Venereol 133:139–143

Polderman MC, Govaert JC, le CS, Pavel S (2003) A double-blind placebo-controlled trial of UVA-1 in the treatment of dyshidrotic eczema. Clin Exp Dermatol 28:584–587

Rosen K, Mobacken H, Swanbeck G (1987) Chronic eczematous dermatitis of the hands: a comparison of PUVA and UVB treatment. Acta Derm Venereol 67:48–54

Ruzicka T, Larsen FG, Galewicz D, Horvath A, Coenraads PJ, Thestrup-Pedersen K, Ortonne JP, Zouboulis CC, Harsch M, Brown TC, Zultak M (2004) Oral alitretinoin (9-cis-retinoic acid) therapy for chronic hand dermatitis in patients refractory to standard therapy: results of a randomized, double-blind, placebo-controlled, multicenter trial. Arch Dermatol 140:1453–1459

Ruzicka T, Lynde CW, Jemec GB, Diepgen T, Berth-Jones J, Coenraads PJ, Kaszuba A, Bissonnette R, Varjonen E, Hollo P, Cambazard F, Lahfa M, Elsner P, Nyberg F, Svensson A, Brown TC, Harsch M, Maares J (2008) Efficacy and safety of oral alitretinoin (9-cis retinoic acid) in patients with severe chronic hand eczema refractory to topical corticosteroids: results of a randomized, double-blind, placebo-controlled, multicentre trial. Br J Dermatol 158:808–817

Scerri L (1999) Azathioprine in dermatological practice. An overview with special emphasis on its use in non-bullous inflammatory dermatoses. Adv Exp Med Biol 455:343–348

Schempp CM, Muller H, Czech W, Schopf E, Simon JC (1997) Treatment of chronic palmoplantar eczema with local bath-PUVA therapy. J Am Acad Dermatol 36:733–737

Schiener R, Gottlober P, Muller B, Williams S, Pillekamp H, Peter RU, Kerscher M (2005) PUVA-gel vs. PUVA-bath therapy for severe recalcitrant palmoplantar dermatoses. A randomized, single-blinded prospective study. Photodermatol Photoimmunol Photomed 21:62–67

Schnopp C, Remling R, Mohrenschlager M, Weigl L, Ring J, Abeck D (2002) Topical tacrolimus (FK506) and mometasone furoate in treatment of dyshidrotic palmar eczema: a randomized, observer-blinded trial. J Am Acad Dermatol 46:73–77

Schurmeyer-Horst F, Luger TA, Bohm M (2007) Long-term efficacy of occlusive therapy with topical pimecrolimus in severe dyshidrosiform hand and foot eczema. Dermatology 214:99–100

Semhoun-Ducloux S, Ducloux D, Miguet JP (2000) Mycophenolate mofetil-induced dyshidrotic eczema. Ann Intern Med 132:417

Sezer E, Etikan I (2007) Local narrowband UVB phototherapy vs. local PUVA in the treatment of chronic hand eczema. Photodermatol Photoimmunol Photomed 23:10–14

Staerkjaer L, Menné T (1990) Nickel allergy and orthodontic treatment. Eur J Orthod 12:284–289

Stambaugh MD, DeNittis AS, Wallner PE, Heymann WR (2000) Complete remission of refractory dyshidrotic eczema with the use of radiation therapy. Cutis 65:211–214

Stojanovic D, Nikic D, Lazarevic K (2004) The level of nickel in smoker's blood and urine. Cent Eur J Public Health 12:187–189

Stuckert J, Nedorost S (2008) Low-cobalt diet for dyshidrotic eczema patients. Contact Dermatitis 59:361–365

Swartling C, Naver H, Lindberg M, Anveden I (2002) Treatment of dyshidrotic hand dermatitis with intradermal botulinum toxin. J Am Acad Dermatol 47:667–671

Thelin I, Agrup G (1985) Pompholyx–a one year series. Acta Derm Venereol 65:214–217

Thyssen JP, Maibach HI (2008) Drug-elicited systemic allergic (contact) dermatitis–update and possible pathomechanisms. Contact Dermatitis 59:195–202

Veien N, Menné T (2000) Acute and recurrent vesicular hand dermatitis (pompholyx). In: Menné T, Maibach H (eds) Hand eczema. CRC Press, Boca Raton, pp 147–164

Veien NK (2009) Acute and recurrent vesicular hand dermatitis. Dermatol Clin 27:337–353, vii

Veien NK, Hattel T, Justesen O, Nørholm A (1983) Oral challenge with metal salts. (I). Vesicular patch-test-negative hand eczema. Contact Dermatitis 9:402–406

Veien NK, Hattel T, Justesen O, Nørholm A (1987) Oral challenge with nickel and cobalt in patients with positive patch tests to nickel and/or cobalt. Acta Derm Venereol 67:321–325

Veien NK, Hattel T, Laurberg G (1994) Chromate-allergic patients challenged orally with potassium dichromate. Contact Dermatitis 31:137–139

Veien NK, Hattel T, Laurberg G (1995) Placebo-controlled oral challenge with cobalt in patients with positive patch tests to cobalt. Contact Dermatitis 33:54–55

Veien NK, Hattel T, Laurberg G (1996) Can oral challenge with balsam of Peru predict possible benefit from a low-balsam diet? Am J Contact Dermat 7:84–87

Veien NK, Hattel T, Laurberg G (2008) Hand eczema: causes, course, and prognosis I. Contact Dermatitis 58:330–334

Veien NK, Kaaber K (1979) Nickel, cobalt and chromium sensitivity in patients with pompholyx (dyshidrotic eczema). Contact Dermatitis 5:371–374

Veien NK, Ølholm LP, Thestrup-Pedersen K, Schou G (1999) Long-term, intermittent treatment of chronic hand eczema with mometasone furoate. Br J Dermatol 140:882–886

Vocks E, Plotz SG, Ring J (1999) The dyshidrotic eczema area and severity index – a score developed for the assessment of dyshidrotic eczema. Dermatology 198:265–269

Volden G (1992) Successful treatment of chronic skin diseases with clobetasol propionate and a hydrocolloid occlusive dressing. Acta Derm Venereol 72:69–71

Wollina U (2008) Pompholyx: what's new? Expert Opin Investig Drugs 17:897–904

Wollina U, Karamfilov T (2002) Adjuvant botulinum toxin A in dyshidrotic hand eczema: a controlled prospective pilot study with left–right comparison. J Eur Acad Dermatol Venereol 16:40–42

Yokozeki H, Katayama I, Nishioka K, Kinoshita M, Nishiyama S (1992) The role of metal allergy and local hyperhidrosis in the pathogenesis of pompholyx. J Dermatol 19:964–967

19 Hyperkeratotic Dermatitis of the Palms

Jacob P. Thyssen · Torkil Menné
Department of Dermato-Allergology, National Allergy Research Centre, Gentofte Hospital, Hellerup, Denmark

Core Messages

- Hyperkeratotic hand eczema is uncommon.
- It is characterized by volar, often bilateral, and symmetric hyperkeratosis of the skin.
- It is typically located centrally or proximally in the palms.
- The hyperkeratotic skin tends to crack which may result in painful fissures.
- First-line treatment options include topical corticosteroids, photochemotherapy, and retinoids.
- Recently, the efficacy of oral alitretionion treatment has been evaluated.

1 Introduction

Hyperkeratotic hand eczema is a relatively rare subtype of hand eczema. This hand eczema subtype is characterized by volar, often bilateral, and symmetric thickening of the skin. The lesions are typically located centrally or proximally in the palms and are less defined than, for example, psoriatic lesions. The thick skin tends to crack which may result in painful fissures. Pruritus is usually weak to moderate. In rare instances, the heels and plantar soles may also be affected. A pioneering study found no association with psoriatic HLA subtypes in 32 (21 women and 11 men) patients with hyperkeratotic hand eczema (Hersle and Mobacken 1982) Also, at 10-year follow-up, only 1 of 32 patients had developed psoriasis and histological examination of skin biopsies in nine patients revealed chronic spongiotic dermatitis (Hersle and Mobacken 1982). These findings support that hyperkeratotic hand eczema is a distinct clinical entity different from, for example, psoriasis (Hersle and Mobacken 1982). Whether it is associated with manual work or not has not been fully elucidated. When a diagnosis of hyperkeratotic hand eczema is made, one needs to exclude allergic and irritant contact dermatitis as well as dermatomycosis. Also, one needs to distinguish this disorder from frictional contact dermatitis which is caused by frictional trauma. Other clinical differential diagnoses include psoriasis, pustulosis palmoplantaris, Bazex syndrome, and lymphoma. In many articles, the term "hyperkeratotic hand eczema" is used to describe hand eczema with hyperkeratosis in general although these morphologically associated subtypes may have a different pathogenesis. This distinction should be taken into account when one interprets the outcome of various treatment regimes.

2 Epidemiology

Only few studies have investigated the prevalence of hyperkeratotic hand eczema. In 1964–1965, Agrup questioned and examined 107,206 subjects from Southern Sweden and found that 33 (2.1%) of 1,551 subjects with inflammatory hand dermatosis had hyperkeratotic hand eczema (Agrup 1969). The disorder was more prevalent among men than women (the female/male ratio was 0.6) (Agrup 1969). Furthermore, hyperkeratotic hand eczema was observed in all age groups but seemed to be most prevalent among 40–69 year olds (Agrup 1969). Among 33 subjects with hyperkeratotic hand eczema, four (12.1%) had occupational relevance, ten (30.3%) had previously been examined at the outpatient department of dermatology in Lund, Sweden, and three (9.1%) had been on sick leave due to their condition (Agrup 1969). In 1982–1983, Meding et al. investigated the epidemiology of hand eczema in Gothenburg, Sweden, and found that 29 (2.3%) subjects had hyperkeratotic hand eczema among a total of 1,238 subjects with hand eczema (Meding and Swanbeck 1989). Two (6.9%) subjects had concomitant allergic contact dermatitis on the hands. The female/male ratio was 0.8 (Meding and Swanbeck 1989). Menné et al. found that 14 (2.5%) of 564 Danish patients under investigation for permanent disability had hyperkeratotic eczema (Menne and Bachmann 1979). The female/male ratio was 0.8 (Menne and Bachmann 1979). Finally, a recent study confirmed the low prevalence of hyperkeratotic hand eczema. Thus, 21 (5.3%) of 319 patients in a European multicenter cross-sectional study had hyperkeratotic hand eczema (Diepgen et al. 2009).

T. Rustemeyer, P. Elsner, S.M. John & H.I. Maibach (eds.), *Kanerva's Occupational Dermatology*,
DOI 10.1007/978-3-642-02035-3_19,

The disease was associated with older age groups, a high hand eczema severity index score (HECSI), and with female gender (Diepgen et al. 2009). Hyperkeratotic hand eczema was mainly located on the palms and fingers and was defined as hyperkeratotic morphology in the palms and absence of relevant contact allergy and irritant exposure and exclusion of atopic dermatitis (Diepgen et al. 2009).

3 Treatment

Treatment options for hyperkeratotic hand eczema are plentiful. The use of emollients is a cornerstone of all treatment protocols. Topical therapy includes application of corticosteroids (Saeki et al. 2009), often applied under occlusion. Intermittent control is necessary to prevent atrophy. Also, the use of topical tar products may be effective. However, no randomized, double-blind, placebo-controlled studies have been performed to investigate their efficacy. Keratolytic therapy with salicylic acid preparation in combination with corticosteroids was excellent at reducing hyperkeratosis and fissures in seven patients (Baden 1974). Topical vitamin A acid treatment was investigated in five patients with hyperkeratotic hand eczema but gave severe inflammation (Gunther 1972). Recently, Egawa applied topical vitamin D3 (calcipotriol 50 µg/g and maxacalcitol 25 µg/g) in five patients with hyperkeratotic hand eczema (Egawa 2005). Lesions improved and almost disappeared within 2–8 weeks in all patients (Egawa 2005). Retreatment was effective at reducing relapses (Egawa 2005). Finally, tarazotene has been anecdotally reported for treatment of hyperkeratotic hand eczema (Warshaw 2004).

Topical and oral psoralen photochemotherapy may also be useful treatment modalities (Mobacken et al. 1983; De Rie et al. 1995; Schempp et al. 1997). Mobacken et al. showed that oral psoralen and UVA irradiation (PUVA) was effective in five patients with hyperkeratotic hand eczema (Mobacken et al. 1983). Furthermore, two patients with hyperkeratotic hand eczema showed partial remission following topical PUVA therapy with psoralen in aqueous gel (De Rie et al. 1995). Among 14 patients with chronic hyperkeratotic palmar or plantar eczema, local bath-PUVA therapy had a good effect in 86% (43% cleared and 43% had substantial improvement) and gave no phototoxic effects (Schempp et al. 1997). In a recent study, a better effect of PUVA-gel than PUVA-bath therapy was observed in one of three patients (Schiener et al. 2005).

Systemic treatment options include oral acitretin and alitretinoin. In a Danish single-blind, placebo-controlled study including 29 patients with hyperkeratotic hand eczema, 14 patients received 30 mg acitretin daily whereas 15 patients received daily placebo treatment (Thestrup-Pedersen et al. 2001). Following 4 weeks of treatment, symptoms such as hyperkeratosis, fissures, scaling, itch, redness, and vesicle count were reduced by 51% among patients that received acitretin in comparison to 9% in the placebo group (Thestrup-Pedersen et al. 2001). No further improvement was observed over another 4 weeks. In a Swiss pilot study, 34 (89%) of 38 patients with chronic refractory hand eczema (of which 22 were diagnosed as having classic hyperkeratotic hand eczema subtype) showed a good or very good response to systemic alitretinoin treatment (20 mg or 40 mg) lasting 1–5 months (Bollag and Ott 1999). "Good" and "very good" were defined as 61–80% and 81–100% reduction of lesions, respectively. All subtypes of hand eczema responded in a similar way. Only mild side effects such as cheilitis, transient headache, and transient flush to the head were recorded. The duration of remission after discontinuation of successful therapy was 1 month to more than 1 year (Bollag and Ott 1999). The above findings were confirmed in a double-blind, randomized, placebo-controlled multicenter study where treatment with oral alitretinoin was performed in 319 patients, of which the majority had hyperkeratotic hand eczema (Ruzicka et al. 2004). However, in this study, "hyperkeratotic hand eczema" was not strictly defined as in the first study using alitretinoin. Treatment with either placebo (n = 78), alitretinoin 10 mg (n = 80), 20 mg (n = 80), or 40 mg (n = 81) was conducted over a 12-week period; 53% of patients who were treated with 40 mg alitretinoin per day and 27% of those who received placebo therapy reported complete or nearly complete disappearance of disease signs and symptoms. Physician's global assessment showed that 12% of patients who received placebo and 43% of patients who received 40 mg alitretinoin per day had clearance of their hand eczema. In general, efficacy seemed to be dose dependent. Adverse effects also seemed to be dose dependent and comprised headache, flushing, elevations in serum lipid level, decreased hemoglobin level, and decreased free thyroxin level (Ruzicka et al. 2004). In a recent randomized, double-blind, placebo-controlled multicenter trial, 1,032 patients with hand eczema (85% hyperkeratotic) were enrolled and randomized to treatment with 10 mg (n = 418) or 30 mg (n = 409) alitretinoin or placebo therapy (n = 205) for up to 24 weeks (Ruzicka et al. 2008). Again, hyperkeratotic hand eczema was not defined. This study also found a dose-dependent effect of alitretinoin therapy as clear or almost clear hands were observed in 17% of those who received placebo and in up to 48% of those who received alitretinoin. Recurrence of 75% of symptoms was observed after typically ½ year (Ruzicka et al. 2008).

References

Agrup G (1969) Hand eczema and other hand dermatosis in South Sweden. Acta Derm Venereol 49:1–91

Baden HP (1974) Treatment of hyperkeratotic dermatitis of the palms. Sequential treatment with a keratolytic gel and corticosteroid ointment. Arch Dermatol 110:737–738

Bollag W, Ott F (1999) Successful treatment of chronic hand eczema with oral 9-cis-retinoic acid. Dermatology 199:308–312

De Rie MA, Van Eendenburg JP, Versnick AC et al (1995) A new psoralen-containing gel for topical PUVA therapy: development, and treatment results in patients with palmoplantar and plaque-type psoriasis, and hyperkeratotic eczema. Br J Dermatol 132:964–969

Diepgen TL, Andersen KE, Brandao FM et al (2009) Hand eczema classification: a cross-sectional, multicentre study of the aetiology and morphology of hand eczema. Br J Dermatol 160:353–358

Egawa K (2005) Topical vitamin D3 derivatives in treating hyperkeratotic palmoplantar eczema: a report of five patients. J Dermatol 32:381–386

Gunther S (1972) Topical administration of vitamin A acid (retinoic acid) in palmar keratoses: callosities, hyperkeratotic eczema, hypertrophic lichen planus, pityriasis rubra pilaris. Dermatologica 145:344–347

Hersle K, Mobacken H (1982) Hyperkeratotic dermatitis of the palms. Br J Dermatol 107:195–201

Meding B, Swanbeck G (1989) Epidemiology of different types of hand eczema in an industrial city. Acta Derm Venereol 69:227–233

Menne T, Bachmann E (1979) Permanent disability from skin diseases. A study of 564 patients registered over a six year period. Derm Beruf Umwelt 27:37–42

Mobacken H, Rosen K, Swanbeck G (1983) Oral psoralen photochemotherapy (PUVA) of hyperkeratotic dermatitis of the palms. Br J Dermatol 109:205–208

Ruzicka T, Larsen FG, Galewicz D et al (2004) Oral alitretinoin (9-cis-retinoic acid) therapy for chronic hand dermatitis in patients refractory to standard therapy: results of a randomized, double-blind, placebo-controlled, multicenter trial. Arch Dermatol 140:1453–1459

Ruzicka T, Lynde CW, Jemec GB et al (2008) Efficacy and safety of oral alitretinoin (9-cis retinoic acid) in patients with severe chronic hand eczema refractory to topical corticosteroids: results of a randomized, double-blind, placebo-controlled, multicentre trial. Br J Dermatol 158:808–817

Saeki H, Watanabe R, Tsunemi Y, Tamaki K (2009) Severe hyperkeratotic palmoplantar eczema (eczema tyloticum). J Dermatol 36:362–363

Schempp CM, Muller H, Czech W et al (1997) Treatment of chronic palmoplantar eczema with local bath-PUVA therapy. J Am Acad Dermatol 36:733–737

Schiener R, Gottlober P, Muller B et al (2005) PUVA-gel vs. PUVA-bath therapy for severe recalcitrant palmoplantar dermatoses. A randomized, single-blinded prospective study. Photodermatol Photoimmunol Photomed 21:62–67

Thestrup-Pedersen K, Andersen KE, Menne T, Veien NK (2001) Treatment of hyperkeratotic dermatitis of the palms (eczema keratoticum) with oral acitretin. A single-blind placebo-controlled study. Acta Derm Venereol 81:353–355

Warshaw EM (2004) Therapeutic options for chronic hand dermatitis. Dermatol Ther 17:240–250

20 Atopic Dermatitis

Kristine Breuer[1] · *Thomas Werfel*[2]
[1]Department of Allergology and Occupational Dermatology, Dermatologikum Hamburg, Hamburg, Germany
[2]Department of Dermatology and Allergy, Hannover Medical School, Hannover, Germany

Core Messages

- Previous atopic hand dermatitis and/or flexural eczema increases the risk of developing irritant contact dermatitis at least twofold in individuals exposed to irritants and wet work.
- In contrast to allergic contact dermatitis to haptens, individuals suffering from atopic dermatitis are prone to protein contact dermatitis and contact urticaria to occupational allergens like food stuff or latex proteins.
- It is often difficult to decide whether occupational exposure or constitutional factors have a greater impact for the development of hand eczema in atopic individuals. The diagnostic workup should therefore lead to a distinct diagnosis and allow to quantify the impact of occupational and nonoccupational factors. An exposure-independent course and persistence of eczema after discontinuation of work suggest a preponderance of atopic skin disposition over occupational exposure.
- With regard to atopy and dependent on the morphology of skin lesions as well as the course of the disease, hand eczema may be classified as chronic irritant contact dermatitis with atopic skin disposition, irritant-induced atopic hand eczema, or atopic hand eczema.
- It is a matter of debate whether "dyshidrotic" vesicular hand eczema without a strict exposure-dependent course, with no relevant contact sensitization and normal IgE levels represents "intrinsic" atopic hand eczema or a distinct entity.
- Since several factors contribute to the development of occupational contact dermatitis, a general exclusion of persons with atopic skin disposition or atopic dermatitis from risk occupations is not effective in terms of primary prevention. Instead, individual advice should rather be given to persons at risk and technical, organizational, and personal protection measures, as well as repeated follow-up examinations have to be considered.

1 Introduction

Atopic dermatitis (AD) is a chronic inflammatory skin disease that commonly begins in early infancy, runs a course of relapses and remissions, and is associated with a characteristic distribution and morphology of skin lesions. Furthermore, pruritus and consequent sleeplessness are hallmarks of AD.

A complex interaction between susceptibility genes, host environments, and specific immunologic responses are involved into the pathogenesis of atopic dermatitis (AD). AD is associated with a deficient epidermal barrier function and irritants play an important role in the initiation and perpetuation of inflammatory lesions. Therefore, AD is often complicated by irritant contact dermatitis in adolescents and adults working in occupations with a continuous exposure to irritants and wet work.

2 Epidemiology, Pathophysiology, and Clinical Features of Atopic Dermatitis

The prevalence of AD has at least doubled in industrialized countries over the past three decades; 15–30% of children and 2–10% of adults suffer from AD (Williams and Flohr 2006). The 12-month prevalence in 11-year-old children ranged from 1% to 20% in the Global International Study of Asthma and Allergies in Childhood trial; prevalence was highest in Northern Europe (Anonymus 1998).

A total of 45% of all cases of AD begin within the first 6 months of life (Kay et al. 1994). Up to 70% of the children suffering from AD have a spontaneous remission before adolescence but may develop occupational irritant contact dermatitis and/or various clinical manifestations of atopic dermatitis in occupationally exposed skin later on (Skudlik and John 2007) (see also ➋ Sect. 6 of this chapter). The clinical presentation of atopic dermatitis is dependent on the age: In infants, erythematous lesions with oozing and crusting are typically located on the cheeks and the scalp. Older children commonly show more chronic lesions with lichenified papules and plaques involving the flexural folds, the wrists, and ankles, but may also have eczema on the hands and feet. In adolescence and adulthood, atopic dermatitis is most frequently located at the face

T. Rustemeyer, P. Elsner, S.M. John & H.I. Maibach (eds.), *Kanerva's Occupational Dermatology*,
DOI 10.1007/978-3-642-02035-3_20,

and neck and the flexural folds. Additionally, the hands and feet are frequently involved in this age group.

Numerous trigger factors have been identified for AD in recent decades. Besides inhalant allergens and food allergens, numerous nonspecific trigger factors have been identified such as irritants (e.g., detergents, textiles, chemicals), climatic factors, and colonization with microorganisms like *Staphylococcus aureus* and *Malassezia furfur.* Moreover, also self-allergens may contribute to the pathophysiology of AD (Akdis et al. 2006; Bieber 2008; Breuer et al. 2006; Werfel and Kapp 1998).

Atopic dermatitis, together with allergic asthma, allergic rhinoconjunctivitis, and IgE-mediated food allergy belongs to the so-called atopic diseases. These diseases are commonly associated with an elevated level of total serum IgE and the presence of specific IgE antibodies directed to inhalant or food allergens. Children with atopic dermatitis are at high risk of developing allergic asthma and allergic rhinitis ("atopic march"). Fifty percent of all children who had AD during the first 2 years of life developed asthma over the subsequent years. A family history of atopy, severe disease, and early sensitization to food allergens were identified as risk factors for asthma in children with AD (Illi et al. 2004; Warner and Esg 2001). However, 20% of all adult patients with atopic dermatitis have normal IgE serum levels. This subtype of AD has been described as "intrinsic" AD, often having a late onset (>20 years of life) and a lack of IgE sensitization against food and inhalant allergens (Schmid-Grendelmeier et al. 2001). In children, a transient form of AD with low serum IgE levels and without any detectable sensitization is observed. Later on, these children show increasing IgE levels and develop IgE sensitizations against inhalant and food allergens ("extrinsic" AD) (Novembre et al. 2001).

A complex interaction between susceptibility genes encoding skin barrier molecules and markers of the inflammatory response, host environments, infectious agents, and specific immunologic responses are involved in the pathophysiology of AD.

Asymptomatic skin in AD differs from normal skin. Lesional but also non-lesional skin of patients with atopic dermatitis has a deficient permeability barrier, and barrier function impairment of uninvolved skin has been related to the severity of atopic dermatitis. This is reflected by an increased transepidermal water loss (TEWL), a decrease in the stratum corneum hydration, and an increased permeation of irritants such as sodium lauryl sulfate (SLS) or polyethylene glycol (Jakasa et al. 2007). Over the last decades, lipid abnormalities and an abnormal differentiation process of keratinocytes have been identified as causes of epidermal barrier defects in atopic dermatitis (Cork et al. 2009; Proksch et al. 2009): Atopic dermatitis has been shown to be associated with a decreased level of ceramides and a reduced sphingomyelinase activity, an impaired metabolism of omega-6-unsaturated fatty acids, and an elevated cholesterol and phospholipid content of the epidermis. In patients with atopic dermatitis, the pH of lesional and non-lesional skin is higher than in normal controls, which may inhibit barrier recovery and facilitate barrier breakdown. In addition, an increased epidermal proliferation was observed, which is associated with a reduced expression of the differentiation keratins K1 and K10, whereas the expression of the basal keratins 5 and 14 and the proliferation-associated keratins 6 and 16 as well as the inflammation-associated keratin 17 is increased. The expression of the cornified envelope proteins involucrin and loricrin and of filaggrin is altered. Recently, it became evident that changes in at least three groups of genes encoding structural proteins, epidermal proteases, and protease inhibitors predispose to a deficient skin barrier and increase the risk of developing atopic dermatitis, mutations of the filaggrin gene being the most relevant. Filaggrin "loss of function" mutations (FLG mutations) were detected in about 30% of patients with atopic dermatitis in European countries. This finding was first published by Palmer et al. (2006) and then confirmed by several groups (see reviews Brown and Mc Lean 2009; O'Regan et al. 2009). According to epidemiological studies, the risk of developing atopic dermatitis is significantly increased for carriers of these mutations – in a recent meta-analysis the odds ratio was calculated to be 4.1 in case-control studies and 2.1 in family studies (Cork et al. 2009; Proksch et al. 2009). Due to FLG mutations, several barrier functions are impaired, such as the formation of the cornified envelope, modeling of the corneocyte shape, moisturization through NMF, and lipid lamellae synthesis, as well as the desquamation process (consequences of the increased pH). The described defects are thought to be causal for the susceptibility to irritant contact dermatitis in patients with atopic dermatitis. Furthermore, microscopic studies revealed a sparse perivascular T cell (Th2) infiltrate in unaffected AD skin that is not seen in normal healthy skin (Leung et al. 1983).

The inflammatory mechanisms and immunological aspects which are specific to AD are reviewed in Werfel 2009. In the circulation of AD patients, a Th2 predominance is found which may partly be due to a genetic background of a general Th2 polarization.

Acute skin lesions are characterized by intensely pruritic, erythematous papules associated with excoriation and oozing exudation. Early events in the AD development are the upregulation of pro-inflammatory mediators such as IL-1α, IL-1β, TNF-α, and GM-CSF; the expression of vascular endothelial cell adhesion molecules which lead to T cell-endothelial interaction; and the production of cytokines and chemokines which attract leucocytes like IL-16, CCL-5 (RANTES), CCL-17 (TARC), CCL-22 (MDC), or CCL-27 (CTACK). There is a marked infiltration of mononuclear cells that is histologically similar to that of allergic contact dermatitis and CD4-positive Th cells dominate the cellular infiltrate. Many intralesional T cells show signs of activation and can further be distinguished by CD45RO, a marker of T-memory cells, suggesting a previous contact with antigen or allergen (e.g., food allergens or inhalant allergens), and by cutaneous lymphocyte-associated antigen (CLA). Mononuclear cells and also eosinophils are mainly found in the dermis. Myeloid dendritic cells (Langerhans cells (LC) and inflammatory dendritic epidermal cells (IDEC)) are found in lesional skin of AD. They act as antigen-presenting cells and express the high-affinity receptor for IgE. Whereas LC play a predominant role in the initiation of the allergic immune response by priming naive T cells into T cells of the Th2 type and produce chemokines, IDECS become more prominent in chronic AD lesions and promote Th1 cytokine production from T cells by release of IL-12 and IL18.

In chronic lesions, tissue remodeling can be observed as thickened plaques with increased skin markings (lichenification), increased collagen disposition in the dermis, and dry fibrotic papules. T cells remain present in the chronic phase, although in smaller numbers than seen in acute AD. The maintenance of chronic AD involves the production of GM-CSF and the Th-1like cytokines as well as several remodeling-associated cytokines, such as IL-11 and TGF-β1.

The cytokine switch from Th2 (IL-4, IL13, IL-31) in the acute phase to Th1 (IFN-γ) in the chronic phase is accepted for AD and is supported by IL-12 and IL-18 produced by antigen-presenting cells. Recently, the Th2 cytokine IL-31, which is overexpressed in itching skin inflammations such as AD, has been shown to be a link between skin-infiltrating T cells and pruritus. Recent studies have identified regulatory T cells (T-reg) which control the activation of autoreactive and T-effector cells in the skin of AD patients and functional differences between AD and normal controls were found. However, the relevance of CD4+ Foxp3+ T-regs for the course of AD is still discussed controversially. Apart from the important role of T cells and dendritic cells, keratinocytes have been shown to be of particular relevance as enhancers of the inflammatory response in AD which act as a source of chemokines and cytokines such as thymic stromal lymphopoetin, CXCL10, CCL17, CCL22, CCL27, or IL-15 and are able to respond to cytokines from T cells.

In addition to dysfunctions of the adaptive immune system, defects in the innate immune response have been identified as causal in AD. Most patients with AD are colonized with Staphylococcus *aureus* and treatment with anti-staphylococcal antiseptics and antibiotics can result in the improvement of the skin condition (Breuer et al. 2002). Recent evidence suggests that a deficiency of the antimicrobial peptides dermcidin, cathelicidin LL-37, human β-defensin (HBD)-2, and HBD-3 contributes to the susceptibility to skin infections. Moreover, pattern recognition receptors like the toll-like receptor (TLR)-2 and TLR-9 have been found to be deficient in AD (reviewed in De Benedetto et al. 2009).

With respect to occupational trigger factors of atopic dermatitis, irritants play a significant role in the initiation and perpetuation of inflammatory lesions. Dependent on the causative agent, irritant-induced atopic dermatitis may become manifest at different localizations but most frequently presents as hand eczema. The high proportion of individuals with atopic skin disposition among patients with occupational contact dermatitis was shown in a previous study, where 38% of nearly 300 patients with severe occupational hand dermatitis suffered from irritant-induced atopic eczema (Skudlik and Schwanitz 2004). Since atopic hand dermatitis has been shown to be associated with long-standing disease and long-lasting sick leave as compared to other forms of hand eczema (Cvetkovski et al. 2005; Veien et al. 2008), preventive measures should specifically consider patients with skin atopy.

3 Atopy as a Risk Factor of Occupational Contact Dermatitis

The definition of "atopy" includes AD, allergic asthma, and allergic rhinoconjunctivitis. The prevalence of atopy in the general population is assumed to be 20–30% (Roberts 1987). Since skin atopy seems to be of higher relevance for a predisposition to occupational irritant contact dermatitis than inhalant atopy and flexural eczema may be absent at the time point of the investigation, diagnostic criteria for the identification of patients with atopic skin disposition are helpful. For the diagnosis of AD, several major and minor clinical features based on traditional clinical experience have been proposed by Hanifin and Rajka (1980). Accordingly, at least three basic and three minor criteria have to be present in a patient in order to diagnose AD. As major criteria, a history of flexural eczema, rhinoconjunctivitis, allergic asthma and a family history of atopy, as well as itch when sweating, were described. In order to develop a scoring system to identify patients with atopic skin disposition, Diepgen et al. have compared the prevalence of these basic and minor features in patients with past or present flexural eczema recruited from their Department of Dermatology and in a normal population (Diepgen et al. 1989). Anamnestic and clinical features which had significantly higher prevalences as compared to the normal population and were more frequent than 20% in AD were included in a score system and weighed according to their statistical significance. Past or present flexural eczema was excluded from the score since it was the selection basis. By using this "Erlangen Atopy Score," patients with past or present flexural eczema and normal individuals could be separated well with minimal overlapping. The authors propose that patients with more than 10 points should be considered to have an atopic skin disposition, and patients with 6–10 points should be suspected to be atopics. According to this study, 7% of the investigated normal population was estimated to have an atopic skin disposition, and a further 19% was suspected to be atopic. The Erlangen Atopy Score was validated in a further study by Diepgen et al. (1991). In the framework of the POSH study (Prevention of Occupational Skin Disease in Hairdressers), Uter et al. have applied the Erlangen Atopy Score in a cohort of hairdressing apprentices (Uter et al. 1999a). Similar to Diepgen et al., the different features of the Erlangen atopy score were associated significantly with past or present flexural eczema, but the association was weaker and the discrimination between individuals with past or present flexural eczema and healthy individuals was worse, which points to a lesser validity of single atopy features. According to the authors, the differing results may be due to clinical distinctions between the investigated cohorts with a higher number of patients with pronounced skin lesions and atopic stigmata in the collective recruited from a dermatologic unit as compared to a working population.

Employees in occupations involving a continuous exposure to irritants and wet work are at high risk of developing occupational irritant contact dermatitis. Among others, the hairdressing trade, health-care professions, cleaning occupations, and the metal industry have an outstanding relevance as risk occupations.

Besides occupational exposure to irritants, several epidemiological studies have identified atopic dermatitis as a relevant risk factor for the development of occupational contact dermatitis, whereas the Erlangen atopy score of Diepgen et al. (1989, 1991) seems to be less relevant. However, due to heterogeneous methods applied in these studies, particularly the definitions of "morbidity" (hand eczema/contact dermatitis), "sensitivity" (atopy), and "exposure," and the statistical measure used to calculate the risk of developing occupational contact dermatitis (Odds Ratio versus Relative Risk versus Prevalence Ratio), the comparison and interpretation of the results is difficult. Moreover, some studies have a retrospective design and no physical examination was done. In most of the studies, patch tests were not performed; therefore, irritant contact dermatitis could not be distinguished clearly from allergic contact dermatitis.

As a part of the Swiss Prospective Metal Worker Eczema Study (PROMETES), Berndt et al. have observed more than 200 healthy male trainee metal workers from the beginning of their apprenticeship over a period of 2.5 years (Berndt et al. 1999a, 2000). Nearly 10% of the study population developed signs of hand dermatitis within 6–8 months after starting the training and the 2.5-year incidence was 23%. Mechanical work and an insufficient amount of skin recovery time increased the risk of hand eczema significantly. A history of flexural eczema was reported by 5% of the study population and could be identified as a relevant risk factor for the development of hand dermatitis within the 2.5 year study period (Odds Ratio, OR 4.2), whereas a preexisting metal sensitivity increased the risk for early onset of hand dermatitis within 6 months (OR 6,96). Interestingly, the risk of developing hand dermatitis was not increased for the 4.5% of trainees who had an Erlangen atopy score indicating atopic skin diathesis (score of 10 and above) and single minor atopic features did not have a significant influence on the development of occupational contact dermatitis.

The Prospective Audi Cohort (PACO) study has investigated the incidence and risk factors of occupational hand dermatitis in more than 2,000 trainees of the German Audi AG, and also white-collar workers were included (Funke et al. 1996, 2001). This study takes a variety of work-related factors into account and demonstrates clearly that irritant exposure at the workplace plays an important role in the development of occupational contact dermatitis. The 1-year and 3-year incidence of hand eczema were 8.6% and 14.1%, respectively, and a particularly high rate of dermatitis occurred within the first 6 months. More than 90% of the cases were diagnosed as irritant contact dermatitis, while allergic contact dermatitis was assumed in about 6%. Within 3 years, blue-collar workers had a significant twofold elevated risk of developing occupational hand dermatitis compared to white-collar occupations. On the basis of the 1-year incidence, previous hand eczema or flexural eczema increased the risk of occupational hand eczema significantly (relative risk, RR 6.0 and 4.8, respectively). Furthermore, private exposure to irritants was identified as a further risk factor. Nearly 1,500 subjects were followed up in the PACO II study (mean follow-up period 13.3 years from the beginning of the apprenticeship) (Apfelbacher et al. 2008). Interestingly, the occurrence of hand eczema dropped after the end of apprenticeship and the cumulative incidence of hand eczema was not significantly different between white- and blue-collar workers which points to the fact that the occupational environment becomes less important in the long run.

The POSH (prevention of occupational skin disease in hairdressers) project, a large prospective population-based study, analyzed the risk associated with constitutional and exposure-related factors of occupational hand eczema in >2,000 hairdressing apprentices (Uter et al. 1995, 1998, 1999b). The point prevalence of hand eczema at the end of the apprenticeship was 55%. While previous flexural or hand dermatitis were associated with an increased risk of occupational contact dermatitis in the first year of training (OR 1.7) (Uter et al. 1995), no association was found at the final follow-up examination and only the rare combination of both factors showed a tendency to being a risk factor. The attributable risk for the development of hand eczema was 4% for previous flexural eczema and 13% for previous hand eczema, which means that most cases of hand eczema were not caused by atopy but by exposition to wet work and irritants. While an elevated atopy-score between 7 and 9.5 points was identified as a significant risk factor, the highest score category (10 points and more) was not associated with an increased risk of developing hand dermatitis. Among the clinical signs of the atopy score, only xerosis and Herthoge sign increased morbidity. Moreover, unprotected wet work of more than 2 h duration was shown to be a major risk factor for irritant hand dermatitis while glove wearing diminished the risk. Low absolute humidity and low outside temperature were identified as significant environmental factors doubling the risk of irritant contact dermatitis.

In a recent retrospective cohort study on Swedish female hairdressers using self-administered questionnaires, the attributable fraction of hand eczema from childhood eczema was 9.6% (Lind et al. 2007). Skin atopy and hairdressing had a synergistic effect on the development of hand dermatitis. For about half of the females with hand eczema, the onset was before the age of 20 years.

Nilsson et al. studied the prevalence and risk factors of occupational hand eczema in 1613 hospital workers and found a period prevalence of 41% over 20 months. Previous atopic dermatitis was identified as a significant risk factor (OR 3). Occupational and domestic wet work further increased the risk (Nilsson et al. 1985).

Few investigators have identified inhalant atopic diseases as risk factors of irritant contact dermatitis. In a prospective study on the development of occupational contact dermatitis in the car manufacturing industry, >1,500 new employees were observed during the first year of employment. Besides previous hand eczema and atopic dermatitis, wool intolerance and hay fever were significantly associated with the occurrence of hand eczema (Kristensen 1992). Since no adjustment for confounders was performed in this study, the data have to be interpreted cautiously. In a small retrospective cohort study which included 111 nurses, Smit et al. identified respiratory atopy as a risk factor for the development of hand dermatitis (Smit and Coenraads 1993). In a cross-sectional study on 1,375 geriatric nurses, a history of allergic rhinitis was associated with an increased risk of hand eczema (OR 1.5), while no association was found for childhood flexural eczema (Skudlik et al. 2009).

Due to the difficulties to define the term "atopy" and the failure of the Erlangen atopy score to predict the development of irritant contact dermatitis, several investigators aimed to identify predictors of individual susceptibility by use of cutaneous bioengineering methods. John et al. followed a cohort of hairdresser apprentices for 3 years (John et al. 2000). Neither the Erlangen atopy score nor the basal bioengineering parameters such as transepidermal water loss (TEWL), microcirculation (laser Doppler flow), capacitance (relative skin moisture), pH, sebum, and temperature measured under standardized circumstances previous to the beginning of the apprenticeship were indicators for the development of occupational contact dermatitis during the follow-up period. Apprentices who later developed irritant contact dermatitis showed a significantly higher increase of TEWL in repetitive measurements of exposed skin areas compared to individuals who did not develop skin lesions. Furthermore, there was no significant association between any of the bioengineering parameters and the atopy score or preexisting atopic dermatitis (hand eczema and/or flexural eczema).

In the framework of PROMETES, different biophysical tests were performed in metalwork trainees and none of the single methods were appropriate to identify individuals at high risk of developing irritant contact dermatitis (Berndt et al. 1999b). A combination of irritation tests with dimethyl sulfoxid (DMSO) and NaOH allowed to identify individuals who developed contact dermatitis during their apprenticeship with a high sensitivity of >90% but a low specificity of <25%. Therefore, the results of cutaneous bioengineering methods are not predictive for the manifestation of occupational skin diseases and do not correlate with preexisting atopic dermatitis or the Erlangen atopy score.

In conclusion, the studies presented above demonstrate that occupational irritant contact dermatitis is a complex disease with a multifactorial pathogenesis involving several constitutional and exogenous risk factors. Wet work performed for at least 2 h daily increases the risk of developing irritant contact dermatitis at least twofold. Furthermore, previous atopic dermatitis (hand dermatitis and/or flexural eczema) is an independent risk factor which adds a further minimum twofold risk to individuals exposed to irritants and wet work. This is a multiplicative effect, which means that the risk of hand eczema in persons with atopic dermatitis who are exposed to occupational irritants is increased at least four times. No association was found with the "minor atopic criteria" or the Erlangen atopy score and only few studies identified inhalant atopy being a significant risk factor. On the other hand, private exposure to irritants and environmental factors (i.e., climate) have been found to be factors increasing the risk of occupational contact dermatitis significantly. Importantly, the impact of atopic dermatitis on the development of occupational hand eczema is dependent on the intensity of occupational exposure to irritants and wet work – in professions associated with an intensive exposure to irritants, a smaller proportion of hand eczema cases will be attributed to atopic dermatitis than in professions with a low or even no exposure to irritants. According to Rystedt et al. (1985), one fourth of individuals with childhood atopic dermatitis working in high-risk professions do not develop hand eczema and two thirds of individuals with childhood atopic dermatitis who have no occupational exposure to irritants suffer from atopic hand dermatitis.

The data suggest that the exclusion of persons with "atopic skin disposition" or atopic dermatitis from risk occupations is not effective in terms of primary prevention and that improvement of working conditions for all employees in risk occupations, individual advice, and use of skin protection measures are of fundamental importance for the prophylaxis of occupational contact dermatitis. Moreover, the relevance of periodical examinations for the prevention of occupational contact dermatitis, specifically in early phases of the apprenticeship is underlined by the study results.

4 Pathogenesis of Occupational Contact Dermatitis in Patients with Atopic Dermatitis

More than half of all patients with active atopic dermatitis exhibit hand involvement dependent on the age (Simpson et al. 2006). With regard to atopic hand eczema, occupational exposure to irritants, specifically wet work, plays an important role in the manifestation and perpetuation of skin lesions.

Patients with altered epidermal barrier function are prone to developing irritant contact dermatitis and existing dermatitis, irrespective of type, enhances reactivity to irritants in other body locations (Slowodnik et al. 2008). This is also the case in patients with atopic dermatitis since the constitutionally deficient epidermal barrier allows the penetration of irritants through the skin, in this way facilitating the interaction with local immune cells. In contrast, individuals with isolated mucosal atopy have a similar barrier function as normal individuals (Conti et al. 1996). This concept is supported by a number of epidemiological studies which have been discussed above.

Cutaneous contact with irritants causes a nonspecific reaction of the skin (Slowodnik et al. 2008): Irritants such as detergents may emulsify the skin surface lipids which are then washed off. Even more important is the increase of the skin pH, leading to an inhibition of enzymes which exhibit a low acid pH optimum and are critical for the synthesis of epidermal lipids such as β-glucocerebrosidase whereas enzymes with a neutral pH optimum such as the serine proteases KLK5 and KLK7 are activated, which play a role in desquamation (Cork et al. 2009). Besides skin barrier dysfunction, direct cellular damage and induction of pro-inflammatory mediators are mechanism which lead to clinical signs of irritant contact dermatitis such as red, dry, scaly, and fissured skin. Keratinocytes play a significant role in the elicitation and perpetuation of irritant contact dermatitis. Skin barrier damage is followed by an upregulation of major histocompatibility complex II antigens and cell adhesion molecules on keratinocytes. Furthermore, pro-inflammatory cytokines such as tumor necrosis factor-alpha (TNF-α), interleukin (IL)-1α, and IL-1β, are released. The chemokine CCL21 is also upregulated and attracts T lymphocytes expressing the CLA antigen to the skin. As shown by Proksch et al., barrier disruption is also followed by an increase of epidermal Langerhans cell density (Proksch et al. 1996). On the basis of these findings, it was postulated that skin barrier disruption alone leads to cytokine production and inflammation.

These processes will likely be facilitated if the skin barrier is constitutionally deficient and inflammatory cells are already increased in the skin as is the case in atopic dermatitis. Indeed, after irritation with SLS, the TEWL was significantly increased in patients with atopic dermatitis as compared to normal controls (Cowley and Farr 1992).

As FLG polymorphisms affect the skin barrier, they may also lead to an increase in the susceptibility to irritants and allergens and to the development of irritant contact and allergic contact dermatitis.

Recently, loss-of-function mutations in the filaggrin gene have found to be associated with an increased susceptibility to chronic irritant contact dermatitis (de Jongh et al. 2008). In a recent study, an association between FLG mutations and combined irritant and allergic contact dermatitis was detected (Molin et al. 2009); however, the methodology used is disputable.

5 The Role of Allergic Contact Dermatitis in Atopic Dermatitis

Irritant allergic contact dermatitis is a risk factor for the development of allergic contact sensitization, and the impaired barrier function in lesional skin as well as the cutaneous inflammatory milieu have been shown to favor the penetration of contact allergens and alleviate type IV sensitization (Smith et al. 2002).

The role of atopic dermatitis as a risk factor for the occurrence of type IV sensitization and contact allergy is still a matter of debate and it has been speculated that the deficient barrier function and the cytokine milieu of atopic skin may alleviate sensitization. Allergic contact dermatitis and atopic dermatitis are both mediated by skin homing T lymphocytes and the cutaneous infiltrate is mainly composed of mononuclear cells. Allergic contact dermatitis is triggered by small allergens (haptens) and occurs at the sites of contact. The clinical presentation of both diseases is similar: acute lesions exhibit papulovesiculae, chronic lesions present with dry, erythematous, and lichenified skin. Atopic dermatitis mainly occurs in early infancy, and concomitant allergic contact dermatitis may also develop in this age (Dotterud and Falk 1994, 1995; Giordano-Labadie et al. 1999), which points to a certain overlap between these diseases. With regard to the pathomechanism, TNF-α polymorphisms were detected in patients with allergic contact dermatitis but not in patients with atopic dermatitis (Reich et al. 2003; Westphal et al. 2003).

In a recent study, Heine et al. have retrospectively analyzed patch test data of nearly 54,000 patients collected by the German Information Network of Departments of Dermatology (IVDK) with respect to the frequency of contact allergic reactions in atopic dermatitis as compared to non-atopic controls (Heine et al. 2006). First, occupational allergic contact dermatitis was diagnosed more often in patients with atopic dermatitis than in control individuals without atopic dermatitis. Second, no significant difference with regard to the number of positive patch test reactions to allergens of the standard series was found between the groups, and the frequencies of single, double, or polyvalent sensitization was nearly identical. Third, the frequency of positive patch test reactions to certain common type IV allergen groups (fragrances, emollients, external drugs, rubbers) were significantly higher in patients with atopic dermatitis than in the control group as was the frequency of sensitization to bufexamac, compositae mix, thiuram mix, and (chloro)-methylisothiazolinone (MCI/MI). Patients with atopic dermatitis and concomitant allergic contact dermatitis were more often employed as office workers and nurses than patients with allergic contact dermatitis without atopy. As allergen sources, external drugs and ointments, fragrances, rubbers and gloves, as well as disinfectants were more often identified in patients with atopic dermatitis. This reflects the higher exposure of atopic dermatitis patients to topical emollients and ointments and the higher proportion of employees of the nursing profession among the patients with atopic dermatitis. In conclusion, a generally increased or decreased risk of atopic dermatitis patients to be sensitized to contact allergens was not found in previous studies and the higher frequency of positive patch test reactions to certain allergens may rather reflect a higher exposure than a greater sensitivity. Vice versa, type IV sensitization may trigger atopic dermatitis by the addition of a contact allergic component to the disease. However, with regard to occupational exposure, the development of irritant contact dermatitis in patients with atopic dermatitis may favor the occurrence of allergic contact dermatitis.

The exposure to volatile occupational allergens such as fragrances, constituents of glues, plastics or rubbers, lubricants, wood or metal dust, as well as pharmaceuticals, may lead to airborne contact dermatitis which presents at uncovered skin areas and has to be differentiated from head-and-neck atopic dermatitis (Breuer et al. 2009; Santos and Goossens 2007).

In contrast to allergic contact dermatitis to haptens, atopic dermatitis is a risk factor for the development of protein contact dermatitis and contact urticaria (von Krogh and Maibach 1981). Protein contact dermatitis usually presents as a chronic eczema with episodic acute exacerbations a few minutes after contact with sources of protein allergens, mainly fruits, vegetables, spices, meat, fish, flour, or plants. Kitchen personnel, bakers, and gardeners are at risk of developing protein contact dermatitis.

With respect to the reading and interpretation of patch tests in patients with atopic dermatitis, irritant reactions which are expected to occur more frequently in patients with atopic dermatitis (Brasch et al. 2003), present at well-demarcated areas, and show a decrescendo phenomenon, have to be distinguished from "true" allergic reactions.

6 Occupational Contact Dermatitis – Clinical Presentations in Atopic Patients

Occupational contact dermatitis is not a homogenous entity, but rather a number of eczema types contributing to different clinical presentations. With regard to atopy, hand eczema may be classified using the following diagnoses (Skudlik and John 2007):

1. *Chronic irritant contact dermatitis with atopic skin disposition* becomes manifest as a consequence of occupational exposure to irritants and shows an exposure-dependent course with fast improvement after discontinuation of exposure. It usually presents with erythema, scaling, and fissures and is located at the back of the hands or the interdigital web spaces. Patients have a history of atopic dermatitis or show a combination of the atopy minor criteria according to Diepgen. Chronic irritant contact dermatitis commonly develops slowly over a period of weeks or months and is the result of multiple subthreshold insults induced by weak irritants (Slowodnik et al. 2008).
2. *Irritant-induced atopic hand eczema* becomes manifest or is significantly deteriorated due to occupational exposure. It often presents at the palmar sides of the hands with itch, vesicles, and erythema. The back of the hands and the volar wrists are frequently involved. Irritant-induced atopic hand eczema shows an exposure-dependent course, but it may also show deterioration in work-free periods. It may persist months after discontinuation of exposure.
3. *Atopic hand eczema* shows similar clinical features as 2., but exacerbations and remissions occur independently from occupational exposures. Nonoccupational trigger factors such as climate, exposition to inhalant or food allergens, domestic wet work and others may lead to exacerbation.

It is a matter of debate whether "dyshidrotic" vesicular hand eczema without a strict exposure-dependent course and with no relevant contact sensitization and normal IgE levels represents "intrinsic" atopic hand eczema or a distinct entity (Diepgen et al. 2009).

In long-standing hand eczema, it is often difficult to differentiate etiological types of dermatitis from each other and from allergic contact dermatitis, since with increasing duration, morphology, localization, and course tend to be similar (Cvetkovski et al. 2005; Diepgen et al. 2009). The fact that different forms of hand eczema may occur in parallel, e.g., irritant-induced atopic hand eczema and subsequent allergic contact eczema, further renders the classification of occupational hand eczema difficult.

Moreover, there are constellations which additionally aggravate the classification of job-related eczema: In patients with previous atopic dermatitis, occupational irritant contact dermatitis of the hands may precipitate a flare of generalized eczema which appears clinically consistent with atopic dermatitis. Many of these patients have not had eczema since childhood, and the pathomechanism beyond this phenomenon is largely unknown (Williams et al. 2007).

After discontinuation of occupational exposure, hand eczema may persist with no obvious present cutaneous exposure. This phenomenon is described as "persistent postoccupational dermatitis" (Sajjachareonpong et al. 2004) and the patients often report initial improvement of the skin condition upon removal from exposure before they develop persistent eczema which clinically resembles endogenous eczema. The pathogenesis of persistent postoccupational dermatitis is poorly understood; severity of preceding eczema, cumulative irritation, and atopic skin diathesis have been suggested as risk factors. However, many patients do not exhibit signs of atopy such as elevated IgE and minor atopic features. It has to be discussed whether postoccupational dermatitis represents a kind of "intrinsic" atopic hand eczema. Irrespective of this aspect, it is difficult to define whether the former occupational exposure still has an influence on the skin condition and skin irritability or whether constitutional factors such as atopic dermatitis or skin atopy are pivotal. Persistent postoccupational dermatitis has a substantial impact on the statutory accident insurances, since months or even years after the approval as occupational skin disease, insurances' compensation payments are reviewed and suspended if the disease is believed to be endogenous due to lack of improvement after cessation of work. Previous long-lasting occupational exposure, a long history of occupational hand eczema, and no evidence of remissions after discontinuation of exposure may suggest a predomination of occupational factors as cause of persistent hand eczema.

Therefore, it may be difficult to decide whether in patients with atopic skin disposition, hand eczema:

1. Has primarily been caused (e.g., become manifest) due to occupational exposure
2. Has been significantly deteriorated due to occupational exposure
3. Has been caused primarily by constitutional factors and not by occupational exposure
4. Is causally linked to former occupational exposure in case of persistent lesions upon discontinuation of work

These aspects are of major importance for the compensation of patients who have lost their occupation due to a skin disease.

Taken together, the classification of occupational hand eczema and the quantification of occupational and constitutional factors in patients with atopic dermatitis/atopic skin disposition are difficult and a standardized classification system is needed. Clinical studies should address this aspect.

7 Management of Occupational Contact Dermatitis in Atopic Dermatitis

When occupational contact dermatitis is suspected in patients with atopic dermatitis, the diagnostic workup should lead to a distinct diagnosis (i.e., irritant contact dermatitis, allergic contact dermatitis) and should allow to quantify the impact of occupational and nonoccupational factors.

The history taking should particularly focus on occupational exposures and the course of disease, i.e., the relationship between deterioration and occupational exposure. In order to quantify competitive factors, private exposure to irritants or allergens and seasonal variation have to be asked for. Clinical investigation should consider atopic minor criteria, and patch testing helps to detect contact sensitization. Besides commercially available contact allergens, the patient's own products should be tested whenever possible.

Eventually, the course of the disease has to be observed over a longer period in order to quantify constitutional and exogenous (occupational) factors.

Avoidance of exposure to irritants and allergens and the use of protective equipment and emollients are basic in the treatment of occupational contact dermatitis.

There are studies showing that the application of potent topical corticosteroids (TCS) results in a decrease in the amount of intercellular lipid lamellae and a reduced number of membrane-coated granules at the stratum granulosum-stratum corneum interface (Kao et al. 2003; Sheu et al. 1997). Moreover, potent corticosteroids induce the expression of serin proteases such as KLK7 which are associated with the skin barrier deficiency in atopic dermatitis (Yousef et al. 2000). Though TCS inhibit cutaneous inflammation, they may also cause further damage to the epidermal barrier and may increase the risk of irritant contact dermatitis in patients with atopic dermatitis. Therefore, the long-term use of potent corticosteroids should be avoided, particularly in adolescents.

Since repetitive UV exposure has been shown to elicit hardening of the skin, to suppress cellular proliferation and to modulate the local immune system by a reduction of the amount of Langerhans cells, phototherapy may be considered in adolescents and young adults (Simons et al. 1997). However, according to current guidelines, phototherapy should not be performed in children younger than 12 years.

8 Prevention

As discussed above, the risk of developing occupational contact dermatitis for individuals with atopic skin disposition is dependent on several factors: first, the degree or severity of atopy, second, the level of exposure to occupational irritants, and third, cofactors like domestic exposures. Among the signs and presentations of atopic skin disposition, a history of hand involvement is a major risk factor for the development of occupational contact dermatitis. Preventive strategies have to consider these aspects.

The general exclusion of persons with "atopic skin disposition" or atopic dermatitis from risk occupations is not effective in terms of primary prevention, since several factors contribute to the risk of occupational contact dermatitis; therefore, individual advice should rather be given to persons at risk.

Preemployment examinations are essential in order to identify individuals at risk of developing occupational contact dermatitis. With regard to the results of epidemiological studies, Coenraads and Diepgen have developed a practical guide for occupational (pre)employment counseling of persons with atopic skin disposition (➋ *Table 20.1*) which allocates persons with distinct symptoms and signs of atopy to certain risk groups (Coenraads and Diepgen 1998). Preventive measures for individuals belonging to these risk groups are suggested. According to this guide, occupations with wet work or other exposure to irritants are not advisable for individuals with atopic dermatitis with hand involvement. Technical, organizational, and personal protection measures as well as repeated follow-up examinations in the first 2 years of employment have to be considered for patients with atopic dermatitis without hand involvement. Similarly, the German occupational organizations have developed guidelines for preemployment advice to aspirants of risk occupations and the frequency of follow-up investigations (G-24) which are, however, not obligatory. In contrast, since 2005 the German Ordinance on Hazardous Substances (Gefahrstoffverordnung) stipulates regular examinations for patients employed in risk professions involving ≥4 h wet work.

Table 20.1

A practical guide for occupational (pre)employment counseling of persons with (possible) atopic dermatitis (AD). According to Coenraads and Diepgen (1998)

Step 1: definition of the occupational risk category	Step 2: occupational counseling for each risk category
First risk category: Moderate to severe AD with hand involvement Chronic hand eczema Change of work due to irritant contact dermatitis	**For the first risk category:** Occupations with wet work or other exposures to irritants not advisable Preemployment medical-occupational and medical advice required
Second risk category: AD without involvement of the hands "Dyshidrosis" (past of pompholyx) Allergic rhinitis or asthma in occupations with increased risk for type I allergies (e.g., bakers)	**For the second risk category:** Technical and organizational protection measures Personal protection measures Repeated follow-up examinations every 3 months in the first year and every 6 months in the second year
Third risk category: Evidence of low threshold for non-specific irritants: Wool intolerance Itch due to sweating Unusually dry skin	**For the third risk category:** Technical and organizational protection measures Personal protection measures Follow-up examinations after 6, 12, and 24 months

References

Akdis CA, Akdis M, Bieber T et al (2006) Diagnosis and treatment of atopic dermatitis in children and adults: European Academy of Allergology and Clinical Immunology/American Academy of Allergy, Asthma and Immunology/PRACTALL Consensus Report. J Allergy Clin Immunol 118:152–169

Anonymous (1998) Worldwide variation in the prevalence of asthma, allergic rhinoconjunctivitis, and atopic eczema: ISAAC. The International Study of Asthma and Allergies in Childhood (ISAAC). Lancet 351:1225–1232

Apfelbacher CJ, Radulescu M, Diepgen TL, Funke U (2008) Occurence and prognosis of hand eczema in the car industry: results from the PACO follow-up study (PACO II). Contact Dermatitis 58:322–329

Berndt U, Hinnen U, Iliev D, Elsner P (1999a) Role of atopy score and of single atopic features as risk factors for the development of hand eczema in trainee metal workers. Br J Dermatol 140:922–924

Berndt U, Hinnen U, Iliev D, Elsner P (1999b) Is occupational irritant contact dermatitis predictable by cutaneous bioengeneering methods? Results of the Swiss Metalworkers' Eczema Study (PROMETES). Dermatology 198:351–354

Berndt U, Hinnen U, Iliev D, Elsner P (2000) Hand eczema in metalworker trainees – an analysis of risk factors. Contact Dermatitis 43:327–332

Bieber T (2008) Mechanisms of disease – atopic dermatitis. N Engl J Med 358:1483–1494

Brasch J, Schnuch A, Uter W (2003) Patch-test reaction patterns in patients with a predisposition to atopic dermatitis. Contact Dermatitis 49:197–201

Breuer K, Haeussler S, Kapp A, Werfel T (2002) *Staphylococcus aureus*: colonizing features and influence of an antibacterial treatment in adults with atopic dermatitis. Br J Dermatol 147:55–61

Breuer K, Werfel T, Kapp A (2006) Allergic manifestations of skin diseases – atopic dermatitis. Chem Immunol Allergy 91:76–86

Breuer K, Worm M, Skudlik C, Schröder C, John SM (2009) Occupational airborne contact dermatitis to tetrazepam in a geriatric nurse. J Dtsch Dermatol Ges 7:896–898

Brown SJ, Mc Lean WH (2009) Eczema genetics: current state of knowledge and future goals. J Invest Dermatol 129:543–552

Coenraads PJ, Diepgen TL (1998) Risk for hand eczema in employees with past or present atopic dermatitis. Int Arch Occup Environ Health 71:7–13

Conti A, Di Nardo A, Seidenary S (1996) No alteration of biophysical parameters in the skin of subjects with respiratory atopy. Dermatology 192:317–320

Cork MJ, Danby SG, Vasilopoulos Y et al (2009) Epidermal barrier dysfunction in atopic dermatitis. J Invest Dermatol 129:1892–1908

Cowley NC, Farr PM (1992) A dose-response study of irritant reactions to sodium lauryl sulfate in patients with seborrhoic dermatitis and atopic eczema. Acta Derm Venereol 72:432–435

Cvetkovski RS, Rothman KJ, Olsen J (2005) Relation between diagnoses on severity, sick leave and loss of job among patients with occupational hand eczema. Br J Dermatol 152:93–98

De Benedetto A, Agnihothri R, Mc Girt LY, Bankova LG, Beck LA (2009) Atopic dermatitis: a disease caused by innate immune defects? J Invest Dermatol 129:14–30

de Jongh CM, Khrenova L, Verberk MM et al (2008) Loss-of-function polymorphisms in the filaggrin gene are associated with an increased susceptibility to chronic irritant contact dermatitis: a case-control study. Br J Dermatol 159:621–627

Diepgen TL, Fartasch M, Hornstein OP (1989) Evaluation and relevance of atopic basic and minor features in patients with atopic dermatitis and in the general population. Acta Derm Venereol (Stockh) Suppl 144:50–54

Diepgen TL, Fartasch M, Hornstein OP (1991) Kriterien zur Beurteilung der atopischen Hautdiathese. Dermatosen 39:79–83

Diepgen TL, Andersen KE, Brandao FM et al (2009) Hand eczema classification: a cross-sectional, multicentre study of the aetiology and morphology of hand eczema. Br J Dermatol 160:353–358

Dotterud LK, Falk ES (1994) Metal allergy in north Norwegian schoolchildren and its relationship with ear piercing and atopy. Contact Dermatitis 31:308–313

Dotterud LK, Falk ES (1995) Contact allergy in relation to hand eczema and atopic diseases in north Norwegian school children. Acta Paediatr 84:402–406

Funke U, Diepgen TL, Fartasch M (1996) Risk-group related prevention of atopic hand eczema at the workplace. Curr Probl Dermatol 25:123–132

Funke U, Fartasch M, Diepgen TL (2001) Incidence of work-related hand eczema during apprenticeship: first results of a prospective cohort study in the car industry. Contact Dermatitis 44:166–172

Giordano-Labadie F, Rancé F, Pellegrin F, Bazex J, Dutau G, Schwarze HP (1999) Frequency of contact allergy in children with atopic dermatitis: results of a prospective study of 137 cases. Contact Dermatitis 40:192–195

Hanifin JM, Rajka G (1980) Diagnostic features of atopic dermatitis. Acta Derm Venereol (Stockh) Suppl 92:44–47

Heine G, Schnuch A, Uter W, Worm M (2006) Type-IV sensitization profile of individuals with atopic eczema: results from the Information Network of Departments of Dermatology (IVDK) and the German Contact Dermatitis Research Group (DKG). Allergy 61:611–616

Illi S, von Mutius E, Lau S et al (2004) The natural course of atopic dermatitis from birth to age 7 years and the association with asthma. J Allergy Clin Immunol 113:925–931

Jakasa I, de Jongh CM, Esposito M, Bos JD, Kezic S (2007) Altered penetration of polyethylene glycol into uninvolved skin of atopic dermatitis patients. J Invest Dermatol 127:129–134

John SM, Uter W, Schwanitz HJ (2000) Relevance of multiparametric skin bioengineering in a prospectively-followed cohort of junior hairdressers. Contact Dermatitis 43:161–168

Kao JS, Fluhr JW, Man MQ et al (2003) Short-term glucocorticosteroid treatment compromises both the barrier homeostasis and stratum corneum integrity: inhibition of epidermal lipid synthesis accounts for functional abnormalities. J Invest Dermatol 120:456–464

Kay J, Gawkrodger DJ, Mortimer MJ, Jaron AG (1994) The prevalence of childhood atopic eczema in a general population. J Am Acad Dermatol 30:35–39

Kristensen O (1992) A prospective study on the development of hand eczema in an automobile manufacturing industry. Contact Dermatitis 26:341–345

Leung DYM, Bhan AK, Schneeberger EE, Geha RS (1983) Characterization of the mononuclear cell infiltrate in atopic dermatitis using monoclonal antibodies. J Allergy Clin Immunol 71:47–56

Lind ML, Albin M, Brisman J et al (2007) Incidence of hand eczema in female Swedish hairdressers. Occup Environ Med 64:191–195

Molin S, Vollmer S, Weiss EH, Ruzicka T, Prinz JC (2009) Filaggrin mutations may confer susceptibility of chronic hand eczema characterized by combined allergic and irritant contact dermatitis. Br J Dermatol 161:801–807

Nilsson E, Mikaelsson B, Andersson S (1985) Atopy, occupation and domestic work as risk factors for hand eczema in hospital workers. Contact Dermatitis 13:216–223

Novembre E, Cianferoni A, Lombardi E, Bernardini R, Pucci N, Vierucci A (2001) Natural history of "intrinsic" atopic dermatitis. Allergy 56:452–453

O'Regan GM, Sandilands A, Mc Lean WH, Irvine AD (2009) Filaggrin in atopic dermatitis. J Allergy Clin Immunol 124(3 Suppl 2):R2–R6

Palmer CN, Irvine AD, Terron-Kwiatkowski A et al (2006) Common loss-of-function variants of the epidermal barrier protein filaggrin are a major predisposing factor for atopic dermatitis. Nat Genet 38:441–446

Proksch E, Brasch J, Sterry W (1996) Integrity of the permeability barrier regulates epidermal Langerhans cell density. Br J Dermatol 134:630–638

Proksch E, Fölster-Holst R, Bräutigam M, Sepehrmanesh M, Pfeiffer S, Jensen J-M (2009) Role of the epidermal barrier in atopic dermatitis. J Dtsch Dermatol Ges 7:899–910

Reich K, Westphal G, Konig IR et al (2003) Cytokine gene polymorphisms in atopic dermatitis. Br J Dermatol 148:1237–1241

Roberts DM (1987) The incidence of atopy in a working population. J Soc Occup Med 37:106–110

Rystedt I (1985) Work-related hand eczema in atopics. Contact Dermatitis 12:164–171

Sajjachareonpong P, Cahill J, Keegel T, Saunders H, Nixon R (2004) Persistent post-occupational dermatitis. Contact Dermatitis 51:278–283

Santos R, Goossens A (2007) An update on airborne contact dermatitis: 2001–2006. Contact Dermatitis 57:353–360

Schmid-Grendelmeier P, Simon D, Simon HU, Akdis CA, Wuthrich B (2001) Epidemiology, clinical features, and immunology of the "intrinsic" (non-IgE-mediated) type of atopic dermatitis (constitutional dermatitis). Allergy 56:841–849

Sheu HM, Lee JYY, Chai CY, Kuo K (1997) Depletion of stratum corneum intercellular lipid lamellae and barrier function abnormalities after long-term topical corticosteroids. Br J Dermatol 136:884–890

Simons JR, Bohnen IJ, van der Valk PG (1997) A left-right comparison of UVB phototherapy and topical photochemotherapy in bilateral chronic hand dermatitis after 6 weeks' treatment. Clin Exp Dermatol 22:7–10

Simpson EL, Thompson MM, Hanifin JM (2006) Prevalence and morphology of hand eczema in patients with atopic dermatitis. Dermatitis 17:123–127

Skudlik C, John SM (2007) Irritativ-provoziertes atopisches Ekzem. In: Fuchs T, Aberer W (eds) Kontaktekzem, 2nd edn. Dustri, München-Deisenhofen, pp 201–211

Skudlik C, Schwanitz HJ (2004) Tertiary prevention of occupational skin disease. J Dtsch Dermatol Ges 2:424–433

Skudlik C, Dulon M, Wendeler D, John SM, Nienhaus A (2009) Hand eczema in geriatric nurses in Germany – prevalence and risk factors. Contact Dermatitis 60:136–143

Slowodnik D, Lee A, Nixon R (2008) Irritant contact dermatitis: a review. Australas J Dermatol 49:1–11

Smit HA, Coenraads PJ (1993) A retrospective cohort study on the incidence of hand dermatitis in nurses. Int Arch Occup Environ Health 64:541–544

Smith HR, Basketter DA, McFadden JP (2002) Irritant dermatitis, irritancy and its role in allergic contact dermatitis. Br J Dermatol 27:138–146

Uter W, Gefeller O, Schwanitz HJ (1995) Occupational dermatitis in hairdressing apprentices – early onset irritant skin damage. Curr Probl Dermatol 23:49–55

Uter W, Pfahlberg A, Gefeller O, Schwanitz HJ (1998) Prevalence and incidence of hand dermatitis in hairdressing apprentices: results of the POSH-study. Int Arch Occup Environ Health 71:487–492

Uter W, Schwanitz HJ, Pfahlberg A, Gefeller O (1999a) Zur Validierung des "Atopie-Score" anhand einer berufsdermatologischen Studienkohorte. Allergo J 8:294–296

Uter W, Pfahlberg A, Gefeller O, Schwanitz HJ (1999b) Hand dermatitis in a prospectively-followed cohort of hairdressing apprentices: final results of the POSH study. Contact Dermatitis 41:280–286

Veien NK, Hattel T, Laurberg G (2008) Hand eczema: causes, course, and prognosis. Contact Dermatitis 58:330–334

von Krogh G, Maibach HI (1981) The contact urticaria syndrome – an updated review. J Am Acad Dermatol 5:328–342

Warner JO, Esg (2001) A double-blinded, randomized, placebo-controlled trial of cetirizine in preventing the onset of asthma in children with atopic dermatitis: 18 months' treatment and 18 months' posttreatment follow-up. J Allergy Clin Immunol 108:929–937

Werfel T (2009) The role of leukocytes, keratinocytes, and allergen-specific IgE in the development of atopic dermatitis. J Invest Dermatol 129:1878–1891

Werfel T, Kapp A (1998) Environmental and other major provocation factors in atopic dermatitis. Allergy 53:731–739

Westphal G, Schnuch A, Moessner R et al (2003) Cytokine gene polymorphisms in allergic contact dermatitis. Contact Dermatitis 48:93–98

Williams H, Flohr C (2006) How epidemiology has challenged 3 prevailing concepts about atopic dermatitis. J Allergy Clin Immunol 118:209–213

Williams J, Cahill J, Nixon R (2007) Occupational autoeczematization or atopic eczema precipitated by occupational contact dermatitis? Contact Dermatitis 56:21–26

Yousef GM, Scorilas A, Magklara A, Soosaipillai A, Diamandis EP (2000) The KLK7 (PRSS6) gene, encoding for the stratum corneum chymotryptic enzyme is a new member of the human kallikrein gene family – genomic characterization, mapping, tissue expression and hormonal regulation. Gene 254:119–128

21 Frictional Trauma/Mechanic Skin Diseases

Klaus E. Andersen
Department of Dermatology and Allergy Centre, Odense University Hospital, University of Southern Denmark, Odense, Denmark

Core Messages

- A multifactorial etiology is common.
- Posttraumatic eczema may persist and recur for a long time.
- Constitutional factors such as psoriasis predispose to development of frictional dermatitis.
- Identification of causing exposure often leads to significant improvement and possibly healing of the eczema.
- Hyperkeratosis and calluses of the hands are common job-related "badge of the trade" with minimal effect on morbidity and quality of life.

1 Introduction

The skin is normally flexible and can resist mechanical trauma to a certain degree. However, excessive friction and superficial skin injuries such as abrasions, pressure, stretching, compressions, and cuts may affect the integrity of the skin and lead to skin changes, which may develop into a disease if not counteracted properly by, that is, glove protection. Multiple handicraft jobs carry a risk of mechanical trauma to the skin and subsequent development of mechanically induced skin disorders.

Eczema patients may complain that their eczema appeared after an injury to the skin. It may be a casual coincidence in some cases. However, mechanical trauma may also precipitate eczema and lead to posttraumatic eczema that persist or recur for long periods of time (Mathias and Morrison 1973; Mathias 1988; Warshaw et al. 2003). Further, patients with preexisting skin disease may experience localized aggravation of the disorder as a consequence of mechanical trauma to the site. If a dynamic relationship between trauma end the development of hand eczema is made probable, and no other cause can be found, then it has important medical implications when the injury is job related. This chapter focuses on occupational skin diseases. Darrell S. Wilkinson reviewed dermatitis from repeated trauma in a broader perspective (Wilkinson 1985) (➋ *Table 21.1*).

1.1 Individual Factors

It is likely that genetic factors play a role in determining the response of the skin to mechanical strain.

Exacerbation of atopic dermatitis and psoriasis (both partly inheritable skin diseases) may occur after mechanical trauma. Physiological factors, such as the hydration of the skin, are important (Pedersen and Jemec 2006). Moderate sweating hydrates the corneal layer and increases the coefficient of friction, whereas dry or wet skin diminishes the friction of resistance. Neurological diseases may impair the withdrawal response to mechanical stimuli and lead to injury of the skin.

1.2 Causes and Frequency of Occupational Skin Injuries

By convention, traumatic injuries result from single and brief episodes of cutaneous exposure and a subsequently rapid onset of skin ailment, whereas irritant cutaneous reactions require multiple and prolonged exposures and show a relatively delayed onset of the disorder. Mechanical stress affects significantly the barrier properties of the skin measured by transepidermal water loss and capacitance (Pedersen and Jemec 2006).

➋ *Figure 21.1* lists the number and distribution of occupational injury and illness cases in the USA. in the private industry in 2006. Skin diseases constitute about 1% while cuts, lacerations, and punctures constitute about 10%.

In most cases, the hands are probably involved, but exact figures are lacking. The lack of a standard definition for skin diseases explains the difficulty in obtaining

T. Rustemeyer, P. Elsner, S.M. John & H.I. Maibach (eds.), *Kanerva's Occupational Dermatology*,
DOI 10.1007/978-3-642-02035-3_21,

accurate epidemiological data. However, several studies have found trends, suggesting both an underestimation of, and regular increase in, the frequency and gravity of observed skin diseases (De Craecker et al. 2008). Common complications of skin injuries include scar formation, infection, persistent pain, and contact dermatitis from topical drugs used for treatment. Further, local eczema may also appear and is common in particular susceptible individuals such as amputees (Lyon et al. 2000).

Table 21.1

Various skin manifestations and conditions resulting from mechanical insults (Adapted from Samitz (1985))

1	Lichenification
2	Hyperpigmentation
3	Hyperkeratosis/calluses
4	Fissuring
5	Blistering/friction injury
6	Increased susceptibility to infection
7	Increased susceptibility to irritants and allergens
8	Development of foreign body reactions
9	Traumatic tattoos
10	Pressure urticaria
11	Scars and keloids
12	Cutaneous neoplasms
13	Koebner's phenomenon (psoriasis) from friction
14	Raynaud's phenomenon from vibration

1.3 Hand Eczema Following a Mechanical Injury

Posttraumatic eczema is a poorly understood complication of skin injuries caused by thermal or chemical burns, lacerations, punctures, abrasions, or chemical injury. The interval between the trauma and the development of eczema is usually a few weeks. Mathias (Mathias 1988) divided posttraumatic eczema into two types. It may occur in association with an underlying endogenous eczema (isomorphic reaction of Koebner's phenomenon) or occur as an isolated idiopathic reaction, when longtime follow-up shows that no new lesions develop on nontraumatized skin.

"Koebner´s phenomenon" is a term applied when the dermatosis develops at the site of trauma. It is well known in relation to psoriasis but also occurs in other conditions, such as lichen planus, vitiligo, Darier's disease, and discoid lupus erythematosus. Isomorphic reactions may also be seen in patients with eczema during its active phases. The isomorphic reaction may be the primary manifestation of an endogenous eczema, and probably more frequently, it occurs as a secondary eczema at the site of trauma. The clinical features of posttraumatic eczema are indistinguishable from typical eczema. Often, it presents within

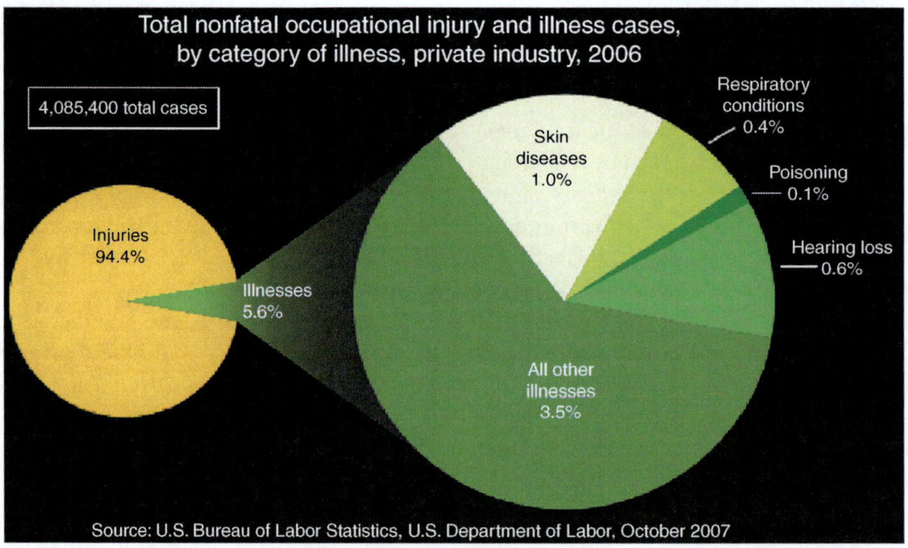

Fig. 21.1

From http://www.bls.gov/iif/oshwc/osh/os/osh06_13.pdf

a few weeks of the acute injury as a discoid or nummular eczema with or without vesicles around the site of trauma. The trauma itself causes obvious damage accompanied by inflammation and regeneration. Fissures, pain, and itching may be pronounced to varying degrees. The posttraumatic eczema may become chronic. The differential diagnosis includes noneczematous skin diseases associated with Koebner's phenomenon, foreign body reactions, bacterial infections, herpes simplex, and secondary allergic contact dermatitis to topical preparations.

1.4 Hand Eczema Following Repeated Friction

Repeated minor mechanical trauma to the skin such as friction, pressure, abrasion, punctures, and shearing forces can cause a variety of skin changes including dermatitis. Dermatitis from friction affects only a small proportion of exposed individuals, depending on constitutional factors and special patterns of exposure. The effects of mechanical forces may be accentuated by other physical agents such as heat and cold.

In a few cases, frictional dermatitis may develop into chronic hand dermatitis. The frictional dermatitis may be elicited by small metal parts, paper and cardboard, driving, fabrics, and other items with a rough surface handled frequently over long periods of time. A Swedish field study among carpet installers revealed that over years, they develop hyperkeratosis on their knuckles and dorsal aspects of the hands as a result of repeated trauma to the skin from friction and pressure (Wahlberg 1985). The scarcity of reports in the literature suggests that hand eczema from repeated mechanical trauma is often mild and that the patients solve the problems themselves by the trial-and-error method. However, frictional dermatitis may often go unrecognized (Paulsen and Andersen 1991; McMullen and Gawkrodger 2006). Mechanical injuries may be an aggravating factor, which together with constitutional factors and exposure to irritants and allergens intensify the degree of hand eczema. Meneghini reported that contact allergy was more prevalent among workers who had sustained cuts, abrasions, and other mechanical injuries compared to those who had not (Meneghini 1985). Further, a Swedish study of 853 hard-metal workers suggested that the traumatic, frictional effect of grinding and etching was an important factor in the development of cobalt allergy (Fischer and Rystedt 1983).

References

De Craecker W, Roskams N, Op de Beeck R (2008) Occupational skin diseases and dermal exposure in the European Union (EU-25): policy and practice overview, vol 6. Office for Official Publications of the European Communities, Luxembourg, pp 7–22

Fischer T, Rystedt I (1983) Cobalt allergy in hard metal workers. Contact Dermatitis 9:115–121

Lyon CC, Kulkarni J, Zimerson E et al (2000) Skin disorders in amputees. J Am Acad Dermatol 42:501–507

Mathias CG (1988) Post-traumatic eczema. Dermatol Clin 6:35–42

Mathias CG, Morrison JH (1973) Occupational skin diseases, United States. Results from the Bureau of Labor Statistics Annual Survey of Occupational Injuries and Illnesses, 1973 through 1984. Arch Dermatol 124:1519–1524

McMullen E, Gawkrodger DJ (2006) Physical friction is under-recognized as an irritant that can cause or contribute to contact dermatitis. Br J Dermatol 154:154–156

Meneghini CL (1985) Sensitization in traumatized skin. Am J Ind Med 8:319–321

Paulsen E, Andersen KE (1991) Irritant contact dermatitis of a gardener's hands caused by handling of fur-covered plant ornaments. Am J Contact Dermat 2:113–116

Pedersen L, Jemec GB (2006) Mechanical properties and barrier function of healthy human skin. Acta Derm Venereol 86:308–311

Samitz MH (1985) Repeated mechanical trauma to the skin: occupational aspects. Am J Ind Med 8:265–271

Wahlberg JE (1985) Occupational hyperkeratoses in carpet installers. Am J Ind Med 8:351–353

Warshaw E, Lee G, Storrs FJ (2003) Hand dermatitis: a review of clinical features, therapeutic options, and long-term outcomes. Am J Contact Dermat 14:119–137

Wilkinson DS (1985) Dermatitis from repeated trauma to the skin. Am J Ind Med 8:307–317

22 Urticaria

Christophe J. Le Coz
Unite Dermato–Allergologie, Hopitaux Universitaires de Strasbourg, Strasbourg, France
Cabinet de Dermatologie, Strasbourg, France
Laboratoire de Dermatochimie, Strasbourg, France

Core Messages

- In occupational contact urticaria, various causative agents have been described, in particular chemicals or proteins.
- The mechanism can be an immunological or non-immunological.
- Natural rubber latex is due to immediatetype.
- Immediate type hypersensitivity reactions to natural latex proteins are well-described causes of occupational contact urticaria, resulting in protein contact dermatitis.
- Identification of occupational contact urticaria, in particular under the clinical picture of protein contact dermatitis is a diagnostic challenge.

1 Introduction

Occupational urticaria (OU) refers to urticaria occurring in work environment. Physical urticaria such as water-induced and cold-induced urticaria can be provoked by occupational activities, but in most circumstances, occupational urticarial symptoms are those of contact urticaria (CU). The term "contact urticaria" was first used by Fisher in 1973 (Wakelin 2001) and then defined by Maibach and Johnson in 1975 as contact urticaria syndrome (CUS) (Maibach and Johnson 1975). Various causative agents can be responsible, chemicals or proteins, with an immunological or non-immunological mechanism. For example, the well-known allergy to natural rubber latex is due to immediate-type hypersensitivity to natural latex proteins, but many other substances and many jobs involving contact with animal and vegetal substances or chemicals can cause CUS. Protein contact dermatitis (PCD) was first described in 1976 (Hjorth and Roed-Petersen 1976), and consists in dermatitis due to immediate-type sensitivity, with frequent acute exacerbation a few minutes after contact of a proteinaceous causative agent. Although less frequent than contact dermatitis, occupational contact urticaria (OCU) may account for almost 30% of occupational allergic skin diseases in Finland (Kanerva et al. 1996).

2 Contact Urticaria

2.1 Clinical Features of CUS and PCD

CUS is a heterogeneous group of skin inflammatory reactions, realizing a transient, wheal-and-flare response at the site of contact with a substance.

CU mainly occurs within minutes after skin or mucosal contact with eliciting agent, and disappears within minutes or hours (<24 h). It consists in erythema and swelling, sometimes angioedema, associated to itching and/or pain, on the site of the contact with the eliciting agent. Spreading of urticarial lesions, generalized urticaria, or extracutaneous symptoms is possible (Von Krogh and Maibach 1981).

Symptoms can be classified in different stages (Ale and Maibach 2000) and are reported in *Table 22.1*. In the first stage, symptoms are localized to the contact area: They can be specific of urticaria (wheal, flare, itching), consist in early signs of protein contact dermatitis, or even be strictly subjective or associated to a discrete erythema (invisible CU). Angioedema, extracutaneous reactions (rhinitis, conjunctivitis, asthma, gastrointestinal symptoms), and even anaphylaxis (and so-called contact anaphylaxis) can occur in severe cases. When the problematic agents are foods, the ingestion can lead to "food contact hypersensitivity syndrome," referring to orally induced food intolerance due to mucosal contact with allergens, which can be sometimes life threatening (Konstantinou and Grattan 2008). Numerous proteinaceous and nonproteinaceous sources have been implicated in CU.

PCD is considered by many authors as a part of CUS (Ale and Maibach 2000; Lachapelle and Maibach 2003). Patients generally have chronic hand dermatitis, mainly located of the hands and the forearms, sometimes on their face. They complain immediate symptoms, occurring with minutes after handling the allergen, with flare of itching, burning, or stinging, accompanied by erythema, swelling (urticaria), or vesicles. Examination after the acute crisis shows chronic or cured hand dermatitis, chronic paronychia, or even fingertip dermatitis (Lachapelle and Maibach 2003). Atopy is more frequent, and irritant

T. Rustemeyer, P. Elsner, S.M. John & H.I. Maibach (eds.), *Kanerva's Occupational Dermatology*,
DOI 10.1007/978-3-642-02035-3_22,

Table 22.1
Stages of CUS according to severity of symptoms

Stages	Symptoms
Stage 1	Localized urticaria, dermatitis, nonspecific symptoms (itching, tingling, burning, etc.)
Stage 2	Generalized urticaria. Cutaneous and extracutaneous reactions
Stage 3	Rhinoconjunctivitis, oro-laryngeal symptoms, asthma, gastrointestinal symptoms
Stage 4	Anaphylaxis

contacts and wet working conditions likely enhance the risk of sensitization and elicitation. PCD is rarely accompanied by anaphylaxis (Willi et al. 2009). Various foods such as fruits, vegetables, meats, and seafood or non-food proteins have been reported as responsible for PCD (Goossens et al. 2007; Amaro and Goossens 2008).

2.2 Physiopathology

CU can be divided into two main types, immunological CU and non-immunological CU, but some substances can induce both types of CU and some situations remain obscure (Bourrain 2006; Doutre 2005; Lachapelle and Maibach 2003; Ale and Maibach 2000).

2.2.1 Immunological CU (ICU)

ICU or allergic CU is an immediate-type (Type 1) hypersensitivity reaction, occurring in patients who have specific IgE against the agent(s) eliciting CU. ICU needs sensitization, and will appear after repeated contacts. ICU is more frequent in people with previous atopic symptoms. The allergen reacts with the IgE at the surface of mast cells and basophiles and provokes release of histamine, except in rare cases in which IgG or IgM responsible for activation of complement has been incriminated.

In such circumstances, symptoms can be severe, with spreading of CU beyond the site of contact, generalized urticaria, and are at higher risk of extracutaneous symptoms and anaphylactic shock. The commonest agents are food proteins (animal or vegetal), animal proteins, and natural rubber latex (Goossens et al. 2007). Some chemicals can also induce immunological CU, contained in drugs, cosmetics, and industrial preparations (Basketter and Lahti 2011; Bourrain 2006; Doutre 2005).

Skin tests such as prick tests are positive, negative in controls, and determination of specific IgE is possible.

2.2.2 Non-immunological CU (NICU)

NICU occurs in people without sensitization to the eliciting agent. Since it needs no sensitization, it can appear during the first contact. The skin penetration of the substance will induce nonspecific release of histamine and other mediators by mast cells, direct effect on dermal vessels by leukotrienes, acetylcholine, prostaglandins, substance P, and other vasoactive amines.

The severity of symptoms, generally restricted to contact area, depends on the amount of skin penetration of the agent: duration of exposure, concentration of the agent, skin permeability, etc. In this situation, severe symptoms like extracutaneous signs and anaphylaxis are generally not expected. Among the numerous substances that can provoke NICU, like plants, animal products, and chemicals, cinnamaldehyde, benzoic acid, sorbic acid, nicotinic acid esters are well-known inducers of NICU (Basketter and Lahti 2011).

Provocation tests are theoretically positive in patients and in controls as well.

2.2.3 Protein Contact Dermatitis

PCD, although clinically presenting as eczema, is mainly defined as a type of dermatitis caused by type I hypersensitivity to protein or proteinaceous materials. However, some combinations of type I and type IV have been discussed (Beck 1982; Matsuo 2010).

2.3 Jobs Exposing to CU

There are extensive lists of proteins and chemicals reported as causing immunological CU (Ale and Maibach 2000; Bourrain 2006; Goossens et al. 2007; Amaro and Goossens 2008; Basketter and Lahti 2011), only a part of them being reported as occupational. Most publications about CU concern case reports or little series and epidemiological studies are scarce. However, some data indicate that CU and PCD are not rare, although frequently underestimated. CU may account for around 30% of occupational allergic skin diseases in Finland (Kanerva et al. 1996), and almost 10% of the total number of patients with occupational skin disease (Williams et al. 2008a). The most frequently affected occupations are farmers, healthcare workers (nurses and dental assistants), veterinarians and domestic animals attendants, bakers and food handlers, and hairdressers. Chemicals (nonproteinaceous allergens) inducing OCU

Table 22.2
Chemicals reported as causing occupational CU immunological (I) type or non-immunological (NI) type (Basketter 2001; Ale and Maibach 2000)

Cosmetic ingredients	Ammonium persulfate (NI, I)
	Basic Blue 99 (I)
	Lawsonia inermis (Henna) (I)
	Myroxylon pereirae (balsam of Peru) (NI, I?)
	Protein hydrolysates (I)
	Para-phenylenediamine (I)
	Ammonium thioglycolate (Shelley et al. 1998)
Industrial and chemical products	Benzonitrile (I) (Li et al. 2004)
	Cyclic acid anhydrides (I) (Helaskoski et al. 2009) such as phthalic, methylhexahydrophthalic, and hexahydrophthalic anhydrides
	di(2-ethylhexyl) phthalate and dibutylphthalate (I) (Sugiura et al. 2002a)
	Diphenylmethane-4-4′-diisocyanate (I) (Valks et al. 2003)
	HATU, HBTU (I) (Yung et al. 2003)
	Methyl Ethyl Ketone (MEK)
	Xylene (I) (Palmer and Rycroft 1993; Weiss and Mowad 1998)
Antibiotics	Cephalosporins: cefotiam (I)
	Penicillins (I): penicillin, amoxicillin, mezlocillin, piperacillin
	Streptomycin (I)
	Beta-lactamase inhibitors: sulbactam (I)
	Macrolides: azithromycin (I)
Fungicides	Albendazole (I) (Macedo et al. 1991)
	Chlorothalonil (I)
Antineoplastic drugs	Cisplatin (I)
Antiparasitic drugs	Pentamidine isethionate (I)
Analgesic antipyretic drugs	Methamizole (I)
Neurop-psychiatric drugs	Levopromazine (I)
	Donepezil (I) (Galvez Lozano et al. 2009)

Table 22.2 (Continued)

Biocides and disinfectants	Chloramine T (I) (Kanerva et al. 1997)
	Chlorhexidine (I)
	Chlorocresol (I, NI)
	Ethanol (NI)
	Formaldehyde (NI, I)
	Phenylmercuric acetate (I)
	Sodium benzoate (NI)
	Didecyl methyl polyoxyethyl ammonium propionate (I)
	Didecyl dimethyl ammonium chloride (I)
Metals and metallic salts	Aluminum (Helgesen and Austad 1997), chromium, cobalt (Krecisz et al. 2009), iridium salts (Bergman et al. 1995), nickel (Estlander et al. 1993; Helgesen and Austad 1997), platinum salts and rhodium (Ale and Maibach 2000), zinc (Farrell 1987)

are listed in *Table 22.2.* Vegetal and animal proteins inducing occupational CU/PCD are reported in *Tables 22.3* and *22.4.*

2.3.1 OCU to Protective Items

Among OCU, natural rubber latex (NRL) remains one of the most frequent agents (Kanerva et al. 1996; Doutre 2005), with a sensitization prevalence of 1–3% in general population and 5–10% in healthcare workers, Europe (Bourrain 2006). Since the 1980s, the wide use of NRL gloves among healthcare workers, in order to prevent blood-borne infections such as viral hepatitis and HIV, has induced the emergence of immediate reactions to NRL protein. NRL gloves are used in various jobs, and nurses, medical or lab technicians, physician's assistants, other clinical professionals, and housekeepers have the highest prevalence of latex glove allergy symptoms (Epling 2011). Other jobs such as hairdressers and glove and dolls manufacturers are at risk (Bourrain 2006). NRL is usually derived from Hevea *brasiliensis* Muell. Arg., family Euphorbiaceae. Among numerous proteins contained in NRL, 13 (named Hev b1 to b13) have been recognized (Doutre 2005, 1987). The risk of sensitization to NRL proteins is highly

Table 22.3

Animal or vegetal products that have caused occupational CU or PCD (Adapted from Ale and Maibach 2000, Basketter and Lahti 2011, and Goossens et al. 2007)

Meat	Beef
	Chicken
	Pork
	Horse
	Calf
	Frog (Goossens et al. 2007)
	Roe deer (Geyer et al. 1998)
Seafood (fishes excepted)	Crab
	Cuttlefish
	Large prawns
	Lobster
	Mussel
	Oysters
	Scallops
	Shrimp
	Squid
Fish	Cod
	Conger eel
	Haddock
	Herring
	Mackerel
	Monkfish
	Perch
	Plaice
	Red mullet
	Salmon
	Sea bream
	Sea perch
	Sole
	Trout
	Tuna
	Whiting
Worms, insects and parasites	*Anisakis simplex* (Scala et al. 2001)
	Cockroaches : *Blaberus giganteus* (Kanerva et al. 1995a) *Periplaneta americana* (Zschunke 1978)
	Chironomus thummi thummi (midge) larvae
	Calliphora vomitoria (maggot)
	Locusta migratoria (African migratory grasshopper) (Lopata et al. 2005)

Table 22.3 (Continued)

	Lumbrinereis impatientis
	Scleroderma domesticum (Lembo and Panariello 2008)
	Tetranychus urticae (spider mite) (Reunala et al. 1983; Jeebhay et al. 2007)
	Tribolium confusum (confused flour beetle) (Alanko et al. 2000)
	Thaumetopoea pityocampa, T. processionea (Ducombs 2007)
	Euproctis chrysorrhoea (Ducombs 2007)
Other animal products	Amniotic fluid
	Blood (calf, pork, cow)
	Cheese (Cheddar, Emmenthal, Parmesan) (Williams et al. 2007a)
	Dander and hair (cow, giraffe, roe deer) (Kanerva and Estlander 1997, Kanerva et al. 1997, Geyer et al. 1998)
	Eggs
	Gut (pork)
	Hair (human, rat, mice)
	Liver (lamb, beef, chicken)
	Mesenteric fat (pork)
	Milk (cow, dog) (Foti et al. 2007)
	Placenta (cow)
	Saliva (calf, cow, rat)
	Serum (amphibian)
	Silk
	Skin (chicken, turkey)
	Sperm (dog) (Krakowiak et al. 2004)
	Urine
	Wools (calf)
Vegetables	Artichoke (Quirce et al. 1996)
	Asparagus (Tabar et al. 2003)
	Beans
	Cabbage
	Carrot
	Castor bean
	Celery
	Chicory (Willi et al. 2009)
	Chive (Alikhan et al. 2009)
	Coffee been (green)
	Cucumber pickles (Weltfriend et al. 1995)
	Endive

Table 22.3 (Continued)

	Garlic (Alikhan et al. 2009)
	Leek (Alikhan et al. 2009)
	Lettuce
	Mustard
	Onion (Alikhan et al. 2009)
	Olives (Williams et al. 2007b)
	Parsley
	Parsnip
	Pepper (red bell p., green bell p., Serrano p., Jalapeno, Pasilla P.) (Alikhan et al. 2009)
	Potato
	Soybean
	Tomato
	Winged bean
Fruits	Apple
	Apricot stone
	Lemon
	Lemon peel
	Lime
	Strawberry (Weltfriend et al. 1995)
	Watermelon
Mushrooms and fungi	Shiitake
	Salami casing molds
Nuts and seeds	Almonds
	Hazelnuts
	Nuts
	Pecan
	Sesam (Keskinen et al. 1991)
Grains and derivatives	Oak
	Corn starch (Fisher 1987)
	Protein hydrolysates
	Barley
	Maize
	Rice
	Rye
	Wheat
Food additives and varia	Beer (Gutgesell and Fuchs 1995)
	Benzaldehyde (Seite-Bellezza 1994)
	Cinnamic aldehyde (Seite-Bellezza 1994)
	Coriander (Ebo et al. 2006)
	Curry
	Paprika (Foti et al. 1997)

Table 22.3 (Continued)

Enzymes	Alpha-amylase
	Cellulase (Tarvainen et al. 1991; Kanerva et al. 1998b)
	Glucoamylase
	Papain (Quiñones et al. 1999)
	Protease (Kanerva and Vanhanen 2001)
	Xylanase (Tarvainen et al. 1991)

enhanced by the use of powdered medical gloves, atopy, and a history of hand dermatitis (Taylor and Praditsuwan 1996; Ale and Maibach 2000). Airborne transmission of the latex allergens is enhanced by their adsorption onto the cornstarch (derived from *Zea mays* L.) used as glove powder (Le Coz et al. 2011). Airborne CU can be associated with rhinitis, conjunctivitis, or asthma. Cross-reactions between NRL proteins and vegetables and fruits or plants have been recognized, mainly tropical fruits, banana, avocado, and chestnuts. The reduction of use of powdered NRL gloves is associated with a decrease in suspected and proved cases of OCU (Allmers et al. 2004).

CU to NRL gloves is exceptionally due to another allergen that latex proteins. A nurse with persistent hand dermatitis strongly reacted to corn, with relevance to cornstarch powder present in many medical examination gloves (Liu and Nixon 2007).

CU to polyethylene gloves was reported in a cook, perhaps due to an antioxidant such as di(2-ethylhexyl) phthalate (DOP) (Sugiura et al. 2002b). DOP used as a plasticizer was implicated in CU from gloves with PVC dots (Sugiura et al. 2000) and was present in work clothes of the same patient, which induced CU as well. He did react to prick tests with DOP and di(2-n-butyl)phthalate (Sugiura et al. 2002a).

CU from nitrile gloves was described in a nurse, with a positive short contact test positive to 2,2'-methylene-bis-(4-methyl-6-tert-butylphenol) used as antioxidant (Horn and Aldridge 2003). Another case of CU induced by nitrile gloves was due to morpholinyl mercaptobenzothiazole (Brehler 1996).

2.3.2 Healthcare Workers

CU from NRL has been largely reported as an occupational problem in health workers with hypersensitivity to latex proteins. Healthcare personnel handle a lot of other sensitizers like antibiotics, antineoplastic drugs, disinfectants, etc. The use of gloves does not always

Table 22.4
Plants and derivatives inducers of OCU/PCD (Ale and Maibach 2000; Goossens et al. 2007; Basketter 2001)

Plants and derivatives	
	Ammi majus (bishop's weed) (Kiistala et al. 1999)
	Camomille (Rudzki et al. 2003)
	Cannabis sativa L. (Williams et al. 2008b)
	Chrysanthemum (Fischer et al. 1999)
	Cinchona (Dooms-Goossens et al. 1986)
	Colophony
	Dianthus caryophillus L.b (carnation) (Vidal and Polo 1998)
	Ficus benjamina (weeping fig) (Kanerva et al. 2001)
	Ficus pumila (creeping fig) (Paulsen et al. 1998)
	Gerbera-Barberton daisy (*Gerbera*) (Estlander et al. 1998; Paulsen et al. 1998)
	Gypsophila paniculata L (Baby's breath) (Vidal and Polo 1998)
	Ivy (Thormann and Paulsen 2008)
	Lilies: *Lilium longiflorum* L. (Vidal and Polo 1998)
	Lime flowers (Rudzki et al. 2003)
	Limonium tataricum (German statice) dried flowers (Quirce et al. 1993)
	Madagascar jasmine (Stephanotis floribunda) (Paulsen et al. 1998)
	Mahogany
	Mentha pulegium (pennyroyal) (Pérez-Calderón et al. 2007)
	Obeche (*Triplochiton scleroxylon*) (Kanerva et al. 1998a)
	Pollens (Uter et al. 2001)
	Poinsettia (*Euphorbia pulcherrima*) (Paulsen et al. 1998)
	Schlumbergera (Christmas cactus) (Paulsen et al. 1997)
	Spathiphyllum wallisii (spathe flower) (Kanerva et al. 2001)
	Tobacco (Tosti et al. 1987)
	Tropical woods (Garcés Sotillos et al. 1995)
	Tulips
	Verbena
	Yucca aloifolia (yucca) (Kanerva et al. 2001)

protect from chemicals, and many substances have been reported as inducers of CU.

Antibiotics include penicillins such as penicillin (Rudzki and Rebandel 1985), amoxicillin (Condé-Salazar et al. 2001), mezlocillin, piperacillin (Kim et al. 2011), cephalosporins such as cefotiam (Shimizu et al. 1996; Miyake et al. 2000), and beta-lactamase inhibitors such as sulbatam (Kwon et al. 2006) streptomycin ().

Cisplatin (Schena et al. 1996), donepezil (Galvez Lozano et al. 2009), pentamidine (Belsito 1993), levopromazine, and methamizole have been reported as well (Warner et al. 1997; Ale and Maibach 2000).

Among disinfectants, quaternary ammonium compounds, a frequent cause of (irritant rather than allergic) contact dermatitis (Lepoittevin 2009), are a rare cause of OCU: didecyl dimethyl ammonium chloride in a catering school (Houtappel et al. 2008) or didecyl methyl polyoxyethyl ammonium propionate in a nurse with a positive prick test at a 1:0.5 × 10^{-4} dilution (Raison-Peyron et al. 2009). Alcohols, and especially ethyl alcohol, can provoke OCU by an immunological or non-immunological mechanism (Ophaswongse and Maibach 1994). Chlorhexidine, widely reported to cause IgE-mediated allergic reactions (from urticaria and angioedema to anaphylaxis) among patients undergoing surgery/invasive procedures, was recently described as occupational IgE-mediated allergen (Nagendran et al. 2009).

2.3.3 Industry Workers

In plastic industry, workers are in contact with highly reacting chemicals, that can be strong sensitizers: epoxy resins (Jolanki et al. 1987; Kanerva et al. 2002), polyfunctional aziridine hardener (Kanerva et al. 1995b; Sartorelli et al. 2003), diphenylmethane-4,4'-diisocyanate (MDI) (Kanerva 1999; Stingeni et al. 2008), (meth)acrylates such as 2-ethylhexyl acrylate (Kanerva et al. 1996). Other chemicals include triphenyl phosphite (Torresani et al. 2003).

Cyclic cid anhydrides are low-molecular-weight chemicals which cause respiratory irritancy and allergy. Phthalic anhydride, methylhexahydrophthalic anhydride, methyltetrahydrophthalic anhydride, and hexahydrophthalic anhydride were responsible for airborne rhinitis and airborne CU in workers (Tarvainen et al. 1995; Kanerva 1999; Yokota et al. 2001; Gutiérrez-Fernández 2007; Helaskoski et al. 2009). Specific IgE were demonstrated to cause them (Helaskoski et al. 2009).

Metals and metallic salts can cause OCU, and aluminum (Helgesen and Austad 1997), chromium, cobalt (Krecisz et al. 2009), iridium salts (Bergman et al. 1995), nickel (Estlander et al. 1993; Helgesen and Austad 1997), platinum salts, and rhodium have been occupationally reported (Ale and Maibach 2000). Among them, platinum salts are important allergens in the catalyst industry and the clinical manifestations may involve both the respiratory system and the skin (Cristaudo et al. 2005). Angioedema and urticaria as acute and late phase reactions to zinc fume exposure were described in a patient who welded zinc at his job (Farrell 1987). In some cases, an immunological mechanism with specific IgE is demonstrated (Estlander et al. 1993).

In pharmaceutical industry (Sherertz 1994), the higher risk of OCU due to the increasing number of sensitizing substances is counterbalanced by the advances of manufacturing technology and primary prevention. OCU has been reported from latex and medicaments, particularly antibiotics such as piperacillin (Moscato et al. 1995) or azithromycin (Milković-Kraus et al. 2007) or to antineoplastic agents such as cisplatin (Warner et al. 1997). The use of volatile or powdered substances can induce airborne CU, as did sodium benzoate (Nethercott et al. 1984) or the antihelminthic drug albendazole (Macedo et al. 1991). In chemistry industry, workers are in contact with highly reactive substances used for synthesis. HBTU (o-(benzotriazol-1-yl)-N,N,N′,N′-tetramethyluronium hexafluorophosphate) and HATU widely used for peptide synthesis induced CU and anaphylaxis (Hannu et al. 2006; Yung et al. 2003).

Among dyes, para-phenylenediamine was the suspected cause of OCU in a doll worker with immediate-type reaction to both PPD and her own black cotton thread (Temesvari 1984).

Formaldehyde was responsible for CU due to leather (Helander 1977).

2.3.4 Hairdressers

Hairdressers are exposed to numerous products causing irritant and allergic contact dermatitis. Occupational CU, although infrequently reported, may occur due to various substances. Ammonium persulfate and other persulfates are used as bleaching agents. They can induce irritant or allergic contact dermatitis, and CU that are most often NICU (Lepoittevin 2009). Generalized CU, rhinitis, asthma, and anaphylactoid reactions have been reported (Ale 2003; Poltronieri et al. 2010) and specific anti-persulfate IgEs have been documented (Aalto-Korte and Mäkinen-Kiljunen 2003).

CU to permanent hair dyes, although rarely and almost exclusively reported in consumers (Le Coz 2007), has been described in a beautician and was due to PPD (Edwards and Edwards 1984).

Protein hydrolysates, formerly collagen or keratin, and recently wheat protein hydrolysates, were responsible from CU in consumers, hairdressers, and beauticians (Niinimäki et al. 1998; Ale and Maibach 2000; Olaiwan et al. 2010).

Some other rare cases have been reported, like immediate hypersensitivity to the acid permanent wave agent glyceryl monothioglycolate (Shelley et al. 1998), to *Lawsonia inermis* – henna (Majoie and Bruynzeel 1996) – or to even human hair and dandruffs (Mikkelsen and Thomsen 1978).

2.3.5 Laboratory Workers and Veterinarians

People working with animals (laboratory workers, scientists, veterinarians, breeders, etc.) have a high risk of allergy to such animals, which was estimated at 20–30% (Ale and Maibach 2000; Aoyama et al. 1992). Other risks concern medicaments and gloves.

Veterinarians are frequently in contact with animal proteins contained in amniotic liquid, placenta, saliva, blood, and animal hair. Obstetric procedures give the higher risk of CU and PCD that is likely enhanced by the repeated hand washing and occlusion due to gloves (Bulcke and Devos 2007; Valsecchi et al. 2003).

Among the numerous animals used for biological research, rat (the most frequently responsible for skin symptoms), mouse, guinea pig, rabbit, hamster, monkey, frog, toads, cats, sheep, and cockroaches have been reported to cause CU, PCD, or extracutaneous symptoms like conjunctivitis, rhinitis, asthma, or even anaphylaxis (Rudzki 1975; Agrup and Sjöstedt 1985; Aoyama et al. 1992; Hesford et al. 1995; Ale and Maibach 2000; Goossens et al. 2007).

2.3.6 Food Industry and Catering

Food industry comprises many activities including farming, food processing, wholesale, and distribution. Workers in food industry and catering are highly exposed to food and food-additives. Such substances are frequently able to induce irritant, allergic dermatitis, contact urticaria, and protein contact dermatitis as well. Moreover, people working in wet environmental conditions are more prone to develop hand eczema. A lot of proteinaceous substances have been reported as inducers of CU and/or PCD. These are listed in ➋ *Table 22.3.*

Epidemiological data are rare, and if the bakers seem to be the most frequently affected by OCU/PCD (Kanerva et al. 1996), cow's dander is the first cause of OCU in Finland (Kanerva and Susitaival 1996; Kanerva et al. 1997).

Chefs, cooks, cold buffet managers, butchers, and sausage makers are in contact with animal proteins in meat, milk, eggs, blood, liver, etc. (Goossens et al. 2007).

Occupational seafood allergy manifests as rhinitis, conjunctivitis, asthma, CU, and PCD (Jeebhay et al. 2001). In the fish industry, prevalence of CU/PCD is 3–11%. One can discern three main groups of causative agents:

- Arthropoda phylum, Crustacea class : crabs, lobsters, prawns, shrimp
- Mollusca phylum, Gastropoda (abalone), Bivalvia (clams, oysters, mussels), and Cephalopoda (squid or cuttlefish) classes
- Pisces phylum (subphylum Chordata), Osteichthyes (bony fish) class: salmon, plaice, tuna, hake, cod, herring, sardine, trout, anchovy, etc.

Among vegetal proteins, numerous fruits, vegetables, plants and plant products, and food additives can induce OCU/PCD. Wheat proteins cause CU and PCD mainly in bakers. Suspected allergens are 27-kD allergen, peroxidase, purple acid phosphatase (Matsuo 2010), and the additive alpha-amylase (Morren et al. 1993).

Some cases are more anecdotal: olives in a pizza worker (Williams et al. 2007b), menthe in a cook (Pérez-Calderón et al. 2007), beer (Garcés Sotillos et al. 1995).

In rare instances, CU/PCD can be due to contaminants such as *Tyrophagus putrescentiae* a storage mite present in ham (Estévez 2006).

Food allergy (food contact hypersensitivity syndrome) after ingestion is possible after occupational sensitization but seems to be rare. Oral syndrome, due to, for example, seafood (Yamaguchi et al. 2007), is a benign situation, but anaphylaxis was reported, for example, in a patient working in a spice factory, who developed urticaria, angioedema, rhinoconjunctivitis, and bronchospasm during handling coriander and fenugreek, and had anaphylaxis from coriander in a meal (Ebo et al. 2006), or generalized urticaria in anaphylaxis in a patient sensitized to Solanaceae and Alliaceae (Alikhan et al. 2009).

2.3.7 Jobs in Contact with Plants and Woods

A lot of workers are concerned by a job with more or less direct contacts with plants: farmers, horticulturists, florists, gardeners, forestry workers, or people in the wood industry.

Numerous plants have been reported as inducers of CU and/or PCD. Some induce CU by an irritant mechanism, while some others lead to immunological CU. Both reactions are possible, as described for tulip (Piirilä et al. 1999).

Probably, the best-known urticant plants are the nettles belonging to family Urticaceae, like *Urtica dioica* L., *U. urens* L., and *U. pilulifera* L. The stinging hairs are disposed on the ventral faces of the leaves, permitting skin penetration of histamine, acetylcholine, and 5-hydroxytryptamine after only a very slight touch (Le Coz et al. 2011). Among other nonprotein substances, plant-derived pharmacological elicitors of urticaria are numerous and include *Myroxylon pereirae* (balsam of Peru) and the cinnamic acid derivatives contained therein, thapsigargin from *Thapsia garganica* L. (family Apiaceae), and capsaicin from different species of capsicum, such as paprika and cayenne (*Capsicum* spp., family Solanaceae). The mechanism by which non-immunological urticant agents elicit their effect (at least for those agents listed above) appears to involve the release of histamine from mast cells.

Most plant and plant products inducing immunological OCU and PCD are listed in ➋ *Table 22.4.* CU and particularly ICU among workers in contact with plant seem underestimated, since in Danish gardeners and greenhouse workers with immediate skin or mucosal reactions to plants, 35 out of 105 people had at least 1 positive reaction likely immunologic to *Schlumbergera cacti, Stephanotis floribunda, Euphorbia pulcherrima* and *Gerbera, Ficus pumila, Gardenia jasminoides, Hibiscus rosasinensis, Campanula, Columnea, Epipremnum aureum, Pelargonium,* and *Primula vulgaris* (Paulsen et al. 1998). A case of OCU with proved sensitization attributable to a gerbera (probably *Gerbera jamesonii* Bolus, family Asteraceae) was published. Conjunctivitis and respiratory symptoms are possible (Estlander et al. 1998). Rhinoconjunctivitis, CU, and dermatitis may occur after handling *Gypsophila paniculata, Dianthus caryophillus,* and *Lilium longiflorum* and were described in a flower supplier with specific IgE (Vidal and Polo 1998). Other plants include *Alstroemeria* (Chan and Oppenheimer 2002). Recently, *Cannabis sativa* has been reported in workers exposed to the plant at work (Williams et al. 2008b).

In general, pollens can induce, in addition to rhinitis, conjunctivitis, and asthma, airborne CU in workers exposed to them, such as florists (Uter et al. 2001). Airborne contact urticaria was reported in a warehouseman as well, resulting from exposure to dust derived from cinchona bark (*Cinchona* spp., family Rubiaceae) (Dooms-Goossens et al. 1986).

In some instances, CU is provoked not by plant themselves, but by several factors present in environment: fungicides or pesticides, wood's parasites, and stinging insects, mainly Lepidoptera with butterflies and caterpillars. Chlorothalonil, a fungicide used for agricultural and horticultural purposes, has been implicated in OCU and anaphylactic symptoms (Dannaker et al. 1993). People in contact with pine processionary moth (*Thaumetopoea pityocampa*) can develop contact urticaria. The larva caterpillar lives usually in pines but also in cedars or larches in Southern Europe and North Africa. CU, frequently associated to airborne and then generalized dermatitis and conjunctivitis, occurs due to urticating hairs containing thaumetopein which induces histamine release, but an immunological mechanism is possible (Ducombs 2007; Vega et al. 2011). *Thaumetopoea processionea* lives in oaks and induces similar manifestation. *Euproctis chrysorrhoea* (browntail moth), present in Europe, North Africa, and Asia, can induce CU as well (Ducombs 2007). Spider mite (*Tetranychus urticae)* can cause CU, and mucosal symptoms and asthma (Reunala et al. 1983; Jeebhay et al. 2007). *Scleroderma domestica* has been implicated in papular CU (although persisting for months) in antique dealers and restorers (Lembo and Panariello 2008). Substances Reported in Occupational CU (Ale and Maibach 2000; Basketter and Lahti 2011; Bourrain 2006).

3 Physical Urticaria

Whatever their mechanism is not occupational, physical urticaria can occur wholly or partly in the workplace (Engel and Lipsker 2009). On can distinguish several syndromes: symptomatic dermographism, delayed pressure urticaria, vibratory, heat, cold, solar and aquagenic urticaria. Every physical urticaria can have occupational consequences.

Symptomatic dermographism is the commonest form of physical urticaria. It combines the triad of erythema, edema, and pruritus, occurring in areas of scratching or friction.

Delayed pressure urticaria is a solid swelling, usually painful, occurring in a several hours delay after heavy and prolonged pressure. Areas most commonly affected are the palms, soles, and buttocks. Systemic manifestations and inflammatory syndrome are possible.

Vibratory urticaria angioedema appears as itchy erythema followed by edema after a vibratory stimulus (e.g., jackhammers).

In ***heat urticaria***, hives appears on areas exposed to heat. It optionally includes mucosal during ingestion of hot foods. This rare situation can be an occupational skin disease as it was in a *churros*-maker (Miranda-Romero et al. 1998).

Cholinergic urticaria consists in numerous pruritic papules, often surrounded by an erythematous halo, appearing during or after exercise with sweating, stress, taking a bath or hot shower, entering a warm store after being in a cold atmosphere, etc. Systemic manifestations are possible.

Aquagenic urticaria occurs at the site of contact with water, with generally follicular papules. The electrolyte composition and temperature of water can influence the occurrence of lesions.

Solar urticaria appears within minutes of sun exposure. Events may extend to the areas covered and accompanied by general signs. A refractory period is generally observed. It may be confounded with photoallergic contact urticaria (Basketter and Lahti 2011).

Cold urticaria is divided into three main sources: familial, acquired idiopathic, and acquired secondary. In familial, autosomal dominant, eruption occurs as erythematous papules and macules, sometimes cyanotic, associated with burning sensations. There are systemic signs such as fever, conjunctivitis, arthralgia, myalgia, and inflammation. The most frequent, idiopathic acquired form consists of superficial or deep lesions after exposure to cold stimuli: water, air, and objects such as ice, cold rain, cold wind, cold water – for example, swimming in sea water or river – ingestion or contact with cold food or drinks. There is a risk of deep edema after ingestion of cold foods, or even shock after swimming in cold water (sometimes only $<20°$). In the acquired secondary form, the manifestations are the same, sometimes associated with necrotic purpura in areas exposed to cold. CU is associated to proteins that precipitate: cryoglobulin, cryofibrinogen, cold agglutinins.

4 Diagnostic

Diagnosis of OCU is based on the patient's previous medical history, chronology, and description of skin symptoms, skin prick tests, and blood determination of specific IgE whenever possible in contact urticaria. In physical urticaria, tests will realize the trauma that induces urticaria (Lachapelle and Maibach 2003).

Patient's past history will focus on atopic symptoms and atypical (invisible CU with subjective signs only, airborne CU) or extracutaneous symptoms.

With exception to substances inducing NICU, skin tests are generally necessary for diagnosis. In suspected ICU, particularly when standardized allergens are not commercially available, and moreover when the patient had severe symptoms (stages 2–4), in vivo tests have to be performed with caution, the resuscitation facilities being immediately available. An order of skin investigations for evaluation of immediate-type responses has been suggested (Ale and Maibach 2000; Lachapelle and Maibach 2003). Each application is done for 15–30 min, and evaluated after removal and further 30 and 60 min. In case of a positive reaction, further evaluation should be discontinued. Positive (histamine) and negative (saline) controls are recommended, in a patient not treated by antihistaminic drug.

1. Open application on unaffected skin
2. Open application on slightly (or previously) affected skin
3. Occlusive application on unaffected skin
4. Occlusive application on slightly (or previously) affected skin
5. Intraepidermal administration (prick test, scratch test, scratch chamber test)
6. Intradermal injection

Actually, the choice of test depends on symptoms and suspected allergen: dilution according to guidelines and case reports, higher dilution when there are serious symptoms, adequate vehicle (water, saline, petrolatum (?)). Prick tests and prick by prick (with raw material such as foods) will be carefully carried out and interpreted. Rub tests and scratch tests.

Determination of specific IgE by RAST will confirm type I hypersensitivity, but their ordinary detection is restricted to some allergens, particularly when they are nonproteinaceous (e.g., formaldehyde) or necessitate specific laboratory. Basophile activation tests are not routinely performed.

5 Management and Prognostic

Although epidemiological data are scarce, occupational CU seems to have a better prognosis than occupational dermatitis. In a 6-month follow-up study of 1,835 patients with occupational skin disease, Mälkönen considers that prognosis was the best in the 155 patients with OCU, of whom 35% cleared-up (Mälkönen et al. 2009). However, 45% had to change work tasks or occupation, or even lost their job. A Danish study on occupational CU indicated similar results, and was rather associated with a risk of prolonged sick leave (Cvetkovski et al. 2006).

Recently, guidelines based on analysis medical literature were published, concerning prevention, identification, and management of contact dermatitis and CU (Nicholson et al. 2010). Data from 119 papers contributed to evidence statements and several key recommendations for OCU.

Employers and safety personnel have to:

- Remove or reduce exposure to agents causing OCU
- Provide appropriate gloves and cotton liners when it is not possible to remove risk of OCU
- Promote use of after-work creams (not prework)
- Provide information and training for workers about health and safety information
- Refer workers with OCU to physicians having expertise for appropriate workplace adjustment

Health practitioners need to:

- Advise atopic workers that they have an increased risk of OCU, and they have to care for and protect their skin
- Take from worker with CU full occupational history about job, materials used at work, location of the rash, and temporal relationship with work
- Confirm objectively (prick test) for a diagnostic of OCU, because of future employment

References

Aalto-Korte K, Mäkinen-Kiljunen S (2003) Specific immunoglobulin E in patients with immediate persulfate hypersensitivity. Contact Dermatitis 49:22–25

Aalto-Korte K, Susitaival P, Kaminska R, Mäkinen-Kiljunen S (2005) Occupational protein contact dermatitis from shiitake mushroom and demonstration of shiitake-specific immunoglobulin E. Contact Dermatitis 53(4):211–213

Agrup G, Sjöstedt L (1985) Contact urticaria in laboratory technicians working with animals. Acta Derm Venereol 65:111–115

Alanko K, Tuomi T, Vanhanen M, Pajari-Backas M, Kanerva L, Havu K, Saarinen K, Bruynzeel DP (2000) Occupational IgE-mediated allergy to Tribolium confusum (confused flour beetle). Allergy 55:879–882

Ale SI, Maibach HI (2000) Occupational contact urticaria. In: Kanerva L, Elsner P, Wahlberg JE, Maibach HI (eds) Handbook of occupational dermatology. Springer, Berlin/Heidelberg/New York, pp 200–216

Alikhan A, Chan HP, Maibach HI (2009) Produce-induced contact urticaria and dermatitis: Solanaceae and Alliaceae. Contact Dermatitis 60:174–176

Allmers H, Schmengler J, John SM (2004) Decreasing incidence of occupational contact urticaria caused by natural rubber latex allergy in German health care workers. J Allergy Clin Immunol 114:347–351

Amaro C, Goossens A (2008) Immunological occupational contact urticaria and contact dermatitis from proteins: a review. Contact Dermatitis 58:67–75

Aoyama K, Ueda A, Manda F, Matsushita T, Ueda T, Yamauchi C (1992) Allergy to laboratory animals: an epidemiological study. Br J Ind Med 49:41–47

Basketter D, Lahti A (2011) Immediate contact reactions. In: Johansen JD, Frosch PJ, Lepoittevin JP (eds) Contact dermatitis, 5th edn. Springer, Berlin/Heidelberg, pp 137–153

Belsito DV (1993) Contact urticaria from pentamidine isethionate. Contact Dermatitis 29:158–159

Bergman A, Svedberg U, Nilsson E (1995) Contact urticaria with anaphylactic reactions caused by occupational exposure to iridium salt. Contact Dermatitis 32:14–17

Bourrain JL (2006) Occupational contact urticaria. Clin Rev Allergy Immunol 30:39–46

Brehler R (1996) Contact urticaria caused by latex-free nitrile gloves. Contact Dermatitis 34:296

Bulcke DM, Devos SA (2007) Hand and forearm dermatoses among veterinarians. J Eur Acad Dermatol Venereol 21:360–363

Chan RY, Oppenheimer JJ (2002) Occupational allergy caused by Peruvian lily (*Alstroemeria*). Ann Allergy Asthma Immunol 88(6):638–639

Condé-Salazar L, Guimaraens D, González MA, Mancebo E (2001) Occupational allergic contact urticaria from amoxicillin. Contact Dermatitis 45:109

Condé-Salazar L, Vazquez-Cortes S, Gonzalez de Olano D, Gonzalez-Guerra E, Raya Aguado C, Martinez Sanchez MJ, Canello Heranz MJ, Canello Heranz MJ, Blancas M, Blancas M, Cuevas M (2005) Occupational contact urticaria caused by seafood handling. Contact Dermatitis 53:178

Cristaudo A, Sera F, Severino V, De Rocco M, Di Lella E, Picardo M (2005) Occupational hypersensitivity to metal salts, including platinum, in the secondary industry. Allergy 60:159–164

Cvetkovski RS, Zachariae R, Jensen H, Olsen J, Johansen JD, Agner T (2006) Prognosis of occupational hand eczema: a follow-up study. Arch Dermatol 142:305–311

Dannaker CJ, Maibach HI, O'Malley M (1993) Contact urticaria and anaphylaxis to the fungicide chlorothalonil. Cutis 52:312–315

Dooms-Goossens A, Deveylder H, Duron C, Dooms M, Degreef H (1986) Airborne contact urticaria due to cinchona. Contact Dermatitis 15:258

Doutre MS (2005) Occupational contact urticaria and protein contact dermatitis. Eur J Dermatol 15:419–424

Ducombs G (2007) Erucisme et papillonite. Progrès en Dermato-Allergologie. John Libbey Eurotext, Paris, pp 79–91

Ebo DG, Bridts CH, Mertens MH, Stevens WJ (2006) Coriander anaphylaxis in a spice grinder with undetected occupational allergy. Acta Clin Belg 61:152–156

Edwards EK Jr, Edwards EK (1984) Contact urticaria and allergic contact dermatitis caused by paraphenylenediamine. Cutis 34:87–88

Engel F, Lipsker D (2009) Urticaires. In: Saurat JH, Lachapelle JM, Lipsker D, Thomas L (eds) Dermatologie et infections sexuellement transmissibles. Elsevier, Masson SAS, pp 327–337

Estévez MD (2006) Occupational contact urticaria-dermatitis by *Tyrophagus putrescentiae*. Contact Dermatitis 55:308–309

Estlander T, Kanerva L, Tupasela O, Keskinen H, Jolanki R (1993) Immediate and delayed allergy to nickel with contact urticaria, rhinitis, asthma and contact dermatitis. Clin Exp Allergy 23:306–310

Estlander T, Kanerva L, Tupasela O, Jolanki R (1998) Occupational contact urticaria and type I sensitization caused by gerbera. Contact Dermatitis 38:118–120

Farrell FJ (1987) Angioedema and urticaria as acute and late phase reactions to zinc fume exposure, with associated metal fume fever-like symptoms. Am J Ind Med 12:331–337

Fisher AA, Stengel F (1977) Allergic occupational hand dermatitis due to calf's liver. An urticarial "immediate" type hypersensitivity. Cutis 19:561–565

Fisher AA (1987) Contact urticaria and anaphylactoid reaction due to corn starch surgical glove powder. Contact Dermatitis 16:224–225

Fischer TW, Bauer A, Hipler UC, Elsner P (1999) Non-immunologic contact urticaria from chrysanthemum confirmed by the CAST method. Complement-activated (C5a) cellular antigen stimulation test. Contact Dermatitis 41:293–295

Foti C, Carino M, Cassano N, Panebianco R, Veña GA, Ambrosi L (1997) Occupational contact urticaria from paprika. Contact Dermatitis 37:135

Foti C, Antelmi A, Mistrello G, Guarneri F, Filotico R (2007) Occupational contact urticaria and rhinoconjunctivitis from dog's milk in a veterinarian. Contact Dermatitis 56:169–171

Galvez Lozano JM, Alcantara M, De San Pedro BS, Quiralte J, Caba I (2009) Occupational contact urticaria caused by donepezil. Contact Dermatitis 61:176

Garcés Sotillos MM, Blanco Carmona JG, Juste Picón S, Rodríguez Gastón P, Pérez Giménez R, Alonso Gil L (1995) Occupational asthma and contact urticaria caused by mukali wood dust (Aningeria robusta). J Investig Allergol Clin Immunol 5:113–114

Geyer E, Kränke B, Derhaschnig J, Aberer W (1998) Contact urticaria from roe deer meat and hair. Contact Dermatitis 39:34

Goossens A, Amaro C, Géraut C (2007) Urticaire et dermatite de contact aux protéines en pathologie professionnelle. Progrès en Dermato-Allergologie. John Libbey Eurotext, Paris, pp 57–70

Gutgesell C, Fuchs T (1995) Contact urticaria from beer. Contact Dermatitis 33:436–437

Gutiérrez-Fernández D, Fuentes-Vallejo MS, Rueda-Ygueravides MD, Bartolomé-Zavala B, Foncubierta Fernández A, León Jiménez A (2007) Contact urticaria to phthalic anhydride. J Investig Allergol Clin Immunol 17:422–423

Hannu T, Alanko K, Keskinen H (2006) Anaphylaxis and allergic contact urticaria from occupational airborne exposure to HBTU. Occup Med (Lond) 56:430–433

Haustein UF (1976) Anaphylactic shock and contact urticaria after the patch test with professional allergens. Allerg Immunol (Leipz) 22(4):349–352

Helander I (1977) Contact urticaria from leather containing formaldehyde. Arch Dermatol 113:1443

Helaskoski E, Kuuliala O, Aalto-Korte K (2009) Occupational contact urticaria caused by cyclic acid anhydrides. Contact Dermatitis 60:214–221

Helgesen AL, Austad J (1997) Contact urticaria from aluminium and nickel in the same patient. Contact Dermatitis 37:303–304

Hesford JD, Platts-Mills TA, Edlich RF (1995) Anaphylaxis after laboratory rat bite: an occupational hazard. J Emerg Med 13:765–768

Hjorth N, Roed-Petersen J (1976) Occupational protein contact dermatitis in food handlers. Contact Dermatitis 2:28–42

Horn HM, Aldridge RD (2003) Contact urticaria due to nitrile gloves. Contact Dermatitis 49:163–164

Houtappel M, Bruijnzeel-Koomen CA, Röckmann H (2008) Immediate-type allergy by occupational exposure to didecyl dimethyl ammonium chloride. Contact Dermatitis 59:116–117

Jeebhay MF, Robins TG, Lehrer SB, Lopata AL (2001) Occupational seafood allergy: a review. Occup Environ Med 58:553–562

Jeebhay MF, Baatjies R, Chang YS, Kim YK, Kim YY, Major V, Lopata AL (2007) Risk factors for allergy due to the two-spotted spider mite (*Tetranychus urticae*) among table grape farm workers. Int Arch Allergy Immunol 144:143–149

Jolanki R, Estlander T, Kanerva L (1987) Occupational contact dermatitis and contact urticaria caused by epoxy resins. Acta Derm Venereol Suppl (Stockh) 134:90–94

Kanerva L, Tarvainen K, Tupasela O, Kaarsalo K, Estlander T (1995a) Occupational allergic contact urticaria caused by cockroach (Blaberus giganteus). Contact Dermatitis 33:445–446

Kanerva L, Estlander T, Jolanki R, Tarvainen K (1995b) Occupational allergic contact dermatitis and contact urticaria caused by polyfunctional aziridine hardener. Contact Dermatitis 33:304–309

Kanerva L, Toikkanen J, Jolanki R, Estlander T (1996) Statistical data on occupational contact urticaria. Contact Dermatitis 35:229–233

Kanerva L, Susitaival P (1996) Cow dander: the most common cause of occupational contact urticaria in Finland. Contact Dermatitis 35:309–310

Kanerva L, Estlander T (1997) Immediate and delayed skin allergy from cow dander. Am J Contact Dermat 8:167–169

Kanerva L, Alanko K, Estlander T, Sihvonen T, Jolanki R (1997) Occupational allergic contact urticaria from chloramine-T solution. Contact Dermatitis 37:180–181

Kanerva L, Tuppurainen M, Keskinen H (1998a) Contact urticaria caused by obeche wood (*Triplochiton scleroxylon*). Contact Dermatitis 38:170–171

Kanerva L, Vanhanen M, Tupasela O (1998b) Occupational contact urticaria from cellulase enzyme. Contact Dermatitis 38:176–177

Kanerva L, Alanko K, Jolanki R, Estlander T (1999a) Airborne allergic contact urticaria from methylhexahydrophthalic anhydride and hexahydrophthalic anhydride. Contact Dermatitis 41:339–341

Kanerva L, Grenquist-Nordén B, Piirilä P (1999b) Occupational IgE-mediated contact urticaria from diphenylmethane-4,4-diisocyanate (MDI). Contact Dermatitis 41:50–51

Kanerva L, Vanhanen M (2001) Occupational allergic contact urticaria and rhinoconjunctivitis from a detergent protease. Contact Dermatitis 45:49–51

Kanerva L, Estlander T, Petman L, Mäkinen-Kiljunen S (2001) Occupational allergic contact urticaria to yucca (*Yucca aloifolia*), weeping fig (*Ficus benjamina*), and spathe flower (*Spathiphyllum wallisii*). Allergy 56:1008–1011

Kanerva L, Pelttari M, Jolanki R, Alanko K, Estlander T, Suhonen R (2002) Occupational contact urticaria from diglycidyl ether of bisphenol A epoxy resin. Allergy 57:1205–1207

Kavli G, Moseng D (1987) Contact urticaria from mustard in fish-stick production. Contact Dermatitis 17:153–155

Keskinen H, Ostman P, Vaheri E, Tarvainen K, Grenquist-Norden B, Karppinen O, Nordman H (1991) A case of occupational asthma, rhinitis and urticaria due to sesame seed. Clin Exp Allergy 21:623–624

Kiistala R, Mäkinen-Kiljunen S, Heikkinen K, Rinne J, Haahtela T (1999) Occupational allergic rhinitis and contact urticaria caused by bishop's weed (Ammi majus). Allergy 54:635–639

Kim JE, Kim SH, Kim JH, Bahn JW, Jin HJ, Ye YM, Park HS (2011) A case of piperacillin-induced occupational anaphylaxis: detection of serum IgE to piperacillin-HSA conjugate. J Korean Med Sci 26:682–685

Konstantinou GN, Grattan CE (2008) Food contact hypersensitivity syndrome: the mucosal contact urticaria paradigm. Clin Exp Dermatol 33:383–389

Krakowiak A, Kowalczyk M, Palczyñski C (2004) Occupational contact urticaria and rhinoconjunctivitis in a veterinarian from bull terrier's seminal fluid. Contact Dermatitis 50:385

Krecisz B, Kiec-Swierczynska M, Krawczyk P, Chomiczewska D, Palczynski C (2009) Cobalt-induced anaphylaxis, contact urticaria, and delayed allergy in a ceramics decorator. Contact Dermatitis 60:173–174

Kwon HJ, Kim MY, Kim HO, Park YM (2006) The simultaneous occurrence of contact urticaria from sulbactam and allergic contact dermatitis from ampicillin in a nurse. Contact Dermatitis 54:176–178

Lachapelle JM, Maibach HI (2003) Patch testing. Prick testing. A practical guide. Springer, Berlin/Heidelberg/New York

Le Coz CJ (2007) Les intolérances aux teintures capillaires et leur mise au point allergologique. Progrès en Dermato-Allergologie. John Libbey Eurotext, Paris, pp 99–129

Lepoittevin JP, Le Coz CJ (2009) Dictionnaire des allergènes de contact. Springer, Paris/Berlin/Heidelberg/New York

Le Coz CJ, Ducombs G, Paulsen E (2011) Plant and plant products. In: Johansen JD, Frosch PJ, Lepoittevin JP (eds) Contact dermatitis, 5th edn. Springer, Berlin/Heidelberg, pp 873–925

Lembo S, Panariello L, D'Errico FP, Lembo G (2008) Professional's and non-professional's papular urticaria caused by Scleroderma domesticum. Contact Dermatitis 58:58–59

Li LF, Sujan SA, Li QX (2004) Contact urticaria syndrome from occupational benzonitrile exposure. Contact Dermatitis 50:377–378

Liu W, Nixon RL (2007) Corn contact urticaria in a nurse. Australas J Dermatol 48:130–131

Lopata AL, Fenemore B, Jeebhay MF, Gäde G, Potter PC (2005) Occupational allergy in laboratory workers caused by the African migratory grasshopper Locusta migratoria. Allergy 60:200–205

Lovell CR, Rycroft RJ (1984) Contact urticaria from winged bean the (Psophocarpus tetragonolobus). Contact Dermatitis 10:314–315

Macedo NA, Piñeyro MI, Carmona C (1991) Contact urticaria and contact dermatitis from albendazole. Contact Dermatitis 25:73–75

Maibach HI, Johnson HL (1975) Contact urticaria syndrome. Contact urticaria to diethyltoluamide (immediate type hypersensitivity). Arch Dermatol 111:726–730

Majoie IM, Bruynzeel DP (1996) Occupational immediate-type hypersensitivity to henna in a hairdresser. Am J Contact Dermat 7:38–40

Mälkönen T, Jolanki R, Alanko K, Luukkonen R, Aalto-Korte K, Lauerma A, Susitaival P (2009) A 6-month follow-up study of 1048 patients diagnosed with an occupational skin disease. Contact Dermatitis 61:261–268

Mendoncafz C, Madan V, Austin S, Beck MH (2005) Occupational contact urticaria from walnut associated with hand eczema. Contact Dermatitis 53:173–174

Mikkelsen F, Thomsen K (1978) Occupational contact dermatitis to human hair. Contact Dermatitis 4:165–166

Milković-Kraus S, Macan J, Kanceljak-Macan B (2007) Occupational allergic contact dermatitis from azithromycin in pharmaceutical workers: a case series. Contact Dermatitis 56:99–102

Miranda-Romero A, Navarro L, Pérez-Oliva N, González-López A, García-Muñoz M (1998) Occupational heat contact urticaria. Contact Dermatitis 38:358–359

Miyake H, Morishima Y, Kishimoto S (2000) Occupational contact urticaria syndrome from cefotiam dihydrochloride in a latex-allergic nurse. Contact Dermatitis 43:230–231

Morren MA, Janssens V, Dooms-Gossens A, Van Hoeyveld E, Cornelis A, De Wolf-Peeters C, Heremans A (1993) alpha-Amylase, a flour additive: an important cause of protein contact dermatitis in bakers. J Am Acad Dermatol 29:723–728

Moscato G, Galdi E, Scibilia J, Dellabianca A, Omodeo P, Vittadini G, Biscaldi GP (1995) Occupational asthma, rhinitis and urticaria due to piperacillin sodium in a pharmaceutical worker. Eur Respir J 8:467–469

Nagendran V, Wicking J, Ekbote A, Onyekwe T, Garvey LH (2009) IgE-mediated chlorhexidine allergy: a new occupational hazard? Occup Med (Lond) 59:270–272

Nethercott JR, Lawrence MJ, Roy AM, Gibson BL (1984) Airborne contact urticaria due to sodium benzoate in a pharmaceutical manufacturing plant. J Occup Med 26:734–736

Nicholson PJ, Llewellyn D, English JS, Guidelines Development Group (2010) Evidence-based guidelines for the prevention, identification and management of occupational contact dermatitis and urticaria. Contact Dermatitis 63:177–186

Niinimäki A, Niinimäki M, Mäkinen-Kiljunen S, Hannuksela M (1998) Contact urticaria from protein hydrolysates in hair conditioners. Allergy 53:1078–1082

Olaiwan A, Pecquet C, Mathelier-Fusade P, Francès C (2010) Contact urticaria induced by hydrolyzed wheat proteins in cosmetics. Ann Dermatol Venereol 137:281–284

Ophaswongse S, Maibach HI (1994) Alcohol dermatitis: allergic contact dermatitis and contact urticaria syndrome. A review. Contact Dermatitis 30:1–6

Palmer KT, Rycroft RJ (1993) Occupational airborne contact urticaria due to xylene. Contact Dermatitis 28:44

Paulsen E, Skov PS, Bindslev-Jensen C, Voitenko V, Poulsen LK (1997) Occupational type I allergy to Christmas cactus (*Schlumbergera*). Allergy 52:656–660

Paulsen E, Skov PS, Andersen KE (1998) Immediate skin and mucosal symptoms from pot plants and vegetables in gardeners and greenhouse workers. Contact Dermatitis 39:16

Pérez-Calderón R, Gonzalo-Garijo A, Bartolomé-Zavala B, Lamilla-Yerga A, Moreno-Gastón I (2007) Occupational contact urticaria due to pennyroyal (*Mentha pulegium*). Contact Dermatitis 57:285–286

Piirilä P, Kanerva L, Alanko K, Estlander T, Keskinen H, Pajari-Backas M, Tuppurainen M (1999) Occupational IgE-mediated asthma, rhinoconjunctivitis, and contact urticaria caused by Easter lily (*Lilium longiflorum*) and tulip. Allergy 54:273–277

Poltronieri A, Patrini L, Pigatto P, Riboldi L, Marsili C, Previdi M, Margonari M, Marraccini P (2010) Occupational allergic "march." Rapid evolution of contact dermatitis to ammonium persulfate into airborne contact dermatitis with rhinitis and asthma in a hairdresser. Med Lav 101:403–408

Quiñones D, Alonso S, López R, Sánchez I, Rodríguez F, Fernández L, Jerez J (1999) Contact urticaria, rhinoconjunctivitis and bronchial asthma from occupational use of papain. Allergol Immunopathol (Madr) 27:273–275

Quirce S, García-Figueroa B, Olaguíbel JM, Muro MD, Tabar AI (1993) Occupational asthma and contact urticaria from dried flowers of *Limonium tataricum*. Allergy 48:285–290

Quirce S, Tabar AI, Olaguibel JM, Cuevas M (1996) Occupational contact urticaria syndrome caused by globe artichoke (*Cynara scolymus*). J Allergy Clin Immunol 97:710–711

Raison-Peyron N, Du Thanh A, Dupuis JC, Guillot B (2009) Occupational immediate-type contact allergy to didecyl methyl polyoxyethyl ammonium propionate. Contact Dermatitis 60: 296–298

Reunala T, Björkstén F, Förström L, Kanerva L (1983) IgE-mediated occupational allergy to a spider mite. Clin Allergy 13:383–388

Rudzki E (1975) Contact urticaria due to hairs from a rat's tail. Contact Dermatitis 1:252

Rudzki E, Rebandel P (1985) Occupational contact urticaria from penicillin. Contact Dermatitis 13:192

Rudzki E, Rapiejko P, Rebandel P (2003) Occupational contact dermatitis, with asthma and rhinitis, from camomile in a cosmetician also with contact urticaria from both camomile and lime flowers. Contact Dermatitis 49:162

Ruiz Oropeza A, Fischer Friis U, Duus Johansen J (2011) Occupational contact urticaria caused by didecyl dimethyl ammonium chloride. Contact Dermatitis 64:297–298

Sartorelli P, Pistolesi P, Cioni F, Napoli R, Sisinni AG, Bellussi L, Passali GC, Cherubini Di Simplicio E, Flori L (2003) Skin and respiratory allergic disease caused by polyfunctional aziridine. Med Lav 94: 285–295

Sasseville D (1998) Contact urticaria from epoxy resin and reactive diluents. Contact Dermatitis 38:57–58

Scala E, Giani M, Pirrotta L, Guerra EC, Cadoni S, Girardelli CR, De Pità O, Puddu P (2001) Occupational generalised urticaria and allergic airborne asthma due to anisakis simplex. Eur J Dermatol 11:249–250

Seite-Bellezza D, el Sayed F, Bazex J (1994) Contact urticaria from cinnamic aldehyde and benzaldehyde in a confectioner. Contact Dermatitis 31:272–273

Shelley WB, Shelley ED, Talanin NY (1998) Urticaria due to occupational exposure to glyceryl monothioglycolate permanent wave solution. Acta Derm Venereol 78:471–472

Schena D, Barba A, Costa G (1996) Occupational contact urticaria due to cisplatin. Contact Dermatitis 34:220–221

Sherertz EF (1994) Occupational skin disease in the pharmaceutical industry. Dermatol Clin 12:533–536

Shimizu S, Chen KR, Miyakawa S (1996) Cefotiam-induced contact urticaria syndrome: an occupational condition in Japanese nurses. Dermatology 192:174–176

Stingeni L, Bellini V, Lisi P (2008) Occupational airborne contact urticaria and asthma: simultaneous immediate and delayed allergy to diphenylmethane-4,4′-diisocyanate. Contact Dermatitis 58:112–113

Sugiura K, Sugiura M, Hayakawa R, Sasaki K (2000) Di(2-ethylhexyl) phthalate (DOP) in the dotted polyvinyl-chloride grip of cotton gloves as a cause of contact urticaria syndrome. Contact Dermatitis 43:237–238

Sugiura K, Sugiura M, Hayakawa R, Shamoto M, Sasaki K (2002a) A case of contact urticaria syndrome due to di(2-ethylhexyl) phthalate (DOP) in work clothes. Contact Dermatitis 46:13–16

Sugiura K, Sugiura M, Shiraki R, Hayakawa R, Shamoto M, Sasaki K, Itoh A (2002b) Contact urticaria due to polyethylene gloves. Contact Dermatitis 46:262–266

Tabar AI, Alvarez MJ, Celay E, López R, de Esteban B, Gómez B (2003) Allergy to asparagus. An Sist Sanit Navar 26(Suppl 2):17–23

Tanaka T, Moriwaki SI, Horio T (1987) Occupational dermatitis with simultaneous immediate and delayed allergy to chrysanthemum. Contact Dermatitis 16:152–154

Tarvainen K, Kanerva L, Tupasela O, Grenquist-Nordén B, Jolanki R, Estlander T, Keskinen H (1991) Allergy from cellulase and xylanase enzymes. Clin Exp Allergy 21:609–615

Tarvainen K, Jolanki R, Estlander T, Tupasela O, Pfäffli P, Kanerva L (1995) Immunologic contact urticaria due to airborne methylhexahydrophthalic and methyltetrahydrophthalic anhydrides. Contact Dermatitis 32(4):204–209

Taylor JS, Praditsuwan P (1996) Latex allergy. Review of 44 cases including outcome and frequent association with allergic hand eczema. Arch Dermatol 132:265–271

Temesvari E (1984) Contact urticaria from paraphenylenediamine. Contact Dermatitis 11:125

Thormann H, Paulsen E (2008) Contact urticaria to common ivy (*Hedera helix* cv. 'Hester') with concomitant immediate sensitivity to the labiate family (Lamiaceae) in a Danish gardener. Contact Dermatitis 59:179–180

Torresani C, Zendri E, Vescovi V, De Panfilis G (2003) Contact urticaria syndrome from occupational triphenyl phosphite exposure. Contact Dermatitis 48:237–238

Tosti A, Melino M, Veronesi S (1987) Contact urticaria to tobacco. Contact Dermatitis 16:225–226

Uter W, Nöhle M, Randerath B, Schwanitz HJ (2001) Occupational contact urticaria and late-phase bronchial asthma caused by compositae pollen in a florist. Am J Contact Dermat 12:182–184

Valks R, Conde-Salazar L, Barrantes OL (2003) Occupational allergic contact urticaria and asthma from diphenylmethane-4,4′-diisocyanatae. Contact Dermatitis 49:166–167

Valsecchi R, Leghissa P, Cortinovis R (2003) Occupational contact dermatitis and contact urticaria in veterinarians. Contact Dermatitis 49:167–168

Vega JM, Moneo I, Ortiz JC, Palla PS, Sanchís ME, Vega J, Gonzalez-Muñoz M, Battisti A, Roques A (2011) Prevalence of cutaneous reactions to the pine processionary moth (*Thaumetopoea pityocampa*) in an adult population. Contact Dermatitis 64:220–228

Vidal C, Polo F (1998) Occupational allergy caused by *Dianthus caryophillus*, *Gypsophila paniculata*, and *Lilium longiflorum*. Allergy 53:995–998

Von Krogh G, Maibach HI (1981) The contact urticaria syndrome. An updated review. J Am Acad Dermatol 5:328–342

Wakelin SH (2001) Contact urticaria. Clin Exp Dermatol 26:132–136

Warner MR, Taylor JS, Leow YH (1997) Agents causing contact urticaria. Clin Dermatol 15:623–635

Weiss RR, Mowad C (1998) Contact urticaria from xylene. Am J Contact Dermat 9:125–127

Weltfriend S, Kwangsukstith C, Maibach HI (1995) Contact urticaria from cucumber pickle and strawberry. Contact Dermatitis 32:173–174

Willi R, Pfab F, Huss-Marp J, Buters JT, Zilker T, Behrendt H, Ring J, Darsow U (2009) Contact anaphylaxis and protein contact dermatitis in a cook handling chicory leaves. Contact Dermatitis 60:226–227

Williams JD, Lee AY, Matheson MC, Frowen KE, Noonan AM, Nixon RL (2008a) Occupational contact urticaria: Australian data. Br J Dermatol 159:125–131

Williams C, Thompstone J, Wilkinson M (2008b) Work-related contact urticaria to *Cannabis sativa*. Contact Dermatitis 58:62–63

Williams JD, Moyle M, Nixon RL (2007a) Occupational contact urticaria from Parmesan cheese. Contact Dermatitis 56:113–114

Williams J, Roberts H, Tate B (2007b) Contact urticaria to olives. Contact Dermatitis 56:52–53

Yamaguchi J, Inomata N, Hirokado M, Shimakura K, Shiomi K, Ikezawa Z (2007) A case of occupational contact urticaria and oral allergy syndrome due to seafood. Arerugi 56:49–53

Yokota K, Johyama Y, Miyaue H, Matsumoto N, Yamaguchi K (2001) Occupational contact urticaria caused by airborne methylhexahydrophthalic anhydride. Ind Health 39:347–352

Yung A, Papworth-Smith J, Wilkinson SM (2003) Occupational contact urticaria from the solid-phase peptide synthesis coupling agents HATU and HBTU. Contact Dermatitis 49:108–109

Zschunke E (1978) Contact urticaria, dermatitis and asthma from cockroaches (*Periplaneta americana*). Contact Dermatitis 4:313–314

23 Biologic Causes of Occupational Dermatoses

Jean-Marie Lachapelle
Unit of Occupational and Environmental Dermatology, Catholic University of Louvain, Montigny-le-Tilleul, Belgium

Core Messages

- Many virus skin infections may be of occupational origin : the most classical are orf, milkers' node, herpes simplex, butchers' warts, and hepatitis B.
- Bacterial skin infections of occupational origin are manifold: staphylococcal, streptococcal, erysipeloid, brucellosis, warty tuberculosis, BCG vaccination complications, anthrax, tularemia, and fish tank granuloma (mycobacteriosis).
- MRSA and CA-MRSA is an emerging problem of prime importance.
- A large variety of mycoses are related to occupational and/or recreational activities. They include most kinds of dermatophytoses, candidiasis, subcutaneous and deep mycoses, the latter being predominantly imported skin diseases.
- Protothecosis is the only occupational skin disease due to an algae, Prototheca, mainly in tropical and subtropical countries.

1 Introduction

Strictly speaking, the biologic agents that cause occupational dermatoses comprise the infections and infestations. It is not always easy to define when a natural hazard becomes an occupational or recreational (e.g., sport activities) hazard. Among infections, it is classical to consider viral, microbial, and mycotic infections (and exceptionally due to algae).

2 Virus Infections

Some virus infections are undoubtedly related to occupational activities. The most important ones have been selected, excluding AIDS, the occurrence of which in occupational life is discussed in another chapter.

2.1 Parapoxvirus Infections

Three parapoxviruses of domestic animals occasionally cause infections in humans: orf virus, normally causing a disease of sheep; pseudocowpox (syn.milkers' nodule, paravaccinia); and bovine pustular stomatitis viruses, normally causing diseases of cattle.

Parapoxviruses (DNA viruses) are ovoid particles that vary from about 260 nm long by 160 nm wide for orf virus to 300 nm long by 190 nm wide for pseudocowpox virus. A tubular, threadlike structure 10–20 nm wide and perhaps 1,000 nm long forms a crisscross pattern on the surface of negatively stained parapoxvirus virions.

2.1.1 Orf

It has been recently demonstrated that orf virus infection provides a vigorous skin immune response. However, the virus has acquired a range of immunomodulatory/pathogenesis-related genes that function to limit (at least transiently) the effectiveness of host immunity. With the advent of the orf virus genome sequence, the study of this dynamic process will provide important insights into virus pathogenesis and the host skin immune response to infection (Haig 2006).

The orf virus may infect sheep (more rarely goats) throughout the world. It affects mainly young lambs, who contract the infection from one another. Ewes that are suckling affected lambs may develop lesions on their udders. Healing occurs in about a month, without scarring. Orf virus remains viable for a long period in dried scabs, and this is important in maintaining enzootic infection in sheep under field conditions. Orf (sometimes called "contagious ecthyma among sheep and goats") remains an economically most important disease (Büttner and Rziha 2002).

Human lesions are caused by direct inoculation of infected material. Various occupations are at risk: shepherds, farmers, and veterinarians are in the first line. Orf is a frequent occupational disease among shearers, of

T. Rustemeyer, P. Elsner, S.M. John & H.I. Maibach (eds.), *Kanerva's Occupational Dermatology*,
DOI 10.1007/978-3-642-02035-3_23,

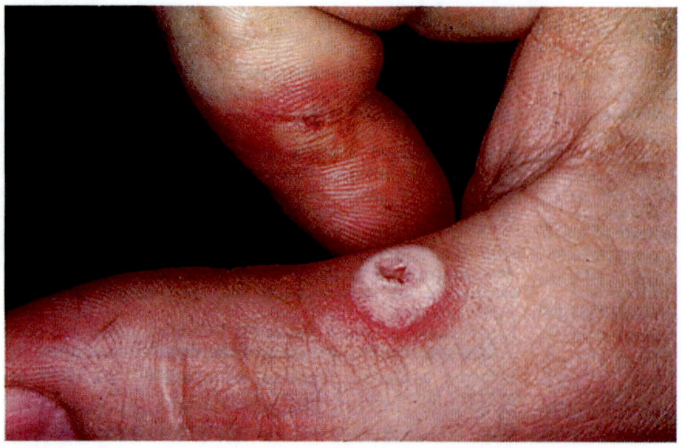

Fig. 23.1
Orf

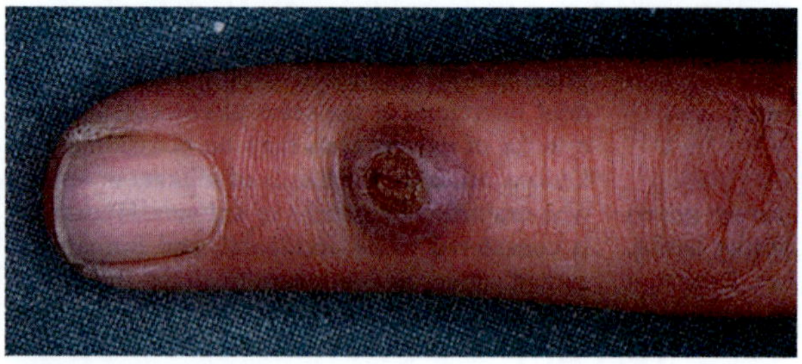

Fig. 23.2
Milkers' node

considerable industrial importance in Australia and New Zealand. More occasionally, butchers and meat porters can be affected from infected carcasses. In Western countries, it is not rare among immigrants from Muslim countries, who work as sheep slaughtermen in unofficial slaughterhouses (Lachapelle et al. 1992). This situation is partly under control in Belgium.

The lesions of orf occurring mainly on fingers (*Fig. 23.1*) are rather large, painful nodules (1–2 cm in diameter), that may be multiple with a vesiculo-pustular roof; the surrounding skin is inflamed. There may be a low fever and swelling of the draining lymph nodes. More rarely, "giant" lesions (as large as 5 cm in diameter) may occur. Secondary infection is not uncommon (Groves et al. 1991). Spontaneous recovery occurs in 3–6 weeks. Second attacks are quite common. Erythema multiforme occasionally develops, typically 10–14 days after the onset of orf (Sterling 2010). Diagnosis is confirmed by examination of collected material (from a vesiculo-pustule or a scab) by negative electron microscopy, which reveals the presence of characteristic virions.

Treatment is limited to prevention and/or cure of secondary infection.

2.1.2 Milkers' Node

Milkers' node (pseudocowpox; paravaccinia). In cattle, two forms of parapox manifestations are commonly observed, the bovine papular stomatitis in young calves and the occurrence of lesions at the udder of cows (Büttner and Rziha 2002).

Man may be occasionally infected. Lesions occur on the hands of milkers or veterinarians who examine the mouths of animals. Human infection is considered accidental and human-to-human spread does not appear to have been recorded. Clinically, the lesions, relatively painless, are hemispherical, cherry-red papules which appear 5–7 days after exposure and gradually enlarge into firm, elastic, purple, smooth hemispherical nodules (*Fig. 23.2*) varying in size up to 2 cm in diameter, and, when fully developed, may be umbilicated. They are highly vascular, which explains the purple color. The lesions disappear after 4–6 weeks (Groves et al. 1991). Negative electron-microscopy examination of biopsy fragments is most useful to confirm diagnosis. There is no treatment available. Milkers' node is considered nowadays less frequent than orf.

2.1.3 Bovine Papular Stomatitis

Human infections with bovine papular stomatitis virus are less common than with the other two parapoxviruses, probably because contacts between animal handlers and lesions of bovine papular stomatitis, clinically similar to milkers' node, are less common than those of shearers and shepherds with orf and milkers with pseudocowpox lesions.

2.2 Orthopoxvirus Infections

Two orthopoxviruses may be very occasionally involved as human offenders in occupational life: the vaccinia virus and the cowpox virus.

Orthopoxviruses are DNA viruses; virions have an ovoid structure, 300 × 250 nm, and are readily identified by negative electron microscopy.

2.2.1 Vaccinia

Vaccinia has barely limited interest in occupational life nowadays. Vaccinia virus can potentially be used as a carrier of genes for protective antigens of other pathogenic microorganisms (recombinant vaccinia viruses) and it is used in some specialized laboratory research. Vaccination has ceased except for investigators at special risk (Sterling 2010). Buffalopox is considered to be a strain of vaccinia virus. It is found in buffalo herds in certain areas in India and may cause bullous or crusted lesions in buffalo farmers (Ramanan et al. 1996).

The geopolitical situation has changed during the last 10 years and this renewed the need for improved vaccinia vaccines. ACAM 2000 is one of the new generation of smallpox vaccines (Handley et al. 2009).

2.2.2 Cowpox

Cowpox is traditionally considered to be a disease of cattle; yet despite the name it appears that cattle are only infected by chance, as are the cat and human (Sterling 2010). Cowpox appears to occur only in Europe; it is uncommon and sporadic.

An occupational source is probable, when professional activities involve contact with infected animals, such as cattle or cats (in the latter case, when skin has been broken by a scratch).

Clinical symptoms can be reported as follows : after an incubation period of 5–7 days, a papule appears and rapidly becomes vesiculo-pustular, hemorrhagic, and later ulcerated. Later on ulceration is covered by a hard black crust, surrounded by a zone of erythema and edema. Lymphangitis and lymphadenitis are usual. Healing takes place in 3 or 4 weeks. Treatment is limited to prevention and/or care of secondary infection.

An epidemic of monkeypox has been reported in the USA (Lewis-Jones 2004) in 2003 from the importation of exotic animal species (occupational cases).

2.3 Butchers' Warts

Virus warts are very common on hands and/or fingers in some occupational groups : meat or poultry handlers (primarily slaughtermen). Fish handlers are another group at risk.

This is not a case of transmission of an animal papillomavirus to man (it has never been mentioned in the literature) but of interhuman transmission, favored by a combination of environmental circumstances. Indeed, several factors acting concomitantly seem to be important for explaining such an occurrence of the disease among selected groups : (a) work at relatively low temperature; (b) constant humidity of the hands; and (c) presence of cuttings and/or repeated minor trauma to the skin (De Peuter et al. 1977; Jablonska et al. 1988). According to our current knowledge, two types of human papillomaviruses (HPV) are preferentially involved. HPV-2 (the cause of common warts) is frequently found in butchers' warts, but HPV-7 is present in up to a third of lesions (Keefe et al. 1994). The clinical features are the following : (a) on the palmar aspect of both fingers and hands, butchers' warts resemble the myrmeciae of HPV-1 infection : endophytic lesions surrounded by a small ring of keratosis with central black dots representing thrombosed capillaries; (b) on the dorsal and/or lateral aspects of fingers and on the backs of hands, virus warts are either of the common type, or may become very exophytic, showing far advanced craggy keratosis (➋ *Fig. 23.3*).

Classical treatments of common warts can be applied to butchers' warts: it is our experience that injections of a bleomycine solution using a Dermo-Jet® do offer better results than liquid nitrogen applications (Lachapelle et al. 1992).

There is no proof that wearing gloves is an efficacious individual preventive method. Recurrence of older lesions and outcome of new lesions is not rare and may represent a real hindrance in terms of quality of life.

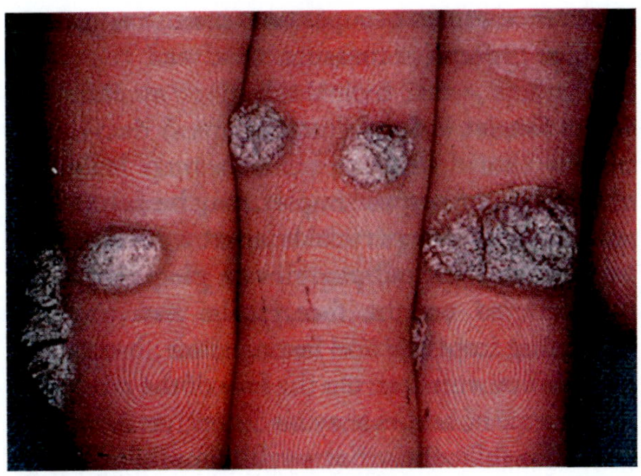

Fig. 23.3
Butchers' warts

2.4 Herpes Simplex

Herpes simplex, caused by *Herpes virus hominis* is one of the commonest infections of humans throughout the world. There are two major antigenic types : type 1 (HSV 1) which is classically associated with facial infection and type 2 (HSV 2), which is typically genital, although there is considerable overlap in disease manifestations. In some circumstances, an occupational origin can be advocated.

2.4.1 Herpes Simplex in Healthcare Workers

It is well-known that trauma facilitates transfer of the virus to fully keratinized skin. Doctors, nurses, dentists, and dental assistants can be infected by contaminated saliva, pharyngeal or laryngotracheal secretions. Primary infection occurs on the extremity of one finger (Gill et al. 1990). Inoculation of the fingertips results in a “herpetic whitlow” in which pruritic and painful deep vesicles coalesce to form a honeycombed appearance or to form a large bulla. The condition is easily confused with pyogenic infection, but virological identification from collected material can be easily achieved nowadays.

Recurrent herpes may occur, presenting as coalescent vesicles gradually transforming to pustules on a very painful erythemato-edematous plaque. Common use of protective gloves has dramatically decreased the occurrence of this occupational disease, and represents the best preventive measure.

2.4.2 Herpes Simplex in Sport Practice

Inoculation herpes simplex may be favored by the practice of some particular sport activities (the so-called herpes gladiatorum). Multiple crops of vesicles and pustules on plaques or erythema and edema on the face, scalp, and upper trunk, simulating impetigo and lasting some 10–12 days have occurred in wrestlers, rugby, or soccer players. On the face of the adult male the appearance of herpes may be deceptive; it may take the form of a folliculitis, but satellite umbilicated vesicles soon suggest the correct diagnosis. Facial contact during rugby is another recognized means of acquiring herpes simplex virus infection (Johnson 2004; Turbeville et al. 2006).

2.4.3 Recurrent Herpes Simplex Triggered by Ultraviolet Radiation

Recurrent facial herpes simplex (and in particular *herpes labialis*) can be triggered by sun exposure. UVB (290–320 nm) seem to play a major role, the mechanisms involved being related to an inhibitory effect on Langerhans cells.

Seasonal workers suffering from recurrent herpes simplex are prone to present reactivation at the beginning of each sun exposure period (➋ *Fig. 23.4*). Skiing, sailing, or swimming instructors are good examples of professions at risk.

Prevention of recurrences is achieved by the use of acyclovir, starting treatment a few days before exposure.

The use of sunscreens is of prime importance during the period of exposure.

2.5 Hepatitis B

The risk of becoming infected with blood-borne pathogens (e.g., hepatitis B) during surgery is real. The degree of risk for perioperative personnel is related to factors that include participating in large numbers of surgical procedures each year; the nature of perioperative work (e.g., use of different types of sharp instruments); exposure to large amounts of blood and body fluids; the prevalence of blood-borne pathogens in the surgical population; the variation in different organisms' ability to be transmitted; the existence of vaccines and the level of vaccination; the availability of postexposure

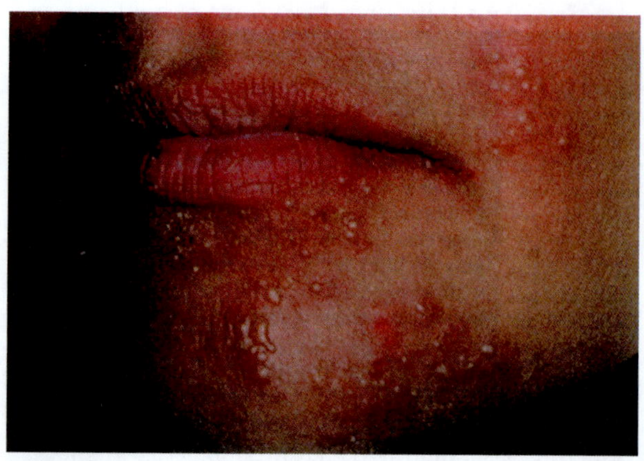

Fig. 23.4
Recurrent herpes simplex in a ski instructor after sun exposure

treatment; and the consequences of acquiring the disease. Controlling risks to perioperative personnel can be accomplished by using the Occupational Safety and Health Administration's three methods of control-redesigning surgical equipment and procedures, changing work practices, and enhancing the personal protection equipment of perioperative personnel (Stringer et al. 2001).

Since hepatitis B vaccination becomes generalized among healthcare personnel in many European countries, some skin side effects may be expected (Grézard et al. 1995). Apart from short-lived local reactions, generalized granuloma annulare has been described (Wolf et al. 1998).

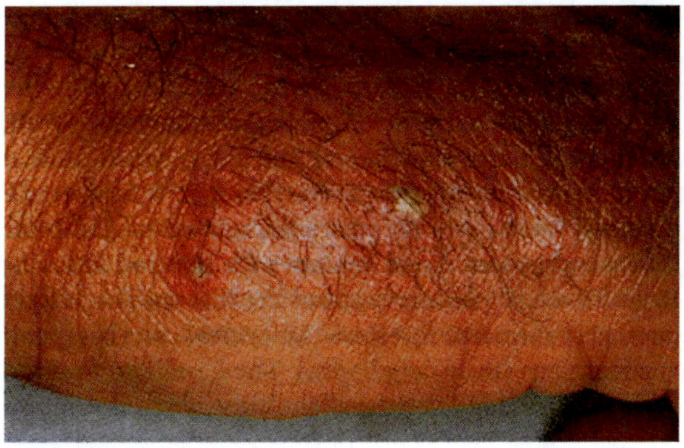

Fig. 23.5
Staphylococcal folliculitis

3 Bacterial Infections

Some occupational bacterial infections are distributed worldwide, whereas others are nowadays limited to certain countries where prevention measures have not been applied.

3.1 Staphylococcal and Streptococcal Infections

The most common staphylococcal and/or streptococcal infections are consecutive to cuttings, abrasions, burns, and/or puncture wounds. Beta-hemolytic *Streptococcus* of group A and *Staphylococcus aureus* or both are the usual bacteria cultured from lesions (Barnham and Neilson 1987). Some occupations are at particular risk : butchers, meat-packers, fish handlers, slaughtermen, etc. The commonest clinical picture is impetigo characterized by erythematous patches covered by a yellowish crust. A variant is ecthyma, mainly observed in tropical countries: it consists of a slow and gradually deepening ulceration surmounted by a thick crust. After healing there is a permanent scar.

Workers in contact with industrial mineral oils, for example, in the metallurgic industry can develop lesions of folliculitis due to *Staphylococcus* spp. (*Fig. 23.5*). Bacteria that may contaminate used oil are not responsible for the infection. In fact, occlusion of hair follicles by cutting, lubrification, and cooling mineral oils may lead to a secondary infection by *Staphylocci* present on the skin of patients. Industrial staphylococcal folliculitis is less frequent nowadays, due to an increased use of soluble oils in industry.

In those conditions, conventional therapy is applied, but secondary prevention of infection is mandatory, requiring in many cases a change of working habits.

3.2 The Problem of MRSA and CA-MRSA Infections

Methicillin-resistant *Staphylococcus aureus* (MRSA) infections have been confirmed to healthcare centers for decades. However, MRSA infections are increasingly seen in young healthy individuals with no exposure to healthcare centers. These community-acquired MRSA (CA-MRSA) differ from healthcare-associated MRSA by the presence of the toxin Panton-Valentine leukocidin. The number of CA-MRSA infections increases in most European countries. Outbreaks with CA-MRSA have occurred in day care centers, athletic teams, and prisons (i.e., groups whose common characteristics appear to be close person-to-person contact). It is therefore a major environmental problem and is considered occupational in pig farmers (or more rarely other farm animals).

The management and control strategies are between the hands of the medical and paramedical staff: nurses, kinesitherapists, pharmacists, etc.

In order to reduce the prevalence of such infections, a more limited use of topical antibiotics such as mupirocin, fusidic acid, and retapamuline is encouraged. They can be replaced advantageously by antiseptics.

The general rules of personal hygiene are of course of prime importance. Information of the care personnel is mandatory (Kieffer et al. 2008; Mempel et al. 2008; Lorette et al. 2009).

3.3 Bacterial Athlete's Foot

The commonest cause of this purely bacterial variant is a mixture of flora comprising both Gram +ve and –ve bacteria. The clinical presentation can be florid, with the entire interdigital web and neighboring skin subject to extensive ulceration with raised, whitish, and macerated margins. It may be associated with small fissures in the clefts providing a portal of entry for erysipelas of the leg. Athlete's foot is a misnomer, as both water sports and occlusive (maceration-promoting) high-ankled trainers also contribute to this environmental dermatosis. It is encountered in occupational life and is considered to be a common problem in sport medicine (Lachapelle et al. 1997). Topical treatment includes potassium permanganate (1/10,000) baths and antibiotic creams. Systemic antibiotics are needed when secondary erysipelas does occur.

Prevention is of prime importance to avoid recurrences; the wearing of shoes provoking minimal occlusion is highly recommended.

3.4 Erysipeloid

Erysipeloid is an acute infection due to *Erysipelothrix rhusiopathiae*, which colonizes a wide variety of animals worldwide, including mammals, birds, fowl, fish, and shellfish. It is a pathogen for many of them, especially for pigs (high prevalence and economic importance).

Human infection is contracted by direct contact, most commonly from carcasses; it is the reason why occupations mainly affected by the disease are slaughtermen, butchers, cooks, fishermen, farmers, veterinarians, and housewifes. Scratches or pricks are the usual mode of incubation. More anecdotically, it has been mentioned among dolphinarium attendants or, in the United States, among crabs fishermen (crab dermatitis).

The clinical symptoms are usually obvious : about 3 days after inoculation, a hot violaceous and tender erythema develops around the inoculation site and extends centrifugally but irregularly, with a sharp and sometimes gyrate border, which may be vesicular. Erysipeloid is in fact a true cellulitis. Most lesions are on the fingers, hands, and forearms. Some lesions have a violaceous hue. Fever and mild general symptoms such as arthralgia are present in only 10% of cases. Without treatment, healing normally occurs spontaneously in 2 weeks without desquamation or suppuration. Other rare clinical forms have been described: a generalized cutaneous form and a septicemic form associated with endocarditis.

Recommended treatment refers to antibiotics: penicillin IM, ciprofloxacin or cephalosporins. Prevention is, as far as pigs are concerned, under the responsibility of the veterinarian : systematic slaughtering of infected animals is mandatory. Reduction of trauma (e.g., in fish processors) can be obtained by constant use of protective gloves.

Two recent reviews (Veraldi et al. 2009; Wang et al. 2010) have been dedicated to erysipeloid, despite the fact that the disease is nowadays less frequent throughout the world.

3.5 Anthrax

Anthrax is a specific infection with *Bacillus anthracis*, a Gram-positive, encapsulated organism which can survive as spores for over 20 years in soil. Herbivores are primarily affected. In endemic countries (some parts of Africa, Pakistan, India, Iran, the Middle East, and parts of Russia), human infections remain a serious problem. In Western Europe or the United States, anthrax often follows occupational exposure during care of livestock or the handling of products. Therefore, most cases occur in the wool, hair, or bristle industries. Unsterilized imported bone meal, or sacks contaminated with it, or even straw remain a potential hazard.

Cutaneous inoculation is favored by minor trauma or preexisting skin lesions. The lesion of cutaneous anthrax, called "the malignant pustule," commonly occurs on exposed skin, and is usually single. One to five days after infection, A papule develops at the site of inoculation. A bulla on a red edematous zone soon follows. The bulla ruptures and forms a hemorrhagic crust. General symptoms of great severity appear and may be life threatening, particularly anthrax meningoencephalitis.

Diagnosis is confirmed by bacteriological examination.

The prevalence of anthrax is decreasing steadily in industrialized countries, but the disease is still endemic in some parts of the world, most always related with agricultural activities.

In recent years, cases of anthrax have been reported from Peru (Maguina et al. 2005), Turkey (Karahocagil et al. 2008), and India (Narayan et al. 2009).

For cutaneous anthrax, oral ciprofloxacin, doxycycline, or amoxicillin may suffice for 7–10 days.

For systemic disease, the treatment of choice is intravenous penicillin G for 7–10 days. Tetracycline or erythromycin can be given in the presence of allergy to penicillin.

Vaccination gives some protection, but prevention should be directed primarily at control of the disease in animals and disinfection of animal products (Hay and Adriaans 2010).

3.6 Brucellosis

Some years ago brucellosis was a common disease in farm animals, due to three *Brucella* organisms: *B. suis* (pigs), *B. abortus* (cattle), and *B. melitensis* (sheep and goats). In recent years, the incidence of the disease has dramatically decreased, due to extensive animal prophylaxis programs, including elimination of infected animals and vaccination of healthy ones; it is well controlled in many European countries, but is still common in some parts of the world.

Farmers, shepherds, veterinarians, and slaughtermen are at risk in endemic areas. Human infection is related to handling of contaminated animals or ingesting milk and cheese that is contaminated and unpasteurized. Occupational injuries are another mode of entry. The skin manifestations are nonspecific and range from a maculopapular eruption to petechiae, which occur in less than 5% of patients. A chronic ulcer may develop at the site of inoculation or injury. Systemic symptoms include chills, high fever, headache, and extreme weakness.

Treatment of choice is a combination of doxycycline (100 mg 2 ×/day) and rifampicin (300 mg 3 ×/day) for 6 weeks.

"Contact brucellosis" refers to urticarial and/or eczematous lesions on the skin sites in contact with infected animals. It is considered to be a protein contact dermatitis to *Brucella* antigens (Lachapelle et al. 1992).

3.7 Tularemia

Tularemia is encountered in the United States, Northern Europe, and Japan. It results from systemic infection with the Gram-negative bacteria, *Francisella tularensis.* Wild rodent (in particular hares) and other small animal populations are the main reservoir of infection. In humans, most cases are sporadic, related to tick bites (*Dermacentor*) or direct contact with infected animals. Shooters are at greatest risk, but the disease also affects butchers, farmers, landscapers, foresters, laboratory workers, and veterinarians (Evans et al. 1985).

An epidemiologic survey has been conducted in France (Vaissaire et al.2005). The authors have demonstrated that the prevalence of the disease is underestimated. They conclude that it is necessary to be increasingly vigilant, for animal cases and human contamination. It is advised to strengthen medical and veterinary supervision especially since *Francisella tularensis* may be used for bioterrorism.

The incubation period varies from 1 to 10 days. The clinical manifestation is usually an ulcerated nodule at the point of inoculation associated with enlargement, and later breakdown of lymph nodes. Systemic symptoms (e.g., meningitis) and toxemia may be severe (Hofinger et al. 2009). Minocycline is considered to be efficacious in most cases (100 mg 2 ×/day during 4 weeks).

3.8 *Pseudomonas aeruginosa* Folliculitis

Epidemics of *Pseudomonas aeruginosa* are now commonly associated with aquatic activities, particularly public jacuzzis (pH > 8 and only 2–3 g free chlorine, which is inadequate at this pH) or inadequately chlorinated swimming pools. *P. aeruginosa* is an organism universally present in humid environments. Sports instructors are of course at risk, but most cases are linked with recreational activities (Lachapelle et al. 1997). The clinical manifestations consist of a papulo-pustular eruption of fulminant onset on the trunk (➔ *Fig. 23.6*). Diagnosis is confirmed by microbiology.

Treatment of first choice is oral ciprofloxacin (500 mg 2 ×/day). Prevention of epidemics is related to usual recommendations in terms of water maintenance (pH between 7.2 and 7.8; adequate chlorination).

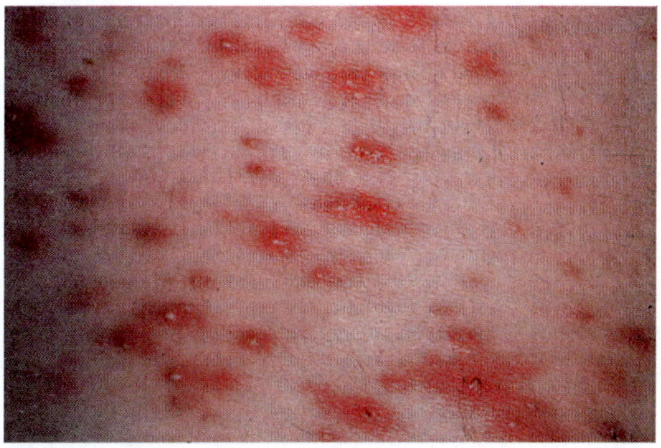

Fig. 23.6
***Pseudomonas aeruginosa* folliculitis**

3.9 Warty Tuberculosis

This variety of tuberculosis occurs as a result of the inoculation of organisms into the skin of a previously infected patient who usually has a moderate or high degree of immunity. In occupational life, the disease occurs by accidental superinfection from extraneous sources : physicians, pathologists, and post-mortem attendants are traditionally at risk. This explains the classical terms used in the past: "anatomist's warts," "prosector's warts" (Lundgren et al. 1987). At the present time, it is an extremely rare disease in Western countries.

The lesion starts as a small, symptomless, indurated warty papule with a slight inflammatory areola. By gradual extension, a verrucose plaque is formed. Its color is purplish, red, or brown. Usual localizations are the hands and fingers. Treatment refers to antibiotic schedules used in other forms of tuberculosis. Wearing of appropriate gloves (resistant to cuttings) is highly recommended in terms of primary prevention.

3.10 BCG: Skin Complications of Vaccination

BCG vaccination is still compulsory for some occupational groups, according to the current legislation applied in each individual country. It is an occasional source of complications that can be summarized as follows : (a) nonspecific reactions including urticaria and erythema multiforme, (b) nonspecific abscess formation generally resulting from an injection made too deeply, and (c) BCGitis that is considered as an attenuated form of tuberculosis (Bellet and Prose 2005).

Treatment is adapted to each individual situation; when BCGitis is confirmed, the use of isoniazid for a period of 6 months is classically prescribed.

3.11 *Mycobacterium marinum* Mycobacteriosis: Fish Tank Granuloma

Mycobacterium marinum is the agent of a cosmopolitan atypical mycobacteriosis, often mentioned in the literature under the name of fish tank granuloma. Its natural habitat is water, particularly enclosures of water that are not often replenished. It is especially prevalent in heated water in temperate climates and in the sea and natural pools in warmer regions.

It can be isolated from diseased fish. Pathogenic only on abraded skin it has been called a "leisure-time pathogen"; in fact, it is mainly observed among people keeping tropical fish. Apart from fish fanciers, pet shop helpers (tropical aquariums) can also be infected, and this represents a true occupational disease.

The portal of entry is a minor wound which may go unnoticed. The lesion presents either as a light-red single nodule (➋ *Fig. 23.7*) which is mildly keratotic or as coalescent purplish red plaques of the fingers or dorsum of the hand (fish tank granuloma). A fairly common clinical variant is the sporotrichoid form (➋ *Fig. 23.8*), in which one or several satellite nodules appear at successive intervals on the forearm along the line of lymph drainage sometimes in association with locoregional lymphadenopathy. Diagnosis seems obvious when considering

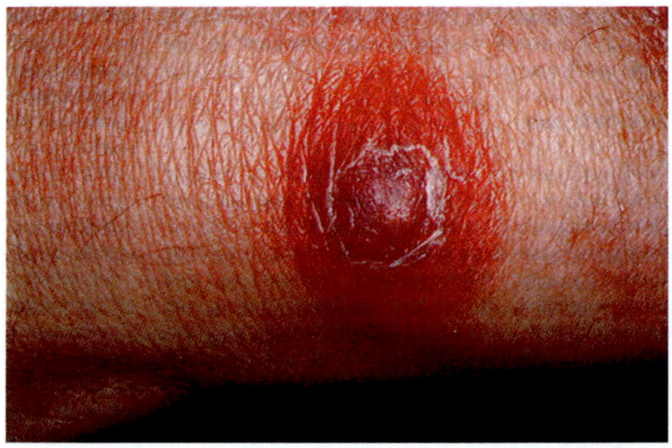

Fig. 23.7
Aquarium granuloma due to *Mycobacterium marinum*

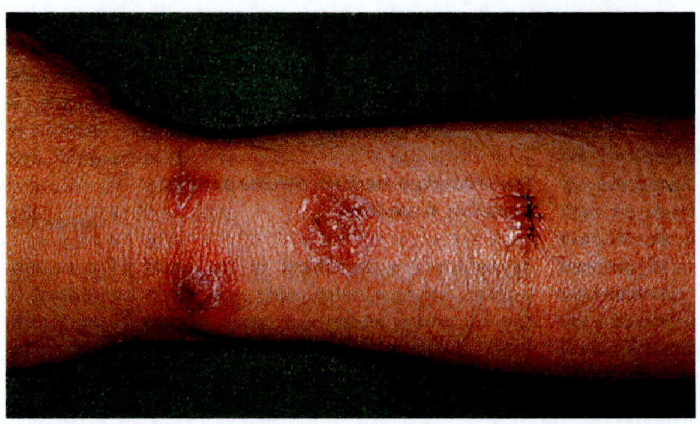

Fig. 23.8
Sporotrichoid form of *Mycobacterium marinum* mycobacteriosis

both anamnestic data and clinical symptoms, and is confirmed in 70% of cases by culture obtained from a skin biopsy (Streit et al. 2008).

Treatment schedules are still debated: combining rifampicin (15 mg/kg/day) and ethambutol (25 mg/kg/day) for 6 months is a classical approach; minocycline (100 mg 2 ×/day) is sometimes but not always efficacious. Excision of the nodule has also been proposed as a reasonable approach.

Simple prevention measures such as the use of gloves could reduce the incidence of infections considerably. Minocycline can be added to fish tank water to eradicate fish infection.

4 Mycotic Infections

Many fungi are able to infect man, provoking common superficial mycoses or subcutaneous and systemic infections. Dermatophytoses, candidosis, and pityriasis versicolor are the most common cutaneous mycoses; systemic mycoses such as cryptococcosis are also of prime importance in some parts of the world. In the following sections, we refer only to mycotic infections that are provoked or significantly worsened by the work environment.

4.1 Dermatophytoses

Dermatophytes are related fungi capable of causing skin changes of the type known as ringworm or dermatophytosis (Hay and Ashbee 2010). Thus defined, the ringworm species are all molds belonging to three asexual genera: *Microsporum, Trichophyton,* and *Epidermophyton.* It is also traditional to group dermatophytes according to their ecological niche: geophilic species originating in the soil, zoophilic species having animal origins, and anthropophilic species, which are largely restricted to human skin. However, these three groups are not always sharply demarcated. It remains classical to describe clinical forms of dermatophytosis, according to the skin sites that are invaded; such a division is useful for epidemiological studies and also for treatment strategies. Diagnostic procedures include (a) direct microscopy of the squames that shows dermatophyte filaments and (b) culture on Sabouraud's medium for the identification of the species involved. The epidemiology of dermatophyte infections has been updated recently (Seebacher et al. 2008).

4.1.1 Tinea Corporis

All known dermatophytes can produce lesions of the glabrous skin. These are perfectly circular erythemato-squamous lesions usually sharply demarcated with a raised edge; in some cases, the center of the lesions is the same color as the normal skin, with a few squames, which means that spontaneous regression is underway. The degree of inflammation is highly variable. This feature depends not only on the species of the fungus and the immune status of the host, but is also roughly proportional to the extent of follicular invasion. In the latter case, ringworm appears as a large, round, infiltrated erythemato-squamous plaque dotted with multiple follicular pustules (➋ *Fig. 23.9*).

The occupational origin of many cases of tinea corporis is obvious and is closely related to the species of the dermatophyte. Among others, the commonest species are *Microsporum canis* (major hosts : cat, dog); *Trichophyton mentagrophytes* (major host : small rodents); *Microsporum persicolor* (major host : voles); *Trichophyton verrucosum* (major host : cattle); and *Trichophyton equinum* (major host : horses). *Microsporum praecox,* living in the horse environment, is a pathogen for human skin. Extensive forms of dermatophytosis, occurring mainly on the trunk and/or buttocks may be due to *Trichophyton rubrum,* an anthropophilic species of dermatophyte.

Not only workers normally in contact with domestic and farm animals but also explorers, surveyors, zoo attendants, and laboratory technicians are at risk. Particular examples include *T. verrucosum* among farmers (or veterinarians) and their families and *T. mentagrophytes* among

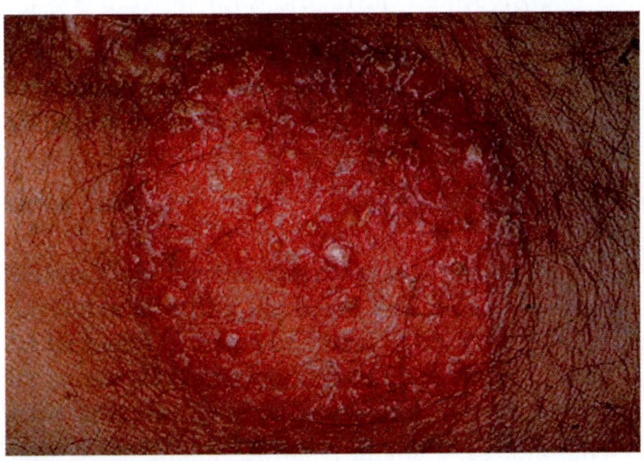

Fig. 23.9
Tinea corporis with follicular pustules

laboratory workers. Pet shop and kennel workers are at risk from *M. canis*. Sportsmen and various categories of workers (e.g., miners) may contract *T. rubrum* infection.

4.1.2 Tinea Cruris

Tinea cruris is due mainly to *Trichophyton rubrum*, *Trichophyton mentagrophytes* var. *interdigitale* and *Epidermophyton floccosum*. It is probably more prevalent in tropical zones and particularly among migrants from temperate countries (Hay and Ashbee 2010). It is also more common in men than in women. The most important feature is the fact that tinea cruris is often combined with tinea pedis: this means that all professional circumstances which favor the onset of tinea pedis can also be of importance for tinea cruris.

Clinically, lesions of tinea cruris are sharply marginated infiltrated erythemato-squamous plaques in the groin. Vesiculation is rare, but dermal nodules forming beading along the edge are commonly found in older lesions. Minute pustules are often present.

4.1.3 Tinea Pedis

Tinea pedis corresponds to an infection of the feet or toes with a dermatophyte. The term athlete's foot, used to imply any form of toe-cleft intertrigo (see ➋ Sect. 3.3) is preferably banned from the dermatologic literature.

Two anthropophilic species, *Trichophyton rubrum* and *Trichophyton mentagrophytes* var. *interdigitale* are together responsible for the vast majority of cases of foot ringworm in Central and Northern Europe. In contrast, in Southern Europe and in Arabic countries, zoophilic dermatophytes such as *Microsporum canis* or *Trichophyton verrucosum* are the most frequently isolated.

It is important to say that tinea pedis is the commonest form of dermatophytosis in most countries. The wearing of shoes and the resultant maceration of toe-cleft predisposes to this condition, usually involving the lateral toe-clefts. About 10% of the total population is considered to be infected; some subjects can be almost asymptomatic. Living in an institution, especially where washing facilities are shared, is likely to increase the chances of infection (English 1969). Prevalence as high as 80% has been reported in some factories or sport institutes. On the other hand, tinea pedis may be equally well transmitted within the family bathroom. Reinfection from the environment is usual (with the same or another species, or with combined species). Maceration of the toe-clefts plays an important role. A simultaneous increase in the bacterial flora may also play a part. Resident bacteria, such as large-colony coryneforms, may be acting as important copathogens. In adolescents and children, attending swimming baths is the major source of infection.

The commonest form of tinea pedis is located in the toe webs. The fourth interdigital web is preferentially infected, but the other webs can also be infected, on one or both feet. The clinical symptoms are characterized by a whitish diffuse maceration in the cleft marginated by a collarette of continuous desquamation (➋ *Fig. 23.10*). In some cases, there is a small painful fissure running along the line of the cleft. The entire area is ulcerative and macerated from microbial superinfection. Itching is usually present. In *Trichophyton rubrum* infections, a squamous hyperkeratotic variety, which is particularly chronic and resistant to treatment and which affects the soles, heels, and sides of the feet ("moccasin foot") is often found (Hay and Ashbee 2010). The dorsal surfaces of the toes and feet are not often affected, but associated onychomycosis is common. Tinea pedis is sometimes associated with reactive plantar pompholyx : extremely pruritic coalescent vesicular eczema is observed. Microscopic examination reveals sometimes the presence of dermatophytic filaments in these "id" reactions.

4.1.4 Tinea Manuum

Infections of the dorsal aspect of the hands resemble ringworm of the glabrous skin. Ringworm of the palmar skin (palm and palmar aspect of the fingers) presents a particular clinical picture. There is dusty desquamation

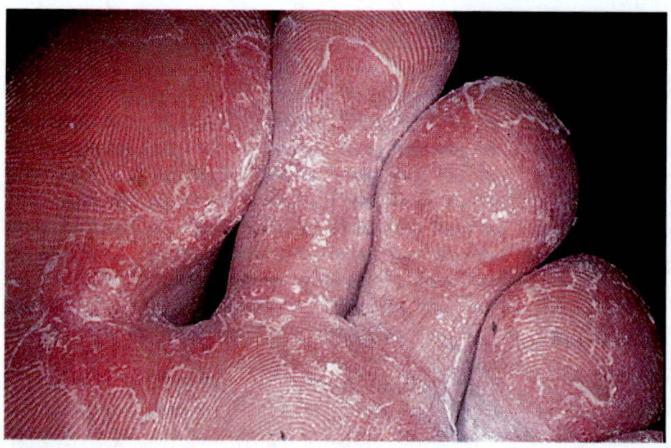

◘ Fig. 23.10
Tinea pedis

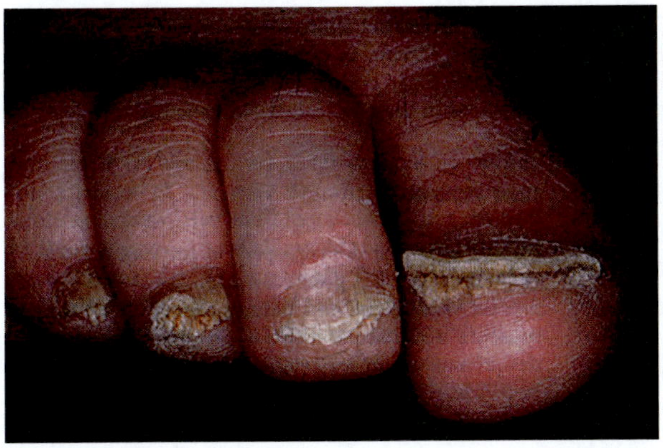

■ Fig. 23.11
Dermatophyte onychomycosis

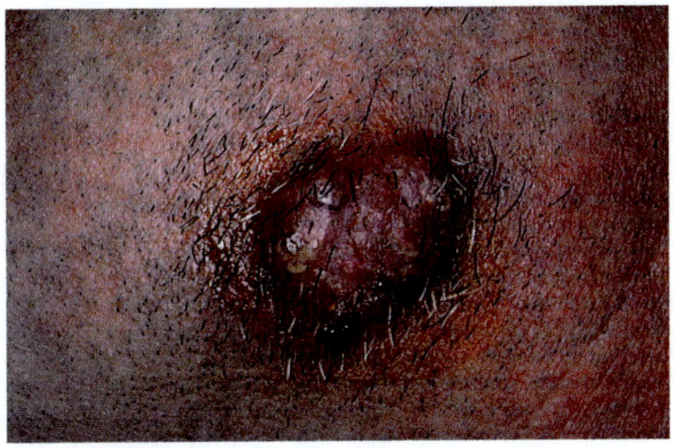

■ Fig. 23.12
Kerion celsi

on an erythematous background with pearl white accentuation of the palmar flexor folds. The appearance is similar to that of some cases of hyperkeratotic palmar eczema, but, in tinea manuum, scraping yields a flurry of disintegrating scabs. In most cases, the organisms concerned are the two anthropophilic species involved in tinea pedis. Zoophilic dermatophytes can also be incriminated. Apart from animal infections, there is preexisting foot infection with or without toenail involvement. In this respect, the occupational origin of tinea manuum can be ascertained in some cases. The "two feet-one hand syndrome" is not uncommon (Daniel et al. 1979). An extensive study of this clinical entity has been carried out (Daniel et al. 1979). From the results, it can be assessed that patients with a high intensity of hand use in their jobs are significantly more likely to develop tinea pedis/onychomycosis and tinea manuum at an earlier age. Tinea pedis precedes in most cases the development of tinea manuum.

4.1.5 Dermatophyte Onychomycosis

This is a frequent condition which may be isolated or associated with tinea pedis and/or tinea manuum. The role of occupational activities is therefore similar to that evoked in tinea pedis. It affects one or more toenails; it is less common on the hands. The infection begins at the distal extremity of the nail bed or nail fold. Onychomycosis may have different clinical characteristics: in some cases, leukonychia affecting part of the distal nail extremity but also extending along a nail fold toward the cuticle is the major symptom. Full thickness, including the superficial plate, accounts for the pearly mat appearance of the infected area. In other cases, massive destruction of the nail does occur, spicules of which being detached all along the free border (➋ *Fig. 23.11*). When irregular pigmentation – whitish at some points and bright yellow at others – does occur, it suggests mixed infection with dermatophytes and opportunistic yeasts, such as *Scopulariopsis brevicaulis.*

4.1.6 Kerion Celsi

Kerion Celsi (or tinea barbae) is a particular form of ringworm, affecting the beard and moustache areas of the face with invasion of coarse hairs. The affected men are commonly farm workers in cases caused by the two main species: *Trichophyton verrucosum* and *Trichophyton mentagrophytes* var. *mentagrophytes.*

The infection is traditionally acquired from contact with cattle, mainly during winter months when keeping cattle in sheds does occur. Veterinarians are also at risk. The clinical picture is that of a highly inflammatory pustular folliculitis. Hairs of the beard or moustache regions are surrounded by red, inflammatory papules or pustules, usually with exudation or crusting (➋ *Fig. 23.12*). Many hairs within the affected areas are loose and easily removed with the forceps without causing pain. It is noteworthy that, without treatment, lesions tend to settle spontaneously, but may persist for some months (Hay and Ashbee 2010).

4.1.7 Treatment and Management of Dermatophytoses

Treatment of dermatophytoses is nowadays straightforward. The topical agents, including various imidazoles (miconazole, econazole, tioconazole, isoconazole, bifonazole, sulconazole, etc.) and/or terbinafine are equally efficient and can be used in all forms of dermatophytosis, except onychomycosis (due to a lack of penetration). One daily application is considered to be adequate for 2–4 weeks. There is a current tendency to use simultaneously systemic antimycotics, even in tinea corporis when multiple lesions are present.

Each type of dermatomycosis requires an adapted schedule of administration. Itraconazole and terbinafine have been more extensively studied for these indications than fluconazole.

In tinea corporis and tinea cruris, the scheme of treatment is as follows: terbinafine – 250 mg/day for 2 weeks; itraconazole – 100 mg/day for 2 weeks; fluconazole – 150 mg once weekly or 50 mg/day for 2–4 weeks.

Tinea manuum and tinea pedis require a longer period of treatment: terbinafine – 250 mg/day for 4 weeks; itraconazole – 100 mg/day for 4 weeks; fluconazole – 150 mg once weekly or 50 mg/day for 4 weeks.

The treatment of dermatophyte onychomycosis has been studied extensively in the last years. The schedules proposed are as follows : terbinafine 250 mg/day for 3–4 months according to the severity of the disease and the response to the treatment; itraconazole is more efficient when a "pulse therapy" is conducted as follows : 100 mg 4×/day during 1 week, followed by 3 weeks of no treatment. Three or four consecutive waves are prescribed following the same schedule (Degreef et al. 1987).

Kerion Celsi also requires a well-defined schedule of treatment: terbinafine 250 mg/day for 6 weeks or itraconazole 100 mg/day for the same period. Fairly long-term follow-up is recommended, and late recurrences undoubtedly occur.

In addition to treatment, some other management measures are generally helpful. The identification of the causative agent is useful, particularly where treatment of infected animals is important, in order to prevent other infections.

4.1.8 Prevention of Dermatophytoses

Specific measures of prevention can be applied to tinea pedis. They include the following:

(a) Frequent washing of changing-room floors and walkways; it will remove infective material in skin scales
(b) Use of imidazole powders to reduce levels of toe-cleft tinea pedis
(c) Prompt treatment of infected people combined with simple hygienic measures such as washing shower-room floors with an antiseptic solution

4.2 Candidiasis

Candidiasis refers to various forms of infection caused by the yeast *Candida albicans*, or occasionally by other species of *Candida*. A limited number of *Candida* infections can be directly related to the work environment.

4.2.1 *Candida* Intertrigo of the Toe Webs

Candidiasis may affect the web spaces of the toes. Marked maceration with a thick, white horny layer is the usual clinical symptom. Gram-negative bacteria are often copathogens. Work circumstances that favor tinea pedis can also play a role in the occurrence of candidiasis of the toe webs.

4.2.2 *Candida* Intertrigo of the Interdigital Folds

An erythematous, glazed, "velvety" maceration area of one or more folds is the usual clinical picture. There is often a collarette of desquamation at the periphery (➋ *Fig. 23.13*). Similar lesions can also develop under the rings. In those cases, it is often considered that candidiasis is triggered by a previous skin irritation, mainly due to detergents and/or to sugar; this could explain the occurrence of the disease in bakeries, confectioner's shops, chocolate-factories or fruit-packing trade, etc. Minor trauma (such as superficial abrasions) could initiate the infection. We may consider that the problem has decreased considerably. A steady decline is related to the introduction of automation in most factories.

4.2.3 *Candida* Paronychia

Candida albicans can be isolated in the majority of cases of chronic paronychia. The yeast has traditionally been considered to play an etiological role in the condition, but bacteria and irritant or allergic contact dermatitis also play a role, although the contribution of each varies from patient to patient. In recent years, a more recent approach is to envisage the primary role of a repeated contact with various kinds of foods. Proteins of foods could induce

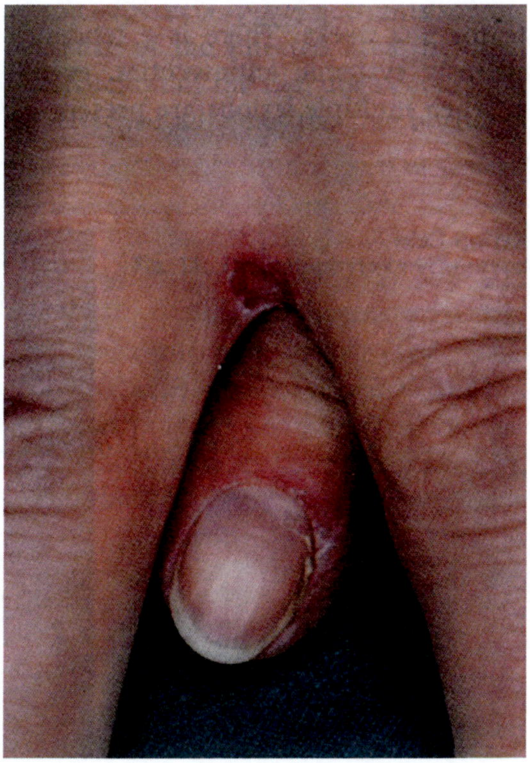

Fig. 23.13
***Candida* intertrigo of an interdigital fold with paronychia**

a protein contact dermatitis (Tosti et al. 1992) and secondarily an infection by *Candida albicans.* When considering this new concept, the primary role of the yeast is therefore minimized. Professions at risk apart from those already quoted as prone to develop *Candida* intertrigo of the interdigital folds include all categories of workers handling food, including cooks and housewives. Clinical symptoms are obvious. Several fingers are usually infected, but one or all may be involved. The nail fold is red and swollen; there is loss of the cuticle, and detachment of the nail fold from the dorsal surface of the nail plate, leading to pocketing (*Fig. 23.13*). Occasionally, thick, white pus may discharge; often force is needed to express it. In more advanced cases, nail dystrophy and onycholysis do occur.

4.2.4 Treatment and Management of Candidiasis

Candida intertrigo requires specific therapy. Topical imidazoles are commonly used for a period of two weeks, but a longer period of treatment is sometimes needed. When the toe webs are involved, attention should be given to treating concomitant bacteria; potassium permanganate soaks (1/10,000) were used in many European countries, but they tend to be replaced nowadays by povidone-iodine or chlorhexidine. In general, systemic treatment is not considered for this indication.

Candida paronychia is often difficult to treat. Topical treatment is insufficient; the best therapeutic approach is intermittent (pulsed) itraconazole or fluconazole, following the schedules indicated in the treatment of dermatophyte onychomycosis. Prevention of candidiasis is straightforward. It implies the avoidance of maceration at work. Chronic paronychia is best prevented by the use of appropriate gloves. The avoidance of contact with foods incriminated in the initiating protein contact dermatitis (assessed by positive prick tests) is mandatory.

4.3 Subcutaneous Mycoses

Subcutaneous mycoses, or mycoses of "implantation" are sporadically occurring infections caused by fungi present in the natural environment, which are directly inoculated into the dermis or subcutaneous tissue through a penetrating injury. They are not common even in endemic countries, and are mainly seen in the tropics (for details see Hay 2006). We have summarized in *Table 23.1* some of the features of the most important subcutaneous mycoses, including occupational sources of infection.

4.4 Systemic Mycoses

The systemic mycoses are fungal infections that involve deep structures and disseminate, usually via the bloodstream, from the original site of infection to different organs, including the skin (for details see Hay 2006). We have summarized in *Table 23.2* some of the features of the most important systemic mycoses, including occupational sources of infection.

5 Skin Protothecosis: A Unique Dermatosis Provoked by Algae

Protothecosis is unique in the world of dermatology. It is provoked by *Prototheca*, a saprophyte algae that can be cultivated on Sabouraud's medium. Skin protothecosis is

Table 23.1
Main subcutaneous mycoses implying occupational sources of infection (after Hay 2006)

Mycosis	Fungus	Endemic areas	Occupational sources of infection
Sporotrichosis	*Sporothrix schenckii*	Cosmopolitan; more frequent in the America and South Africa than in Europe	Inoculation by trauma (thorns, splinters, etc.); common among South African miners; sporadic among foresting workers, florists, or gardeners
Mycetoma	Various species of fungi or actinomycetes	Tropical and subtropical countries	Inoculation by trauma (thorns, splinters, etc.)
			Agricultural workers
Chromoblastomycosis	Various species of fungi	Various countries throughout the world; rare in Europe (imported cases mostly)	Inoculation by trauma
			Agricultural workers

Table 23.2
Main systemic mycoses implying occupational sources of infection (after Hay 2006)

Mycosis	Fungus	Endemic areas	Occupational sources of infection
Histoplasmosis	*Histoplasma capsulatum*	Cosmopolitan, but very rare in Europe	Soil contaminated with chicken feathers or dippings (occasionally bats)
			Airborne conidia
			Cleaners, laboratory workers, speleologists
Blastomycosis	*Blastomyces dermatitidis*	North and Central America, Middle East, India, Poland, Zimbabwe	Wood debris and soil close to rivers
			Agricultural workers
Coccidioidomycosis	*Coccidioides immitis*	Southwestern states of USA, Central and South America	Inhalation of airborne spores
			Travellers in endemic areas
			Agricultural workers
Paracoccidioidomycosis	*Paracoccidioides brasiliensis*	Latin American countries	Inhalation of airborne spores
			Agricultural workers

a rare disease, ubiquitous, but mainly encountered in tropical countries, particularly in Southeast Asia (Vietnam, Cambodge, etc.). It is observed mainly, but not exclusively, in immunocompromised patients. Skin lesions are provoked by an inoculation due to microtraumas (work in the rice plantations, mud banks, drainage systems, and waste products of nutrition). In these countries, it can be considered an occupational disease. For our European countries it is a good example of "imported skin disease" (Arrese et al. 2003; Laurent 2008).

Three types of clinical manifestations are described: papules and squamo-crusted plaques (mimicking pyodermatitis), olecranon bursitis (25% of cases), and systemic protothecosis.

The histopathological features are characteristic: spherulated PAS + organites (4–15 μm in diameter) in the epidermis and dermis, free or engulfed in giant cells. Sporulation leads to the formation of endospores and morula ("sporangia") typical of the disease.

Treatment is successful: systemic antifungals such as amphotericin B, ketoconazole, itraconazole, or fluconazole.

References

Arrese JE, Quatresooz P, Piérard-Franchimont C et al (2003) Protothécose cutanée chez deux adultes de retour d'Extrême-Orient. Dermatologie Actualité (Brussels) 77:27–29

Barnham M, Neilson DJ (1987) Group 2 beta haemolytic streptococcal infection in meat handlers: another streptococcal zoonosis ? Epidemiol Infect 99:257–264

Bellet JS, Prose NS (2005) Skin complications of Bacillus Calmette-Guérin immunization. Curr Opin Infect Dis 18:97–100

Büttner M, Rziha HJ (2002) Parapoxviruses: from the lesion to the viral genome. J Vet Med B Infect Dis Vet Public Health 49:7–16

Daniel CR, Gupta AK, Daniel MP et al (1979) Two feet – one hand syndrome: a retrospective multicenter survey. Int J Dermatol 36:658–660

De Peuter M, De Clercq B, Minette A et al (1977) An epidemiological survey of virus warts of the hands among butchers. Br J Dermatol 97:48–52

Degreef H, Marien K, De Veylder H et al (1987) Itraconazole in the treatment of dermatophytoses: a comparison of two daily dosages. Rev Infect Dis 9(Suppl 1):104–108

English MP (1969) Tinea pedis as a public health problem. Br J Dermatol 81:705–707

Evans ME, Gregory DW, Schaffner W et al (1985) Tularemia: a 30-year experience with 88 cases. Medicine 54:252–269

Gill MJ, Arlette J, Buchan KA (1990) Herpes simplex virus infection of the hand. J Am Acad Dermatol 22:111–116

Grézard P, Philippot V, Perrot H (1995) Incidents et accidents de la vaccination contre l'hépatite B. J Med Lyon 1502:1133–1136

Groves RW, Wilson-Jones E, Mac Donald DM (1991) Human orf and milkers' nodule: a clinicopathological study. J Am Acad Dermatol 25:706–711

Haig DM (2006) Orf virus infection and host immunity. Curr Opin Infect Dis 19:127–131

Handley L, Buller RM, Frey SE et al (2009) The new ACAM 2000 vaccine and other therapies to control orthopoxvirus outbreaks and bioterror attacks. Expert Rev Vaccines 8:841–850

Hay RJ (2006) Fungal infections. In: Faber WR, Hay RJ, Naafs B (eds) Imported skin diseases. Elsevier, Maarssen, pp 55–71

Hay RJ, Adriaans BM (2010) Anthrax. In: Burns T, Breathnach S, Cox N, Griffiths C (eds) Rook's textbook of dermatology, 8th edn. Blackwell, Oxford, pp 30–40, 30–41

Hay RJ, Ashbee HR (2010) Mycology. In: Burns T, Breathnach S, Cox N, Griffiths C (eds) Rook's textbook of dermatology, 8th edn. Blackwell, Oxford, pp 36.1–36.93

Hofinger DM, Cardona L, Mertz GJ et al (2009) Tularemic meningitis in the United States. Arch Neurol 66:523–527

Jablonska S, Obalek S, Golebiowska A et al (1988) Epidemiology of butchers' warts. Arch Dermatol Res 280(Suppl):24–28

Johnson R (2004) Herpes gladiatorum and other skin diseases. Clin Sports Med 23:473–484

Karahocagil MK, Akdeniz N, Akdeniz H et al (2008) Cutaneous anthrax in eastern Turkey: a review of 85 cases. Clin Exp Dermatol 33:406–411

Keefe M, Al-Ghamdi A, Coggon D et al (1994) Cutaneous warts in butchers. Br J Dermatol 130:9–14

Kieffer C, Cribier B, Prevost G et al (2008) Community-acquired methicillin-resistant *Staphylococcus aureus*. Ann Dermatol Venereol 135:263–270

Lachapelle JM, Frimat P, Tennstedt D et al (1992) Précis de dermatologie professionnelle et de l'environnement. Masson, Paris, 400 pp

Lachapelle JM, Tennstedt D, Marot L (1997) Atlas of environmental dermatology UCB pharma. Braine-l'Alleud, Belgium, p 166

Laurent R (2008) L'Hôpital Français de Hanoï (HFH). La protothécose cutanée. Dermatologie Actualité (Brussels) 108:16–21

Lewis-Jones S (2004) Zoonotic poxvirus infections in humans. Curr Opin Infect Dis 17:81–89

Lorette G, Beaulieu P, Allaert FA et al (2009) Superficial community-acquired skin infections: prevalence of bacteria and antibiotic susceptibility in France. J Eur Acad Dermatol Venereol 23:1423–1426

Lundgren R, Normann E, Asberg I (1987) Tuberculosis infection transmitted by autopsy. Tubercule 68:147–150

Maguina C, Flores Del Pozo J, Terashima A et al (2005) Cutaneous anthrax in Lima, Peru: retrospective analysis of 71 cases, including form with a meningoencephalic complication. Rev Int Med Trop Sao Paulo 47:25–30

Mempel M, Kerzl R, Ring J (2008) Methicillin-resistant *Staphylococcus aureus* (MRSA). Relevance in dermatology. Hautartz 59: 659–665

Narayan SK, Sreelakshmi M, Sujatha S et al (2009) Anthrax meningoencephalitis – declining trends in an uncommon but catastrophic CNS infection in rural Tamil Nadu, South India. J Neurol Sci 28:41–45

Ramanan C, Ghorpade A, Kalra SK et al (1996) Buffalopox. Int J Dermatol 35:128–130

Seebacher C, Bouchara JP, Mignon B (2008) Updates on the epidemiology of dermatophyte infections. Mycopathologia 166:335–352

Sterling JC (2010) Orf. In: Burns T, Breathnach S, Cox N, Griffiths C (eds) Rook's textbook of dermatology, 8th edn. Blackwell, Oxford, pp 33.8–33.10

Streit M, Bregenzer T, Heinzer I (2008) Cutaneous infections due to atypical mycobacteria. Hautarzt 59:59–70

Stringer B, Infante-Rivard C, Hanley J (2001) Quantifying and reducing the risk of bloodborne pathogen exposure. AORN J 16:1135–1140; 1142–1143; 1145–1146; 1147–1148; 1151–1154

Tosti A, Guerra L, Morelli R et al (1992) Role of foods in the pathogenesis of chronic paronychia. J Am Acad Dermatol 27: 706–710

Turbeville SD, Cowan LD, Greenfield RA (2006) Infectious disease outbreaks in competitive sports: a review of the literature. Am J Sports Med 34:1860–1865

Vaissaire J, Mendy C, Le Doujet C et al (2005) Tularemia. The disease and its epidemiology in France. Med Mal Infect 35:273–280

Veraldi S, Girgenti V, Dassoni F et al (2009) Erysipeloid: a review. Clin Exp Dermatol 34:859–862

Wang Q, Chang BJ, Riley TV (2010) Erysipelothrix rhusiopathiae. Vet Microbiol 140:405–417

Wolf F, Grézard P, Bérard F et al (1998) Generalized granuloma annulare and hepatitis B vaccination. Eur J Dermatol 8:435–436

24 Occupation-Induced Skin Cancer

Anand N. Patel · John S. C. English
Department of Dermatology, Queen's Medical Centre Nottingham University Hospital, Nottingham, UK

Core Messages

- Occupational skin cancer occurs years after exposure.
- Due to improvements of industrial processes, there has been a decline in occupational skin cancers.
- Common carcinogens are polycyclic aromatic hydrocarbons, ionizing radiation, and arsenic.
- Skin malignancy induction is usually due to mutation of the p53 gene by the carcinogen.
- There is an increasing frequency of melanoma among the aviation crew.

Nonmelanoma skin cancers are the most common form of skin cancers that occur worldwide, namely, basal cell carcinoma and squamous cell carcinoma. They are also an important category of skin disease due to occupation. The link between skin cancer and occupation was first made in 1775 when a London surgeon, Sir Percival Pott, made an affiliation between skin cancer and chimney sweeps. The industrial revolution brought exposure to tar and pitch and thus an increase in cutaneous malignancy. Now in the twenty-first century, the culprits of induced skin cancer are: UV radiation and chemicals such as arsenic and shale oil, ionizing radiation, and X-rays used in medicine and dentistry (Adams et al. 1999).

Miller and Weinstock (1994) estimated that there were between 900,000 and 1.2 million new nonmelanoma skin cancers in the USA in the year of 1994; this equaled the total number of cancers reported in all other organs of the body. The national cancer institute published data from 2009 that reported more than one million new cases of nonmelanoma skin cancer in the USA and 100,000 new cases in the UK per year.

In the USA in 2007 (Tung and Vidimos 2009), the annual incidence of basal cell carcinoma (BCC) was approximately 900,000 cases (550,000 in men, 350,000 in women). The age-adjusted incidence per 100,000 white individuals is 475 cases in men and 250 cases in women. The estimated lifetime risk of BCC in the white population is 33–39% in men and 23–28% in women.

The annual incidence of SCC in the USA is 250,000 new cases per year (http://www.skincancer.org/squamous/squamous-cell-carcinoma.html) ranging from 81 to 136 cases per 100,000 population for men and from 26 to 59 cases per 100,000 population for women (Miller and Weinstock 1994). Whereas in the UK, 100,000 nonmelanoma skin cancers were reported in 2006, 20% of which were squamous cell carcinomas (SCCs) (Cancer Research UK) (http://www.info.cancerresearchuk.org/cancerstats/types/skin).

Prevalence rates of squamous cell carcinoma vary in different countries. The highest incidence occurs in Australia, where the age-adjusted incidence has been calculated to be 1,332 cases per 100,000 population for men and 755 cases per 100,000 population for women. Again, this is likely due to large numbers of light-skinned people in this region who have had extensive sun exposure (Buettner and Raasch 1998). It has been difficult to determine the exact role of chemical carcinogens on those patients with SCC due to the fact that these patients also have experienced daily UV light exposure.

Determining the true incidence of skin cancer is difficult because health registries exclude nonmelanoma skin cancer (including squamous cell carcinoma) from their databases, due to the high number of cases and limited resources to collect data and because the rate of squamous cell carcinoma varies based on geographic location.

Malignant melanoma makes up 5–10% of all reported skin cancer and 95% of deaths from skin cancer. More than 11,000 people in the UK are diagnosed with melanoma each year (http://www.macmillan.org.uk/Cancerinformation/Cancertypes/Skin/Aboutskincancer/Typesofskincancer.aspx). The number of cases has about doubled in the last 20 years or so (http://www.patient.co.uk/health/Cancer-of-the-Skin-Melanoma.htm). It is rather unlikely that chemical carcinogens are a major contributor in the development of malignant melanoma. However, an association with pesticides is reported (Mackie et al. 2009). A strong association is held with UV exposure. A progressive change from predominantly occupational to predominantly recreational patterns of sun exposure is the most likely cause of increasing real incidence of melanoma in populations over the last few decades (Armstrong and Kricker 1994). In the past, few studies have demonstrated a correlation between nonsolar radiation and a significantly increased risk of melanoma. Examples of this are workers exposed to printing lights, welding torchlights

T. Rustemeyer, P. Elsner, S.M. John & H.I. Maibach (eds.), *Kanerva's Occupational Dermatology*,
DOI 10.1007/978-3-642-02035-3_24, © Springer-Verlag Berlin Heidelberg 2012

(Elwood et al. 1986), and fluorescent lights (Walter et al. 1992). However, more recently, there are more studies looking at nonsolar radiation and its association with melanoma. A study from Spain in 2004 showed risk ratios of melanoma and its site with occupation. Apart from UV exposure and artificial sources, risk excesses were seen in fur tailors/tanners/dressers, patternmakers/cutters, electric fitters/wiremen, telephone/telegraph installers/repairmen, and some glass/pottery/tile workers. Specific risk excesses were seen with rolling mill workers in head and neck melanoma, for chimney sweeps in the upper limbs, and for aircraft pilots/navigators/flight engineers in the lower limbs. It was also found that artificial UV sources did not confine melanoma to exposed sites and that the trunk was most affected in these cases (Perez-Gomez et al. 2004).

A study carried out in 2009 examined the relationship between occupational physical activity and risk of melanoma with adjustment for occupational and recreational sun exposure. The data showed an elevated risk for cutaneous malignant melanoma among those with higher levels of physical activity (Lee et al. 2009).

In the UK over a period of 6 years, 1,608 cases of skin cancer thought to be occupation related were reported to a surveillance scheme (Cherry et al. 2000). In the current era, the relationship between skin cancer and occupation is usually linked with sun exposure from leisure activity, as more people have more leisure time available to them. Alongside this is the fashion for having a suntan, or working outdoors.

The rising incidence of cutaneous carcinoma may be due to an increase in sun exposure to the general population. Some postulate that ozone depletion may be intensifying UV exposure (Gray et al. 1997). Other factors that may contribute to the increased incidence include the advancing age of the population, earlier and more frequent diagnosis of skin malignancy due to enhanced public awareness of skin cancer, and more frequent skin examinations by physicians and public health drive.

In addition, the number of patients on immunosuppressive therapy, used in solid organ transplantation and various rheumatologic and dermatologic conditions, is increasing. Mainly squamous cell carcinoma formation has been associated with immunosuppressive drug therapy in solid organ transplantation patients, who have a markedly elevated risk. Metastasis also may be more common in this group (Hampton 2005).

It is thought that skin cancers are the result of carcinogens inducing mutations to genes, in specific the p53 gene. The p53 gene is a tumor suppressor gene and it is found to be mutated in more than 50% of all tumors (Hollstein et al. 1996).

In this chapter, occupational skin cancer will be defined as skin cancers induced by chemical carcinogens and radiation in the workplace. There have been numerous studies that have probed the relationship between sunlight-induced skin malignancy and outdoor occupation. Lear et al. showed a strong correlation between outdoor work and skin cancer in the UK (Lear et al. 1998), whereas other studies by Green et al. (1996) and Freedman et al. (1997) showed the opposite. For this reason, we will not include outdoor work as a form of occupational skin cancer.

Skin tumors can result from exposure to substances such as polycyclic hydrocarbons, inorganic metals, and arsenicals (Nixon 1998; Alam and Ratner 2001). These lesions can also develop because of trauma, burns, and exposure to ultraviolet light or ionizing radiation, particularly in developing countries (Nixon 1998; Alam and Ratner 2001). Co-carcinogenesis, such as the interaction of sunlight and tar, is often implicated. Frequently skin tumors do not appear until two or three decades after the exposure (Jerant et al. 2000).

The results of a case-control study, looking at occupation and skin cancer published in 2007, showed that the frequency of BCC proved higher among railway engine drivers, firemen, salesmen, and specialized farmers in addition to miners, quarrymen, and secondary education teachers. The occupations that showed higher risk of SCC were those involving contact with livestock, construction workers, stationary engine and related equipment operators, and masons (Saurez et al. 2007).

Establishment of an occupational etiology for skin tumors is complicated because of the mobile work force, numerous job changes by individual workers, and exposures that occur both at work and away from the job. All patients should be provided with information on how to prevent skin cancer.

1 Arsenic

Chronic exposure to inorganic arsenic increases the risk of developing arsenical keratoses, Bowen's disease (SCC in situ), BCC, and SCC (Yu et al. 2006). Arsenic enhances ultraviolet carcinogenesis (Burns et al. 2004). It is a cocarcinogen with UVR and is able to induce large chromosomal mutations by this means (Hei et al. 1999). Chronic liver disease and malnutrition (Hsueh et al. 1995) may increase the risk of skin cancer in arsenic-exposed individuals.

Contaminated drinking water is the commonest source of arsenic exposure (Knobeloch et al. 2006) and thus exposure is usually via GI absorption rather than a transdermal means.

Industries which may use arsenic include glass production and manufacture of semiconductors; it may be found in some pesticides and herbicides (potential risk for farmers) (Blair and Freeman 2009), and may occur as a by-product in the smelting of copper, lead, and zinc (Gawkrodger 2004). Workforce may also come into contact with arsenic in its mining and smelting. Arsenical keratoses are clinical signs of exposure, and they may progress to basal cell cancers or squamous cell cancers (Gou et al. 2001).

Arsenic is a puzzling carcinogen as it does not cause cancer in laboratory animals. Studies have associated arsenic with an induction of gene amplification, an inhibition of DNA repair, a cessation of cells in mitosis, and an expression of heme oxygenase, the oxidative stress protein, and the c-fos gene (Lee et al. 1988; Keyse et al. 1990; Vega et al. 1995). A report in 1998 by Hei et al. (1998) found that arsenic is in fact a strong mutagen that causes large chromosomal mutations.

2 Polycyclic Aromatic Hydrocarbons (PAHs)

PAH are made up of two or more benzene rings and comprise of a large group of chemical carcinogens found in the work environment. They are formed by a pyrolytic process such as the combustion of organic compounds. Exposure is mainly by inhalation or skin contact (Bofetta et al. 1997). PAHs are the main carcinogens found in coal tar products, including tar, pitch, soot, and raw paraffin.

Exposure to polycyclic aromatic hydrocarbons may result from gas production from coal, coke plants, aluminum production, steel and iron foundries, and exposure to diesel engine exhaust fumes. As well as this PAH in shale oil, creosote, asphalt, coal tar products, chimney soot have been associated with an increased risk of tar keratoses, BCC, SCC, and keratoacanthomas (Letzel and Drexler 1998).

UVR may work in tandem with PAH to increase the risk of skin cancer (Millard 1986). Its effect on the p53 tumor suppressor gene for the causation of skin cancer remains unknown.

PAHs are complicated in the fact that they may be found in mixtures with other carcinogens. To add to this, a lot of the data previously used was mortality data. This data underestimates the potency of PAHs as a carcinogen due to low mortality rates for BCC and SCC (Bofetta et al. 1997).

3 Tar

In the late 1990s, an employer's insurance company in Germany reported 15 accepted cases of skin cancer due to tar, soot, raw paraffin, hard coal, pitch, and similar materials. This was an increase from nine reported the previous year. These numbers are most likely underestimated as physicians are not required to ask about potential occupational exposure. The main carcinogen in tar is PAH. However, it is also thought that tar-induced skin cancer is also affected by UV exposure (Millard 1986). Tar-induced skin cancers are most commonly found on sun-exposed sites, with the exception of a high incidence of cancers on the scrotum Korting (1981).

A study in 2005 showed increased risk of SCC with use of coal tar and dandruff shampoos (Mitropoulos and Norman 2005).

4 Welding

Even in the twenty-first century, welding is still a common occupation (Meo and Al-Khlaiwi 2003). The hazardous agents associated with the welding processes are acetylene, carbon monoxide, oxides of nitrogen, ozone, phosgene, tungsten, arsenic, beryllium, cadmium, chromium, cobalt, copper, iron, lead, manganese, nickel, silver, tin, and zinc. Inhalation of these chemicals may lead to respiratory disease as well as nonmelanocytic skin cancer and melanoma (Meo and Al-Khlaiwi 2003).

Arc welding can also produce a full spectrum of UVR which in turn can increase risk of skin malignancy.

5 UV and Ionizing Radiation

Ultraviolet radiation is usually encountered in the form of sunrays; however, occupational exposure could occur from ultraviolet tubes. UV exposure was believed to be the main causative agent in skin cancer. A study carried out by Cherry et al. in 2000 showed that UV exposure was believed to be the cause of 96% of skin cancers from a population of 1,608 over 6 years (Cherry et al. 2000).

Epidemiological studies over recent years have found circumstantial evidence on the causative role of the sun in the induction of skin cancer (Turner et al. 2007). Studies confirming the relationship as well as determining dose responses, energy requirements, relationship to chemical stimuli, immune responsiveness, oncogene expression, and tumor suppressor gene inactivity have been solely down to experiments using animal models due to impropriety of such experimentation on humans and practicality. Such tumor induction would need roughly 20 years of recurrent closely monitored exposures. A study published in 2009 looks at a population in Bavaria during the period 2001 until 2005. The data was provided by the cancer registry of this district, and it essentially confirmed previous reports of increased risk in BCC and SCC in outdoor workers compared to indoor workers (Radespiel-Troger et al. 2009). Natural and artificial ultraviolet radiation exposure has been shown to be a risk factor for the development of invasive cutaneous melanoma (Mackie et al. 2009).

Ionizing radiation is well recognized to potentially cause skin cancer, especially squamous cell cancer of the skin and premalignant changes. The time period elapsing between exposure and occurrence of skin malignancy maybe several decades. This phenomenon was discovered from previous physicians and physicists who used X-rays and radiation (Piérard et al. 2009). Thus, this is now well controlled and supervised. Occupations like radiography are not thought to yield an excess of skin malignancy due to the appropriate measures being adopted. However, a report in 2003 showed a higher risk of malignant melanoma in radiological technicians who had first worked before 1950 and in those who did not use the standard lead protection regularly when they first started (Freedman et al. 2003). A review in 2005 looked at seven categories of exposure to ionizing radiation and its link with melanoma. These categories included: (1) The Canadian radiation dose registry, (2) nuclear industry workers, (3) subjects near nuclear test blasts, (4) survivors of atomic bombings of Japan, (5) airline pilots and cabin attendants, (6) recipients of medical radiation, and (7) radiological technicians. Relative risk for leukemia in each of these studies was used to confirm the likelihood to exposure to ionizing radiation. Generally, it was found that groups with elevated relative risks of leukemia had proportionately elevated relative risks of melanoma, suggesting that ionizing radiation is indeed a risk factor for melanoma (Fink and Bates 2005).

UV radiation is known to induce mutations into the p53 tumor suppressor gene (Ziegler et al. 1993) and this is one of the mechanisms by which it may be carcinogenic.

6 Pilots and Aircrew

Skin cancers among commercial airline pilots have been reported to occur at increased rates in pilot populations worldwide. The reasoning behind this is unclear but postulated factors include ionizing radiation, leisure sun exposure, and circadian disruption (Nicholas et al. 2009). A study undertaken in the USA in 2009 showed that pilots who had been working for less than 20 years had similar risk factors to developing skin cancer as the normal population, i.e., skin type, family history, and childhood skin burns. Among pilots who had greater than 20 years flight time, the same risk factors were present with the addition of flight time at high latitude (Nicholas et al. 2009) which increased the risk of skin cancer. Another study in 2006 performed a Medline database search looking at cosmic radiation in aviation and found that seven out of eight studies showed an increased risk for aviators to develop malignant melanoma, basalioma, and other kinds of skin cancer (Ott and Huber 2006). However, there is some controversy with this and other studies due to the lack of scientific evidence to support the hypotheses solely as well as other factors like lifestyle not being incorporated. One study from Iceland in 2003 concluded that there was no substantial correlation between commercial pilots and the general population with respect to prevalence of risk factors for malignant melanoma. Thus, they concluded that it is unlikely that the increased incidence of malignant melanoma found in previous studies of aircrew can be solely explained by excessive sun exposure at high altitude (Rafnsson et al. 2003). An analysis on published data by Buja et al. (2005) believed that as well as the cosmic ionizing radiation that was inflicted upon pilots and aircrew, other factors like chemicals (jet fuel, engine exhausts, cabin air pollutants), electromagnetic fields from cockpit instruments, and disrupted sleep patterns may play a role in the development of skin cancer in this profession.

7 Trauma

Skin cancer may occasionally follow an injury caused in industry such as burns from hot metal or from welding. The cancer will usually develop in the scar and is usually a BCC (Dix 1960). The cancer will usually take several years to develop. A report in 2009 describes a spindle cell melanoma developing in an old scar caused by a burn (Sheff and Pane 2009).

Arsenic	Polycyclic hydrocarbons	Ultraviolet radiation	Ionizing radiation	Burn
Manufacture of insecticide or herbicide	Distillation of coal tar	Outdoor work, e.g., agriculture, driving, fishing, and construction	Nuclear plant operations	Welding
Agricultural exposure to pesticide	Manufacture of coal gas	Welding	Diagnostic X-ray work	
Mining of arsenic	Working with shale oil, creosote, asphalt, and chimney soot	Laser exposure	Uranium mining	
		Certain printing processes	Airline staff	
		Airline staff		

8 The p53 Tumor Suppressor Gene

The p53 gene controls cell growth and metastasis from malignant cells. It has also been associated with several cellular functions including DNA repair, programmed cell death, cell cycle control, differentiation, and genomic plasticity (Trappey et al. 2010).

Molecular epidemiology will allow scientists to investigate cancer risk factors at a more specific level. It has already achieved this for cigarette smoke in lung cancer and UV radiation in skin cancer. Carcinogens like tar and UV light can damage DNA and cause specific genetic mutations regarding the type and location in cancer-related genes. Reports have identified the p53 genetic marker for UV-induced skin cancer (Moles et al. 1993). The DNA mutations encountered from UV exposure occur when UV radiation is absorbed by the DNA and pyrimidine photoproducts are produced. The mis-repair of the photoproducts causes transition mutations (Mitchell et al. 1992). CC to TT transition mutations in the p53 gene have been identified as the unique marker for UV-light-induced skin cancer (Brash et al. 1996). It was reported that 90% of SCCs contained the genetic marker for UV light compared to 50% of BCCs being found to have specific UV-induced mutations of p53 (Rass and Reichrath 2008). This is most likely due to the difference in biology between the two tumors. Mutations in p53 have only been found in 5% of melanomas (Brash et al. 1996). There is a major gap in our current knowledge of how UV initiates melanoma. However, the components of the retinoblastoma (Rb) pathway, and the p53 and p16 pathways are considered the major targets of UV-induced NMSC and melanoma, respectively (Trappey et al. 2010).

9 Conclusions

Improvements in industrial processes alongside a decrease in the amount of distilling of coal tar and its products have resulted in a reduction in risk of occupation-induced cutaneous neoplasm. Increased care in handling sources of ionizing radiation and a better understanding of the risks has also augmented this decrease. The risk from exposure of natural solar UV radiation is largely disregarded as a predisposing factor except in Australia where skin cancer is a public health target (Gawkrodger 2004). Educating outdoor workers with regard to covering up bare skin with clothing and the use of sun creams as well as earlier recognition, management, and public awareness of skin malignancies continues to be the best means of prevention.

Molecular epidemiological techniques can be used to explore the association between UV light- and tar-induced skin cancer, and this will allow risk stratification in further detail. Occupational skin cancer is an important social and public health problem especially in equatorial countries which necessitates further investigation into the most efficient method of assessment (Callahan et al. 2000).

References

Adams RM, Ormsby A, Epstein JH (1999) Occupational skin cancer. In: Adams RM (ed) Occupational skin disease, 3rd edn. WB Saunders, Philadelphia, pp 142–164. ISBN 0-7216-7037-7

Alam M, Ratner D (2001) Cutaneous squamous-cell carcinoma. N Engl J Med 344:975–983

Armstrong BK, Kricker A (1994) Cutaneous melanoma. Cancer Surv 20:219–240

Blair A, Freeman LB (2009) Epidemiologic studies in agricultural populations: observations and future directions. J Agromedicine 14:125–131

Bofetta P, Jourenkova N, Gustavsson P (1997) Cancer risk from occupational and environmental exposure to polycyclic aromatic hydrocarbons. Cancer Causes Control 8:444–472

Brash DE, Ziegler A, Jonason AS, Simon JA, Kunala S, Leffell DJ (1996) Sunlight and sunburn in human skin cancer: p53, apoptosis and tumour promotion. J Invest Dermatol Symp Proc 1:136–142

Buettner PG, Raasch BA (1998) Incidence rates of skin cancer in Townsville, Australia. Int J Cancer 78:587–593

Buja A, Lange JH, Perissinotto E, Rausa G, Grigoletto F, Canova C, Mastrangelo G (2005) Cancer incidence among male military and civil pilots and flight attendants: an analysis on published data. Toxicol Ind Health 21:273–282

Burns FJ, Uddin AN, Wu F et al (2004) Arsenic-induced enhancement of ultraviolet radiation carcinogenesis in mouse skin: a dose response study. Environ Health Perspect 112:599–603

Callahan CP, Merk HF, Blomeke B (2000) Occupational skin cancer and tumours. In: Kanerva L (ed) Handbook of occupational dermatology. Springer, Heidelberg, pp 248–253. ISBN 3-540-64046-0

Cherry N, Meyer JD et al (2000) Surveillance of occupational skin disease: EPIDERM &OPRA. Br J Dermatol 142:1128–1134

Dix CR (1960) Occupational trauma and skin cancer. Plast Reconst Surg 26:546–554

Elwood JM, Williamson C, Stapleton PJ (1986) Malignant melanoma in relation to moles, pigmentation and exposure to fluorescent and other light sources. Br J Cancer 53:65–74

Fink CA, Bates MN (2005) Melanoma and ionizing radiation: is there a causal relationship? Radiat Res 164:701–710

Freedman DM, Zahm SH, Dosemeci M (1997) Residential and occupational exposure to sunlight and mortality from non-Hodgkin's lymphoma: composite case control study. Brit Med J 314:1451–1455

Freedman DM, Sigurdson A, Roa RS et al (2003) Risk of melanoma among radiology technologists in the United States. Int J Cancer 103:559–562

Gawkrodger DJ (2004) Occupational skin cancers. Occup Med 54:458–463

Gou HR, Yu HS, Hu H, Monson RR (2001) Arsenic in drinking water and skin cancers: cell type specificity. Cancer Causes Control 12:909–916

Gray DT, Suman VJ, Su WP, Clay RP, Harmsen WS, Roenigk RK (1997) Trends in the population-based incidence of squamous cell carcinoma of the skin first diagnosed between 1984 and 1992. Arch Dermatol 133:735–740

Green A, Battistutta D, Hart V, Leslie D, Weedon D, Nmabour Study Group (1996) Skin cancer in a subtropical Australian population: incidence and lack of association with occupation. Am J Epidemiol 144:1034–1040

Hampton T (2005) Skin cancer's ranks rise: immunosuppression to blame. JAMA 294:1476–1480

Hei TK, Liu SX, Waldren C (1998) Mutagenicity of arsenic in mammalian cells: role of reactive oxygen species. Proc Natl Acad Sci USA 95:8103–8107

Hollstein M, Rice K, Greenblatt MS, Soussi T, Fuchs R, Sorlie T (1996) p53 data base. Nucleic Acids Res 22:3547–3551

Hsueh YM, Cheng GS, Wu HS et al (1995) Multiple risk factors associated with arsenic-induced skin cancer: effects of chronic liver disease and malnutritional status. Br J Cancer 71:109–114

http://info.cancerresearchuk.org/cancerstats/types/skin. Skin Cancer Statistics-UK. Cancer Research. Accessed 8 Dec 2011

http://www.macmillan.org.uk/Cancerinformation/Cancertypes/Skin/Aboutskincancer/Typesofskincancer.aspx. Types of skin Cancer. Macmillan Cancer Support. Accessed 1 Sep 2011

http://www.patient.co.uk/health/Cancer-of-the-Skin-Melanoma.htm. Patient.co.uk. Reviewed July 2009. Accessed January 2010.

http://www.skincancer.org/skin-cancer-information/squamous-cell-carcinoma. Skin Cancer Foundation. Accessed January 2010

Jerant AF, Johnson JT, Sheridan CD, Caffrey TJ (2000) Early detection and treatment of skin cancer. Am Fam Physician 62:357–368, 375–376, 381–382

Keyse SM, Applegate LA, Tyrell RM (1990) Oxidant stress leads to transcriptional activation of the human heme oxygenase gene in skin fibroblasts. Mol Cell Biol 10:4967–4972

Knobeloch LM, Zierold KM, Anderson HA (2006) Association of arsenic-contaminated drinking water with prevalence of skin cancer in Wisconsin's Fox River Valley. J Health Popul Nutr 24:206–213

Korting GW (1979–1981) Dermatologie in Praxis und Klinik. Bd. I-IV, Thieme, Stuttgart

Lear JT, Tan BB, Smith AG, Jones PW, Fryer AA (1998) A comparison of risk factors for malignant melanoma, squamous cell and basal cell carcinoma in the UK. Int J Clin Pract 52:145–149

Lee TC, Tanaka N, Lamb PW (1988) Induction of gene amplification by arsenic. Science 241:79–81

Lee TK, MacArthur AC, Gallagher RP, Elwood MJ (2009) Occupational physical activity and risk of malignant melanoma: the Western Canada melanoma study. Melanoma Res 19:260–266

Letzel S, Drexler H (1998) Occupationally related tumours in tar refinery workers. J Am Acad Dermatol 39:712–720

Mackie RM, Hauschild A, Eggermont AM (2009) Epidemiology of invasive cutaneous melanoma. Ann Oncol 20(Suppl 6):vi1–7

Meo SA, Al-Khlaiwi T (2003) Health hazards of welding fumes. Saudi Med J 24:1176–1182

Millard LG (1986) Multiple pigmented papular basal cell carcinomas: a new pattern of industrial tar-induced skin tumours. Br J Ind Med 43:143–146

Miller DL, Weinstock MA (1994) Nonmelanoma skin cancer in the United States: incidence. J Am Acad Dermatol 30:774–778

Mitchell DL, Jen J, Cleaver JE (1992) Sequence specificity of cyclobutane pyrimidine dimmers in DNA treated with solar radiation. Nuceic Acids Res 20:225–229

Mitropoulos P, Norman R (2005) Occupational non-solar risk factors of squamous cell carcinoma of the skin: a population based case controlled study. Dermatol Online J 11:5

Moles JP, Moyret C, Guillot B, Jeanteur P, Guilhou JJ, Theillet C, Basset Sanguin N (1993) p53 gene mutations in human epithelial skin cancers. Oncogene 8:583–588

Nicholas JS, Swearingen CJ, Kilmer JB (2009) Predictors of skin cancer in commercial airline pilots. Occup Med (Lond) 59:434–436

Nixon R (1998) Occupational skin cancer. In: English JSC (ed) A colour handbook of occupational dermatology. Manson, London, pp 135–146

Ott C, Huber S (2006) The clinical significance of cosmic radiation in aviation. Praxis (Bern 1994) 95:99–106

Perez-Gomez B, Pollan M, Gustavsson P, Plato N, Aragones N, Lopez-Abente G (2004) Cutaneous melanoma: hints from occupational risks by anatomic site in Swedish men. Occup Environ Med 61:117–126

Piérard GE, Piérard-Franchimont C, Paquet P, Quatresooz P (2009) Emerging therapies for ionizing radiation-associated skin field carcinogenesis. Expert Opin Pharmacother 10:813–821

Radespiel-Troger M, Meyer M, Pfahlberg A, Lausen B, Uter W, Gefeller O (2009) Outdoor work and skin cancer incidence: a registry-based study in Bavaria. Int Arch Occup Environ Health 82:357–363

Rafnsson V, Hrafnkelsson J, Tulinius H, Sigurgeirsson B, Olafsson JH (2003) Risk factors for cutaneous malignant melanoma among aircrews and a random sample of the population. Occup Environ Med 60:815–820

Rass K, Reichrath J (2008) UV damage and DNA repair in malignant melanoma and non-melanoma skin cancer. J Adv Exp Med Biol 624:162–178

Saurez B, Lopez-Abente G, Martinez C, Navarro C, Tormo MJ, Rosso S, Schraub S, Gafa L, Sancho-Garnier H, Wechsler J, Zanetti R (2007) Occupation and skin cancer: the results of the HELIOS-I multicenter case-control study. BMC Public Health 7:180

Sheff JS, Pane TA (2009) Spindle cell melanoma arising from decades-old burn scar. Plast Reconstr Surg 124:274e–275e

Trappey A, Fernando A, Gaur R, Raj M, Ouhtit A (2010) The shady side of sunlight: current understanding of the mechanisms underlying UV-induction of skin cancers. Front Biosci (Schol Ed) 2:11–17

Tung R, Vidimos A (2009). Non Melanoma Skin Cancer: http://www.clevelandclinicmeded.com/medicalpubs/diseasemanagement/dermatology/nonmelanoma-skin-cancer

Turner S, Carder M, van Tongeren M et al (2007) The incidence of occupational skin disease as reported to The Health and Occupation Reporting (THOR) network between 2002 and 2005. Brit J Dermatol 157:713–722

Vega L, Gonsebatt ME, Ostrosky-Wegman P (1995) Aneugenic effect of sodium arsenite on human lymphocytes in vitro: an individual susceptibility effect detected. Mutat Res 334:365–373

Walter SD, Marrett LD, Shannon HS, From L, Hertzman C (1992) The assoc of cutaneous malignant melanoma and fluorescent light exposure. Am J Epidemol 135:749–762

Yu HS, Liao WT, Chai CY (2006) Arsenic carcinogenesis in the skin. J Biomed Sci 13:657–666

Ziegler A, Leffell DJ, Kunala S, Sharma HW, Gailani M, Simon JA, Halperin AJ, Baden HP, Shapiro PE, Bale AE, Brash DE (1993) Mutation hotspots due to sunlight in the p53 gene of non-melanoma skin cancers. Proc Natl Acad Sci USA 90:4216–4220

25 Occupational Nail Disorders

Robert Baran
Nail Disease Center, Cannes, France

Core Messages
To assess nail disorders:

- Rule out nail involvement leading to a "false-positive" diagnosis in the absence of a thorough history and test laboratory.
- Determine, whether it may be exacerbated or just revealed by occupational trauma.
- Visualize what the hands do at work.
- Look for functional distribution of the lesions.
- Look for occupational stigmata on the nails.
- Examine the whole skin surface and mucous membranes.

1 Introduction

1.1 Anatomy

The nail plate is the product of constantly differentiating ectodermal tissue. Its normal appearance and growth depend on the integrity of: (1) the four epidermal structures (matrix, nail bed, hyponychium and proximal nail fold) and (2) the bony phalanx that forms part of the nail apparatus. The nail is set into proximal and lateral nail grooves formed by invaginations in the corresponding nail folds. The periungual tissue and, above all, the distal bony phalanx determine its gross form.

Study of the local anatomy reveals four areas which are particularly vulnerable to trauma. The nail plate emerges from beneath the proximal nail fold, which adheres closely to the nail for a short distance and forms a transverse strip of desquamating tissue, the cuticle (first area of weakness), which seals the cul-de-sac, the matrix from which the nail is derived extends approximately 6 mm under the proximal nail fold, but its most distal part is visible as the white semicircular lunula. For most of its length, the nail plate, which is loosely attached to the matrix, lies distally on a firmly adherent nail bed of highly vascular connective tissue containing glomus organs. It is colorless but translucent, transmitting the pink color of the underlying nail bed. The nail bed epithelium presents with parallel longitudinal rete ridges. The subepithelial capillaries run longitudinally at different but parallel levels. Distally adjacent to the nail bed, the hyponychium, which is an extension of the epidermis under the nail plate, ends at the distal groove. The hyponychium (second area of weakness of the nail apparatus) marks the point at which the nail plate separates from the underlying tissue. There is very little space between the nail and the bone of the distal phalanx, and this space is solely occupied by the nonkeratinizing nail epidermis and mesenchyme. There is no subcutaneous tissue.

The functions of the nail are multiple: (1) to protect the normal nail bed, (2) to act as a weapon or as a tool for scraping or gripping small objects, and (3) to provide counter-pressure for the pulp, which is essential to the tactile sensation involving the fingers. Fingernails grow at a rate of 0.1 mm/day; toenails grow much more slowly.

1.2 Definition

Occupational nail diseases are abnormalities of one or more of the structures of the nail apparatus, produced or aggravated by the working environment.

In assessing a nail condition suspected of being occupational, one should:

1. Rule out nail involvement produced by dermatoses, such as psoriasis, atopic dermatitis, onychomycosis, and lichen planus, which may present with an isolated symptom and lead to a "false-positive" diagnosis (Bennet 1975) in the absence of a thorough history and laboratory tests.
2. Determine whether it may be exacerbated, precipitated, or revealed by occupational trauma (Baran and Levy 1992; Fisher and Baran 1992).
3. Visualize what the hands do at work.
4. Look for functional distribution of the lesions; for example, the first three fingers of the dominant hand are commonly involved in occupational disease.
5. Look for occupational stigmata on the nails (Ronchese 1962a).
6. Examine the whole skin surface and mucous membranes.

T. Rustemeyer, P. Elsner, S.M. John & H.I. Maibach (eds.), *Kanerva's Occupational Dermatology*,
DOI 10.1007/978-3-642-02035-3_25, © Springer-Verlag Berlin Heidelberg 2012

2 Clinical Reaction Patterns

Clinical reaction patterns mainly include:

1. Variations in the contour or micro-contour of the nail including modification of the shape, such as clubbing and koilonychia, and alteration of the surface, such as longitudinal or transverse ridging, brittleness, and pitting.
2. Modifications of the nail plate and soft tissue attachments. This may give rise to paronychia with disappearance of the cuticle and the creation of a pocket between the ventral aspect of the proximal nail fold and the dorsum of the nail plate. Spontaneous separation of the nail plate from the matrix, called onychomadesis, may appear. Acute trauma may result in dorsal or even ventral (distal) pterygium. Onycholysis refers to the detachment of the nail from its bed at its distal and lateral end. Occasionally, epithelial hyperplasia of the subungual tissues may result from exudative skin diseases and produce subungual hyperkeratosis.
3. Variations in the color of the nail or subungual tissue.
4. Distal bony phalanx anomalies. Some physical hazards are mentioned in ➋ *Table 25.1.*

3 Occupational Traumatic Abnormalities

Occupational traumatic abnormalities in the nail area represent one of the most important chapters in this field. This includes major trauma, repeated microtrauma, and injury caused by foreign body.

◘ Table 25.1
Physical hazards

Burns (onycholysis, pterygium)
Cold (Beau's line, nail shedding, koilonychia)
Dishwashers using heavy rubber gloves (subungual hemorrhages)
Foreign bodies
Ionizing radiation (De Dulanto and Camacho 1979)
Trauma
Vibrating power tools (discoloration, ridging, nail shedding, carpal tunnel syndrome and Raynaud's phenomenon, also observed in typists, violinists and pianists)

3.1 Major Trauma

The impairment of the normal functional anatomy of the tip and perionychium will depend on the various levels at which fingertip injuries are sustained, for example, distal to the bony phalanx; distal to the lunula; and proximal to the distal end of the lunula. The place of injury will determine the most suitable approach to the reconstruction of the pedicle. The level of nail bed injury is the critical factor in deciding the requirement for nail bed management. Nail stability requires at least 5 mm of healthy nail bed distal to the lunula for nail adherence (Rosenthal 1983) (➋ *Tables 25.2–25.9*).

3.2 Variations in Color

The term chromonychia indicates an abnormality in color of the substance and surface of the nail plate and/or subungual tissues. Abnormalities of color depend on the transparency of the nail, its attachment to the underlying tissues and the character of the latter. Examination of the abnormal nails should be studied with the fingers completely relaxed and not pressed against any surface. The fingertips should be blanched to see whether the pigmented abnormality is grossly altered; this may help to differentiate between discoloration of the nail plate itself and discoloration of the vascular nail bed. If the abnormality lies in the latter, it usually disappears. Further information may be gleaned by transillumination of the nail using a pen-torch (light) placed against the pulp. If the discoloration is in the subungual soft tissues, its exact position can be identified more easily.

When discoloration results from abnormalities at the nail plate-nail bed attachment, leading to onycholysis and/or subungual hyperkeratosis, the history of the condition will help in diagnosis. Chemicals, wet occupation, trauma or infection may be implicated. Thus, history of the condition may, for example, confirm the traumatic origin of

◘ Table 25.2
Acute injuries (Baran and Dawber 2001)

May be associated with:
Partial or total hematoma
Lacerating wounds
Fractures of the terminal phalanx
Denudation of the terminal phalanx

Table 25.3
Delayed post-acute traumatic deformities (Baran and Dawber 2001)

Onycholysis
Split nail deformity
Pterygium
Various nail dystrophies
Hooked nail

Table 25.4
Repeated microtrauma associated with koilonychia. In time, nail changes may become irreversible

Automotive workers
Cabinet makers
Cement workers
Chimney sweeps
Coil winders
Glass workers
Hairdressers (thioglycolates)
Homemakers
Mushroom growers
Oil burner repairers
Organic chemists (organic solvents)
Pin threaders
Rickshaw pullers (feet)
Slaughterhouse workers

a hematoma. However, the possibility of malignant melanoma following trauma to a nail as a coincidental or causal event should be kept in mind (Roberts 1984). When the discoloration is confined to the nail plate, neither fingertip pressure producing blanching nor the pen-torch placed against the pulp will alter the pigmentation.

When there is nail contact with occupationally derived agents, or topical application of therapeutic agents, the discoloration often follows the shape of the proximal nail fold, and it can be removed by scraping the nail plate or cleaning it with a solvent such as acetone. To determine whether the color is within the nail plate, a piece of nail should be cut off and examined while immersed in water. When specimens are allowed to dry, their true color may be obscured by the scattering of the transmitted light.

Table 25.5
Repeated microtrauma associated with fingernail fragility. This leads to a gradual destruction of the nail plate, which becomes brittle and atrophic. Nail fragility may occur in isolation or associated with paronychia and/or onycholysis

Bean shellers and potato peelers (paronychia)
Butchers
Cement workers
Chemists and laboratory workers (paronychia)
Dentists (onycholysis, subungual hyperkeratosis, dermatitis)
Engravers (paronychia)
Etchers (paronychia)
File makers
Glaziers (paronychia)
Hat cleaners (paronychia)
Multiple myxoid cysts (pushing a garment into an embroidery mold)
Nurses
Optical glass handlers
Packers
Painters (paronychia)
Photographers (paronychia, discoloration)
Plasterers (corroded nails)
Porcelain workers (serrated nails)
Pottery workers
Radio workers (paronychia and nail loss)
Rope workers
Shoe shiners
Shoemakers (onycholysis and paronychia)
Silk weavers (Ronchese 1955)
Tea-picker (thumbnail lamellar splitting)
Weeder thumb. Bilateral distal subungual hematoma
Wet work (paronychia)
Wine growers (subungual splinter hemorrhages)
Woodworkers (paronychia and stains)
Workers exposed to microwave radiation (onycholysis)
Workers handling small instruments
Workers repeatedly lifting heavy plastic bags (Schubert et al. 1977)

When the pigmentation involves all the digits, it results from the systemic absorption of a chemical.

1. When the route of systemic absorption is oral, the discoloration is more likely to correspond to the

Table 25.6
Repeated microtrauma associated with toenail dystrophy

Dancers (exostosis) (Sebastian 1977)
Rickshaw pullers (koilonychia)
Miners (onychomycosis) (Gugnani and Oyeka 1989)
Sportsmen (hematoma; nail shedding)
Athletes
Joggers
Walkers
Squash players
Soccer players
Tennis players

Table 25.7
Repeated microtrauma associated with onycholysis of mechanical origin (Ronchese 1962b; Somov et al. 1976)

Chicken processing plant workers
Cropping
Fur workers
Housewives (chemical and physical problems) (Sharquie et al. 2005)
Milking
Nut cracking
Poultry plucking
Separating meat from bone
Scraping
Shell casing
Destalking mushrooms

shape of the lunula. Transverse leukonychia might occur, for example, in arsenic or thallium poisoning.

2. When systemic absorption of a chemical through the lung or the skin produces dyschromia, there are two possibilities:
   (a) Disappearance of the pigmentation on the nail bed blanching test means that the pigment originates from the blood vessels. Methemoglobinemia, as an example, manifests as a bluish discoloration of the terminal digits and should be looked for in an otherwise asymptomatic worker, that is, following exposure to aromatic nitro and amino compounds that can penetrate all glove materials. The color disappears within 16 h of leaving work, as opposed to sulfhemoglobinemia, which presents with the same distal discoloration as an early warning sign of intoxication (Pinkus et al. 1963) but which only disappears with the normal life span of the red blood cell, that is, 4 months (Kern 1990).
   (b) If the pigmentation is not altered on the nail blanching test, it may be obliterated by the pen-torch pressed against the pulp. This means that the pigment is deposited in the nail bed, as observed in the blue nails of silver refinery workers (*Tables 25.10–25.12*).

Table 25.8
Repeated microtrauma associated with onycholysis caused by foreign bodies. This may be associated with an acute trauma (metal) or repeated microtrauma (hairdressers, for example). Occupational onycholysis is most frequently due to chemical irritants or sensitizers. In addition, there are infective causes, which tend to be limited to medical personnel and occupations which entail prolonged soaking of the hands (*Candida* and *Pseudomonas*)

Animal (bristles, sea urchin, oyster shell)
Metal, glass, fiber glass, plastic. They may also produce paronychia
Splinters of hair (Buendia-Eisman et al. 1997; De Berker et al. 1994) and bacterial infection sometimes associated with subungual manifestation of barber hair signs (Nagtzaam et al. 2007)
Vegetable (thorn, splinter, hyacinth and narcissus bulbs raphide cells with crystals of calcium oxalate)

3.3 Bacterial Infections

The usual microorganisms that may develop in abrasions or lacerations of the nail area are: coagulase-positive staphylococci and various streptococci (Barnham et al. 1980; Barnham and Kerby 1984). Pseudomonas; infection is responsible for the green nail syndrome. Such infected nails (in health care personnel) may then be a source of nosocomial infections, especially from nurses with artificial nails where Serratia, Acinobacter, and Pseudomonas have been found.

Acute paronychia frequently occurs in meat handlers (Barnham and Kerby 1984). Erysipeloid infection is rare and can be observed in meat and fish handlers. Prosector's wart (tuberculosis verruca cutis [Goette et al. 1978]) has its source in a tuberculous-infected cadaver. It may be seen in pathologists, morgue attendants, and other hospital personnel.

Table 25.9
Occupational paronychia

Occupational paronychia
Agricultural workers
Automotive workers (sulfuric acid exposure from batteries)
Bakers and pastry cooks
Barbers and hairdressers (onycholysis)
Bartenders
Bean shellers
Book binders (paste)
Bricklayers (limes, cement, mortar)
Builders and carpenters (including glass fiber)
Button makers
Cement workers
Chemists and laboratory workers
Chicken factory workers
Confectioners
Cooks
Cosmetic workers
Dentists (Kanerva et al. 1997b)
Dyers (aniline dyes, producing stains and necrosis)
Engravers, glass etchers (brittle nail)
Fishermen
Fishmongers
Florist and gardeners (onycholysis) (hyacinth, narcissus
bulbs, tulip fingers) (fungal infection)
Glaziers (brittle nail)
Ground keepers
Hairdressers
Janitorial and domestic workers
Meat handlers
Mechanics
Milkers (onycholysis from bristle)
Oil-rig workers
Painters
Photographic developers (brittle nail, discoloration)
Pianists
Physicians, dentists' nurses
Potato peelers
Radio workers (methanol, causing pigmentation and nail loss)
Salt plant workers (ulcers)
Shoes workers (brittle nails)
Tanners (whitlow)
Textile workers (threads of fabric)
Violinists (nail dystrophy)
Woodworkers (brittle nails, stains)
Wool workers (wool thread)

Table 25.10
Variations in color of the nail plate

Sign	Workers affected
Leuconychia	Arsenic workers
	Butchers
	Keypunchers
	Salt plant workers and contact with salted intestines (Frenk and Leu 1966)
	Weedkillers (paraquat) (Dobbelaere and Bouffioux 1974)
	Workers manufacturing thallium rodenticides
	Fly tyer's finger (apparent leuconychia) (MacAulay 1990)
Blue	Anodisers
	Local argyria
	Auto mechanics (oxalic acid in radiators)
	Cyanosis from methemoglobinemia or sulfhemoglobinemia-
	Dye makers
	Electroplaters
	Gold plasterers
	Metal cleaners, metal patina solution
	Ink makers
	Paint removers
	Photographers
	Rust removers
	Silver protein as a disinfection medicine (generalized argyria)
	Silver workers (presenting generalized argyria) (Sakai et al. 2006)
	Textile workers
Brown/Black	Cigar makers
	Coffee bean workers
	Cooks and bakers (burnt sugar)
	Electric bulb cleaners (hydrochloric acid)
	Gunsmiths
	Hairdressers

Table 25.10 (Continued)

Sign	Workers affected
	Photographers
	Roadway pavers
	Shoe reparers
	Shoe shiners
	Vintners (red wine)
	Walnut pickers (pecans)
	Woodworkers (varnish)
	Woodworkers (ebony, mahogany)
Green (usually caused by *Pseudomonas* infection)	
	Bartenders
	Dishwashers
	Electricians
	Fruit handlers
	Laundry workers
	Metallurgists
	Restaurant workers
	Sugar factory workers
Yellow	Epoxy system handlers
	Metaphenylenediamine and 4,4′-methylenedianiline (Cohen 1985)
	Flower handlers
	Pesticide workers : diquat, paraquat, dinitro-orthocresol dinobuton (Wahlberg 1974)
	Workers handling chromium salts
	Workers handling dyestuffs: dinitro-salicylic acid (Fregert and Trulson 1980), dinitrobenzene, dinitrotoluene and trinitrotoluene

Mycobacterium marinum infection (Califano et al. 1998), called fish-tank granuloma or swimming pool granuloma, the association of skin infection with aquariums and tropical fish has been noted. A prick from a rose thorn might also cause the infection. This is characterized by the presence of a papule, nodule, or erythematous plaque with a verrucous surface on the dorsum of the distal phalanx of the finger.

Pasteurella tularensis is transmitted to man by direct contact with infected wildlife (wild rabbits are the principal reservoirs of tularemia). Over half of the patients with an cutaneous ulcers, present with multiple lesions including shallow erosions into the subungual tissues (Young et al. 1969).

3.4 Viral Infections

Viral infections involving the distal digit include (➲ *Tables 25.13–25.15*):

1. Foot and mouth disease (pustular paronychia) (Armstrong et al. 1967).
2. Herpes simplex infection. This is the most frequent viral infection. It occurs in dentists (Rames et al. 1984), nurses (Kanaar 1967), anesthesiologists (Rosato et al. 1970) and pathologists (Haedicke et al. 1989), and tends to frequently recur in these professions.
3. Human Orf can assume a target-like appearance on the dorsum of the right index finger which is the most commonly affected (Amichai et al. 1993).
4. Milker's nodule is clinically similar to human Orf and mostly involves agricultural workers and veterinarians (Groves et al. 1991).
5. Viral warts are more common in butchers (Jablonska et al. 1987; Aloi et al. 1988; Keefe et al. 1994), poultry handlers (Moragon et al. 1987), and fish handlers (Rüdlinger et al. 1984).

4 Final Comments

There are often pitfalls in diagnosis such as:

1. Where the presentation of cutaneous disease is restricted to an isolated sign involving the nail
2. Where dual pathology exists, such as fungal infection combined with any of the previously mentioned conditions
3. Where there is an isomorphic reaction, for example, in a psoriasis which may not yet be evident, can even be overlooked, or might be latent

The main goals when handling occupational nail disorders are: (1) long-term management and (2) prevention. Management must take into account the patient's continuing occupation; for example, protective gloves might be effective when handling epoxy resins, as these chemicals have probably caused more instances of occupational dermatitis than any other chemicals introduced in recent years. However, the gloves might impair the persons manual dexterity. Furthermore, rubber gloves are penetrated by acrylic

Table 25.11
Some contact sensitizers according to the cause

Contact sensitization occurring through the nail plate is probably rare. Usually sensitizers alter the distal sub- and periungual tissue	
Flowers and plants	Alstroemeria (onycholysis) (Rycroft and Calnan 1981; Marks 1988)
	Hydrangea (paronychia)
	Nasturtium (finger tip dermatitis) (Derrick and Darley 1997)
	Tabernaemontana coronaria (finger tip dermatitis) (Bajaj et al. 1996)
	Tulip fingers (painful onycholysis and fissured keratotic eczema)
	Rhus dermatitis from poison ivy, oak and sumac (onycholysis, yellowish discoloration of the nail)
Chemicals	Acrylic resins[a] (Kanerva et al. 1997c, d) beauticians specializing in nail sculpturing (Lazarov 2007) photobonded acrylic gel nails (occupational airborne dermatitis (Cravo et al. 2008)
	"Cain" (local anesthetics) and propanidid (Castelain and Piriou 1980)
	Cement dermatitis from dichromate content (koilonychia, fissures)
	Codein (onycholysis, subungual hyperkeratosis, nail atrophy) (Romaguera and Grimalt 1983)
	Ethyl cyanoacrylate (Shelley and Shelley 1988)
	Epoxy resin (Castelain et al. 1992)
	Hydroxyethyl dimethacrylate in cow hoof trimmers (McGrath et al. 2009)
	Hydroxylamine (onycholysis, paronychia) (Baran 1991)
	1-methylquinoxalinium-*p*-toluene sulfonate (periungual dermatitis)
	Mydriatic agents containing tropicamide and phenylephrine hydrochloride (nurses)
	Nonoxynol-6 (transverse nail dystrophy)
	Propolis in dental technician (pulpitis fingertip and nail eczema localized in the right thumb and index finger. (Langan and English, 2007)
	Quaternium 15 (subungual hyperkeratosis, onycholysis) (Marren et al. 1991)
	p-Tertiary butyl phenol formaldehyde (onycholysis subungual hyperkeratosis, nail atrophy, periungual dermatitis) (Rycroft et al. 1980)
	Thiourea (Dooms-Goossens et al. 1988)
	Turpentine (periungal dermatitis, subungual hyperkeratosis)
Protein contact dermatitis	Baits (onycholysis, paronychia) (Montel and Gouyer 1957)
	Food animal origin (food handlers) (Tosti et al. 1992)
	Vegetable origin

[a]Acrylic dermatitis usually starts from the fingertips. Fingertips paresthesia (dental nurses, orthopedic surgeons) can be seen Kanerva et al. 1998). Most of the analyzed acrylate products contain undeclared highly sensitizing acrylics up to 46% (Kanerva et al. 1997c). Acrylic tri-cure glass ionomer produces fingertip dermatitis (dental nurses) (Kanerva et al. 1997a)

monomers and this is relevant for orthopedic surgeons, nurses, or dental personnel. The overall aims should include:

1. Efficacy of treatment
2. Prevention of continuing cause
3. Cleanliness
4. Hand comfort
5. Facilitation of continued manual dexterity
6. Above all, ease of application in the treatment and the preventive measures

Table 25.12
Chemical irritants

Chemical irritants
Alkalis
Alkaline chlorine-containing compounds (Coskey 1974)
Aminoethylethanolamine-containing soldering flux (onycholysis, periungual dermatitis) (Goh 1985)
Detergents (onycholysis, subungual bleeding ulcerations) (Göthe et al. 1972)
Formaldehyde
Gold potassium cyanide (purplish-brown discoloration, onycholysis) in electroplaters, electronic workers (Budden and Wilkinson 1978)
Hydrofluoric acid (excruciating pain, onycholysis) (Shewmake and Anderson 1979)
Organic solvents and motor oils (onycholysis, subungual hyperkeratosis, nail softening)
Oxalic acid (bluish discoloration, brittle nails)

Table 25.13
Fungal infections

Candida fungal infection of the nail area is a common condition involving occupations that require the hands to be wet for prolonged periods	
Candida spp. (onycholysis paronychia)	Dishwashers, poultry and fish handlers
Dermatophytic toenail infection	
Trichophyton rubrum is the most common dermatophyte, sometimes responsible for the one hand-two-foot tinea syndrome	Increased prevalence in coal miners and others who work in hot, humid environment
Trichophyton mentagrophytes var. *interdigitale*	Washing facilities
Molds, especially *Scytalidium* spp. involves the toenails	Miners
Onychomycosis	Dental nurses (Alandko et al. 1997)

Table 25.14
Individuals at risk of fungal infections (Baran 1997)

Individuals at risk
Athletes
Carpet weaving (Kaçar et al. 2009)
Dustmen
Employees of indoor swimming pools
Excavation workers
Green tea leaf pluckers (*Scytalidium dimidiatum*) (Barua-Purnima et al. 2007)
Mine workers
Rubber industry workers
Sewer workers
Soldiers
Steel and furnace workers
Woodcutters

Table 25.15
Occupational systemic conditions

Clubbing (resulting from pneumoconiotic lung diseases)	Exposure to:
	Asbestos (Petry 1966)
	Talc
	Beryllium (Kern 1990)
	Silica
	Cobalt (Desoille et al. 1962)
	Tungsten (Desoille et al. 1962)
Pseudoclubbing (systemic sclerosis with acroosteolysis)	Vinyl chloride monomer
Cutaneous hemangioendothelioma	Polyvinyl chloride (Davis et al. 1990)
Collagen diseases:	
Systemic sclerosis	Vinyl chloride monomer
	Epoxy resin (vapors)
	Trichlorethylene, trichlorethane
	Silica (Rustin et al. 1989)
Sclerodactyly (nail-fold capillary changes, Raynaud's phenomenon, acroosteolysis) (Bachurzewska and Boruka 1986; Flindt-Hansen and Isager 1987)	
Lupus eythematosus-like erythema and periungual telangiectasia	Coffee plantation workers (Narahari et al. 1990)

Acknowledgments

We would like to thank the publisher for the permission to reproduce some of the tables which appeared in (Rycroft and Baran R 2001).

References

Alandko K, Kanerva L, Estlander T et al (1997) Hairdresser's koilonychia. An J Contact dermatitis 8:177–178

Aloi FG, Molinero A, Passera A et al (1988) Viral warts in butchers. Clinical and statistical study. G Ital Dermatol Venereol 123:341–344

Amichai B, Grunwald MH, Abraham A et al (1993) Tense bullous lesions on fingers. Arch Dermatol 129:1043–1048

Armstrong R, Davie J, Hedger RS (1967) Foot and mouth disease in man. BMJ 4:529–530

Bachurzewska B, Boruka I (1986) Dermatosen in Beruf und Umwelt. Occup Environ Dermatol 34:77–79

Bajaj AK, Pasricha JS, Gupta S et al (1996) Tabernaemontana coronaria causing fingertip dermatitis. Contact Dermatitis 35:104–105

Baran R (1991) Onycholysis from hydroxylamine. Contact Dermatitis 24:158

Baran R (1997) Epidemiology and prevention of onycholysis. In: Grob JJ, Stern RS, Mackie RM, Weinstock WA (eds) Epidemiology, causes and prevention of skin diseases. Blackwell Science, Oxford, pp 276–278

Baran R, Dawber RPR (2001) Nail diseases and their management. Blackwell Science, Oxford

Baran R, Levy JL (1992) Onychopathies et travail. Rev Med Travail 19:47–49

Barnham M, Kerby J (1984) A profile of skin sepsis in meat handlers. J Infect 9:43–50

Barnham M, Kerby J, Skillin J (1980) An outbreak of streptococcal infection in a chicken factory. J Hyg Camb 84:71–75

Barua-Purnima BS, Borkakoty B et al (2007) Onychomycosis by *Scytalidium dimidiatum* in green tea leaf pluckers: report of two cases. Mycopathologia 164:193–195

Bennet JH (1975) The "false positive" diagnosis: skin disorders that mimic an occupational dermatitis. Cutis 15:410–411

Budden MG, Wilkinson DS (1978) Skin and nail lesions from gold potassium cyanide. Contact Dermatitis 4:172–173

Buendia-Eisman A, Serrano-Ortegas O, del Olmo RM (1997) Hair fragments as a subungual foreign body. Eur J Dermatol 7:517–518

Califano L, Cannavo SP, Malara G et al (1998) Verrucous nodule of the finger. Arch Dermatol 134:365–366

Castelain PY, Piriou A (1980) Contact dermatitis due to propanidid in an anesthetist. Contact Dermatitis 6:360

Castelain PY, Com J, Castelain M (1992) Occupational dermatitis in the aircraft industry: 35 years of progress. Contact Dermatitis 27:311–316

Cohen SR (1985) Yellow staining caused by 4,4'-methylenedianiline exposure. Arch Dermatol 121:1022–1027

Coskey RJ (1974) Onycholysis from sodium hypochlorite. Arch Dermatol 109:96

Cravo M, Cardoso JC, Gonçalo M et al (2008) Allergic contact dermatitis from photobonded acrylic gel nails: a review of four cases. Contact Dermatitis 59:250–251

Davis MFP, Curtis M, Howat JMT (1990) Cutaneous hemangioendothelioma: possible link with chronic exposure to vinyl chloride. Br J Ind Med 47:65–67

De Berker D, Dawber R, Wojnarowska F (1994) Subungual hair implantation in hairdressers. Br J Dermatol 130:400–401

Derrick E, Darley C (1997) Contact dermatitis to nasturtium. Br J Dermatol 136:287–299

Desoille H, Brouet G, Assouly M et al (1962) Diffuse pulmonary fibrosis in a subject exposed to cobalt and tungsten carbide dusts (heavy metal industry). Discussion of a simple coincidence or an ultimate relation of cause and effect. Arch Mal Prof 23:570–578

Dobbelaere F, Bouffioux J (1974) Leuconychie en bandes due au paraquat. Arch Dermatol 30:283–384

Dooms-Goossens A, Dubusschère K, Morren M et al (1988) Silver polish: another source of contact dermatitis reactions to thiourea. Contact Dermatitis 19:133–135

Dulanto (De) F, Camacho F (1979) Radiodermatitis. Acta Derm Sif 70:67–94

Fisher AA, Baran R (1992) Occupational nail disorders with a reference to Koebner's phenomenon. Am J Contact Dermat 3:404–406

Flindt-Hansen H, Isager H (1987) Scleroderma after occupational exposure to trichlorethylen et trichloretane. Acta Derm Venereol 67:263–264

Fregert S, Trulson L (1980) Yellow stained skin from dinitrosalicylic acid. Contact Dermatitis 6:362

Frenk F, Leu F (1966) Leukonychie durch beruflichn Kontakt mit gesalzenen Da'rmen. Hautarzt 17:233–235

Goette DK, Jacobson KW, Doty RD (1978) Primary inoculation tuberculosis of the skin. Prosector's paronychia. Arch Dermatol 114:567

Goh CI (1985) Occupational dermatitis from soldering flux among workers in electronic industry. Contact Dermatitis 13:85–90

Göthe CJ, Nilzen A, Holmgren A et al (1972) Medical problems in the detergent industry caused by proteolytic enzymes from bacillus subtilis. Acta Allergol 1:63–86

Groves RW, Wilson-Jones E, MacDonald DM (1991) Human Orf and milkers nodules: a clinico pathologic study. J Am Acad Dermatol 25:706–711

Gugnani HC, Oyeka CA (1989) Foot infections due to hendersonula toruloidea and scytalidium hyalinun in coal miners. J Med Vet Mycol 27:169–179

Haedicke GJ, Crossman JAI, Fisher AE (1989) Herpetic whitlow of the digits. J Hand Surg Br 14:443–446

Jablonska S, Obalek S, Favre M et al (1987) The morphology of butcher's warts as related to papilloma-virus types. Arch Dermatol Res 279:566–572

Kaçar N, Ergin S, Ergin C et al (2009) Carpet weaving: an occupational risk for onychomycosis? J Eur Acad Dermatol Venereol 24(3):353–355

Kanaar P (1967) Primary herpes simplex infection of fingers in nurses. Dermatologica 134:346

Kanerva L, Estlander T, Jolanki R (1997a) Occupational allergic contact dermatitis caused by acrylic tri-cure glass ionomer. Contact Dermatitis 37:49–50

Kanerva L, Henriks-Eckerman ML, Estlander T et al (1997b) Dentists' occupational allergic paronychia and contact dermatitis caused by acrylics. Eur J Dermatol 7:177–180

Kanerva L, Henricks-Eckerman ML, Jolanki R et al (1997c) Plastics/acrylics: material safety data sheets need to be improved. Clin Dermatol 15:533–546

Kanerva L, Jolanki R, Estlander T (1997d) Ten years of patch testing with the (meth)acrylate series. Contact Dermatitis 37:255–258

Kanerva L, Mikola H, Henriks-Eckerman ML et al (1998) Fingertip paresthesia and occupational allergic contact dermatitis caused by acrylics in a dental nurse. Contact Dermatitis 38:114–116

Keefe M, Ghamdi A, Coggon D et al (1994) Cutaneous warts in butchers. Br J Dermatol 130:9–14

Kern DG (1990) Occupational disease. In: Scher R, Daniel C (eds) Nails: therapy, diagnosis, surgery. W.B. Saunders, Philadelphia, pp 224–243
Langan MS, English JS (2007) Occupational contact dermatitis from propolis in a dental technician. Contact Dermatitis 52:43
Lazarov A (2007) Sensitization to acrylates is a common adverse reaction to artificial fingernails. J Eur Acad Dermatol Venereol 21:169–174
MacAulay JC (1990) Fly tiers finger. Can J Dermatol 2:67
Marks JG (1988) Allergic contact dermatitis to alstroemeria. Arch Dermatol 124:914–916
Marren P, de Berker D, Dawber R et al (1991) Occupational contact dermatitis due to quaternium 15 presenting as nail dystrophy. Contact Dermatitis 25:253–255
McGrath EJ, Darvay A, Lovell CR (2009) Nail dystrophy and fingertip dermatitis as a manifestation of methyl methacrylate allergic contact dermatitis in a cow hoof trimmer. Contact Dermatitis 60:344
Montel MI, Gouyer E (1957) L'Escavenite. Bull Soc Fr Dermatol Syphiligr 64:672
Moragon M, Ibanez MD, San Juan L et al (1987) L'incidence des verrues vulgaireschez les travailleurs d'abattoirs industriels de volaille de la province de Valence. Arch Mal Prof 48:41–43
Nagtzaam IF, Van der Velden JJAJ, Kelleners-Smeets NWJ et al (2007) Onycholysis associated with subungual manifestation of barber's hair sinus. Int J Dermatol 46:48–49
Narahari SR, Skiniva CR, Kelkar SK (1990) L.E.-like erythema and periungual telangiectesia among coffee plantations workers. Contact Dermatitis 22:296–297
Petry H (1966) Uhrglasnagel und Trommelschlegelfinger bei Asbestose. Int Arch Geweberpath, Gewerberghyg 22:55–59
Pinkus J, Djadetti M, Joshua H et al (1963) Sulfhemoglobinemia and acute hemolytic anemia with Heinz bodies following contact with a fungicide - zinc ethylene bisdithiocarbamate in a subject with glucose-6-phosphate dehydrogenase deficiency and hypocatalasemia. Blood 21:484–494
Rames S, Folkmar T, Roed-Petersen B (1984) Herpes simplex as a possible occupational disease in dentists of the county of Aarhus, Denmark. Acta Derm Venereol 64:163–165
Roberts AHN (1984) Subungual melanoma following a single injury. J Hand Surg Br 9:328–330
Romaguera C, Grimalt F (1983) Dermatitis de contacto professional por codeina. Bol Inform GEIDC 5:21–23
Ronchese F (1955) Peculiar silk weavers nails. A new type of artefacts. Arch Dermatol 71:525–526
Ronchese F (1962a) Nails: injuries and disease in traumatic medicine and surgery for the attorney, vol 6. Butterworth, Washington, pp 626–639
Ronchese F (1962b) Nail defect and occupational trauma. Arch Dermatol 85:404
Rosato FE, Rosato EF, Plotkin SA (1970) Herpetic paronychia, an occupational hazard of medical personnel. N Engl J Med 282: 804–805
Rosenthal EA (1983) Treatment of fingertip and nail bed injuries. Orthop Clin North Am 14:675–697
Rüdlinger R, Bunney MH, Grab R et al (1984) Warts in fish handlers. Br J Dermatol 120:375–381
Rustin MHA, Bull HA, Ziegler V et al (1989) Silica exposure and silica-associated systemic sclerosis. Br J Dermatol 121(Suppl 34): 29–30
Rycroft RJG, Baran R (2001) Occupational abnormalities and contact dermatitis. In: Baran R, Dawber RPR (eds) Diseases of the nails and their management, 3rd edn. Blackwell Science, Oxford, Chap 7, pp 330–357
Rycroft RJG, Calnan CD (1981) Alstroemeria dermatitis. Contact Dermatitis 7:284
Rycroft RJG, Wilkinson JD, Homes R et al (1980) Contact sensitization to p-tertiary butylphenol (PTBP) resin in plastic nail adhesive. Contact Dermatitis 5:441–445
Sakai N, Aoki M, Miyazawa S et al (2006) A case of generalized argyria caused by the use of silver protein as a disinfection medicine. Acta Derm Venereol 86:186–187
Sebastian G (1977) Subungual Exostose der Grosszche, Berufsstigma bei Tänzern. Derm Monatsschr 163:998–1000
Schubert B, Minard JJ, Bara R et al (1977) Onychopathie de champignonnistes. Ann Dermatol Venereol 104:627–630
Sharquie IK, Al-Faham M, Karhoot JM et al (2005) Housewife onycholysis. Saudi Med J 26:1439–1441
Shelley DE, Shelley WB (1988) Nail dystrophy and periungual dermatitis due to cyanoacrylate glue sensitivity. J Am Acad Dermatol 19:574–575
Shewmake SW, Anderson BG (1979) Hydrofluoric acid burns. Arch Dermatol 115:593–596
Somov BA, Lipets ME, Ivanov VV et al (1976) Occupational onycholysis. Vestn Derm Venereol 2:51–55
Tosti A, Guerra L, Morelli R et al (1992) Role of foods in the pathogenesis of chronic paronychia. J Am Acad Dermatol 27:706–710
Wahlberg JE (1974) Yellow staining of hair and nails and contact sensitivity to dinobuton. Contact Dermatitis Newslett 16:481
Young IS, Bicknell DS, Archer BG et al (1969) Tularemia epidermic: Vermont 1968. Forty-seven cases linked to contact with muskrats. N Engl J Med 280:1253

26 Hair Disorders Induced by External Factors

Marcel C. Pasch
Department of Dermatology, Radboud University Nijmegen Medical Centre, Nijmegen, The Netherlands

Core Messages

- External factors may result in hair loss, increased hair growth, or changes in the color and texture of the hair.
- External factors responsible for hair loss are drugs, radiation, traction, fungi, pesticides, plant toxins, heavy metals and several other chemicals.
- Several groups of drugs may be responsible for unintentional induction of hair growth.
- Texture and color of hair may be changed by drugs, metals, and ultraviolet and other radiation.
- Full recovery is the rule after elimination of the responsible factor.

1 Introduction

Hair has many useful biologic functions, including protection from the elements and dispersion of sweat-gland products. It also has psychosocial importance in our society, and patients with hair loss (alopecia) or excessive hair growth (hypertrichosis or hirsutism) often suffer tremendously. Not surprisingly, patients being confronted with hair disorders will seek for medical care in order to find the cause of their hair disorder. Hair disorders have a high incidence in the general population. Most of them can be explained by aging (male and female pattern hair loss), factors concerning general health (e.g., thyroid dysfunction, pregnancy, and malnutrition), use of medication, and inflammatory and infectious scalp disorders. Occupational and environmental factors belong to the more rare causes of hair disorders. However, not considering them and only focusing on the more common causes of hair disorders will result in persistence of situations which may lead to expanding the problem to larger groups of people. On the other hand, some causes of hair loss have such a high prevalence in the general population that involved coworker might assume causality with their working environment and exposition to chemicals. However, the incidence of alopecia areata was reported to be 1.7% and male or female pattern hair loss is ubiquitous (Safavi et al. 1995). Confusion about occupational or external factors involved in development of alopecia areata and pattern hair loss is understandable but has never been convincingly documented.

This chapter focuses on hair diseases and external factors which may play a role in their pathogenesis.

2 Anatomy and Hair Cycle

Hair follicles cover almost the entire surface of the body. Only the palms, soles, glans penis, and labia minora are devoid of them. The scalp possesses the greatest density of hair follicles with a range of 300–500 hair follicles/cm^2. Approximately five million hair follicles are on the body, with 100,000 on the scalp.

The hair producing matrix cells of the follicular bulb constitute a pool of undifferentiated transit amplifying cells that have intense metabolic activity. This metabolic activity is greater than of any other tissue, except the bone marrow, making them vulnerable for cell cycle inhibiting factors like fever, endocrine abnormalities, parturition, major surgery, anemia, and malnutrition. Also drugs, radiation, and external toxic factors, which are the focus of this chapter, easily can inhibit cell cycle in the follicular bulb, resulting in hair loss. Regulation of hair growth and details on the biology of the hair follicle are complex processes which are beyond the scope of this chapter. Furthermore, one should realize that the hair follicle has more functions than producing a hair fiber. For example, the hair follicle acts as a sensory organ and immunologic sentinel of the skin.

2.1 The Hair

The hair fiber is about 50–100 μm in diameter and consists of a cuticle, cortex, and medulla. The cortex provides the majority of hair fiber mass, is responsible for its strength, and contains melanin pigment. It is made from cells which are tightly packed together. It contains keratins with a high level of sulfur-containing amino acids. Cross-linking of

T. Rustemeyer, P. Elsner, S.M. John & H.I. Maibach (eds.), *Kanerva's Occupational Dermatology*,
DOI 10.1007/978-3-642-02035-3_26, © Springer-Verlag Berlin Heidelberg 2012

these amino acids results in formation of disulfide bonds which give the hair most of its great tensile strength. The cuticle covers the cortex and consists of layers of scales, each about 0.5 μm thick, which overlap in a roofing tile manner. The cuticle protects the underlying cortex and acts as a barrier against the external environment. The medulla of the hair is only present in thick terminal hairs. It consists of air space containing specialized cells, which may have a function in the thermal insulation of the body.

2.2 Hair Cycle

Cyclic growth is a typical characteristic of the hair follicle. Each hair follicle perpetually goes through three stages: growth (anagen), involution (catagen), and rest (telogen). The release of dead hair is sometimes called exogen. The exogen coincides with the end of the telogen stage and the entrance to the anagen phase of the next hair cycle.

Normally, each human hair follicle cycles independently, so that while some hairs are growing, others are resting and others are shedding. Thus, under normal circumstances there is a balance between hair growth and hair shedding. Since most people are born with about 80,000–150,000 scalp hairs, and normally a hair cycle lasts about up to 8 years, shedding of 50–150 telogen hairs per day is normal. Loss of anagen hair is always pathological. Hair loss and unwanted hair growth reflects aberrations of the hair-follicle cycling, except for rare congenital hair defects, caused by mutations in keratins or other structural proteins, and "scarring" alopecias. Thus, in principle, hair loss and unwanted hair growth are reversible phenomena.

2.2.1 Anagen

Anagen is the stage of active hair growth. In this stage, which can last 2–8 years on the scalp or beard areas, each hair follicle will produce monthly about 10 mm of hair fiber. Other areas of the human body have hair follicles with shorter anagen stages. The anagen stage on the brows or trunk does not exceed 6 months. Because of the differences in duration of the anagen stage, the maximum length of a hair differs between the scalp and, for example, the eyebrow and the pubic hairs. The maximum length of an untrimmed hair is proportional to the duration of the anagen cycle. Cell division rates are highest in anagen hair follicles. Therefore, areas with a high percentage of anagen follicles, such as scalp or beard, will be more susceptible to factors affecting rapidly dividing cells. Areas with a high percentage of telogen follicles, such as eyebrows, will be more resistant to these factors. This difference explains why hair loss during chemotherapy or due to exposure to toxic substances is often solely located on the scalp and beard and does not comprise other body hairs.

2.2.2 Catagen

Anagen is followed by an involutional stage called catagen, which last an couple of weeks. During this stage hair follicles go through a process of involution that largely reflects a burst of programmed cell death (apoptosis) in the majority of follicular keratinocytes and cessation of follicular cell division.

2.2.3 Telogen

The catagen stage is followed by a resting or telogen stage. In this stage the hair remains loosely attached in the dormant follicle. The hair shaft matures into a club hair, which is eventually shed from the follicle, usually during washing or combing. The time between entering the telogen stage and the shedding of the hair is 2–4 months and is independent from the anatomical region. It is unknown whether shedding is an active, regulated process or a passive event that occurs at the onset of the next anagen stage, as a new hair grows in. Under normal circumstances all hairs which are shed are telogen hairs.

2.3 Occupational Hair Disorders

Occupational hair disorders are abnormalities of structures of the hair follicle caused or aggravated by the working environment. Alopecia is not an uncommon phenomenon in toxicological animal studies. The relevance for humans is frequently not clear. Therefore, only substances with proven or likely effects on hairs in humans will be discussed.

The most common acquired hair disorder is hair loss or thinning. The first, but often difficult, task in diagnosing hair disorders is to distinguish between true disorders and subjective complaints. After having diagnosed a true disorder the elucidation of the nature of the hair disease may be even more challenging. However, before focusing on occupational and other external factors one should realize that hair disorders have a high incidence in the general population, so common causes of hair disorders need to be ruled out.

2.4 Evaluation of Hair Loss

Hair diagnostic tools in a dermatologic or occupational medicine consultation comprise a thorough clinical history, physical examination including the skin of the scalp, a hair pull test, and often microscopic examination of hair shafts and hair roots. A scalp biopsy is only indicated in selected cases.

2.4.1 Clinical History

The thorough clinical history always will facilitate making the correct diagnosis. The duration of hair shedding, the character (episodic or continuous), a subjective estimation of percentage of hair loss, recent surgery, fever, illness, childbirth, or physiological stress needs to be addressed. Also the presence of chronic disease, malignancy, infection, autoimmune disease, and liver or renal disease requires attention. The role of mental stress is not clear but may also play a role. Particular attention should be paid to the time between a potential cause and the actual begin of the hair loss. Few simple questions may rule out the presence of thyroid disease, while presence of hirsutism, acne, seborrhea, irregular cycle or infertility may be indications for high androgen levels. Of particular importance is a meticulous history of drugs used in the past months, including over-the-counter drugs, vitamin A, and botanicals. Incidental, acute, or chronic (occupational) exposure to chemicals, animals, heavy metals, or radiation needs to be addressed. Most effluvium is loss of telogen hairs caused by a premature disruption of the anagen phase of hair cycle and entrance to the telogen phase. After entering the telogen phase, hair shedding will follow after completing this phase. So hair shedding after exposure to a causing factor mostly will follow 2–3 months later. However, after exposure to many antimitotic agents, too high doses of radiation, or to toxins an acute anagen effluvium may occur within days to few weeks.

2.4.2 Physical Examination

The physical examination of the scalp will show the severity, a potential pattern of the hair loss and the presence of scalp disorders. As a rule of thumb one may take into account that hair loss of less than 25–50% may not be visible for outsiders. The pattern will reveal whether the hair loss is diffuse or localized, or has a distinctive clinical distribution like in male or female androgenetic alopecia. Physical examination of the scalp may show the presence of an inflammatory or infectious skin disorder. Scalp psoriasis, dermatitis, fungal infections, but also rare primary or secondary cicatricial alopecias will present with both hair loss and abnormal skin of the scalp.

2.4.3 Hair Pull Test

The hair pull test is a simple test to determine the ongoing activity and severity of any kind of hair loss. To perform the hair pull test a bundle of about 50 hairs is grasped between the thumb, index finger, and middle finger near the scalp. The hair is firmly tugged away from the scalp as fingers slide along the hair shaft. This procedure is repeated in the left and right parietal area, the frontal area, and the occipital area. Hair that can be detached from the hair follicle in the hair pull test was only loosely attached to the hair follicle. Extraction of no more than 10%, so five to six hairs, is considered physiological. Extraction of more hairs constitutes a positive pull test, implying active hair shedding. Despite it simplicity, this test has some major draw backs. The interobserver variability is very high and the result greatly depends on hair care habits of the patient. Recent washing, the use of sticky hair cosmetics, like hair spray, gel, wax, or extensive brushing will influence the outcome of this test. Therefore, patients are asked not to wash their hair and to avoid sticky hair cosmetics in the 5 days before the examination. Nevertheless, the hair pull test is only a rough approach, which appears to be useful only for acute and more severe phases of hair loss.

The nature of the extracted hairs can be analyzed by light microscopy to narrow the differential diagnosis. In case of telogen hair loss the hair roots will have the typical club-like characteristics of telogen hair (➋ *Fig. 26.1a*), in alopecia areata there will be both telogen and tapered broken anagen hairs (➋ *Fig. 26.1b*), and in acute anagen effluvium increased numbers of tapered anagen hairs or anagen hair (➋ *Fig. 26.1c*) can be seen.

After clinical evaluation a first estimation can be made of the extent, clinical diagnosis, and origin of the hair loss.

2.5 Diffuse Hair Loss

Diffuse hair loss can be defined as a positive hair pull test in both the vertex area and margins of the scalp. It is further classified by the types of hairs that are shed: are they anagen, dystrophic anagen, or telogen?

Chemicals, drugs, or radiation may either cause excessive hair shedding by precipitating telogen development,

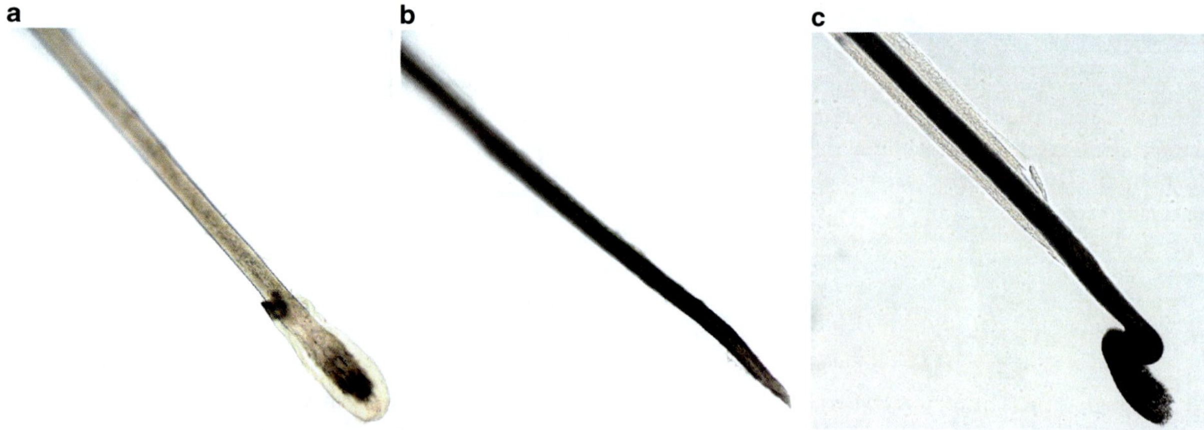

Fig. 26.1
(a) Telogen hair obtained by hair pull. (b) Tapered broken anagen hair from a alopecia areata patient. (c) Anagen hair obtained by plucking

directly poison the anagen root, or work in a undetermined way. Precipitation of telogen development results in telogen hair loss occurring 2–4 months after the insult, reflecting the time required for the full telogen state to be accomplished. Direct poisoning of the anagen hair may result in rapidly occurring hair loss, only days to few weeks after the insult.

2.6 Anagen Hair Loss

Two types of anagen hair loss can be recognized. Dystrophic anagen effluvium and loose anagen syndrome. The loose anagen syndrome is beyond the scope of this chapter, because it is predominantly described in children and no external or occupational factors have been recognized in this disorder.

Dystrophic anagen hair loss is the result of interruption of the anagen phase of hair cycle. It presents as abrupt anagen hair shedding with severe and diffuse scalp alopecia. Since the loss affects the anagen hairs but not the telogen hairs, eyebrow and body hair is relatively spared. The time course for anagen hair loss is usually rapid after the insult to the hair follicles. All causative factors share one characteristic: they abruptly stop normal cell division of rapidly dividing hair matrix cells in the hair bulb. Important causative factors are antineoplastic drugs, radiation, environmental or occupational exposure to toxins, and diffuse alopecia areata. The common time frame is an onset within days to weeks after exposure to the causative factor. So hair loss commences fast after exposure but a rapid reversal within weeks to few months after withdrawal of the exposure is another hallmark of dystrophic anagen hair loss.

2.6.1 Diagnosis

Anagen hair loss is the consequence of a directly toxic effect on the hair matrix cells. This leads to hair loss in two ways. If the matrix itself suffers a severe and prolonged insult, then much of the follicle is affected, and immediate anagen hair loss will occur in which there is an *immediate release of dystrophic hairs.* At the pull test the hairs are easily removed with a necrotic anagen sheath adhering to them (➋ *Fig. 26.1c*). If the insult is less severe or of a short duration, then mitotic activity will decrease only temporally. There will be *hair damage without anagen release:* the hair will continue growing but has developed a weak constricted area in the shaft. As soon as this constricted area grows above the surface of the skin, a minor trauma can cause a fracture of the hair, resulting in shedding. Under the microscope a tapered hair is visible, which is characteristic of anagen hair loss (➋ *Fig. 26.1b*) and may be seen in alopecia areata as well.

2.6.2 Treatment

Hair loss commences fast after exposure and once the insult is removed, regrowth is usually prompt because normal anagen growth has been only temporarily interrupted. So a rapid and generally complete clinical reversal within weeks to few months after withdrawal of the exposure is a hallmark of anagen hair loss, with only few exceptions. Additional treatment is neither effective nor necessary.

2.6.3 Causes of Anagen Hair Loss

External and occupational factors able to cause anagen hair loss will be discussed in detail below. Chemotherapy-induced alopecia is the most frequent of them. It occurs with an estimated incidence of 65% in cancer patients. Forty-seven percent of female cancer patients consider it the most traumatic aspect of chemotherapy (Trueb 2009). It has been reported several times that health workers involved in preparation and administration of antineoplastic drugs have a fivefold to sevenfold increased risk of developing hair loss (Krstev et al. 2003). Hair loss is also part of the radiation sickness. Public and medical interests have been stimulated following the poisoning incident of the Russian dissident Alexander Litvinenko with the radioactive compound Polonium-210 in 2006. Exposure to heavy metals is a well known cause for anagen hair loss and still might play a role in hair loss in occupational medicine. The same is true for other anagen hair loss inducing chemicals, such as boric acid and selenium.

Anagen Hair Loss Induced by Chemotherapy and Other Cytostatic Drugs

The three major toxicities of antineoplastic drugs are gastrointestinal disturbances, bone marrow suppression, and alopecia. They all are the result of direct toxic effects on the rapidly dividing cells of the gastrointestinal tract, the bone marrow, and the cells of the hair matrix.

Hair loss can be induced by all traditional antineoplastic drugs: alkylating agents, alkaloids, and antimetabolites, but also several monoclonal antibodies may have this distressing side effect. It is more common and severe with combination therapy than with the use of only a single drug, but major differences exist between individual antineoplastic drugs (➋ *Table 26.1*). Hair starts to fall out usually few weeks after exposure to the antineoplastic drug. Complete baldness may have developed 1 or 2 months later. Usually antineoplastic drug-induced hair loss is reversible. Regrowth will occur 2–6 month after discontinuation of the therapy, indicating that the empty hair follicle has to run through the complete telogen phase before a new and normal anagen hair will start growing. Full regrowth may be the rule, but permanent changes in texture or density of hair may become apparent. Particularly regimens containing busulfan are known to cause permanent damage to the hair follicles but permanent

Table 26.1
Cytotoxic drugs and hair loss

Cytotoxic agents that usually do cause hair loss	Adriamycin
	Cyclophosphamide
	Daunorubicin
	Docetaxel
	Epirubicin
	Etoposide
	Ifosfamide
	Irinotecan
	Sorafenib
	Teniposide
	Topotecan
	Vindesine
	Vinorelbine
Cytotoxic agents that sometimes cause hair loss	Amsacrine
	Bleomycin
	Busulfan
	Cytarabine
	Dacarbazine
	Doxifluridine
	Erlotinib
	5-Fluorouracil
	Gefitinib
	Gemcitabine
	Interferon-α2b
	Ixabepilone
	Lomustine
	Paclitaxel
	Sunitinib
	Temozolomide
	Thiotepa
	Thioguanine
	Trastuzumab
	Vinblastine
	Vincristine
Cytotoxic agents that rarely cause hair loss	Capecitabine
	Carboplatin
	Carmustine
	Cisplatin
	Doxorubicin
	Fludarabine
	Hydroxyurea
	6-mercaptopurine
	Methotrexate

Table 26.1 (Continued)

	Mitomycin C
	Mitoxantrone
	Procarbazine
	Raltitrexed
	Streptozotocin

Abele et al. 1983; Akerley 1996; Cascinu et al. 1997; Rajkumar et al. 2000; Stafford-Fox and Guindon 2000; Hamilton et al. 2002; Kumar et al. 2002; Leyland-Jones et al. 2003; Herrlinger et al. 2003; Muggiano et al. 2004; Cohen et al. 2005; Conlin and Vahdat 2006; Autier et al. 2008; Trueb 2009; Hartmann et al. 2009; Lee et al. 2009; Forde et al. 2011

baldness has also been observed after other high-dose chemotherapy regimens, like with cyclophosphamide, thiotepa, and carboplatin (CTC) (Prussick 1996; de Jonge et al. 2002). Partial or total permanent alopecia occurs in about half of the patients receiving busulfan. Possible explanations for follicular disappearance can be either stem cell destruction or acute damage of the matrix keratinocytes that die in the hypodermis instead of entering the catagen phase (Tosti et al. 2005).

Treatment Great improvement has been achieved in development of strategies to manage chemotherapy-induced gastrointestinal disturbances and suppression of the bone marrow. However, no effective pharmacologic treatment is available for the third major toxicity of chemotherapy, alopecia. Research into overcoming chemotherapy-induced alopecia has been hampered due to lack of clinically relevant models.

Since the 1970s scalp cooling has been used and studied. In most of these studies a significant decrease in hair loss was observed with scalp cooling, most evident when anthracyclines or taxanes were used (Grevelman and Breed 2005). Concerns have been expressed about the risk of scalp metastases after cooling. It is considered contraindicated for those with hematological malignancies and its use is controversial in patients with nonhematological malignancies who undergo curative chemotherapy (Trueb 2009).

Anagen Hair Loss Induced by Radiation

Humans can be exposed to several sources of radioactivity. Natural background radiation, exposure to medical sources of radiation, radiation from consumer goods, nuclear energy derived, occupational or accidental exposure, and poisoning. Background radioactivity is everywhere in our environment. The main source of human exposure to radiation is caused by medical actions, like X-rays, radioactive drugs, and radiation therapy. Consumer goods responsible for additional exposure to radiation are tobacco (Polonium-210), building materials (radium and radon), fuels (gas, oil), television sets, X-rays at airports, and starters for fluorescent tubes. The nuclear energy industry causes only limited additional exposure to radiation, but this has never been measured reliably. Occupational exposure to radioactivity may occur in nuclear power stations, industrial quality control procedures, scientific procedures, hospital workers, airline staff, military working with depleted uranium, and during food irradiation to destroy microorganisms, bacteria, viruses, or insects. The best known example of intentional radioactive poisoning concerns the Russian dissident Alexander Litvinenko with the radioactive compound Polonium-210.

Radiation describes any process in which energy travels through a medium or through space, ultimately to be absorbed by another body. The energy can be emitted as waves (electromagnetic radiation) or as particles, for example, α-radiation or β-radiation. α-Particles will cause severe damage if ingested. However, they have little energy and a low range; typically, α-particles can be stopped with a sheet of paper (or skin). Therefore, the cutaneous radiation syndrome, which is associated with high-dose irradiation of the skin, is not a feature of exposure to α-emitters, such as polonium, plutonium, and uranium. However, decay products of α-particles may emit β- and γ-radiation. External contamination with α-emitters can be eliminated through undressing, careful hand-washing, and showering. α-Emitters may be responsible for acute or chronic radiation sickness after entering the body through eating or drinking contaminated material, breathing contaminated air, or through an open wound. β-Radiation is less ionizing than α-radiation, but more than γ-radiation and can be stopped with a few centimeters of metal. γ-Radiation has high penetrating power. X-rays have higher energy than visible light or ultraviolet but with lower energy than γ-radiation.

Hair disorders are not directly induced by nonionizing radiation (i.e., thermal, radio waves, microwaves, terahertz radiation, infrared light, and visible light) but thermal destruction of the skin may result in scar formation with corresponding focal hair loss.

Skin Changes Following Exposition to Radiation A wide variety of expressions of radiation-induced skin effects have been described after exposure to external high-dose ionizing radiation (Geleijns and Wondergem 2005). There are four clinical stages in acute radiation sickness after systemic exposure to radioactivity. The first is the "prodromal" phase, in which there is nausea, vomiting, anorexia and, if the exposure is high enough, diarrhea. Following the prodromal illness, there may be a "latent" phase. This phase may last from a couple of days to few weeks. The patient usually looks better. Subsequently, the "manifest illness" stage develops with bone marrow, GI, cardiovascular, and skin symptoms, including hair loss. Of course, systemic signs of radiation sickness will often be absent in the cutaneous radiation syndrome which is associated with high-dose external irradiation of the skin.

Early transient erythema occurs a few hours after irradiation and reaches a peak value within 1 day. A second and more severe erythema, accompanied by a sensation of heat and itching, develops after a latent period of 8–10 days. The maximum severity is reached in 14–16 days and it subsides after 4 weeks. Dry desquamation may take place during subsidence and the skin may become pigmented. Depending on the dose, radiodermatitis, induced by killing of basal layer cells, may progress from dry desquamation to the exudative phase of moist desquamation. Damage to skin appendages may become apparent during the second or third week, resulting in loss of sweat and sebaceous glands, as well as in hair loss.

Recovery of skin commences after the desquamation reaches a peak value and starts from islands of epidermal stem cells in the hair follicle or interfollicular epidermis. The recovered skin may be hypoplastic/atrophic, show both hyperpigmentation and hypopigmentation, and can be devoid of any appendages. Disappearance of sebaceous glands may result in a dry skin and increasing numbers of telangiectasia may become visible as a late sign of radiation of the skin. Another late injury to the skin includes development of chronic skin fibrosis, skin contraction, and in rare cases even dermal necrosis owing to vascular damage and resulting in chronic ulcers. Development of squamous cell carcinoma might be a serious late complication of exposure of the skin to irradiation.

Hair Loss Following Exposition to Radiation Radiation has a dose-dependent effect on hair follicles. The response may vary from temporary anagen hair loss after exposure to low doses of radiation, via telogen hair loss after intermediate doses of radiation, to permanent hair loss following high doses of radiation. In general, temporary epilation begins 8–10 days after a single dose of irradiation and continues for 2–3 weeks, with full hair regrowth from surviving cells in the germinal matrix by 8–12 weeks (Sinclair et al. 2003). The doses required to induce epilation vary between different areas of the body. Scalp hair is much more sensitive to radiation than axillary hair, beard hair, pubic hair, and eyelashes. The dose of radiation necessary to cause alopecia will also depend on the quantum energy of the respective type of radiation. The threshold for damage to hair follicles is lower than that for erythema. A dose of 3–5 Gy of low-LET radiation (X-rays of γ-rays) delivered in a single, brief exposure can cause temporary epilation. The threshold for permanent epilation is higher; i.e., about 7 Gy in a single exposure or 50–60 Gy fractionated over several weeks (Rubin and Casarett 1968; UNSCEAR 1982; Geleijns and Wondergem 2005). In clinical radiotherapy dose fractioning is employed. Epilation is then dependent on both the daily dose and the time interval between doses. Radiation to the skull for oncological indications characteristically ranges from 20 to 50 Gy in divided doses. These patients develop alopecia which ought to be temporary.

Incomplete regrowth or regrowth of hair with a different texture or color may happen occasionally. The hair may become grey or white, effects which are usually associated with the killing or inactivation of melanocytes. The depigmentation effect is permanent. In contrast, increased pigmentation that involves the hair follicles occurs only with photon and particle radiation (Geleijns and Wondergem 2005).

Hair Loss After Occupational Exposure to Radiation X-rays used in intervention radiology or cardiology may expose patients to relatively high doses of radiation of up to 6 Gy. Also occupational exposure to X-rays may reach high levels since interventional radiology techniques are being used by an increasing number of clinicians. Not all are adequately trained in radiation safety and radiobiology. Skin and hair abnormalities in staff and physicians performing interventional procedures have been observed after cumulative radiation dose of 10–12 Gy (Wiper et al. 2005).

Depleted uranium is a waste product of the manufacture of nuclear fuel and has several civilian and military applications. It has low specific radioactivity with dominance of α-radiation above β- or γ-radiation. Therefore, no acute risk is attributed to external exposure to depleted uranium. Claims of causing health effects among troops and local populations who were present at locations where depleted uranium ammunition had been used during conflicts appear to be unfounded and hair loss has never been claimed (Bleise et al. 2003). Also ingestion of drinking water containing high natural concentrations of uranium or inhalation of depleted uranium particles does not represent an acute risk, even though uranium miners have a well documented risk of lung cancer (Saccomanno et al. 1996).

Anagen Hair Loss Induced by Heavy Metals

Formation of the hair shaft may be disrupted by many heavy metals. Almost all causative factors able to induce anagen hair loss share one characteristic: they abruptly stop normal cell division of rapidly dividing hair matrix cells in the hair bulb. However, the mechanism by which heavy metals are responsible for hair loss is different. Physiologically, the major binding power within keratin is sulfhydryl groups. Heavy metals weaken these bonds by formation of covalent bonds with the sulfhydryl groups, resulting in abnormal development of the hair shaft. In consequence, the hair shaft becomes increasingly sensitive to fragmentation. The binding of heavy metals not only weakens the hair shaft but also provides a lasting record of the long-term exposure to these substances. Just like the nail plate the hair shaft may serve as a recoverable memory for exposure to heavy metals in the past months to years.

Many metals have the capability of causing hair loss. A couple of them are particularly notorious for inducing hair loss because of a more frequent exposure to them. In the past, thallium, mercury, and arsenic were the heavy metals most commonly responsible for causing hair loss. However, also copper, cadmium, and bismuth have been reported to cause alopecia in human in isolated cases (Sinclair et al. 2003). No reports exist on negative effects of lead on hair growth.

Anagen Hair Loss Induced by Thallium Thallium is an odorless, colorless, and tasteless heavy metal formerly used in rodenticides and still used in some manufacturing processes. It is used in the manufacture of optical lenses, semiconductors, scintillation counters, low temperature thermometers and switching devices, green colored fireworks, and imitation jewelery, and as chemical catalyst. Up to the 1940s the metal has been used for depilation of children with tinea capitis, and hair loss has been described in those with dermal exposure to thallium-containing pesticides. Thallium is still used as a pesticide in Africa and was found to be a contaminant in some Chinese herbal medications. Occupational exposure and toxicity has been described in the vicinity of a cement plant due to emission of thallium-containing dust. The major route of intake was found to be the consumption of vegetables and fruit grown in the vicinity of the cement plant. However, in the cases no positive correlation was found between the thallium levels in hair and urine and the prevalence of hair loss (Brockhaus et al. 1981). Another industrial case of chronic occupational exposure to thallium-containing dust in a glass manufacturing company was published in 1998. In this patient alopecia was the first sign of thallium poisoning, followed by other signs of intoxication (Hirata et al. 1998).

Thallium is toxic by cumulative intake; it can be absorbed through the skin, respiratory, and gastrointestinal tract. Poisoning can cause extensive hair loss, which usually develops 1–3 weeks after an acute exposure but may begin after months in chronic thallotoxicosis. The hair loss affects the scalp, temporal parts of the eyebrows, the eyelashes, the limbs, and sometimes the axillary regions (Tromme et al. 1998). Regrowth of hair will be complete and starts 1–2 months later. Since thallium has been banned from use as a household rodenticide more than 30 years ago, reports of thallium poisoning suggest that nowadays exposure usually results from criminal and suicidal behavior or from unintentional or occupational exposure. Most cases of thallium toxicity occur after oral ingestion but severe toxicity has been reported after inhalation of contaminated dust from pyrite burners, in zinc and lead smelting, and in the manufacture of cadmium, and after dermal absorption through protective rubber gloves (Moore et al. 1993; Hirata et al. 1998; Atsmon et al. 2000).

Initial features of thallium poisoning may occur within several hours or can be delayed by 12–14 h after ingestion. The initial symptoms are nonspecific: gastrointestinal disturbances (nausea, vomiting, epigastric pain, diarrhea). Fluid loss can be substantial. Within few days neurological manifestations are apparent, involving the peripheral (sensorimotor neuropathy, characterized by severe hyperesthesia, primarily of the soles and palms) and/or central (confusion, disorientation, lethargy, thirst, convulsions, psychosis, choreiform movements, and cerebral edema with central respiratory failure) and/or autonomic (tachycardia, hypertension, salivation, hyperhidrosis, dry skin) nervous systems. Skin lesions are commonly present as a chronic effect of thallium poisoning, appearing few weeks after exposure. Not only hair loss is characteristic but also erythematous rashes on the cheeks and perioral region, acneiform and pustular eruptions, scaling as well as hyperkeratosis of the palms and soles, stomatitis and glossitis. Late skin signs are follicular plugging and the development of white transverse lines on the nail plate (Mees' lines) (Tromme et al. 1998; Lu et al. 2007). In severe cases, cranial nerve involvement may also be present. The prognosis for acute thallium toxicity is serious, having a mortality rate of 6–15%. Among survivors 33–50% will have neurological or ocular sequelae. The lost hair always regrows and there are no dermatological sequelae (Tromme et al. 1998).

2.6.4 Diagnosis

Physicians who see a sudden onset of painful peripheral neuropathy and hair loss in patients should prompt consider thallium exposure. A high concentration in the serum and urine may confirm clinical suspicion. Exposure to thallium weeks to months earlier can be detected by analysis of hairs and nails, since this metal is stored in these appendages after ingestion (Daniel et al. 2004).

Microscopic examination of the hair roots by polarized light shows a distinctive but not specific pattern. The tapered, distorted anagen roots are described as black and visible from the fourth day after poisoning. If poisoning occurs in successive doses, several black zones are found, corresponding to the growth of the surviving hair. Their intensity directly corresponds to the degree of severity of the intoxication. However, their specificity is insufficient to allow either the early diagnosis or the chronology of thallium absorption. Whether the black color is caused by light diffracting gaseous inclusions or hyperpigmentations is not clear (Tromme et al. 1998).

2.6.5 Treatment

The treatment options for thallium poisoning are rather limited and have not evolved due to its relatively rare occurrence. Activated charcoal has been reported to be effective in vitro in adsorbing thallium and may in vivo interrupt its enterohepatic and enteroenteric recirculation. However, the effectiveness is controversial, as well as the usefulness of hemodialysis, hemoperfusion, and forced diuresis. Currently, Prussian blue (or "Berlin blue"), a crystal blue lattice of potassium ferric ferrocyanide, is regarded as treatment of choice for thallium poisoning. It acts by forming a nonabsorbable complex with thallium, thus interrupting its enterohepatic recycling and increasing its excretion.

Anagen Hair Loss Induced by Mercury

Mercury is a silvery-white heavy metal that exists as a liquid at room temperature. It exists in a variety of inorganic and organic forms that exhibit variable absorption, excretion, and toxicity. Exposure to mercury can lead to balding, which is ironic considering many who were first discovered to be victims of mercury poisoning were "hatters" of the nineteenth century. A hatter was a person who used the toxin to cure fur from which they made hats. These workers inhaled mercuric vapors, which not only led to hair loss but the development of dementia, thus the term "mad hatter." More recent victims of mercury poisoning include those who ingest large amounts of seafood, as methylmercury is abundant in shellfish and in many types of fishes including king mackerel, swordfish, and shark (Brodkin et al. 2007).

Exposure to mercury in industrial processes may occur in mercury recycling factories, mining for mercury, gold (where mercury is used to form an amalgam before being burnt off), and other metals, such as copper, zinc, and silver, as well as from refining operations. Chronic exposure to metallic mercury vapor appeared to be responsible for hair loss in workers in a thermometer factory. Other complains were headache, irritability, and wrist and ankle pain (Richter et al. 1982).

Most of the mercury in the environment results from human activity, particularly from coal-fired power stations, residential heating systems and incinerators of (medical) waste. Significant releases of mercury to the environment result from the use of thermometers and blood pressure monitors. Health-care facilities may be responsible for as much as 5% of all mercury released in wastewater.

Dental amalgam is a potentially significant source of exposure since it can contain up to 50% elemental mercury. It is released as vapor, ions, or fine particles and may be inhaled or ingested. Although no adverse health effects have been proven, use of dental amalgam is declining rapidly. Amalgam may represent an occupational risk for dentists and can cause release of mercury to the atmosphere during cremation.

Thiomersal (sodium ethylmercurythiosalicyclate or thimerosal), which contains 49.6% ethylmercury, has been used as a vaccine preservative since the 1930s. As ethylmercury does not accumulate and is actively excreted via the gut, the health risk from this exposure is low. Cinnabar, which contains mercury sulfide, has been used in Chinese traditional medicines and is a widely unrecognized source for mercury intoxication.

Diagnosis Contrary to thallium poisoning hair loss is a much rarer phenomenon in mercury poisoning. The few publications that exist do not allow a detailed clinical description. Some publications mention patchy alopecia, while others do not specify the type of alopecia. The time frame between exposure to the poison and onset of the alopecia is not clear, but likely depends on the dose of the exposure (Richter et al. 1982; Schrallhammer-Benkler et al. 1992; Haas et al. 2003).

Neurological and behavioral disorders may be observed after inhalation, ingestion, or dermal application of different mercury compounds. Elemental and methylmercury are toxic to the central and peripheral nervous system. The inhalation of mercury vapor can produce harmful effects on the nervous, digestive and immune systems, lungs and kidneys, and may be fatal. The inorganic salts of mercury are corrosive to the skin, eyes, and gastrointestinal tract, and may induce kidney toxicity if ingested. Symptoms include tremors, insomnia, memory loss, neuromuscular effects, headaches, and cognitive and motor dysfunction. Mild subclinical signs of central nervous system toxicity can be seen in workers exposed to an elemental mercury level in the air of 20 μg/m^3 or more for several years. Kidney and immune effects have been reported. There is no conclusive evidence linking mercury exposure to cancer in humans.

Children are especially vulnerable and may be exposed directly by eating contaminated fish. Methylmercury bioaccumulated in fish and consumed by pregnant women may lead to neurodevelopmental problems in the developing fetus. Transplacental exposure is the most dangerous, as the fetal brain is very sensitive. Neurological symptoms include mental retardation, seizures, vision and hearing loss, delayed development, language disorders, and memory loss. In children, a syndrome characterized by red and painful extremities called acrodynia has been reported to result from chronic mercury exposure. Also some autism spectrum disorders might be the result of mercury exposure (Kazantzis 2002; Brodkin et al. 2007).

Biological measurement of mercury, for example, in hair and blood, allows exposure to be quantified and is linked to possible health effects. Mercury levels in hair can be used as an indicator of environmental exposure and may reflect chronic exposure to this heavy metal.

Anagen Hair Loss Induced by Arsenic

Arsenic is a metalloid widely distributed in the earth's crust. Arsenic and its compounds are used as pesticides, herbicides, insecticides, and in various alloys. Elemental arsenic is not soluble in water but arsenic salts exhibit a wide range of solubility. Inorganic arsenic of geological origin is found in groundwater used as drinking water in several parts of the world. Arsenic trioxide is produced as a by-product of metal smelting operations. It has been estimated that 70% of the world arsenic production is used in timber treatment as copper chrome arsenate, 22% in agricultural chemicals, and the remainder in glass, pharmaceuticals and nonferrous alloys. Mining, smelting of nonferrous metals and burning of fossil fuels are the major industrial processes that contribute to anthropogenic arsenic contamination of air, water, and soil. Historically, use of arsenic-containing pesticides has left large tracts of agricultural land contaminated. The use of arsenic in the preservation of timber has also led to contamination of the environment. Arsenic is emitted into the atmosphere by high-temperature processes such as coal-fired power generation plants, burning vegetation, and volcanism (WHO (World Health Organization) 2010).

Soluble inorganic arsenic is acutely toxic, and ingestion of large doses leads to acute gastrointestinal symptoms, disturbances of cardiovascular and nervous system functions, and eventually death. In survivors, bone marrow depression, hemolysis, hepatomegaly, melanosis, polyneuropathy, and encephalopathy may be observed.

Chronic arsenic exposure to humans mainly occurs from the ingestion of arsenic contaminated water and food and is responsible for various types of skin lesions such as melanosis, leucomelanosis, and keratosis. While the skin is most susceptible for the chronic effects of arsenic, other organs may also become intoxicated by chronic exposure to arsenic. Other manifestations include neurological effects, obstetric problems, high blood pressure, diabetes mellitus, diseases of the respiratory system and of blood vessels including cardiovascular, and cancers typically involving the skin, lung, and bladder (Rahman et al. 2009).

Arsenic levels in both hair and nails are elevated within one to a few weeks after poisoning, and return to background levels within a few months. Toxic effects of arsenic on hair are frequently repeated in literature, but evidence and reports are rare, indicating that hair loss is not an important feature of arsenic poisoning (Wakhlu et al. 2003; Amster et al. 2007).

Anagen Hair Loss Induced by Boric Acid

The element Boron is a normal constituent of the diet and is frequently used in commercial products such as boric acid or the sodium salts of tetra-coordinated borates. These include the anhydrous, pentahydrate, and decahydrate sodium tetra-coordinated borates. Borax is the commonly used name for decahydrate sodium tetraborate. Although the medical uses of boric acid have gradually dropped, it is still widely used in multiple industries including laundering, fireproofing wood and fabric, manufacturing leather, and producing pottery glazed and enamel. It is also sold commercially as a household pesticide (Sinclair et al. 2003).

In several reports acute systemic poisoning from ingestion of boric acid has been recognized as a cause of hair loss among other skin, gastrointestinal, and renal symptoms after suicide attempts with boric acid powder and medications but also with chronic exposure to consumer products such as mouth washer (Stein et al. 1973; Schillinger et al. 1982; Beckett et al. 2001). Hair loss occurs 10–14 days after ingestion of the toxin and may be complete, indicating anagen hair loss as the nature of the alopecia. The skin symptoms are intense erythema, desquamation, and exfoliation and is sometimes referred to as a "boiled lobster" appearance. Also psoriasiform lesions and bullae may appear (Schillinger et al. 1982). In case of chronic exposure hair loss may also occur but is generally milder in nature but sometimes is the most obvious presentation of chronic boric acid intoxication (Tan 1970).

Ingestion is the most common cause of borate intoxication. However, boric acid in solutions can also be absorbed through the intact skin of humans. Cases of systemic toxicity in children, some with alopecia, from medical application of boric acid-containing compounds as wound treatments have been described in the 1960s (Skipworth et al. 1967).

Although industrial boron compounds have a high toxicity and have been used for decades as an additive to metal working fluids, antifreeze/coolants, and other industrial materials it has only infrequently been reported to cause toxic alopecia in the workplace. Occupational alopecia from long-term skin and possibly inhalant exposure to borax containing washing powder has been reported (Tan 1970). The development of patchy alopecia from acute exposure to boric acid–containing fluids has been suggested but causality was heavily disputed by others (Beckett et al. 2001; Tosti et al. 2002). Direct skin contact with borax in the dry or powdered form, such as in borax mining or processing has not been associated with hair disorders.

Diagnosis The diagnosis can be made by measuring blood boric acid levels: normal values are up to 0.3 mg per 100 ml blood as boron. The acute lethal dose of boric acid ingestion appears to be 18–20 g in adults and 5–6 g in children.

Treatment One reason that boric acid poisoning, particularly the acute form, is so serious is that there is no effective antidote for it. Spontaneous or induced vomiting and diarrhea aid in emptying the intestinal tract of the substance. To speed up the removal of the boric acid before irreversible damage has been done, exchange blood transfusions have been utilized with success. Both peritoneal dialysis and hemodialysis may be effective. Symptomatic treatment is advised for the skin exfoliation as well as maintenance of a good fluid balance. Despite these measures, boric acid poisoning carries a high mortality rate (Schillinger et al. 1982; Sinclair et al. 2003).

Anagen Hair Loss Induced by Selenium

Selenium is a nonmetal element that serves vital roles in normal physiologic function. Substantial toxicity can occur with excessive selenium consumption. Hair loss may occur few weeks after ingestion of high doses of selenium, which often is preceded by gastrointestinal complaints. Also muscle cramps, joint pain, fatigue, paresthesias, and difficulty with concentration have been reported, similar to those associated with arsenic and other metal toxicities. Massive hair loss as well as discoloration of fingernails, nail loss, and Mees' lines have been attributed to acute selenium poisoning from ingestion of paradise nuts (Muller and Desel 2010), chronic intoxication with nutritional supplements (Sutter et al. 2008) but also from occupational exposure to a selenium alloy used for the manufacture and maintenance of drums used in photocopy machines (Srivastava et al. 1995). An endemic chronic selenium intoxication was reported from China where vegetables were contaminated with water soluble coal-derived selenium in the soil (Yang et al. 1983). Clinically, the diffuse hair loss resembles alopecia areata but the Mees' lines in the nails are typically for an intoxication.

Hair loss has been attributed to the disruption of structural proteins in keratin. Similar to alopecia induced by heavy metals selenium is thought to interpolate into disulfide bridges, causing structural weakness that leads to hair loss. The hair loss is completely reversible and regrowth will start few months after discontinuation of the intoxication.

Diagnosis Selenium levels can be determined in hair, blood, and urine (Yang et al. 1983).

3 Telogen Hair Loss

Telogen hair loss is the result of a premature conversion of a growing anagen hair into a resting telogen hair, which will be shed few months later. Recognized factors able to induce telogen are thyroid dysfunction, pregnancy, hormonal contraception, hormone replacement therapy, weight loss, deficiency of essential fatty acids, iron, zinc or biotin. Also physiological stress like fever, systemic illness, surgery, and extreme psychological stress are inducers of telogen hair loss.

Many drugs have been reported to cause hair loss. Antineoplastic drug commonly are responsible for predictable acute anagen hair loss which commences about 2 weeks after onset of the therapy (see above). Other drugs may force the growing anagen hair to enter the telogen phase, resulting in telogen hair loss several months after the medication was started. The prevalence and severity of alopecia depend on the drug as well as on individual predisposition. Some drugs cause hair loss so uniformly that the relationship is convincing. Other drugs have been reported only occasionally to be able to induce telogen hair loss and the causal relationship sometimes is doubtful. Transient shedding typically begins 2–5 months after the inciting event and after discontinuation of the responsible drug the hair cycle will be normalized only several months later because the hairs that already have entered the telogen phase will be shed before clinical normalization can occur (Paus and Cotsarelis 1999). Antimitotic agents given in high doses usually induce anagen hair loss; however, some follicles may later show a telogen effluvium. Sometimes low dose of antimitotic agents methotrexate and colchicines induce telogen hair loss instead of anagen hair loss (Van Dooren-Greebe et al. 1994).

The list of drugs accused of being responsible for hair loss is almost infinitively and not the primary scope of this chapter. Frequently used drugs with relatively high frequency of hair loss are ACE inhibitors, amiodarone, amantadine, anticoagulants of all kinds, anticonvulsants, antiestrogens and aromatase inhibitors, antiretroviral drugs, antithyroid drugs, β-blockers, cholesterol-lowering drugs, cimetidine, colchicine, some cytokines, etretinate and vitamine A, heavy metals, hormones, isotretinoine, interferons, ketoconazole, leflunomide, lithium, penecillamine, propranolol, thiamphenicol, and valproic acid (Tosti and Pazzaglia 2007; Tosti et al. 1994; Kimyai-Asadi et al. 1999; Scott et al. 2001; Trefzer et al. 2003; Luther and Glesby 2007; Litt 2007). If all these drugs cause telogen type of hair loss has not been studied. Possibly other mechanisms resulting in effluvium may also be involved.

3.1 Diagnosis

Determining the etiology of diffuse alopecia is always time consuming. Diagnostic tools for clinical evaluation of hair loss have been discussed above and apply unrestrained for telogen hair loss. The mechanism involved in developing telogen hair loss is forcing growing anagen hair into resting telogen hair. The fate of these telogen hair is the normal fate of any telogen hair: shedding after 2–5 months. Therefore, a clinical history should start months before the shedding has started and is the cornerstone leading toward a correct diagnosis. At the pull test an increased number of hair can be detached from the hair follicles. In normal circumstances the number of extracted hairs will not exceed five to six and analysis by light microscopy will reveal that all of these hairs are telogen (➋ *Fig. 26.1a*). In case of a positive pull test the absence of anagen hair with a necrotic anagen sheath adhering to them and the absence of tapered hair allows to differentiate telogen hair loss from anagen hair loss (➋ *Fig. 26.1c*). However, the hair pull test is only a rough approach, which appears to be useful only in acute and more severe phases of hair loss.

3.2 Treatment

In general, the prognosis for regrowth is excellent if the provoking factor can be assigned and eliminated. After cessation of the provoking factor regrowth may take several months because shedding of telogen hairs is determined months before, at the moment the hair follicle leaves the growing anagen phase and enters the resting telogen phase.

4 Mixed Types or Undetermined Types of Hair Loss

4.1 Hair Loss Induced by Pesticides

Acute poisoning with pesticides is a global public health problem and accounts for as many as 300,000 death worldwide every year, mostly occurring in rural areas of the Asia Pacific region, where easy access to highly toxic pesticides turns many impulsive acts of self-poisoning into suicide (Eddleston and Phillips 2004). Not only suicide attempts but also unintentional exposures to pesticides are responsible for intoxications (Spiewak 2001). Intoxications with pesticides have a broad spectrum of clinical manifestations, including dermatological symptoms and hair loss. Pesticides are classified into insecticides, herbicides, fungicides, molluscicides, rodenticides, and insect repellants.

The insecticide albendazole is known to induce reversible hair loss but these reports derive from its therapeutic use in humans and not from occupational exposure (Saimot 2001). Pyrethroids are the most frequently used indoor insecticides. Exposure following indoor treatments with a dog flea powder was reported to lead to hair loss, most likely alopecia areata, and gastrointestinal symptoms in one patient (Schulze et al. 2002). Considering the fact that this patient already had had a period of complete baldness before exposure to the insecticide, one might doubt about the role the pyrethroids did play is this case. No hair loss has been reported relating to human exposure to organophosphate or organochlorine insecticides. Dichlorodiphenyltrichloroethane (DDT) was used worldwide until the 1970s, when concerns about its toxic effects, its environmental persistence, and its concentration in the food supply led to use restrictions and prohibition. DDT continues to be used for malaria control in several African and Asian countries. Hair diseases are rarely promoted by DDT, however possibly pesticide-related diffuse hair loss was described in a farmer spraying DDT (Spiewak 2001).

Hair loss due to exposure to dipyridyl herbicides paraquat and diquat has not been reported in humans. Local overexposure to paraquat may cause reversible leukonychia of the nail plate and irritative skin reactions.

The fungicides with substituted benzene, chloroneb, and chlorothalonil are well known to cause local irritant dermatitis. No reports exist on any role thiocarbamates may play in induction of hair loss. Occupational exposure to organomercurial fungicides may play a role in development of hair loss, because methylmercury and phenylmercuric acid contain mercury. This topic is discussed in detail above.

Metaldehyde, a cyclic tetramer of acetaldehyde, is a widely used molluscicide. Intoxication with metaldehyde is exceptional and toxicity from metaldehyde is largely mild but the clinical course of metaldehyde poisoning may be rapidly deteriorating and fatal on rare occasions. However, alopecia does not appear to be one of the features of acute metaldehyde intoxication in humans. Chronic metaldehyde intoxication induces some alopecia in rats (Verschuuren et al. 1975).

Many chemically unrelated rodenticides are used worldwide. Rodenticides containing the heavy metal thallium are very well known to be able to induce massive alopecia. This topic is extensively discussed above. Aluminum phosphide and zinc phosphide are highly toxic rodenticides but without reported alopecia inducing capacities. Warfarin and superwarfarin are rodenticide compounds with anticoagulative effects. Used as a drug, coumarins are reported to induce telogen hair loss in a high proportion of users (Leong 2008). Occupational exposure to coumarins leading to hair loss has never been reported. The rodenticide yellow phosphorus does not appear to be able to induce hair loss. June 2007, 2,484 persons were exposed to fume of yellow phosphorus due to an accident of a Ukraine freight train. Alopecia turned out to be no typical feature of exposure to this fume (Badiugin 2009). Also reports of suicide attempts with oral ingestion of yellow phosphorus do not mention development of hair loss (Tafur et al. 2004).

The frequently used insect repellent diethyl toluamide (DEET) may have several dermal side effects, like hives, rash, itching, redness, and swelling. However, hair loss has never been attributed to the use of this compound (Osimitz et al. 2010).

4.2 Hair Loss by Plant Toxins

Hair loss has been reported after poisoning with several plants. Hair loss after acute poisoning with autumn crocus, also known as meadow saffron or *Colchicum autumnale*, is the result of colchicine intoxication (Brvar et al. 2004). Colchicine is a highly active alkaloid which is also used in the treatment of gouty arthritis, pseudogout, familial Mediterranean fever, and Behçet's disease. Colchicine poisoning is a rare event which is characterized by multiorgan involvement and a poor prognosis. Hair loss is not the predominant feature but will occur in course of the history if the patient survives. The course typically shows three phases: initially gastrointestinal symptoms predominate, and in the second phase multiorgan failure may occur possibly leading to death. In case the patient survives, the third phase of recovery follows in which the patient always presents with hair loss (Bismuth et al. 1977). This hair loss may occur weeks to months after the intoxication, indicating telogen hair loss. However also cases with hair loss 1–2 weeks after the poisoning have been reported, indicating acute disruption of hair shaft formation, so anagen hair loss (Atas et al. 2004; Bicer et al. 2007).

Ingestion of the nut of coco de mono (*Couroupita nicaraguensis*) is an even rarer cause of alopecia than autumn crocus; this wooly plant is on the red list of threatened species. It belongs to the Lecythidaceae family and can only be found in Colombia, Costa Rica, Ecuador, El Salvador, Nicaragua, Panama, and Puerto Rico (Kerdel-Vegas 1964; Sinclair et al. 2003).

St John's Wort (*Hypericum perforatum*) is widely consumed since it has been proven to relieve symptoms associated with mild to moderate depression. One case of hair loss has been attributed to the consumption of this popular herb, occurring several months after initiating St John's Wort. Microscopic analysis of hairs revealed a mixed telogen and anagen morphology that suggests rather a drug reaction than a newly developed alopecia areata (➋ *Fig. 26.1*) (Parker et al. 2001).

Hair loss has also been described after the consumption of *Leucaena leucocephala*. This is a species of small Mimosoid tree that is native to southern Mexico and northern Central America (Belize and Guatemala). Common names include White Leadtree, Jumbay, and White Popinac. Responsible for hair loss appears to be the alkaloid, β-3-hydroxy-4pyridone amino acid leucenol, also known as leucenine or mimosine, which can be found in growing tips, young leaves, and seeds of this plant (Crounse et al. 1962; Luo et al. 2000).

Cinnamon is the bark of the *Cinnamomum zeylanicum* tree. True cinnamon is a native of Sri Lanka and grows almost exclusively in this country. It contains cinnamic aldehyde, which is an irritant. Workers processing cinnamon are exposed to much cinnamon dust. Uragoda investigated 40 cinnamon workers. Thirty-five of them had symptoms, 26 complained of loss of weight, 9 having asthma, 20 skin irritation, and 9 smarting of the eyes while at work. Loss of hair was present in 15, so 37.5%, much more in women (57%) than in men (21%) (Uragoda 1984). The hair loss was mild and "did not alter their appearance." A control group was not investigated, so the relative contribution of the cinnamon dust to the hair loss, as well as the mechanism involved remains to be illuminated.

4.3 Hair Loss in Semiconductor Workers

In 1995, McCurdy et al. published a cross-sectional survey among 3,175 semiconductor industry workers. Alopecia was not defined properly, but was reported to be more common in the fabrication room than in the nonfabrication room workers (RR = 2.44). Alopecia showed a dose–response relationship with isopropanolol and fluoride, although the authors concluded that the relationship between work exposures and alopecia was not obvious (McCurdy et al. 1995).

4.4 Hair Loss Induced by Sanitary Cleaners

Exposition to drain and sanitary cleansing vapors containing sodium hypochlorite and sodium hydroxide was reported to provoke alopecia on the scalp and beard region within 3–4 days after exposure which lasted for a period of 4 weeks. The alopecia was preceded by dermatitis of the scalp. The prerequisite for the exposure was the improper use of cleansing agents and other conditions which lead to intense exposition of the scalp to sodium hypochlorite vapor. A possible chemical reaction between cleansing agent and dirt may have been responsible. Hair loss was caused by breakage of the hair fiber within the hair follicle. Additional genital hair loss arose after sodium hydroxide use. Body and scalp hair was completely restored after 1 year (Stuttgen et al. 1982).

4.5 Hair Loss in Toxic Oil Syndrome

In the spring and summer of 1981, an epidemic of a new illness occurred in central and northwestern Spain, resulting in some 20,000 cases, 12,000 hospital admissions and more than 300 deaths in the first year of the epidemic. The initial onset of illness was usually acute and patients presented primarily with a respiratory syndrome. Half of patients recovered from this phase without apparent sequelae, the remaining patients developed an intermediate of chronic phase of illness involving severe myalgia, eosinophilia, peripheral nerve damage, sclerodermiform skin lesions, sicca syndrome, joint contractures, and alopecia (Kilbourne et al. 1991). The presence of alopecia turned out to be predictive of outcome (Kaufman et al. 1995).

The toxic oil syndrome has been linked to the ingestion of oil mixtures containing rapeseed oil denatured with aniline. Aniline itself did not cause the illness, but putative etiologic agents of toxic oil syndrome are 3-(N-phenylamino)-1,2-propanediol 1,2-dioleoyl ester, 3-(N-phenylamino)-1,2-propanediol 1-oleoyl ester, N-(5-vinyl-1,3-thiazolidin-2-ylidene)phenylamine, and 1-phenyl-5-vinyl-2-imidazolidinethione. However, the precise identity of the etiologic agent has never been identified.

4.6 Localized Hair Loss

4.6.1 Alopecia Areata

Alopecia areata commonly presents as localized patches of baldness. However, also diffuse alopecia areata may occur. Clinically, the latter resembles anagen or telogen hair loss, but the hair pull test contains both telogen and tapered dystrophic anagen hairs (➋ *Fig. 26.1*). It is generally assumed that alopecia areata is an immune mediated form of hair loss in which an autoimmune lymphocytic attack on the hair bulb takes place. The antigen which triggers the immune system remains unidentified. Several factors have been shown to play a role in disease susceptibility and severity. Genetic factors like an atopic diathesis, a positive family history for alopecia areata or Down syndrome increase susceptibility to develop alopecia areata and may indicate a protracted course. Also environmental triggers may be important in disease expression but are partly speculative. Infections, vaccinations, desensitizations, emotional stress, and anxiety have all been implicated (Madani and Shapiro 2000).

Alopecia Areata as an Occupational Disease

Whether occupational exposure to chemicals can induce alopecia areata or not is a matter of dispute. Alopecia areata is common in 1.7% of the studied population

(Safavi et al. 1995). Therefore, it is not easy to prove an assumed cause and effect relationship between a factor and the development of alopecia areata. Occupation exposure to an acrylamide-like substance in a paper factory and to a selenium alloy have been suggested to play a role in development of the disease (Srivastava et al. 1995; Roselino et al. 1996). Acrylamide is used as a water treatment agent and in the manufacture of adhesives, dyes, and fabrics. Beckett at al. reported an association between alopecia areata and occupational topical exposure to borax-containing solutions but many experts in the field disagreed with their conclusion (Beckett et al. 2001; Tosti et al. 2002).

4.6.2 Tinea Capitis

The introduction of griseofulvin in the late 1950s resulted in a largely disappearance of ringworm of the head, tinea capitis, from the Western world. Over the past years a large increase has been noted in tinea capitis in Europe and North America. Alopecia resulting from infectious causes is most commonly focal and patchy. The predominant fungi causing tinea capitis in a given area of the world depend on the dermatophyte species that are circulating among the people or animals in that area or are present in the soil. Most cases of tinea capitis occur in prepubertal children, but its incidence among adults is increasing, in particular among patients over 60 years of age.

Depending on geographical region *Trichophyton tonsurans* (USA, UK, and Brazil) or *Microsporon canis* (Central and Southern Europe) are the most relevant causes for tinea capitis among human (Fuller 2009). *Trichophyton tonsurans* spreads directly from child to child at home, school, or the hairdresser. However, *Microsporon* organisms and *Trichophyton verrucosum* are the most relevant fungi responsible for occupational tinea capitis, because they are transmitted primarily from animal to human (zoophilic). *Microsporon canis* can be transferred by an infected puppy or, more often, kitten. *Trichophyton verrucosum* can be obtained from infected cattle. Spontaneous resolution in humans is the rule; however, transfer to other people may occur and damage to the scalp may be permanent, so hairless areas may remain bald forever.

Tinea Capitis as an Occupational Disease

Tinea capitis and tinea barbae have been reported to be transferred by cattle and horses, especially animals under 2 years of age raised in stables. *Trichophyton verrucosum* is the usual cause of ringworm in cattle throughout the temperate regions of the world and has been reported in parts of Europe including England, the USA, Canada, Iran, Australia, and New Zealand. There have been reports of isolations from horses, sheep, dog, donkeys, an ass, a dromedary and a goat (Maslen 2000). Authors from Italy, Iran and Australia reported several cases of infection due to *Trichophyton verrucosum* after working with horses and cattle (Maslen 2000; Roman et al. 2001; Aghamirian and Ghiasian 2011). In 2009 Aghamirian and Ghiasian reported a prevalence of dermatophytosis in over 20% in Iranian herdsmen, mostly with the zoophilic *Trichophyton verrucosum* as the prevalent causative agent, confirming previous studies (Chadeganipour et al. 1997; Aghamirian and Ghiasian 2011). So *Trichophyton verrucosum* is a common cause of human ringworm and tinea capitis in rural areas and infections are contracted directly or indirectly from cattle. Not only dairy and cattle farmers and their family can be involved but also slaughtermen who work in an abattoir, laboratory assistants working with infected calves and even *Trichophyton verrucosum* infection in a veterinary tutor has been reported. Apart from an epidemic reported in 47 cattle keepers in Finland, infections generally are sporadic (Lehenkari and Silvennoinen-Kassinen 1995). Infection among animals can be largely controlled by vaccines. Occupational mycoses caused by other *Trichophyton species, Trichophyton mentagrophytes,* and *Trichophyton quinckeanum*, with mice as vector, were found in Eastern Europe (Balabanoff 1985).

Clinical features The morbidity of tinea capitis is significant. It may cause local symptoms of inflammation, hair loss, pain, pruritus, and kerion formation. Also constitutional symptoms, social embarrassment, and secondary bacterial infections can be found.

The skin of the scalp may be red, swollen, tender, and warm as signs of local inflammation but clinical diagnosis can be difficult as signs of inflammation may be missing. Therefore, the diagnosis may be overlooked by inexperienced clinicians. The presenting features can be divided into six main patterns (Fuller et al. 2003).

Grey type: Circular patches of alopecia with marked scaling.

Black dot: Swollen stubs of broken off hairs are visible within the patch of alopecia. The hair shafts break off because they become vulnerable through invasion by the dermatophyte.

Kerion: Boggy, localized swelling occurs due to an aggressive inflammatory response to the fungus. Concomitant cervical lymphadenopathy is common.

Diffuse scale: Clinically resembles dandruff which covers the whole scalp.

Moth eaten: Patchy hair loss. In contrast to luetic alopecia the scalp may be generally scaly.

Diffuse pustular pattern: This type is hardest to diagnose with its widespread scattered pustules on the scalp, its brisk inflammatory response but only sparse presence of fungus. Similar to kerion, a simultaneous cervical lymphadenopathy is common. It often is misdiagnosed as a bacterial infection.

Diagnosis Traditionally, the Wood's lamp is used to diagnose fungal infections of the skin and its appendages. The Wood's lamp shines ultraviolet light onto the skin of the patient. In many fungal infections fluorescence becomes visible. *Microsporon* infections can be detected this way, since the fungal spores form a sheath on the outside of the hair shaft and light green upon exposure to ultraviolet radiation. In contrast to these so-called ectothrix infections of the hair, no fluorescence can be detected in endothrix infections with *Trichophyoton tonsurans*, where the spores reside inside the hair shaft and there is no fluorescence (Fuller 2009).

Since absence of fluorescence after shining with the Wood's light does not rule out a tinea capitis, the diagnosis often relies upon mycological analysis of scales and broken off infected hairs. Material for analysis can be collected by scraping off scales or brushing with a toothbrush or cytobrush. Both microscopy with 10% potassium hydroxide (KOH) and culture can be used to detect the fungus. Microscopy will allow immediate identification of the spores and hyphae and thus confirms the diagnosis of tinea capitis. Only culturing will allow definitive determination of the species and its potential resistance for antifungal treatments. However, this may take several weeks.

Treatment Spontaneous remission of *Microsporon Canis* and kerions has been recognized. However, treatment of all forms of tinea capitis is general accepted because of the morbidity involved and risk of transmission (Seebacher et al. 2004; Gupta et al. 2005; Fuller 2009). Topical antifungal preparations are unable to penetrate the hair shaft sufficiently to clear the infection. Therefore, systemic treatment for 6–12 weeks is unavoidable. Oral griseofulvin in a daily dose of 10–25 mg/kg per day is the classical treatment but there is evidence of emerging resistance. *Microsporon audouinii, Microsporon canis*, and *Trichophyton violaceum* appear to be more sensitive to griseofulvin than *Trichophyton tonsurans*. The latter may need the higher advised daily dose.

In the 1980s new oral antifungal drugs were introduced. The oral azoles ketoconazole (200–400 mg daily in adults), fluconazole (6–8 mg/kg daily), and itraconazole (100–200 mg daily in adults) were found to be effective for dermatophyte infections. The oral allylamine terbinafine (250 mg daily in adults) is effective against all dermatophytes, although moderately so for *Microsporon* species. While fungistatic treatment with oral griseofulvin may take several months, azoles and terbinafine are fungicidal and commonly are used for 1–2 months. Termination of treatment must always depend on mycological cure. None of the newer antifungal drugs is specifically EMEA or FDA approved for tinea capitis and only fluconazole is FDA approved for use in children.

The parallel use of antifungal creams or shampoos is often advised to reduce the risk of progression and transmission while waiting for the onset of action of the oral treatment. Most commonly ketoconazole shampoo or selenium sulfide is used for daily adjunctive therapy for a period of 2 months. Preventive daily use of ketoconozole shampoo is a recommended topical therapy for close contacts and an appropriate health measure. It is also important to discard or disinfect with bleach objects that may support fungal conidia, such as combs, hats, pillow, blankets, and scissors.

Nurse's Cap Alopecia

Prolonged traction due to religious or traditional customs and cosmetic hairstyles imposes physical stress on the hair follicle, and result in a well-delineated form of traumatic alopecia known as traction alopecia. Traction alopecia associated with the nurse's cap is a form of occupational hair loss which should be taken into consideration in the differential diagnosis of patchy alopecia. In countries where wearing a nurse cap is the rule an incidence of 3.5% has been described (Hwang et al. 1999).

Clinically it is characterized by circumscribes, rectangular, symmetric, and bilateral hair loss on the parieto-occipital scalp where the nurse cap is secured. On close inspection, the lesions show a decrease in density of follicular orifices. Perifollicular erythema, follicular hemorrhage, follicular pustules, scales, and diffuse erythematous swelling may also be observed. Avoidance of traction will only result in partial improvement, because the number of hair follicles is reduced due to persistent traction.

4.7 Hair Disorders with Increased Hair Growth

4.7.1 Trichomegaly

Trichomegaly means excessively large eyelashes. This may be part of a congenital syndrome or HIV infection, but also was reported to be induced by epidermal growth factor receptor (EGFR) inhibitors erlotinib, cetuximab, and panitumumab. Hair abnormalities were reported in almost 90% of patients using EGFR inhibitors. Trichomegaly was found in 62% of patients, male pattern-like alopecia appeared in 44% of patients, diffuse alopecia in 19%, and over 80% complains of changes in the texture of their hair: more brittle, finer, curlier, unruly, or straighter (Osio et al. 2009). Trichomegaly may also be induced by latanoprost, interferon alpha-2b, bimatoprost, cyclosporin, and tacrolimus (Jayamanne et al. 1996; Woo and Francis 2001; Hernandez-Nunez et al. 2002; Herane and Urbina 2004; Ward et al. 2006).

4.7.2 Hypertrichosis and Hirsutism

Hirsutism and hypertrichosis are characterized by an excess of terminal hair. In hypertrichosis this excess is localized or generalized, while in hirsutism there is excess of terminal hair in females and children with an adult male pattern of distribution. Hirsutism is a distressing and relatively common problem, affecting 5–10% of women in the reproductive age group. It is usually a sign of androgen excess, the commonest cause being the polycystic ovarian syndrome. Both hirsutism and hypertrichosis may be associated with drug administration. Drugs most commonly responsible for the development of hirsutism include testosterone, danazol, ACTH, metyrapone, anabolic steroids, and glucocorticoids (Hosea et al. 1980; Tosti and Pazzaglia 2007). Hypertrichosis is a common adverse event of cyclosporine, prostaglandin analogs, minoxidil and diazoxide (Tosti and Pazzaglia 2007).

4.7.3 Hair Changes Caused by Ultraviolet Radiation

Exposure to ultraviolet radiation damages hair fiber. Dryness, reduced strength, rough surface texture, loss of color, decreased luster, stiffness, and brittleness of hair are caused by sun exposure. Photochemical degradation of hair results in attack on both hair proteins and melanin. Destruction of hair protein is thought to be the result of UVB-induced oxidation of sulfur-containing molecules within the hair shaft (Santos Nogueira and Joekes 2004). Destruction of melanin within the cortex of the hair has been studied extensively in wool, where it is known as photoyellowing and is more pronounced for light colored hairs. It appears to be caused by UVA through oxidation of the amide carbon of polypeptide chains producing carbonyl groups (Muller et al. 2003; Nogueira et al. 2004; Santos Nogueira and Joekes 2004).

Trüeb postulated in 2003 that androgenetica alopecia might be a photoaggravated dermatosis (Trueb 2003). Definite evidence, however, is still lacking.

4.7.4 Changes in Hair Color

Hair color changes result not only from alterations of melanin production but also from changes in the hair structure itself, altering its optical properties. A variety of genetic, metabolic, nutritional, and acquired disorders result in hair color changes. Most drug-induced changes in hair color result in lighter hair color, although PABA and some chemotherapy regimens have darkened hair (Cline 1988). Exposure to copper from domestic water or cosmetics may result in green discoloration in blond, grey, or white hair. In those who develop this from swimming pools, the copper can be from copper-based algaecides, corrosion of pipes, and/or a low pH that allows leaching from copper pipes (Mascaro et al. 1995). An outbreak of green hair was reported secondary to fluoridation tap water that lowered the water pH from 8.0 to 5.8. Copper was liberated from household piping by the acidified water. Electrical grounds connected to copper pipes can also cause leakage of copper into the water (Nordlund et al. 1977). Metal exposure in cobalt workers may result in blue discoloration of the hair (Daniel et al. 2004).

References

Abele R, Alberto P, Kaplan S, Siegenthaler P, Hofmann V, Ryssel HJ, Hartmann D, Holdener EE, Cavalli F (1983) Phase II study of doxifluridine in advanced colorectal adenocarcinoma. J Clin Oncol 1:750–754

Aghamirian MR, Ghiasian SA (2011) Dermatophytes as a cause of epizoonoses in dairy cattle and humans in Iran: epidemiological and clinical aspects. Mycoses 54:e52–e56

Akerley W (1996) Phase I/II trial of weekly paclitaxel in patients with advanced lung cancer. Semin Oncol 23:55–58

Amster E, Tiwary A, Schenker MB (2007) Case report: potential arsenic toxicosis secondary to herbal kelp supplement. Environ Health Perspect 115:606–608

Atas B, Caksen H, Tuncer O, Kirimi E, Akgun C, Odabas D (2004) Four children with colchicine poisoning. Hum Exp Toxicol 23:353–356

Atsmon J, Taliansky E, Landau M, Neufeld MY (2000) Thallium poisoning in Israel. Am J Med Sci 320:327–330

Autier J, Escudier B, Wechsler J, Spatz A, Robert C (2008) Prospective study of the cutaneous adverse effects of sorafenib, a novel multikinase inhibitor. Arch Dermatol 144:886–892

Badiugin IS (2009) Incendiary and toxic characteristics of phosphorus. Lessons learned from the accident in L'vov. Voen Med Zh 330:20–26

Balabanoff VA (1985) Berufliche Dermatomykosen zoophilen Ursprungs in Bulgarien. Derm Beruf Umwelt 33:170–174

Beckett WS, Oskvig R, Gaynor ME, Goldgeier MH (2001) Association of reversible alopecia with occupational topical exposure to common borax-containing solutions. J Am Acad Dermatol 44:599–602

Bicer S, Soysal DD, Ctak A, Ucsel R, Karabocuoglu M, Uzel N (2007) Acute colchicine intoxication in a child: a case report. Pediatr Emerg Care 23:314–317

Bismuth C, Gaultier M, Conso F (1977) Aplasie médullaire aprés intoxication aiguë à la colchicine. Nouv Presse Med 6:1625–1629

Bleise A, Danesi PR, Burkart W (2003) Properties, use and health effects of depleted uranium (DU): a general overview. J Environ Radioact 64:93–112

Brockhaus A, Dolgner R, Ewers U, Kramer U, Soddemann H, Wiegand H (1981) Intake and health effects of thallium among a population living in the vicinity of a cement plant emitting thallium containing dust. Int Arch Occup Environ Health 48:375–389

Brodkin E, Copes R, Mattman A, Kennedy J, Kling R, Yassi A (2007) Lead and mercury exposures: interpretation and action. Can Med Assoc J 176:59–63

Brvar M, Kozelj G, Mozina M, Bunc M (2004) Acute poisoning with autumn crocus (Colchicum autumnale L.). Wien Klin Wochenschr 116:205–208

Cascinu S, Del FE, Ligi M, Graziano F, Catalano G (1997) The clinical impact of teniposide in the treatment of elderly patients with small-cell lung cancer. Am J Clin Oncol 20:477–478

Chadeganipour M, Shadzi S, Dehghan P, Movahed M (1997) Prevalence and aetiology of dermatophytoses in Isfahan, Iran. Mycoses 40:321–324

Cline DJ (1988) Changes in hair color. Dermatol Clin 6:295–303

Cohen MH, Johnson JR, Pazdur R (2005) Food and Drug Administration Drug approval summary: temozolomide plus radiation therapy for the treatment of newly diagnosed glioblastoma multiforme. Clin Cancer Res 11:6767–6771

Conlin AK, Vahdat L (2006) Dermatological toxicity of ixabepilone. Anticancer Res 26:2279–2280

Crounse RG, Maxwell JD, Blank H (1962) Inhibition of growth of hair by mimosine. Nature 194:694–695

Daniel CR III, Piraccini BM, Tosti A (2004) The nail and hair in forensic science. J Am Acad Dermatol 50:258–261

de Jonge ME, Mathot RA, Dalesio O, Huitema AD, Rodenhuis S, Beijnen JH (2002) Relationship between irreversible alopecia and exposure to cyclophosphamide, thiotepa and carboplatin (CTC) in high-dose chemotherapy. Bone Marrow Transplant 30:593–597

Eddleston M, Phillips MR (2004) Self poisoning with pesticides. BMJ 328:42–44

Forde P, Murphy C, O'Sullivan C, Carney D (2011) Triad of trichomegaly, alopecia and male-pattern hair growth during treatment with erlotinib in non-small-cell lung cancer. Ir J Med Sci 180:283–284

Fuller LC (2009) Changing face of Tinea capitis in Europe. Curr Opin Infect Dis 22:115–118

Fuller LC, Child FJ, Midgley G, Higgins EM (2003) Diagnosis and management of scalp ringworm. BMJ 326:539–541

Geleijns J, Wondergem J (2005) X-ray imaging and the skin: radiation biology, patient dosimetry and observed effects. Radiat Prot Dosimetry 114:121–125

Grevelman EG, Breed WP (2005) Prevention of chemotherapy-induced hair loss by scalp cooling. Ann Oncol 16:352–358

Gupta AK, Ryder JE, Chow M, Cooper EA (2005) Dermatophytosis: the management of fungal infections. Skinmed 4:305–310

Haas NS, Shih R, Gochfeld M (2003) A patient with postoperative mercury contamination of the peritoneum. J Toxicol Clin Toxicol 41:175–180

Hamilton A, Biganzoli L, Coleman R, Mauriac L, Hennebert P, Awada A, Nooij M, Beex L, Piccart M, Van Hoorebeeck I, Bruning P, de Valeriola D (2002) EORTC 10968: a phase I clinical and pharmacokinetic study of polyethylene glycol liposomal doxorubicin (Caelyx, Doxil) at a 6-week interval in patients with metastatic breast cancer. European Organization for Research and Treatment of Cancer. Ann Oncol 13:910–918

Hartmann JT, Haap M, Kopp HG, Lipp HP (2009) Tyrosine kinase inhibitors: a review on pharmacology, metabolism and side effects. Curr Drug Metab 10:470–481

Herane MI, Urbina F (2004) Acquired trichomegaly of the eyelashes and hypertrichosis induced by bimatoprost. J Eur Acad Dermatol Venereol 18:644–645

Hernandez-Nunez A, Fernandez-Herrera J, Buceta LR, Garcia-Diez A (2002) Trichomegaly following treatment with interferon alpha-2b. Lancet 359:1107

Herrlinger KR, Kreisel W, Schwab M, Schoelmerich J, Fleig WE, Ruhl A, Reinshagen M, Deibert P, Fellermann K, Greinwald R, Stange EF (2003) 6-thioguanine–efficacy and safety in chronic active Crohn's disease. Aliment Pharmacol Ther 17:503–508

Hirata M, Taoda K, Ono-Ogasawara M, Takaya M, Hisanaga N (1998) A probable case of chronic occupational thallium poisoning in a glass factory. Ind Health 36:300–303

Hosea SW, Santaella ML, Brown EJ, Berger M, Katusha K, Frank MM (1980) Long-term therapy of hereditary angioedema with danazol. Ann Intern Med 93:809–812

Hwang SM, Lee WS, Choi EH, Lee SH, Ahn SK (1999) Nurse's cap alopecia. Int J Dermatol 38:187–191

Jayamanne DG, Dayan MR, Porter R (1996) Cyclosporin-induced trichomegaly of accessory lashes as a cause of ocular irritation. Nephrol Dial Transplant 11:1159–1161

Kaufman LD, Izquierdo MM, Serrano JM, Gomez-Reino JJ (1995) 12-year follow-up study of epidemic Spanish toxic oil syndrome. J Rheumatol 22:282–288

Kazantzis G (2002) Mercury exposure and early effects: an overview. Med Lav 93:139–147

Kerdel-Vegas F (1964) Generalized hair loss due to the ingestion of "coco de mono" (*Lecythis ollaria*). J Invest Dermatol 42:91–94

Kilbourne EM, de la Posada PM, Abaitua Borda I, Diez Ruiz-Navarro M, Philen RM, Falk H (1991) Toxic oil syndrome: a current clinical and epidemiologic summary, including comparisons with the eosinophilia–myalgia syndrome. J Am Coll Cardiol 18:711–717

Kimyai-Asadi A, Harris JC, Nousari HC (1999) Critical overview: adverse cutaneous reactions to psychotropic medications. J Clin Psychiatry 60:714–725

Krstev S, Perunicic B, Vidakovic A (2003) Work practice and some adverse health effects in nurses handling antineoplastic drugs. Med Lav 94:432–439

Kumar B, Saraswat A, Kaur I (2002) Mucocutaneous adverse effects of hydroxyurea: a prospective study of 30 psoriasis patients. Clin Exp Dermatol 27:8–13

Lee WJ, Lee JL, Chang SE, Lee MW, Kang YK, Choi JH, Moon KC, Koh JK (2009) Cutaneous adverse effects in patients treated with the multitargeted kinase inhibitors sorafenib and sunitinib. Br J Dermatol 161:1045–1051

Lehenkari E, Silvennoinen-Kassinen S (1995) Dermatophytes in northern Finland in 1982–90. Mycoses 38:411–414

Leong WA (2008) Case studies in anticoagulation management. J Thromb Thrombolysis 25:78–84

Leyland-Jones B, Gelmon K, Ayoub JP, Arnold A, Verma S, Dias R, Ghahramani P (2003) Pharmacokinetics, safety, and efficacy of trastuzumab administered every three weeks in combination with paclitaxel. J Clin Oncol 21:3965–3971

Litt JZ (2007) Drug eruption reference manual, 13th edn. Informa Healthcare, London

Lu CI, Huang CC, Chang YC, Tsai YT, Kuo HC, Chuang YH, Shih TS (2007) Short-term thallium intoxication: dermatological findings correlated with thallium concentration. Arch Dermatol 143:93–98

Luo J, Litherland AJ, Sahlu T, Puchala R, Lachica M, Goetsch AL (2000) Effects of mimosine on fiber shedding, follicle activity, and fiber regrowth in Spanish goats. J Anim Sci 78:1551–1555

Luther J, Glesby MJ (2007) Dermatologic adverse effects of antiretroviral therapy: recognition and management. Am J Clin Dermatol 8:221–233

Madani S, Shapiro J (2000) Alopecia areata update. J Am Acad Dermatol 42:549–566

Mascaro JM Jr, Ferrando J, Fontarnau R, Torras H, Dominguez A, Mascaro JM (1995) Green hair. Cutis 56:37–40

Maslen MM (2000) Human cases of cattle ringworm due to *Trichophyton verrucosum* in Victoria, Australia. Australas J Dermatol 41:90–94

McCurdy SA, Pocekay D, Hammond SK, Woskie SR, Samuels SJ, Schenker MB (1995) A cross-sectional survey of respiratory and general health outcomes among semiconductor industry workers. Am J Ind Med 28:847–860

Moore D, House I, Dixon A (1993) Thallium poisoning. Diagnosis may be elusive but alopecia is the clue. BMJ 306:1527–1529

Muggiano A, Mulas C, Fiori B, Liciardi G, Pintus M, Tanca L, Tedde A, Turno R, Desogus A (2004) Feasibility of high-dose interferon-alpha2b adjuvant therapy for high-risk resected cutaneous melanoma. Melanoma Res 14:S1–S7

Muller D, Desel H (2010) Acute selenium poisoning by paradise nuts (*Lecythis ollaria*). Hum Exp Toxicol 29:431–434

Muller U, Ratzsch M, Schwanninger M, Steiner M, Zobl H (2003) Yellowing and IR-changes of spruce wood as result of UV-irradiation. J Photochem Photobiol B 69:97–105

Nogueira AC, Nakano AK, Joekes I (2004) Impairment of hair mechanical properties by sun exposure and bleaching treatments. J Cosmet Sci 55:533–537

Nordlund JJ, Hartley C, Fister J (1977) On the cause of green hair. Arch Dermatol 113:1700

Osimitz TG, Murphy JV, Fell LA, Page B (2010) Adverse events associated with the use of insect repellents containing N, N-diethyl-m-toluamide (DEET). Regul Toxicol Pharmacol 56:93–99

Osio A, Mateus C, Soria JC, Massard C, Malka D, Boige V, Besse B, Robert C (2009) Cutaneous side-effects in patients on long-term treatment with epidermal growth factor receptor inhibitors. Br J Dermatol 161: 515–521

Parker V, Wong AH, Boon HS, Seeman MV (2001) Adverse reactions to St John's Wort. Can J Psychiatry 46:77–79

Paus R, Cotsarelis G (1999) The biology of hair follicles. N Engl J Med 341:491–497

Prussick R (1996) Adverse cutaneous reactions to chemotherapeutic agents and cytokine therapy. Semin Cutan Med Surg 15:267–276

Rahman MM, Ng JC, Naidu R (2009) Chronic exposure of arsenic via drinking water and its adverse health impacts on humans. Environ Geochem Health 31(Suppl 1):189–200

Rajkumar SV, Reid JM, Novotny PJ, Safgren SL, Scheithauer BW, Johnson PS, Nair S, Morton RF, Hatfield AK, Krook JE, Ames MM, Buckner JC (2000) A randomized phase II and pharmacokinetic study of dacarbazine in patients with recurrent glioma. J Neurooncol 49:255–261

Richter ED, Peled N, Luria M (1982) Mercury exposure and effects at a thermometer factory. Scand J Work Environ Health 8(Suppl 1): 161–166

Roman C, Massai L, Gianni C, Crosti C (2001) Case reports. Six cases of infection due to *Trichophyton verrucosum*. Mycoses 44:334–337

Roselino AM, Almeida AM, Hippolito MA, Cerqueira BC, Maffei CM, Menezes JB, Vieira RE, Assis SL, Ali SA (1996) Clinical-epidemiologic study of alopecia areata. Int J Dermatol 35:181–184

Rubin P, Casarett GW (1968) Clinical radiation pathology as applied to curative radiotherapy. Cancer 22:767–778

Saccomanno G, Auerbach O, Kuschner M, Harley NH, Michels RY, Anderson MW, Bechtel JJ (1996) A comparison between the localization of lung tumors in uranium miners and in nonminers from 1947 to 1991. Cancer 77:1278–1283

Safavi KH, Muller SA, Suman VJ, Moshell AN, Melton LJ III (1995) Incidence of alopecia areata in Olmsted County, Minnesota, 1975 through 1989. Mayo Clin Proc 70:628–633

Saimot AG (2001) Medical treatment of liver hydatidosis. World J Surg 25:15–20

Santos Nogueira AC, Joekes I (2004) Hair color changes and protein damage caused by ultraviolet radiation. J Photochem Photobiol B 74:109–117

Schillinger BM, Berstein M, Goldberg LA, Shalita AR (1982) Boric acid poisoning. J Am Acad Dermatol 7:667–673

Schrallhammer-Benkler K, Ring J, Przybilla B, Meurer M, Landthaler M (1992) Acute mercury intoxication with lichenoid drug eruption followed by mercury contact allergy and development of antinuclear antibodies. Acta Derm Venereol 72:294–296

Schulze M, Helber B, Hardt J, Ehret W (2002) Pyrethroidbelastung durch Parasitenprophylaxe beim Hund. Dtsch Med Wochenschr 127:616–618

Scott DL, Smolen JS, Kalden JR, van de Putte LB, Larsen A, Kvien TK, Schattenkirchner M, Nash P, Oed C, Loew-Friedrich I (2001) Treatment of active rheumatoid arthritis with leflunomide: two year follow up of a double blind, placebo controlled trial versus sulfasalazine. Ann Rheum Dis 60:913–923

Seebacher C, Abeck D, Brasch J, Daeschlein G, Effendy I, Ginter-Hanselmayer G, Haake N, Hamm G, Hof H, Korting HC, Kramer A, Mayser P, Schlacke KH, Tietz HJ (2004) Tinea capitis. J Dtsch Dermatol Ges 2:462–468

Sinclair R, Grossman KL, Kvedar JC (2003) Anagen hair loss. In: Olsen EA (ed) Disorders of hair growth: diagnosis and treatments, 2nd edn. McGraw-Hill, New York, pp 275–302

Skipworth GB, Goldstein N, McBride WP (1967) Boric acid intoxication from "medicated talcum powder". Arch Dermatol 95:83–86

Spiewak R (2001) Pesticides as a cause of occupational skin diseases in farmers. Ann Agric Environ Med 8:1–5

Srivastava AK, Gupta BN, Bihari V, Gaur JS (1995) Generalized hair loss and selenium exposure. Vet Hum Toxicol 37:468–469

Stafford-Fox V, Guindon KM (2000) Cutaneous reactions associated with alpha interferon therapy. Clin J Oncol Nurs 4:164–168

Stein KM, Odom RB, Justice GR, Martin GC (1973) Toxic alopecia from ingestion of boric acid. Arch Dermatol 108:95–97

Stuttgen G, Haas N, Mittelbach F, Zesch A (1982) Toxischer akuter reversibler Haarausfall durch Dampf/Dunst-Kontakt mit

Natriumhypochlorid bzw. Natriumhydroxid enthaltenden Abfluss- und Sanitärreinigers. Wien Klin Wochenschr 94:479–484

Sutter ME, Thomas JD, Brown J, Morgan B (2008) Selenium toxicity: a case of selenosis caused by a nutritional supplement. Ann Intern Med 148:970–971

Tafur AJ, Zapatier JA, Idrovo LA, Oliveros JW, Garces JC (2004) Bone marrow toxicity after yellow phosphorus ingestion. Emerg Med J 21:259–260

Tan TG (1970) Occupational toxic alopecia due to borax. Acta Derm Venereol 50:55–58

Tosti A, Pazzaglia M (2007) Drug reactions affecting hair: diagnosis. Dermatol Clin 25:223–231, vii

Tosti A, Misciali C, Piraccini BM, Peluso AM, Bardazzi F (1994) Drug-induced hair loss and hair growth. Incidence, management and avoidance. Drug Saf 10:310–317

Tosti A, Piraccini BM, Bergfeld W, Camacho F, Dawber RPR, Happle R, Olsen EA, Price V, Rebora A, Shapiro J, Sinclair R, VanNeste D, Whiting DA (2002) Occupational alopecia or alopecia areata? J Am Acad Dermatol 47:636–637

Tosti A, Piraccini BM, Vincenzi C, Misciali C (2005) Permanent alopecia after busulfan chemotherapy. Br J Dermatol 152:1056–1058

Trefzer U, Hofmann M, Sterry W (2003) Kutane Nebenwirkungen klinisch relevanter Zytokintherapien. Dtsch Med Wochenschr 128:1782–1787

Tromme I, Van ND, Dobbelaere F, Bouffioux B, Courtin C, Dugernier T, Pierre P, Dupuis M (1998) Skin signs in the diagnosis of thallium poisoning. Br J Dermatol 138:321–325

Trueb RM (2003) Is androgenetic alopecia a photoaggravated dermatosis? Dermatology 207:343–348

Trueb RM (2009) Chemotherapy-induced alopecia. Semin Cutan Med Surg 28:11–14

UNSCEAR (United Nations Scientific Committee on the Effects of Atomic Radiation) (1982) Ionizingradiation: sources and biological effects, United Nations ed., New York, E.82.IX.8

Uragoda CG (1984) Asthma and other symptoms in cinnamon workers. Br J Ind Med 41:224–227

Van Dooren-Greebe RJ, Kuijpers AL, Mulder J, De BT, Van de Kerkhof PC (1994) Methotrexate revisited: effects of long-term treatment in psoriasis. Br J Dermatol 130:204–210

Verschuuren HG, Kroes R, Den Tonkelaar EM, Berkvens JM, Helleman PW, Van Esch GJ (1975) Long-tern toxicity and reproduction studies with metaldehyde in rats. Toxicology 4:97–115

Wakhlu A, Aggarwal A, Misra R (2003) Chronic arsenic poisoning mimicking Gottron's rash. J Rheumatol 30:415–416

Ward KM, Barnett C, Fox LP, Grossman ME (2006) Eyelash trichomegaly associated with systemic tacrolimus. Arch Dermatol 142:248

WHO (World Health Organization) (2010) Environmental Health Criteria 224: arsenic and arsenic compounds

Wiper A, Katira R, Roberts DH (2005) Images in cardiology. Interventional cardiology: it's a hairy business. Heart 91:1432

Woo TL, Francis IC (2001) Intermittent blurred vision and trichomegaly due to latanoprost. Clin Experiment Ophthalmol 29:272–273

Yang GQ, Wang SZ, Zhou RH, Sun SZ (1983) Endemic selenium intoxication of humans in China. Am J Clin Nutr 37:872–881

27 Pigment Disorders

J. P. Wietze van der Veen · Maryam Yazdani
Netherlands Institute for Pigment Disorders and Department of Dermatology, Academic Medical Centre University of Amsterdam, Amsterdam, The Netherlands

Core Messages

- Darker skin types are more prone to exogenous pigmentary changes
- The most common exogenous hyperpigmentation is post-inflammatory
- Occupational pigmentary changes predominantly consist of chemically induced hypo-/depigmentations
- Occupational leukoderma/vitiligo is rare in western countries but quite common in developing countries

1 Introduction

1.1 The Epidermal Melanin Unit

Skin color largely is determined by many factors (➋ *Table 27.1*) of which melanocyte derived epidermal melanin is the most important. The melanocyte is a dendritic cell present in the basal layer of the epidermis with no desmosomes or tonofilaments. Melanocytes arise from the neural crest as melanoblasts and migrate to the dermis, hair follicles, leptomeninges, uveal tract, and retina. By the eighth week of intrauterine life, they start to migrate from the dermis to the epidermis. Although full melanocyte migration is normally completed prior to birth, residual dermal melanocytes are sometimes left, as can be seen in mongoloid spots and Ota nevi.

In 1963, Fitzpatrick and Breathnach proposed the concept of the epidermal melanin unit, which described the interplay of epidermal melanocytes and keratinocytes in constituting the color of the skin. One melanocyte produces melanin for approximately 36 surrounding keratinocytes by delivering to their neighboring cells melanosomes, cell membrane enveloped organelles in which melanin was produced and stored (Nordlund et al. 2006; Nordlund and Ortonne 2006; Nordlund 2007; Ansty 2010).

The genetically determined basal state is called constitutive pigmentation. By UV-induced tanning facultative pigmentation is being formed. Nowadays, it is believed that also epidermal Langerhans cells are important in the cellular interplay regulating melanogenesis. Probably all epidermal cells cooperate in the defense against noxious environmental stimuli and the concept of the keratinocyte-Langerhans-melanocyte (KLM) unit has been proposed (Nordlund 2007). The close interplay by all epidermal cells in all aspects of protection is supported by data showing that depigmented vitiligo patches (1) have a lack of inflammatory response to contact allergens and (2) do have a lower but still significant protection against sunburn correlating with the UVB sensitivity of their healthy skin (Caron-Schreinemachers et al. 2005).

1.1.1 Melanogenesis

Melanogenesis, the production of melanin within melanocytes takes place in cell organelles called melanosomes. Basically two types of melanin can be produced, the black-brown eumelanin predominant in darker skin types, and the red-yellow pheomelanin, predominant in very light skin. The enzyme tyrosinase plays a key role in producing both types of melanin.

The hormone α-MSH is very important in the regulation of melanogenesis. It is classically considered to be produced by the pituitary but we now know that it is produced in most cells of the body including keratinocytes, Langerhans cells, and melanocytes. α-MSH not only stimulates melanogenesis and transfer of melanosomes but also has anti-inflammatory properties and stimulates DNA synthesis in keratinocytes. In this way, (hyper) pigmentation is linked to epidermal tissue repair explaining the often found post-inflammatory hyperpigmentation (see below) (Bolognia 2003; Ansty 2010).

1.1.2 Skin Types and Ethnic Skin

A classic way to classify skin types is proposed by Fitzpatrick and is based on reaction of the skin to sun exposure (➋ *Table 27.2*) (Nordlund and Ortonne 2006). Though roughly corresponding to pigmentation and certainly useful for clinical purposes such as phototherapy, it does not cover ethnic aspects of skin that bear clinical significance as well.

As opposed to white skin, colored skin has larger and more dendritic melanocytes, with larger melanosomes,

T. Rustemeyer, P. Elsner, S.M. John & H.I. Maibach (eds.), *Kanerva's Occupational Dermatology*,
DOI 10.1007/978-3-642-02035-3_27,

which are being transferred in larger amounts to the epidermal keratinocytes. The highly productive melanogenesis is more sensitive to noxious stimuli as can be seen in post-inflammatory hyper- and hypopigmentations.

Apart from these very common but temporary melanogenetic dysregulations, colored skin can show several physiological pigment patterns (➋ *Table 27.3*) that should be recognized as such (Van der Veen et al. 2006). Other differences between white and colored skin include the clinical expression of erythema which is hardly or not visible in black skin, the larger cohesion of keratinocytes in colored skin giving the vesicular dermatoses of white skin a more papular appearance in the colored, the greater tendency for acne-like eruptions and subsequent hyperpigmentations, and sometimes keloid formation in people with a black-African skin type and the greater risk for skin cancer in the white (Naafs 2006).

Table 27.1
Determinants contributing to color of skin

Melanin associated	Others
Melanin:	Capillary blood flow and its components variation:
Eumelanin (Black-brown)	Oxyhemoglobin, Reduced hemoglobin
Pheomelanin (Red-yellow)	Collagen
In:	Carotene or lycopene
Melanocytes	Chemicals or drugs
Keratinocytes	Others factors:
Dermal macrphages (melanophages)	Transparency of stratum corneum and epidermis
	Light reflection, refraction, and absorption to skin

2 Hyperpigmentations

2.1 Post-inflammatory Hyperpigmentation

Post-inflammatory hyperpigmentation (PIH) is one of the most common pigmentary disorders specifically in dark skin. Inflammatory skin conditions like infection, (occupational) chemical irritation, or repetitive trauma can cause increased pigmentation. The two processes involved are an epidermal inflammatory response and incontinentia pigmenti (➋ *Fig. 27.1*).

The epidermal inflammatory response consists of an increased synthesis of melanin, resulting in an epidermal melanosis. The final common pathway of chemicals like prostoglandines, leucotrienes, and α-MSH released during inflammatory processes has an effect on cyclic AMP, which stimulate pigment synthesis.

Incontinentia pigmenti occurs after disruption of the epidermal basal cell layer causing dermal melanosis. Apoptosis of the pigment cells due to inflammatory reaction will cause melanosomes leak to the dermis, which will be accumulated in macrophages called melanophages. In lighter skin types, epidermal hyperpigmentation can be differentiated from pure dermal hyperpigmentation by Woods lamp illumination. Under

Table 27.2
Skin phototypes

Skin type and history		Examples	
I	Always burns, never tans	Very light/Celtic	Red hair and freckles, green, gray, or blue eyes
II	Always burns, tans minimally	Light/light skinned European	Light or dark hair, Blue, brown, or gray eyes
III	Burns moderately, tans gradually	Light intermediate/dark- skinned European	Brown hair, blue, green hazel eyes
IV	Rarely burns, tans well	Dark intermediate/Mediterranean	Black to brown hair, brown, or dark brown eyes
V	Burns minimally, tans well	Dark/Brown type/Middle Eastern. Latin American, Orientals	Black hair and brown or dark brown eyes
VI	Never burns, deeply brown	Very dark/"Black" type/African/Australian natives	Black hair and dark brown eyes, with minor variations

Table 27.3
Normal pigmentary variations in ethnic skin

	Description	Area	Remarks
Voigt's or Futcher's lines	Lines of demarcation between darker and lighter skin areas	Posterior portion of the lower limb, presternal area, posteromedial area of the spine, bilateral aspect of the chest, upper arm anteromedially	75% of the African(- American) population
Hyperpigmentation	Macular hyperpigmentations, varying in shape or mottled	Palmar/plantar	Differential diagnosis: palmar/plantar lesion of syphilis, ephelides, nevi, melanoma
	Fairly circumscribed macules	Extensor side of the joints	Caused by stretching of the skin at the joints
Nail pigmentation	Longitudinal linear dark bands in the nail plates	Mostly thumb and index finger	Mostly in black with a very dark complexion. Absent at birth and increases with age
Familial periorbital hyperpigmentation		Childhood: lower eyelids	Autosomal dominant hereditary disorder. Starting in childhood and progressing with age
		Adult: entire periorbital area	
Linea nigra		A line between the xyphoid process and the symphysis	Darkens during pregnancy
Oral pigmentation		Usually: on the gingivae	
		Less common: hard palate, buccal mucosa, tongue	
Mongolian spot	Gray- blue macular lesions varying in size but usually	Sacrum buttocks and back	Most common congenital hyperpigmentation, 80–100% of the Asian and black newborns, dermal melanocytosis due to arresting of the fetal mealnocytes migration to the epidermis from the neural crest
	<5% of the body surface		

this light epidermal pigment becomes more accentuated, while deep dermal pigment is hardly visible.

Dermal hyperpigmentation can take years to fade away to normal, whereas epidermal melanosis usually disappears in 6–12 month. Sun exposure, chemicals, and certain drugs can aggravate PIH. Epidermal hyperpigmentation can be influenced by topical agents like retinoids, corticosteroids, and hydroquinone, but deeper hyperpigmentations are very therapy-resistant (Van der Veen et al. 2006).

3 Hypopigmentations

3.1 Post-inflammatory Hypopigmentation

In dark skin, even minor triggers of an inflammatory response can lead to hypopigmentation. Triggers can be common inflammatory skin disorders like psoriasis, any kind of dermatitis (seborrheic, atopic, contact- etc.), or repetitive trauma or irritation (*Fig. 27.2*).

The prognosis is favorable and in due time, when the trigger can be avoided and regular sun exposure is possible, repigmentation within months is possible (Van der Veen et al. 2006). In general, post-inflammatory hyperpigmentation is seen much more frequently and poses a larger therapeutical challenge than its hypopigmented counterpart.

4 Bleaching Products

Modern humans probably all stem from black-skinned ancestors with curly hair. In moderate climates adaptation of skin color took place and this new white-skinned variant appeared to be very successful in the ages to come. A classic example of white-skinned domination can be

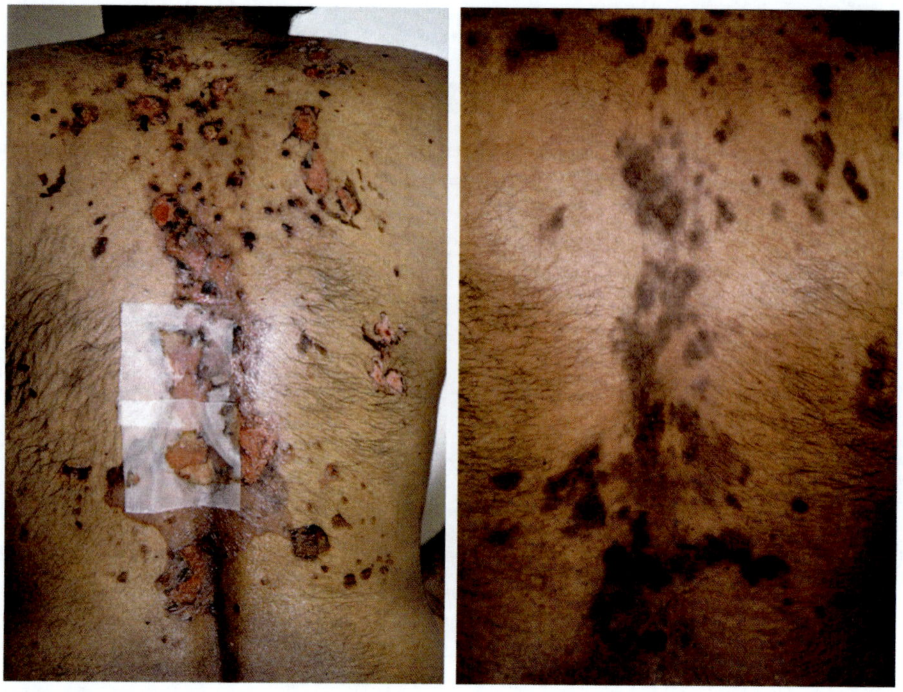

Fig. 27.1
Post-inflammatory hyperpigmentation after a blistering skin disease

found in India, where the ruling white elite stems from white-skinned ancestors who invaded the Indian subcontinent more than 5,000 years ago.

Nowadays, lots of people all over the world try to lighten their skin in order to be more successful in society (Westerhof 2007). To this end, many products have been developed by the cosmetic industry. These over the counter creams contain compounds like arbutin, licorice extract, mulberry, kojic acid, magnesium L-ascorbyl-2-phosphate, alpha-tocopherol, *n*-acetyl-D-glucosamine, or carvacrol. Most of these compounds work through inhibition of tyrosinase. For medical purposes such as the treatment of melasma hydroquinone, retinoic acid, and azelaic acid are currently being used in several prescriptions often combining different compounds, for example, hydroquinone, tretinoin, and a corticosteroid. Though effective in downregulating melanogenesis these prescriptions often induce irritation which in dark skin always comes with the hazard of post-inflammatory hyperpigmentation as a paradoxal side-effect. The more effective prescription only compounds are illegally available on a large scale and can be very harmful because uncontrolled prolonged use can give rise to unwanted pigmentary changes like ochronosis and leukoderma en confetti (hydroquinone), chemical vitiligo (monobenzone), skin atrophy, and Cushing syndrome (corticosteroids).

Strong bleaching agents with melanocytotoxic properties like monobenzone and 4-methoxyphenol can be used in treating patients with universal vitiligo to remove disfiguring areas with remnant pigmentation (➋ *Fig. 27.3*).

5 Vitiligo

Vitiligo probably is the best known pigment disorder as it has a worldwide prevalence of approximately 1% and can be very conspicuous, especially in dark skin (Taiëb and Picardo 2009). It is an acquired disorder characterized by the development of white patches due to a progressive loss of melanocytes (➋ *Fig. 27.4*). Vitiligo often runs in families and is associated with autoimmune endocrinopathies of which thyroid disease (20–30% prevalence) is the most important. In half of the cases, the first symptoms already start before the age of 20 and the disease runs a chronic course with exacerbations and relapses, eventually leading to more and larger white areas that can be found in different patterns. Important is to differentiate between

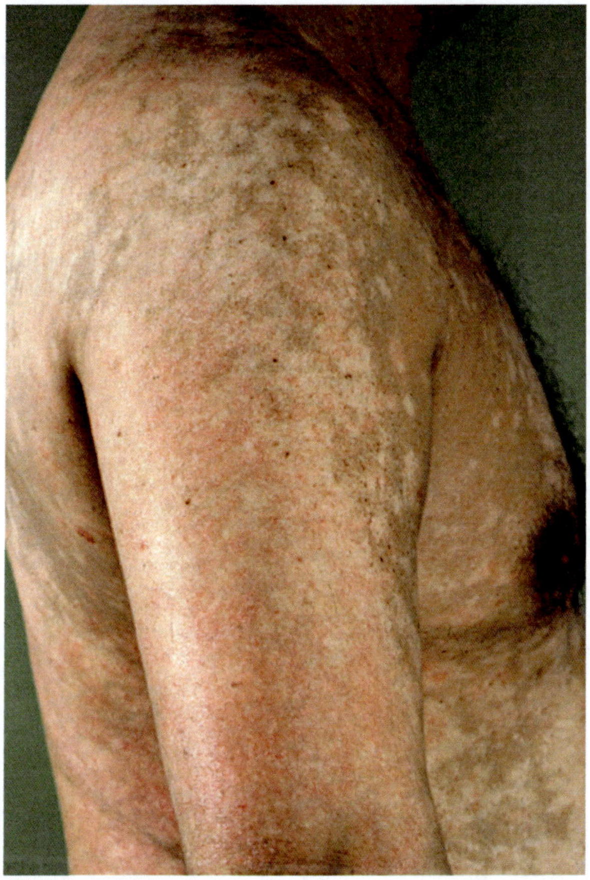

Fig. 27.2
Post-inflammatory hypopigmentation after psoriasis

non-segmental versus segmental vitiligo (➋ *Fig. 27.5*), the latter being a disease on its own with a different presentation, a different therapy, and probably a different pathogenesis (➋ *Table 27.4*). Both types of vitiligo can start with focal vitiligo, characterized by a small affected area (<15 cm^2). Very rare is universal vitiligo, in which >85% of the body surface is affected and the familial disposition is greater, as is the association with other autoimmune diseases (Linthorst Homan et al. 2008).

We will focus here on non-segmental also called generalized vitiligo, accounting for 85–90% of adult cases, which has a lot in common and can overlap with occupational (chemical) vitiligo.

5.1 Diagnosis

The observation of depigmentations distributed in a characteristic pattern together with a carefully taken (family) history leads to an easy diagnosis in most of the cases. In patients with a very light skin type depigmentations sometimes are difficult to judge by the naked eye and Woods lamp examination can be helpful in these cases. Other diagnoses to be ruled out include: piebaldism, nevus anemicus, progressive macular hypomelanosis, post-inflammatory hypopigmentation, post-traumatic leukoderma (burns), pityriasis alba, and melanoma-associated leukoderma.

5.2 Impact of the Disease

Vitiligo should be considered as a serious disease. There certainly are cultural differences regarding the social acceptance of the disease. An association with leprosy has always played a role in some regions, whereas in some societies vitiligo is a legally accepted reason for divorce, and marital prospects for vitiligo patients are very poor.

Nevertheless, vitiligo can profoundly influence the life of patients in any society.

A striking example of the burden of vitiligo was given by a (white) patient suffering from both type 1 diabetes and vitiligo. Though well aware of the physical threats imposed by his diabetes, he judged the vitiligo to be more devastating for his quality of life (Austin 2004).

In general however, vitiligo has more impact on dark skinned people than on whites in terms of quality of life (Linthorst Homan et al. 2009).

5.3 Pathogenesis

Different pathogenic mechanisms appear to play a role in vitiligo and their exact interplay is still under debate (Westerhof and d'Ischia 2007).

Of importance seem biochemical factors interfering with melanogenesis in genetically susceptible individuals, leading to the formation of auto-antigens triggering an autoimmune reaction. The biochemical factors mentioned above, may be external as in occupational vitiligo or intrinsic, due to a defective free-radical defense affecting melanin content and synthesis (Dell'Anna and Picardo 2006). In the end, the immune response takes the lead and propagates the depigmentation process independent from the original trigger.

5.4 Koebner Phenomenon

An important aetio-pathogenetic factor in vitiligo is the Koebner phenomenon, which can be defined as

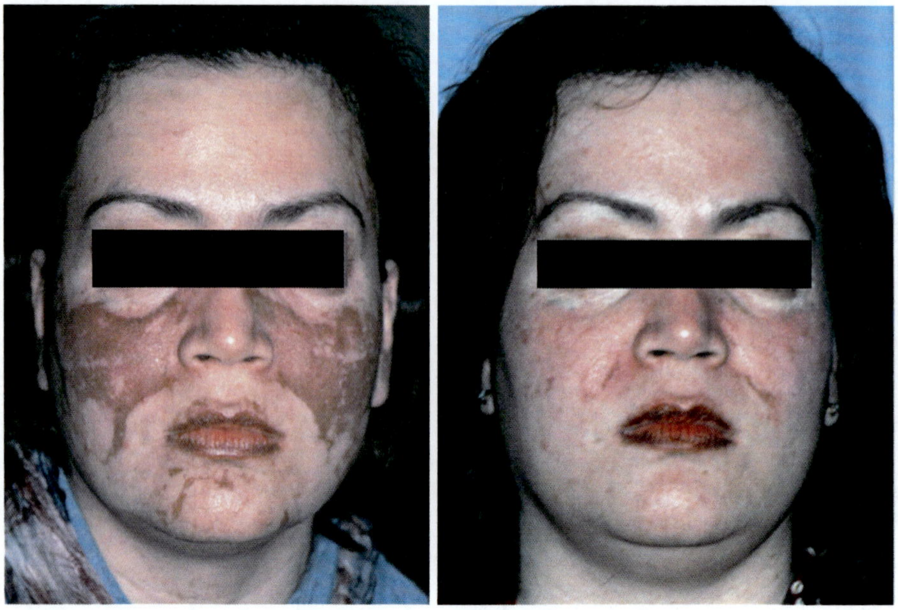

Fig. 27.3
Effects of bleaching with monobenzone in a patient with universal vitiligo

a cutaneous disease-specific response to a nonspecific, usually traumatic stimulus such as pressure or friction (Taieb and Picardo 2006). Local loss of melanocytes could be found 24 h after the mechanical stimulus suggesting an intrinsic vulnerability of the melanocytes.

This Koebner phenomenon can easily explain the distribution of vitiligo in many patients and can play a role in nonchemical occupational vitiligo.

5.5 Chemical (Occupational) Vitiligo and Leukoderma

Occupational vitiligo can essentially comprise vitiligo patches elicited by mechanical trauma in a work situation or vitiligo induced by contact with chemicals during work.

Moreover, also contact with chemicals on other occasions can play a role. Here, we will speak about chemical vitiligo/leukoderma in general.

Chemical leukoderma is characterized by depigmentation on the area of contact with a chemical. In patients with a genetic predisposition for vitiligo or with preexisting non-segmental vitiligo the depigmentation spreads beyond the areas of contact and here we can speak of chemical vitiligo (Boissy and Manga 2004).

A list of compounds associated with occupational chemical leukoderma/vitiligo is given in *Table 27.5* and professions prone to have contact with these chemicals are listed in *Table 27.6*.

Many of these compounds are phenolic/catecholic derivates and most research has been done on 4-*tert*-butylphenol (4-TBP). These compounds have chemical similarity with tyrosine and dopa, the endogenous substrates of the melanocyte- specific enzyme tyrosinase. Apart from downregulating melanogenesis by competition, these compounds clearly are able to be melanocytotoxic. Recent data indicate that immune destruction of melanocytes preceded by haptenation of tyrosinase by binding to oxidation products of the involved compounds probably plays the main role (Westerhof and d'Ischia 2007).

A prototype of such a reaction can be seen during treatment of patients with universal vitiligo. Many of these patients ask for bleaching of their often disfiguring remaining pigmented skin areas and to this end monobenzone is employed.

These patients develop a dermatitis strictly limited to their pigmented skin resulting in depigmentation, also in areas that have not been treated. Histologically, the inflammation is characterized by a dense infiltrate of T-lymphocytes and macrophages at the derm–epidermal junction (Westerhof and d'Ischia 2007). The end result is complete depigmentation of the affected area.

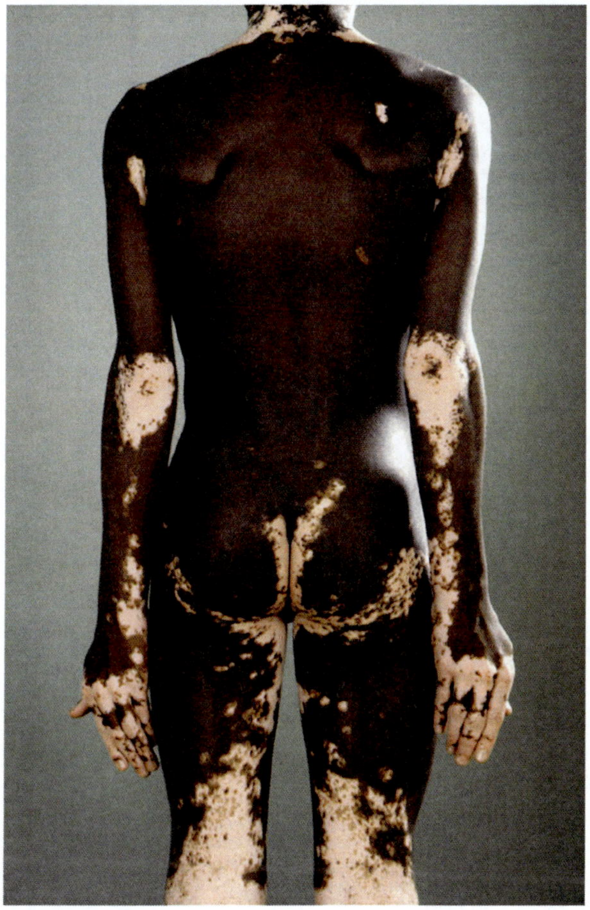

■ Fig. 27.4
Generalized vitiligo

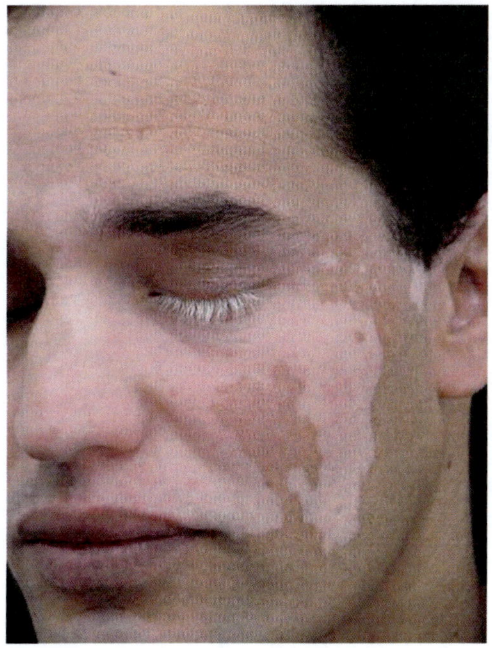

■ Fig. 27.5
Segmental vitiligo

■ Table 27.4
Segmental versus non-segmental vitiligo (Adapted from Taiëb and Picardo 2009)

Segmental vitiligo	Non-segmental vitiligo
Often begins in childhood	Can begin in childhood, but later onset is more common
Has rapid onset and stabilizes	Is progressive, with flare-ups
Involves hair compartment soon after onset	Involves hair compartment in later stages
No association with autoimmune disease	Is often associated with personal or family history of autoimmunity
Unilateral	Bilateral, often symmetrical
Most common on the face	Commonly at sites sensitive to pressure, friction or trauma
Excellent response to surgery	Variable results with surgical therapy

Chemical vitiligo seems to be seen very rarely in Western countries. The National Registration for Occupational Diseases in the Netherlands speaks of only one patient since 2002. In a retrospective study performed at the Netherlands Institute for Pigment Disorders on 1,264 vitiligo patients seen in the period 2003–2007, six patients reported chemicals as elicitating factors, but upon scrutinizing their history by an occupational health specialist in only three a chemical vitiligo could be proven. One of these patients mentioned several colleagues having the same skin problems, but none of them sought medical advice or was willing to stop exposure (unpublished results).

On the other hand in developing countries like India, chemical leukoderma is seen far more frequently and here predominantly induced by common domestic products (Ghosh and Mukhopadhyay 2009). In a series of 864 cases, two-third had developed de novo leukoderma with spread to remote areas in 26.3%, while one-third had a history of preexisting vitiligo. The chemicals involved

Table 27.5
Chemicals associated with vitiligo

Phenolic and Catecholic derivates	Alkylphenol
	Butylphenol
	Amylphenol
	Butylhydoxytoluene
	Dihydoxyphenylbutane
	Hydroquinone
	Monobenzyl ether of hydoquinone
	Monomethyl ether of hydroquinone
	Catechol
	Methylcatechol
	p-tert-Butylcatechol
	p-tert-Butylphenol
	p-tert-Amylphenol
	4-Isopropylcatechol
	4-Hydroxy-anisol
Sulfhydryls	Bèta-mercapto-ethylamine hydrochloride
	3-Mercaptopropylamine hydrochloride
	Sulfanolic acid
	N-2-mercapto-ethyldimethylamine hydrochloride
Others	Mercurials
	Arsenic
	Benzyl alcohol
	Chloroquine
	Cinnamic aldehyde
	Corticosteroids
	Guanonitrofuracin
	Fluphenazine
	Triethylene-thiophosphoramide
	Physostigmine
	Para-phenylene diamine
	Azaleic acid
	Kojic acid
	Squaric acid dibutylester

included para-phenylene diamine, para-tertiary butyl phenol, monobenzone and azo dyes. *Table 27.7* gives a list with consumer products associated with chemical leukoderma/vitiligo.

Table 27.6
Professional fields at risk for occupational vitiligo

Production workers in contact with: antioxidants, bacteriostatic agents, organic chemicals, glues, dyes, rubber, plastic stabilizer
Beauticians, hairdressers
Health workers
Workers in contact with paints, glues, photographic chemicals, printing ink, motor oil additives
Farmers

Table 27.7
Consumer products associated with chemical leukoderma/vitiligo

Acrylic derivatives	Photo development products
Nylon, plastic	Rubber
Bindi	Synthetic leather
Adhesive tapes	Medication
Latex gloves	Deodorants
Germicides	Toothpaste
Insecticides	Cosmetics
Soap antioxidants	

References

Ansty AV (2010) Disorders of skin colour. In: Burns T et al (eds) Rook's textbook of dermatology, 8th edn. Wiley-Blackwell, Chichester

Austin M (2004) Fighting and living with vitiligo. J Am Acad Dermatol 51:57–58

Boissy RE, Manga P (2004) On the etiology of contact/occupational vitiligo. Pigment Cell Res 17:208–214

Bolognia JL (2003) Melanocyte biology. In: Bolognia JL et al (eds) Dermatology, 1st edn. Mosby, London

Caron-Schreinemachers AL et al (2005) UVB 311 nm tolerance of vitiligo skin increases with skin phototype. Acta Derm Venereol 85:24–26

Dell'Anna ML, Picardo M (2006) A review and a new hypothesis for non-immunological pathogenetic mechanisms in vitiligo. Pigment Cell Res 19:406–411

Ghosh S, Mukhopadhyay S (2009) Chemical leucoderma: a clinico-aetiological study of 864 cases in the perspective of a developing country. Br J Dermatol 160:40–47

Linthorst Homan MW et al (2008) Characteristics of patients with universal vitiligo and health-related quality of life. Arch Dermatol 144:1062–1064

Linthorst Homan MW et al (2009) The burden of vitiligo. Patient characteristics associated with quality of life. J Am Acad Dermatol 61:411–420

Naafs B (2006) Coloured versus white skin. In: Faber WR et al (eds) Imported skin diseases. Elsevier, Maarssen

Nordlund JJ (2007) The melanocyte and the epidermal melanin unit: an expanded concept. In: Lotti T (ed) Dermatological clinics. Pigmentary disorders. W.B. Saunders, Philadelphia

Nordlund JJ, Ortonne JP (2006) The normal color of human skin. In: Nordlund JJ et al (eds) The pigmentary system, 2nd edn. Blackwell, Malden

Nordlund JJ et al (2006) A More precise lexion for pigmentation, pigmentary disorders, and "chromatic" abnormalities. In: Nordlund JJ et al (eds) The pigmentary system, 2nd edn. Blackwell, Malden

Taiëb A, Picardo M (2009) Vitiligo. N Engl J Med 360:160–169

Van der Veen JPW et al (2006) Pigmentary disorders in black skin. In: Faber WR et al (eds) Imported skin diseases. Elsevier, Maarssen

Westerhof W (2007) Evolutionary, biologic, and social aspects of skin color. In: Lotti T (ed) Dermatological clinics. Pigmentary disorders. W.B. Saunders, Philadelphia

Westerhof W, d'Ischia M (2007) Vitiligo puzzle: the pieces fall in place. Pigment Cell Res 20:345–359

28 Noneczematous Occupational Contact Reactions

Chee Leok Goh
National Skin Centre, Singapore

Core Messages

- Allergic contact dermatitis may present as noneczematous lesions.
- Patch tests often produce an eczematous reaction.
- EM-like eruption can occur with woods, plants, metals, and chemicals.
- Purpuric eruption can occur with IPPD containing rubber products.
- Lichen-planus-like can occur with color developers.
- Papular and nodular eruption can occur with gold salts.
- Granulomatous reaction can occur with gold and beryllium salt.
- Pustular eruption can occur with metallic salt.
- Erythema and exfoliation can occur with TCE.
- Pseudoscleroderma can occur with chlorinated hydrocarbon and solvents.

1 Introduction

1.1 Patch Test

Contact reactions may present as noneczematous lesions. A variety of noneczematous occupational contact reactions have been described. The exact pathomechanism of these reactions is unknown. The following noneczematous contact reactions have been described:

1. Erythema-multiforme-like eruption [urticarial papules and plaque eruptions (UPPE)]
2. Purpuric eruption
3. Lichen-planus-like eruption
4. Papular and nodular eruption
5. Granulomatous reaction
6. Pustular eruption
7. Erythema and exfoliation
8. Pseudoscleroderma

2 Erythema-Multiforme-like Reaction (UPPEs)

Several contact allergens, e.g., metal, topical medicaments, wood, and industrial chemicals, have been reported to cause "erythema-multiforme-like" eruptions. These allergic contact reactions can be confirmed by positive patch-test reactions. The morphology of these reactions includes target-like erythemacular and urticarial lesions. Such eruptions have been described as UPPE to distinguish them from the classical erythema multiforme (Goh 1989).

2.1 Clinical Features

The characteristic presentation is usually an eczematous lesion on the primary contact site. Within a few days, urticarial papular and plaque lesions appear on the primary contact site, spreading to adjacent skin and occasionally distant sites. The urticarial eruptions persist longer than the primary eczematous lesions and tend to persist after the disappearance of the initial dermatitis.

In all cases, a positive patch test to the contact allergen can be elicited. The patch-test reaction is always eczematous and often severe.

2.2 Histology

The epidermis is normal or shows mild spongiosis with upper dermal edema and perivascular lymphohistiocytic infiltrate. Vacuolar degeneration of the basal cells is occasionally present. The classical features of erythema multiforme are absent. The morphology, clinical course, and histology of the eruptions are not characteristic of classical erythema multiforme.

The pathomechanism of these papular and urticarial eruptions is unknown. An immune complex reaction may be the basis of the clinical manifestation here. Goh postulated that the allergen is absorbed percutaneously and

T. Rustemeyer, P. Elsner, S.M. John & H.I. Maibach (eds.), *Kanerva's Occupational Dermatology*,
DOI 10.1007/978-3-642-02035-3_28,

evoked an allergic contact dermatitis at the primary site, while concurrently forming immune complexes with a circulating antibody (Goh 1989). The immune complexes were probably deposited in the microvasculature and triggered by an inflammatory process that led to the UPPE. Occupational allergens reported to cause UPPE include woods and/or plants and chemicals.

2.3 Woods and Plants

Hoist et al. (1976) described three carpenters who developed erythema-multiforme-like eruption from contact allergy to three different tropical woods – Rio rosewood (Dalbergia nigra), pao ferro (Mackerium scleroxylon), and Eucalyptus saligna. The antigen in pao ferro was R-3, 4-dimethoxy-dalbergione. A wooden bracelet (Fisher 1986a) and pendant (Fisher and Bikowski 1981) made from Dalbergia nigra were also reported to cause erythema-multiforme-like eruption. The specific chemical antigen was identified as quinone R-4-methoxy-dalbergione (Hausen 1981). Nonoccupational causes have also been reported. Irvine et al. (1988) reported such reaction to pao ferro (Mackerium scleroxylon) in a hobbyist handling the wood. Plants reported to cause erythema-multiforme-like eruption include poison ivy (Toxicodendron) (Schwartz and Downham 1981; Mallory et al. 1982), primula *(Primula obconica)* (Hjorth 1966), and mugwort *(Artemesia vulgaris)* (Kurz and Rapaport 1979). Mallory et al. (1982) reported urticarial eruptions with black deposits on the skin of four patients with *Toxicodendron radicans* dermatitis. Urticaria, erythema-multiforme-like eruptions, in a patient from Rhus dermatitis was reported by Schwartz and Downham (1981). They recommended that patients with such reactions should be screened for systemic involvement as previous reports have shown that nephritis can be an associated feature (Meneghini and Angelini 1981; Fisher 1986b).

2.4 Metals and Chemicals

Metals and several industrial chemicals have been reported to cause UPPE in sensitized patients. Nonoccupational UPPE from nickel was first described by Calnan (1956). Cook also reported UPPE in a 13-year-old girl due to allergic contact dermatitis from nickel and cobalt from the metal studs in her jeans (Cook 1982). Friedman and Perry (1985) described a garment worker who developed UPPE from nickel dermatitis on her hands from her scissors. Patch test revealed allergy to nickel and paraphenylenediamine. During patch testing, there was exacerbation of the worker's hand dermatitis and UPPE. Similar eruption appeared when the worker was patch tested to nickel alone.

2.5 Laboratory Chemicals

De Feo reported chemistry students who developed UPPE while synthesizing 9-bromofluorene in the laboratory (De Feo 1966). Roed-Petersen reported of a 22-year-old chemistry student who developed UPPE on the exposed parts from a phenyl sulfone derivative which he was synthesizing. Patch test gave a strong positive reaction to the compound (Roed-Petersen 1975). Tjiu et al. (2004) reported on a 22-year-old female chemistry student who developed widespread erythema-multiforme-like lesions after local contact with 1,2-ethanedithiol. The patient had a positive patch test to 1,2-ethanedithiol.

2.6 Industrial Chemicals

Nethercott et al. (1982) reported of four men working with printed circuit boards who developed erythema multiforme. Liver involvement was documented in three cases. Formaldehyde was suspected to be the cause of the eruption since two of the workers gave a positive reaction to formaldehyde. However, these workers were also exposed to other substances, including trichloroethylene. Trichloroethylene was suspected to cause erythema multiforme in five workers in an electronic factory. The liver was involved in three workers, and one died of liver failure. Patch test to trichloroethylene on one worker was negative. The reaction was suspected to be due to a hypersensitivity reaction from percutaneous and/or transrespiratory tract absorption of trichloroethylene (Phoon et al. 1984).

Goh (1988) reported erythema-multiforme-like eruption in a worker with contact allergy to trinitrotoluene who was employed at an ammunition factory. The systemic absorption of trinitrotoluene appeared low as its urinary metabolite, dinitroaminotoluene, was not detected. Patch test to trinitrotoluene gave a strong eczematous reaction.

Recently, contact dermatitis to natural rubber latex was also reported to present with features of erythema-multiforme-like eruptions (Bourrain et al. 1996). Contact with laurel oil was recently reported to cause erythema-multiforme-like eruption (Athanasiadis et al. 2007).

Airborne erythema-multiforme-like eruption was also reported in individuals exposed to pyrethrum (Garcia-Bravo et al. 1995).

3 Pigmented Purpuric Reaction

Occupational contact allergy occasionally presents as purpuric eruption. The eruption may or may not be preceded by erythema or itch. The exact mechanism of the reaction is unknown. It appears to represent an immune complex disease. Percutaneous absorption of contact allergens appears to form immune complexes with a circulating antibody that becomes deposited in the microvasculature, producing the vasculitic lesions. However, such immune complexes cannot be identified (Calnan and Peachey 1971). Purpuric eruption associated with allergic contact dermatitis to rubber chemical N-phenyl-n-isopropyl PPD (IPPD) in clothing was described by Batschvarov and Minkov in 1968 (Batschvaros and Minkow 1968). Allergic contact dermatitis to IPPD, which is used in the manufacture of some types of rubber in rubber boots, was also reported to cause purpuric eruption (Calnan and Peachey (1971). Fisher (1974) reported similar eruptions in three patients caused by a rubber diving suit, elasticized shorts, and a rubberized support bandage. Romaguera and Grimalt (1977) also reported similar eruption from IPPD in a rubberized brassiere due to nonoccupational cause. Shmunes (1978) reported a woman with purpuric allergic contact dermatitis to paraphenylenediamine from black hats she was handling as a saleswoman.

4 Lichen-Planus-like and Lichenoid Reaction

Occupational allergic contact dermatitis to some color developers may manifest as lichen-planus-like eruptions. Such eruptions often present as itchy, dusky, or violaceous papules or plaques on areas of skin exposed to the allergen. The eruptions behave like any allergic contact dermatitis and tend to clear when the allergen is removed.

The histological features of patients with lichen-planus-like eruptions from color developer pose an interesting feature. Buckley (1958), Canizares (1959), and Hyman and Berger (1959) reported the histology as compatible with lichen planus in a number of instances, but some authors reported nonspecific chronic dermatitis changes. Fry reported that only two of five patients' biopsies showed histology suggestive of lichen planus (Fry 1965). Histology of the lesions may show nonspecific superficial perivascular dermatitis or lichenoid infiltrate in the upper dermis.

There is controversy about the etiology of the lichen-planus-like eruption from color developers. Color developers are known to cause lichen-planus-like eruptions. Kodak CD2 (*4-N,* N-diethyl-2 methylphenylenediamine), Kodak CD3 (4-N-ethyl-N-2-methanesulfonylamino-ethyl 2 methyl-phenylenediamine sesquisulfate mono-hydrate), Agfa TSS (4-amino-N-diethylanilinesulfate), Ilford MI 210 (N-ethyl-N[5-hydroxy-amyl] paraphenylenediamine hydrogen sulfate), and Kodak CD4 (2-amino-5-N-ethyl-N-[beta-hydroxyethyl] amino toluene sulfate) are reported allergens (Goh et al. 1984).

Recently, lichen-planus-like eruptions have been reported from contact with methacrylic acid esters. The patient presented with lichen-planus-like lesions on sites repeatedly exposed to methacrylic acid esters used in the car industry. Histologically, the lesions showed all the features of classical lichen planus. Patch testing revealed positive reactions to methacrylic acid esters in concentrations (Kawamura et al. 1996).

5 Nodular and Papular Reactions

Contact allergy to gold has been reported to cause papular and nodular eruptions (Shelly and Epstein 1963). These occurred peculiarly on the earlobes after ear piercing with gold earrings. Similar eruptions have been observed on the hands and forearms of gold electroplaters who develop contact allergy to gold salts. The eruptions characteristically persist for months after the patients have avoided contact with metallic gold (Petros and Macmillan 1973). In some patients, the patch test also evokes an unusual reaction, the reaction being infiltrative, and tends to persist for months (Monti et al. 1983). In most of these patients, the patch test produced strong positive and persistent delayed-type hypersensitivity reaction to gold compounds. The reaction to gold in these individuals appeared to provoke lymphoplasia. Histology of such eruptions or its patch-test reaction may show dense lymphomonocytic infiltrate in the dermis (Iwatsuki et al. 1982).

6 Granulomatous Reaction

Contact reactions to metals and metallic salts can manifest as granulomatous lesions. Skin injury from zirconium, silica, magnesium, and beryllium may cause granulomas (Rubin 1956). Some reactions are due to delayed-type allergic reaction, and some are nonallergic reactions. Clinically, the granulomatous eruptions appear as inflamed papules. Eczema is usually present, but pruritus is usually minimal. The histology shows epithelioid cells and may be indistinguishable from sarcoid.

Contact with sheep wool has been reported to cause granulomatous eruptions. An unusual case of cutaneous foreign body granulomas was provoked by sheep wool. The patient presented, within 1 year, two episodes of a papular eruption on her neck and limbs. She was working as a farmer's wife, and each episode occurred after preparing the ewes for coupling. She had to keep a tight hold on the ewes while the farmer introduced warm and moist compresses in the genitals of the animals. Each diseased skin area was closely related to the tight contact with the sheep's wool, and on histological slides, each granuloma was centered by a tiny ply of wool (Lambert et al. 1995).

7 Pustular Reaction

Pustular reaction to contactant was first observed in patch-test reaction. The pustules are sterile and are transient. Fisher et al. (1959) reported that metallic salts, e.g., nickel, copper, arsenic, and mercurial salts, may produce pustular reaction. Stone and Johnson explained that such reactions may represent an enhanced reaction of prior inflammation, rather than an irritant or allergic reaction, because such a reaction can be elicited in non-nickel-sensitive patients on skin sites previously injected with heat-killed corynebacterial acne organisms (Stone and Johnson 1967). Hjorth reported that atopics are more predisposed to such reactions (Hjorth 1977). The significance of such reaction remains controversial. Wahlberg and Maibach believed that such pustular reactions are usually irritant in nature but may also be a manifestation of allergic reactions (Wahlberg and Maibach 1981).

Conde-Salazar reported a subcorneal pustular eruption in a patient with trichioroethylene exposure (Conde-Salazar et al. 1983). The patient reacted systemically upon cutaneous challenge test made by exposing only the right leg to an environment saturated with trichloroethylene (to avoid inhalation) with reappearance of erythema on the exposed area within a few hours and fleeting exanthema on the trunk and in the flank.

8 Erythema and Exfoliation

Exposure to some industrial organic chemicals, e.g., trichloroethylene, appears to cause localized or generalized erythema with or without papular and/or vesicular eruption to be followed by skin exfoliation. The skin eruptions usually take several weeks to clear. In most of cases, the skin reaction was believed to be a toxic or allergic reaction from percutaneous or mucosal absorption of the chemicals.

8.1 Trichloroethylene

Generalized erythema followed by exfoliation after exposure to trichloroethylene was reported by Schwartz et al. (1957). It was believed to be due to systemic sensitization to trichloroethylene. The route of entry may be inhalation of the vapor or percutaneous penetration or a combination of both. Similar eruption was also documented by Bauer and Rabens (1977).

Nakayama et al. (1988) also reported a generalized erythema and exfoliation with mucous membrane involvement in a patient exposed to trichloroethylene. The patient gave positive patch-test reaction to trichloroethylene and trichloroethanol (its metabolite). It was believed that the reaction was mediated by delayed-type hypersensitivity. In their patient, the skin eruption continued to appear after cessation of exposure to trichloroethylene. This was explained by the action of trichloroethylene and its metabolites accumulated in the fatty tissue and released from there. Trichloroethylene appears to have an affinity for adipose tissue.

Goh and Ng (1988) reported of a patient with recurrent localized erythematous xerotic plaques, which became parched and fissured on the arms and trunk of a patient with trichloroethylene. Biopsy showed superficial perivascular lymphohistiocytic infiltrate. The epidermis shows parakeratosis. The route of entry of trichloroethylene was from the respiratory tract, and it was believed to be a form of systemic trichloroethylene toxicity in a sensitized individual.

8.2 Methyl Bromide

Exposure to methyl bromide was reported to cause sharply demarcated erythema with vesiculation in six workers during fumigation work by Hezemans-Boer et al. (1988). Plasma bromide levels after exposure strongly suggested percutaneous absorption of methyl bromide. The lesions were especially more prominent on skin that was relatively moist or subject to mechanical pressure, such as axillae, groin, and abdomen. Microscopically, early skin lesions revealed necrosis of keratinocytes, severe edema of the upper dermis, subepidermal blistering, and diffuse infiltration of neutrophils. The skin lesions were believed to be due to the direct toxic effect of methyl bromide as an alkylating agent.

9 Scleroderma-like Reaction

Solvents have been reported as predisposing or eliciting factors in some patients with scleroderma-like reaction. The reaction is suspected to result from repeated cutaneous contact with the solvent. The pathogenic mechanism is unknown. Walder (1983) reported six scleroderma patients who had close contact with aromatic hydrocarbon solvents, such as benzene, toluene, and white spirit. Unlike chlorinated hydrocarbons, these aromatic hydrocarbons do not produce multisystem disease resembling vinyl chloride disease. The associated scleroderma is limited to the skin of hands and feet where the direct contact took place.

Yamakage and Ishikawa (1982) also reported that various aliphatic hydrocarbons, such as naphtha, n-hexane, and hexachloroethane, can induce a generalized morphea-like sclerosis either by vapor exposure or by direct contact.

In a recent report of an analysis of 28 men suffering from systemic sclerosis collated over a 25-year period, 21 (75%) were suspected to be associated with occupational scleroderma. The exposures were revealed by patients' files, reports to health authorities, and interviews and/or answers to questionnaires. The most frequent chemical exposure was to organic solvents. This was found in 13 of the patients (46%). A significant difference was found between scleroderma patients and control patients not suffering from connective tissue diseases in relation to total number of subjects exposed to one or several of the agents in question (Zachariae et al. 1997).

References

Athanasiadis GI, Pfab F, Klein A, Braun-Falco M, Ring J, Ollert M (2007) Erythema multiforme due to contact with laurel oil. Contact Dermatitis 57:116–118

Batschvaros B, Minkow DM (1968) Dermatitis and purpura from rubber in clothing. Trans St Johns Hosp Dermatol Soc 54:73–78

Bauer M, Rabens SF (1977) Trichloroethylene toxicity. Int J Dermatol 16:113–116

Bourrain JL, Woodward C, Dumas V, Caperan D, Beani JC, Amblard P (1996) Natural rubber latex contact dermatitis with features of erythema multiforme. Contact Dermatitis 35:55–56

Buckley WR (1958) Lichenoid eruptions following contact dermatitis. Arch Dermatol 78:454–457

Calnan CD (1956) Nickel dermatitis. Br J Dermatol 68:229–232

Calnan CD, Peachey RDG (1971) Allergic contact purpura. Clin Allergy 1:287–290

Canizares O (1959) Lichen planus-like eruption caused by color developer. Arch Dermatol 80:81–86

Conde-Salazar L, Guimaraens D, Romero LV, Yus ES (1983) Subcorneal pustular eruption and erythema from occupational exposure to trichloroethylene. Contact Dermatitis 9:235–237

Cook U (1982) Associated nickel and cobalt contact dermatitis presenting as erythema multiforme. Contact Dermatitis 8:280–281

De Feo CP (1966) Erythema multiforme bullosum caused by 9-bromofluorene. Arch Dermatol 94:545–551

Fisher AA (1974) Allergic petechial and purpuric rubber dermatitis. The PPPP syndrome. Cutis 14:25–27

Fisher AA (1986a) Erythema multiforme-like eruptions due to exotic woods and ordinary plants: part I. Cutis 37:101–104

Fisher AA (1986b) Erythema multiforme-like eruptions due to topical medications: part II. Cutis 37:158–161

Fisher AA, Bikowski J (1981) Allergic contact dermatitis due to wooden cross made of Dalbergia nigra. Contact Dermatitis 7:45–46

Fisher AA, Chargrin L, Fleischmayer R et al (1959) Pustular patch test reactions. Arch Dermatol 80:742–752

Friedman SF, Perry HO (1985) Erythema multiforme associated with contact dermatitis. Contact Dermatitis 12:21–23

Fry L (1965) Skin disease from color developers. Br J Dermatol 77:456–461

Garcia-Bravo B, Rodriguez-Pichardo A, de-Pierola SF, Camacho F (1995) Airborne erythema-multiforme-like eruption due to pyrethrum. Contact Dermatitis 33:433

Goh CL (1988) Erythema multiforme-like eruption from trinitrotoluene allergy. Int J Dermatol 27:650–651

Goh CL (1989) Urticarial papular and plaque eruption. A manifestation of allergic contact dermatitis. Int J Dermatol 28:172–176

Goh CL, Ng SK (1988) A cutaneous manifestation of trichloroethylene toxicity. Contact Dermatitis 18:59–60

Goh CL, Kwok SF, Rajan VS (1984) Cross sensitivity in color developers. Contact Dermatitis 10:280–285

Hausen BM (1981) Woods injurious to human health. Walter de Gruyter, Berlin, p 59

Hezemans-Boer M, Toonstra J, Meulenbelt J, Zwaveling JH, Sangster B, van Vioten WA (1988) Skin lesions due to exposure to methylbromide. Arch Dermatol 124:917–921

Hjorth N (1966) Primula dermatitis. Trans St Johns Hosp Dermatol Soc 52:207–219

Hjorth N (1977) Diagnostic patch testing. In: Marzulli F, Maibach HI (eds) Dermatoxicology and pharmacology. Wiley, New York, p 344

Hoist R, Kirby J, Magnuson B (1976) Sensitization to tropical woods giving erythema multiforme-iike eruptions. Contact Dermatitis 2:295–296

Hyman AB, Berger RA (1959) Lichenoid eruption due to color developer. Arch Dermatol 80:243–244

Irvine C, Reynolds A, Finlay AY (1988) Erythema multiforme-like reaction to "rosewood". Contact Dermatitis 19:224–225

Iwatsuki K, Tagami H, Moriguchi T, Yamada M (1982) Lymphoadenoid structure induced by gold hypersensitivity. Arch Dermatol 118:608–611

Kawamura T, Fukuda S, Ohtake N, Furue M, Tamaki K (1996) Lichen planus-like contact dermatitis due to methacrylic acid esters. Br J Dermatol 134:358–360

Kurz G, Rapaport MJ (1979) External/internal allergy to plants (Artemesia). Contact Dermatitis 5:407–417

Lambert D, Terrussot MC, Dalac S, Boulitrop-Morvan C (1995) Granuloma la lame de brebis. Ann Dermatol Venereol 122:534–535

Mallory SB, Miller OF, Tyler WB (1982) Toxicodendron radicans dermatitis with black lacquer deposit on the skin. J Am Acad Dermatol 6:363–368

Meneghini CL, Angelini G (1981) Secondary polymorphic erupt- ions in allergic contact dermatitis. Dermatologica 163:63–70

Monti M, Berti E, Cavicchini S, Sala F (1983) Unusual cutaneous reaction after gold chloride patch test. Contact Dermatitis 9:150–151

Nakayama H, Bobayashi M, Takahashi M, Ageishi Y, Takano T (1988) Generalized eruption with severe liver dysfunction associated with occupational exposure to trichloroethylene. Contact Dermatitis 19:48–51

Nethercott JR, Albers J, Gurguis S et al (1982) Erythema multiforme exudativum linked to the manufacture of printed circuit boards. Contact Dermatitis 3:314–322

Petros H, Macmillan AL (1973) Allergic contact sensitivity to gold with unusual features. Br J Dermatol 88:505–508

Phoon WH, Chan MOY, Rajan VS et al (1984) Stevens-Johnson syndrome associated with occupational exposure to trichloroethylene. Contact Dermatitis 10:270–276

Roed-Petersen J (1975) Erythema multiforme as an expression of contact dermatitis. Contact Dermatitis 1:270–271

Romaguera C, Grimalt F (1977) PPPP syndrome. Contact Dermatitis 3:102–103

Rubin L (1956) Granulomas of axillae caused by deodorants. JAMA 162:953–955

Schwartz RS, Downham TF (1981) Erythema multiforme associated with Rhus contact dermatitis. Contact Dermatitis 27:85–86

Schwartz L, Tulipan L, Birmingham A (1957) Occupational disease of the skin, 3rd edn. Lea & Febiger, Philadelphia, p 771

Shelly WB, Epstein E (1963) Contact-sensitivity to gold as a chronic papular eruption. Arch Dermatol 87:388–391

Shmunes E (1978) Purpuric allergic contact dermatitis to paraphenylenediamine. Contact Dermatitis 4:225–229

Stone OJ, Johnson DA (1967) Pustular patch test – experimentally induced. Arch Dermatol 95:618–619

Tjiu JW, Chu CY, Sun CC (2004) 1,2-Ethanedithiol-induced erythema multiforme-like contact dermatitis. Acta Derm Venereol 84:393–396

Wahlberg JE, Maibach HI (1981) Sterile cutaneous pustules – a manifestation of primary irritancy? J Invest Dermatol 76:381–383

Walder BK (1983) Do solvents cause scleroderma? Int J Dermatol 22:157–158

Yamakage A, Ishikawa H (1982) Generalized morphea-like scleroderma occurring in people exposed to organic solvents. Dermatologica 165:186–193

Zachariae H, Bjerring P, Sondergaard KH, Halkier-Sorensen L (1997) Occupational systemic sclerosis in men. Ugeskr Laeger 28:2687–2689

29 Occupational Connective Tissue Disorders

Uwe-Frithjof Haustein · B. Lietzberg
Department of Dermatology, Venerology and Allergology, University of Leipzig, Leipzig, Germany

Core Messages

- Systemic sclerosis (SSc) can be induced by long-term silica exposure.
- In terms of clinical and laboratory features, this silica-induced scleroderma is indistinguishable from idiopathic scleroderma.
- Silica is able to trigger the immune system, vasculature, as well as fibroblasts on the basis of an increased genetic susceptibility.
- Silica can also contribute to the pathogenesis of other autoimmune diseases such as (systemic) lupus erythematosus, dermatomyositis, rheumatoid arthritis, overlap syndromes, and Sjögren's syndrome.
- If silica exposure has been long enough and its concentration high enough under occupational conditions, SSc should be acknowledged as an occupational disease and financially compensated.
- Silicon (breast augmentation) does not induce the so-called adjuvant disease.
- Organic solvents such as (chlorinated) aliphatic and aromatic hydrocarbons can trigger scleroderma-like diseases (SLDs) characterized by scleroderma and, in addition, toxic effects to liver, kidney, nervous system, sometimes absence of autoantibodies and to some extent reversibility of the disease.

Connective tissue disorders involving occupational factors are, first of all, systemic sclerosis (SSc), probably also lupus erythematosus (LE) and very rarely dermatomyositis, mixed connective tissue disease (MCTD), rheumatoid arthritis (RA), and Sjögren's syndrome (Zschunke et al. 1990; Koeger et al. 1991).

1 Systemic Sclerosis

1.1 Introduction

SSc, characterized by fibrosis of the skin and internal organs, is a disease of unknown etiology with a pathogenesis that is still vague. The prevalence in a Caucasian population is estimated at 0.3–1.9/100,000 (Haustein and Albrecht 1993). Women are affected three to six times more frequently (Medsger and Masi 1971; Sluis-Cremer et al. 1985). In recent years, some environmental substances have been reported as inducing factors in SSc and in so-called scleroderma-like diseases (SLDs) (➋ *Table 29.1*).

1.2 Silica (Quartz)

Next to oxygen, silicon is the most common substance in the environment. Silicon has never been found in its elementary state. In nature, it exclusively occurs in compounds derived from silicon dioxide (silica = SiO_2). Silica is a regular constituent part in about 92% of all sorts of rock.

The three important crystalline structures of silica are quartz, tridymite, and cristobalite. These compounds are also called "free silica" to distinguish them from the silicates, minerals containing silica bound to one or more metallic cations (American Thoracic Society 1997).

From the chemical point of view, quartz is an extremely inert material. It cannot be destroyed by water or solvents. Only hydrofluoric acid is capable of dissolving quartz. It may easily be detected by crystallographic methods, e.g., X-ray diffractometry and polarization microscopy, but it is difficult to trace by chemical analysis.

1.3 Epidemiological and Clinical Aspects

In 1914, the Scottish physician Bramwell reported a coincidence between "sclerodermia" and occupations involving exposure to silica dust. Five of the nine patients who reported diffuse SSc worked as stonemasons. Bramwell supposed that holding the chisel and working under cold-weather outdoor conditions might be work-associated causative factors (Bramwell 1914).

Erasmus (1957) observed 17 cases of SSc among 8,000 underground miners in South Africa, 6 of them with silicosis. In order to get an impression about the morbidity of SSc, he examined 25,000 male and 27,000 female

T. Rustemeyer, P. Elsner, S.M. John & H.I. Maibach (eds.), *Kanerva's Occupational Dermatology*,
DOI 10.1007/978-3-642-02035-3_29, © Springer-Verlag Berlin Heidelberg 2012

Table 29.1
Factors inducing systemic sclerosis (SSc) or scleroderma-like diseases (SLDs), respectively

SSc	SLDs
Mineral	**Chemical compounds**
Silica	**Plastics**
Solvents	Vinyl chloride
Chlorinated hydrocarbons	Epoxy resins (bis(4-amino-3-methylcyclohexyl)methane)
Aromatic hydrocarbons	**Solvents**
	Chlorinated hydrocarbons
	Aromatic hydrocarbons
	Aliphatic hydrocarbons
	Pesticides
	Drugs (e.g., bleomycin, pentazocine)
	Others
	Aniline and fatty acid anilides (oleylanilides)
	Paraffin, silicon

infirmary patients. He found one male patient (also a miner) and nine female patients with SSc and suggested a greater incidence among miners than among nonminers. In the following years (from 1960 until 1969), 29 additional cases of SSc were registered in miners who had been working in the South African gold mines. That corresponds to an incidence of 7.7 cases per 100,000 miners per year in contrast with an incidence of 0.33 in 100,000 in a control group consisting of railway and harbor workers. From 1955 to 1984, a total of 79 definite or probable cases of SSc in miners were registered. These investigations were related exclusively to Caucasian individuals (Sluis-Cremer et al. 1985). Cowie (1987) analyzed the occurrence of SSc in a native South African male population. Among miners, he found an incidence of 8.2/100,000 versus merely 0.3/100,000 among inhabitants serving as a control group. In the Republic of South Africa, SSc has been acknowledged since 1974 as an occupational disease in miners that has to be compensated by law (Sluis-Cremer et al. 1985).

In the United States, Rodnan and colleagues (1967) analyzed the occupations of 60 male patients with SSc. They reported that 26 of them had been coal miners and 10 of them had been foundry workers exposed to quartz sand. In eight of the patients, SSc was associated with silicosis of the lungs. This association between SSc and silicosis has been confirmed by other groups (Beck et al. 1976; Ziegler et al. 1982).

One report on the increased prevalence of SSc in workers exposed to silica dust, mainly in the mining of ores in the former German Democratic Republic, was published in 1976 by Zschunke, whose findings initiated a study that appears to be the most extensive evaluation until now (Zschunke 1976). A first analysis, which included all SSc patients of the whole country, was performed by Ziegler and colleagues in 1981 and revealed that 77% of all male patients with SSc had been exposed to silica dust in the workplace. In addition, half of the patients showed simultaneous silicosis of the lungs (Ziegler et al. 1981, 1982, 1986; Haustein and Ziegler 1985). Continuing this evaluation, records are currently available on 137 male patients with SSc. Silica dust exposure was established in 111 of these patients, and silicosis was found in 57 of them (Haustein and Herrmann 1994). The comparable occupational silica exposure in the general population of an industrial area is estimated as being 10% or less. Utilizing epidemiological tools, the following risk was calculated. The likelihood (odds ratio) that SSc will develop in men with silicosis who are older than 40 years of age is 12 times higher than in workers who are the same age but not exposed to silica dust. Ten female patients with SSc were also exposed to silica dust in the workplace. One of them had also developed silicosis. In contrast to the male patients, the epidemiologic research concerning females lacks evidence, probably due to their small numbers.

All the patients fulfilled the criteria of the American College of Rheumatology (ACR). The average time of exposure was 13.6 years. The delay in symptomatic disease (from beginning of exposure to onset of SSc) was 24.3 years on average. In some cases, the silica exposure lasted until the onset of SSc. The majority of pulmonary silicosis started before SSc in 41 of 57 (72%); the reverse was true in a minor fraction (19%). In 9%, both diseases were detected at the same time. From the remaining 54 SSc patients without silicosis, 25 (46%) developed lung fibrosis within 2 years. Raynaud's phenomenon was observed as a preceding or concurrent symptom in 107 of the 111 silica-dust-exposed SSc patients (96%). Skin involvement occurred before pulmonary symptoms in 36 of 111 (32%), at the same time in 5 of 111 (5%), after silicosis in 41 of 111 (37%), and in 29 of 111 (26%) patients no respiratory disorders were observed.

The occupations of the silica-exposed SSc patients are listed in ➋ *Table 29.2*. Fifty-seven of the 77 miners were exclusively exposed through uranium mining, 8 through coal mining, and 12 through both. Forty-two of the

Table 29.2
Occupations of systemic sclerosis patients of the Leipzig group with verified silica dust exposure (n = 111)

Occupation	Number of patients
Miner	77
Foundry worker	10
Quarryman	6
Sandblaster	5
Dental mechanic	4
Sandstone sculptor	3
Glass grinder	3
Cast polisher	3

111 patients have never worked in uranium mines. Twelve of these 42 suffered from silicosis. The odds ratio of the 42 patients who never worked in uranium mines to develop SSc was still 3.9. Since uranium mines were shut down between 1980 and 1989, only the sequelae of this exposure could be followed up. Today, only a few patients are still alive or have been recently diagnosed.

It is possible that sclerosis of the lungs, fibrosis due to nonspecific dust impact, and genuine silicosis might be confused in several cases; however, fibrosis of the lungs accompanied by SSc obviously occurs in subjects exposed to silica dust rather than in those who have not been exposed in such a way. The rate of silicosis in the male patients with SSc presented in this group is higher than the number reported by Erasmus (1957) and Rodnan et al. (1967). This difference might be explained by regional variations in defining silicosis in the past, by differences in the composition of the rocks, and at least in several cases by the radioactivity of the uranium. Progress in the differential diagnosis has been achieved by high-resolution computer tomography.

Sluis-Cremer et al. (1985) suggested that a brief exposure to dust with high silica content causes SSc without simultaneous silicosis. This would imply that the mode of exposure determines whether SSc with or without silicosis might develop. Haustein and colleagues (1986) do not share the opinion that SSc in these patients is not idiopathic SSc, but rather should be labeled as SLD (Siegel 1977). The symptomatic criteria for diagnosing SSc (compiled by the ACR; Masi 1980) have been fulfilled by almost all patients investigated (*Table 29.3*). According to this view, Rodnan et al. (1967), Rustin et al. (1990), and Gabay and Kahn (1992) emphasized the lack of differences between so-called idiopathic SSc and SSc in patients with silicosis.

Table 29.3
Clinical features and laboratory findings of systemic sclerosis patients associated with silicosis (n = 37), limited: diffuse form = 22:15

Symptoms/laboratory findings	Number of patients	Limited form	Diffuse form
Raynaud's phenomenon	36	21	15
Fingertip ulcers	28	15	13
Arthralgia	28	13	12
Lung involvement	37	22	15
Esophagus involvement	29	16	13
Heart involvement	11	3	8
Muscle involvement	9	2	7
Kidney involvement	5	0	5
Antinuclear antibodies (ANAs)	35	20	15
Anti-topoisomerase antibodies (ATAs)	13	1	12
Anti-centromere antibodies (ACAs)	9	8	1
Platelet factor 4	27	14	13
β-thromboglobulin	27	15	12
Endothelin	17	7	10

Typical workplaces in which exposure to silica dust must be taken into account are listed in *Table 29.4*. However, numerous hidden sources of silica exposure exist, e.g., cleansers used in housekeeping (Mehlhorn et al. 1990; Koeger et al. 1992) and polishes used in various jobs. Even fondant powders contained quartz in the past and were found to be a cause of silicosis (Beck and Irmscher 1974). Silicosis was also observed in female laundry workers washing dust-contaminated clothes (Evans and Posner 1971). One anecdote refers to a husband and his wife who both developed SSc, the husband after silica exposure and his wife probably by inhaling dust from his clothes (Christy and Rodnan 1984). Koeger et al. (1992) reported of two patients who developed edematous scleroderma and subluxing arthropathy, respectively, after applying aerosolic silicon glaze on cables over a 20-year period.

Yamamoto et al. (1994) described an SSc patient with high levels of serum immonoglobulin E who developed multiple papules in an area of nonsclerotic skin. He had been working on polishing watches with an abrasive agent composed mainly of aluminum, chromium dioxide, and silica. Histological examination of a biopsy of the papules

Table 29.4
Workplaces associated with silica dust exposure (According to Zschunke et al. 1990)

Mining industry	Underground workers
Extracting and processing of stones (sandstone, granite, slate, fluorspar, mica)	Quarrymen, crushers, sculptors, stonemasons, workers producing slate pencils, workers handling slate powder, e.g., as a carrier for hexachlorocyclohexane insecticides, workers producing roof paper
Producing and processing of chamotte blast furnace-lining bricklayers	Grinders, mixers, stove fitters
Foundry industry	Molders, coremakers, casters, cast dressers
Tire industry and industries producing other products made from natural or synthetic rubber, e.g., cables contaminated by silica	Workers handling talc that is sometimes heavily
Industries producing pottery including glassware	Workers handling raw material, in particular sand and kaolin; the latter also regularly contains considerable quantities of silica
Dental technical laboratories (polishing and embedding materials)	Dental technicians

revealed the typical features of scleroderma. This seems to be the first report of nodular scleroderma that occurred in the course of SSc being associated with chemical agents.

It is also known that dental technicians are exposed to various particulate matters including silica, alloys, and acrylic plastics which may induce pneumoconiosis and probably other occupational lung diseases (Choudat 1994). The prevalence of pneumoconiosis is very high and related to the duration of exposure: Three epidemiological studies have reported a prevalence of pneumoconiosis 1/0 or greater of about 15% in technicians with 20 or more years of exposure. However, silica is probably not the sole causative agent. Since pneumoconiosis is a frequent risk among dental technicians, compensation should be paid to those suffering from this work-related disease (Choudat 1994).

Yanez-Diaz et al. (1992) presented two male patients with SSc and pulmonary silicosis after occupational exposure to silica and one of them to trichloroethylene as a degreasing agent. The clinical and analytical findings could not be distinguished from those present in idiopathic SSc except the chest X-ray with interstitial images featuring calcified hilar lymph nodes suggestive of pulmonary silicosis.

Gabay and Kahn (1992) have analyzed 202 SSc patients diagnosed at the Rheumatology Department, University Bichat (Paris), since 1976. Among them were 39 male patients (women/men = 4.2/1). Twenty-five men were included in a subsequent study, 14 of them with a high occupational risk and a duration of exposure between 4 and 33 years (mean ± SD 14.5 ± 11.4 years). Eleven of them had been exposed to silica dust (as miners, foundry workers, or bricklayers), one to solvents (as a painter), and two to both. The mean age at onset of disease was 50.4 ± 10.19 years (range 31–72 years) with Raynaud's phenomenon before onset of disease in 24 cases (mean duration 6 months). The delay between the beginning of exposure and onset of disease was 24.4 ± 12.2 years (range 4–45 years). Clinical manifestations included lung diseases in 18 patients, gastrointestinal tract diseases (13 patients), joint problems (5 patients), diseases of the serosa (4 patients), myositis (4 patients), Sjögren's syndrome (3 patients), arterial pulmonary hypertension (2 patients), cardiomyopathy (1 patient), impotence (1 patient), and subcutaneous nodules (1 patient). There were no significant differences between the two groups (induced SSc versus "primitive" SSc) regarding age at onset of disease, mortality, systemic manifestations except myositis (which occurred only in the "primitive" group), therapy, antinuclear antibodies (ANAs), and anti-Scl-70 antibodies [anti-topoisomerase antibodies (ATAs)]. Among the 163 female patients, there was no silica-induced case.

In an Australian population-based case-control study Englert et al. (2000) found 60 out of 160 SSc patients with silica exposure (odds ratio 3.93) including a long latency and clinical characteristics indistinguishable from idiopathic disease. Maitre et al. (2004) reported on 93 SSc patients (10 men, 83 women). Construction workers were at higher risk (odds ratio = 4.01). This was not strictly related to silica exposure rather than due to various other offenders simultaneously.

Recently, Smith et al. (2008) reported on a tenfold higher prevalence of construction-related professions in males with SSc than in the general working population preferentially in electricians in 91 patients, 20 of them males in Belgium.

Surprisingly, the occupational analysis of 56 men with SSc in the United Kingdom showed no evidence of silica exposure implicated in the onset of the disease (Silman and Jones 1992). In addition, odds ratios were nonsignificantly increased among Michigan woman potentially exposed to "silica dust, sand or other silica products" (Burns et al. 1996) and among crystalline silica exposed men from Italy (Bovenzi et al. 1995).

In a meta-analysis of Medline, Toxline, BIOS, and Embase (1949 and 2009), McCormic et al. (2010) calculated the combined estimator of relative risk (CERR) of occupational silica exposure for scleroderma as 3.20 (95% confidence interval 1.89–5.43), for males 3.02 (95% CI 1.24–7.35) and for females 1.03 (95% CI 0.74–1.44). In the case-control studies it was 2.24 (95% CI 1.65–3.31) and in the cohort studies 15.49 (95% CI 4.54–52.87).

Case reports and epidemiological studies reporting on patients suffering from SSc and silicosis are summarized in ➋ *Table 29.5.*

1.4 Silica and Other Autoimmune Diseases

Evaluating 764 patients with connective tissue disease (CTD) hospitalized in the clinic of the University Pitiè/Salpétière/Paris, Koeger et al. (1995) found 24 (3%) patients with silica-associated CTD. Eight of them had SSc, in four cases in association with Sjögren's syndrome, and in three cases in association with silicosis. RA has been found in five patients (four in association with Sjögren's syndrome), systemic LE in four patients (three with silicosis), discoid LE in one patient, and dermatomyositis in association with Sjögren's syndrome in three patients. The last three patients had erosive polyarthritis and Sjögren's syndrome, Grave disease, and inflammatory polyarthralgia. Three additional cases of autoimmune diseases after unusual exposure to silica or silicons have been reported by the same authors (Koeger et al. 1992). A woman who had extensively used an abrasive cleansing powder rich in silica for 12 years developed a CTD consisting of destructive inflammatory oligoarthritis, Gougerot-Sjögren's syndrome, Raynaud's syndrome, ANA, and hypocomplementemia. Another woman, who had sprayed silicon glaze on cables for 15 years, suffered from edematous SSc. A man who had applied the same silicon glaze on cables over a 20-year period developed a subluxing arthropathy. The authors pointed out that these means of exposure have not been reported previously and merit recognition in the name of future prevention.

Steenland and Brown (1995) updated a study of 3,328 gold miners who worked underground for at least 1 year between 1940 and 1965 in South Dakota. Multiple-cause analysis revealed significant excesses of arthritis, musculoskeletal diseases, and various cutaneous disorders (including SSc and systemic LE).

Evidence that occupational exposure to silica is also associated with autoimmunity was reinforced by the observation that workers from a factory that produced scouring powder with an increased silica content (70–90% powdered quartz) exhibited a high prevalence of clinical and biological autoimmune manifestations (➋ *Table 29.6*). Among a group of 50 workers, Sanchez-Roman et al. (1993) demonstrated symptoms of systemic illness in 32 (64%) and ANA in 36 (72%) of them.

Wichmann et al. (1996) showed that individuals chronically exposed to silica, independent of whether they are suffering from CTD, have antibodies to myeloperoxidase (MPO) as detected by enzyme-linked immunosorbent assay (ELISA) in a range higher than the normal population and in the same range as systemic diseases not induced by silica (i.e., systemic LE, SSc).

In 9 of 11 patients with silica exposure and renal involvement with systemic vasculitis, Chevalier et al. (working in Angers) found various antibodies indicative of autoimmunity, such as MPO-anti-neutrophil cytoplasmic antibodies (ANCAs) and ANA at low titers, with anti-RO/Sjögren's syndrome A in two patients, but without anti-double-stranded DNA (dsDNA) (Conrad et al. 1997).

Conrad et al. (1997) demonstrated that uranium miners with heavy exposure to silica run a higher risk of developing SSc and systemic LE than miners with slight or no exposure, because they showed a higher frequency of SSc-specific autoantibodies [anti-centromere antibodies (ACAs), ATAs, antinucleolar antibodies] related to the intensity of the silica exposure and to preceding symptoms of SSc (Raynaud's phenomenon, diffuse interstitial lung fibrosis).

By summarizing various studies and case reports, Gregorini (working in Brescia) showed that extrapulmonary silicotic lesions and/or autoimmune processes may play a role in kidney diseases after silica exposure, more specifically MPO-ANCA-positive microscopic polyangiitis and its renal-limited form of "idiopathic," rapidly progressive glomerulonephritis (Conrad et al. 1997).

In conclusion, silica may induce systemic diseases with various clinical and serological manifestations: systemic sclerosis with ACA, ATA, or antinucleolar antibodies, systemic LE and systemic LE-like diseases with anti-dsDNA and/or anti-RO/SS-A and anti-cardiolipin antibodies, and necrotizing systemic vasculitis with renal involvement and MPO-ANCA (Conrad et al. 1997).

Table 29.5
Published cases of systemic sclerosis (SSc) in association with silica exposure and silicosis, respectively

Year	Author	Cases	Diagnosis	Occupation	Exposure
1914	Bramwell	5	Diffuse scleroderma	Stonemasons	Silica dust
1957	Erasmus	17	SSc, six with silicosis	Underground miners	Silica dust
1959	Francia et al.	6	SSc and silicosis		
1967	Rodnan et al.	36	SSc, eight with silicosis	26 Coal miners, 10 foundry workers	Silica dust (coal miners), quartz sand (foundry workers)
1955–1984	Sluis-Cremer et al. (including the cases of Erasmus 1957)	79	SSc	Gold miners	Silica dust
1987	Cowie	10	SSc, six with silicosis	Gold miners	Silica dust
1981–1997	Haustein and Herrmann (1994) (some of these patients were also reported by Ziegler et al. 1986; Baur 1994; Mehlhorn 1994)	111	SSc, 57 with silicosis	Uranium mining (57), coal mining (8), both (12)	Silica dust (uranium)
1984	Christy and Rodnan	2	SSc	The husband developed SSc after silica exposure and his wife probably by inhaling dust from his clothes	Silica dust
1990	Mehlhorn et al.	1	SSc	Cleaning woman	Scouring powder containing crystalline silica
1992	Koeger et al.	1	Edematous scleroderma	Sprayed silicon glaze on cables	Silicon glaze
1992	Yánez-Díaz et al.	1	SSc, silicosis	Lead mine	Silica dust
1992	Yánez-Díaz et al.	1	SSc, silicosis	Lead mine	Fiberglass, (trichloroethylene)
1992	Gabay and Kahn	11	SSc	Miner, foundry worker, bricklayer	Silica dust
1992	Gabay and Kahn	2	SSc	Miner, foundry worker, bricklayer	Silica and solvents
1994	Yamamoto et al.	1	Multiple papules in an area of nonsclerotic skin in SSc	Polishing watches	Abrasive agent (aluminum, chromium dioxide, silica)
1995	Koeger et al.	8	SSc, three with silicosis	Underground worker, sand molder, dental prosthetist, foundry engineer, marble sculptor, miner, sandblaster, mason, sandstonecutter	Silica dust

Table 29.5 (Continued)

Year	Author	Cases	Diagnosis	Occupation	Exposure
1996	Wichmann et al. (including the patients reported by Sanchez-Roman et al. 1993)	12	SSc	Scouring powder	Silica content: 70–90% powdered quartz
		Total = 287			
2000	Englert et al.	60 of 160	SSc	Population-based study	Odds ratio 3.93
2002	Diot et al.	10	SSc	Case-control study	Odds ratio 3.74
2003	Calvert et al.	2 of 2,895 death certificates	SSc	US National occupational mortal surveillance	Mortality odds ratio 2.00
2004	Maitre et al.	4 of 93 (10 men, 83 women)	SSc	Case-control study	
2004	Bovenzi et al.	3	SSc	Worker in the pottery industry,	Ceramic materials
2008	Smith et al.	10 of 20	SSc	Construction-related occupations	Prevalence tenfold higher
		Total = 300			

Table 29.6
Autoimmune diseases in association with silica exposure (According to Sanchez-Roman et al. 1993; Wichmann et al. 1996)

	Sanchez-Roman et al. (1993), 50 workers; number (%)	Wichmann et al. (1996), 52 workers, same factory; number (%)
Systemic sclerosis (SSc)	5 (10)	12 (23)
Systemic lupus erythematosus (SLE)	3 (6)	16 (31)
Polymyositis (PM)		1 (2)
Overlap syndrome (SLE/SSc)	5 (10)	7 (14) (Included in SLE, SSc, PM, and undefined collagen disease)
Secondary Sjögren's syndrome	6 (12) (Included in the three first clinical diagnosis)	
Undefined collagen disease	19 (38) (Including three cases of primary Sjögren's syndrome)	15 (29)
Asymptomatic subjects	19 (38)	15 (29)

1.5 Silicon

For many years, controversial discussions continued concerning whether silicon breast implants performed for augmentation mammaplasty are able to cause autoimmune disease and SSc. The term "human adjuvant disease" was introduced by Miyoshi et al. in 1964, who reported two patients with CTD after direct injections of paraffin and silicon to augment breast size. Later, implantable cushions of silicon gel or saline were applied. After a delay of approximately 20 years, 50 of 85 subjects treated in this way suffered from a definite CTD, including 25 patients with SSc, 13 with RA, 8 with systemic LE, and 4 with MCTD (Hochberg 1993). In addition, corresponding autoantibodies, including anti-silicon antibodies, were detected. Apart from leakage in the surrounding tissue followed by foreign body granuloma, connective tissue formation, and fibrosis, the current scientific literature no longer supports the idea of systemic autoimmune diseases, due to a lack of convincing evidence that implants are a major risk to the integrity of the immune system.

This is confirmed by a retrospective cohort study evaluating 395,543 women via a questionnaire. The self-reported data indicated that the relative risk of any CTD among the women with implants was 1.24 (Hennekens et al. 1996). Similar results were reported from three university-based tertiary-care scleroderma research centers with 837 women and 2,507 race-matched local control individuals. The adjusted odds ratio was 1.07 versus 1.11 (no significant difference) (Hochberg et al. 1996).

In addition, Burns et al. (1996) reported on a population-based case-control study among 274 female patients with SSc and 1,184 controls in Michigan. They found no increased risk of SSc among women with silicon breast implants, equivocal evidence of risk from other silicon exposures, and no evidence of risk from silica exposure. In an US retrospective cohort study between 1960 and 1996, Brinton et al. (2003) showed that the results of self-reports of connective tissue disorders are influenced by reporting and surveillance biases.

The meta-analyses of nine cohort studies, nine case-control studies, and two cross-sectional studies did not give evidence that breast implants were associated with a significant increase in the summary adjusted relative risk of individual connective tissue disease. Nor was there any evidence of significantly increased risk in the adjusted analysis restricted to silicon-gel-filled implants. This meta-analysis was conducted both with and without adjustment for confounding factors (Janowsky et al. 2000). Kjoller et al. (2001) came to similar conclusion for 2,761 Danish women with cosmetic silicon breast implants (8,807 control subjects) Karlson et al. (2001) did not found signs of activation of the immune system such as elevated levels of C3, C4, or antinuclear antibodies.

Finally, it is doubtful whether silica can be released from silicon. Using electron-probe microanalysis, however, it has been shown that silicon or even silica may escape from breast implants (even without frank rupture) and may migrate beyond the capsule to regional lymph nodes and distant sites where inflammatory and fibrotic processes can take place, triggered by vacuolated, silica-incorporating macrophages (Varga et al. 1989; Silver et al. 1993).

1.6 Pathogenesis

Silica-associated SSc is clinically, serologically, and immunologically indistinguishable from idiopathic SSc (Haustein and Ziegler 1985; Rustin et al. 1990; Gabay and Kahn 1992).

Quartz is absorbed both via inhalation and percutaneously. Silicosis of the lung is caused by particles with a diameter of less than 5 μm. The orifice of the sebaceous glands in healthy individuals is approximately 24 times wider than the particle size relevant for silicosis. At the extremities, there are up to 50 follicles per square centimeter (Plewig and Kligman 1978). Miners experience microinjuries of their hands and forearms quite frequently. Therefore, it is not surprising that about 150 particles of quartz between 1 and 20 μm could be traced in a single biopsy specimen (Ziegler et al. 1988).

Table 29.7
Silica in exposed skin areas

Subjects	Positive/total
Silica-induced SSc	24/26
Silicosis	4/5
Silica-exposed miners (without SSc/silicosis)	3/5
Nonexposed controls	1/6

In several patients, Ziegler and colleagues (1988) determined the silica content in skin specimens obtained from fingers, dorsum of the hand, and lower arms by polarization and phase-contrast microscopy, and in two cases by electron spectroscopy for chemical analysis. As shown in *Table 29.7*, silica crystals can be found in a high percentage of silica-exposed subjects. In the majority of occupations, the mechanical forces (e.g., in air or compressed air, drilling, or hewing) are substantial and may promote the penetration of silica crystals by microwounding. However, these data do not distinguish patients from silica-exposed miners without skin and lung diseases.

This mechanism of penetration might serve as an explanation for the observation that symptoms start at the distal portions of extremities in the majority of cases.

Silica particles are ingested by macrophages (*Fig. 29.1*), e.g., in the lung or skin, and can be transported to extrapulmonary sites (Holt 1981). Subsequently, activated macrophages release enhanced amounts of interleukin (IL)-1α and β (Oghiso and Kubota 1986). Similarly, silica-stimulated monocytes can release fibroblast-proliferation-inducing factors (Schmidt et al. 1984), leading to stimulation of collagen production by fibroblasts, too. The spontaneous secretion of IL-1 from silicotic rat alveolar macrophages can be inhibited by anti-Ia antibodies (Struhar and Harbeck 1989). Furthermore, silica added to antigen- or mitogen-stimulated lymphocyte cultures increases the number of immunoglobulin-secreting cells (Moseley et al. 1988). IL-1α and β also affect T-helper lymphocytes promoting production and release of IL-2. IL-2 may stimulate B lymphocytes synthesizing immunoglobulins and (auto) antibodies. Activated T lymphocytes also produce other lymphokines (e.g., macrophage-activating factors) which are capable of stimulating macrophages and fibroblasts.

These mechanisms are continuously triggered by silica, which is not chemically reactive and remains in the

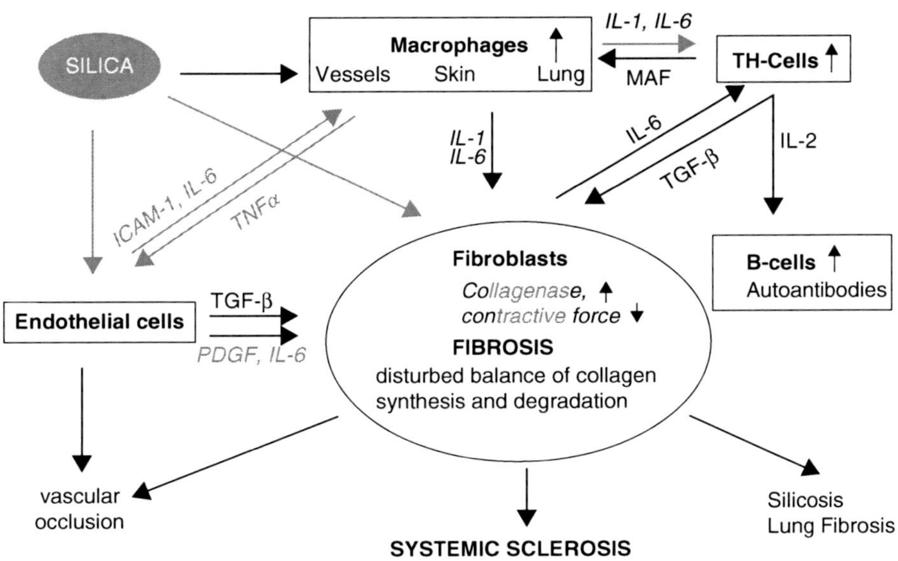

Fig. 29.1
Silica can activate various cell types involved in the pathophysiology of systemic sclerosis (SSc). Macrophages activated by silica in vitro liberate the same cytokines and growth factors known to be active in the pathophysiology of idiopathic SSc. Microvascular endothelium is involved in silica-induced as well as idiopathic SSc with similar activation patterns in vitro and in vivo. Dermal fibroblasts are affected by silica in vitro, and fibroblasts are the cells producing large amounts of extracellular matrix in vivo. In vitro, the synthesizing capacity of fibroblasts depends greatly on culture conditions. All these effects are based on the in vitro experiments with silica shown in italic. These effects are similar to pathophysiological events known from idiopathic SSc

tissue over an extended period. Nevertheless, it has toxic effects on macrophages in a dose-dependent manner. After phagocytosis and destruction of these cells, silica is set free in the tissue, and the process of ingestion through phagocytosis might start again. In this way, a vicious cycle of a dysfunctional inflammatory response is established (Haustein and Herrmann 1994).

However, Adamson et al. (1989) have shown that silica and irradiation are each able to enhance the number of interstitial cells in the lung. In addition, the content of cells, protein, and hydroxyproline is increased in bronchoalveolar lavage fluids. Taken together, irradiation plus silica exposure might lead to a synergistic enhancement of their effects.

Obviously, the endothelial cell damage occurs early, before systemic symptoms appear. This is suggested by the observation that Raynaud's phenomenon often precedes SSc and by elevated levels of von Willebrand factor and circulating immune complexes not only in silica-induced SSc, but also in healthy silica-exposed miners.

Concerning the involvement of blood vessels, Dowd and Ziegler (1987) demonstrated decreased formation of prostacyclin, a vasodilating lipid mediator originating from endothelial cells. The lack of prostacyclin formation was shown in patients with Raynaud's phenomenon as well in patients with SSc who had been exposed to silica. Furthermore, there are certain patterns of ultrastructural changes of the endothelial layer which seem to be characteristic of SSc (Haustein and Klug 1975; Haustein et al. 1986). Accordingly, subintimal fibrosis of small arteries has been described by Fleischmajer et al. (1983).

Silica seems to be a potent activator of endothelial cells in vitro, too. Incubation of human dermal microvascular endothelial cells (HDMECs) with silica at nontoxic concentrations increased the steady-state levels of the messenger RNA (mRNA) for intercellular adhesion molecule 1 (ICAM-1), and also increased the corresponding levels of this cell-surface protein as shown by fluorescence-activated cell-sorter (FACS) analysis; the incubation also increased the level of soluble protein in the culture fluid, as shown by means of ELISA, in a dose- and time-dependent manner. Additionally, increased levels of IL-6 in the culture supernatants have been found. In addition, a significant increase in collagenase I mRNA in HDMEC has been demonstrated (Anderegg et al. 1997).

The intratracheal instillation of silica crystals (α quartz) into the lungs of C57Bl/6 mice resulted in a significant increase in levels of ICAM-1 in lung tissue and bronchoalveolar lavage fluids (Nario and Hubbard 1996).

In patients with SSc, Frank et al. (1993) found a slight decrease of IL-1 basal secretion from monocytes in comparison with healthy volunteers, and no changes in IL-6 and tumor necrosis factor α (TNF α) production. In monocyte-enriched cultures from healthy donors, a dose-dependent modulation of the cytokine pattern (IL1 α, IL-1 β, IL-6, TNFα) could be demonstrated after silica phagocytosis. Using titanium dioxide for phagocytosis, no comparable effects were observed. The impact of silica on cytokine secretion of monocytes might explain inflammatory tissue reactions and increased collagen synthesis in silica-associated SSc.

The incubation of fibroblasts in culture with silica demonstrated the induction of interstitial collagenase I mRNA and protein in the monolayer and a decreased ability to contract collagen fibers in a three-dimensional gel. Unexpectedly, Anderegg and colleagues (1996) could not find an increase in the expression of collagen I or III mRNA.

Taken together, the enhanced expression of ICAM-1 by endothelial cells might cause enhanced adhesion of activated (and activating) mononuclear cells to the microvascular wall. Together with increased collagenase activities originated from endothelial cells and the neighboring dermal fibroblasts, the extravasation of monocytes into the surrounding tissue could be realized. The resulting perivascular infiltrate may take part again in the activation of fibroblasts to produce more collagen and matrix proteins in skin or lung tissue. The mechanism of SSc due to silica is summarized in ➋ *Fig. 29.1.*

Recent studies discuss the induction of CD 69 expression in peripheral blood mononuclear cells on silica exposure (Wu et al. 2004), alterations of Fas and Fas-related molecules, in particular alternatively spliced variant messages of Fas gene, and attenuated function of the CD4+CD25+ T cell function due to silica (Otsuki et al. 2000, 2007). In addition, Brown et al. (2004a, b) reviewed in detail the effect of silica on Fas/Fas-ligand, caspase activation, TNFα, protein kinase C, as well as on T and B lymphocytes, thereby explaining the progression from an autoimmune response into systemic autoimmune disease and helping to understand the etiology of environmental autoimmune disease process (Yoshida and Gershwin 1993). Finally, Xiong et al. (2008) found in a state-space model for the regulatory network that TGFβ pathway under perturbation of silica shows significant differences in dynamic properties between normal and scleroderma fibroblasts.

In an experimental study with 20 brown Norway rats, Al-Mogairen (2010) has shown that subcutaneous sodium silicate administration (3 mg) induced serum ANA and anti-RNP, but neither Scl 70 nor ACA antibodies after 7 and 14 weeks, respectively, i.e., to some extent scleroderma-related autoantibodies, but no sclerodermatous lesions. The histology of the injected areas has not been investigated.

1.7 Vibration

Vibrations caused by pneumatic tools are known to induce Raynaud's phenomenon, which regresses after cessation of the exposure. To what extent vibration hammers, which are often used in mining and treating stones, take part in promotion of SSc is still vague (Blair et al. 1974). However, it is extremely unlikely that some of the patients, such as sandblasters, glass grinders, cast polishers, and stove fitters, have ever worked with pneumatic tools. Increased incidences of Raynaud's phenomenon, sclerodactyly, and edema of the hands were observed in chainsaw workers and in individuals operating jackhammers (Nagata et al. 1993). In two case-control studies in the provinces Trento (n = 21) and Verona (n = 55), Bovenci et al. (2001), did not show a significant association between scleroderma and hand-transmitted vibration probably owing to the rarity of the disease and the small number of cases.

1.8 Human Lymphocyte Antigen Association

The association of immunological disorders to certain human lymphocyte antigen (HLA) alleles emphasizes the role of genetic factors determining susceptibility to environmental factors (➋ *Table 29.8*). Rihs et al. (1994) analyzed the association of circulating autoantibodies and HLA alleles in 71 uranium miners and 1 cleaning woman. They could show a positive correlation of anti-Scl-70 to DR3 (1*0300) and DQ2 (1*0201) as well as of ACA to DR1 (1*0101-1*0103), DR8 (1*0801-1*0804), and DQ4 (1*0400). Significant differences between affected and unaffected miners have not been observed.

In addition, Rihs et al. (1996) studied the genetic association of HLA-DPB1 alleles in 54 patients with idiopathic SSc, 26 uranium miners with SSc, and 70 unrelated, healthy control subjects. SSc patients with and without former employment in mines were assigned to two subgroups according to their scleroderma-specific autoantibody pattern – anti-Scl-70 positive and ACA positive – and a third subgroup comprising the rest. Statistical analysis revealed a significantly increased frequency of DPB1*1301, DPB1*0601, and DPB1*1701 ($p = 0.0001$, corrected $p = 0.011$) in idiopathic anti-Scl-70-positive SSc cases when

Table 29.8
Association between human lymphocyte antigen (HLA) alleles and several subgroups of systemic sclerosis (SSc) patients (According to Rihs et al. 1994, 1996; Baur et al. 1996; Conrad et al. 1997)

Circulating autoantibody	SSc patient subgroup	HLA alleles
Anti-Scl-70/ anti-topoisomerase antibodies	Uranium miner	DR 3 (DRB 1*0300), DQ2 (DQB 1*0201)
	Silica-associated SSc	DRB 1*0301, DQB 1*0201
	Idiopathic SSc	DPB 1 (1*1301, *0601, *1701)
Anti-centromere	Uranium miners	DR 1 (1*0100, *0101-*0103), DR 8 (1*0800, *0801-*0804), DQ (1*0400)
	Silica-associated SSc	DRB 1*0800, DQB 1*0402

compared with unexposed controls. Since these three alleles contain the genetic information encoding a glutamic acid residue in position 69 of DPB1, a strong association of this residue with anti-Scl-70 expression was observed in idiopathic SSc patients when compared with anti-Scl-70-negative idiopathic SSc patients ($p = 0.0009$) or unrelated controls ($p = 0.0007$). ACA expression was not associated with the presence of any DPB1 allele tested. The data show that anti-Scl-70 expression in idiopathic SSc patients is linked with DPB1*1301, whereas anti-Scl-70-positive miners do not exhibit such a DPB1 association. Furthermore, the data indicate that glutamate at position 69 of DPB1 might be involved in the susceptibility to idiopathic anti-Scl-70 expression.

Additionally, DRB1*0301 and DQB1*0201 were significantly increased in ATA-positive, silica-associated SSc patients, and DRB1*0800 and DQB1*0402 were elevated in ACA-positive, silica-associated SSc patients compared with unrelated controls and the idiopathic SSc group studied (Conrad et al. 1997).

One TNFα2 allele (associated with an increased TNF production capacity) was only increased in silica-associated SSc, independently of any DRB alleles. The prevalence of TNFα2 in ATA responders was significantly different between idiopathic SSc (decreased compared with controls) and silica-associated SSc patients (increased). A similar result was found with TNFα-308A. The results of this study reinforce the idea that not only structural conditions of antigen binding encoded by major histocompatibility class-II genes, but also an association to a certain TNF region, may be important for the generation of an immune response through regulation of TNF production, which is modified in silica-associated SSc patients due to continuous ingestion of silica by macrophages (Conrad et al. 1997). In Japan, Ueki et al. (2001) found a different distribution of HLA class II alleles in anti-topoisomerase I antibody responders between silicosis and systemic sclerosis patients, with a common distinct amino acid sequence in the HLA-DQB1 domain.

1.9 Conclusion

As silica cannot be removed from the body once it is incorporated, its deleterious precipitating effect is unavoidable. This indicates that the clinical course of silica-induced disorders is quite similar to classical autoimmune diseases or SSc, characterized by progressions and remissions. The subsequent therapy should take these findings into account and has to be adjusted according to the criteria for the extent, organ involvement, and clinical activity of the disease. The best way to prevent this type of SSc is to minimize the exposure to silica.

However, continuous efforts are still required to encourage acknowledgment of SSc as an occupational disease after long-term silica exposure. Individual decisions by clinical experts should provide the basis enabling social and financial support to reduce the harm caused by silica-induced SSc.

2 Scleroderma-Like Diseases

In contrast to silica and several solvents, a whole variety of substances is reported to induce SLD, which can be distinguished from SSc using the following criteria:

- Type of skin manifestation, in particular acrosclerosis, circumscribed and generalized morphea, fibrotic nodules, or joint contractures
- Visceral involvement due to toxic damage of liver, kidney, nervous system, and muscles, or angiosarcoma of the liver
- Laboratory findings, discrete thrombocytopenia, and absence of autoantibodies
- Cessation or reversal of the disease process after early discontinuation of exposure
- Female preponderance for idiopathic SSc is often not observed in occupationally induced SLD

2.1 Vinyl Chloride

Individuals cleaning or inspecting autoclaves for polymerization of vinyl chloride (VC) to polyvinyl chloride (PVC) are in danger of developing SLD with high incidence (Lelbach and Marsteller 1981; Ostlere et al. 1992). Cleaning is usually performed by scraping and water splashing. In this way, workers are exposed to the remnants of the monomer.

The first large study was conducted in Rumania in 1963, where 168 PVC workers had been observed over 4 years (Suciu et al. 1963). The symptoms included pruritus of the arms and face, and scleroderma-like lesions which mostly disappeared after removal from the workplace. Later on, the disease was described in detail and labeled as occupational acro-osteolysis (OAOL) in England, France, and the United States (Cordier et al. 1966; Harris and Adams 1967; Wilson et al. 1967; Dinman et al. 1971; Markowitz et al. 1972). The disease is characterized by Raynaud's phenomenon, papular-fibrotic skin lesions on the wrist and dorsa of the hands, and osteolysis in the middle of the distal phalanges (bullet holes), mainly of the first three fingers, which became shortened and shapeless. OAOL occurred only in those workers who had been exposed to the VC monomer and was most common in reactor cleaners (Lelbach and Marsteller 1981).

Histopathological examination of scleroderma-like lesions showed distended collagen fibers, shrinkage of elastic fibers, interstitial edema, sometimes perivascular lymphocytic infiltrates, swollen endothelial cells of the enlarged capillaries, and marked acanthosis in the epidermal layer (Czernielewski et al. 1979).

In 1974, Lange et al. reported of a systemic form of VC disease (Lange et al. 1974). Changes included skin sclerosis, pulmonary fibrosis, fibrosis of the liver and spleen, and disturbances in the capillary vascular system, joints, and musculature. Further manifestations are paresthesia, thrombocytopenia, leukopenia, and splenomegaly (Bachner et al. 1974). Capillary microscopy reveals that abnormalities of the nail fold in VC workers are similar but less pronounced than those found in SSc (Maricq et al. 1976). Distal pitting scars, esophageal dysmotility, renal disease, and cardiac disease are generally absent.

Leukopenia, as well as angiosarcoma of the liver, drew attention to the carcinogenic and mutagenic properties of VC. Whether other kinds of malignancies are caused by VC was questioned by Fox and Collier (1977) based on an extensive epidemiological study. The relationship between VC disease and SSc is shown in ➋ *Table 29.9.*

Finally, common symptoms of VC-related diseases such as fatigue, cold, burning pain, emotional instability, loss of libido, and impotence should be mentioned (Penin et al. 1975; Veltman 1980). After discontinued exposure, skin lesions, capillary abnormalities, and acro-osteolytic lesions will revert to an almost normal status (Veltman 1980). VC is a volatile gas. It is not quite clear to what extent inhalation of VC might induce skin lesions; however, remnants of the gaseous monomer VC have been demonstrated in the polymer PVC. VC is stored and metabolized by the organism. One of its metabolites, thiodiglycolic acid, can easily be detected in urine samples, even when levels of VC in the atmosphere are considerably lower (Mueller et al. 1978). So-called activated metabolites of VC (➋ *Fig. 29.2*) may participate in the pathogenesis. Other mechanisms might affect the individual's cellular immune response, especially in workers exposed to the small molecules of VC (Kohanka 1982). Circulating immune complexes were found to be increased (Milford 1976). However, autoantibodies – particularly ANA, ATA, and ACA – could not be traced (Black et al. 1983). HLAs of the pattern HLA DR5, HLA DR3, HLA A1, HLA B8, and HLA B3 prevail in patients with VC disease. The genetic background, together with the impairment of cellular immune functions, might lead to an increased

▪ Table 29.9

Relationship between vinyl chloride (VC) disease and systemic sclerosis (SSc) (According to Veltman 1980; Haustein and Ziegler 1985)

Features of VC disease resembling SSc	Percentage
Raynaud's phenomenon	33–74
Fibrotic skin, sclerodactyly	10
Resorption of bone at the distal phalanges	11
Pulmonary fibrosis	13
Esophageal variation	23
Skin capillary abnormalities	23
Arthralgia	82
Myalgia	16
Features of VC disease different from SSc	Percentage
Paresthesia	80
Thrombocytopenia	76
Splenomegaly	48
Reticulocytosis	35
Central nervous system symptoms	17
Leukopenia	8
Angiosarcoma of the liver	6
No calcinosis	

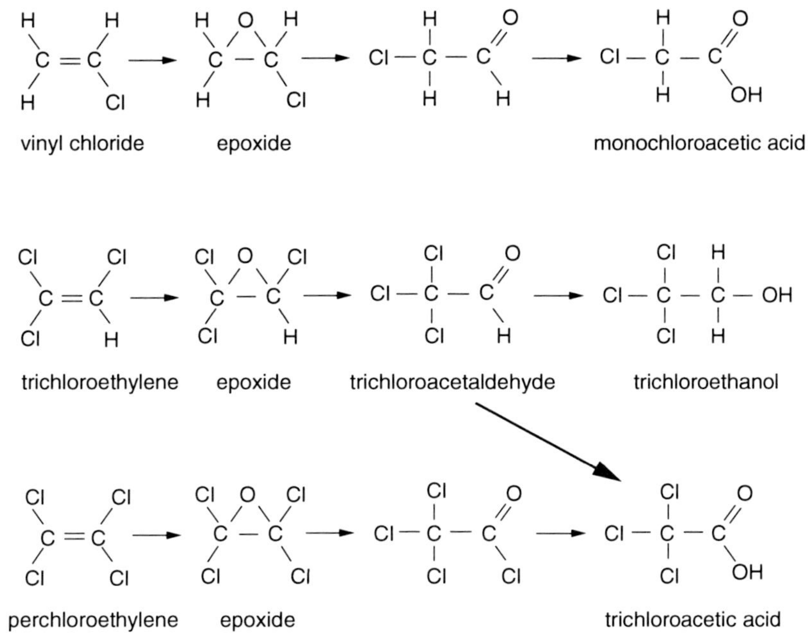

Fig. 29.2
Metabolism of chlorinated ethylenes (According to Bolt et al. 1982)

susceptibility to the disorder (Black et al. 1983). One of the main targets of VC-inducible effects seems to be microvascular tissues. Fibrosis of the vessel wall results in fibrosis of other organ systems. Patients with VC disease have fewer capillary abnormalities of their fingers than patients with SSc, but they have more than healthy controls (Maricq 1981).

In rats fed for 2 years with 30 mg VC per kilogram of body weight, thickening of the skin with collagen deposition as well as an increase in glycosylated lysine and hydroxylysine have been described, indicating an increased collagen synthesis (Knight and Gibbons 1987).

Reducing maximum concentrations in the workplace from 500 ppm to negligible levels (<5 ppm) by automation and contact-free technology will subsequently decrease the number of reported cases.

2.2 PVC Dust

Recently, a case of MCTD in a male patient occupationally exposed to PVC and other toxic agents was presented. Clinical symptoms consisted of typical signs of systemic LE, rheumatoid arthritis, and lupoid hepatitis. MCTD diagnosis was confirmed serologically by the presence of u 1-ribonucleoprotein-autoantibodies. Prednisone, 60 mg daily, produced remission (Panaszek et al. 1993). Studnicka et al. (1995) presented a 58-year-old patient exposed to thermoplastic dusts, mainly PVC, for 10 years. He developed pneumoconiosis and secondary SSc.

2.3 Bis(4-Amino-3-Methylcyclohexyl) Methane (Polymerization of Epoxy Resins)

Two male patients (of 233 workers) with a newly diagnosed SLD induced by epoxy resins were reported from Japan in 1980 (Yamakage et al. 1980). Ishikawa et al. (1995) described the clinical and laboratory findings of these patients after a 17-year follow-up from 1976 to 1993. Both patients have been employed by a chemical factory since May 1975 and were continuously exposed to a polymerization process of epoxy resins. First symptoms appeared after 1 month (patient 1) and 1.5 months (patient 2). After this brief exposure, the patients developed erythema and edema, which evolved to generalized dermal sclerosis and alopecia, weakness, and muscle atrophy, but no Raynaud's phenomenon or ANA. Treatment was started with a small dose of prednisolone and discontinued in 1980. The hair loss recovered in 1977, the sclerotic skin changes disappeared by 1980, and the sclerodactyly recovered in 1993. Bis(4-amino-3-methylcyclohexyl)methane (BAMM), a new type of plasticizer

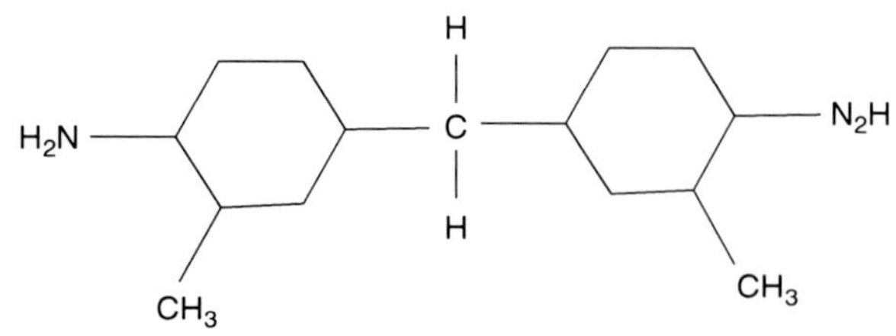

Fig. 29.3
Bis(4-amino-3-methylcyclohexyl)methane

belonging to the cyclohexamines (Fig. 29.3), was suspected as the causative agent from the list of chemical substances used.

BAMM may interfere with the amine metabolism which has been suggested to be disturbed in SSc patients (Stachow et al. 1979). In addition, oligomers of epoxy resins, being strong sensitizers, might induce dysfunctional immune responses (Thorgeirsson et al. 1978). Using SSc-inducing glycosaminoglycans in lymphocyte transformation tests, splenocytes of mice experimentally treated with BAMM showed a positive response (Ishikawa et al. 1982). Intraperitoneal injections of one compound produced skin sclerosis in a murine model (Yamakage et al. 1980).

A 33-year-old man developed SSc without scleroderma while working and being exposed from age 20 to 30 years to epoxy resin polymerization during surfboard manufacturing (Inachi et al. 1996). The symptoms included a shortening of the frenulum linguae, diffuse hyperpigmentation and facial telangiectasia, positive ANA, and pulmonary dysfunction, but no acrosclerosis or sclerodactylia. Modest dermal collagen proliferation in the forearm skin confirmed SSc without scleroderma.

2.4 Chlorinated Hydrocarbons, Aliphatic Hydrocarbons

The chlorinated hydrocarbons trichloroethylene and perchloroethylene (Fig. 29.2) are widely used as solvents and cleaners. They may be considered closely related to VC because of the clinical similarity of the disorders caused by these compounds to VC disease. Trichloroethylene is more volatile (boiling point 87.2°C) and much more toxic than perchloroethylene (boiling point 121.1°C). It penetrates the skin and, in its vaporous state, is also absorbed by the alveolar capillaries. Prolonged contact with the skin will induce irritative dermatitis (Schirren 1971; Bauer and Rabens 1977). Besides the well-described toxic effects in the nervous system, liver, kidney, and bone marrow, several reports on SLD resembling VC disease have been published (Reinl 1957; Saihan et al. 1978). Sparrow (1977) observed a SLD similar to VC disease, probably caused by perchloroethylene.

Recently, Flindt-Hansen and Isager (1987) reported three cases of SSc after occupational, prolonged (4–12 years), and intensive exposure to trichloroethane and/or trichloroethylene during metal-cleaning procedures. According to the ACR-criteria, all three cases could be classified as definite SSc.

Another case of SSc after working with trichloroethylene (Czirjak et al. 1993) was observed in a female patient after inhalation for 2 years (beginning at the age of 40 years). At the age of 43 years, she developed Raynaud's phenomenon, acrosclerosis, and joint symptoms. A serious involvement of the lower esophagus was found from the age of 47 years. Thirteen years later, congestive heart failure, thrombocytopenia, and renal involvement were detected. Two years later, the patient died suddenly due to cardiac arrest. Indirect immunofluorescence showed a speckled ANA pattern on Hep-2 cell monolayers. In addition, Griffin et al. (2002) demonstrated the acceleration of a nonspecific autoimmune response (Th1, CD44) in MRL +/+ mice including trichloroethylene-specific immune response after long-term trichloroethylene exposure.

Lockey et al. (1987) described a 47-year-old woman with previously excellent health who developed fatal SSc after a single 2.5 h predominantly dermal exposure to trichloroethylene. During a period of 10 months, the patient developed proximal scleroderma, reflux esophagitis, microangiopathic hemolytic anemia, restrictive pulmonary disease, pericarditis with effusion, and renal insufficiency with severe hypertension. Renal and skin biopsies were consistent with SSc. An additional case of SSc in a 51-year-old female worker has been presented, who developed SSc after 15 years of exposure to perchloroethylene (Szeimies et al. 1992).

A 26-year-old woman with localized scleroderma after 1 year of exposure to various organic solvents, including trichloroethylene, tetrachloroethylene, acetone, benzene, isopropyl alcohol, dimethyl phthalate, methoxyethanol, polyethylene glycol, polyvinyl alcohol, polyvinyl acetate, xylene, and phenol, has been presented by Czirjak et al. (1994). Disseminated circumscribed scleroderma (morphea) has been described in a painter exposed to perchloroethylene (Hinnen et al. 1995).

Recently, two cases of fasciitis (no scleroderma) with eosinophilia associated with prolonged exposure to trichloroethylene were reported: The first case (a 63-year-old woman) by drinking contaminated water from a residential well, and the second (a 65-year-old man) through occupational exposure (Waller et al. 1994).

Czirjak et al. (1987) analyzed 21 female patients with SSc. In eight of them, occupationally hazardous agents were considered: trichloroethylene in one, organic solvents in six, and polyethylene and possibly its derivatives in the last. Another patient had been heavily exposed to trichloromethane during 13 years of work renovating carburetors in Israel (Tibon-Fisher et al. 1992).

The analysis of 61 patients with SSc (Czirjak et al. 1989) revealed a female-to-male ratio of 60:1. Prior occupational exposure to chemicals (mainly organic solvents) was found in 17 (28%) of the patients, with a mean age of 49 ± 8 years. The exposure preceded the onset of disease by 9 ± 7 years. The mode of exposure was mainly through inhalation, with a duration of 6.3 ± 6.5 years. Features from patients with exposure to organic solvents were clinically indistinguishable from the other cases studied (Czirjak and Kumanovics 2002).

As mentioned by Yamakage and Ishikawa (1982), various aliphatic hydrocarbons, such as naphtha and *n*-hexane, are able to induce generalized morphea-like sclerosis, either by exposure to vapor or by direct skin contact with the liquid substance. Further features of the induced disorder are sclerodactyly, Raynaud's phenomenon, esophageal dysfunction, and fibrosis of the lung. The disease could be reproduced by chronic intraperitoneal injection of these organic compounds in animal experiments.

A 41-year-old male foundry worker with exposure to trichloroethane, xylene, trimethylbenzene, and naphthalene for 15 years developed following symptoms: sclerodactyly, digital pitting scars, Raynaud's phenomenon, impotence, reflux esophagitis, and ANA titers of 1:320 (Brasington and Thorpe-Swenson 1991).

Trichloroethylene elicits acute pulmonary cytotoxicity in mice, which involves Clara cells of bronchioles. Forkert and Forkert (1994) examined the effects of a single dose of trichloroethylene in lungs of mice and showed that structural and functional abnormalities progress for at least 3 months. Pulmonary fibrosis was first detected at 15 days and was ongoing which diffuses in the alveolar zone, resulting in thickening of alveolar septa and destruction of lung structure. The fibrosis was most pronounced at 90 days. Levels of total lung hydroxyproline content were not significantly different in control and treated mice at days 30 and 60, but were significantly increased at day 90, while the proline content remained unchanged. The increase in collagen deposition at 90 days coincided with a significant increase in lung elastic recoil (Forkert and Forkert 1994).

As shown in ➔ *Fig. 29.2*, chlorinated hydrocarbons such as VC, perchloroethylene, and trichloroethylene are metabolized in similar pathways (Lockey et al. 1987). However, the significance of the P 450 system for metabolization and in the detoxification of putative SSc-inducing environmental toxins has not been studied so far.

2.5 Aromatic Hydrocarbons

In 1983, Walder reported of six patients with limited scleroderma who were exposed to aromatic hydrocarbon solvents, such as benzene, toluene, xylene, white spirit, and diesel oil (Walder 1983). Unlike chlorinated hydrocarbons, these aromatic hydrocarbons do not cause systemic disorders. The scleroderma-like lesions were limited to hands and feet, body parts directly exposed.

Recently, however, a sclerodermatous syndrome with unusual features and visceral involvement has been reported following prolonged occupational exposure (32 years) to a wide variety of organic solvents (including benzene in various forms, toluenes, toluidines, xylenes, xylidenes, aniline compounds, and ethanolamine and its derivatives) (Bottomley et al. 1993). Associated functional changes include cold sensitivity, restrictive pulmonary disease, peripheral neuropathy, esophageal dysfunction, labile hypertension, and a monoclonal paraproteinemia.

Garcia-Zamalloa et al. (1994) described a 56-year-old patient who developed SSc with skin, lung, and pericardial affections after he had worked in a rubber transformation section of a tire factory for 23 years. He had been exposed to toluene (an aromatic hydrocarbon), heptane (an aliphatic hydrocarbon), dimethylbuthylphenyldiamine (an aromatic amine), and octhyphenol formaldehyde (a formaldehyde derivative), cutaneously and by inhalation. Exposure to nonchlorinated hydrocarbon and sulfated substances was also assessed. Two male patients developed SLD after occupational exposure to various chemicals (meta-phenylenediamine, VC, and silicon tetrachloride, respectively) in the same building. One patient had been exposed to VC, a known cause of SLD. Because of the prolonged delay between the VC exposure and the onset of scleroderma, the authors excluded this agent as the causative one. In addition, both patients were intermittently exposed to silicon tetrachloride, which yields hydrochloric acid and free silica upon chemical breakdown. It might be speculated that the disease described therein was precipitated by an unusual indirect exposure to silica, which seems unlikely. The most attractive candidate for a potential causative agent in this SLD is meta-phenylenediamine (Owens and Medsger 1988).

In their clinical practice, Haustein and Albrecht (1996) examined a 58-year-old painter who had been exposed to a wide variety of organic solvents for 30 years. He developed a SLD of the skin, esophagus, and lung, with polyneuropathy and chronic hepatosis and elevated titers of ANA and Scl-70-antibodies. The second patient was a 49-year-old woman who had sewn leather in an oil bath containing various oils and organic solvents for 12 years. She suffered from an acrosclerosis of the hands, lung fibrosis and kidney involvement, chronic hepatitis, and peripheral neuropathy including positive ANA and ACA titers.

Bovenzi et al. (1995) examined 21 patients (16 women, 5 men) with SSc or localized variants of scleroderma. A significant association was found between exposure to organic solvents (aromatic hydrocarbons) and SSc (three men, one woman). Among the male subjects, an increased odds ratio for SSc was observed for exposure to organic solvents, silica dust, and hand-transmitted vibration. Exposure to solvents and other chemicals was associated, albeit not significantly, with SSc among the women.

Finally, SLD has also been reported in a 53-year-old man after exposure to LOC, a domestic detergent widely used in Japan. Its constituents are polyoxyethylene alkyl ether and fatty acid alkanol amide (Tanaka et al. 1993).

In a recently performed occupational analysis of 56 men with SSc in the United Kingdom showing no evidence of silica exposure implicated in the onset of the disease, only exposure to organic solvents were reported to any extent. No significant increase in exposure to organic solvents was found in a case-control analysis (Silman and Jones 1992).

2.6 Solvents in General

Recent reports did not specify the different solvents; their studies are related to solvents in general. In the majority of reports, case-control studies have been conducted and relative risks (odds ratio) have been calculated. Nietert et al. (1998) reported on a high cumulative intensity score (odds ratio 2.9) and a high maximum intensity score (OR 2.9) for any solvent exposure in 37 men with preference to anti-Scl-70 autoantibody positive patients. Garabrant et al. (2002) investigated 660 female SSc patients from Michigan and Ohio in a case-control study and concluded that exposures to paint thinners and removers were associated with scleroderma in woman but showed no evidence of increasing risk with increasing duration. Other petroleum distillates such as gasoline and mineral spirits were not significantly associated with scleroderma in multivariable analyses.

Diot et al. (2002) conducted a case-control study of 80 SSc patients in Tours (France) from 1998 to 2000. They calculated an exposure score for each subject based on probability, intensity, daily frequency, and duration of exposure for each period of employment. They found among other known associations also one for welding fumes. Maitre et al. (2004) found significantly increased risk for workers with cleaning products (odds ratio = 1.66) and with solvents (odds ratio = 3.23).

In a new meta-analysis conducted by Kettaneh et al. (2007), the risk of SSc associated with organic solvent exposure was variable among 11 studies (1,291 pat, 3,435 controls), there was an overrepresentation in smaller studies suggesting "publication bias" with an average odds ratio of 2.4 and 1.8 after adjusting of bias, respectively. The relative risk was higher in man (OR 3.0) than in woman (OR 1.8), whereas women were predominantly affected by SSc in general.

In terms of gene-environment interaction, Povey et al. (2001) found that cytochrome P2 polymorphisms may be involved in the increasing susceptibility to SSc among subjects who have been exposed to organic solvents. All seven patients carry the 2C19EM genotype and the 2E1*3 allele was found in two of seven patients.

Cooper et al. (2009) reported on autoimmune-related effects of trichloroethylene exposure in mice ($MRL^{+/+}$ lupus mice) such as increased antinuclear antibodies, interferon y, decreased IL-4 and autoimmune hepatitis and in humans they described symptoms such as increased interferon y, IL-2, decreased IL-4, as well as hepatitis.

➲ *Table 29.10* summarizes data on patients with SSc or SLD in association with exposure to organic solvents.

2.7 Pesticides/Herbicides

Dunnill and Black (1994) reported a case of generalized cutaneous sclerosis associated with prominent myositis and esophageal involvement in a patient exposed to herbicides containing bromocil, diuron, and aminotriazole. There was no evidence of lung involvement, and antibody titers were in the normal range. Treatment with oral prednisolone resulted in modest improvement of the cutaneous changes, particularly of the face, trunk, and proximal limbs. The considerable exposure to chemicals, time course, and unusual pattern of organ involvement were suggestive for the diagnosis of occupational scleroderma.

Another case of sclerodermiform lesions after use of various herbicides has been described by Poskitt et al. (1994). A 53-year-old man developed chloracne, palmoplantar keratoderma, and scleroderma after many years of exposure to a variety of chloracnegens. Chloracne is a rare but important acneiform eruption associated with

Table 29.10

Cases of systemic sclerosis (SSc) and scleroderma-like diseases (SLDs) in association with exposure to solvents

Author	Number	Clinical symptoms	Exposure
Sparrow (1977)	1	SLD	Perchloroethylene
Walder (1983)	6	SLD	Benzene, toluene, xylene, white spirits, diesel oil
Czirjak et al. (1987)	8	SSc	Trichloroethylene (1), organic solvents (6), polyethylene (1)
Lockey et al. (1987)	1	SSc	Trichloroethylene
Flindt-Hansen and Isager (1987)	3	SSc	Trichloroethylene, trichloroethane
Owens and Medsger (1988)	2	SLD	Meta-phenylenediamine, silicon tetrachloride (hydrochloric acid and free silica), meta-phenylenediamine, vinyl chloride, and silicon tetrachloride
Czirjak et al. (1989)	17	SSc	Benzene and petroleum-derived crude solvents (3), organic solvents (isopropyl alcohol, terpene derivatives) (4), ethyl acetate and other solvents (3), organic solvents (not well defined) (4), silica dust, paints, and solvents (1), ethylene derivatives (1), trichloroethylene (1)
Szeimies et al. (1992)	1	SSc	Perchloroethylene
Brasington and Thorpe-Swenson (1991)	1	SSc	Trichloroethane, xylene, naphthalene, trimethylbenzene
Yanez-Diaz et al. (1992)	1	SSc, silicosis	Trichloroethylene, fiberglass
Tibon-Fisher et al. (1992)	1	SSc	Trichloromethane
Gabay and Kahn (1992)	3	SSc	Solvents (1), solvents and silica dust (2)
Czirjak et al. (1993)	1	SSc	Trichloroethylene
Tanaka et al. (1993)	1	SLD	LOC (domestic detergent, constituents: polyoxyethylene alkyl ether, fatty acid alkanol amide)
Bottomley et al. (1993)	1	SLD	Organic solvents (including benzene in various forms, toluenes, toluidines, xylenes, xylidenes, aniline compounds, and ethanolamine and its derivatives)
Waller et al. (1994)	2	Fasciitis, eosinophilia	Trichloroethylene
Czirjak et al. (1994)	1	Localized scleroderma	Trichloroethylene, tetrachloroethylene, acetone, benzene, isopropyl alcohol, dimethyl phthalate, methoxyethanol, polyethylene glycol, polyvinyl alcohol, polyvinyl acetate, xylene, phenol
Garcia-Zamalloa et al. (1994)	1	SSc	Toluene, heptane, dimethylbutylphenyldiamine, and octyphenol formaldehyde, exposure to nonchlorinated hydrocarbon and sulfated substances was also assessed
Hinnen et al. (1995)	1	Disseminated morphea	Perchloroethylene
Bovenzi et al. (1995)	4	Scleroderma	Organic solvents (aromatic hydrocarbons)
Haustein and Albrecht (1996)	2	SLD	Wide variety of organic solvents (for 30 years), various oils and organic solvents (for 12 years)
Nietert et al. (1998)	37	Scleroderma	Trichlorethylene, trichloroethane, carbon tetrachloride, benzene
Povey et al. (2001)	7	Scleroderma	Organic solvents

Table 29.10 (Continued)

Author	Number	Clinical symptoms	Exposure
Czirjak and Kumanovics (2002)	16	Scleroderma	Solvents
Diot et al. (2002)	57?	Systemic sclerosis	Solvents: trichloroethylene, chlorinated solvents toluene, aromatic solvents, ketones, white spirit
Garabrant et al. (2002)	Among 660 pat.?	Scleroderma	Solvents
Bovenzi et al. (2004)	11	Systemic sclerosis	Solvents
Maitre et al. (2004)	28	Systemic sclerosis	Solvents, OR = 3.23
	32	Systemic sclerosis	Cleaning products, OR = 1.66
Kettaneh et al. (2007)	Meta-analysis of 11 studies!	Systemic sclerosis	Solvents
	Detailed figures and odds ratios!		

exposure to halogenated aromatic compounds used primarily in agriculture. However, to the authors' knowledge, the association of palmoplantar keratoderma and scleroderma with exposure to chloracnegens has not been previously reported.

Dermatohistopathological changes, selected as an example of highly organized connective tissue, were studied by eight different staining and histochemical techniques in 896 biopsies of macroscopically uninvolved skin from the gluteal region of 56 patients with acute phospho-organic pesticide intoxication between days 2 and 15 after intoxication (Tashev and Tsonev 1990). Two hundred and seventy-two biopsies from 17 healthy individuals and published data served as controls. Nonspecific changes affecting mainly the elastic and collagen components were found, in some cases paralleled with the severity of intoxication. The reticular net, vessels, matrix, and cell elements were far less affected, indicating their relative stability to the pesticides' toxicity.

2.8 Mercury Chloride

Mean urinary Hg levels were significantly elevated in the antifibrillarin antibody-positive SSc patients (Arnett et al. 2000). Mercury chloride induces a strong immune activation and dysregulation, but does not accelerate the development of dermal fibrosis in tight skin 1 mice (Hanson and Abedi-Valugerdi 2002). Therefore, the potential occult exposure to Hg has to be considered in antifibrillarin-positive SSc patients in future until further epidemiological and basic research studies can prove or refute this observation.

3 Mixed Connective Tissue Disease

Vincent et al. (1996) reported a 25-year-old woman who developed Sharp's syndrome 5 years after diagnosis of acute silicosis due to inhalation of the scouring powder Ajax (Colgate Palmolive Co.), containing 95% silica, 2% alkylbenzosulphonate, and 3% trichlorocyanuric acid. MCTD due to PVC dust is mentioned above (Panaszek et al. 1993).

4 Sjögren's Syndrome

Three cases of primary Sjögren's syndrome were described by Puisieux et al. (1994) in silicotic coal miners. All patients fulfilled the diagnostic criteria for Sjögren's syndrome recently established by the European Community study group. One patient had cryoglobulinemia and polyneuritis. Another had Raynaud's phenomenon, arthralgia, purpura, and polyneuritis. Capillary microscopy revealed normal findings in all three patients. ANA were detected only in one patient, who also had anti-SS-A (RO) and anti-SS-B (LA) antibodies. Although the prevalence of SSc, RA, and probably systemic LE is significantly higher after long-standing occupational exposure to silica, so far no case of Sjögren's syndrome has been described in the course of pulmonary silicosis.

5 Lupus Erythematosus

Silica-induced LE is a chronic multiorgan system autoimmune disease with frequent exacerbations and remissions similar to the natural course of mixed connective tissue disease. The pathomechanism of LE is not yet completely understood. Based on a genetic background, a major role seems to be played by disturbances of immune regulation, such as T-cell abnormalities, including T-cell cytokine network, polyclonal B-cell stimulation, immune complex formation, defects in the clearance of immune complexes, and dysregulation of apoptosis. Various environmental factors have been discussed, such as drugs, solvents, and silica. In lupus-prone New Zealand mixed mice, the exposure of silica induced significantly higher levels of immune complexes, antinuclear, as well as antihistone autoantibodies, increased number of CD4+ T cells and B1a B cells, increased TNFa, thus altogether accelerating systemic autoimmune disease (Brown et al. 2003; 2004a, b).

There is only scant knowledge with reference to occupational influences on LE. Exposure to heat, cold, and wind were cited in the past (Warde 1903). Sunlight was frequently considered an eliciting factor for the primary manifestations and the exacerbations as well (Baer and Harber 1965; Epstein et al. 1965; Diezel et al. 1977). However, among 236 patients examined, only six showed an improvement after the patients moved from an outdoor job to an indoor workplace. In this study, no relationship between occupation and LE could be confirmed (Nebe and Lenz 1971). In terms of association with silicosis of the lung in the former German Democratic Republic, 193 male infirmary patients were examined, with three cases of coincidental silicosis among them (Ziegler et al. 1987).

Further reports exist about the association of LE with silicosis (Hatron et al. 1982) or with occupational silica exposure (Ebihara and Kawami 1985). In addition, Mehlhorn and Gerlach (1990) and Ziegler and colleagues (1991) demonstrated several cases in the uranium-mining industry in East Germany. The former author observed 37 patients with LE exposed to quartz over many years (Mehlhorn and Gerlach 1990). Thirty of them suffered from silicosis. In a survey of 877 male LE patients (592 systemic LE, 279 discoid LE), Ziegler and colleagues (1991) only found seven patients with silicosis out of 428 systemic LE patients over 40 years of age. Recently, Haustein (1998)reported of four additional male systemic LE patients with long-term silica exposure (12–23 years) and silicosis. In 1996, Wichmann et al. published a study of 16 systemic LE patients among a group of 52 workers occupationally exposed to silica (Wichmann et al. 1996).

Siebels et al. (1993) presented case histories of five patients with silicosis who had developed systemic LE and microscopic polyarteritis in two cases each, and rapidly progressive glomerulonephritis (limited Wegener's granulomatosis) in one case. Recently, a male patient who had worked as a stonecutter and had developed silicosis and systemic LE was also reported by Siebels et al. (1995).

Koeger et al. (1995) observed four patients with systemic LE (three with silicosis) and one with discoid LE among 24 cases of silica-associated CTD.

Conrad et al. (1996) described 28 definite and 15 likely systemic LE patients among 15,000 heavily silica-exposed miners, probably part of the same group analyzed by Mehlhorn and Gerlach (1990). Therefore, the prevalence of systemic LE in the population of highly quartz-dust-exposed uranium miners may be estimated at up to 93 of 100,000. ANA could be detected in all definite and in 72.9% of probable patients having systemic LE. Middle-to-high-titred ANAs were present in 94.4% of definite and in 54.7% of probable patients having systemic LE. In patients exhibiting definite systemic LE, clear positive results were obtained for anti-dsDNA in 38.9%, anti-RO/SSA in 38.9%, and anti-LA/SSB in 11.1%. In uranium miners without systemic LE, the prevalence of ANA was significantly higher than the age- and gender-related control group. Furthermore, an increase in ANA titers in heavily rather than slightly exposed uranium miners could be detected. ➲ *Table 29.11* comprises data of patients with LE in association with silica exposure.

An ANA profile suggestive of Sjögren's syndrome or systemic LE without symptoms of either disease occurred in a patient with chronic obstructive pulmonary disease. He worked for less than 5 years as a maintenance mechanic in a plant in South Carolina manufacturing silica flour and industrial sand (Johnson and Busnardo 1993). Excessive occupational exposure to free silica by inhalation was documented. An open-lung biopsy revealed an early stage of silicosis characterized by perivascular and peribronchial accumulation of macrophages, as well as early granuloma formation.

Table 29.11
Lupus erythematosus (LE) in association with silica exposure

Author	Cases	Diagnosis	Exposure (occupation)
Ziegler et al. (1987)	3	Systemic LE and silicosis	Silica
Mehlhorn and Gerlach (1990)	37	Twenty-five systemic LE and silicosis, 5 discoid LE and silicosis, 4 systemic LE, 3 discoid LE	Silica (36 ore miners, 1 foundry worker)
Ziegler et al. (1991)	30	LE, five with silicosis	Silica (16 ore miners, 3 foundry workers, 2 underground workers, 2 enamellers, 1 sandblaster, quarry worker, stove bricklayer, grindstone maker, well driller, glass industry worker)
Siebels et al. (1993)	2	Systemic LE and silicosis	Silica
Siebels et al. (1995)	1	Systemic LE and silicosis	Silica (stonecutter)
Koeger et al. (1995)	5	Four systemic LE (three with silicosis), one discoid LE	Silica (mason, miner, dental prosthetist, scouring and tooth powder worker)
Wichmann et al. (1996)	16	Systemic LE	Silica (scouring powder factory)
Haustein and Albrecht (1996)	1	Systemic LE and silicosis	Silica (uranium hewer)
Conrad et al. (1996) (partially the same group as analyzed by Mehlhorn and Gerlach 1990)	43	Twenty-eight systemic LE, 15 probable systemic LE	Silica (uranium miners)
Haustein (1998)	4	Systemic LE and silicosis	Silica (uranium hewer, cast polisher, stone mason, uranium driller)
Ueki and Omori (2001)	1	Discoid LE, left cheek	Fine fragments of windshield glass embedded after automobile accident 8 years before
Parks et al. (2002)	19 of 265 (case control)	SLE	Medium (OR 2.1) or high (OR 4.6) exposure

In a population-based case-control study, Parks et al. (2002) calculated the risk for SLE after medium silica exposure as 2.4 (odds ratio) and after high exposure 4.6, respectively (n = 19 of 265 SLE patients). However, specific task-based questions must be included to assess the full potential of occupational silica exposure. Thus, the assessment of all work at least 2 weeks 9% of SLE patients were classified as medium or high silica exposed (odds ratio 2.9) whereas, in contrast, at least 12 months occupational exposure provided a much lower risk among the same group of patients (odds ratio 0.4) (Parks et al. 2004).

Certain chemical contaminants in well water have been implicated in the etiology of rheumatic disorders. Kilburn and Warshaw (1992) found an association between the prevalence of symptoms of systemic LE and ANA with chronic exposure to trichloroethylene and other chemicals in well water in the Tucson, Arizona area. Beer et al. (1994) presented two patients with insecticide-induced LE after use of two "bug-bombs" containing 1,1,1-trichloroethane, propane, *S*-methoprene, and permethrin in the patients' trailer home.

6 Dermatomyositis

Few reports are available on dermatomyositis after occupational exposure. Koeger et al. (1991) described dermatopolymyositis in two men and one woman after 5, 16, and 21 years of occupational exposure to silica. Pulmonary involvement was present as diffuse interstitial fibrosis in two patients whose lung biopsies revealed high particulate silica contents. Another patient with

Table 29.12

Exposure to crystalline silica or organic solvents and the risk of systemic sclerosis (According to Kettaneh et al. 2007)

Study	Exposure	Controls	N	Odds ratio	(Confidence interval)
Haustein (1998)	Silica	HC	111	5.7	(1.72–8.54)
	Silicosis	HC	57	12.0	(5.23–19.29)
Englert et al. (2000)	Silica	CC	60	3.93	(1.84–8.54)
Diot et al. (2002)	Silica	CC?	10	3.74	(1.06–13.18)
Smith et al. (2008)	Silica	BNIS	10	Tenfold	Higher prevalence
Czirjak et al. (1989)	Solvents	CC	51	23.18	(2.97–180.79)
Silman et al. (1992)	Solvents	CC	56	2.23	(1.04–4.80)
Bovenzi et al. (1995)	Solvents	HC	21	9.65	(1.00–92.73)
Goldman (1996)	Solvents	CD	33	5.82	(2.53–13.39)
Zachariae et al. (1997)	Solvents	HC	28	3.18	(0.99–10.23)
Nietert et al. (1998)	Solvents	HC	178	1.28	(0.65–2.50)
Diot et al. (2002)	Solvents	HC	80	2.66	(1.35–5.23)
Czirjak et al. (2002)	Solvents	HC	63	2.60	(1.11–6.06)
Garabrant et al. (2003)	Solvents	CC	623	1.53	(1.24–1.89)
Bovenzi et al. (2004)	Solvents	HC	55	2.13	(0.93–4.83)
Maitre et al. (2004)	Solvents (in general)	CC	28	3.23	(1.58–6.63)
	Cleaning products		32	1.66	(0.90–3.08)
Overall for solvents			1,281	2.41	(1.73–3.37)

CC community controls, *HC* hospital controls, *CD* patients with other connective tissue diseases, confidence interval 95%, *BNIS* Belgian National Institute occupational list

polymyositis among 52 workers from a factory producing scouring powder with an increased silica content (70–90% powdered quartz) was described by Wichmann et al. (1996). Among 24 patients with silica-associated CTD, three patients have been diagnosed with dermatomyositis and Sjögren's syndrome (Koeger et al. 1995).

Yang et al. (2001) reported seven patients (one female, six male) suffering from polymyositis/dermatomyositis associated with silicosis in a retrospective review.

7 Rheumatoid Arthritis

Rosenman and Zhu (1995) found an association between silicosis and RA using hospital discharge data from Michigan between the years 1990 and 1991, examining potential associations between pneumoconiosis and pulmonary hypertension, lung cancer, obstructive lung disease, and connective tissue disease among both male and female patients. In an updated multivariate analysis of 3,328 gold miners who worked underground for at least 1 year in South Dakota between 1940 and 1965, an extended follow-up from 1977 to 1990 revealed significant excesses of arthritis, musculoskeletal diseases, and skin conditions including systemic LE and SSc, in addition to silicosis and tuberculosis, but without lung cancer (Steenland and Brown 1995). The study of Koeger et al. (1995) presented five patients with RA (four in association with Sjögren's syndrome). Calvert et al. (2003) calculated a mortality odds ratio of 1.19 for rheumatoid arthritis after silica exposure (among 18,335 patients in total) and a mortality odds ratio of 3.75 for RA patients with silicosis (n = 15). Olsson et al. (2004) found a twofold increased risk of rheumatoid arthritis among male metalworkers or in jobs that involved cleaning metal from Sweden.

8 Conclusion

Connective tissue disorders such as SSc, LE, Sjögren's syndrome, dermatomyositis, and RA can be induced by occupational exposure to silica, solvents, and other chemical offenders. An enhanced genetic susceptibility seems to favor these disorders. SSc is the most frequent and best-studied disease. While silica precipitates SSc, the other offenders induce scleroderma-like diseases with different clinical and laboratory findings than with SSc. Taking a careful case history of patients with SSc will help to identify the occupational causes. The best way to prevent this type of connective tissue disease is to minimize the exposure to occupational substances. However, efforts in the form of individual expert decisions have to be made in order to acknowledge these disorders as occupational diseases and provide some social and financial support to patients and reduce the harm caused by these disorders. In France, however, SSc is recognized as an occupational disease, in patients with former or present exposure to crystalline silica (Maitre et al. 2004), and by the way, even in Germany, polyneuropathy and encephalopathy due to organic solvents or their mixtures are recognized as an occupational disease (number 1,317). Calculated odds ratios between 3.74 and 5.7 for crystalline silica and 2.41 for organic solvents are an important argument for the existence of occupationally induced systemic sclerosis and other connective tissue diseases (➋ *Table 29.12*).

References

Adamson IYR, Letourneau HL, Bowden DH (1989) Enhanced macrophage fibroblast interactions in the pulmonary interstitium increases fibrosis after silica injection to monocyte-depleted mice. Am J Pathol 134:411–418

Al-Mogairen SM (2010) Role of sodium silicate in induction of scleroderma-related autoantibodies in brown Norway rats through oral and subcutaneous administration. Rheumatol Int. doi:10.1007/s00296-009-1327-3

American Thoracic Society (1997) Adverse effects of crystalline silica exposure. Am J Respir Crit Care Med 155:761–765

Anderegg U, Vorberg S, Herrmann K, Haustein UF (1996) Increased expression of interstitial collagenase in silica-treated fibroblasts. Eur J Dermatol 6:51–55

Anderegg U, Vorberg S, Herrmann K, Haustein UF (1997) Silica directly induces intercellular adhesion molecule 1 (ICAM-1) expression in cultured endothelial cells. Eur J Dermatol 7:27–31

Arnett FC, Fritzler MJ, Ahn C, Holian A (2000) Urinary mercury levels in patients with autoantibodies to U3-RNP (fibrillarin). J Rheumatol 27:405–410

Bachner U, Etzel F, Lange CE, Marsteller HJ, Veltman G (1974) Haemostaseologische Aspekte bei der Vinylchlorid-Krankheit. Dtsch Med Wochenschr 99:2409–2410

Baer RL, Harber LC (1965) Photobiology of lupus erythematosus. Arch Dermatol 92:124–128

Bauer M, Rabens SF (1977) Trichloroethylene toxicity. Int J Dermatol 16:113–116

Baur X (1994) Systemische Sklerodermie im Uranerzbergbau der ehemaligen SDAG Wismut. Arbeitsmed Sozialmed Umweltmed Sonderheft 22:5–7

Baur X, Rihs HP, Altmeyer P, Degens P, Conrad K, Mehlhorn J, Weber K, Wiebe V (1996) Systemic sclerosis in German uranium miners under special consideration of autoantibody subsets and HLA class II alleles. Respiration 63:368–375

Beck B, Irmscher G (1974) Silikosen durch weniger bekannte Expositionsarten. Z Erkr Atmungsorgane 140:282–293

Beck B, Irmscher G, Zschunke E (1976) Sklerodermie und Silikose – Versuch einer Synopsis. Z Gesamte Inn Med 31:493–496

Beer KR, Lorincz AL, Medenica MM, Albertini J, Baron J, Drinkard L, Swartz T (1994) Insecticide-induced lupus erythematosus. Int J Dermatol 33:860–862

Black CM, Welsh KI, Walker AE, Bernstein RM, Catoggio LJ, McGregor AR, Jones JK (1983) Genetic susceptibility to scleroderma-like syndrome induced by vinyl chloride. Lancet 1:53–55

Blair HM, Headington JT, Lynch PJ (1974) Occupational trauma, Raynaud's phenomenon and sclerodactylia. Arch Environ Health 28:80–81

Bolt HM, Laib RJ, Filser JG (1982) Reactive metabolites and carcinogenicity of halogenated ethylenes. Biochem Pharmacol 31:1–4

Bottomley WW, Sheehan-Dare RA, Hughes P, Cuncliffe WJ (1993) A sclerodermatous syndrome with unusual features following prolonged occupational exposure to organic solvents. Br J Dermatol 128:203–206

Bovenci M, Barbone F, Pisa FE, Betta A, Romeo L (2001) Scleroderma and occupational exposure to hand-transmitted vibration. Int Arch Occup Environ Health 74:579–582

Bovenzi M, Barbone F, Betta A, Tommasini M, Versini W (1995) Scleroderma and occupational exposure. Scand J Work Environ Health 21:289–292

Bovenzi M, Barbone F, Pia FE, Betta A, Romeo L, Tonello A, Biasi D, Caramaschi P (2004) A case-control study of occupational exposures and systemic sclerosis. Int Arch Occup Environ Health 77:10–16

Bramwell B (1914) Diffuse sclerodermia: its frequency; its occurrence in stone-masons; its treatment by fibrolysin injections – elevations of temperature due to fibrolysin. Edinburgh J Med 12:387–401

Brasington RD, Thorpe-Swenson AJ (1991) Systemic sclerosis associated with cutaneous exposure to solvent: case report and review of the literature. Arthritis Rheum 34:631–633

Brinton LA, Buckley LM, Dvorkina O, Lubin JH, Colton T, Murray MC, Hoover RN (2003) Risk of connective tissue disorders among breast implant patients. Am J Epidemiol 160:619–627

Brown JM, Archer AJ, Pfau JC, Holian A (2003) Silica accelerated systemic autoimmune disease in lupus-prone New Zealand mixed mice. Clin Exp Immunol 131:415–421

Brown JM, Pfau JC, Holian A (2004a) Immunoglobulin and lymphocyte responses following silica exposure in New Zealand Mixed mice. Inhalat Toxicol 16:133–139

Brown JM, Pfau JC, Pershouse MA, Holian A (2004b) Silica, apoptosis, and autoimmunity. J Immunotoxicol 1:177–187

Burns CJ, Laing TJ, Gillespie BW, Heeringa SG, Alcser KH, Mayes MD, Wasko MCM, Cooper BC, Garabrant DH, Schottenfeld D (1996) The epidemiology of scleroderma among women: assessment of risk from exposure to silicone and silica. J Rheumatol 23:1904–1911

Calvert GM, Rice FL, Boiano JM, Sheehy JW, Sanderson WT (2003) Occupational silica exposure and risk of various diseases: an analysis using death certificates from 27 states of the United States. Occup Environ Med 60:122–129

Choudat D (1994) Occupational lung diseases among dental technicians. Tuber Lung Dis 75:99–104

Christy WC, Rodnan GP (1984) Conjugal progressive systemic sclerosis (scleroderma): report of the disease in husband and wife. Arthritis Rheum 27:1180–1182

Conrad K, Mehlhorn J, Lüthke K, Dörner T, Frank KH (1996) Systemic lupus erythematosus after heavy exposure to quartz dust in uranium mines: clinical and serological characteristics. Lupus 5:62–69

Conrad K, Humbel RL, Tan EM, Shoenfeld Y (1997) Autoantibodies – diagnostic, pathogenetic and prognostic relevance. Clin Exp Rheumatol 15:457–465

Cooper GS, Makris SL, Nietert PJ, Jinot J (2009) Evidence of autoimmune-related effects of trichloroethylene exposure from studies in mice and humans. Environ Health Perspect 117:696–702

Cordier JH, Fieviez C, Lefevre MJ, Sevrin A (1966) Acroosteolyse et lesions cutanees chez deux ouvriers affectees au nettoyage d'autoclaves. Can Med Travail 4:3

Cowie RL (1987) Silica-dust-exposed mine workers with scleroderma (systemic sclerosis). Chest 92:260–262

Czernielewski A, Swierczynska-Kiec M, Gluszcz M (1979) Dermatological aspects of so called vinyl chloride monomer disease. Derm Beruf Umwelt 27:108–112

Czirjak L, Kumanovics G (2002) Exposure to solvents in female patients with scleroderma. Clin Rheumatol 21:114–118

Czirjak L, Danko K, Schlammadinger J, Suranyi P, Tamasi L, Szegedi GY (1987) Progressive systemic sclerosis occurring in patients exposed to chemicals. Int J Dermatol 26:374–378

Czirjak L, Bokk A, Csontos G, Lörincz G, Szegedi G (1989) Clinical findings in 61 patients with progressive systemic sclerosis. Acta Derm Venereol 69:533–536

Czirjak L, Schlammadinger J, Szegedi G (1993) Systemic sclerosis and exposure to trichloroethylene. Dermatology 186:236–237

Czirjak L, Pocs E, Szegedi G (1994) Localized scleroderma after exposure to organic solvents. Dermatology 189:399–401

Diezel W, Meffert H, Günther W, Huse K, Sönnichsen N (1977) Exazerbation des Lupus erythematodes visceralis infolge UV-Bestrahlung. Dermatol Monatsschr 163:290–295

Dinman BD, Cook WA, Whitehouse WM, Magnuson HJ, Ditcheck T (1971) Occupational acroosteolysis: an epidemiological study. Arch Environ Health 22:61–65

Diot E, Guilmot JL, Metzger MD, Pilore R, Rogier S, Stadler M, Diot P, Lemarie E, Lasfargues G (2002) Systemic sclerosis and occupational risk factors: a case-control study. Occup Environ Med 59:545–549

Dowd PM, Ziegler V (1987) Endothelial cell cultures in silica induced systemic sclerosis. In: Abstr Sympos Aktuel Probl Arbeitsderm, Leipzig, p 51

Dunnill MG, Black MM (1994) Sclerodermatous syndrome after occupational exposure to herbicides-response to systemic steroids. Clin Exp Dermatol 19:518–520

Ebihara I, Kawami M (1985) Health hazards of mineral dust with special reference to the causation of immuno-pathologic systemic diseases. J Sci Labour 61:1–31

Englert H, Small-McMahon J, Davis K, O'Connor H, Chambers P, Brooks P (2000) Male systemic sclerosis and occupational silica exposure – a population-based study. Aust NZ J Med 30:215–220

Epstein IH, Tuffanelli DL, Dubois EL (1965) Light sensitivity and lupus erythematosus. Arch Dermatol 91:483–485

Erasmus LD (1957) Scleroderma in gold-miners on the Witwatersrand with particular reference to pulmonary manifestations. S Afr J Lab Clin Med 3:209–231

Evans DJ, Posner E (1971) Pneumoconiosis in laundry workers. Environ Res 4:127–128

Fleischmajer R, Perlish IS, Duncan M (1983) Scleroderma: a model for fibrosis. Arch Dermatol 119:957–962

Flindt-Hansen H, Isager H (1987) Scleroderma after occupational exposure to _ssociazione_lene and trichlorethane. Acta Derm Venereol 67:263–264

Forkert PG, Forkert L (1994) Trichloroethylene induces pulmonary fibrosis in mice. Can J Physiol Pharmacol 72:205–210

Fox AJ, Collier PF (1977) Mortality experience of workers exposed to vinyl chloride monomer in the manufacture of polyvinyl chloride in Great Britain. Br J Ind Med 34:1–10

Francia A, Monarca A, Cavallot A (1959) Osservazioni clinico-roentgenologiche soll _ssociazione silicosi-sclerodermia. Med Lav 50:523

Frank R, Giese T, Dummer R, Walther T, Rytter M, Ziegler V, Haustein UF (1993) Silica-induced cytokine release in human monocyte cultures and its possible involvement in the pathophysiology of silica-associated scleroderma. Eur J Dermatol 3:304–309

Gabay C, Kahn MF (1992) Les sclerodermies masculines role de l'exposition professionelle. Schweiz Med Wochenschr 122:1746–1752

Garabrant DH, Lacey JV, Laing TJ, Gillespie BW, Mayes MD, Cooper BC, Schottenfeld D (2002) Scleroderma and solvent exposure among woman. Am J Epidemiol 157:493–500

Garcia-Zamalloa AM, Ojeda E, Gonzalez-Beneitez C, Goni J, Garrido A (1994) Systemic sclerosis and organic solvents: early diagnosis in industry. Ann Rheum Dis 53:618

Goldman JA (1996) Connective tissue diseases in peoble exposed to organic chemical solvents. Systemic sclerosis (scleroderma) in dry cleaning plants and aircraft industry workers. J Clin Rheumatol 2:185–190

Griffin JM, Blossom SJ, Jackson SK, Gilbert KM, Pumford NR (2002) Trichlorethylene accelates an autoimmune response by Th1 T cell activation in MRL +/+ mice. Immunopharmacology 46:123–137

Hanson M, Abedi-Valugerdi M (2002) Mercury chloride induces a strong immune activation, but does not accelerate the development of dermal fibrosis in tight skin 1 mice. Scand J Immunol 59:469–477

Harris DK, Adams WGF (1967) Acroosteolysis occurring in men engaged in the polymerisation of vinyl chloride. BMJ 3:712–714

Hatron PY, Plouvier B, Francois M (1982) Assoziation von systemischem Lupus erythematodes und Silikose. Kasuistik (5 Pat.). Rev Med Intern 3:245–246

Haustein UF (1998) Silica-induced lupus erythematosus. Acta Derm Venereol 78:73–74

Haustein UF, Albrecht M (1993) Zur Epidemiologie und Klinik der systemischen Sklerodermie. Z Haut Geschlechtskr 68:651–658

Haustein UF, Albrecht M (1996) Berufsbedingte progressive Sklerodermie, Pseudosklerodermie und systemischer Lupus erythematodes. Derm Beruf Umwelt 44:77–80

Haustein UF, Herrmann K (1994) Environmental scleroderma. Clin Dermatol 12:467–473

Haustein UF, Klug H (1975) Zur Ultrastruktur der Hautkapillaren bei Lupus eythematodes, Dermatomyositis und progressiver Sklerodermie. Dermatol Monatsschr 161:353–363

Haustein UF, Ziegler V (1985) Environmentally induced systemic sclerosis-like disorders. Int J Dermatol 24:147–151

Haustein UF, Herrmann K, Boehme HJ (1986) Pathogenesis of progressive systemic sclerosis. Int J Derm 25:286–293

Hennekens CH, Lee IM, Cook NR, Hebert PR, Karlson EW, LaMotte F, Manson JE, Buring JE (1996) Self-reported breast implants and connective-tissue diseases in female health professionals. JAMA 275:616–621

Hinnen U, Schmid-Grendelmeier P, Muller E, Elsner P (1995) Exposure to solvents in scleroderma: disseminated circumscribed scleroderma (morphea) in a painter exposed to perchloroethylene (in German). Schweiz Med Wochenschr 125:2433–2437

Hochberg MC (1993) Cosmetic surgical procedures and connective tissue disease: the Cleopatra syndrome revisited. Ann Intern Med 118:981–983

Hochberg MC, Perlmutter DL, Medsger TA, Nguyen K, Steen V, Weisman MH, White B, Wigley FM (1996) Lack of association between augmentation mammoplasty and systemic sclerosis (scleroderma). Arthritis Rheum 39:1125–1131

Holt PF (1981) Transport of inhaled dust to extrapulmonary sites. J Pathol 133:123–129

Inachi S, Mizutani H, Ando Y, Shimizu M (1996) Progressive systemic sclerosis sine scleroderma which developed after exposure to epoxy resin polymerization. J Dermatol 23:344–346

Ishikawa H, Yamakage A, Tamura T et al (1982) Scleroderma induced by epoxy resins with special reference to experimental scleroderma with Bis (4-amino-3-methylcyclohexyl) methane as the probable causative agent. J UOEH 4:225–235

Ishikawa O, Warita S, Tamura A, Miyachi Y (1995) Occupational scleroderma. A 17-year follow-up study. Br J Dermatol 133:786–789

Janowsky EC, Kupper LL, Hulka BS (2000) Meta-analysis of the relation between silicone breast implants and the risk of connective tissue diseases. New Engl J Med 342:781–790

Johnson WM, Busnardo MS (1993) Silicosis following employment in the manufacture of silica flour and industrial sand. J Occup Med 35:716–719

Karlson EW, Lee I-M, Cook NR, Buring JE, Hennekens C, Bloch KJ (2001) Serologic evaluation of woman exposed to breast implants. J Rheumatol 28:1523–1530

Kettaneh A, Moufti OA, Tiev KP, Chayet C, Toledano C, Fabre B, Fardet L, Cabane J (2007) Occupational exposure to solvents and gender-related risk of systemic sclerosis: meta-analysis of case-control studies. J Rheumatol 34:97–103

Kilburn KH, Warshaw RH (1992) Prevalence of symptoms of systemic lupus erythematosus (SLE) and of fluorescent antinuclear antibodies associated with chronic exposure to trichloroethylene and other chemicals in well water. Environ Res 57:1–9

Kjoller K, Friis S, Mellenkjaer L, McLaughlin JK, Winther JF, Lipworth L, Blot WJ, Frycek J, Olsen JH (2001) Connective tissue disease and other rheumatic conditions following cosmetic breast implantation in Denmark. Arch Intern Med 161:973–979

Knight KR, Gibbons R (1987) Increased collagen synthesis and cross-link formation in the skin of rats exposed to vinyl chloride monomer. Clin Sci (Colch) 72:673–678

Koeger AC, Alcaix D, Rozenberg S, Bourgeois P (1991) Occupational exposure to silicon and dermatopolymyositis. 3 cases (in French). Ann Med Interne 142:409–413

Koeger AC, Marre JP, Rozenberg S, Gutmann L, Bourgeois P (1992) Autoimmune diseases after unusual exposure to silica or silicones. 3 cases. (in French). Ann Med Interne 143:165–170

Koeger AC, Lang T, Alcaix D, Milleron B, Rozenberg S, Chaibi P, Arnaud J, Mayaud C, Camus JP, Bourgeois P (1995) Silica-associated connective tissue disease. A study of 24 cases. Medicine (Baltimore) 74: 221–237

Kohanka V (1982) Epidemiologic studies of the delayed-type immunity in workers exposed to vinyl chloride monomers (in German). Boerg Vener Szemle 58:145–149

Lange GE, Juehe S, Veltman G (1974) Ueber das Auftreten von Angiosarkomen der Leber bei zwei Arbeitern der PVC-herstellenden Industrie. Dtsch Med Wochenschr 99:1598–1599

Lelbach WK, Marsteller HJ (1981) Vinyl chloride-associated disease. Ergeb Inn Med Kinderheilkd 47:1–110

Lockey JE, Kelly CR, Cannon GW, Colby TV, Aldrich V, Livingston GK (1987) Progressive systemic sclerosis associated with exposure to trichloroethylene. J Occup Med 29:493–496

Maitre A, Hours M, Bonneterre V (2004) Systemic sclerosis and occupational risk factors: role of solvents and cleaning products. J Rheumatol 31:2395–2401

Maricq HR (1981) Vinyl chloride disease. In: International conference on progressive systemic sclerosis, Austin, 9 Oct 1981

Maricq HR, Johnson MN, Whetstone CL, LeRoy EC (1976) Capillary abnormalities in polyvinyl chloride production workers. Examination by in vivo microscopy. JAMA 236:1368–1371

Markowitz SS, McDonald CJ, Fethiere W (1972) Occupational acroosteolysis. Arch Dermatol 106:219–233

Masi AT (1980) Preliminary criteria for the classification of systemic sclerosis. Arthritis Rheum 23:581–590

McCormic ZD, Khuder SS, Aryal BK, Ames AL, Khuder SA (2010) Occupational silica exposure as a risk factor for scleroderma: a meta-analysis. Int Arch Occup Environ Health. doi:10.1007/s00420-009-0505-7

Medsger TA, Masi AT (1971) Epidemiology of systemic sclerosis. Ann Intern Med 74:714–721

Mehlhorn J (1994) "Qarzinduzierte" Progressive Systemische Sklerodermie – Exposition, Klinische Beobachtungen, Lungenfunktion. Arbeitsmed Sozialmed Umweltmed Sonderheft 22:8–11

Mehlhorn J, Gerlach C (1990) Gemeinsames Auftreten von Silikose und Lupus erythematodes. Z Erkr Atmungsorgane 175:38–41

Mehlhorn J, Gerlach C, Ziegler V (1990) Berufsbedingte progressive systemische Sklerodermie durch ein quarzhaltiges Scheuermittel. Derm Beruf Umwelt 38:180–184

Milford WA (1976) Evidence of an immune complex disorder in vinyl chloride workers. Proc R Soc Med 69:289–291

Miyoshi K, Miyaoka T, Kobayashi Y, Itahura T, Nishijo K, Hagashitara M, Shiragami H, Ohno F (1964) Hypergammaglobulinemia by prolonged adjuvanticity in man: disorders developed after augmentation mammoplasty. Ijishimpo 2122:9–14

Moseley PL, Monick M, Hunninghake GW (1988) Divergent effects of silica on lymphocyte proliferation and immunoglobulin production. J Appl Physiol 65:350–357

Mueller G, Norpoth K, Kusters E (1978) Determination of thiodiglycolic acid in urine specimens of vinyl chloride exposed workers. Int Arch Occup Environ Health 41:199–205

Nagata C, Yoshida H, Mirbod SM, Komura Y, Fujita S, Inaba R, Iwata H, Maeda M, Shikano Y, Ichiki Y et al (1993) Cutaneous signs (Raynaud's phenomenon, sclerodactylia and edema of the hands) and hand-arm vibration exposure. Int Arch Occup Environ Health 64:587–591

Nario RC, Hubbard AK (1996) Silica exposure increases expression of pulmonary intercellular adhesion molecule-1 (ICAM-1) in C57Bl/6 mice. J Toxicol Environ Health 49:599–617

Nebe H, Lenz U (1971) Untersuchungen ueber berufliche Noxen beim Lupus erythematodes. Dermatol Monatsschr 157:500–504

Nietert PJ, Sutherland SE, Silver RM, Pandey JP, Knapp RG, Hoel DG, Dosemeci M (1998) Is occupational organic solvent exposure a risk factor for scleroderma? Arthrit Rheumat 41:1111–1118

Oghiso Y, Kubota Y (1986) Enhanced interleukin 1 production by alveolar macrophages and increase in Ia-positive lung cells in silica-exposed rats. Microbiol Immunol 30:1189–1198

Olsson AR, Skogh T, Axelson O, Wingren G (2004) Occupations and exposures in the work environment for rheumatoid arthritis. Occup Environ Med 61:233–238

Ostlere LS, Harris D, Buckley C, Black C, Rustin MH (1992) Atypical systemic sclerosis following exposure to vinyl chloride monomer. A case report and review of the cutaneous aspects of vinyl chloride disease. Clin Exp Dermatol 17:208–210

Otsuki T, Sakagchi H, Tomokuni A, Aikoh T, Matsuki T, Isozaki Y, Hyodoh F, Kawakami Y, Kusaka M, Kita S, Ueki A (2000) Detection of alternatively spliced variant messages of Fas gene and mutational screening of Fas and Fas ligand coding regions in peripheral blood mononuclear cells derived from silicosis patients. Immunol Lett 72:137–143

Otsuki T, Maeda M, Murakami S, Hayashi H, Miura Y, Kusaka M, Nakano T, Fukuoka K, Kishimoto T, Hyodoh F, Ueki A, Nishimura Y (2007) Immunological effects of silica and asbestosis. Cell Mol Immunol 4:261–268

Owens GR, Medsger TA (1988) Systemic sclerosis secondary to occupational exposure. Am J Med 85:114–116

Panaszek B, Malolepszy J, Wrzyszcz M, Jutel M, Machaj Z (1993) Mixed connective tissue disease in a male patient chronically exposed to toxic chemicals (in Polish). Pol Tyg Lek 48:430–432

Parks CG, Cooper GS, Nylander-French LA, Sanderson WT, Dement JM, Cohen PL, Dooley MA, Treadwell EL, StClair EW, Gilkeson GS, Hoppin JA, Savitz DA (2002) Occupational exposure to crystalline silica and risk of systemic lupus erythematosus. Arthritis Rheum 48:1840–1850

Parks CG, Cooper GS, Nylander-French LA, Hoppin JA, Sanderson WT, Dement JM (2004) Comparing questionaire-based methods to assess occupational silica exposure. Epidemiology 15:433–441

Penin H, Sager G, Lange GE et al (1975) Neurologisch-psychiatrische und elektroenzephalographische Befunde bei Patienten mit Vinylchlorid-Krankheit. In: Proc. 15. Jahrestagung Dt Gesellschaft Arb Med, Gentner, Stuttgart, pp 299–304

Plewig G, Kligman A (1978) Acne. Springer, Berlin/Heidelberg/New York

Poskitt LB, Duffill MB, Rademaker M (1994) Chloracne, palmoplantar keratoderma and localized scleroderma in a weed sprayer. Clin Exp Dermatol 19:264–267

Povey A, Guppy MJ, Wood M, Knight C, Black CM, Silman AJ (2001) Cytochrome P2 polymorphisms and susceptibility to scleroderma following exposure to organic solvents. Arthritis Rheum 44:662–665

Puisieux F, Hachulla E, Brouillard M, Hatron PY, Devulder B (1994) Silicosis and primary Gougerot-Sjogren syndrome (in French). Rev Med Intern 15:575–579

Reinl W (1957) Sklerodermie durch Trichloraethyleneinwirkung? Zentralbl Arbeitsmed 7:58–60

Rihs HP, Conrad K, Mehlhorn J, May-Taube K, Welticke B, Frank KH, Baur X (1994) Association between HLA-D alleles and scleroderma-specific autoantibodies in quartz dust exposed persons (in German). Z Arztl Fortbild (Jena) 88:513–518

Rihs HP, Conrad K, Mehlhorn J, May-Taube K, Welticke B, Frank KH, Baur X (1996) Molecular analysis of HLA-DPB1 alleles in idiopathic systemic sclerosis patients and uranium miners with systemic sclerosis. Int Arch Allergy Immunol 109:216–222

Rodnan GP, Benedek TG, Medsger TA, Cammarata RJ (1967) The association of progressive systemic sclerosis (scleroderma) with coal miners pneumoconiosis and other forms of silicosis. Ann Intern Med 66:323–334

Rosenman KD, Zhu Z (1995) Pneumoconiosis and associated medical conditions. Am J Ind Med 27:107–113

Rustin MHA, Bull HA, Ziegler V, Mehlhorn J, Haustein UF, Maddison PJ, James J, Dowd PM (1990) Silica-associated systemic sclerosis is clinically, serologically indistinguishable from idiopathic systemic sclerosis. Br J Dermatol 123:725–734

Saihan EM, Burton JL, Heaton KW (1978) A new syndrome with pigmentation scleroderma, gynaecomastia, Raynaud's phenomenon and neuropathy. Br J Dermatol 99:437–441

Sanchez-Roman J, Wichmann I, Salaberri J, Varela JM, Nunez-Roldan A (1993) Multiple clinical and biological autoimmune manifestations in 50 workers after occupational exposure to silica. Ann Rheum Dis 52:534–538

Schirren SM (1971) Skin lesions caused by trichloroethylene in a metal working plant. Berufsdermatosen 19:240–245

Schmidt JA, Oliver CN, Lepe-Zuniga JL, Green I, Gery I (1984) Silica-stimulated monocytes release fibroblast proliferation factors identical to interleukin 1. J Clin Invest 73:1462–1472

Siebels M, Schulz V, Andrassy K (1993) Silicosis and systemic diseases (in German). Immun Infekt 21:53–54

Siebels M, Schulz V, Andrassy K (1995) Systemic lupus erythematosus and silicosis (in German). Dtsch Med Wochenschr 120:214–218

Siegel RC (1977) Scleroderma. Med Clin North Am 61:283–296

Silman AJ, Jones S (1992) What is the contribution of occupational environmental factors to the occurrence of scleroderma in men? Ann Rheum Dis 51:1322–1324

Silver RM, Sahn EE, Allen JA, Sahn S, Greene W, Maize JC, Garen PD (1993) Demonstration of silicon in sites of connective tissue disease in patients with silicone-gel breast implants. Arch Dermatol 129:63–68

Sluis-Cremer GK, Hessel PA, Hnizdo E, Churchill AR, Zeiss EA (1985) Silica, silicosis and progressive systemic sclerosis. Br J Ind Med 42:838–843

Smith V, Vanthuyne M, Vander Cruissen B, Van Praet J, Vermeiren F, Smets H, Houssiau F, DeKeyser F (2008) Over-representaion of construction-related occupations in male patients with systemic sclerosis. Ann Rheum Dis 67:1448–1450

Sparrow GP (1977) A connective tissue disorder similar to vinyl chloride disease in a patient exposed to perchloroethylene. Clin Dermatol 2:17–22

Stachow A, Jablonska S, Skiendzielewska A (1979) Biogenic amines derived from tryptophan in systemic and cutaneous scleroderma. Acta Derm Venereol 59:1–5

Steenland K, Brown D (1995) Mortality study of gold miners exposed to silica and nonasbestiform amphibole minerals: an update with 14 more years of follow-up. Am J Ind Med 27:217–229

Struhar D, Harbeck RJ (1989) Anti-Ia antibodies inhibit the spontaneous secretion of IL-1 from silicotic rat alveolar macrophages. Immunol Lett 23:31–33

Studnicka MJ, Menzinger G, Drlicek M, Maruna H, Neumann MG (1995) Pneumoconiosis and systemic sclerosis following 10 years of exposure to polyvinyl chloride dust. Thorax 50:583–585

Suciu I, Drejman I, Valaskai M (1963) Contributii la studiul imbolnavirilor produse de clorina de vinil. Med Int 15:967–978

Szeimies RM, Lissner A, Meurer M (1992) Perchlorethylen-induzierte systemische Sklerodermie. Derm Beruf Umwelt 40:66–69

Tanaka M, Niizeki H, Shimizu S, Miyakawa S (1993) Scleroderma after exposure to domestic detergent LOC. J Rheumatol 20:1993–1994

Tashev TS, Tsonev I (1990) The connective tissue changes in patients with acute poisonings by organophosphate pesticides (in Bulgarian). Vutr Boles 29:83–87

Thorgeirsson A, Fregert S, Ramnaes O (1978) Sensitization capacity of epoxy resin oligomers in the guinea pig. Acta Derm Venereol 58:17–21

Tibon-Fisher O, Heller E, Ribak J (1992) Occupational scleroderma due to organic solvent exposure. Harefuah 122(530–532):551

Ueki H, Omori K (2001) Dscoid lupus erythematosus developing in areas where fragments of windshield glass had become embedded in the skin. Eur J Dermatol 11:127–130

Ueki A, Isozaki Y, Tomakuni A, Ueki H, Kusaka M, Tanaka S, Otsuki T, Sakaguchi H, Hyodoh F (2001) Different distribution of HLA Class II alleles in anti-topoisomerase I autoantibody responders between silicosis and systemic sclerosis patients, with a common distinct amino acid sequence in the HLA-DQB1 domain. Immunobiology 204:458–465

Varga J, Schumacher R, Jimenez SA (1989) Systemic sclerosis after augmentation mammoplasty with silicone implants. Ann Intern Med 111:377–383

Veltman G (1980) Klinische Befunde und arbeitsmedizinische Aspekte der Vinylchlorid-Krankheit. Dermatol Monatsschr 166:705–712

Vincent M, Pouchelle C, Martinon S, Gerard F, Arthaud Y (1996) Connective tissue disease due to intentional inhalation of scouring powder. Eur Respir J 9:2688–2690

Walder WB (1983) Do solvents cause scleroderma? Int J Dermatol 22:157–158

Waller PA, Clauw D, Cupps T, Metcalf JS, Silver RM, Leroy EC (1994) Fasciitis (not scleroderma) following prolonged exposure to an organic solvent. J Rheumatol 21:1567–1570

Warde WB (1903) Lupus erythematosus: some illustrative cases. Br J Dermatol 15:161–168

Wichmann I, Sanchez-Roman J, Morales J, Castillo MJ, Ocana C, Nunez-Roldan A (1996) Antimyeloperoxidase antibodies in individuals with occupational exposure to silica. Ann Rheum Dis 55:205–207

Wilson RH, McCormick WE, Tatum CF, Greech JL (1967) Occupational acroosteolysis: report of 31 cases. JAMA 201:577–580

Wu P, Hyodoh F, Hatayama T, Sakaguchi H, Hatada S, Miura Y, Takata-Tomokuni A, Katsuyama H, Otsuki T (2004) Induction of CD 69 antigen expression in peripheral blood mononuclear cells on exposure to silica, but not by asbestos/chrysotile-A. Immunol Lett 98:145–152

Xiong M, Arnett FC, Guo X, Zhou X (2008) Differential dynamic properties of scleroderma fibroblasts in response to perturbation of environmental stimuli. PLoS ONE 3(2):e1693

Yamakage A, Ishikawa H (1982) Generalized morphea-like scleroderma occurring in people exposed to organic solvents. Dermatologica 165:186–193

Yamakage A, Ishikawa H, Saito Y, Hattori A (1980) Occupational scleroderma-like disorder in men engaged in the polymerization of epoxy resins. Dermatologica 161:33–44

Yamamoto T, Furuse Y, Katayama I, Nishioka K (1994) Nodular scleroderma in a worker using a silica-containing abrasive. J Dermatol 21:751–754

Yanez-Diaz S, Moran M, Unamuno P, Armijo M (1992) Silica and trichloroethylene-induced progressive systemic sclerosis. Dermatology 184:98–102

Yang Y, Fujita J, Tokuda M, Bandoh S, Dobashi H, Okada T, Okahara M, Kishimoto T, Ishida T, Takahara J (2001) Clinical features of polymyositis/dermatomyositis associated with silicosis and review of the literature. Rheumatol Int 20:235–238

Yoshida S, Gershwin ME (1993) Autoimmunity and selected environmental factors of disease induction. Semin Arthritis Rheum 22:399–419

Zachariae H, Bjerring P, Sondergaarrd KH, Halkier-Sorensen L (1997) Arbejdsbetinget systemisk sklerodermi hos maend. Ugeskr Laeger 195:2687–2689

Ziegler V, Köpping H, Münzberger H, Haustein UF, Löschke K (1981) Arbeitsmedizinische Aspekte der progressiven Sklerodermie. Wiss Z Karl Marx Univ Leipzig 30:478–482

Ziegler V, Pampel W, Zschunke E, Münzberger H, Mährlein W, Köpping H (1982) Kristalliner Quarz – (eine) Ursache der progressiven Sklerodermie? Dermatol Monatsschr 168:398–401

Ziegler V, Haustein UF, Mehlhorn J, Münzberger H, Rennau H (1986) Quarzinduzierte Sklerodermie, sklerodermie-aehnliches Syndrom oder echte Sklerodermie? Dermatol Monatsschr 172:86–90

Ziegler V, Kipping D, Herrmann K, Haustein UF, Löschke K (1987) Quarz – seine Relevanz für die Dermatologie. Derm Beruf Umwelt 35:199–204

Ziegler V, Keyn J, Mehlhorn J, Kipping D, Haustein UF (1988) Qarznachweis in Sklerodermiehaut. Dermatol Monatsschr 174:688–689

Ziegler V, Pfeil B, Haustein UF (1991) Berufliche Quarzstaubexposition – Progressive Sklerodermie und Lupus erythematodes. Z Haut Geschlechtskr 66:968–970

Zschunke E (1976) Dermatologische Probleme in der Arbeitsmedizin. Dermatol Monatsschr 162:454–458

Zschunke E, Ziegler V, Haustein UF (1990) Occupationally induced connective tissue disorders. In: Adams RM (ed) Occupational skin disease. Saunders, Philadelphia

30 Systemic Diseases by Absorption Through the Skin

Hans Drexler
Institute and Outpatient Clinic for Occupational, Social and Environmental Medicine, Friedrich-Alexander-University, Erlangen, Germany

Core Messages

- The relevance to health of percutaneous absorption of hazardous substances is often underestimated. The transdermal absorption of hazardous substances or pharmaceuticals usually requires exposure to just a few square centimeters of skin in order to administer a effective dose to the body. Skin contamination can occur in the workplace or in the general environment. The systemic effects (acute intoxication, chronic intoxication, cancer) of substances are in principal independent of the uptake path.

1 Introduction

The relevance to health of percutaneous absorption of hazardous substances is often still underestimated. Impurities can be inhaled into the body through the respiratory tract, ingested through the gastrointestinal tract, and absorbed through the skin. But only two of these paths are monitored sensorially. The nose is as sensitive as a gas chromatograph and this enables people to avoid exposure to hazardous substances. Ingestion by the gastrointestinal tract is also sensorially controlled. However, a comparable sensory organ for absorption through the skin (percutaneous absorption) is missing as this plays a subordinate role in nature. In contamination of the skin by toxic substances, it is sometimes awareness of the danger that is absent and sometimes it is the sensory organ to notice that something is being absorbed by the skin. In addition, in percutaneous absorption, as opposed to ingestion, the first-pass effect by the liver is missing, because of which in the case of certain hazardous substances, detoxification may be held up.

The clinical significance of absorption through the skin is obvious when the effect of transdermal therapeutic systems (TTS) is studied. The transdermal absorption of systemic pharmaceuticals usually requires exposure to just a few square centimeters of skin in order to administer a pharmacologically effective dose to the body. These transdermal therapeutic systems often contain penetration enhancers to accelerate absorption. The penetration-enhancing effect is due mainly to changes in intercellular lipid layers (deformities, alterations, etc.), but interactions with desmosomes and proteins, and keratin fibers in the corneocytes or improvement in the solubility of the active substance and its distribution in the stratum corneum (keratinous layer) are equally under discussion. Dimethyl sulfoxide, fatty acid esters, tensides, essential oils, amides, and various alcohols are typical penetration-enhancing substances (Wellner et al. 2006). Taking these into consideration is therefore of particular significance, as intensive decontamination using appropriate substances is often attempted following exposure.

2 Characterization of Hazardous Substances Absorbable Through the Skin

The extent of percutaneous absorption through an intact epidermis depends on:

- The lipophilicity and water solubility of the penetrating molecule
- The molecular size and structure
- The aggregate or the concentration of the substance
- The characteristics of the skin (area of the body, skin disease, etc.)

The ability of a molecule to permeate the skin increases with its water solubility and lipophilicity and diminishes with the molecular size. Therefore, small amphiphilic molecules in particular penetrate the skin easily. These substances can be solid, liquid, or gaseous, the last one being significant when respiratory protective masks are worn. To draw attention to the danger of absorption through the skin in the workplace, substances which are absorbable through the skin are labeled as such (S = Skin, H = Haut, HUIT). The criteria for assignment of a skin notation vary however. For example, the American Conference of Governmental Industrial Hygienists in the USA uses the dermal LD50 as a criterion for assigning the notation Skin (Kennedy et al. 1993). The

T. Rustemeyer, P. Elsner, S.M. John & H.I. Maibach (eds.), *Kanerva's Occupational Dermatology*,
DOI 10.1007/978-3-642-02035-3_30, © Springer-Verlag Berlin Heidelberg 2012

problem with this is that carcinogenic and long-term effects are underestimated. When labeling a substance as absorbable through the skin, the toxic potential of the compound as well as the permeability of the skin must be considered. The German Commission for the Investigation of Health Hazards of Chemical Compounds in the Work Area labels a substance as absorbable through the skin when the skin contamination endangers the person exposed to it and when one of the following criteria is fulfilled:

Percutaneous absorption is relevant if adherence to the stipulated MAK value alone no longer gives sufficient protection against damage to health.

A substance is classified as absorbable by the skin, if one of the following criteria is fulfilled:

I. Classification on the basis of investigations in man

   Field studies or scientifically based case studies show that percutaneous absorption after contact with the substance in question is of practical relevance:

   Percutaneous absorption is without doubt responsible for part of the internal exposure and this exposure can lead to toxic effects.

II. Classification on the basis of investigations in animals

   Animal experiments were able to show percutaneous absorption and this exposure can lead to toxic effects.

III. Classification on the basis of in vitro investigations

   Relevant percutaneous absorption was quantified using recognized methods. The "flux" through the skin was determined and the permeability constant was calculated or will be calculated, or there are data available on the percentage absorption of the applied dose (percentage absorbed per unit of time and surface area).

IV. Classification on the basis of theoretical models

   Relevant percutaneous absorption can be assumed on the basis of analogy or mathematical model calculations.

   Criteria I to IV are arranged in order of importance with the data from man being the most important (Drexler 1998). About one third of all substances are classified as absorbable through the skin according to these criteria.

3 Dermal Exposure

Skin contamination can occur in the workplace or in the general environment as the result of an accident, for example, when the skin or clothing is contaminated by leakage from a container or explosion of a substance which is absorbable through the skin. Large-scale contamination is more easily noticed than small-scale contamination, as from a splash.

The danger of contamination and absorption through the skin always exists where skin-absorbable substances are employed. Skin contact can occur directly, for example, from a splash, an aerosol, seepage through clothing, or result indirectly from soiled clothing or contaminated surfaces. The extent of the skin contact is established by measuring the area of the body part involved and the frequency and intensity of the contact. The duration of the skin contact and the frequency is also significant. The fact that the skin forms a depot for many foreign substances allowing percutaneous absorption to take place hours after the contamination and that the highest internal doses develop after a time lapse is also significant. Furthermore, a series of physical and chemical factors can change the condition of the skin and thus influence percutaneous absorption. In addition, the simultaneous impact of substances or preparations, which damage the skin directly (corrosive, sensitizing, or an irritant), increases the percutaneous absorption of systemically active substances. Moreover, during or following an activity, which empirically causes microlesions to the skin, increased absorption through the skin must be assumed. Where there is simultaneous or previous damage to the skin by substances which influence the structure of the skin, there is also increased danger, as loss of skin integrity favors increased absorption. This also includes solvents such as acetone, methanol, diethyl ether, and hexane. Detergents such as soap can also destroy the integrity of the skin and act as an absorption promoter. Raising the epidermal water content can cause swelling of the corneal layer of the skin, which also favors percutaneous absorption of substances (occlusion). Wearing gloves can lead to direct skin contact of the allegedly protected areas, firstly because of permeation through the glove material and secondly because of the collection of perspiration and liquid substances from unprotected areas, for example, sweat from uncovered lower arms and the parts of the arm inside the gloves. Therefore, increased dermal penetration must be taken into account under such occlusive circumstances. The protective effect of any gloves used must be checked carefully before they are recommended. Where substances which enhance blood circulation are being used, there is a simultaneous local effect so it must also be assumed that there is an increased health hazard.

In addition to accidental or operational contamination, there is also intentional contamination of the skin with substances which are absorbable through the skin.

The use of cosmetics and transdermal therapeutic systems and the military deployment of warfare agents in particular must be mentioned here.

4 Systemic Illnesses Following Percutaneous Absorption

The systemic effect of a substance is in principal independent of the uptake path, with the exception that when it is ingested, the first-pass effect takes place in the liver, which can lead to either poisoning or detoxification of the substance. When inhaled, the foreign substances enter the systemic circulation quickly and are therefore not metabolized immediately. In percutaneous absorption, metabolism can take place in the skin like in the liver. The skin is a metabolically active organ like the liver, but the enzyme activity is lower.

In acute intoxication, the uptake path can often be unequivocally described, for example, absorption primarily through the skin or primarily inhaled. In the case of chronic intoxication or cancer, simultaneous inhalation and absorption through the skin can generally be surmised as particles of the dangerous substance can also be detected in the breath. Even in purely airborne exposure, percutaneous absorption is paramount, that is, the gaseous substance is absorbed into the body more through the skin than through the lungs (Johanson and Boman 1991; Bader et al. 2008).

If absorption through the skin could have been the cause of the illness, then whether the symptoms of the illness fit the toxic profile of the substance in question and whether the substance is able to penetrate the skin to a sufficient extent must be proved first of all. Systemic illnesses are shown as examples of percutaneous absorption below.

5 Systemic Illnesses from Percutaneous Absorption

5.1 Acute Intoxication Following Dermal Absorption in an Industrial Accident

N,N-Dimethylformamide is an organic solvent which is produced in large quantities worldwide. It is used industrially as a solvent, a chemical intermediate, and an additive. In many cases, dermal exposure happened accidentally to workers when their clothes were soaked with dimethylformamide due to a technical fault. Within hours, the affected workers developed abdominal pain as the first sign of toxic hepatitis. They also suffered from dizziness, nausea, anorexia, vomiting, and alcohol intolerance. Liver dysfunction was proven in the clinical laboratory. The affected persons recovered within 2–3 weeks (IPCS 1991). Dimethylformamide is absorbed almost completely through intact skin, so the high internal contamination, which caused the clinical symptoms, was absorbed primarily through the skin. The impairment of liver metabolism and alcohol intolerance are the typical symptoms of intoxication with dimethylformamide (Schaller and Drexler 1995).

5.2 Acute Intoxication by Percutaneous Absorption Due to Inadequate Safety Procedures

Many pesticides, primarily the organophosphates, penetrate human skin quickly. Poisoning by pesticides frequently affects agricultural workers, particularly in Third World countries. Poisoning through percutaneous absorption of pesticides is a major health problem in these countries (Kesavachandran et al. 2009). The danger of percutaneous absorption of pesticides, which are not being used professionally, is not sufficiently heeded, as the following casuistry from Wu and Deng (2009) shows. A 54-year-old man treated his dog with trichlorfon. Trichlorfon is used as an insecticide in agriculture, veterinary medicine, and in the household. The dog was supposed to be cleared of parasites. Half an hour after the treatment, the dog died. The description of the symptoms indicated acetylcholinesterase poisoning. The man suffered from cramping stomach pains. A little later, he developed severe nausea, vomiting, shivering, a high temperature, and cold sweats. This was followed by hemolysis with renal impairment.

5.3 Acute Intoxication Following Intentional Application to the Skin

Intentional contamination of the skin with skin-absorbable hazardous substances can happen during military action. Warfare agents such as the organophosphorus compound "VX" are viscous fluids with low vapor pressure whose preferred uptake path is through the skin. In transdermal therapeutic systems, the percutaneous introduction of foreign substances leads to effects which are pharmacologically desired.

Cosmetics too can contain substances which are absorbed through the skin. Of particular toxicological significance with ensuing clinically obvious intoxication are preparations for external use which contain mercury.

Mercury preparations have been applied to the skin for almost 500 years in order to bleach it. A raised level of mercury contamination is detectable in the user (Sin and Tsang 2003). Used correctly, concentrations which would cause acute intoxication are never reached. If there has been an error during manufacturing however, where too high a concentration was used, lethal doses of mercury can be absorbed percutaneously. A 77-year-old woman used a gel on her breast to treat eczema. This gel contained a high concentration of mercury bromide. Due to an error in the manufacture of the preparation, mercury bromide was used instead of talcum powder. Two days into the treatment with the product, clinical intoxication manifested itself. Locally the skin became necrotic and retention of urine resulted from acute renal failure. The patient was disoriented and agitated. Four days after admission to hospital, an extremely high level of mercury was detected in the blood (4,836 mg/l, which corresponds to about 1,000 times the concentration of mercury normally found). Despite hemodialysis, the patient died 7 days later (Triunfante et al. 2009).

6 Chronic Intoxication Following Accidental Exposure

A 48-year-old professor of chemistry was admitted to the hospital complaining of increasing loss of balance, uncertain gait, and speech disorder. She had lost 6.8 kg weight within 2 months without dieting. The patient remembered that 5 months prior to hospitalization, while working in the laboratory, transferring dimethylmercury from a container to a capillary tube using a pipette, she got a few drops of the liquid on the back of her hand which was protected by a latex glove. She said that she had removed the drops and changed the protective gloves. The neurological symptoms were paramount. Otherwise, she appeared healthy. The routine blood counts were within normal parameters. Because of the history of potential methyl mercury contamination, blood and urine were tested for mercury. One hundred and fifty-four days after the contamination, a concentration of over 1,000 μg/l mercury was still detectable. Despite intensive treatment including using a chelating agent to accelerate the elimination of the mercury, the neurological symptoms were clinically progressive. The patient died 298 days after this single contamination. A postmortem showed 1,000 times the normal concentration of mercury in the brain. Organic metallic compounds such as dimethylmercury are able to penetrate the blood-brain barrier relatively well. The resulting mercury ions released intracerebrally do not penetrate the blood-brain barrier well, so that even after a single contamination, chronic intracerebral contamination results (Nierenberg et al. 1998).

7 Chronic Intoxication by Dermal Absorption When Handling Skin-Absorbable Substances

If a worker falls ill years after contact with a skin-absorbable substance, then generally speaking contamination through the skin and the lungs has taken place. Compounds with low vapor pressure can be inhaled as dust-borne particles and thus contribute to toxic contamination. There are however several substances, particularly those with low vapor pressure or solid substances, whose absorption through the skin is paramount in causing internal contamination. Dinitrobenzene, for example, has been used in munitions manufacturing since the nineteenth century and leads repeatedly to intoxication. Poisoning takes place predominantly by absorption through the skin (soiled clothing and dusty skin). The known spectrum of intoxication extends from discomfort, loss of appetite, gastrointestinal disorders, severe headaches, and anemia to irreparable damage resulting in death.

8 Cancer Caused Through Dermal Absorption When Handling Skin-Absorbable Carcinogens

Cancer occurs mostly after many years of latency. Establishing facts about the exposure, which caused the cancer, retrospectively, is exceedingly difficult. If records quantifying the contamination by hazardous substances exist at all, they concern primarily air monitoring. In epidemiological studies, therefore, the cancer risk of a product is calculated from the air concentration (in mg/m^3 or ppm) and the duration of exposure in years. Only in recent years has the additional absorption through the skin, which contributes significantly to internal contamination and thus to the cause of cancer, been taken into consideration. This is demonstrated by two examples of carcinogenic substances relevant to industrial medicine.

Aromatic amines are a group of chemicals used in a variety of ways as a base or intermediate product, particularly in the manufacture of dyes, pigments, and insecticides. Several exponents have been identified as human carcinogens. The main organ affected by the carcinogenic effect of aromatic amines on humans is the urinary bladder.

Aromatic amines have a low vapor pressure and penetrate the skin easily. The extent of absorption through the skin is influenced by the condition of the skin. A field study proved that persons with a damaged skin barrier caused by skin disease or workers who used skin creams at work, had a raised internal contamination (Korinth et al. 2007). Acceleration of the penetration of aromatic amines could – experimentally – be affected by using hand cream (Wellner et al. 2008). Therefore, when an investigation to establish the cause of a carcinoma of the bladder is carried out, and it concentrates solely on air contamination, the occupational hazard is significantly underestimated. The significance of absorption through the skin in occupational carcinoma of the bladder caused by aromatic amines has been acknowledged for a long time and is generally accepted.

In the case of substances with a high vapor pressure, generally only the inhaled contamination is taken into consideration. Benzene is a hemotoxic solvent and causes malignant disease of the blood formation system. The connection between exposure to benzene and leukemia has been known since the beginning of the twentieth century. In addition, exposure to benzene is regarded as a cause of malignant non-Hodgkin's lymphoma (NHL). There are several epidemiological studies in existence in which this risk has been proven. The logging of the exposure is always carried out using the results of air monitoring, formation of the product, and duration of the exposure (known as ppm years). Taking dermal exposure into consideration, therefore, would appear to be very important, not only for retrospective estimation after the illness has broken out, but also because it is of major significance in prevention.

The significance of the absorption of benzene through the skin is controversial (Nies and Korinth 2008). It is agreed that benzene can penetrate the skin even though inhalation is usually clinically more relevant. Absorption through the skin from the atmosphere however plays a subordinate role when respiratory protection is worn. Percutaneous absorption is of significance, however, where there has been direct skin contact. Direct skin contact with liquid benzene or benzene mixtures can occur when painters or car mechanics clean their hands of oil by using benzene or when they have contact with work pieces which are wet with benzene (e.g., when servicing cars or planes). Indirect contact with liquid benzene occurs when clothing or gloves are wet with benzene. As opposed to percutaneous absorption from the atmosphere, percutaneous absorption on direct skin contact can no longer be ignored. In an estimation of exposure, it was shown that 3-minute handwashing with an organic solvent containing 0.5% benzene, contaminates the body with benzene to the same extent as 8 h inhaling air with an average benzene concentration of 0.05 mg/m^3 in the air breathed (Nies et al. 2005).

References

Bader M, Wrbitzky R, Blaszkewicz M, Schäper M, van Thriel C (2008) Human volunteer study on the inhalational and dermal absorption of N-methyl-2-pyrrolidone (NMP) from the vapour phase. Arch Toxicol 82(1):13–20

Drexler H (1998) Assignment of the skin notation for MAK values and its legal consequences in Germany. Int Arch Occup Environm Health 71:503–505

IPCS (1991) Environmental health criteria 114 dimethylformamid. WHO, Geneva

Johanson G, Boman A (1991) Percutaneous absorption of 2-butoxyethanol vapour in human subjects. Br J Ind Med 48:788–792

Kennedy GL, Brock JW Jr, Banerjee AK (1993) Assignment of skin notation for threshold limit values chemicals based on acute dermal toxicity. Appl Occup Environ Hyg 8:26–30

Kesavachandran CN, Fareed M, Pathak MK, Bihari V, Mathur N, Srivastava AK (2009) Adverse health effects of pesticides in agrarian populations of developing countries. Rev Environ Contam Toxicol 200:33–52

Korinth G, Weiss T, Penkert S, Schaller KH, Angerer J, Drexler H (2007) Percutaneous absorption of aromatic amines in rubber industry workers: impact of impaired skin and skin barrier creams. Occup Environ Med 64:366–372

Nierenberg DW, Nordgren RE, Chang MB, Siegler RW, Blayney MB, Hochberg F, Toribara TY, Cernichiari E, Clarkson T (1998) Delayed cerebellar disease and death after accidental exposure to dimethylmercury. N Engl J Med 338(23):1672–1676

Nies E, Korinth G (2008) Commentary on "Penetration of benzene, toluene and xylenes contained in gasolines through human adominal skin in vitro". Toxicol In Vitro 21:275–277

Nies E, Barrot R, Drexler H, Hallier E, Kalberlah F, Prager HM, Schaller KH, Westphal G, Korinth G (2005) Perkutane aufnahme von benzol – folgerungen für die retrospektive expositionsabschätzung. Arbeitsmed Sozialmed Umweltmed 40:585–594

Schaller KH, Drexler H (1995) N, N-Dimethylformamid. In: Greim H, Lehnert G (eds) Biological exposure values for occupational toxicants and cancerogene, vol 2. VCH, Weinheim, pp 51–57

Sin KW, Tsang HF (2003) Large-scale mercury exposure due to a cream cosmetic: community-wide case series. Hong Kong Med J 9(5):329–334

Triunfante P, Soares ME, Santos A, Tavares S, Carmo H, de Lourdes Bastos M (2009) Mercury fatal intoxication: two case reports. Forensic Sci Int 184(1–3):e1–e6

Wellner T, Göen TH, Drexler H (2006) Systemische therapie durch dermale applikation: transdermale therapeutische systeme (TTS). Dermatologie Beruf Umwelt 54:13–18

Wellner T, Lüersen L, Schaller KH, Angerer J, Drexler H, Korinth G (2008) Percutaneous absorption of aromatic amines – a contribution for human health risk assessment. Food Chem Toxicol 46(6):1960–1968

Wu ML, Deng JF (2009) Acute hemolysis caused by incidental trichlorofon exposure. J Chin Med Assoc 72(4):214–218

31 Occupational and Environmental Acne

Penpun Wattanakrai[1] · *James S. Taylor*[2]
[1]Division of Dermatology, Department of Medicine, Mahidol University, Ramathibodi Hospital, Bangkok, Thailand
[2]Department of Dermatology, Desk A-61, Dermatology-Plastic Surgery Institute Cleveland Clinic, Cleveland, OH, USA

Core Messages

- Occupational and environmental acne includes oil acne, coal-tar and pitch acne, acne cosmetica, acne aestivalis (from sun), acne mechanica, tropical acne, and chloracne.
- Chloracne is a refractory acneiform eruption clinically characterized by comedones and straw-colored cysts. The comedones predominantly affect the malar region of the cheek and the retroauricular areas.
- Although chloracne is rare, it is a sensitive indicator of chemical exposure to certain polyaromatic halogenated hydrocarbons and may be associated with internal poisoning that should be recognized by physicians treating occupational skin disease.
- Patients with the cutaneous manifestations of chloracne should be carefully investigated for systemic complications (such as hepatic, ophthalmic, neurologic, lipoprotein, and endocrine abnormalities).

1 Introduction

Occupational and environmental acne is a variety of acne venenata, resulting from various chemical exposures and from a variety of environmental, physical, and mechanical factors, usually encountered in the workplace but occasionally seen in nonoccupational settings. The eruption may be mild, involving localized exposure or covered areas of the body, or severe, explosive and disseminated with the involvement of almost every follicular orifice. Additionally, chloracne almost always represents a cutaneous sign of systemic exposure to highly toxic chemicals. Occupational and environmental acne comprises oil acne, coal-tar and pitch acne, acne cosmetica, acne aestivalis (from sun), acne mechanica, tropical acne, drug-induced acne, and chloracne (➋ *Table 31.1*). This listing serves as a useful paradigm and includes the most common causes of occupational and environmental acne.

2 Oil Acne

Oil acne or oil folliculitis is the most common form of occupational acne and consists of numerous follicular papules and pustules occurring in areas with heavy oil exposure, such as the thighs and forearms. Oil acne is most commonly observed in workers employed in the machine tooling trades. Other workers likely to be affected may include machinists, auto, airplane and truck mechanics, roofers, oil well drillers, petroleum refiners, rubber workers, textile mill workers, and road pavers. The incidence of oil acne has declined in recent years because of decreased use of pure cutting oils and improved industrial and personal hygiene practices (Kokelj 1992).

Cutting oils, especially insoluble (straight) oils, and semisynthetic coolants have been the most commonly incriminated oil acnegens (Taylor 1987). In mechanics, prolonged exposure to grease, lubricating oils, and kerosene may induce oil acne (Upreti et al. 1989). An anecdotal report of acne observed in young fast-food workers exposed to grease and fat while frying hamburgers has been termed "McDonald's acne" (Litt 1974), although there is no other evidence that this is a separate entity.

Prolonged oil exposure produces a reactive follicular hyperkeratosis and results in sebum retention. This manifests clinically as multiple open comedones, inflammatory folliculitis, and microcystic lesions caused by the oil itself. Lesions are distributed primarily over exposed areas, such as the dorsal hands and extensor forearms. Oil-soaked clothing may produce lesions on the thighs, lower abdomen, and buttocks (Kokelj 1992). The face may be involved from wiping the brow with an oil-contaminated sleeve. Although the lesions are commonly referred to as oil boils, they usually do not develop from bacteria present in the oils (Taylor 1986). The inflammatory lesions, larger furuncular and carbuncular lesions may form, are more prominent than in chloracne and may mimic conglobate cystic acne.

T. Rustemeyer, P. Elsner, S.M. John & H.I. Maibach (eds.), *Kanerva's Occupational Dermatology*,
DOI 10.1007/978-3-642-02035-3_31,

Table 31.1
List of types and etiologies of occupational and environmental acne

Type	Etiology	Occupations/other sources
Oil acne	Cutting oils, semisynthetic coolants, grease, fat, lubricating oils and kerosene	Machinists working with oil-based cutting fluids; auto, airplane and truck mechanics; roofers; oil well drillers; petroleum refiners; rubber workers; textile mill workers; and road pavers
Pitch/coal-tar acne	Coal-tar oils, creosote and pitch	Coal-tar plant, road maintenance and construction workers; roofers
Cosmetic acne	Greasy, oily makeup or grooming substances, pomade	Actors, actresses, models, and cosmetologists
Acne aestivalis	Sun exposure; ultraviolet and fluorescent lighting; and ionizing radiation	Performing artists; occupations with heavy sun exposure; and those who work under florescent lighting
Acne mechanica	Pressure; friction on dependent areas; repeated or prolonged physical insults to the skin; and tight fitting work clothes	Truck drivers; professional/amateur athletes; fiddlers/violinists; those who wear face masks, hats or helmets and use telephones
Tropical acne	Hot or humid environments	Soldiers stationed in tropical climates
Drug-induced acne	Anabolic steroids (e.g., danazol, testosterone); corticosteroids, corticotropin, phenytoin, lithium, isoniazid, iodides, bromides, and epidermal growth factor receptor (EGFR) inhibitors	Exposure to certain medications, supplements or medical procedures
Chloracne	Specific halogenated aromatic hydrocarbons; wood preservatives, herbicides, and pesticides; pollutants of industrial production processes and during waste incineration	Chemical production workers; manufacture of pesticides and wood preservatives

Acquired perforating (transepidermal elimination) disease has been reported in oil field workers exposed to drilling fluids. The fluids contain many additives, including calcium chloride. Histopathologic examination revealed transepidermal elimination of calcium with minimal involvement of hair follicles (Knox et al. 1986).

Oil acne is treated with the usual acne vulgaris modalities, such as topical benzoyl peroxide and retinoic acid. Systemic treatment is often needed with tetracycline, erythromycin or minocycline, or with isotretinoin in severe cases. The key factor is avoiding contact with oils and grease and the practice of good hygiene. Work clothes should be changed daily and frequent cleansing of the skin with soap and water is advised.

3 Pitch or Coal-Tar Acne

Coal-tar oils, creosote and pitch can produce a comedonal type of acne, which shows a predilection for exposed areas, particularly the malar regions (Bartolini 1989) and periorbital areas in individuals exposed to pitch tar (Adams et al. 2000). Coal-tar plant workers, roofers, road maintenance workers, and construction workers are among those at risk. Coal-tar derivatives have been reported to be not only acnegenic, but also carcinogenic and photosensitizing (Adams et al. 2000). Therefore coal-tar acne may be complicated by phototoxic reactions affecting both the skin and the eyes and resulting in hyperpigmentation known as coal-tar melanosis. Late complications include the development of pitch and tar papillomas, keratoses, and acanthomas (Taylor 1987). Pitch acne responds to treatment much better than chloracne. Prevention of pitch acne includes showers and available cleansers at work facilities, clean uniforms, protective coverings, and exhaust ventilation systems (Adams et al. 2000).

4 Acne Cosmetica

In 1972, Kligman and Mills described acne cosmetica consisting chiefly of small, scattered comedones occurring mainly in women in the age range 20–50 years. These women, who were using a variety of cosmetics for prolonged periods of time, developed comedonal lesions exclusively on the face, predominantly on the chin.

Acne cosmetica may develop in actors and models who are often required to wear heavy, greasy makeup; cosmetologists may also be affected (Kligman and Mills 1972). Acne cosmetica consists of essentially noninflammatory, small, closed comedones and a few intermittent papules, and pustules. When superimposed upon acne vulgaris, the clinical picture may be obscured (Kligman and Mills 1972).

Animal models were originally used to determine the comedogenic potential of raw materials with the assumption that finished formulations containing these ingredients would also be comedogenic. Cosmetic ingredients found experimentally to be comedogenic include : isopropyl palmitate, isopropyl myristate, butyl stearate, isopropyl isostearate, decyl oleate, isostearyl neopentanoate, isocetyl stearate, myristle myristate, cocoa butter, cetyl alcohol, paraffin, stearyl alcohol, sodium lauryl sulfate (SLS), and petrolatum (Nguyen et al. 2007). Despite the fact that finished products using comedogenic ingredients are not necessarily comedogenic (Draelos and DiNardo 2006) many of these substances are avoided or modified by cosmetic manufacturers and cosmetics are frequently advertised as noncomedogenic.

Acneiform eruptions with predominantly deep-seated nodules and a few comedones situated mainly on the cheeks can occur after facial massage beauty treatment. This eruption is unlike classic acne cosmetica in being inflammatory, indolent, and often occurring a few weeks after facial massage (Khanna and Gupta 1999).

5 Acne Aestivalis (Mallorca Acne)

Acne aestivalis is a rare, infrequently described, generally, nonoccupational eruption, which can also affect performing artists. Typically, it affects women in the age range of 25–40 years and involves the cheeks, sides of the neck, chest, shoulders, and upper arms. Typical lesions are monomorphic popular, round, hard, and small lesions reported to develop after sun exposure. Comedones and pustules are absent or scarce. Lesions involute in the fall without scar formation.

The eruption is due to sun exposure, ultraviolet radiation, mainly UVA, and florescent light exposure (Plewig and Jansen 1998; Zugerman 1990). PUVA therapy and ionizing radiation are also potentially acnegenic. Acne aestivalis responds to topical retinoic acid or benzoyl peroxide but not to antibiotics (Hjorth et al. 1972). Prophylactic treatment has been reported by gradually increasing exposure to artificial UV radiation (UVB, UVA or PUVA) prior to the first exposure to natural sunlight (Plewig and Jansen 1998).

Actinic follicuitis a rare photodermatosis presenting with recurrent pustular facial eruptions, typically appearing 4–6 h after exposure to sunlight falls into the same spectrum as acne aestivalis and actinic superficial folliculitis (Veysey and George 2005).

6 Acne Mechanica

In 1975, Mills and Kligman defined acne mechanica as a process in which mechanical factors such as pressure, occlusion, friction, rubbing, or heat provoke acne lesions by inducing the rupture of microcomedones. Repeated or prolonged physical insults to the skin may produce an acneiform eruption that can be strikingly inflammatory in nature. An example is the local pressure and rubbing against seat covers which occurs in truck drivers. Acne mechanica is specifically related to sporting activities. Occupational causes of acne mechanica include the use of face masks (as in hospital workers or clean-room workers in the semiconductor industry), belts, straps, tight-fitting work clothing, football shoulder pads, football helmets, hats, and telephones (Mills and Kligman 1975). Fiddler's neck (Brun and Baran 1984) and violinists neck is also a variant of acne mechanica (Omohundro and Taylor 1998).

Clinically, crops of inflammatory papules and pustules appear in affected areas of skin. Deep, inflammatory nodules may result from prolonged pressure. It has been emphasized that acne mechanica is a complication of acne vulgaris and that external physical forces merely exacerbate the underlying disease focally (Mills and Kligman 1975). Improvement of mechanical acne may occur promptly after removing the source of mechanical and physical factors. Skin washing and use of topical cleansing agents may reduce the risk of acne mechanica.

7 Tropical Acne

Tropical acne may result from exposure to excessively hot or humid environments and, when such exposure is required in the performance of the patient's job, may be considered to be a form of occupational acne. Tropical acne has been observed most commonly in soldiers stationed in tropical climates, but variants may result from chronic exposure to other hot and/or humid environments as can be found in foundries (Mathias 1994).

Onset is explosive in nature and typically occurs several months after entering the hot, humid environment.

This is a severely inflammatory condition, with the development of papules, pustules, nodules, and draining sinuses as in acne conglobata. Patients often feel quite ill, and acute-phase reactants may be elevated. There is characteristic involvement of the buttocks and upper thighs, but lesions may be extensive, with the neck, arms, and trunk being affected. The face is usually spared (Sperling 1994).

Cultures have not identified a consistent pathogen, and the role of bacterial infection is felt to be unimportant. Antibiotic therapy is without significant benefit. The only effective therapeutic measure is to remove the patient from the precipitating environment (Sperling 1994).

8 Drug-Induced Acne

Eruptive acneiform lesions or acneiform folliculitis can be seen as a side effect of medications, commonly known including: anabolic steroids (e.g., danazol, testosterone), corticosteroids, corticotropin, phenytoin, lithium, isoniazid, iodides, and bromides. Less often, azathioprine, cyclosporine, tetracyclines, vitamins B1, B6, B12, and D2, phenobarbital, PUVA, propylthiouracil, disulfiram, or quinidine have been incriminated. Clinically drug-induced acne presents as an abrupt, monomorphous eruption of inflammatory papules and pustules in contrast to the heterogeneous morphology of lesions of acne vulgaris (Zaenglein and Thiboutot 2008).

The inhibitors of the epidermal growth factor receptor (EGFR) erlotinib, cetuximab, and panitumumab are well-known to induce head and neck acneiform folliculitis (Osio et al. 2009). This acneiform "EGFR-inhibitor like" cutaneous side effect has also been reported with other drugs including the tyrosine kinase inhibitor imatinib mesylate (Demirci et al. 2010; Martín et al. 2006), sirolimus, thalidomide, and lenalidomide (Michot et al. 2010).

9 Chloracne

Chloracne is an acneiform dermatosis, often refractory to treatment, which results from environmental exposure to certain halogenated aromatic hydrocarbons. It is characterized by comedones with pale yellow cysts predominantly affecting the malar region of the cheek and the retroauricular areas. In more severe cases, lesions may spread to the trunk and genitalia and inflammatory lesions are found. Skin involvement in chloracne is considered one of the most sensitive indicators of biological response to these chemicals and it occurs regardless of whether chemical exposure has occurred via skin contact – the usual route, inhalation, or ingestion (Crow and Puhvel 1991).

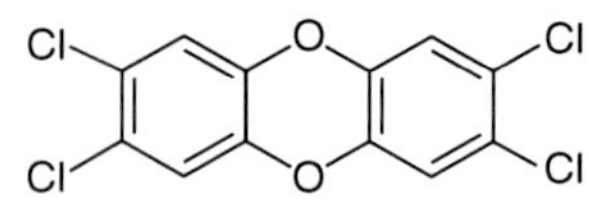

Fig. 31.1
2,3,7,8-tetrachlorodibenzo-*p*-dioxin (TCDD) – a halogenated aromatic compound – is highly toxic and causes chloracne

Chloracne was first reported by Von Bettman in 1897. In (Herxheimer 1899) used the term chloracne to describe four cases of severe acne resulting from environmental contact with electrolytically produced potassium hypochlorite. Since that time, various chloracnegenic chemicals have been identified. Chloronapthalenes and polychlorinated biphenyls (PCBs) were the causative agents in the pre-World-War-II era. Since then, trace contaminants formed during the manufacture of PCBs and other polyhalogenatcd compounds, especially herbicides and insecticides, have been the major causes of chloracne. These include polyhalogenated dibenzofurans, polychlorinated dibenzo-*p*-dioxins, and chlorinated phenols, azo- and azoxy benzenes.

When it occurs, chloracne tends to be sporadic. It is caused primarily by exposure to chloracnegenic agents in industrial or agricultural settings. Chloracne has also been caused by nonoccupational exposures via accidental environmental pollutions and in food contaminations. A decreasing incidence of chloracne may be attributed to the advent of plastics, the substitution of chlorinated hydrocarbons with synthetic resins and the restriction of the use of polychlorinated biphenyls to only closed-system formulations (Kokelj 1992). However, the recent attempt to poison Ukrainian president, Viktor Yushenko with dioxins in 2004 raised the public attention regarding these toxic chemicals (Sterling and Hanke 2005; Sorg et al. 2009).

Chloracnegenic compounds are structurally similar (Table 31.1), sharing relative molecular planarity and containing two benzene rings with halogen atoms occupying at least three of the lateral ring positions. The degree of halogenation does not necessarily determine toxicity, whereas the position of halogen atoms on the outside of the molecule seems to be crucial as reduced biological activity results from halogen substitution into positions that lead to molecular nonplanarity (Crow 1981; Kokelj 1992). The main groups of chloracnegens include dioxins, naphthalenes, biphenyls, dibenzofurans, azobenzenes, and azoxybenzenes, with the chloracnegenic potential being closely correlated with the potential to induce the enzyme aryl hydrocarbon hydroxylase (Poland et al. 1976).

9.1 Chloracne-Producing Chemicals and Sources of Exposure

Table 31.2 classifies the chemical causes of chloracne. Of related interest, *Table 31.3* provides a partial list of past and present sources of the various chloracnegens. The majority of chloracne cases have resulted from occupational exposure during chemical manufacturing or rarely from end-product use.

Table 31.2
Chloracne-producing chemicals

Polyhalogenated naphthalenes:[a]
Polychloronaphthalenes
Polybromonaphthalenes[b,c]
Polyhalogenated biphenyls:
Polychlorobiphenyls (PCBs)
Polybromodiphenyls (PBBs)
Polyhalogenated dibenzofurans:[a]
Polychlorodibenzofurans, especially tri-, tetra-, penta- and hexachlorodibenzofuran
Polybromodibenzofurans, especially tetrabromodibenzofuran
Contaminants of polychlorophenol compounds, especially Herbicides (2,4,5-T and pentachlorophenol) and herbicide intermediates (2,4,5-trichlorophenol):
2,3,7,8-Tetrachlorodibenzo-*p*-dioxin (TCDD)
Hexachlorodibenzo-*p*-doxin
Tetrachlorodibenzofuran
Contaminants of 3,4-dichloroaniline and related herbicides:
3,4,3,4,-Tetrachloroazoxybenzene (TCAOB)
3,4,3,4-Tetrachloroazobenzene (TCAB)
Other:
Dihydrotrifluoromethylphenylbenzothipyrazolone (Sceeri et al. 1995)
1,2,3,4-Tetrachlorobenzene (experimental)
Dichlobenil, a herbicide (clinical only)
DDT (crude trichlorobenzene)
Triazoloquinoxalines; most recent chloracnegens (Gawkrodger et al. 2009)

[a]The polychlorodibenzofurans and hexachlonaphthalenes may occur as contaminants in some PCBs
[b]The polybromonaphthalenes may occur as contaminants in some PBBs
[c]Not confirmed as chloracnegens

9.2 Occupational Exposure

Selected outbreaks will be discussed as classified by chemical cause.

9.2.1 Dioxins

Polychlorinated dibenzo-p-dioxins (PCDDs), commonly known as *dioxins*, are produced as byproduct pollutants of manufacturing processes that utilize chlorine, such as in the manufacturing of herbicides, paper, and pulp bleaching; in industrial production processes and during incineration (e.g., of waste). High levels of dioxins are also emitted from metallurgical industries including copper smelters, electric furnaces in steel mills, and wire reclamation incinerators. Trace levels are detectable in emissions from motor vehicles using leaded gasoline or diesel fuel, in forest fires, and in residential wood burning. These

Table 31.3
Partial list of past and present sources of chloracnegens

Chloracnegen	Source
Polychloronaphthalenes	Electrical insulators; fire-resistant materials; Wood preservative; boat hull coatings (antimagnetic properties); and high-pressure additives for lubricants
Polychlorobiphenyls (PCBs)	Hydraulic fluids; plastics; adhesives; fire retardants in transformers; and sealants
Polychlorodibenzofurans (PCDFs)	Contaminants of PCBs and various chlorinated phenols
Polyclorinated phenols, Pentachlorophenols (PCP)	Wood preservatives; leather; paper industry applications; herbicides; pesticides; fungicides; algicides; insecticides; and disinfectants
Dioxins	Contaminant of agent orange, formed during production of chlorinated organic solvents (hexachlorophene and the herbicide 2,4,5,-T); and products of combustion
Azo- and azoxybenzenes	Herbicide intermediates
Triazoloquinoxalines	Intermediates discovered during novel drug synthesis by pharmaceutical discovery chemists

chemicals are extremely stable in the environment, are highly lipophilic and accumulate in animal fat and plant tissues (Mukerjee 1998; Pelclova et al. 2006). Dioxins contaminate polychlorophenols, especially the herbicides 2,4,5-T and pentachlorophenol (PCP) and herbicide intermediates (2,4,5-trichlorophenol).

Of the hundreds of dioxins, *2,3,7,8-tetrachlorodibenzo-p-dioxin* (*TCDD*) is the paradigm for chemicals causing chloracne and also for the biological importance of trace industrial contaminants. TCDD is one of the most toxic small molecules known to man. It is also one of the best-studied toxic chemicals, largely after intense scrutiny over its use as the main component in the herbicide Agent Orange used during the Vietnam War to clear vegetation and expose the enemy. The elimination half-life of 2,3,7,8-tetrachlorodibenzo-p-dioxin (TCDD) in humans is approximately 7–11 years (Mukerjee 1998). TCDD currently serves no commercial purpose. Pure TCDD must be manufactured in a laboratory. It is made in labs in Europe, Russia, and the United States for use as a control for measuring dioxin levels (Sterling and Hanke 2005).

In 1949, the first descriptions of human exposure to 2,3,7,8-tetrachlorodibenzo-*p*-dioxin (2,3,7,8-TCDD)-contaminated chemicals were reported after a trichlorophenol reactor explosion in Nitro, West Virginia, Unites State (Sweeney and Mocarelli 2000). More than 20 outbreaks of dioxin chloracne, as well as its other health effects, have been reviewed (Taylor et al. 1977; Tindall 1985; Mukerjee 1998). Follow-up studies have shown persistence of chloracne up to 20 years from the exposure (Baccarelli et al. 2005). These studies identified an increased risk of soft-tissue sarcoma from end-product use in Sweden, occupational exposure in the Unites States and nonoccupational environmental exposure in Seveso, Italy. Although these conclusions are controversial, the International Agency for Research on Cancer has concluded that TCDD is a human carcinogen (Mukerjee 1998).

Occupational exposures to TCDD in herbicide and chemical plants were much greater than from most other nonoccupational exposures. Exposure would sometimes begin as a caustic chemical burn when the trichlorophenol reactors would over heat. These workers showed the earliest and most severe chloracne (Taylor 1979; Tindall 1985).

Chloracne is the hallmark of dioxin exposure in man; however, its absence does not exclude dioxin exposure. There is no apparent dose-response model for chloracne in exposed human populations and lesions may develop weeks or months after exposure. In Germany, six workers who developed chloracne after an industrial accident had an estimated mean TCDD body burden of 44 μg (range 9.7–124 μg) shortly after the accident. Thus, a body burden of 9.7 μg, as measured in adipose tissue, may be the lowest observable effect level for TCDD-related chloracne in humans. Thirty-two years after exposure, these German workers still had detectable levels of TCDD in adipose tissue, and one still had chloracne (Agency for Toxic Effects of Chemical Substances 1993). In a follow-up study after the Seveso accident in 1976, which resulted in one of the largest ever-reported environmental outbreaks of chloracne, residents of communities contaminated with TCDD still had elevated levels of plasma TCDD up to 20–30 years after exposure (Baccarelli et al. 2005).

A case of palmoplantar keratoderma, scleroderma, and chloracne was reported in an agricultural worker who had been a weed sprayer for 5 years. He had used 2,4,5-trichlorophenoxyacetic acid and/or 2,4 dichlorophenoxyacetic acid, both of which may contain chlorinated dibenzodioxins as impurities. He also had been chronically exposed to multiple other, non-chloracne associated herbicides, some of which have been associated with scleroderma. Safety equipment was not utilized (Poskitt et al. 1994).

Pentachlorophenol (*PCP*) is frequently used as a wood preservative, herbicide, and fungicide. It has additional uses in the leather and paper industry and an estimated 17,000 workers are exposed to PCP in the United States (O'Malley et al. 1990). Pentachlorophenol (PCP) is a stable and persistent compound. In humans, it is readily absorbed by ingestion and inhalation but is less well absorbed dermally. Severe exposure by any route may result in an acute and occasionally fatal illness that bears all the hallmarks of being mediated by uncoupling of oxidative phosphorylation. Tachycardia, tachypnea, sweating, altered consciousness, hyperthermia, convulsions, and early onset of marked rigor (if death occurs) are the most notable features. Pulmonary edema, intravascular hemolysis, pancreatitis, jaundice, and acute renal failure have been reported. There is no antidote and no adequate data to support the use of repeat-dose oral cholestyramine, forced diuresis or urine alkalinization as effective methods of enhancing PCP elimination in poisoned humans. Supportive care and vigorous management of hyperthermia should produce a satisfactory outcome. Chronic occupational exposure to PCP may produce a syndrome similar to acute systemic poisoning, together with conjunctivitis and irritation of the upper respiratory and oral mucosa. Long-term exposure has also been reported to result in chronic fatigue or neuropsychiatric features in combination with skin manifestations (including chloracne), chronic respiratory symptoms, neuralgic pains in the legs, and impaired fertility and hypothyroidism secondary to endocrine disruption (Proudfoot 2003).

A retrospective review of 648 medical and personnel records from individuals manufacturing PCP between 1938 and 1978 demonstrated 47 cases of chloracne occurring in a 25-year period. These workers were exposed only to PCP for 2 years prior to their diagnosis. PCP was produced by direct chlorination of phenol, monochlorophenol, dichlorophenol and/or 2,4,6-trichlorophenol in the presence of an aluminum catalyst. During the commercial synthesis of PCP, varying amounts of polychlorinated aromatic by-products, including dioxins, are produced (O'Malley et al. 1990). Russian workers who manufactured phenoxy herbicides and related compounds in the 1960s in the city of Ufa, Bashkortostan, a republic of the former Soviet Union, were studied for exposure to polychlorinated dibenzo-*p*-dioxins (PCDDs) and dibenzofurans. The patterns of the PCDDs and dibenzofurans (as defined by the specific congeners and their relative amounts) were distinctive for the type of chemical produced, with notable contributions to the TCDD toxic equivalents from the 2,3,7,8-TCDD and 1,2,3,7,8-pentachloro-p-dioxin (PnCDD) congeners.

No correlation was found between chloracne status in 1965–1967 and TCDD or toxic equivalent blood lipid concentrations in 1992. These Russian phenoxy herbicide and related chemical producers have some of the highest occupational exposure to dioxins of any cohort studied to date and seem to be unique with respect to the presence of appreciable amounts of 1,2,3,7,8-PnCDD (Ryan and Schecter 2000).

Cole et al. (1986) reported an unusual case of occupational chloracne that developed in a carpenter who assembled piers for small boat marinas using.

PCP-treated lumber. The worker, wearing only shorts and shoes, took measurements for extended periods of time while laying atop the treated lumber. After 9 months of this activity, he noted the onset of a papular acneiform eruption. Multiple small yellow-white papules were present involving the malar regions of the face, post auricular area, trunk, buttocks, thighs, and lower legs. Samples of treated lumber were tested for octachlorodibenzodioxin (OCD) and contained 1,040 times the amount of OCD than untreated wood. The yellow residue from treated wood contained 400 ppm OCD compared with technical grade PCP which contained 1600 ppm OCD. This case is unusual because the only source of PCP exposure was pressure-treated lumber; chloracne developing from this type of exposure is unusual. In the United States, the Environmental Protection Agency oversees the use of wood preservatives. In 1986, the agency proposed a level of hexachloro-*p*-dioxin no greater than 15 ppm, which was to be reduced to 1 ppm within 18 months (Cole et al. 1986).

9.2.2 Polyhalogenated Naphthalenes (PCNs)

Polychlorinated naphthalenes (PCNs) have a wax like consistency and have been used since the early 1900s in the electronics industry, as a dielectric material for condensers, as wire insulation, on boat hulls, as a lubricant, and as a wood preservative. Chloronaphthalenes were sold under the trademark Halowax by Koppers Company until the 1970s, but many potential uses have now been taken over by plastic and silicone. Their manufacture has been greatly curtailed (Adams).

Industrial use of the polyhalogenated naphthalenes (PCNs), occupational chloracne outbreaks and experimental human and animal studies have been reviewed. No occupational cases of PCN chloracne have been reported since 1972. Trace contamination of polychlorinated biphenyls (PCBs) with hexachloronaphthalenes and of polybrominated biphenyls (PBBs) with polybromonaphthalenes are potential current, but unlikely, sources of exposure (Taylor 1979).

9.2.3 Polyhalogenated Biphenyls (Polychlorinated Biphenyls PCBs, Polybrominatedted Biphenyls PBBs)

Chloracne has also been ascribed to exposure to *polychlorinated biphenyls* (*PCBs*), but most cases are probably due to a contamination of the PCBs with the above mentioned dioxins and dibenzofuranes. Polychlorinated biphenyls (PCBs) have been in use since 1929, and only over the last few decades have been recognized as environmental contaminants. Their use has now been confined to closed-system applications, such as in electrical capacitors and transformers. Other previous uses, such as in paints, in sealants, and in printing, have been eliminated (Zugerman 1990). Chloracne from PCBs has been demonstrated in reports in capacitor workers (Taylor et al. 1977; Tindall 1985) and in other workers (Longnecker et al. 1997). Cutaneous hyperpigmentation, eye discharge, and palpebral edema have also been reported (Taylor et al. 1977).

The greatest mass poisoning with PCBs occurred in nonoccupation settings of "oil-poisoning" in Yusho, Japan 1968 and Yu-Cheng, Taiwan 1979 when thousands of persons were affected after eating rice-based cooking oil that had been contaminated with large amounts of PCBs as described in detail below.

In 1973, *polybrominated biphenyls (PBBs)* were accidentally introduced into cattle feed as a result of a shipping error in Michigan. Thousands of dairy animals died or were destroyed, and farm workers were exposed to significant levels of these chemicals. Three percent of the exposed farm workers developed chloracne, but abnormal sweating and nonscarring alopecia were the more common complaints (Zugerman 1990).

9.2.4 Polyhalogenated Dibenzofurans (PHDFs)

Polychlorinated dibenzofurans were used as recently as 1974 in flame retardants; but due to their extreme toxicity they are no longer manufactured. Since polyhalogenated dibenzofuans (PHDFs) may occur as contaminants of PCBs and polyhalogenated phenols, their cutaneous effects are discussed under those headings.

9.2.5 Azo and Azoxybenzenes

We first documented cases of chloracne from a chlorobenzene compound tetrachloroazoxybenzene (TCAOB) in 1977. Tetrachloroazobenzene (TCAB) was also produced during the synthesis of 3,4-dichloro aniline or during its further conversion to herbicides. More than 90% of 41 workers in a small chemical plant developed chloracne from direct skin contact, but inhalation and ingestion were also possible routes. Family members of four workers, none of whom had been in the plant, also developed chloracne, probably from exposure at home to contaminated tools or work clothes (Taylor et al. 1977). No systemic reactions were found in any individuals. Eight years later, three of five workers with chloracne still had some evidence of chloracne and scarring. Two children who had chloracne were clear, except for mild scarring; one had acne vulgaris when seen again (Taylor and Lloyd 1982). Similar episodes of chloracne have been reported in workers exposed to TCAOB from the production of the pesticide-herbicide Proponil in Arkansas in 1977. A 38% incidence of chloracne developed among the 102 workers in the plant, and 11% were hospitalized for acute illness related to chemical exposure.

We are aware of other reports of TCAB and TCAOB chloracne in the United States and England in the 1970s and 1980s (Taylor and Lloyd 1982).

An outbreak of chloracne in 17 workers from a British plant manufacturing dichloro-aniline-derived herbicides was reported in 1993. TCAB and TCAOB were the acnegens. Comedones evolved 6–12 weeks after exposure to these chloracnegenic contaminants. Cutaneous xerosis and folliculitis on the trunk, limbs, thighs, and buttocks, previously uncommonly described, were present in 50% of exposed workers. Affected follicles were surrounded by a collarette of scale and frequently the hair shaft was twisted or broken. The pathogenesis of these lesions is unclear but may involve a disorder of keratinization. A direct toxic effect on epidermal keratinocytes or a secondary effect due to a perifollicular inflammatory reaction has been theorized (McDonough et al. 1993). They suggested that folliculitis and xerosis should be included in the clinical spectrum of chloracne.

In 1996, nine workers from a Mexican chemical plant were evaluated for the efftects of chronic exposure to chlorobenzenes (mono-, ortho- and paradichlorobenzenes). They had a mean exposure of 24 working years and worked in all stages of chemical production. Safety equipment was not used, and direct contact with the chlorobenzenes occurred via the skin and respiratory tract. The nine workers had a polymorphic acneiform eruption consisting mainly of comedones and cysts. All had comedones on the face, predominately in the malar area; lesions on the nose, axillae, chest, shoulders, arms, buttocks, and thighs were also present. Yellow cysts (2–5 mm in diameter) were found on the malar area of the face, eyelids, penis, scrotum, chest, axilla, and ears. Abnormal hyperpigmentation of the face, oral cavity, or diffuse hyperpigmentation was also observed in all patients. Chlorobenzenes were measured in the water at a concentration of 15 ppm. All workers reported chronic conjunctivitis with thick secretions from meibomian glands similar to those seen in Yusho. Hepatic involvement including elevated serum alkaline phosphatase and lower extremity peripheral neuropathy were also evident (Vazquez et al. 1996).

9.2.6 Triazoloquinoxalines

In 2009, a new chloracnegen was reported from the United Kingdom in an outbreak of chloracne among seven male pharmaceutical discovery chemists who synthesized novel polycyclic halogenated chemical compounds which were classified as triazoloquinoxalines (Gawkrodger et al. 2009). Comedones developed on the face, malar area, postauricular, periauricular, and preauricular areas with occasional inflammatory papules, pustules, and cysts. Other findings on examination included dry skin on the back and papular folliculitis on the thighs. A clinical diagnosis of chloracne was made. One subject had slightly raised serum level of alanine aminotransferase. There were no other signs of systemic toxicity. Toxicological investigations of the synthesized compounds found that the triazoloquinoxalines which showed high activity in the chemically activated luciferase gene expression (CALUX) cell bioassay for estimation of dioxin-like activity, were several times more chloracnegenic than dioxins on a weight for weight basis. Triazoloquinoxalines were synthetic intermediates in the project, being synthesized in small scale (mg g^{-1}) quantities. Triazoloquinoxalines were not previously known as chloracnegens however, they showed the basic structural features and physiochemical properties that are typical of chloracnegens, such as high metabolic stability, a polycyclic structure, a lipophilic nature, and the potential to be halogenated (Gawkrodger et al. 2009). The chloracne in subjects mostly resolved within 18–24 months although on examination about 3 years later, five of the seven still showed minor changes of chloracne.

9.3 Nonoccupational Exposure

Nonoccupational chloracne has resulted from industrial accidents, contaminated industrial waste, and poisoned food products. A well-publicized example was the extensive environmental contamination with by 2,3,7,8-tetrachlorodibenzo-*p*-dioxin (TCDD), which occurred on 10 July, 1976, at the ICMESA chemical plant near Seveso, Italy. An explosion occurred during the manufacturing of trichlorophenol that resulted in the formation and ultimate discharge into the atmosphere of an estimated 2 kg of TCDD. The contaminated area encompassed more than 200 acres of land, and 135 cases of chloracne, mostly in children, were confirmed among the 2000 area inhabitants. The toxic cloud caused the death of hundreds of fowl in the first days after the explosion; the development of chloracne occurred after different time periods. Aside from chloracne, some cases of subclinical neurological damage were reported (Pocchiari et al. 1979).

In a long-term follow-up study of health status and plasma dioxin levels in chloracne cases 20 years after exposure, residents of the Seveso communities contaminated with industrial effluent dioxin levels still had elevated levels of TCDD in plasma and adipose tissues; particularly in females, in subjects who had eaten home-grown animals, and in individuals with older age, higher body mass index, and residence near the accident site. However, the health conditions of chloracne cases were similar to those of controls from the Seveso area. There was also a strong association between plasma TCDD levels and chloracne occurrence, which appeared related to younger age and light hair color (Baccarelli et al. 2005). The Seveso cancer incidence was updated to cover the 20 years period from 1977–1996 which confirmed an excess risk of lymphatic and hematopoietic tissue neoplasms in the most exposed zones. There was also elevated risk of breast cancer in very high contaminated zone females after 15 years since the accident. No cases of soft tissue sarcomas occurred (Pesatori et al. 2009).

Ingestion alone of PCBs and their thermally degraded polychlorinated dibenzofurans (PCDFs) played a major role in two mass "oil-poisoning" episodes Yusho in Japan in 1968 and Yu-Cheng in Taiwan in 1979, the largest epidemics of chloracne to date. In both countries, several thousand persons were affected after eating rice-based cooking oil that had been accidentally contaminated with large amounts of tetrachlorobiphenyl. Most clinical manifestations were observed in patients who had directly ingested the oil. Dermatologic manifestations in typical Yusho and Yucheng cases having high PCB and PCDF concentrations in blood included acneiform eruptions, hyperpigmentation, fingernail abnormalities, and hypersecretion of conjunctival meibomian glands which recovered very slowly after several years. However, elevated serum triglycerides and serum thyroxin, immunoglobulin disorders, goiter, decreased sperm mobility, dental abnormalities joint inflammation, decreased IQ score in children, headache, and numbness were persisting 30 years later (Masuda 2001).

PCBs and PCDFs can persist in human tissues with the median half-life of 2.9 years in the first 15 years after onset and 7.7 years in the next stage of 15 years (Masuda 2001) (similar dioxins have half-lives in humans of about 7 years). The offspring of exposed females are described as cola babies because of their dark color. Generalized hyperpigmentation, meibomian gland enlargement with eye discharge, and nail deformities occurred in congenitally exposed individuals. Severe chloracne scars were observed 11 years postcongenital exposure in some affected individuals in Taiwan (Hsu et al. 1995).

We studied 128 children who were transplacentally exposed to PCBs and dibenzofurans in Taiwan, their parents and siblings who were directly exposed, and 115 control children. Direct exposure of the mothers stopped in 1979 and the children were born as late as 1985. At birth, the exposed children had increased rates of hyperpigmentation, eyelid swelling and discharge, deformed nails, acne, natal teeth, and swollen gums unlike controls. On cutaneous examination in 1985, key findings were a much higher rate of dystrophic fingernails and pigmented or dystrophic toe nails than in controls. Increased rates of hyperpigmentation and acne were also seen in the exposed groups. The cutaneous findings were part of a transplacental neuroectodermal dysplasia, with dental abnormalities, a growth deficit, developmental delay, and a behavior disorder. Transplacental dermatotoxins are rare (minoxidil, phenytoin, carbamazepine and hexachlorobenzene). This syndrome is one of very few documented to result from transplacental exposure to pollutant chemicals (Rogan et al. 1988). On reexamination 6 years later, nail changes were still present and suggested prenatal injury to the nail matrix (Hsu et al. 1995). The findings in transplacentally exposed children differ from those seen in people directly exposed, particularly the higher prevalence of acne in the latter group (Rogan et al. 1988; Gladen et al. 1990; Hsu et al. 1995).

In 1982, eight members of a Spanish family were poisoned by consumption of olive oil contaminated with PCDDs and PCDFs. The entire family had varying degrees of acneform lesions, including papules, pustules, cysts, comedones, and scars located on the face, axilla, neck, trunk, groin, and genitals. Hyperpigmentation of the face was also reported. These lesions are comparable in severity to those described in the Yusho incident. The olive oil consumed was stored in a plastic container, which had presumably stored hexachlorobenzene and pentachlorophenol prior to the oil. The causative agents were identified as PCDDs, PCDFs, and PCP, each of which was recovered from the cooking oil. There were high serum levels of PCDDs and PCDFs, which returned to normal when measured 5 years after oil consumption ceased (Rodriguez-Pichardo et al. 1991).

In 1981, an electrical transformer fire occurred in Binghamton, New York. The fire began in the basement mechanical room of an 18-story office building. Approximately 180 gallons of Askarel, a dielectric fluid composed of 65% PCBs (Aroclor 1254) and 35% polychlorinated benzenes leaked from a transformer.

The fire originated in the switch gear of the secondary electrical power distribution system. Pyrolysis of the Askarel led to the formation of a fine oily soot containing PCBs, dibenzo-*p*-dioxins, and dibenzofurans, which spread to all areas of the building through ventilation shafts. Three-year post-exposure serum PCB concentrations increased with the degree of potential exposure, but 98% of samples tested had values similar to those found in unexposed populations. One-third of the fire fighters and other persons who were in the building for 25 h or more reported "rash" or itching.

However, no cases of chloracne, liver disease or neurological disorders were identified in the exposed individuals (Fitzgerald et al. 1989).

10 Cutaneous Manifestations

Clinical features of chloracne include multiple closed comedones and straw-colored cysts distributed primarily over the malar crescents and retroauricular folds, typically sparing the nose. This pattern of distribution is of significant diagnostic importance. Inflammatory lesions occur but are less frequent than in other forms of acne. As severity increases, the posterior neck, trunk and extremities, buttocks, scrotum, and penis may become involved. The axillae are most likely to be involved in those who ingest chloracnegens, such as in Japan's Yusho poisoning in 1968 or in those at Seveso, Italy in 1976, who were exposed in toxic cloud (Jirasek et al. 1973).

Associated with the classic lesions of chloracne is a relatively dry appearance of the skin. Metaplasia of sebaceous epithelium occurs, with subsequent atrophy of sebaceous and meibomian glands leading to xerosis of the facial skin, skin of the chest and back and the reduction in sebum excretion seen in chloracne (Zugerman 1990; Gawkrodger et al. 2009).

Hyperpigmentation may also occur and is usually confined to the face, although in severe cases it can be generalized. Hyperpigmentation has also affected the nails, mucous membranes, lips, and mouth in those involved in Yusho and Yuchng poisoning in Japan and Taiwan respectively. Individuals exposed to chlorobenzenes and industrial polychlorinated biphenyl (PCB) poisoning may lead to similar pigmentation.

Eye involvement is relatively common and is termed "ophthalmic acne " (Taylor 1974; Crow and Puhvel 1991). Conjunctivitis with meibomian gland involvement may be seen in severe cases of poisoning from chloracnegens, especially in the Yusho poisoning. The Yusho victims demonstrated extreme eye findings when their meibomian glands were converted to squamous cysts filled with a cheesy keratinous substance; the unusual oral route of entry and absorption of PCBs may have been an essential part of the syndrome (Tindall 1985).

Dermatologic observations associated with chloracne, which may lead to identification of specific exposures, include hyperpigmentation of the skin (PCBs, TCDD), mucous membrane and nail hyperpigmentation (PCBs), follicular hyperkeratosis (PCBs, TCDD [Seveso]), conjunctivitis and meibomian gland changes (PCBs), facial erythema and edema (trichlorophenol, hypertrichosis

(TCDD), hyperhidrosis of the palms and soles (TCDD, PCBs), folliculitis and xerosis (TCAB, TCAOB), and actinic elastosis (TCDD). Erythema and edema of the exposed face and extremities associated with trichlorophenol production was also seen in the Seveso cases. These "pre-chloracne" lesions were also accompanied by vesiculobullous and necrotic lesions on finger tips and palms, and papulonodular lesions, all of which resolved within a few weeks. Hyperkeratotic, infiltrative erythematous granuloma annulare, or erythema elevatum diutinum-like lesions were also seen in association with chloracne 2 months after the explosion. Axillary involvement and follicular hyperkeratosis are linked with inhalation or ingestion of chloracnegens (Taylor 1979; Tindall 1985).

Hypertrichosis in association with chloracne has been mainly confined to the temples and may rarely be a sign of hepatic porphyria. However, hypertrichosis has also been described in chloracne patients with normal uroporphyrin levels (Jirasek et al. 1973; Crow and Puhvel 1991).

Punctate keratoderma-like lesions on the palms and soles clinically and histologically indistinguishable from keratosis punctata palmaris et plantaris (KPPP) was reported to occur in a female patient with dioxin intoxication (Geusau et al. 2000). In addition to chloracne, she also exhibited acral granuloma annulare-like lesions, distal onycholysis, hypertrichosis, and brownish-gray hyperpigmentation of the face.

Scarring may occur in the end stage of moderate to severe chloracne. It may appear as fine pits seen in atrophodermia vermiculata, or may resemble scars caused by severe acne vulgaris (Zugerman 1990).

Chloracne may occur in relatives of workers exposed at home to contaminated work clothing and tools (Taylor et al. 1977).

10.1 Onset and Duration

The clinical course of chloracne varies. After exposure to a chloracnegenic agent, there usually is a delay of 2–4 weeks until the development of chloracne. However, the onset can be delayed up to months. Lesions tend to persist for decades even without additional contact and are refractory to treatment (Crow and Puhvel 1991; Sterling and Hanke 2005).

11 Non-cutaneous Manifestations

Chloracnegen exposures to humans have been associated with increased risk of severe skin lesions such as chloracne and hyperpigmentation, altered liver function, hypertriglyceridemia, hypercholesterolemia, general weakness, weight loss, depression of the immune system, increased risk for diabetes and cardiovascular disease, various hormonal alterations, nervous-system abnormalities, effects on reproduction, impaired developmental, neurological, and cognitive function in infants. It is a potent teratogenic and fetotoxic chemical in animals. Other systemic disorders reported with chloracne include bronchitis, renal, and pancreatic involvement (Taylor 1987). Patients with chloracne should have appropriate physical examination and laboratory evaluations to exclude systemic involvement.

Epidemiologic data suggesting that high-level dioxin exposure causes liver function abnormalities and chloracne are incontrovertible (Longnecker et al. 1997). In Seveso, a transient rise in values of hepatic enzymes that reflected hepatocellular damage, that is, gamma-glutamyl transferase and alanine amino transferase occurred. Alkaline phosphatase and serum bilirubin levels were not elevated and jaundice or other signs of hepatic injury were not appreciated. Crow and Puhvel (1991) suggested that the degree of hepatic injury was dependent on the specificity of the toxicant involved, rather than as a consistent consequence of all forms of chloracnegen exposure.

Porphyria cutanea tarda (PCT) has been reported in humans following TCDD exposure (Bleiberg et al. 1964). Both normal urine porphyrin levels have been observed from individuals with severe chloracne (Strik 1979) and higher levels of urine porphyrins in workers exposed to pentachlorophenol pesticide exposure (Hryhorczuk et al. 1998). TCDD is a porphyrinogen in animal models and inhibits uroporphyrinogen decarboxylase, the enzyme precipitating PCT in some patients (Mukerjee 1998).

Peripheral neuropathy with pain and numbness may be observed, especially in persons severely exposured to chlorinated hydrocarbons (Thomke et al. 1999). Neuropathy has been confirmed by delayed nerve conduction velocity. In the 1968 Japanese epidemic of chloracne caused by ingestion of contaminated cooking oil (Yusho), these neurologic symptoms were especially apparent.

The long-term health effects of dioxin exposure in humans have not been conclusively proven. Carcinogenesis, teratogenicity, and immunosuppressive effects of these compounds are extremely controversial areas. Although animal studies with TCDD have strongly suggested that this material is carcinogenic in animal systems, these findings cannot necessarily be extrapolated to humans. Anecdotal information has pointed to TCDD as being a human carcinogen. Populations occupationally or accidentally exposed to chemicals contaminated with dioxin may have an increased incidence of soft-tissue sarcomas and non-Hodgkin's lymphoma (Mukerjee 1998). In a long-term cohort of 2,187 male workers exposed to dioxin Bodner found no increased cancer risk from dioxin exposure and concluded that there is a wide range of cancer rates and the lack of consistency across dioxin studies (Bodner et al. 2003). However, mortality and morbidity findings during the 20-year period following the accident showed increased risk of lymphatic and hematopoietic tissue neoplasms, digestive system cancer (rectum in males, and biliary tract among females, in particular), and respiratory system cancer (lung, among males). There was also elevated risk of breast cancer in females in very high contaminated zones (Pesatori et al. 2003, 2009). In the incidence analyses, thyroid and pleural cancer were suggestively increased (Hardell and Sandstrom 1979). Soft tissue sarcomas showed an increase in the largest, yet least exposed, exposure sub-cohort (Pesatori et al. 2003). Because of the long-term persistence of TCDD in the human body, atherosclerosis, hypertension, diabetes and various hormonal alterations, vascular, ocular changes, effects on reproduction, neural system damage, including neuropsychological impairment, neurological, and cognitive impairments in infants can be present several decades after exposure. Such chronic effects are nonspecific, multifactorial, and may be causally linked to TCDD (Sweeney and Mocarelli 2000; Pelclova et al. 2006). Continuous long-term surveillance and follow-up is warranted to cover the long time period, even decades, often elapsing from exposure to carcinogenic chemicals and occurrence of disease.

11.1 Mechanism

The mechanism involved in the initiation of chloracne remains unknown. The interference of halogenated biphenyls, dibenzo-*p*-dioxins, dibenzofurans, and azo and azoxybenzenes in vitamin A metabolism and function may offer an explanation about the acnegenic effects of these compounds on human skin (Chen et al. 1992; den Besten et al. 1993; Coenraads et al. 1994). Coenraads and coworkers (1994) found that retinol concentrations in skin biopsies from nine PCP-exposed workers with chloracne were much lower in comparison with controls. This suggests that the chemicals may affect vitamin A metabolism and hence influence pilosebaceous units and the epidermis.

A reduction in sebum excretion is a hallmark of chloracne, and fewer *Propionibacterium* acnes organisms are present in follicles of those with chloracne than of those with acne vulgaris (Cunliffe et al. 1975). Dioxins, for example, TCDD have been shown to impede androgen action possibly through interfering with androgen receptors (Gawkrodger et al. 2009). The biological mechanisms of chloracne induction are still debated but it was suggested that dioxins have their chloracnegenic effect by activating skin stem cells and shifting the differentiation commitment of the stem cell progeny (Panteleyev and Bickers 2006).

The molecular mechanisms of dioxin-mediated chloracne have not been clarified. The action of dioxins resembles that of hormones, since their toxicity is mostly receptor-mediated. The degree of affinity of various chloracnegens for the binding protein designated as the aryl hydrocarbon (Ah) receptor (for aromatic hydrocarbons) correlated with their biological efficacy (Poland et al. 1976). One of the most important initial steps in prerequisite of chloracne pathogenesis and toxicity of dioxins is the activation of a the aryl hydrocarbon receptor a transcription factor that binds to the Ah receptor nuclear translocator (ARNT) to regulate the transcription of numerous genes, including cytochrome P450 CYP1A1, GSTA1, and TGF-alpha. The changes of genes expression may disturb normal proliferation and differentiation of human epidermis cells, and then lead to chloracne (Furness and Whelan 2009; Tang et al. 2008).

In cultures of normal human epidermal keratinocytes dioxin accelerates cell differentiation, as measured by the formation of cornified envelopes. This acceleration is mediated by the aryl hydrocarbon receptor AHR; also, dioxin increases the expression of several genes known to be regulated by Ah receptor nuclear translocator (ARNT), which have critical roles in the cornification and epidermal barrier function of the skin. It has been demonstrated that all of these responses are opposed by ligand-activation of the EGF receptor (R), an important regulator of keratinocyte cell fate. Epidermal growth factor (EGF) represses the dioxin-mediated gene transcription induction of CYP1A1 in cultured normal human keratinocytes by inhibiting the recruitment of the transcriptional coactivator protein p300 to the *CYP1A1* gene. EGF also inhibits the dioxin-dependent induction of certain parameters in keratinocytes that are reflective of dioxin-induced chloracne. This epidermal growth factor receptor signaling may modulate the incidence and severity of chloracne and be of potential therapeutic relevance to human poisonings by dioxin (Sutter et al. 2009; Hankinson 2009).

11.2 Histopathology

In 1957, Hambrick studied the pathology of chloracne. Histologic changes in the skin may begin within 5 days of severe exposure to chloracnegenic chemicals (Hambrick 1957). The primary lesion of chloracne appears to be keratotic plugging of the hair follicle with collection of keratinous material in the follicular orifice. The follicular epithelium thickens, followed by atrophy of sebaceous glands and their replacement by keratinous cysts. Inflammation is minimal or absent. Histological features of chloracne are characterized by noninflammatory keratinization of pilosebaceous units with comedones and dilated infundibulum (Coenraads et al. 1994) but the specificity of these findings is unclear. A characteristic of chloracne is the rapid transformation of sebaceous glands into comedones. This appears to be pathognomic for chloracne poisoning. Biopsies from Seveso showed eccrine duct metaplasia with possible acrosyringeal cyst formation. Foreign body granulomas around detached walls of eccrine gland excretory ducts may also be present (Omohundro and Taylor 1998).

Hyperpigmentation of the lesions in chloracne has been demonstrated to result from hyperproduction of melanin by a normal number of melanocytes along the basal layer of the epidermis and infundibular epithelium.

11.3 Diagnosis

In 1984, a diagnostic criteria for chloracne was established by the Veterans Administration Chloracne Task Force including (1) exposure to a chloracnegen; (2) aggravation or onset within weeks to 2 months of exposure; (3) predominance of open comedones and straw-colored cysts; (4) atypical distribution, that is, malar crescent and "crow's-foot" area of the face; (5) compatible histology; and (6) inflammatory cysts and abscesses on the face, behind the ears, and on the neck, buttocks, scrotum, and thighs (Veterans Administration Chloracne Task Force 1984). The diagnosis of chloracne entails a compatible clinical picture with distribution of comedones and noninflammatory cysts beyond the typical locations of acne vulgaris. It is characterized by open and closed comedones with straw-colored cysts found predominantly in the malar region, postauricular area, axilla, and scrotum. Documentation of significant exposure to known chloracnegens and the absence of other external causes is also required.

Based on cutaneous findings alone or in novel settings, it may be very difficult to differentiate chloracne from acne vulgaris and other types of environmental acne – oil folliculitis, pitch acne, and tropical acne – is listed in *Tables 31.4* and *31.5.* Senile (solar) comedones of the Favre-Racouchot syndrome and Dowling-Degos' disease also can be considered in the clinical differential diagnosis (Kersevovich et al. 1992).

Table 31.4
Clinical features of acne vulgaris compared with chloracne (After Peter Pochi, MD with permission)

Clinical features	Acne vulgaris	Chloracne
Exposure to chloracnegen	Absent	Present
Usual age	Teenage	Any age
Comedones	Present	Many (if absent, not chloracne)
Straw-colored cysts	Rare	Pathognomonic
Temporal comedones	Rare	Diagnostic
Inflammatory papules, cysts	Common	Uncommon
Retroauricular involvement	Uncommon	Common
Nose involvement	Often spared	Often spared
Axillary, genital involvement	Rare	Maybe
Eye involvement	Absent	Present
Sebaceous glands	Active	Atrophic, with dry xerotic skin
Associated systemic findings	Rare	Common

11.4 Treatment

Chloracne tends to resolve slowly upon cessation of chemical exposure. Its duration correlates with the severity of the disease which usually reflects the degree and extent of exposure. Dioxins are highly lipophilic, have a long half-life in fat tissue and low turnover rate in the body. If exposure ceases, the lesions will gradually improve over many years or decades. The severely exposed victims of Yusho in 1968 had characteristic chloracne lesions that continued to develop for as long as 14 years postexposure.

Treatment of chloracne is usually unsatisfactory as the modalities that are useful in acne vulgaris are often ineffective in chloracne. Topical application of retinoic acid (0.005–0.3% concentration) or of tretinoin (Retin-A) gel or cream is of some benefit in controlling comedones, but other topical agents are of little use (Caputo et al. 1988). A combination of tetracycline and

Table 31.5
Differential diagnosis of various forms of occupational and environmental acne

	Etiology	Location	Lesions
Chloracne	Halogenated aromatics	Malar, retroauricular, mandibular	Comedones, straw-colored cysts (0.1–1.0 cm)
Oil folliculitis	Oil	Arms, thighs, buttocks	Comedones, inflammatory papules, pustules
Pitch acne	Tar/pitch	Exposed facial areas, malar, periorbital	Open comedones
Tropical acne	Heat/humidity	Buttocks, thighs	Inflammatory nodules, cysts
		Face spared	

short courses of orally administered prednisone helped with severe inflammatory cases. A trial regimen of methotrexate, 25 mg every 10 days for several months was unsuccessful (Taylor et al. 1977; Scerri et al. 1995).

There are anecdotal reports of both unsuccessful use (Sterling and Hanke 2005) and efficacious use of oral 13-*cis*-retinoic acid (isotretinoin) which, if instituted early, may prevent cyst formation. Isotretenoin 0.3–1 mg/kg/day may be indicated in severe cases for a course of 20 weeks. The drug should be administered only by those experienced in its use and in strict accordance with current prescribing instructions. The hepatotoxicity and lipid abnormalities sometimes associated with chloracne are theoretical reasons to avoid isotretinoin. Isotretinoin is a potent teratogen with other potentially significant side effects that require close monitoring (Gawkrodger 1991).

Local therapy with acne surgery and dermabrasion has been reported. Light cautery following topical anesthesia with EMLA cream has been used successfully in six patients with resistant chloracne lesions (Yip et al. 1993).

A promising new approach to lowering blood dioxin levels employed the use of Olestra, a nonabsorbable, nondigestible, lipophilic dietary fat substitute has been reported to accelerate the patients' intestinal excretion of TCDD by eight to ten fold. This is sufficient to reduce the normally observed elimination half-life of TCDD from about 7 years to 1–2 years (Geusau et al. 1999).

References

Adams BB, Chetty VB, Mutasim DF (2000) Periorbital comedones and their relationship to pitch tar: a cross-sectional analysis and a review of the literature. J Am Acad Dermatol 42(4):624–627

Agency for Toxic Substances and Disease Registry (1993) Dioxin toxicity. Am Fam Physician 47:855–861

Baccarelli A, Pesatori AC, Consonni D et al (2005) Health status and plasma dioxin levels in chloracne cases 20 years after the Seveso, Italy accident. Br J Dermatol 152(3):459–465

Bartolini R (1989) Acne. A summary of the occupational health concern. Canadian Centre for Occupational Health and Safety, Hamilton. Report No. F89-1E:I-7

Bleiberg I, Wallen M, Brodken R et al (1964) Industrial acquired porphyria. Arch Dermatol 89:793–797

Bodner KM, Collins JJ, Bloemen LJ et al (2003) Cancer risk for chemical workers exposed to 2,3,7,8-tetrachlorodibenzo-*p*-dioxin. Occup Environ Med 60(9):672–675

Brun P, Baran R (1984) A special type of mechanical acne: fiddler's neck dermatitis. Ann Dermatol Venereol 111(3):241–245

Caputo R, Monti M, Ermacora E et al (1988) Cutaneous manifestations of tetrachlorodibenzo-*p*-dioxin in children and adolescents. J Am Acad Dermatol 19:812–819

Chen LC, Berberian I, Koch B et al (1992) Polychlorinated and polybrominated biphenyl congeners and retinoid levels in rat tissues: structure-activity relationships. Toxicol Appl Pharmacol 114:47–55

Coenraads PI, Brouwer A, Olie K, Tang N (1994) Chloracne. Some recent issues. Dermatol Clin 12:569–576

Cole GW, Stone O, Gates D, Culver D (1986) Chloracne from pentachlorphenol – preserved wood. Contact Dermatitis 15:164–168

Crow KD (1981) Chloracne and its potential clinical implications. Clin Exp Dermatol 6:243–257

Crow KD, Puhvel MS (1991) Chloracne (halogen acne). In: Manulli FN, Maibach HI (eds) Dermatoxicology. Hemisphere, New York, pp 647–667

Cunliffe WJ, Williams M, Edwards JC et al (1975) An explanation for chloracne-an industrial hazard. Acta Derm Venereol (Stockh) 55:211–214

Demirci U, Coskun U, Erdem O, Ozturk B, Yilmaz IB, Benekli M, Buyukberber S (2010) Acne rosacea associated imatinib mesylate in a gastrointestinal stromal tumor patient. J Oncol Pharm Pract [Epub ahead of print]

den Besten C, Bennik MHJ, Bruggeman I et al (1993) The role of oxidative metabolism in hexchlorobenzene induced porphyria and thyroid hormone homeostasis: a comparison with pentachlorobenzene in a 13-week feeding study. Toxicol Appl Pharmacol 119:181–194

Draelos ZD, DiNardo JC (2006) A re-evaluation of the comedogenicity concept. J Am Acad Dermatol 54(3):507–512

Fitzgerald EF, Weinstein AL, Youngblood LG et al (1989) Health effects three years after potential exposure to the toxic contaminants of an electrical transformer fire. Arch Environ Health 44:214–221

Furness SG, Whelan F (2009) The pleiotropy of dioxin toxicity–xenobiotic misappropriation of the aryl hydrocarbon receptor's alternative physiological roles. Pharmacol Ther 124(3):336–353

Gawkrodger DJ (1991) Chloracne: causation, diagnosis and treatment. J Derm Treat 2:73–76

Gawkrodger DJ, Harris G, Bojar RA (2009) Chloracne in seven organic chemists exposed to novel polycyclic halogenated chemical compounds (triazoloquinoxalines). Br J Dermatol 161(4): 939–943

Geusau A, Tschachler E, Meixner M et al (1999) Olestra increases faecal excretion of 2,3,7,8-tetrachlorodibenzo-*p*-dioxin. Lancet 354: 1266–1269

Geusau A, Jurecka W, Nahavandi H et al (2000) Punctate keratoderma-like lesions on the palms and soles in a patient with chloracne: a new clinical manifestation of dioxin intoxication? Br J Dermatol 143(5):1067–1071

Gladen BC, Taylor JS, Wu YC, Ragan NB, Rogan WJ, Hsu CC (1990) Dermatologic findings in children exposed transplacentally to heat-degraded polychlorinated biphenyls in Taiwan. Br J Dermatol 122:799–808

Hambrick GS (1957) The effects of substituted napthalenes on the pilosebacious apparatus of rabbit and man. J Invest Dermatol 28:29–103

Hankinson O (2009) Repression of aryl hydrocarbon receptor transcriptional activity by epidermal growth factor. Mol Interv 9(3): 116–118

Hardell L, Sandstrom A (1979) Case-control study: soft tissue sarcoma and exposure to phenoxy-acetic acids or chlorophenols. Br J Cancer 39:711–717

Herxheimer K (1899) Ueber chlorakne. Munch Med Wochenschr 46:278

Hjorth N, Sjolin KE, Sylvest B et al (1972) Acne aestivalis: Mallorca acne. Acta Derm Venereol 52:61–63

Hryhorczuk DO, Wallace WH, Persky V et al (1998) A morbidity study of former pentachlorophenol-production workers. Environ Health Perspect 106(7):401–408

Hsu MM-L, Mak C-P, Hsu C-C (1995) Follow up of skin manifestations in Yu-Cheng children. Br J Dermatol 122:799–808

Jirasek L, Kalensky J, Kubec K (1973) Acne chlorina and porphyria cutanea tarda during the manufacturing of herbicides Part I. Cesk Dermatol 48:306–317

Kersevovich J, Langenberg A, Odom RB et al (1992) Dowling-Degos' disease mimicking chloracne. J Am Acad Dermatol 27:345–348

Khanna N, Gupta SD (1999) Acneiform eruptions after facial beauty treatment. Int J Dermatol 38(3):196–199

Kligman AM, Mills OH (1972) Acne cosmetica. Arch Dermatol 106: 843–850

Knox JM, Dinehart SM et al (1986) Acquired perforating disease in oil field workers. J Am Acad Dermatol 14:605–611

Kokelj F (1992) Occupational acne. Clin Dermatol 10:213–217

Litt JZ (1974) McDonald's acne. Arch Dermatol 110:956

Longnecker MP, Rogan WJ, Lucier G (1997) The human health effects of DDT (dichlorodiphenyltrichloroethane) and PCBs (polychlorinated biphenyls) and overview of organochlorines in public health. Annu Rev Public Health 18:211–244

Martín JM, Jordá E, Monteagudo C, Alonso V, García L, Villalón G (2006) Follicular acneiform eruption induced by imatinib. J Eur Acad Dermatol Venereol 20(10):1368–1370

Masuda Y (2001) Fate of PCDF/PCB congeners and change of clinical symptoms in patients with Yusho PCB poisoning for 30 years. Chemosphere 43(4–7):925–930

Mathias CGT (1994) Occupational dermatoses. In: Zenz C, Dickerson OB, Horvath EP (eds) Occupational medicine, 3rd edn. Mosby, St. Louis, pp 93–131

McDonough AI, Gawkrodger DJ, Walker AE (1993) Chloracne study of an outbreak with new clinical observations. Clin Exp Dermatol 18:523–525

Michot C, Guillot B, Dereure O (2010) Lenalidomide-induced acute acneiform folliculitis of the head and neck: not only the anti-EGF receptor agents. Dermatology 220(1):49–50

Mills OH, Kligman A (1975) Acne mechanica. Arch Dermatol 111:481–483

Mukerjee D (1998) Health impact of polychlorinated dibenzo-*p*-dioxins: a critical review. J Air Waste Manag Assoc 48:157–165

Nguyen SH, Dang TP, Maibach HI (2007) Comedogenicity in rabbit: some cosmetic ingredients/vehicles. Cutan Ocul Toxicol 26(4):287–292

O'Malley MS, Carpenter AV, Sweeney MH, Fingerhut MA et al (1990) Chloracne associated with employment in the production of pentachlorophenol. Am J Ind Med 17:411–421

Omohundro C, Taylor JS (1998) Occupational acne. In: English JSC (ed) A colour handbook of occupational dermatology. Manson, London, pp 121–134

Osio A, Mateus C, Soria JC, Massard C, Malka D, Boige V, Besse B, Robert C (2009) Cutaneous side-effects in patients on long-term treatment with epidermal growth factor receptor inhibitors. Br J Dermatol 161(3):515–521

Panteleyev AA, Bickers DR (2006) Dioxin-induced chloracne – reconstructing the cellular and molecular mechanisms of a classic environmental disease. Exp Dermatol 15:705–730

Pelclova D, Urban P, Preiss J et al (2006) Adverse health effects in humans exposed to 2,3,7,8-tetrachlorodibenzo-*p*-dioxin (TCDD). Rev Environ Health 21(2):119–138

Pesatori AC, Consonni D, Bachetti S et al (2003) Short- and long-term morbidity and mortality in the population exposed to dioxin after the "Seveso accident". Ind Health 41(3):127–138

Pesatori AC, Consonni D, Rubagotti M et al (2009) Cancer incidence in the population exposed to dioxin after the "Seveso accident": twenty years of follow-up. Environ Health 8:39

Plewig G, Jansen T (1998) Acneiform dermatoses. Dermatology 196: 102–107

Pocchiari F, Silano V, Zampieri A (1979) Human health effects from accidental release of tetrachlorodibenzo-*p*-dioxin (TCDD) at Seveso, Italy. Ann NY Acad Sci 320:311–320

Poland A, Glover E, Kende AS (1976) Stereo-specific high affinity binding of 2,3,7,8-tetrachlorodibenzo-*p*-dioxin by hepatic cytosol. J Biol Chem 251:4936–4946

Poskitt LB, Duffill MB, Rademaker M (1994) Chloracne, palmoplantar keratoderma and localized scleroderma in a weed sprayer. Clin Exp Dermatol 19:264–267

Proudfoot AT (2003) Pentachlorophenol poisoning. Toxicol Rev 22(1):3–11

Rodriguez-Pichardo A, Camacho F, Rappe C, Hansson M, Smith AG, Greig IB (1991) Chloracne caused by ingestion of olive oil contaminated with PCDDs and PCDFs. Hum Exp Toxicol 10: 311–322

Rogan WJ, Gladen BC, Hung K-L, Koong S-L, Shih L-Y, Taylor JS (1988) Congenital poisoning by polychlorinated biphenyls and their contaminants in Taiwan. Science 241:334–336

Ryan JJ, Schecter A (2000) Exposure of Russian phenoxy herbicide producers to dioxins. J Occup Environ Med 42(9):861–870

Scerri L, Zaki I, Millard LG (1995) Severe halogen acne due to a trifluoromethylpyrazole derivative and its resistance to isotretinoin. Br J Dermatol 132:l44–l148

Sorg O, Zennegg M, Schmid P, Fedosyuk R, Valikhnovskyi R, Gaide O, Kniazevych V, Saurat JH (2009) 2,3,7,8-tetrachlorodibenzo-*p*-dioxin (TCDD) poisoning in Victor Yushchenko: Identification and measurement of TCDD metabolites. Lancet 374:1179–1185

Sperling L (1994) Skin disease associated with excessive heat, humidity, and sunlight. In: Zajtchuk R (ed) Textbook of military medicine, part III. Sergent General, Department of the Army, Washington DC, pp 44–45

Sterling JB, Hanke CW (2005) Dioxin toxicity and chloracne in the Ukraine. J Drugs Dermatol 4(2):148–150

Strik JJ (1979) Porphyrins in urine as an indicator of exposure to chlorinated hydrocarbons. Ann NY Acad Sci 320:308–310

Sutter CH, Yin H, Li Y et al (2009) EGF receptor signaling blocks aryl hydrocarbon receptor-mediated transcription and cell differentiation in human epidermal keratinocytes. Proc Natl Acad Sci USA 106(11):4266–4271

Sweeney MH, Mocarelli P (2000) Human health effects after exposure to 2,3,7,8-TCDD. Food Addit Contam 17(4):303–316

Tang NJ, Liu J, Coenraads PJ et al (2008) Expression of AhR, CYP1A1, GSTA1, c-fos and TGF-alpha in skin lesions from dioxin-exposed humans with chloracne. Toxicol Lett 177(3):182–187

Taylor JS (1974) Chloracne, a continuing problem. Cutis 13:585–591

Taylor JS (1979) Envionmental chloracne: update and overview. Ann NY Acad Sci 320:295–307

Taylor JS (1986) Occupational dermatoses. In: Conn HF (ed) Current therapy. Saunders, Philadelphia, pp 686–688

Taylor JS (1987) Pilosebaceous unit. In: Maibach HI (ed) Occupational and industrial dermatology. Year Book Medical Publishers, Chicago, pp 105–120

Taylor JS, Lloyd KM (1982) Chloracne from 3.3',4,4' -tetrachloroazoxybenzene and 3.3',4,4'-tetrachloroazobenzene: update and review. In: Hutzinger O (ed) Chlorinated dioxins and related compounds. Pergamon, Oxford, pp 535–544

Taylor JS, Wuthrich RC, Lloyd KM, Poland A (1977) Chloracne from manufacture of a new herbicide. Arch Dermatol 113:616–619

Thomke F, Jung D, Besser R et al (1999) Increased risk of sensory neuropathy in workers with chloracne after exposure to 2,3,7,8-polychlorinated dioxins and furans. Acta Neurol Scand 100(1):1–5

Tindall JP (1985) Chloracne and chloracnegens. J Am Acad Dermatol 13:539–558

Upreti RK, Das M, Shanker R (1989) Dermal exposure to kerosene. Vet Hum Toxicol 31:16–20

Vazquez ER, Macias PC, Tirado IG, Solana CG, Casanova A, Moncada IF (1996) Chloracne in the 1990s. Int J Dermatol 35:643–645

Veterans Administration Chloracne Task Force (1984) Guidelines for the Diagnosis of Chloracne. U.S. Veterans Administration, Washington, DC, USA

Veysey EC, George S (2005) Actinic folliculitis. Clin Exp Dermatol 30(6):659–661

Yip J, Peppall L, Gawkrodger DJ, Cunliff WJ (1993) Light cautery and EMLA in the treatment of chloracne lesions. Br J Dermatol 128:313–316

Zaenglein AL, Thiboutot DM (2008) Acne vulgaris. In: Bolognia JL, Jorizzo JL, Rapini RP (eds) Dermatology, 2nd edn. Mosby, London, pp 495–508

Zugerman C (1990) Chloracne, chloracnegenesis, and other forms of environmental acne. In: Adams RM (ed) Adams occupational skin disease, 2nd edn. WB Saunders, Philadelphia, pp 127–135

32 Psoriasis and Work

Christoph Skudlik · Swen-Malte John
Department of Dermatology, Environmental Medicine and Health Theory, University of Osnabrueck, Osnabrueck, Germany

Core Messages

- Psoriasis is a constitutional disease, but may be triggered by occupational factors.
- The frequency of occupationally triggered Psoriasis in patients with occupational skin diseases has been reported to be between 1.2% and 6.5%.
- In addition to adequate therapy, special skin protection measures, such as anti-impaction gloves and the avoidance of irritant and mechanical influences are pivotal in terms of adequate prevention

1 Introduction

Psoriasis is a common and often chronic inflammatory skin disease. It is characterized by variable clinical features. Psoriasis vulgaris is the most common type of psoriasis. Circular plaques are predominant on the elbows, knees, lower back, and the retroauricular areas of the scalp, whereas eruptive (guttate) lesions are often confined to the trunk and proximal extremities. Palmar psoriasis is also a frequent manifestation. Some authors have indicated that in a number of cases there is an overlapping between psoriasis and eczema (Ancona et al. 1986; Maibach and Epstein 1983). This form of psoriasis is sometimes difficult to distinguish clinically and histologically from hyperkeratotic hand eczema.

So palmar psoriasis is often confused with chronic hyperkeratotic hand eczema, skin biopsies often show nonspecific changes of eczema rather than those of psoriasis, and the histological findings often do not help to confirm the diagnosis.

The incidence of psoriasis vulgaris in industrialized western countries is 1.5–2% (Nevitt and Hutchinson 1996). Psoriasis vulgaris shows a multifactorial, polygenetic pattern of inheritance. A number of susceptibility genes predispose a person to the disease. The psoriatic tissue reaction is an extremely complex cutaneous immune reaction with a pronounced inflammatory component and epidermal hyperproliferation. By means of an antigen or auto-antigen through antigen-presenting cells, specific T cells are activated and migrated into the skin. Homing factors include the cutaneous lymphocyte–associated antigen (CLA). Infiltration of the papillary dermis and epidermis leads to activation of the resident cells. Here, by means of central mediators (e.g., TNF-α) endothelial cells, fibroblasts, and keratinocytes are stimulated. Keratinocyte stimulation and proliferation lead to increased epidermal turnover and parakeratosis. Keratinocytes in patients with psoriasis react more strongly to the local release of mediators. Phenomena observed with psoriasis such as the isomorphous irritation effect (Koebner phenomenon) also indicate this predisposition (Boehncke and Sterry 2009; Nast et al. 2007).

2 Koebner Phenomenon

In the case of an occupational cause of psoriasis, usually the so-called Koebner phenomenon plays an important role. Heinrich Koebner (1834–1904) was one of the leading dermatologists of the nineteenth century. He was the Director of the Breslau University, Head of the Breslau School of Dermatology and the first President of the Berlin dermatological society. In 1872, he described a patient who, 5 years after developing psoriasis, noted that various traumatic insults of his skin resulted in lesions of psoriasis (Rubin and Stiller 2002). Today the Koebner phenomenon is defined as a nonspecific traumatic skin stimulus eliciting a disease-specific skin reaction, especially in psoriasis. The Koebner phenomenon is also known as an "isomorphic response."

3 Incidence

Compared to the epidemiological data regarding occupational hand eczema, there are only few data available on the incidence of occupationally induced psoriasis.

In a Swedish investigation of 246 patients with occupational hand dermatitis, psoriasis of the hands were diagnosed in 16 cases (n = 6.5%) (Agrup 1969).

An Italian study reported that occupationally induced psoriasis accounted for 1.2% of all occupational dermatoses observed (n = 3,000) (Moroni et al. 1988). Only 10% of the cases with occupationally derived psoriasis suffered

T. Rustemeyer, P. Elsner, S.M. John & H.I. Maibach (eds.), *Kanerva's Occupational Dermatology*,
DOI 10.1007/978-3-642-02035-3_32, © Springer-Verlag Berlin Heidelberg 2012

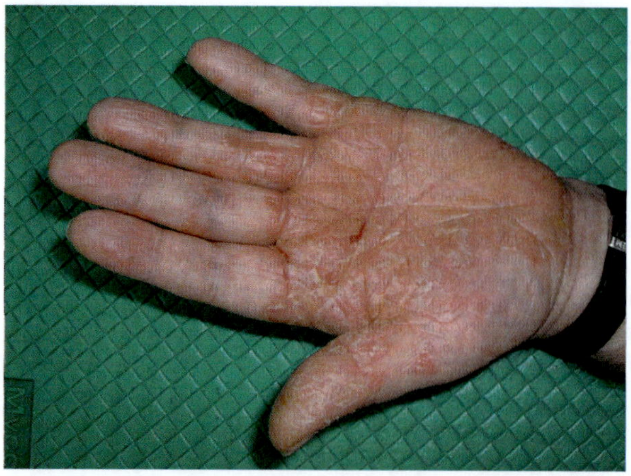

Fig. 32.1
Occupational psoriasis of the hand of a masseur (palmar) (Note: Clinical similarity to hyperkeratotic hand eczema, but in contrast to this type of an eczema sharp demarcation of the erythematous lesions)

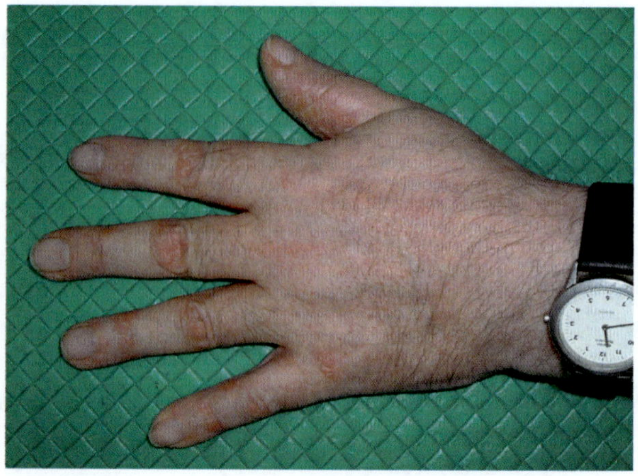

Fig. 32.2
Occupational psoriasis of the hand of a masseur (back of the hand) (Note: Typically plaques at the knuckles)

from classical and typically localized lesions. Most of the patients with occupationally induced psoriasis in this study had mechanical effects on the skin during their work activities (e.g., packaging workers, construction workers, mechanics, etc.) (Moroni et al. 1988).

Psoriasis of the hands was diagnosed in 73 of 1,901 patients (3.8%) who took part in an interdisciplinary inpatient rehabilitation measure for recalcitrant occupational skin disease in Germany (Skudlik et al. 2008). In 42 cases (2.2%) of this, a professional context of psoriasis of the hands was observed. This was due to mechanical effects in 10 cases, wet work in 7 cases, a combination of mechanical effects and wet work in 24 cases, and micro-injuries in 1 case (unpublished data).

4 Diagnostics

Occupationally induced psoriasis of the hands is rare in comparison to occupational hand eczema.

A family background of psoriasis and the presence of psoriasis lesions on typical predilection areas can be helpful for the diagnosis.

Furthermore nail changes (pits in the nail plate, yellowish macules beneath the nail plate or severe onychodystrophy) may be indicative. In contrast to hand eczema in most cases psoriasis of the hands showed raised, erythematous plaques with layers of silvery scales (which are sharply demarcated).

Psoriasis palmaris can persist several weeks or month after avoiding the occupational cause.

Clinically and histologically distinction between psoriasis of the hands and hand dermatitis can be difficult (*Figs. 32.1* and *32.2*). Especially the differential diagnosis to hyperkeratotic hand eczema may sometimes be difficult, but widespread lesions are not found in hyperkeratotic eczema (Agner 2011).

Although psoriasis of the hands is not an allergic skin disease, patch testing with occupational and non-occupational (e.g., domestic) allergens should be performed in all patients with psoriasis of the hands because of the clinical similarity and a relevant overlap with hand eczema in many cases.

5 Occupational Contact Psoriasis

Occupational psoriasis palmaris is usually caused by mechanical or physical trauma, friction or contact with irritants (see Chap. 78, "Mechanical Causes of Occupational Skin Disease," by R. Brans and S.M. John). Such constellations are published for various occupations, for example, baker, barkeeper, bookbinder, bus driver (from the pressure of the steering wheel), cashier, cleaner, construction worker, dentist (caused by the pressure of various instruments), draftsman, electrician, joiner, manufacturing/packaging worker, masseur, mechanic (e.g., from gripping tools), newspaper-vendor, pharmacist (from twirling finger movements while handling bottle caps), seamstress and tailor (Fisher 1979; Maibach and Epstein 1983; Menne and Hjorth 1984; Ancona et al. 1986; Moroni et al. 1988; Kanerva et al. 1998; Kanerva and Estlander 2001) (*Figs. 32.3* and *32.4*).

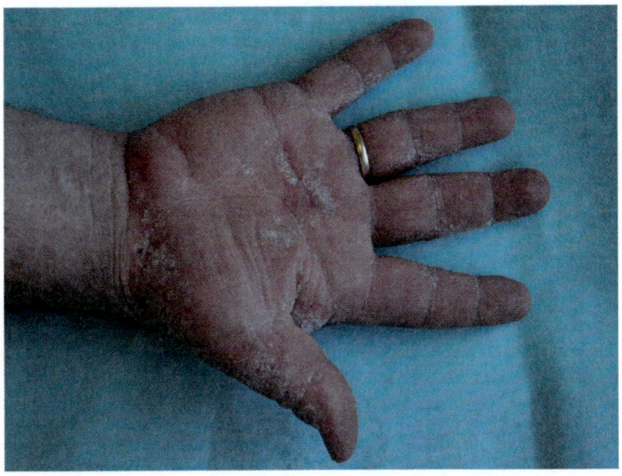

◘ Fig. 32.3
Occupational psoriasis of the hand due to regular contact to a handle of packaging tool (Note: There is no presence of psoriasis lesions on other areas except the *right hand*)

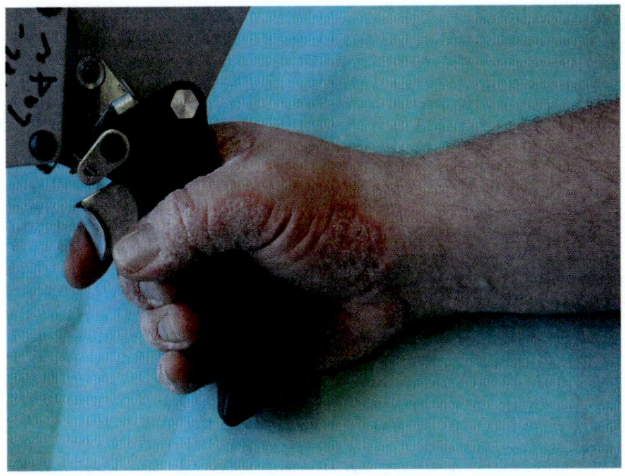

◘ Fig. 32.4
Occupational psoriasis of the hand due to regular contact to a handle of packaging tool: Holding the tool (same patient as in ➋ *Fig. 32.3*). Lesions subsided after proper therapy and use of anti-impaction gloves and anti-impaction grip

Koebner reactions may rarely also be triggered by allergic processes. Such a constellation has recently been reported in a metalworker who developed severe allergic contact dermatitis against ingredients of water-based cutting fluids (colophony). After the replacement of the contact allergen the dermatitis healed but for the first time a psoriatic plaque formed in this area (back of hands and palmar). He had no psoriasis lesions before or later on other areas of the body (Ebisch et al. 2009). Other publications report psoriasis of the hands elicited by allergic occupational contact dermatitis from thiuram in a nurse and a farmer wearing rubber gloves (Hill and Ostlere 1998; Spiewak 2004).

6 Prevention

On the level of primary prevention it is important to advise young people with psoriasis on adequate skin protection measures before starting job training in a risk profession (e.g., mechanical trauma, wet work, etc.) (Wulfhorst et al. 2011). Trainees with severe psoriasis palmaris should not choose a risk profession.

On the level of secondary and tertiary prevention it is important for the physician to consider the diagnosis of occupationally triggered psoriasis of the hands and to distinguish this diagnosis from occupational hand eczema. In the same way, it is essential to ensure that the patient understands the precise diagnosis and its consequences.

All necessary therapeutic options should be taken according to the severity of the disease (Nast et al. 2007). This comprises basic treatment (skin care program and moisturizers), topical therapy (e.g., salicylic acid, anthralin, vitamin-D_3 analogues, tazarotene, tar, topical Glucocorticoids), physical therapy (e.g., photochemotherapy [topical PUVA of the hands], balneophototherapy, selective UVB-therapy), and systemic therapy (e.g., retinoids, methotrexate, fumaric acid esters, biologicals).

It is equally important to remove or reduce the potential triggers. Therefore, the working conditions should be altered as far as possible. Concerning this from central importance are technical or work organization measures to reduce mechanical or physical trauma, friction, or contact with irritants (and allergens). In addition, the padding of contact materials, as for example handheld tools (soft grips etc.) and the use of anti-impaction gloves, before return to work are pivotal (Kwok et al. 2009; Wulfhorst et al. 2011). To the social insurance system the work relatedness of the disease needs specific explanation, if possible tailored preventive support for the patients should be made available by the occupational accident insurances, including skin protection seminars (see ➋ Chap. 108, "Prevention and Rehabilitation," by C. Skudlik and S.M. John). If preventive measures fail, job retraining and compensation will be required, if psoriasis was occupationally triggered (Frosch et al. 2011).

References

Agner T (2011) Hand eczema. In: Duus Johansen J, Frosch PJ, Lepoittevin JP (eds) Contact dermatitis, 5th edn. Springer, Berlin/Heidelberg, pp 395–406

Agrup G (1969) Hand eczema and other hand dermatoses in south Sweden. Acta Derm Venereol 49(suppl 61):59–61

Ancona A, Fernandez-Diez J, Bellamy C (1986) Occupationally induced psoriasis. Dermatosen 34:71–73

Boehncke WH, Sterry W (2009) Psoriasis - a systemic inflammatory disorder: clinic, pathogenesis and therapeutic perspectives. JDDG 7:946–952

Ebisch MA, Skudlik C, John SM (2009) Berufsbedingte Psoriasis Palmaris: Köbner-Phänomen, induziert durch allergisches Kontaktekzem bei Kontakt zu Kühlschmiermitteln. Dermatol Beruf Umwelt/Occup Environ Dermatol 57:158–162

Fisher AA (1979) Occupational palmar psoriasis due to safety prescription container. Contact Dermatitis 5:56

Frosch PJ, Aberer W, Agner T et al (2011) International comparison of legal aspects of worker's compensation for occupational contact dermatitis. In: Duus Johansen J, Frosch PJ, Lepoittevin JP (eds) Contact dermatitis, 5th edn. Springer, Berlin/Heidelberg, pp 1029–1051

Hill VA, Ostlere LS (1998) Psoriasis of the hands köbnerizing in contact dermatitis. Contact Dermatitis 39:194

Kanerva L, Estlander T (2001) Occupational post-traumatic psoriasis. Contact Dermatitis 44:317–318

Kanerva L, Talvi A, Estlander T (1998) Occupational contact psoriasis. Eur J Dermatol 8:217–218

Kwok T, Arrandale V, Skotnicki-Grant S (2009) Repeated mechanical trauma to the hands: the use of anti-impaction gloves for treatment and return to work. Dermatitis 20:278–283

Maibach HI, Epstein E (1983) Eczematous psoriasis. Semin Dermatol 2:45–50

Menne T, Hjorth N (1984) Mechanically provoked contact dermatitis and psoriasis. Z Hautkr 59:647–653

Moroni P, Cazzaniga R, Pierini F et al (1988) Occupational contact psoriasis. Dermatosen 36:163–164

Nast A, Kopp IB, Augustin M et al (2007) Evidence-based (S3) guidelines for the treatment of psoriasis vulgaris. JDDG 5(Suppl 3):1–77

Nevitt GJ, Hutchinson PE (1996) Psoriasis in the community: prevalence, severity and patient's beliefs and attitudes towards the disease. Br J Dermatol 135:533–537

Rubin AI, Stiller MJ (2002) A listing of skin conditions exhibiting the Koebner and Pseudo-Koebner Phenomena with eliciting stimuli. J Cutan Med Surg 6(1):29–34

Skudlik C, Wulfhorst B, Gediga G et al (2008) Tertiary individual prevention of occupational skin diseases – a decade's experience with recalcitrant occupational dermatitis. Int Arch Occup Environ Health 81(8):1045–1058

Spiewak R (2004) Köbnerizing occupational contact allergy to thiuram in a farmer with psoriasis. Contact Dermatitis 51:214–215

Wulfhorst B, Bock M, Skudlik C et al (2011) Prevention of hand eczema – gloves, barrier creams and workers' education. In: Duus Johansen J, Frosch PJ, Lepoittevin JP (eds) Contact dermatitis, 5th edn. Springer, Berlin/Heidelberg, pp 985–1028

33 Physical Causes – Heat, Cold, and Other Atmospheric Factors

Wolfgang Uter[1] · *Lasse Kanerva*[2]
[1]Department of Medical Informatics, Biometry and Epidemiology, University of Erlangen/Nürnberg, Erlangen, Germany
[2]Section of Dermatology, Finnish Institute of Occupational Health, Helsinki, Finland

Core Messages

- Heat induces skin damage not only directly in terms of thermal or electrical burns, but also via infrared radiation or prolonged direct exposure to moderate heat (erythema ab igne).
- Sweat retention in different layers of the eccrine sweat glands may cause miliaria.
- Cold has considerable systemic effects and can cause frostbite or, if only moderate, perniosis (chilblains).
- Prolonged wetness of the feet and lower legs, especially if combined with low temperature, can cause "immersion foot" as a nonfreezing cold injury.
- Both low outdoor and (subsequent) low indoor air humidity may cause skin irritation and favors irritation by other agents, e.g., wet work.

1 Introduction

Injuries by some of the physical factors mentioned in this chapter are among the most ancient health risks of mankind, and, indeed, of all living objects. Other factors have been introduced by man. Partly, these produce the same morbidity, such as Erythema ab igne not caused by open fires, from caves to castles, but by holding lap top computers on the thighs for prolonged periods. However, in a few instances man-made physical factors may produce novel skin changes, such as thermal effects of microwave radiation or low humidity dermatoses in "clean rooms." The following chapter will present the most important types of injury in a systematic way.

2 Heat

2.1 Thermal Burns

Burns result from exposure to extremes of heat. The lowest temperature at which a burn can occur has been estimated to be 44°C (111°F) (Moritz and Henriques 1947). Burns may be of industrial, domestic, or environmental origin. Industrial burns are common (Cason 1981) and may have characteristic occupational patterns (Renz and Sherman 1994; Woods et al. 1996). They may be caused by direct contact with hot objects, radiation heat (infrared, IR) or hot steam, or air, e.g., emitted by improperly handled heat torches. Moreover, accidental exposure to laser energy may cause thermal destruction through absorption by skin chromophores such as melanin and hemoglobin, well known from the therapeutic application of different lasers in dermatology. Classification of burns is based on the depth of the burn as first, second, or third degree (➋ *Table 33.1*) (Burke and Bondoc 1993).

Although in many countries dermatologists are often not involved in the acute-phase treatment of more severe burns, they frequently are requested to evaluate impairment of patients with healed burns. Pigmentation, vascularity, pliability, and scar height are the main parameters (Sullivan et al. 1990) for dermatological evaluation. Sometimes, scarring is extensive enough to limit joint mobility or muscle strength (Jonsson et al. 1997) in addition to producing varying degrees of disfigurement. Squamous cell carcinoma arising from burn scars was described by Marjolin in 1828; the frequency of this complication is unknown (Kennedy 1992). The criteria established by Ewing (1935) for associating a carcinoma with a previous burn are still considered valid.

Burns may cause either hyperpigmentation or hypopigmentation. When total loss of pigment occurs, it denotes deeper burns with destruction of melanocytes, and recovery of skin color is doubtful. With more superficial burns, hyperpigmentation may result depending on the depth of the burn and the genetic background of the patient. Blacks and other dark skinned persons show the greatest hyperpigmentation, which on the face and other exposed areas may be very disfiguring. Fading occurs

T. Rustemeyer, P. Elsner, S.M. John & H.I. Maibach (eds.), *Kanerva's Occupational Dermatology*,
DOI 10.1007/978-3-642-02035-3_33, © Springer-Verlag Berlin Heidelberg 2012

Table 33.1
Classification of burns based on the depth of the burns (From Burke and Bondoc 1993)

Classification of burns	Surface appearance	Sensation	Outcome/prognosis
First-degree	Dry, erythematous, no blisters	Painful, hypersensitive	Complete healing within 1 week; no scar
Second-degree (superficial)	Blisters, red oozing base, good capillary refill, blanching on pressure	Painful, extremely sensitive to pinprick	Complete healing within 3 weeks; may be erythematous early after healing
Second-degree (deep)	Blisters may be present; pale, indurated areas; some areas red	Some insensitive areas; many areas anesthetic to pinprick	Firm, thick scar with loss of hair follicles, sweat glands, and skin pigmentation; healing may take 1 month
Third-degree	Pearly white or brown opaque gray; firm leathery, dry	No sensation	Total skin loss includes all appendages; heals by scar formation if small

slowly; a final evaluation of permanency should not be made until 18–24 months after the burn has completely healed.

2.2 Electrical Burns

These occur from environmental, domestic, and industrial sources. Out of 290 fatal factory accidents in Great Britain, 21 were due to electric shock; a larger number died from burns after contact with domestic 240 V alternating current (50 Hz) current (Cason 1981). The lesions are due to heat and direct injury by electricity, the severity depending, e.g., on current voltage, thickness and wetness of the skin, and duration of contact (Kennedy 1992). High-voltage burns are severe while low-voltage burns are milder, but penetrating more deeply than is apparent following nerves and vessels, extending some distance away from the edge of the visible wound. Even 24 V may produce deep injury (Benmeir et al. 1993). Late rupture of blood vessels can occur even as long as 2 weeks after the electrical burn (Kennedy 1992). Electrothermal burns may be caused by touching a heated electrical element. Burns from cardiac defibrillators have caused local skin ulcers. The depth of electric flash burns depends on the temperature of the agent and the duration of contact. Recently, Campbell and coworkers (1996) reported high-voltage electrical injury in two hang-glider pilots from 11,000 V power lines. Magnetic resonance imaging (MRI) is a valuable diagnostic aid in the care of high-voltage electrical burns (Nettelblad et al. 1996).

Burns from lightning cause a bizarre, superficial erythema which Bartholome et al. (1975) considered pathognomonic. The skin shows numerous erythematous macules arranged in a streaked feather- or fern-like pattern. Blanching on diascopy does not occur, and in those persons who survive fading occurs in 24–48 h. The condition is probably due to the transmission of static electricity along the superficial vessels, similar to that occurring when an electrodessiccating current is used to destroy small angiomas. Lightning injuries are occupational risk of outdoor workers such as railroad and highway construction workers, surveyors, geologists, foresters, and agricultural workers.

2.3 Erythema ab igne

Infrared radiation, composed of wavelengths of 800–170,000 nm, results in thermal burns at temperatures over 44°C (Zalar and Harber 1985). Chronic exposure to heat can result in erythema ab igne and skin cancer. It is characterized by a mottled, reticulate hyperemia with melanoderma and telangiectasia and sometimes superficial epidermal atrophy and subepidermal blistering. Erythema ab igne occurs after prolonged exposure to heat, i.e., infrared radiation, which is usually insufficient to produce burn. At one time, the condition was common on the anterior legs and inner thighs of women who sat for long periods before an open fire, and on the abdomens of patients with chronical abdominal pain who applied heating pads for hours at a time. New cases are now being seen as heating with wood fires has become more common again. Heater cushions still cause erythema ab igne (Dvoretzky and Silverman 1991). Erythema ab igne may be a sign leading one to suspect hypothyroidism (Kennedy 1992). It has also been reported as a marker of chronic pancreatitis (Mok and Blumgart 1984).

Workers who may develop erythema ab igne include stokers, blacksmiths, glassblowers, bakers (especially those using old-fashioned brick-lined ovens), and cooks and others working over a heat source. Schwartz et al. (1957) described the condition in stenographers who sit very close to radiators in cold weather. According to Kennedy (1992), it also occurs in the face of silversmiths and jewelers and on the arms of foundry men. A more recent source of erythema ab igne mediated by contact, and not radiation, are laptop computers, if held for many hours and days (several case reports published, e.g., Bachmeyer et al. 2009). In mentally disturbed patients with thermophilia, bizarre areas of erythema ab igne have been encountered (Kennedy 1992).

After an interval of up to over 30 years, thermal skin injury and erythema ab igne may proceed to cancer (Kaplan 1987). Several variants, mostly depending on a certain geographical influence or habit, have been described (Kanerva 1999). Infrared radiation (IR) may significantly enhance aging and carcinogenic effects of ultraviolet radiation (Kligman and Kligman 1984).

Table 33.2
Workers potentially exposed to excessive heat

Animal rendering workers
Asphalt workers
Bakers
Bitumen workers
Boiler heaters
Cannery workers
Chemical plant operators working near hot containers and furnaces
Cleaners
Coke oven operators
Cooks and other kitchen workers
Firemen
Foundry workers
Glass manufacturing workers
Greenhouse workers
Kiln workers
Miners in deep mines
Outdoor workers during hot weather
Sailors passing hot climatic zones
Shipyard workers when cleaning cargo holds
Smelter workers
Steel and metal forges
Textile manufacturing workers (weaving, dyeing)
Maintenance workers in nuclear plants
Tight protective clothing (all occupations)
Tire (rubber) manufacturing workers

2.4 Erythermalgia

Erythermalgia is a syndrome of bilateral symmetric burning and redness of the lower, or sometimes upper, extremities. Symptoms can be initiated by exercise or exposure to heat, while rest and cold bring relief (Heller Page and Shear 1993; Drenth and Michiels 1994; Gaur and Koroscil 2009). Thus, occupational factors may aggravate symptoms (*Table 33.2*). Primary erythermalgia usually arises in childhood. Secondary erythermalgia develops in adult age in association or without an apparent underlying disorder. Aspirin (Heller Page and Shear 1993) or avoidance of triggering situations by lifestyle modification (Gaur and Koroscil 2009) has given the best results, but treatment may be difficult, and symptoms may persist throughout life. Secondary erythermalgia can arise as a side effect of drugs but otherwise the etiology is yet unknown (Drenth and Michiels 1994; Drenth et al. 1997).

2.5 Miliaria

Miliaria is caused by sweat retention. Heat causes swelling of the keratin within sweat ducts, resulting in poral closure and rupture of the ducts immediately beneath the obstruction. If the obstruction occurs within the stratum corneum, miliaria crystallina (sudamina) results. This produces small, clear vesicles that soon rupture and lead to desquamation. Cutaneous bacteria, particularly *Staphylococci* seem to play a role in the pathogenesis of miliaria (Mowad et al. 1995). The skin surface may or may not be faintly erythematous. It is most commonly seen after mild nonspecific damage to the epidermis and/or profuse sweating. While miliaria crystallina is usually asymptomatic, patients may become concerned when they suddenly notice the entire palm is desquamating (Lobitz 1962). Widespread involvement may in rare cases interfere with thermoregulation.

When closure occurs somewhat deeper in the epidermis, in the granular layer, firm vesicles are formed accompanied by marked pruritus. Called miliaria rubra, or prickly heat it is easily confused with contact dermatitis. This condition is more troublesome than miliaria crystallina because the eruption may be quite extensive and accompanied by paroxysms of burning and itching. The lesions are small erythematous macules and vesicles unassociated with follicular openings; a hand lens aids in visualization. The lesions may appear a few days after exposure to hot, humid environment, but most commonly appear after one to several months (Lillywhite 1992).

The trunk and intertriginous areas are particularly involved, while the palms and soles are spared. When poral closure is severe, hyperpyrexia and heat exhaustion occur, causing a decrease in work efficiency. The lesions that later develop may be pustular from infiltration of inflammatory cells and may be complicated by secondary bacterial infection.

If obstruction is even deeper, i.e., in the dermo-epidermal junction zone, miliaria profunda results (Kirk et al. 1996), producing deep-seated asymptomatic vesicles, that appear much like gooseflesh, but close examination shows that they spare the follicles. The lesions consist of pale white papules 1–3 mm in diameter, which are most prominent on the trunk. Erythema and pruritus are mild or absent. This serious condition is caused by widespread inactivation of sweat glands from prolonged exposure to a hot environment. It usually follows an extended period of miliaria rubra. Heat exhaustion and collapse are common sequelae. A condition called tropical anhidrotic asthenia with acute fatigue, nausea, dizziness, palpitations, tachycardia, and malaise has been observed among military personnel during wartime in very hot, humid environments. Tropical anhidrotic asthenia is secondary to widespread miliaria profunda in particularly adverse conditions (Cage et al. 1987).

Treatment of miliaria consists of cooling the patient to reduce sweating. Mild, nonocclusive lotions may be used. In miliaria crystallina, removal of the damaged area by mechanical means or by natural sloughing stops the process. In miliaria rubra, a week of rest from the inciting factors allows removal of the damaged portion of the epidermis by natural desquamation while in miliaria profunda rest in cool surroundings for several weeks is needed for complete recovery. Systemic and topical steroids are not helpful.

Occupations where excessive heat exposure can occur are listed in ➋ *Table 33.2*; in addition, work in the tropics may be inadvisable for very susceptible persons.

2.6 Intertrigo

A macerated, erythematous eruption in body folds – intertrigo – can occur from excessive sweating, especially in obese persons. Friction between opposing surfaces in addition to sweat retention are important etiologic factors. Secondary bacterial or *Candida* infection commonly accompanies intertrigo. The groin, axillae, and interdigital areas are favored sites. In particular, the interdigital space between the third and fourth fingers is a common site for intertrigo and secondary *Candida* infection among cannery workers, bartenders, medical and dental personnel, and others performing wet work for prolonged periods. Cooks, swimming instructors, nurses, and others exposed to moisture are also disposed to this condition. An important differential diagnosis, if finger web spaces are affected, is interdigital dermatitis as a common, early type of irritant contact dermatitis in wet work occupations (Schwanitz and Uter 2000). This will, however, show scaling and probably fissuring without maceration and should respond well to emollient treatment and improved skin protection measures.

2.7 Miscellaneous Conditions

Acne vulgaris and rosacea can be aggravated by prolonged chronic exposure to heat, especially intense heat from ovens, steam, open furnaces, or heat torches. Herpes simplex may be triggered by sudden blasts of heat. Prolonged exposure to excessive heat also increases irritability, decreases workers' ability to concentrate, and results in a generally lower level of efficiency.

3 Cold

The effect of coldness is the result of a complex interaction of climatic factors (air temperature, mean radiant temperature, humidity, and wind), protection (clothing), and metabolic heat production (activity). The nature of cooling encompasses (1) whole-body cooling, (2) extremity cooling, (3) convective cooling (wind chill), (4) conductive cooling (contact), and (5) airway cooling (Holmer 1993). Cooling the brain leads to confusion and later to incoordination, while cooling the limbs results in numbness and clumsiness, making the performance of intricate tasks difficult.

Local cooling in most cases produces discomfort and harmful effects, before more significant whole-body cooling develops. With strong wind or exposure to very low temperature, frostbite of unprotected skin may quickly develop (see below). However, as digit cooling largely depends on whole-body heat balance, it is important to control body cooling by selection and use of appropriate protective clothing (Holmer 1993).

Everybody reacts to cold, but in addition to physiologic responses to cold, abnormal reactions may occur in some individuals. Chilblains may result from chronic exposure to moderate cold. Cold plays an important role in, e.g., Raynaud's phenomenon, cryoglobulinemia, and cold urticaria. Cutaneous reactions to cold can be divided into reactions to abnormal cold and abnormal reactions to "normal" cold. The diseases caused or aggravated by cold are listed in ➋ *Table 33.3.*

3.1 Frostbite

There are three stages of freezing cold injury: (1) massive vasoconstriction causing a rapid fall in skin temperature; (2) the hunting phenomenon, i.e., transient cyclic vasodilatation by the opening of arteriovenous anastomoses causing a cyclic rise and fall in skin temperature; and (3) if cold exposure continues, freezing, as the skin temperature falls to approach ambient temperature (Kulka 1965; Heller Page and Shear 1993).

Table 33.3
Diseases caused or aggravated by cold

I. Reactions to abnormal cold	1. Cold injury
	2. Frostbite
	3. Nonfreezing cold injury a. Immersion or trench foot b. Immersion foot c. Tropical immersion foot
II. Abnormal reactions to cold	1. Perniosis
	2. Pulling boat hands
	3. Acrocyanosis
	4. Erythrocyanosis
	5. Livedo reticularis
	6. Cold urticaria
	7. Cold erythema
	8. Cold panniculitis
	9. Sclerema neonatorum
	10. Subcutaneous fat necrosis of the newborn
	11. Cryoglobulinemia
	12. Raynaud's phenomenon

The events that follow freezing and nonfreezing cold injury are similar and include: (1) arterial and arteriolar vasoconstriction, (2) excessive venular and capillary vasodilatation, (3) increased endothelial leakage, (4) erythrostasis, (5) arteriovenous shunting, (6) segmental vascular necrosis, and (7) massive thrombosis (Heller Page and Shear 1993).

The degree of cellular injury depends on (1) the minimum temperature, (2) the duration of time at that temperature, (3) the cooling rate, with rapid cooling causing more destructive intracellular ice crystal formation, and hence more destruction as is obvious from cryotherapy, (4) rewarming rate. In slow rewarming, intracellular ice crystals become larger and more lethal for the cell and (5) finally, repeated freeze-thaw cycles lead to greater injury. Different cell types vary in their susceptibility to cold. Melanocytes are very sensitive, and damage occurs at −4°C to −7°C (25–19°F). Accordingly, cryotherapy causes hypopigmentation (Heller Page and Shear 1993).

Low air temperatures and high wind speeds ("wind chill") are associated with an increased risk of freezing of the exposed skin. As the skin surface temperature falls from −4.8°C to −7.8°C, the risk of frostbite increases from 5% to 95% (Danielsson 1996). Frostbite additionally causes impairment of circulation due to slowly progressing vasoconstriction.

In its mildest form only redness and pain are present. In more severe cases, tissue destruction and blistering occur and this may be superficial, full thickness or involve deep tissues analogous to the burns (see ➋ *Table 33.1*). In its most extreme form, gangrene and loss of limb may result. Exposed parts, i.e., toes, feet, fingers, ears, nose, and cheeks are most often affected.

As tissue temperature falls, the area becomes numb, and the initial redness is gradually replaced by a white, waxy appearance with blistering and later necrosis; the affected part becomes deceptively anesthetic. In the early stages, it is difficult to predict the extent of tissue loss becoming perceivable after rewarming, especially concerning deeper structures like muscle and bone. Accurate estimation may clinically not be possible for several weeks (Knize et al. 1969), however, magnetic resonance imaging (MRI) and angiography (MRA) provide for early recognition of damaged tissue (Barker et al. 1997). The more superficial the injury, the better the prognosis, especially if infection is absent. However, even without loss of tissue, long-term effects may include telangiectasia

(Huh et al. 1996), vasomotor instability with Raynaud-like changes, paresthesia and hyperhidrosis. This is attributed to damage to the blood vessels and sympathetic nerves. Squamous cell carcinoma may arise in the old scars (Rossis et al. 1982).

In slow rewarming, intracellular ice crystals become larger and more lethal for the cells. Therefore, treatment entails rapidly rewarming the part for which a whirlpool or water bath, or warm air for 20 min (until the most distal part is flushed) is useful. A temperature no higher than blood temperature (Daniels 1987) or 42°C (Heller Page and Shear 1993) has been recommended, e.g., employing warm baths for some 20 min (Champion 1992). Thereafter, the affected part is rested at usual room temperature. Rewarming is painful and causes an increase in erythema and blistering. The pain should be relieved with analgesics. The damaged part should be elevated and blisters left intact. Infection must be treated vigorously. Early application of heparin or infusion of low molecular weight dextran may be of some additional benefit (Champion 1992). The popular old idea of rubbing the affected part with snow has an adverse, even disastrous effect.

Historically, the persons at greatest risk of frostbite have been military personnel. Nearly 200,000 cold casualties occurred during World Wars I and II and the Korean conflict (Daniels 1987). Today, many cases are associated with alcohol consumption, homelessness in urban centers, and car breakdown (Miller and Chasmar 1980). Frostbite also occurs in winter sports to, e.g., cross country skiers or backpackers. Workers at risk include oil pipeline workers in northern regions; utility maintenance personnel, sailors, especially those working on icebreakers, fishermen, firefighters, mail delivery persons, rescue personnel, researchers in cold laboratories and polar areas, and others who work outdoors in cold regions (➋ *Table 33.4*).

Table 33.4
Workers potentially exposed to excessive cold

Workers
Cooling room workers
Divers
Dry ice workers
Firefighters
Ice makers
Liquefied gas workers
Outdoor workers during cold weather
Packing house workers
Refrigerated warehouse workers
Refrigeration workers
Winter sports instructors

3.2 Immersion Foot/Nonfreezing Cold Injury

Formerly called trench foot, immersion foot results from exposure to cold temperatures above freezing for several days. In the presence of moisture and constrictive clothing, however, continuous exposure for as little as 19 h may be sufficient (Rietschel and Allen 1976). Immersion foot is less severe than frostbite and develops in three stages: initial erythema, edema, and tenderness (stage I); followed within 24 h by paresthesia, marked edema, numbness, and sometimes bullae (stage II); and progressing to gangrene (stage III). Gangrene does not develop unless there is infection. Convalescence may be prolonged for several weeks or months, during which time there is cold sensitivity, vasomotor instability, hyperemia, and hyperhidrosis. Rest, analgesics, and antibiotics are the mainstays of treatment, which is the same as for frostbite.

During the Korean and Vietnam Wars thousands of cases occurred, and immersion foot became the major cause of disability. In industries, in which workers are required to stand for long periods in cold wet mud or water, as when excavating foundations for new construction, immersion-type injuries may be frequent (Schwartz et al. 1957). Street and sewer workers as well as golf caddies walking for hours on wet grass are also at risk (Chow et al. 1980). For the homeless, immersion foot can be a major health problem (Wrenn 1991), aggravated by lack of care. Interestingly, immersion foot can also develop in warm water (Humphrey and Ellyson 1997), including the tropics (tropical immersion foot, ➋ *Table 33.3*).

3.3 Chilblains (Perniosis)

The mildest form of cold injury, chilblains or perniosis, occur as an abnormal reaction to cold in the temperate humid climate of Great Britain and northwestern Europe, where there is a lack of central heating (Heller Page and Shear 1993). Chilblains are less often seen in continental cold climates such as Finland, where well-heated houses and warm clothing are essential. The lesions are reddish blue discolorations that become swollen and boggy, with tense bullae and later ulcerations that may result in scarring. Often, chilblains are superimposed on a background of acrocyanosis or erythrocyanosis. Lesions occur especially on the dorsa of the proximal phalanges of the fingers and toes, heels, lower legs, thighs, nose, and ears. The shiny red plaques itch and burn severely. Chilblains are particularly frequent in children, where they tend to start at the beginning of winter. In adults who work outdoors, chilblains often seem to start in the spring months (Champion 1992). Genetic factors are often apparent, e.g., acrocyanosis as an underlying factor. Differential diagnoses of idiopathic perniones include chilblain lupus erythematosus (Millard and Rowell 1978), sarcoidosis, and several other entities which have to be considered clinically, histologically, and serologically (Crowson and Magro 1997).

The most important point in management is prophylaxis with warm housing, warm clothing, and regular exercise. Once chilblain has appeared, treatment is mainly symptomatic with local application of an antipruritic. Some patients may benefit from ultraviolet radiation (Champion 1992). This therapy may relieve chronic vasospasm believed to occur in chilblains (Heller Page and Shear 1993). Nifedipine may be effective in the treatment of severe recurrent perniosis (Dowd et al. 1986). In 7 of 10 patients, clearing ranged from 8 days for lesions of the hands to 23 days for foot lesions (Dowd et al. 1986).

3.4 Pulling Boat Hands

This dermatosis has been described from coastal New England (Toback et al. 1985). Erythematous macules and plaques developed on the dorsa of the hands and fingers of instructors and students after 3–14 days aboard a pulling boat. Later, small vesicles appeared, accompanied by itching, burning, and tenderness. Subjects had been exposed to high humidity, cool air, and wind. This was considered an ideal setting for the development of this nonfreezing type dermatosis. Hours of vigorous rowing provided additional repetitive trauma. Some of the patients also had a history of frostbite and Raynaud's phenomenon. This syndrome may be caused by a combination of nonfreezing cold and the mechanical effects of rowing (Toback et al. 1985).

3.5 Other Reactions to Cold

Cold urticaria and Raynaud's phenomenon are dealt with later in this book. The reader interested in other types of abnormal reactions to cold (➋ *Table 33.3*) is referred to major textbooks of dermatology, e.g., the article of Heller Page and Shear (1993).

4 Other Atmospheric Factors

A low water content of ambient air may cause, or contribute to, occupational dermatoses, as emphasized by Rycroft and coworkers (Rycroft and Smith 1980; White and Rycroft 1982; Rycroft 1984, 1985), see below. In addition, low temperature, wind, electromagnetic fields, or electrostatic charge have been claimed to be ambient factors important to some skin conditions.

4.1 Low Outdoor Humidity

The following two measures are most commonly used to quantify the humidity of air: absolute humidity (AH) is the mass of water vapor present in a unit volume of the atmosphere and is mostly measured as mg/l. Relative humidity (RH) is the ratio of the quantity of water vapor present in the atmosphere to the quantity which would saturate it at the existing temperature (expressed as percentage). Thus, with a given quantity of water per air volume (AH), RH depends on the temperature: the higher the temperature, the greater the water-holding capacity of the atmosphere and the lower the RH, and vice versa.

Low humidity of the air is believed to cause dehydration of the horny layer and impairment of the epidermal barrier function (Agner and Serup 1989), i.e., increased irritability of the skin. Subclinical xerotic changes may occur within hours of exposure and are more pronounced in atopics (Eberlein-König et al. 1996).

Persons working and living in (sub-) polar or even temperate climates with a strong continental influence (prolonged periods of dry, frosty weather in winter) are regularly exposed to low atmospheric humidity, such as 10 mg/l or less. Clinical experience from these countries gives a strong hint on the contributing role to irritant hand dermatitis of these meteorological condition (Kavli and Föde 1984), which has recently been confirmed by an epidemiological study (Uter et al. 1998) and is in good accordance with some experimental data (partially reviewed by Uter et al. 1998).

Interestingly, unexposed skin displays an impaired epidermal barrier function also (Agner and Serup 1989), which may indicate that even the wearing of protective (warm, wind-tight) gloves may not completely be able to abolish the effect of low humidity on the skin of the hands. The hands may additionally be exposed to a variety of occupational irritants or to wet work. Thus, as (sub-) clinical irritation is known to often be a multifactorial process (Malten 1981), this fairly inalterable environmental condition puts extra emphasis on the necessity of adequate skin protection, be it domestic or occupational.

4.2 Other Ambient Factors

Several authors of experimental studies have attributed negative effects on epidermal properties to low temperature. However, absolute humidity is always also low with low temperature, according to the functional relationship mentioned above, and absolute humidity has not been considered in most of these older studies. At present, the effect of temperature concerning irritant damage can most likely be regarded as indirect.

Wind speed had been found to be a significant risk factor of the occurrence of "dry flaking" facial skin (Cooper et al. 1992). Parish (1992), who exposed the hands of volunteers to "a cold dry wind" 3 h daily, found visible alteration (roughness, desquamation) and impaired lipid and enzyme composition of the epidermis after a few days.

In addition to natural environmental conditions, anthropogenic factors may lead to occupational (skin) disease:

- During work on a television mast, exposure to high levels of ultrahigh frequency radiofrequency radiation (UHF, 785 MHz mean frequency) caused an immediate sensation of intense heating and later transient erythema, malaise, numbness, and pain (Schilling 1997).
- Similarly, microwave radiation (1–30 GHz) has been reported as a cause of more or less severe burns, lesser injury being followed by paraesthesia (Kennedy 1992).

4.3 Low Indoor Humidity

Below a water content of 10%, the stratum corneum loses its softness and pliability (Blank 1952). The water content of the horny layer remains below 10% when the relative humidity is less than 50% at room temperature (Rycroft 1985). High temperature and air flow accentuates the drying of the horny layer. An open-plan office next to or under the ventilation system, where warm, un-humidified air is introduced into the room is a typical working site, where the risk of low humidity dermatosis is apparent. Low humidity dermatoses can be accentuated by small irritant or hygroscopic airborne particles, such as textile particles, dust from ceramics, small particles from paper cutting, and fine angular, hygroscopic particles, as in a soft lens factory (Rycroft 1984, 1985). Domestic and general climatic conditions can potentiate low humidity occupational dermatoses: Air-conditioned buildings have a low relative (and absolute) humidity, and in temperate areas such as Scandinavia, the low humidity/high temperature indoor environment is accompanied by low humidity/low temperature outdoor climate during the winters, which also has a drying effect on the stratum corneum (see above). The empirical threshold value of 40% relative humidity reported by White and Rycroft (1982) corresponds at a temperature of around 20°C well with a threshold value of 9–10 mg/l absolute humidity as significant outdoor risk factor (Uter et al. 1998). Some of the occupations where low humidity dermatoses have been reported are listed in ➋ *Table 33.5*.

These dermatoses are far more distressing than their comparative paucity of physical signs might suggest (Rycroft 1985). Pruritus and burning can be the only sign of low humidity. Puffiness of the cheeks and eyelids has been observed. The skin lesions evolve through dryness of the skin to erythema and round or oval patches of eczema. Erythema has been accompanied by urticarial whealing possibly secondary to scratching pruritic skin. In some cases, areas covered by clothing have been predominantly involved, while facial itching with diffuse superficial scaling on the cheeks, forehead, and neck have been the main anatomical areas in other instances. Patchy erythema on the shaved face of male employees has been observed. Fair skinned individuals are at higher risk. Both atopics and nonatopics have been affected.

Differential diagnosis includes a wide variety of possibilities that have to be considered such as inhalable and ingestible allergens, irritant or allergic airborne contact dermatitis, psychological causes, menopausal hot flashes, rosacea and seborrheic eczema, or scabies.

Treatment should include routine use of emollients and increasing the relative humidity indoors to about 50% during the whole low humidity (winter) season.

Table 33.5
Reported low humidity risk occupations

1	Office work
2	Soft contact lens manufacturing
3	Silicon chip manufacturing
4	Cabin crew of long distance airplanes
5	Resident staff in hospitals and hotels
6	Traveling salesmen (from automobile heaters)

4.4 Visual Display Units

In some countries, patients often complain of skin symptoms from work with visual display units (VDU; Lidén and Wahlberg 1985; Berg 1989; Eriksson and Stenberg 2006). A study from Sweden among 353 routine office workers showed an increased tendency for seborrheic eczema and nonspecific erythema. Organizational conditions during VDU work, such as high work load, and inability to take rest breaks, were found to be associated with the reported skin symptoms. A low relative humidity was associated with a diagnosis of seborrheic eczema. However, no associations were found between current field levels of electric or magnetic field and skin diseases/signs or reported symptoms (Bergqvist and Wahlberg 1994). Accordingly, a reduction of electric fields was only weakly associated with an improvement of symptoms attributed to VDU work (Oftedal et al. 1995). Possibly independent from the initial cause of skin problems, psychological conditioning may lead to a perpetuation of symptoms even without exposure, as illustrated by experiments with affected office workers (Swanbeck and Bleeker 1989). In some cases, perceived symptoms, attributed to VDU work or other indoor factors, may be part of the ill-defined "sick building syndrome" (Stenberg et al. 1994; Norbäck 2009).

References

Agner T, Serup J (1989) Seasonal variation of skin resistance to irritants. Br J Dermatol 121:323–328

Bachmeyer C, Bensaid P, Bégon E (2009) Laptop computer as a modern cause of erythema ab igne. J Eur Acad Dermatol Venereol 23:736–737

Barker JR, Haws MJ, Brown RE et al (1997) Magnetic resonance imaging of severe frostbite injuries. Ann Plast Surg 38:275–279

Bartholome CW, Jacoby WD, Ramchand SC (1975) Cutaneous manifestations of lightning injury. Arch Dermatol 111:1466–1468

Benmeir P, Lusthaus S, Ad-El D, Neuman A et al (1993) Very deep burns of the hand due to low voltage electrical laboratory equipment: a potential hazard for scientists. Burns 19:450–451

Berg M (1989) Facial skin complaints and work at visual display units. Epidemiological, clinical and histopathological studies. Acta Derm-Venereol (Stockh) Suppl 150:1–40

Bergqvist U, Wahlberg JE (1994) Skin symptoms during work with visual display terminals. Contact Dermatitis 30:193–196

Blank IH (1952) Factors which influence the water content of the stratum corneum. J Invest Dermatol 18:433–440

Burke JF, Bondoc CC (1993) Burns: the management and evaluation of the thermally injured patient. In: Fitzpatrick TB, Eisen AZ, Wolff K et al (eds) Dermatology in general medicine, 4th edn. McGraw-Hill, New York, pp 1592–1598

Cage GW, Sato K, Schwachman H (1987) Eccrine glands. The management and evaluation of the thermally injured patient. In: Fitzpatrick TB, Eisen AZ, Wolff K et al (eds) Dermatology in general medicine, 3rd edn. McGraw-Hill, New York, pp 691–704

Campbell DC, Nano T, Pegg SP (1996) Pattern of burn injury in hang-glider pilots. Burns 22:328–330

Cason JS (1981) Treatment of burns. Chapman & Hall, London, pp 205–220

Champion RH (1992) Reactions to cold. In: Rook A, Wilkinson DS, Ebling FJG et al (eds) Textbook of dermatology, 5th edn. Blackwell Scientific, Oxford, pp 833–847

Chow S, Westfried M, Lynfield Y (1980) Immersion foot: an occupational disease. Cutis 25:662

Cooper MD, Jardine H, Ferguson J (1992) Seasonal influence on the occurrence of dry flaking facial skin. In: Marks RG, Plewig G (eds) The environmental threat to the skin. M. Dunitz, London, pp 159–164

Crowson AN, Magro CM (1997) Idiopathic perniosis and its mimics: a clinical and histological study of 38 cases. Hum Pathol 28:478–784

Daniels F (1987) Physiologic factors in the skin's reactions to heat and cold. In: Fitzpatrick TB, Eisen AZ, Wolff K et al (eds) Dermatology in general medicine, 3rd edn. McGraw-Hill, New York, pp 1412–1424

Danielsson U (1996) Windchill and the risk of tissue freezing. J Appl Physiol 81:2666–2673

Dowd PM, Rustin MHA, Lanigan S (1986) Nifedipine in the treatment of chilblains. Br Med J 293:923–924

Drenth JPH, Michiels JJ (1994) Erythromelalgia and erythermalgia: diagnostic differentiation. Int J Dermatol 33:393–397

Drenth JPH, Michiels JJ, Van Joost Th (1997) Substance P is not involved in primary and secondary erythermalgia. Acta Derm Venereol (Stockh) 77:325–326

Dvoretzky I, Silverman NR (1991) Reticular erythema of the lower back. Arch Dermatol 127:405–410

Eberlein-König B, Spiegl A, Przybilla B (1996) Change of skin roughness due to lowering air humidity in climate chamber. Acta Derm Venerol 76:447–449

Eriksson NM, Stenberg BG (2006) Baseline prevalence of symptoms related to indoor environment. Scand J Public Health 34:387–396

Ewing J (1935) Modern attitude toward traumatic cancer. Arch Pathol 19:690–728

Gaur S, Koroscil T (2009) Late-onset erythromelalgia in a previously healthy young woman: a case report and review of the literature. J Med Case Rep 3:106

Heller Page E, Shear NH (1993) Disorders due to physical factors. In: Fitzpatrick TB, Eisen AZ, Wolff K et al (eds) Dermatology in general medicine, 4th edn. McGraw-Hill, New York, pp 1581–1592

Holmer I (1993) Work in the cold. Review of methods for assessment of cold exposure. Int Arch Occup Environ Health 65:147–155

Huh J, Wright R, Gregory N (1996) Localized facial telangiectasias following frostbite injury. Cutis 57:97–98

Humphrey W, Ellyson R (1997) Warm water immersion foot: still a threat to the soldier. Mil Med 162:610–611

Jonsson CE, Schuldt K, Linder J et al (1997) Rehabilitative, psychiatric, functional and aesthetic problems in patients treated for burn injuries–a preliminary follow-up study. Acta Chir Plast 39:3–8

Kanerva L (1999) Physical causes of occupational skin disease. In: Adams RM (ed) Occupational skin disease, 3rd edn. W.B. Saunders, Philadelphia, pp 35–68

Kaplan RP (1987) Cancer complicating chronic ulcerative and scarifying mucocutaneous disorders. Adv Dermatol 2:19–46

Kavli G, Föde OH (1984) Hand dermatoses in Tromsö. Contact Dermatitis 10:174–177

Kennedy CTC (1992) Reactions to mechanical and thermal injury. In: Rook A, Wilkinson DS, Ebling FJG et al (eds) Textbook of dermatology, 5th edn. Blackwell Scientific, Oxford, pp 777–832

Kirk JF, Wilson BB, Chun W et al (1996) Miliaria profunda. J Am Acad Dermatol 35:854–856

Kligman LH, Kligman AM (1984) Reflections on heat. Br J Dermatol 110:369–375

Knize DM, Weatherley-White LCA, Paton BC et al (1969) Prognostic factors in the management of frostbite. J Trauma 9:749–759

Kulka JP (1965) Cold injury of the skin. Arch Environ Health 38:484

Lidén C, Wahlberg JE (1985) Does visual display terminal work provoke rosacea? Contact Dermatitis 13:235–241

Lillywhite LP (1992) Investigation into the environmental factors associated with the incidence of skin disease following an outbreak of Miliaria rubra at a coal mine. Occup Med (Oxf) 42:183–187

Lobitz WC (1962) Sweat retention syndrome. In: Rees RB (ed) Dermatoses due to environmental and physical factors. Charles C Thomas, Springfield, pp 146–156

Malten KE (1981) Thoughts on irritant contact dermatitis. Contact Dermatitis 7:238–247

Millard LG, Rowell NR (1978) Chilblain lupus erythematodes (Hutchinson). A clinical and laboratory study of 17 patients. Br J Dermatol 98:497–506

Miller BJ, Chasmar LR (1980) Forstbite in Saskatoon: a review of 10 winters. Can J Surg 23:423–426

Mok DWH, Blumgart LH (1984) Erythema ab igne in chronic pancreatic pain: a diagnostic sign. J R Soc Med 77:299–301

Moritz AR, Henriques FC Jr (1947) Studies in thermal injuries. II. The relative importance of time and surface temperature in the causation of cutaneous burns. Am J Pathol 23:695–720

Mowad CM, McGinley KJ, Foglia A et al (1995) The role of extracellular polysaccharide substance produced by *Staphylococcus epidermidis* in miliaria. J Am Acad Dermatol 33:729–733

Nettelblad H, Thuomas KA, Sjöberg F (1996) Magnetic resonance imaging: a new diagnostic aid in the care of high-voltage burns. Burns 22:117–119

Norbäck D (2009) An update on sick building syndrome. Curr Opin Allergy Clin Immunol 9:55–59

Oftedal G, Vistnes AI, Rygge K (1995) Skin symptoms after the reduction of electric fields from visual display units. Scand J Work Environ Health 21:335–344

Parish WE (1992) Chemical irritation and predisposing environmental stress (cold wind and hard water). In: Marks RG, Plewig G (eds) The environmental threat to the skin. M. Dunitz, London, pp 185–193

Renz BM, Sherman R (1994) Hot tar burns: twenty-seven hospitalized cases. J Burn Care Rehabil 15:341–345

Rietschel RL, Allen AM (1976) Immersion foot: a method for studying the effects of protracted water exposure on human skin. Mil Med 141:778–780

Rossis CG, Yiacoumettis AM, Elemenoglou J (1982) Squamous cell carcinoma of the heel developing at site of previous frostbite. J Roy Soc Med 75:715–718

Rycroft RJG (1984) Low humidity occupational dermatoses. Dermatol Clin 2:553–557

Rycroft RJG (1985) Low humidity and microtrauma. Am J Ind Med 8:371–373

Rycroft RJG, Smith WDL (1980) Low humidity occupational dermatoses. Contact Dermatitis 6:488–492

Schilling CJ (1997) Effects of acute exposure to ultrahigh radiofrequency radiation on three antenna engineers. Occup Environ Med 54:281–284

Schwanitz HJ, Uter W (2000) Interdigital dermatitis: sentinel skin damage in hairdressers. Br J Dermatol 142:1011–1012

Schwartz L, Tulipan L, Birmingham DJ (1957) Occupational diseases of the skin. Lea & Febiger, Philadelphia

Stenberg B, Eriksson N, Hoog J et al (1994) The stick building syndrome (SBS) in office workers. A case-referent study of personal, psychosocial and building-related risk indicators. Int J Epidemiol 23:1190–1197

Sullivan T, Smith J, Kermode J et al (1990) Rating the burn scar. J Burn Care Rehabil 11:256–260

Swanbeck G, Bleeker T (1989) Skin problems from visual display units – provocation of skin symptoms under experimental conditions. Acta Derm Venereol (Stockh) 69:46–51

Toback AC, Korson R, Krusinski PA (1985) Pulling boat hands: a unique dermatosis from coastal New England. J Am Acad Dermatol 12:649–655

Uter W, Gefeller O, Schwanitz HJ (1998) An epidemiological study of the influence of season (cold and dry air) on the occurrence of irritant skin changes of the hands. Br J Dermatol 138:266–272

White IR, Rycroft RJG (1982) Low humidity occupational dermatosis-an epidemic. Contact Dermatitis 8:287–290

Woods JA, Cobb AT, Drake DB et al (1996) Steam press hand burns: a serious burn injury. J Emerg Med 14:357–360

Wrenn K (1991) Immersion foot. A problem of the homeless in the 1990s. Arch Intern Med 151:785–788

Zalar GL, Harber LC (1985) Reactions to physical agents. In: Moschella SL, Hurley HJ (eds) Dermatology, 2nd edn. W.B. Saunders, Philadelphia, pp 1672–1690

34 Chronic Venous Insufficiency and Occupation

Edith M. de Boer
Department of Dermatology, VU Medisch Centrum, Amsterdam, The Netherlands

Core Messages

- Chronic venous disease is an often-trivialized common multifactorial slowly progressive disease, increasing with age and influenced by obesity, parity, heredity, and lifestyle.
- Comparison of studies on chronic venous disease and occupation is hampered by lack of uniformity of definition of venous disease, working position, sample size, etc.
- Exact data on the influence of work on the development/progression of venous disease and vice versa lack.
- Ambulatory hypertension due to hampered venous return occurs with inactivity of the calf muscle pump, such as in prolonged standing.
- Evening edema is physiological and can be prevented by low-pressure (10–20 mmHg) medical elastic stockings. The use of low-pressure elastic below-knee stockings should be considered for each worker with a predominantly standing or sitting position at work.
- With a short questionnaire and a simple physical examination, (the risk for) venous disease can be easily established.
- Medical elastic stockings are the devices of choice for the prevention of venous disease, for relief of complaints, and for slowing down progression. They are an indispensible part of the treatment of subjects with venous disease. The choice of stocking requires knowledge of the subscriber of both the properties of the individual worker and of stockings.

1 Introduction

Chronic venous disorders are one of the most common ailments affecting mankind in the world today. In the Netherlands, government authorities do not record the instance of venous disorders in a way that provides data for epidemiologic interpretation. In other countries, the situation is often similar, meaning that exact numerical data are not available.

In contrast to other chronic conditions, patients and physicians alike often trivialize the presence and severity of venous disorders. This might be attributed to the fact that varicose veins are common and that progression takes place slowly. Many workers with venous disorders, even with progressed forms, never consult a doctor (Krijnen et al. 1997a). Literature shows indications that venous disorders lead to incapacity to work in about 2% (Krijnen et al. 1997a). In our study, we found that 7% of almost 400 male workers with a standing profession had been temporarily unfit for work due to phlebological disorders (Krijnen et al. 1997a).

2 Chronic Venous Insufficiency: Epidemiology, Symptoms and Risk Factors, Treatment

In the pathogenesis of venous disorders, the elevated venous pressure due to hampered venous return is crucial. The term "chronic venous insufficiency" (CVI) refers to an array of symptoms resulting from venous hypertension. Subjective complaints of varicose veins and CVI often include a feeling of heaviness and pain, a sensation of swelling of the legs, nighttime calf cramps, and restless legs. Complaints increase during the course of the day, especially after prolonged standing and also after sitting. Edema, ankle flare, and corona paraplantaris phlebectatica and varices in all sizes are the first objective signs of venous incompetence. Subsequently, hyperpigmentation, lipodermatosclerosis, white atrophy, eczema, phlebitis, thrombosis, or ulcerations may develop. For a useful classification for comparison between investigations, an international system has been accepted and modified, called CEAP (Eklöf et al. 2004), based on *C*linical signs, *E*tiology, *A*natomy, and *P*athology. Apart from the clinical evaluation, duplex ultrasound investigation is required for this classification. In many studies, a (complete) classification is not used.

From many large epidemiological studies among the general population, it is evident that venous disorders are

T. Rustemeyer, P. Elsner, S.M. John & H.I. Maibach (eds.), *Kanerva's Occupational Dermatology*,
DOI 10.1007/978-3-642-02035-3_34,

common, even more often present than absent. In a large study among 2,211 individuals in San Diego (40–79 years) using duplex investigation, a modified CEAP classification was made. Only about 15% among the general white population had no visible signs (Criqui et al. 2003, 2007). Among Hispanics, Afro-Americans, and Asians these data were about 20–30%. Subjective complaints were also not unusual, varying from painful legs in 18% and tired heavy legs in about 13% (Criqui et al. 2003, 2007). In the representative randomized sample of 1,566 individuals from the general population, 18–64 years in Edinburgh a questionnaire, clinical investigation and duplex examination were performed (Evans et al. 1999; Ruckley 2002). C1 telangiectasias and reticular veins occurred in over 80% and the more severe chronic venous insufficiency (CVI) occurs in somewhat less than 10%, increasing with age.

In the large epidemiological Bonn Vein Study, 49% of males and 62% of females reported subjective venous complaints, increasing with age (Rabe et al. 2003, 2009; Rabe and Pannier 2009a, b; Pannier-Fischer and Rabe 2003). Among more than 3,000 participants, less than 10% showed no sign of venous disease, 60% had telangiectasias or reticular veins, 14% varicose veins, 13% edema, and 3% skin changes. Only 0.6% had healed venous ulceration (C5) and 0.1% present ulceration of the leg (C6 in CEAP classification).

In a longitudinal study among schoolchildren it appeared that varicose veins occur not often before puberty. From puberty on varicose veins evolve to occur at the age of 20 years in 30%, increasing to 80% small caliber intracutaneous varices at 30 years. At that age, 29% had already real larger varices (C2 in CEAP classification) and almost 4% skin changes (C4) (Schultz-Ehrenburg et al. 1989, 2009). In the first years of this lasting study, children were, in addition to a clinical investigation, examined by Doppler ultrasound, but in the more recent follow-ups, duplex investigation was performed.

In the most recent epidemiological studies, the presence of rather severe CVI is declining to 2–4% (Rabe et al. 2003; Evans et al. 1999) compared to about 10% in older studies (Fischer 1980; Widmer et al. 1981). The modern approach of earlier interventions seems to bear fruit and prevent the beginning stages of venous disease to develop to full-blown CVI and ulceration. There is evidence of venous disease in the majority of leg ulcers.

The epidemiological studies have cited a number of *risk factors* for venous disease. Age is a major risk factor (Carpentier et al. 2004; Criqui et al. 2007; Ruckley 2002; Maurins 2008; Rabe et al. 2003, 2009; Rabe and Pannier 2009a, b and many others).

Gender is another factor which is often mentioned. However, though clinically less important side branch and intracutaneous varices occur more often in females, more severe varices and advanced CVI have about the same prevalence in males and females (Criqui et al. 2007; Rabe et al. 2003). During pregnancy, hormonal changes cause relaxation of smooth muscle and increased venous distensibility. Higher prevalences of varicose veins are seen in women having had pregnancies, related to the number of pregnancies, compared to women without pregnancies (Evans et al. 1999; Carpentier et al. 2004).

Obesity is proven to be a clear risk factor, especially for the development of more severe CVI (Maurins 2008; Criqui et al. 2007; Rabe et al. 2003; Schultz-Ehrenburg et al. 2009; van Rij et al. 2008). Also an urban life was mentioned to be a risk factor (Rabe et al. 2003; Rabe and Pannier 2009a). Heredity is an often-cited risk factor, but family history is not always very reliable and family members are seldom investigated for objectivation.

In the daily patient-related practice, a physical examination of the patient standing erect is performed, supplemented with ultrasound examination. In the near past, this was usually a continuous-wave Doppler, but nowadays duplex scanning is widely available. This noninvasive technique based on echo-Doppler enabling visualization of both the superficial and the deep venous systems and blood flow measurements for the determination of refluxes.

There are several *treatments* available for venous diseases. The main objective is to normalize venous physiology. In case of superficial varices, more invasive techniques like stripping of the superficial stem veins is more and more replaced by less invasive intravascular ablations using lasers, radiofrequency, or steam. Ambulatory phlebectomy by mini-incisions and sclerocompression therapy with sclerosing injections (fluids and foams) are widely performed. In case of deep venous insufficiency, compression therapy is the only option. This compression therapy remains the cornerstone of venous therapy, and is mostly realized by medical elastic stockings, which support the function of the calf muscle pump, thus improving venous hemodynamics by lowering the ambulatory venous hypertension. Adequate compression intents to overcome the effect of gravity. Medical elastic stockings exert pressure on the leg. This so-called interface pressure changes with posture (van der Wegen-Franken 2009). The pressure exerted by a stocking changes during movements, causing pressure pulsations. The maximum pressure called working pressure and the minimum pressure called resting pressure are dependent on the characteristics elasticity, stiffness, and hysteresis. The importance of this dynamic stiffness, next to the static stiffness for the effectivity for medical elastic stockings, is demonstrated only recently (van der Wegen-Franken 2009). For an optimal choice of compression stockings, knowledge of the properties of both the patient and the stocking are required.

3 Risk Inventarisation

Risk inventarisation may focus on general and individual aspects. The occupational physician has access to the workplace of a given worker. By observing the physical activity, he is provided with information of the use of the calf muscle pump. Workers with static standing or sitting duties do not use their muscle pump, making them prone to increased venous pressure. Furthermore, individuals should be examined in terms of their own personal risk factors, focusing on CVI and restrictions of the locomotor system, particularly the lower extremities.

As there are many factors of influence on the development and progression of venous disease, both known factors and unknown influences and as venous disease progresses gradually and slowly, it is difficult to determine the deteriorating influence of work. In the years or decennia of life spent working, venous disease may also increase due to the natural process of aging and may decrease due to the nowadays more often applied interventions. In the Bonn Vein Study, it appeared that 13% of males and 31% of females had been treated by surgery or sclerotherapy and/or medical elastic stockings (Rabe et al. 2003). A history of interventions in the past increased with age. Of the males, 7.5% had now or in the past elastic stockings and 20% of females. Individuals appreciated these stockings as successful and the compliance was 50% (Rabe and Pannier 2009c). Other individual risk factors may change as well, such as body weight, parity, and locomotor factors, especially in ankles, knees, and hips. Furthermore, working environments may change in the course of a career. Not to neglect is the difficulty of ascertaining an individual's posture at work by questionnaire, as has been done in most studies. A minority of studies describe the inspection of the investigator of the working environment of the individuals included in a study (Krijnen et al. 1997a, epidemiology). Not quantifiable is the interaction of venous disease and ability to work. Data on absence of work, disqualification, or change of jobs due to venous disease are not known and therefore not taken into account in studies. Preexistent presence of varicose veins, early onset beginning CVI, or subjective complaints may influence the choice of profession. The influence of work/occupation on the development of venous disorders has been a challenge to many investigators.

4 Studies on Occupation and Venous Disease

Comparing data from different authors is often confusing, not equivocal. Some epidemiological studies confirm to the CEAP criteria, others use data from medical records. Definitions of varices, venous disease, edema, and subjective complaints vary in studies. Some studies are focused on venous disease, others register venous disease as an extra above the real goal of the study. Some studies describe the general population, some special groups of patients, and some select on age or gender. Most of the larger studies just register professions and ask participants about their main position at work, relying on the accuracy of workers to describe their body posture at work, often over long periods of time. There are only a few studies that mainly focus on the relation between occupation and venous disease.

For effective venous return from the legs, interaction of the heart, a pressure gradient, venous muscle pumps in the leg, and competent valves in the veins are obligatory (Meissner et al. 2007). During prolonged orthostasis, the calf muscle pump function, "the peripheral heart," is diminished. In prolonged standing, the hydrostatic pressure increases as the valves in the veins allow retrograde flow. The weight of the entire column of blood causes a huge pressure. During standing without skeletal-muscle activity, venous pressures in the legs are determined by the hydrostatic component and capillary flow, reaching up to 90 mmHg (Bergan et al. 2006). In the presence of competent valves, minor leg movements provide sufficient pumping, resulting in a decrease of intravenous pressure to about 20 mmHg. In case of impairment of the venous system, e.g., due to incompetent valves in veins, high pressures in the superficial system and the microcirculation occur, known as ambulatory venous hypertension, as the calf muscle contractions are not able to reduce venous hypertension. Prolonged high pressure causes disturbed venous flow patterns (changes in shear stress), inducing inflammation and the production of free reactive radicals (Bergan et al. 2006). So prolonged standing results in venous hypertension in the lower legs, activating inflammatory mechanisms and enhancing the development of CVI. In a study among 200 female surgery room nurses and outpatient department nurses, the production of reactive oxygen species (ROS) was measured before and after work. It appeared that ROS increased during standing work and did not return to prework levels as compared to actively walking nurses. Thus, enhanced oxidative stress was demonstrated in these standing workers, putting them at risk for the development of CVI due to damage of the endothelium, but possibly also for other cardiovascular and systemic disease (Flore et al. 2004). The same group demonstrated lower limb venous pressure increases in workers having a standing position, but also in controls having more mobile work. The standing operating theater nurses showed additionally higher levels of ROS (Flore et al. 2007). While wearing class 1 elastic stockings (18–21 mmHg) venous pressures and ROS did not increase in both groups of workers.

A representative random sample of 8,664 (being the 90% response rate) working individuals below 60 years in Denmark was interviewed over the telephone (Tüchsen et al. 2005) about their work and lifestyle. During 12 years, data from the national hospital register were combined with governmental information about occupation. It appeared that the relative risk for being hospitalized for varicose veins was 1.8 in employees with prolonged standing or walking at work, both for men and women. Data were adjusted for other variables. It was calculated that this risk excess accounted for more than 20% of all cases at the working age. In this study, which was also not primarily focused on occupation, individuals were not investigated and all outpatient treatments were left out of consideration.

In a study among 204 hospital employees of all varieties in Vienna, chronic venous disease was present in 34%, predominantly women (Ziegler et al. 2003). The prevalence was highest among those working in a standing position or in high temperatures and humidity. Chronic venous disease was classified according to CEAP criteria. All kinds of risk factors were registered and taken into account. Regular evaluation and primary preventive measures were advocated.

In the Edinburgh Vein Study (Evans et al. 1999), performed among a group of 1,566 individuals below 54 years from a randomized sample of 12 general practices, the prevalence of varicose veins tended to be clearly lower in those who spent their working time sitting and higher in those who worked standing compared to the general population. A questionnaire, clinical investigation, and duplex investigation were used for CEAP classification.

In the longitudinal Framingham study, in contrary, people leading a sedentary life were more at risk for developing varicose veins (Brand et al. 1988).

In a study especially focused on the relationship between working posture and venous disease, 28 symptom-free male vascular surgeons without a history of venous treatment were compared to 25 male controls leading flexible lives. Duplex examination showed in 52% of surgeons reflux in the superficial venous system compared to 32% in the volunteers (Labropoulos et al. 1995). In over 75%, reflux was present in the long saphenous vein. The likelihood of venous reflux was significantly higher in symptom-free surgeons.

In a multicenter cross-sectional study in Poland, over 40,000 individuals (16–97 years) were assigned the clinical severity of venous disease (C classification according to CEAP) based on medical records. No association of chronic venous disease and spending a long time in the sitting position was documented (Jawien et al. 2003 Phlebology). There was a significantly higher proportion of men and women having a standing occupation in the group with CVI compared to the group without CVI ($p < 0.001$). A lack of physical activity was strongly associated with CVI in women (Jawien 2003, Angiology). Leg complaints were reported by 81% of people having varicose veins and by 35% without. No single visible sign was reported present in 51%. This extraordinary low figure might indicate that doctors not especially trained in/focused on phlebology might diagnose less signs of venous disorder.

In a study in Bulgarian general practitioners, in rural and urban areas, each selected 50 consecutive patients over 18 years and assigned them in the C classification of CEAP, based on a questionnaire and a clinical investigation. Over 2,600 individuals were included and 400 subjects of these were seen by specialists for re-diagnosis. As a risk factor in this subgroup, 34% of the individuals indicated a prolonged standing position and 38% a prolonged sitting position (Zahariev et al. 2009).

In our department, we performed a study in 387 males having a strictly standing position at work. We inspected the work environment, took a questionnaire, performed physical examination, Doppler investigation, light reflection rheography (LRR), and optical leg volume measurements. CVI was present in 29% of the subjects and correlated with age, body weight, and the duration of standing work. Complaints of the legs were reported by 81% of the individuals with CVI, but also by 63% of the subjects without CVI (Krijnen et al. 1997a). Several screening methods were compared and evaluated. It appeared that a short questionnaire in combination with physical examination (inspection and palpation of the legs in a standing subject) had a predictive value of 87% (sensitivity 85%, specificity 88%).The questionnaire consisted of only four items: age, body weight, history of treatment for phlebologic disorders, and a tired feeling in the legs. Age and weight appeared to be the most important risk factors, age being the dominant factor. The value of LRR measurements as a predictive tool was low with a predictive value of 73% (sensitivity 11%, specificity 95%) (Krijnen et al. 1997a).

Also others evaluated screening instruments for the screening on venous disease. In a large car factory, a venous checkup was offered to 9,600 employees. In the response group of 1,460 males and 370 females, a questionnaire was compared with the outcomes of the determination of venous refilling time by photoplethysmography (Stücker et al. 2009). Subjects having a pathological refilling time were considered to be venous morbid. The prevalence was 32% of cases, increasing with age. The self-administered survey referring to venous disease in the parents, thrombophlebitis, leg swelling, leg heaviness, hyperpigmentation, and visible varicosities was able to distinguish between persons with physiological and pathological venous refilling time, acquiring a specificity of over 90% if symptoms were characterized as marked or repeatedly.

From the combination of both studies (Krijnen et al. 1997a, b; Stücker et al. 2009), it can be concluded that a simple *questionnaire* provides a good tool for the screening for venous disease or proneness to venous disease. A questionnaire should contain questions about age and body weight, family history of varices, previous venous interventions, thrombophlebitis, a tired feeling or heaviness in the legs, the presence of hyperpigmentation of the lower legs, and of visible varicose veins. A simple physical inspection of the standing subjects on signs of venous disease has additional value. In this way, an alert physician can adequately screen for venous disease and select individuals for preventive measures and referral to a specialist, using simple means and without any equipment.

5 Preventive Measures

Early intervention in order to prevent venous hypertension and venous reflux, and thus chronic inflammation, is the basis of prevention of, or reducing the progression of chronic venous disease. Of course, the most ideal situation would be to ban working postures that require long-standing inactivity of the calf muscle pump. By the way, what about hobbies? The most easy device for intervention are medical elastic stockings.

Evening edema of the legs is a physiologic phenomenon occurring after sitting and standing caused by extravasation of fluid from venules due to increased venous pressure. In healthy individuals, subjective hinder may occur, but the swelling is disappeared after a night's rest. In case of failing of the calf pump function for instance due to dysfunctioning of the ankle joint (orthopedic, neurologic, immobility) or incompetent venous valves, this edema may become irreversible, leading to chronic inflammation. Using an opto-electronic device (de Boer et al. 1999) or different types of water displacement devices (Partsch et al. 2004) to determine the leg volume in the morning and after a full working day showed this physiological diurnal volume increase.

In a study in our department on 387 healthy male workers with a standing position at work, we inspected the work environment, took a questionnaire, performed physical examination, Doppler investigation, and light reflection rheography. With opto-electronical volume measurements, the diurnal changes in volume of the lower legs were monitored several days. A mean diurnal volume increase in the lower leg +1.6%, distributed as a Gaussian curve (Krijnen et al. 1998), not associated with subjective symptoms or clinically evident edema in 197 healthy workers was confirmed. With the same opto-electronic device, a mean higher diurnal volume increase in individuals having CVI compared to healthy workers was demonstrated (Krijnen et al. 1997b). In male workers with "minor CVI," this mean volume increase was +2.6% and in more severs CVI +3.6%. As a predictor of CVI, isolated volume measurements appeared nondiscriminative because of overlap with the distribution of volume increase in healthy individuals. These volume increases in case of CVI were associated with complaints.

In healthy individuals also other studies could not demonstrate a correlation with subjective complaints and volume increase (de Boer et al. 1999; Partsch et al. 2004). Both authors showed an increase in volume of the lower legs in the course of a working day in healthy individuals. Intervention with compression stockings is able to reduce evening edema significantly. A meta-analysis of randomized controlled trials that compared stockings exerting an ankle pressure of 10–20 mmHg with placebo or no treatment and with stockings exerting a pressure of over 20 mmHg among healthy individuals and patients with CVI was performed (Amsler and Blättler 2008). Included often small studies reported occupational symptoms and edema and were performed among varying groups of standing volunteers, workers in factories or hospitals, flight attendants, etc. It appeared that compression with 10–20 mmHg had a clear effect on edema and on symptoms as compared to stockings exerting lower pressures or no stockings. A benefit of higher pressure was not demonstrated. As edema in these studies was not differentiated, the overall conclusion must be restricted to subjects with symptoms of mild venous insufficiency.

The cause of occasional pain in the legs and reported edema in apparently healthy individuals remains unknown. Medical elastic stockings of 15 mmHg effectively relieve the symptoms resembling venous insufficiency, prevent edema, and are well tolerated (Blättler et al. 2008). Stockings providing <10 mmHg were ineffective and those providing >19 mmHg not well tolerated.

In our group of almost 400 male workers with a standing profession, only the individuals having CVI ($n = 114$) were provided with class 2 stockings (30–32 mmHg), randomly assigned in comparison with rubber floor mats and no intervention. These semi-bouncy, uneven mats cause slight changes in the position of the angle of the foot, resulting in lower leg muscle contractions, theoretically stimulating the calf muscle pump, especially in case of high resilient rubber mats. The group of individuals treated with stockings experienced significant reduction of subjective complaints and of the development of edema, while both other groups remained unchanged (Krijnen et al. 1997a, b, c). Patients suffering from more severe CVI, with more prominent edema, need adaptation of therapy with stronger compression.

References

Amsler F, Blättler W (2008) Compression therapy for occupational leg symptoms and chronic venous disorders – a meta-analysis of randomized contolled trials. Eur J Vasc Endovasc Surg 35(3):366–372

Bergan JJ, Schmid-Schönbein GW, Coleridge Smith PD, Nicolaides AN, Boisseau MR, Eklöf B (2006) Chronic venous disease. N Engl J Med 355:488–498

Blättler W, Kreis N, Lun B, Winiger J, Amsler F (2008) Leg symptoms of healthy people and their treatment with compression hosiery. Phlebology 23:214–221

Brand FN, Dannenberg AL, Abbott RD et al (1988) The epidemiology of varicose veins: the Framingham study. Am J Prev Med 4:96–101

Carpentier PH, Maricq HR, Biro C, Poncot-Makinen CO, Franco A (2004) Prevalence, risk factors, and clinical patterns of chronic venous disorders of lower limbs: a population-based study in France. J Vasc Surg 40:650–659

Criqui MH, Jamosmos M, Fronek A, Denenberg JO, Langer RD, Bergan J et al (2003) Chronic venous disease in an ethnically diverse population: the San Diego population study. Am J Epidemiol 158:448–456

Criqui MH, Denenberg JO, Langer RD, Kaplan RM, Fronek A (2007) Epidemiology of chronic peripheral venous disease. In: Bergan JJ (ed) The vein book. Elsevier/Academic, Amsterdam/Boston

de Boer EM, Broekhuijsen RW, Nieboer C, Bezemer PD (1999) Lycra support tights: are they effective? Phlebology 14:162–166

Eklöf B, Rutherford RB, Bergan JJ, Carpentier P, Gloviczki P, Kistner RL, for the American Venous Forum International Ad Hoc Committee for Revision of the CEAP classification et al (2004) Revision of the CEAP classification for chronic venous disorders: consensus statement. J Vasc Surg 40:1248–1252

Evans CJ, Fowkes FRG, Ruckley VC, Lee AJ (1999) Prevalence of varicose veins and chronic venous insufficiency in men and women in the general population. Edinburgh vein study. J Epidemiol Community Health 53:149–153

Fischer H (1980) Sozioepidemiologische studie über die venenleiden bei einer erwachsenen wohnbevölkerung in der bundesrepublik Deutschland. Phlebol Proktol 9:147–152

Flore R, Gerardino L, Santoliquido A, Pola R, Flex A, Di Campli C, Pola P, Tondi P (2004) Enhanced oxidative stress in workers with a standing occupation. Occup Environ Med 61:548–550

Flore R, Gerardino L, Santoliquido A, Catananti C, Pola P, Tondi P (2007) Reduction of oxidative stress by compression stockings in standing workers. Occup Med 57:337–341

Jawien A (2003) The influence of environmental factors in chronic venous insufficiency. Angiology 54(Suppl 1):19–31

Jawien A, Grzla T, Ochwat A (2003) Prevalence of chronic venous insufficiency (CVI) in men and women in Poland: multicenter cross-sectional study in 40,095 patients. Phlebology 18:110–121

Krijnen RMA, de Boer EM, Adèr HJ, Bruynzeel DP (1997a) Venous insufficiency in male workers with a standing profession. Part I. Epidemiology. Dermatology 194:111–120

Krijnen RMA, de Boer EM, Adèr HJ, Bruynzeel DP (1997b) Venous insufficiency in male workers with a standing profession. Part II. Dermatology 194:121–126

Krijnen RMA, de Boer EM, Adèr HJ, Osinga DSC, Bruynzeel DP (1997c) Compression stockings and rubber floor mats: do they benefit workers with CVI and a standing profession? J Occup Dermatol 39:889–894

Krijnen RMA, de Boer EM, Adèr HJ, Bruynzeel DP (1998) Diurnal volume changes of the lower legs in healthy males with a profession that requires standing. Skin Res Technol 4:18–23

Labropoulos N, Delis KT, Nicolaides AN (1995) Venous reflux in symptom-free vascular surgeons. J Vasc Surg 22:150–154

Meissner MH, Moneta G, Burnand K, Gloviczki P, Lurie F, Mattos MA, McLafferty RB, Mozes G et al (2007) The hemodynamics and diagnosis of venous disease. J Vasc Surg 46:4S–24S

Pannier-Fischer F, Rabe E (2003) Epidemiologie der chronischen venenerkrankungen. Hautartz 54:1037–1044

Partsch H, Winiger J, Lun B (2004) Compression stockings reduce occupational leg swelling. Dermatol Surg 30:737–743

Rabe E, Pannier F (2009a) Epidemiology of chronic venous disease. In: Abstract book XVI world meeting of the UIP 2009, Monte Carlo, p 72

Rabe E, Pannier F (2009b) Epidemiology of chronic venous disorders. In: Gloviczki P et al (eds) Handbook of venous disorders, 3rd edn. Hodder Arnold, London

Rabe E, Pannier F (2009c) Use of MCS in the general population – data from the Bonn vein study. In: Abstractbook XVI world meeting of the UIP 2009, Monte Carlo, p 178

Rabe E, Pannier-Fischer F, Bromen K, Schuldt K, Stang A, Poncar Ch, Wittenhorst M, Bock E, Weber S, Jöckel K-H (2003) Bonner venenstudie der deutschen gesellschaft für phlebologie. Epidemiologische untersuchung zur frage der häufigkeit und ausprägung von chronischen venenkrankheiten in der städtischen und ländlichen wohnbevölkerung. Phlebologie 32:1–14

Rabe E, Ko A, Berboth G, Pannier F, Hofmann B, Hertel S (2009) Incidence of varicose veins and CVI in the Bonn vein study II. In: Abstract book XVI world meeting of the UIP 2009, Monte Carlo, p 154

Schultz-Ehrenburg U, Weindorf N, von Uslar D et al (1989) Prospective epidemiologische studie die entstehungsweise der krampfadern bei kindern und jugendlichen (Bochumer studie I und II). Phlebol Proktol 18:3–11

Schultz-Ehrenburg U, Reich-Schupke S, Robak-Pawelczyk B, Rudolph T, Moll C, Weindorf N, Hirche H, Altmeyer P, Stücker M (2009)

Prospective epidemiological study on the beginning of varicose veins. Bochum study I-IV. Phlebologie 38:17–25

Stücker M, Puyn S, Rabe E, Altmeyer P, Reich-Schupke S (2009) Evaluation eines standardisierten fragebogens als screening-instrument fuer venenerkrankungen. Hautarzt:1–7

Tüchsen F, Hannerz H, Burr KN (2005) Prolonged standing at work and hospitalisation due to varicose veins: a 12 year prospective study of the Danish population. Occup Environ Med 62:847–850

van der Wegen-Franken K (2009) Medical elastic stockings. Thesis, Rotterdam

van Rij AM, De Alwis CS, Jiang P, Christie RA, Hill GB, Dutton SJ, Thomson IA (2008) Obesity and impaired venous function. Eur J Vasc Endovasc Surg 35:739–744

Widmer LK, Stähelin HB, Nissen C, da Silva A (1981) Venen-, Arterien-Krankheiten, koronare Herzkrankheit bei Berufstätigen, Prospektiv-epidemiologische Untersuchung (Basler Studie I-II). Hans Huber, Bern

Zahariev T, Anastassov V, Girov K, Goranova E, Grodzinski L, Kniajev V, Stankev S (2009) The prevalence of primary chronic venous disease: the Bulgarian experience. Int Angiol 28:303–310

Ziegler S, Eckhardt G, Stöger R, Machula J, Rüdiger HW (2003) High prevalence of chronic venous disease in hospital employees. Wien Klin Wochenschr 115(15–16):549–551

35 Dermatitis Artefacta

Wolfgang Harth
Chefarzt, Klinik für Dermatologie und Allergologie Vivantes Klinikum Spandau,
Berlin, Germany

Core Messages

- Factitious Disorders are self-inflicted skin lesions and includes the creation of physical or psychiatric symptoms in oneself or other reference persons. In dermatology, frequently there are mechanical injuries by pressures, friction, occlusion, biting, cutting, stabbing, thermal burns or self-inflicted infections with wound-healing impairment, abscesses, mutilations or damages by acids, and other toxic to the skin.
- The current classification differentiates between four groups: (1) Dermatitis artefacta syndrome in the narrower sense as unconscious/dissociated self-injury, (2) Dermatitis paraartefacta syndrome: Disorders of impulse control, often as manipulation of an existing specific dermatosis (often semiconscious, admitted – self-injury), (3) Malingering: consciously simulated injuries and diseases to obtain material gain, (4) special forms, such as the Gardner-Diamond Syndrome, Münchhausen Syndrome and Münchhausen-by-Proxy Syndrome.
- This categorization is helpful in understanding the different pathogenic mechanisms and the psychodynamics involved, as well as in developing various therapeutic avenues and determining the prognosis.

1 Introduction

Self-inflicted Dermatitis reflects a variety of conditions that share the common finding of automutilating behavior resulting in trauma to the skin. They represent a spectrum that spans from conscious manipulation of skin and appendages all the way to a delusional psychosis. The degree of severity is mostly determined by the progressive loss of awareness of the process (Gupta et al. 1987).

2 Definition

Self-inflicted skin lesions (Factitious Disorders) includes the creation of physical or psychiatric symptoms in oneself or other reference persons. Factitious disorders (ICD-10: F68.1, L98.1) is the term to describe self-mutilating actions (DSM-IV 300.16/300.19), which lead directly or indirectly to clinically relevant damage to the organism, without the direct intention of committing suicide. In dermatology, frequently there are mechanical injuries by pressures, friction, occlusion, biting, cutting, stabbing, thermal burns or self-inflicted infections with wound-healing impairment, abscesses, mutilations or damages by acids, and other toxic to the skin (➋ *Table 35.1*) (Harth and Gieler 2006). These are the direct consequences of psychological or psychiatric disorders.

The current classification differentiates between four groups (➋ *Table 35.2*): (1) Dermatitis artefacta syndrome in the narrower sense as unconscious/dissociated self-injury, (2) Dermatitis paraartefacta syndrome: Disorders of impulse control, often as manipulation of an existing specific dermatosis (often semiconscious, admitted – self-injury), (3) Malingering: consciously simulated injuries and diseases to obtain material gain, (4) special forms, such as the Gardner-Diamond Syndrome, Münchhausen Syndrome and Münchhausen-by-Proxy Syndrome (Harth et al. 2009)

This categorization is helpful in understanding the different pathogenic mechanisms and the psychodynamics involved, as well as in developing various therapeutic avenues and determining the prognosis.

3 Prevalence/Incidence

The prevalence of Self-inflicted Dermatitis is estimated at 0.05–0.4% in the population (Gieler 2004). Although the disorder can be seen in any clinical discipline, the prevalence of factitious disorders seems to be highest in dermatology patients. A survey of doctors in various specialties found that dermatologists reported factitious disorder among 2% of all patients in clinical dermatology units. Self-harming behaviors are 3–8 times more common among women, with the exception of malingering which is more common among men.

T. Rustemeyer, P. Elsner, S.M. John & H.I. Maibach (eds.), *Kanerva's Occupational Dermatology*,
DOI 10.1007/978-3-642-02035-3_35,

Table 35.1
Genesis of the dermatitis artefacta

Mechanical	Pressures
	Friction
	Occlusion
	Biting
	Cutting
	Stabbing
	Mutilations
Toxic damage	Acids
	Alkali
	Thermal (burns, scalding)
Self-inflicted infections	Wound-healing impairments
	Abscesses
Medications (covert taking of pharmaceuticals)	Heparin injections
	Insulin

Table 35.2
Self inflicted skin diseases

Dermatitis artefacta syndrome	In the narrow sense, unconscious self-harm
Dermatitis paraartefacta syndrome	Impulse control disorders, often manipulation of existing skin lesions
	Often partly conscious, admitted self-injury, also known as skin-picking syndrome
Malingering	Willful deception by feigning injury or disease in order to gain something
Special forms	Gardner-Diamond syndrome
	Münchhausen syndrome
	Münchhausen-by-proxy syndrome

4 Dermatitis Artefacta Syndrome (DAS)

The clinical appearance of dermatitis artefacta syndrome (ICD-10 F 68.1, unintentional L98.1) depends on the type of manipulation used. In principle, the appearance of artificially produced symptoms can mimic any skin disorder. "Atypical appearances are typical," that is, patients with dermatitis artefacta syndrome often have lesions at atypical sites or with an atypical morphology, histology, or disease that relapses for reasons that are unclear. Physicians should be alert to the presence of foreign, toxic, or infectious substances. The consequences are serious when the patient's deception leads to harmful or unnecessary procedures being performed by a physician based on the patient's feigned symptoms.

4.1 Psychiatric Symptoms

Dermatitis Artefacta is a syndrome (DAS) caused by unconscious/dissociated self-injury. DAS in the narrower sense as dissociated self-injury may express a reactivation of injuries suffered in childhood based on a serious psychiatric disorder from earlier times, and may contain a nonverbal connotation.

The damaging behavior usually occurs covertly, often in dissociative states, without the patient is being able to remember or emotionally comprehend the event (*Fig. 35.1a, b*).

The so-called hollow history (van Moffaert 2003) is characteristically often found in taking the history of patients with DAS. This refers to the fact that unclear, vague statements are made about the onset of disease, which suddenly appeared without any warning or symptoms.

Typically, the patients themselves appear astonished by the skin changes and cannot give clear statements or details about the first occurrence or appearance and course of development. The history remains unclear. The patients are conspicuously emotionally uninvolved while they relate the history of their disease, as though they were not affected themselves when details of the often disfiguring lesions are related. Pain that would be medically expected resulting from the lesions is also often not reported. The family, on the other hand, is often enraged and accusatory, complaining of the physicians incompetence to reach an appropriate diagnosis and treatment.

There is a heterogeneous psychopathological spectrum among patients with DAS (*Table 35.3*). There are often serious personality disorders (mainly emotionally unstable personality disorders of the borderline type, ICD-10: F60.31; DSM-IV-TR: 301.83 Borderline Personality Disorder) or other of the disorders described below (*Fig. 35.2*).

Two thirds of patients report traumatizing experiences, such as sexual and physical abuse and deprivation situations in the anamnesis (Harth and Linse 2000).

Mild forms of factitious disorders result from conflicts of adolescence or alcohol, medications, and drug abuse.

In addition, DAS occurs as a comorbidity in depressive, anxiety, and compulsive disorders, as well as in posttraumatic stress disorders. Dissociative amnesias and

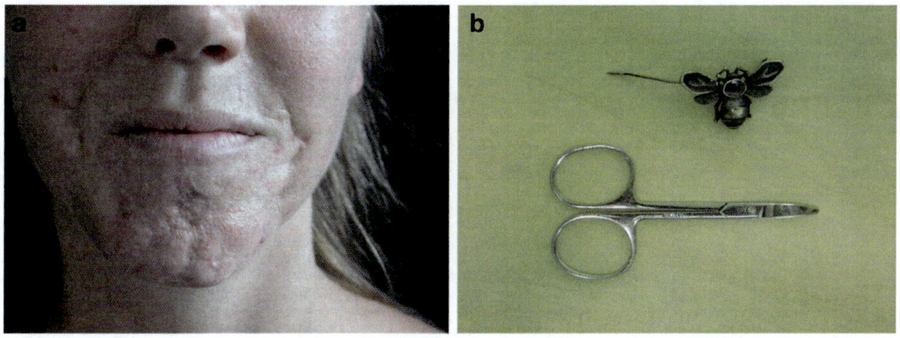

◘ Fig. 35.1
(a) DAS: Extensive scars, self-inflicted dermatosis in the face. (b) DAS: Instruments for self-manipulation

◘ Table 35.3
Frequent psychiatric disorders in self inflicted dermatosis

Frequent psychiatric disorders in self-inflicted dermatosis
Early personality disorders
Emotionally unstable personality disorders of the borderline type
Narcissistic personality disorders
Histrionic personality disorders
Antisocial personality disorders
Dependency personality disorders
Depressive disorders
Anxiety disorders
Compulsive disorders
Posttraumatic stress disorders

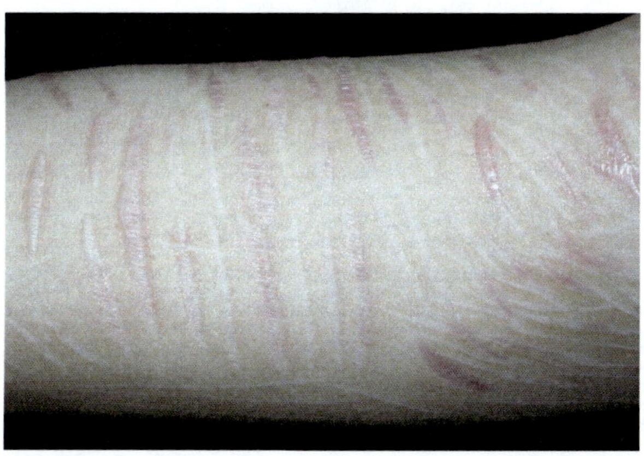

◘ Fig. 35.2
DAS: 26-year-old woman with borderline syndrome

serious depersonalization states may occur in connection with self-mutilating behavior.

The autoaggressive behavior of DAS patients manifests in other conspicuous incidents, so that the connection between artifacts and suicidal behavior should be emphasized, a point that is highlighted in the literature, to the extent that DAS may represent a masked suicidal behavior.

Very often, the patients report being under great pressure and tension prior to self-injury and feel relieved following it, which releases tension and acts as a form of "tranquilizer" (Janus 1972).

Overt self-damaging behavior or conscious DAS may represent the desire for secondary gain from illness, or show blurred transitions to dermatitis paraartefacta syndrome.

4.2 Differential Diagnosis in Dermatitis Artefacta Syndrome

At the time of the self-damaging acts, manifest psychotic illness may be in the foreground, within whose framework the self-injury occurs. The illnesses listed in the following overview belong in this category (➋ *Table 35.4*).

The underlying co-occurring psychiatric conditions need to be enumerated as well as other medical conditions triggering or co-occurring with the skin condition or generating additional psychiatric/psychological burden.

5 Dermatitis Paraartefacta Syndrome (DPS)

In Dermatitis paraartefacta, the most common underlying psychiatric condition is an impairment of impulse control

Table 35.4
Differential diagnosis in DAS

Differential diagnosis in dermatitis artefacta syndrome	
Emotionally unstable personality disorders of the borderline type	
Schizophrenias, schizotype, and delusional disorders	
Affective disorders with psychotic symptoms, juvenile autism	
Hypochondriacal delusion	
Delusion of Parasitosis	
Monosymptomatic psychosis	
Acute intoxications, psychotropic substances, withdrawal syndrome	
Brain-organic psychosyndrome	
Seizures	
Cultural-religious acts	
Sexual acts	
Suicidal intent	
Comorbidity with organic diseases	Lesh-Nyhan Syndrome
	Cornelia de Lange Syndrome
	Rett Syndrome
	Chronic encephalitis, neurolues, temporal-lobe epilepsy
	Oligophrenia
	Dementia syndrome (F00-F04)

(ICD-10:F63.9; DSM-IV-TR: 312.30 Impulse-Control Disorder), but other psychiatric conditions may underlie this syndrome. The patients have lost control over the manipulation of their skin. Often in dermatology, a minimal primary lesion is characteristically excessively traumatized, leading to pronounced, serious clinical findings.

The patterns of disease listed in the following summary belongs to DPS (➋ *Table 35.5*).

Differential diagnostics should also consider paraartefacts in the Köbner-phenomenon.

Table 35.5
Pattern of diseases in Dermatitis paraartefacta

Dermatitis paraartefacta syndrome (DPS)	
Skin/mucosa	Skin-picking syndrome (epidermotillomania, neurotic excoriations)
	Acne excoriée
	Pseudo-knuckle pads
	Morsicatio buccarum
	Cheilitis factitia
Integuments	Onychophagia, onychotillomania, onychotemnomania
	Trichotillomania, trichotemnomania, trichoteiromania

5.1 Clinical Presentation

The clinical presentation of DPS is characterized by the following specifically-defined dermatoses:

5.1.1 Skin-Picking Syndrome (Neurotic Excoriations)

In skin-picking syndrome DPS formerly termed neurotic excoriations is most often facilitated by impairment of impulse control, resulting in self-injury to the skin or mucosa and usually serving to reduce underlying emotional tension (Koblenzer 1996).

5.1.2 Clinical Findings

The skin-picking syndrome (neurotic excoriations) (ICD-10: F63.9; DSM-IV-TR 312.30) is characterized by excoriations, erosions, crusting in addition to atrophic, and hyperpigmentated scarring secondary to self-inflicted trauma (➋ *Fig. 35.3a, b*).

Most commonly localized on arms and legs, the skin-picking syndrome may also occur in the face, where it is frequently referred to as Acne excoriée.

5.2 Psychiatric Symptoms

The psychiatric disorder is characterized by an impairment of impulse control with repeated inability to resist

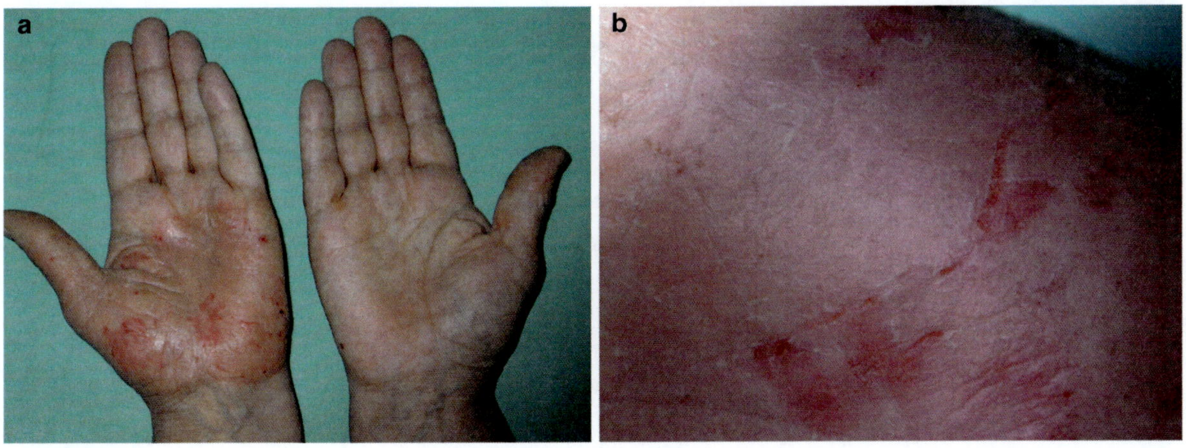

Fig. 35.3
(a, b) DPS: Skin-picking syndrome with manipulation during psychosocial stress situation

the impulse to scratch. In some cases, there is an urgency to suppress or destroy a skin lesion perceived as disfiguring. At the beginning of the skin-picking behavior, there is a progressive buildup of a feeling of tension, in a circular process of lack of impulse control, picking and subsequently phase feeling of relief and satisfaction, and a progressive concern and guilt about the new lesion created. The syndrome is often accompanied by comorbid depressive and anxiety disorders. When diagnosing an impulse control disorder, the presence of obsessive-compulsive disorder should be ruled out in the differential diagnosis.

5.3 Differential Diagnosis

The psychiatric and somatic differential diagnosis includes Lichen Simplex Chronicus, whereby most compulsive disorders are in the foreground of the psychiatric symptoms. Clinically, there are chronically lichenified areas.

5.3.1 Acne Excoriée

A special form of the skin-picking syndrome is Acne excoriée (ICD-10: F68.1, L70.5; F68.1; DSM-IV-TR 312.30), which is characterized and defined by its localization in the face.

In Acne excoriée often there is minimal acne and usually minimal lesions are extensively manipulated by squeezing and pressing, usually with the fingernails or sharp instruments (Bach and Bach 1993). This results in excoriations, erosions, or even ulcerations healing with stellate discolored scarring. Often the patients cannot resist the impulse to perform these acts, but justify the manipulations with the argument that they are removing infectious material.

5.3.2 Morsicatio Buccarum

Morsicatio buccarum (ICD-10: F68.1, K13.1; F68.1; DSM-IV-TR 312.30) are benign sharply demarcated usually leukodermic lesions around the tooth base and buccal mucosa. The changes may result from continuous, unconscious sucking, and chewing on the oral mucosa. The diagnostic criteria of impaired impulse control are in the foreground of the psychiatric symptoms.

Compulsive disorders may also be in the underlying psychiatric condition.

Morsicatio buccarum is found more often among denture wearers without other psychiatric symptoms. Lichen Planus can be ruled out by a biopsy in cases of doubt.

5.3.3 Cheilitis Factitia

Cheilitis factitia (ICD-10: F68.1, K13.0; F68.1; DSM-IV-TR 312.30) is compulsive licking (Lip Licker's dermatitis) and the basis of the pathogenesis. It results in an irritant contact dermatitis, leading to eczematous skin changes and a predisposition to secondary impetigenization. The licking usually affects discrete, symmetric, sharply delineated areas beyond the outline of the lips, frequently associated to traumatizing lip-chewing.

Psychopathologically, impaired impulse control is in the foreground, which often goes unnoticed. Frequently, the patients are children, and following diagnosis, and careful explanation of the causes to parents and patients, full healing is achieved by controlling the eliciting mechanism

5.3.4 Pseudo-knuckle Pads

Pseudo-knuckle pads (ICD-10: F68.1, M72.1; F68.1; DSM-IV-TR 312.30) occur due to trauma (rubbing, massaging, chewing, sucking) to the finger joints and are clinically characterized by hypertrophic, pad-like, rough, and slightly scaly skin lesions. Mental retardation may be common. Real knuckle pads are due to a genodermatosis, form without mechanical trauma and are characterized histologically by cell-rich fibrosis.

5.3.5 Onychophagia, Onychotillomania, Onychotemnomania

Onychophagia

Onychophagia (ICD-10: F68.1, F98.8; DSM-IV-TR 312.30) is nail-biting or nail-chewing, usually with swallowing of nail fragments. A combination with thumb-sucking is also frequent.

Nevertheless bacterial or fungal infections, inflammation, bleeding, and malformations may arise or be triggered by the repeated trauma with shortening of the distal nail plate. Onychophagia usually occurs as part of unresolved conflicts or tension and is observed especially in adolescence.

The frequency is cited at up to 45% of adolescents, so certainly not every patient with onychophagia has a serious personality disorder or urgently requires psychotherapy.

The central causality factor is inappropriate dealing with stressful situations.

Onychotillomania

In onychotillomania constant manipulation, "picking" and removal of the cuticle and/or nail or trauma of the paronychium is seen as the elicitor of self-induced nail diseases. This may range from onychodystrophy to serious paronychias.

Onychotemnomania

Cutting nails too short leads to traumatization of the nail body or nail fold.

5.3.6 Trichotillomania, Trichotemnomania, Trichoteiromania

Trichotillomania

Trichotillomania is the best-investigated DPS disorder, whereby women are thought to be especially affected with a prevalence of up to 3.5% (Muller and Winkelmann 1972; Wichel et al. 1992). The disease occurs often at younger ages.

Trichotillomania (ICD-10: F63.3, F68.1; DSM-IV-TR 312.30) is based on pulling out the hair, resulting in marked hair loss.

Clinically, there is a typical three-phase zone presentation with:

Zone 1: long hair (unremarkable, not affected, normal hair/haircut)
Zone 2: missing hair (fresh alopecia due to pulling)
Zone 3: regrowth of hair, shorter and less regular than the normal hair (older, former alopecia areas with irregular hair regrowth after intermittent pulling)

The cause of the three-zone presentation is that normal healthy long hair (Zone 1) can be easily grasped and then pulled.

Around the torn hair, there is a hairless Zone 2, whereby isolated hemorrhages can be found in the area of the pulled-out hair in the fresh tear area.

In addition, the older areas show regrowth (Zone 3), with shorter hair that cannot be grasped and pulled yet. If such a three-zone presentation is found, the diagnosis of trichotillomania is confirmed.

If alopecia areata is considered in the differential diagnosis, a trichogram may be helpful. In alopecia areata, hair is seen in the telogen phase while in patients with trichotillomania, hair is usually pulled out in the telogen phase and thus most of the hair is in the anagen phase (➲ *Table 35.5*). Very rarely, after pulling the hair out, it is swallowed, sometimes leading to trichobezoar with ileus symptoms. There are only a few case reports of this happening, however.

Transient tearing of hair in early childhood can be viewed as a nonmalignant habit which will spontaneously stop later on. The diagnosis of trichotillomania should be made only with pronounced findings and persistence of the disorder over a period of months. However, the symptoms, especially in adulthood, may last for decades and anamneses show a high proportion of episodes in childhood or adolescence.

Psychiatric Symptoms

Trichotillomania is based psychopathologically on impairment of impulse control characterized by buildup

Table 35.6
Hair and DPS

	Trichotillomania	Trichotemnomania	Trichoteiromania
Pattern of harm	Hair-pulling	Cutting hair	Breaking off of hair by rubbing and scratching
Clinical appearance	Typical triple-zone appearance with long, missing, and re-growing hair	Pseudoalopecia with what appears to be stubble	Pseudoalopecia with broken-off hairs, normal thickness, stubble with white, frizzy ends
Trichogramm	Reduced number of hairs in telogen phase	Normal hair root pattern	Dystrophic hair root pattern, partly reduced telogen component

of tension prior to pulling, followed often by a feeling of pleasure, satisfaction, or relaxation upon the removal of the hair.

Many people twist and play with their hair due to increased anxiety or under stress in certain situations with greater concentration, without suffering trichotillomania.

Differential diagnosis includes compulsive disorder. Tearing out hair as a stereotype (ICD-10: F98.4) must also be delineated, whereby this is a psychiatric illness with skin reference.

Trichotemnomania

Trichotemnomania is a rare form of hair damage, whereby the hair is intentionally cut off. This form of hair damage is classified as an artifact/malingering.

Trichoteiromania

In this variant of self-inflicted hair loss, there is physical damage to the hair by rubbing and scratching the scalp, resulting in pseudoalopecia. In trichoteiromania (teiro Greek.: I scratch) there are macroscopic whitish hair tips with split ends, corresponding under the light microscope to brush-like hair breaks or trichoptilosis (Reich and Trüeb 2003).

Casuistic case reports state in trichoteiromania that the patients complain additionally of trichodynia with dysesthesias and pruritus.

The differences between the three paraartefacts affecting the hair are presented in *Table 35.6.*

5.4 Summary Psychiatric Symptoms of DPS

The main characteristic of paraartefacts is impairment of impulse control and thus the failure to resist impulsive urges or temptation to perform a repeated act without reasonable motivation, which is damaging to the person or to others. In questioning, however, the patient can often admit the manipulation, denoting the presence of a semiconscious impairment (*Table 35.7*).

Often, a minimal primary lesion is excessively manipulated, which only then leads to a pronounced, serious finding. A classical example is manipulation of acne in the morning in front of the mirror, whereby the urge to manipulate cannot be resisted. Emotionally tense situations or unresolved conflicts and an ungovernable urge to self-manipulation may be present as the cause. Compulsive disorders often play a causal role.

6 Malingering

6.1 Clinical Findings

Malingering (ICD-10: Z76.5) V65.2 in DSM-IV-TR are defined as an intentional and conscious creation and elicitation of physical or psychiatric symptoms.

In Malingerings, too, mechanical injuries from pressing, rubbing, biting, cutting, stabbing, burning or self-inflicted infections with wound-healing impairments, abscesses, mutilations, acid burns or other toxic damages to the skin are in the foreground. Hematological symptoms may occur due to occlusion of extremities, creation of petechias and additional covert taking of pharmaceuticals, as well as by heparin injections.

Malingerings provide another focus in dermatology in the framework of expert opinions of occupational illnesses and disability procedures (*Fig. 35.4*). Additionally, there are manipulations of epicutaneous tests during evaluation procedures and simulation of serious symptoms to obtain workman's compensation certification. In intentional provocation of contact allergies, the patient is usually familiar with the causative allergen, but does not admit this to the doctor.

Table 35.7
Diagnostic criteria of paraartefacts

Diagnostic criteria of paraartefacts (DSM IV)
Repeated inability to resist impulses
Increasing feeling of tension prior to the act
Pleasure, satisfaction or feeling of relaxation during the act
No causal relationship to other somatic or psychiatric diseases
The impairment is accompanied by clinically-significant suffering

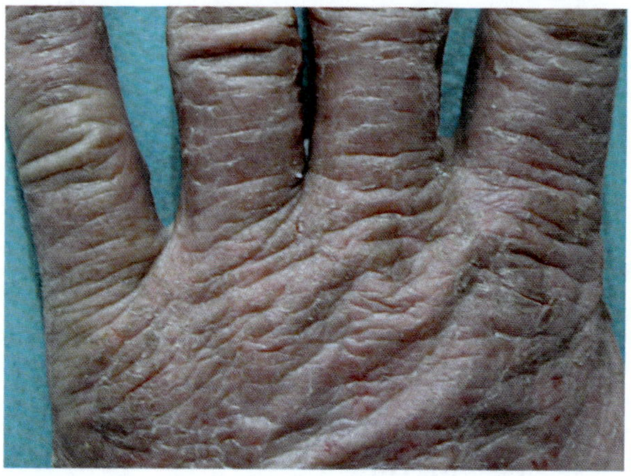

Fig. 35.4
Malingering: 44-year-old construction worker with skin lesions due to of constant intentional immersing of the hands in liquid cement without protective gloves. Numerous periods of disability certified by various doctors and desire for disability

6.2 Psychiatric Symptoms

Malingerings are conscious, intentional self-injurious behavior by the patient in order to obtain an apparent material advantage from the illness (V65.2 Malingerings in DSM-IV-TR). They may also be characterized by another social advantage, such as another secondary gain by eliciting attention and care by the family as in Factitious Disorder (300.10 and 300.19 DSM-IV-TR, ICD-10 F68.1) in which the physician is intentionally deceived.

Among the psychosocial motivations for malingerings are to avoid criminal prosecution, obtain narcotics, avoid military service, or obtain financial advantages. The advantage may lie in higher disability pensions and other financial compensations. Intentional and conscious simulations are hardly amenable to psychotherapeutic measures, since there is no patient motivation for therapy.

7 Special Forms

7.1 Gardner-Diamond Syndrome

Definition: The Gardner-Diamond Syndrome (ICD-10: F68.1; F68.1) is characterized by periodically-occurring painful infiltrated blue patches, multiple physical complaints, and characteristic psychiatric symptoms. Synonyms are painful ecchymoses syndrome, psychogenic purpura, and painful bruising syndrome. The Gardner-Diamond Syndrome occurs mostly in young women (Gardner and Diamond 1955; Behrendt et al. 2001).

7.1.1 Pathogenesis

Initially, the first descriptions supported the assumption of an autoimmune process after injection of autologous blood, in the sense of an autoerythrocytic sensitization syndrome. Currently, an artificial genesis is accepted as most likely (Ivanov et al. 2009).

7.1.2 Clinic

As prodrome, there is initially itching, feeling of tension or burning pains, usually in the extremities, most often the legs. Then edematous erythemas develop with ecchymoses, which heal within 1–2 weeks (*Fig. 35.5*). Characteristically, the course is in periodic attacks and heals without scarring.

Systemic symptoms include attacks of abdominal pain, nausea, vomiting, diarrhea, weight loss, headache, blurred vision, paresthesias, and other neurological symptoms, as well as hematuria, hematemesis, metrorrhagias, and amenorrhea.

7.1.3 Psychiatric Symptoms

The personality structure of the patients presents classical features of dissociative disorders, including conversion disorders, masochism, depressiveness, anxiety, and inhibition in emotional expression feelings (aggression inhibition) (Ivanov et al. 2009).

The differential diagnosis includes the spectrum of artifact diseases.

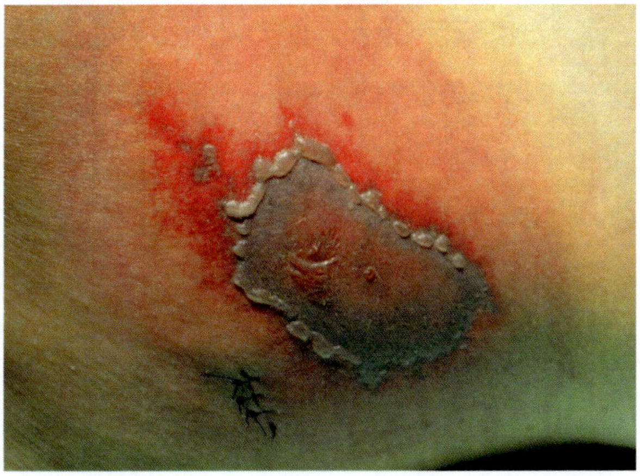

Fig. 35.5
Woman with Gardner-Diamond syndrome

7.2 Münchhausen Syndrome

The Münchhausen syndrome (ICD10: F68.1; DSM-IV-TR 300.16 & 19) is characterized by the triad: hospital wandering, pathological lying, and self-injury (Oostendorp and Rakoski 1993).

In 1951, Richard Asher, a London physician reported the first cases and features of three female patients with self-induced disease, coining the term Münchhausen Syndrome (Asher 1951), in reference to Baron Karl Friedrich Hieronymus von Münchhausen (1720–1797). This disease denotes malingering/simulation of acute diseases with demonstrative dramatic description of complaints and false information about the anamnesis, and includes numerous hospitalizations and surgical procedures, sometimes with visible multiple scars. Frequently it is based on a borderline disorder.

Characteristically, patients often display splitting of the environment into good and bad in the same fashion as seen in subjects with borderline personality disorder.

A pathological doctor–patient relationship is frequently present, making these subjects the most difficult problem patients to treat in medicine (Rothenhausler and Kapfhammer 2002).

7.3 Münchhausen-By-Proxy Syndrome

In the Münchhausen-by-proxy syndrome (ICD-10: F74.8; DSM-IV-TR 300.16 & 19), it is usually children who are injured by their primary caretakers in order to establish contact with medical caregivers. Thus, the Münchhausen-by-proxy syndrome is a special form of child abuse.

Two cases of Münchhausen-by-proxy syndrome were published for the first time in 1977 by an English pediatrician (Meadow 1977). The term was coined because the mothers systematically deceived the doctor with fictitious stories about the disease, but instead of their own bodies, abused the body of the children (by proxy). This observation was followed by numerous publications of case reports.

In most cases, a "detectivesque" elucidation is necessary. In 98%, women are the perpetrators, and of these 90% are the biological mother, with the rest stepmothers or day-care providers.

Bleeding, seizures, clouding of consciousness up to and including respiratory arrest, diarrhea, vomiting or fever, as well as also skin changes with scratching, acid burns, or occlusions may be caused.

Based on individual case reports, from the psychodynamic point of view there appears to be a bizarre split in the mothers in relation to their children. On the one hand, the child is experienced as a threat, whereby the mother thinks the child would take from her everything she herself needs to live (Thomas 2003).

By injury or abuse, the child is placed in a completely dependent situation, in which the mother devotes herself to the illusion of a perfect, caring, and ideal mother. Characteristically, the patients appear to the nursing personnel as particularly zealous and engaged.

Breaking through the vicious circle of violence is primary in the psychotherapeutic process, since the violence will be repeated until it can be made conscious, worked through, verbalized, and thus integrated in the therapeutic process.

8 Therapy

Therapy of self-inflicted dermatoses is one of the greatest challenges for the dermatologist, especially when the patient comes to the specialist primarily with purely somatic concepts and expectations without insight compared to other dermatological skin diseases (Gieler et al. 1987; Koo and Lee 2003; Harth 2007).

DAS is especially therapy-resistant, because these conditions either arise unconsciously and cannot be recalled by the patient or is malingering created by the patient with intentional calculation (Koblenzer 2000). So, on the one hand, clear delineation must be drawn in

Table 35.8
Therapy of self inflicted skin diseases

Therapy	Dermatitis artefacta syndrome	Dermatitis paraartefacta syndrome	Malingering
Psychosomatic care (diary of symptoms)	+++	+++	+
Psychoeducation	+++	+++	+
Behavioral therapy	+	+++	–
Depth psychology/psychoanalysis	+++	+	–
Psychopharmaceuticals	++	+	–
Confrontation	– – –	+/–	+++

+++ Very common indication, ++ Common indication, + Rare indication, +/– Questionable indication, – possible contraindication, – – – absolute contraindication

malingering, while on the other hand, confronting the patient too soon with the unconscious artificial genesis may lead to termination of the doctor-patient relationship and even end in suicide or attempted suicide (*Table 35.8*).

8.1 Dermatitis Artefacta Syndrome

Somatic or monocausal therapy alone often does not achieve healing in DAS patients and may lead to frustrations and even to bilateral open aggression in treatment. The therapy of DAS is usually long-term, lasting for years.

At the beginning of therapy, careful (non-accusatory) development of a therapeutic relationship is the primary task. Local measures to aid wound healing should be undertaken with mild therapies for self-induced lesions, for example, for excoriations on the lower legs zinc oxide paste may be used (Harth et al. 2009).

In dermatitis artefacta syndrome, patients may not understand their unconscious physical manipulation and may not be able to talk about it since it often occurs in a dissociative state. Premature confrontation or embarrassing accusations should be avoided as these threaten to end the doctor-patient relationship and can lead to further autoaggressive behavior, including suicidal impulses, or to a "physician odyssey". Psychotherapy is usually necessary. Psychodynamic therapy can help stabilize the personality. These measures generally require long-term hospitalization.

The treating physician should accompany the patient until he or she can switch to a specific outpatient therapy or be referred to a psychosomatic clinic or be motivated to begin psychopharmacotherapy. The patient should only be confronted with the need for psychiatric care or psychotherapy after a stable relationship of trust has been established between the doctor and the patient.

8.2 Dermatitis Paraartefacta Syndrome

The prognosis for dermatitis paraartefacta syndrome is generally better because the disorder is "semiconsciously." Behavioral-therapeutic measures for impulse control are particularly indicated and successful in this condition, including methods to improve self-management with promotion of self-observation, cognitive restructuring, and relaxation techniques (Vitulano et al. 1992).

An explanatory consultation (psychoeducation) with the patient (or parents in case of children) may be the first step toward making the offending mechanism apparent, laying the foundation for regaining impulse control. Subsequent self-observations or outsider observation and control of the action can often achieve healing. If this is not sufficient, keeping a pulling diary (trichotillomania) or manipulation diary (skin picking) may enable better analysis and control. In addition to the date, time of day and duration of the manipulation, the place, and emotions associated with the situation as well as any special features should be recorded.

Moreover, psychoeducation taking the environment (family) into account is helpful from the perspective of psychosomatic primary care. For example, in pediatric trichotillomania, a session of psychoeducation with the parents is often successful. This is frequently a psychoreactive disorder and a self-limiting course with spontaneous healing is achieved by attentive observation of the impaired impulse control and appropriate support in the environment.

Measures to divert tension by replacing pulling of the hair or skin-picking with other motor acts like clutching and squeezing stress balls, may be successfully used in the next step and are well-accepted by patients, as are relaxation measures.

In longer courses, introduction of a behavioral therapy is important. The habit-reversal technique has proven valuable as a behavioral-therapeutic measure.

The basis begins with the conscious recognition of the impulse to self-injury, followed by interruption of the acts with internal warning signals, and lastly achieving and remaining in a relaxation phase.

In courses lasting several years, high-grade conditioning of the actions or additional serious personality disorders, in-hospital psychotherapy may be indicated along with the use of psychopharmaceuticals. Initiation of psychotherapy is determined by the comorbidities.

8.3 Malingering

Due to a lack of therapy motivation, malingering is difficult or impossible to treat psychotherapeutically. Primary is the structuring of the doctor–patient relationship, with clear, often purely somatic reports and confrontation, also in cooperation with health insurance. Special attention should, however, also be paid to depressive or suicidal tendencies, which may be in the foreground in emotionally-conspicuous patients with simulations and thus easily overlooked if the clinical presentation changes.

8.4 Psychopharmacotherapy in Dermatitis Artefacta

Psychopharmaceuticals have proven valuable in the stabilization of the usually massive affects and must be applied with appropriate expert knowledge (Harth et al. 2007). Symptomatic therapy with low-strength neuroleptics to relieve states of tension or antidepressants to relieve concurrent psychopathological symptoms, such as depressive disorders, may be helpful.

In DPS such as trichotillomania, therapy with SSRIs may be indicated under the aspect of impaired impulse control (Koo and Lee 2003). Fluoxetine and clomipramine have been successfully used in recalcitrant forms of trichotillomania, taking comorbidities into account (Wichel et al. 1992).

In dissociative artifacts, low-strength neuroleptics are usually more effective and are preferred.

DPS, a combination therapy with drugs and behavioral therapy has been found beneficial.

9 Prognosis

The prognosis for patients with self-injuries depends on the severity of the symptoms; it is good in mild forms, but even with appropriate treatment, it is moderate to poor in serious forms, and in particular patients with "Münchhausen's Syndrome" have a bad prognosis.

There is acute danger for the patient himself – or for others – and at the same time a lack of treatment motivation, a legal intervention may become necessary for admission to a psychiatric hospital in cooperation with a psychiatrist.

References

Asher R (1951) Munchhausen's syndrome. Lancet 1:339–341

Bach M, Bach D (1993) Psychiatric and psychometric issues in acne excoriee. Psychother Psychosom 60(3–4):207–210

Behrendt C, Goos M, Thiel H, Hengge UR (2001) Painful-bruising-syndrome. Hautarzt 52:634–637

Gardner FH, Diamond LK (1955) Auto-erythrocyte sensitization. A form of purpura producing painful bruising following auto-sensitization to red bloodcells in certain women. Blood 10:675–690

Gieler U (2004) Leitlinien in der psychotherapeutischen medizin: artifizielle störungen. J Dtsch Dermatol Ges 2(1):66–73

Gieler U, Effendy I, Stangier U (1987) Kutane artefakte: möglichkeiten der behandlung und ihre grenzen. Z Hautkr 62:882–890

Gupta MA, Gupta AK, Habermann HF (1987) The self-inflicted dermatoses: a critical review. Gen Hosp Psychiatry 9(1):45–52

Harth W (2007) Leitlinie psychosomatische dermatologie (psychodermatologie). In: Korting HC, Callies R, Reusch M, Schlaeger M, Sterry W (eds) Dermatologische qualitätssicherung leitlinien und empfehlungen, 5th edn. ABW Wissenschaftsverlag, Berlin, pp 411–428

Harth W, Gieler U (2006) Psychosomatische dermatologie. Lehrbuch und bildatlas. Springer, Heidelberg/Berlin, pp S1–S330

Harth W, Linse R (2000) Dermatological symptoms and sexual abuse: a review and case reports. J Eur Acad Dermatol Venereol 14(6):489–494

Harth W, Seikowski K, Gieler U, Niemeier V, Hillert A (2007) Psychopharmakologische behandlung dermatologischer patienten – wenn reden allein nicht hilft. J Dtsch Dermatol Ges 5:1101–1106

Harth W, Gieler U, Kusnir D, Tausk F (2009) Clinical management in psychodermatology. Springer, New York

Ivanov OL, Lvov AN, Michenko AV, Künzel J, Mayser P, Gieler U (2009) Autoerythrocyte sensitization syndrome (Gardner-Diamond syndrome): review of the literature. J Eur Acad Dermatol Venereol 23(5):499–504

Janus L (1972) Personality structure and psychodynamics in dermatological artefacts. Z Psychosom Med Psychoanal 18(1):21–28

Koblenzer CS (1996) Neurotic excoriations and dermatitis artefacta. Dermatol Clin 14(3):447–455

Koblenzer CS (2000) Dermatitis artefacta. Clinical features and approaches to treatment. Am J Clin Dermatol 1:47–55

Koo J, Lee CS (2003) Psychocutaneous medicine. Dekker, New York/Basel

Meadow R (1977) Munchhausen syndrome by proxy: the hinterland of child abuse. Lancet 2:343–345

Muller SA, Winkelmann RK (1972) Trichotillomania. A clinicopathologic study of 24 cases. Arch Dermatol 105:535–540

Oostendorp I, Rakoski J (1993) Münchausen-Syndrome. Artefakte in der Dermatologie. Hautarzt 44:86–90

Reich S, Trüeb RM (2003) Trichoteiromanie. J Dtsch Dermatol Ges 1:22–28

Rothenhausler HB, Kapfhammer HP (2002) Munchhausen patients in general hospitals – clinical features and treatment approaches in C-L psychiatry settings. Psychiatr Prax 29(7):381–387

Thomas K (2003) Munchausen syndrome by proxy: identification and diagnosis. J Pediatr Nurs 18:174–180

van Moffaert M (2003) The spectrum of dermatological self mutilation and self destruction including dermatitis artefacta and neurotic excoriations. In: Koo J, Lee C-S (eds) Psychocutaneous medicine. Marcel Dekker, New York/Basel

Vitulano LA, King RA, Scahill L, Cohen DJ (1992) Behavioral treatment of children and adolescents with trichotillomania. J Am Acad Child Adolesc Psychiatry 31:139–146

Wichel RM, Jones JS, Stanley B, Molcho A, Stanley M (1992) Clinical characteristics of trichotillomania and response to fluoxetine. J Clin Psychiatry 53:304–308

Section 3

Causative Factors

36 Antiseptics and Disinfectants

Jean-Marie Lachapelle
Unit of Occupational and Environmental Dermatology, Catholic University of Louvain, Montigny-le-Tilleul, Belgium

Core Messages

- Antiseptics and disinfectants (see definitions) share common skin side effects, i.e., irritation, allergic contact dermatitis, and eventually immunological contact urticaria.
- Some antiseptics fall into disuse, due to their lack of efficacy (dyes) or their strong allergic properties (mercurials), except thiomersal, the indications of which remain important.
- Current antiseptics (i.e., povidone-iodine or chlorhexidine) are of great importance, due to the emergence of MRSA and CA-MRSA, leading to a decrease in the use of topical antibiotics to which Gram-positive and Gram-negative bacteria are more and more resistant.
- Silver-based wound and burn dressings may lead to new cases of allergic contact dermatitis, mainly related to the incorporation of new antiseptics, such as octenidine or PHMB.
- Disinfectants are a common source of occupational irritant and/or allergic contact dermatitis.
- Aldehydes are widely used as disinfectants. Formaldehyde, glutaraldehyde, and glyoxal are responsible for many cases of allergic contact dermatitis.
- Quaternary ammonium compounds, and particularly benzalkonium chloride, are disinfectants provoking irritant and/or allergic contact dermatitis. The interpretation of patch tests is difficult, and the use of ROAT's is advised.

1 Introduction

Antiseptics and disinfectants are largely present in our modern environment. Antiseptics are mainly, but not exclusively, used in relation with medical and nursing activities.

Disinfectants have a very broad field of indications in daily life.

Both antiseptics and disinfectants are not devoid of some side effects which are of great concern in occupational dermatology.

2 Definitions and General Considerations

2.1 Antiseptics

2.1.1 Preliminary Remarks

Antiseptics are – by definition – substances that inhibit the growth and development of microorganisms (without necessarily killing them) in living tissue. Their indications are varied, such as cleansing of preoperative skin, cleansing of acute and chronic wounds, and also, on some occasions, treatment of skin infections.

Some qualities are required for a suitable use of antiseptics (➋ *Table 36.1*).

The emergence of methicillin-resistant *Staphylococcus aureus* (MRSA) infections has been confirmed in healthcare centers for decades. More recently, MRSA infections have been increasingly observed in healthy individuals with no exposure to healthcare centers (community-acquired MRSA or CA-MRSA).

The management of such infections is the responsibility of the medical and paramedical staff: nurses, kinesitherapists, etc.

In order to reduce the prevalence of such infections, a very important (sometimes neglected) measure is to reduce the use of topical antibiotics such as bacitracin, mupirocin, fusidic acid, and retapamuline. They can be replaced advantageously by antiseptics that do not induce resistance. The inevitable corollary is an increased use of antiseptics, not only at the hospital, but also in different communities and even now at home (Upton et al. 2003; Gosbell 2004; Osterlund et al. 2006).

The general rules of personal hygiene are of course of prime importance (Lorette et al. 2009).

T. Rustemeyer, P. Elsner, S.M. John & H.I. Maibach (eds.), *Kanerva's Occupational Dermatology*,
DOI 10.1007/978-3-642-02035-3_36, © Springer-Verlag Berlin Heidelberg 2012

2.1.2 An Overview of Antiseptics of Common Use Nowadays

Many different antiseptics have been used in the past; some of them have been almost abandoned in most countries, due to either their high allergenic properties (e.g., mercury compounds) or their limited antiseptic activity (e.g., dyes).

A list of antiseptics of common use nowadays, including their in vitro spectrum of activity against Gram-positive and Gram-negative bacteria, is presented in ➋ *Table 36.2.*

Table 36.1
Qualities of antiseptics required for a suitable use

Broad spectrum of activity
Low irritancy
Low allergenicity
Good tolerance
No (or very low) cytotoxicity
Fast and long-lasting efficacy
No (or very limited) inhibition by organic matter
No propensity to select bacterial resistance

Table 36.2
Antiseptics of common use and their in vitro spectrum of activity against Gram-positive and Gram-negative bacteria[a]

Antiseptics	Bacteria	
	Gram-positive	Gram-negative
Ethanol	xx	xx
Povidone-iodine (PVP-I)	xxx	xxx
Hydrogen peroxide	x	x
Chlorines (ex.Dakin)	xxx	xx
Chlorhexidine	xxx	xx
Quaternary ammonium compounds (ex.cetrimide)	xx	x
Hexamidine	x	x/0
Hexetidine	x	x/0
Silver salts	x	x
Phenols (ex.triclosan)	xx	xx

[a]After Teot et al. 2004
xxx: very strong; xx: strong; x: weak; 0: no activity

2.2 Disinfectants

Disinfectants refer, by definition, to substances designed to destroy pathogens in the environment (e.g., on working surfaces or operating materials). They are very diversified, with different chemical structures.

3 Skin Side Effects of Antiseptics and Disinfectants

Antiseptics and disinfectants share common skin side effects. These are of course particularly important for antiseptics, which are designed to be in direct contact with the skin.

3.1 Irritant Reactions

The most common side effect of antiseptics and disinfectants is irritation. There is a common sentence in the literature that "an antiseptic or a disinfectant devoid of any irritant properties does not exist." It is roughly true, but irritant reactions depend upon several factors, which are listed in ➋ *Table 36.3.*

Health workers can be affected when they do not apply protective measures for the hands, when using antiseptics. In those conditions, irritant hand dermatitis is not a rare event.

On the other hand, irritant reactions to disinfectants are a major problem in occupational dermatology. Preventive measures are of prime importance in this respect.

Table 36.3
Factors influencing the irritancy of antiseptics

Concentration of antiseptic
Vehicle
Application under occlusion or non-occlusion
Repeated applications (cumulative effect)
Site of application on the skin (e.g., folds, scrotum, vulva, eyelids, mucosae are more susceptible to irritant effects)
Excited skin syndrome (in case of active eczematous reaction)
Atopic background (mainly, but not exclusively on clinically affected areas of skin)

3.2 Allergic Contact Dermatitis Reactions

The allergenic properties of antiseptics and disinfectants can differ considerably from a substance to another.

It is generally accepted that they are not very frequent nowadays with the products on the market, contrary to the situation observed in the past decades.

They are reviewed in the following sections, and discussed individually for each antiseptic and/or disinfectant.

3.3 Other Reactions

Other types of reactions can occur, such as immunological contact urticaria and, very rarely, anaphylactic reactions.

4 The Repertoire of Skin Side Effects of Antiseptics

The repertoire of skin side effects of antiseptics is broad. In this section, the common (or uncommon) use of antiseptics is not taken into account.

Referring to patch test procedures, if not specifically mentioned, concentrations and vehicles are derived from de Groot's textbook 2008.

4.1 Alcohols

Probably the most widely used antiseptics are the lower aliphatic alcohols, ethanol and isopropanol. The bactericidal activity of the aliphatic alcohols increases with their molecular weight. Alcohols are considered less irritating than aldehydes.

The irritancy of an alcohol compound decreases as the molecular size of the compound increases.

Alcohols are known to delipidize and dehydrate the upper part of the stratum corneum, thereby impairing the barrier function of the epidermis.

4.1.1 Ethyl Alcohol (Ethanol)

Irritant contact dermatitis is the most common skin side effect due to ethanol. It results most often in the cumulative irritant contact type, and, in rare cases, in the acute irritant type (Tupker et al. 1997).

The current advices (in terms of antisepsis) given to the members of the hospital staff, i.e., frequent washing of the hands with a 70% ethanol solution (Mc Donnell and Russell 1999) may lead to an increase in the number of cumulative irritant contact dermatitis. It is therefore a problem of occupational dermatology of great actuality.

Ethanol dermatitis may take the form of an eczematous eruption.

More rarely, an urticarial reaction has been noticed at the exposed site (Fregert et al. 1963).

Undiluted ethanol (95%) causes a short-lasting sharp stinging sensation in most individuals in sensitive skin regions (face and neck, genital areas). If the skin has slight abrasions, e.g., due to shaving, this phenomenon is experienced by everybody (Frosch and John 2006).

Allergic contact dermatitis to ethanol has been very rarely reported (Patruno et al. 1994; Ophaswongse and Maibach 1994).

Patch testing: 10% aq.

4.1.2 Isopropyl Alcohol (Isopropanol)

Skin side effects due to isopropanol are less documented, but, by extrapolation, are comparable to reactions to ethanol with a lesser irritant effect. For instance, cases of contact urticaria have been reported (de Groot 2008).

Patch testing: 10% aq.

4.2 Iodine Compounds

4.2.1 Iodoform

Iodoform (tri-iodomethane) released iodine under the influence of light and temperature. It was considered an irritant and a strong contact allergen. The first cases were described by Bruno Bloch 1911 under the term "idiosyncrasies," very popular in the first years of the twentieth century. It is almost beyond doubt that it is not in use nowadays.

Patch testing: 5% pet.

4.2.2 Iodine Tincture

Iodine tincture (alcoholic solution) has been used extensively in the past, either at a 5% concentration for human use (against bacteria and ringworm) and a 10% concentration for veterinary use (e.g., ringworm of cattle). In past years, it was considered a gold standard for many infections. It was a strong irritant and cases of allergic contact dermatitis were not infrequent among medical personnel, nurses, veterinarians, and farmers, mainly due to a total lack of protection of the hands.

As iodine tincture is a strong irritant, it is advised to test it by the "open method" as is (Mathelier-Fusade 1994; Lee et al. 2005).

4.2.3 Povidone-Iodine

(Polyvinylpyrrolidone-iodine; PVP-iodine)

Povidone-iodine has replaced since many years other iodine compounds, such as iodoform or iodine tincture.

Povidone-iodine is an iodophor, used as a topical antiseptic, on a very large scale, throughout the world, under several trade names (the most common is Betadine®). A 10% povidone-iodine solution contains 1% available iodine, but free-iodine is at 0.1% concentration.

It is well demonstrated nowadays that skin exposure causes irritant rather than allergic contact dermatitis. It is therefore advised not to use povidone-iodine on damaged skin (e.g., eczematous lesions of atopic dermatitis, perilesional irritated skin, encountered in various types of wounds or stomas). Povidone-iodine is intended to be used on intact skin. It has been shown that povidone-iodine could be used for the treatment of a large variety of skin superficial infections (Lachapelle and de Prost 2007).

Cases of allergic contact dermatitis to povidone-iodine have been reported in the literature. An epidemic of occupational allergic contact dermatitis of the hands has been reported in a pig slaughterhouse (Lachapelle 1984). Slaughterers worked barehanded and suffered from frequent cuttings. They washed their hands many times daily with a povidone-iodine solution.

Other cases have been reported (Tosti et al. 1990; Erdmann et al. 1999; Pecquet 2003).

The results of patch tests to PVP-I (10% pet, i.e., 1% free-iodine), considered positive in the literature, can be in some cases false positives, due to an irritation to PVP-I (under occlusion). In a recent study (Lachapelle 2005), 500 consecutive patients were patch tested with PVP-I. Fourteen had a positive patch test (2.8%). In a second step, the 14 patients were tested again, in a different way: The PVP-I aqueous solution was applied twice daily (without occlusion) at the flexor aspect of the forearm (5 × 5 cm) during 7 days, i.e., 14 open applications (ROAT test, after Hannuksela and Salo 1986). At day 7, 2 patients only had a positive ROAT test and 12 a negative ROAT test. Therefore, it means that only 2 out of 500 patients were allergic to PVP-I (prevalence: 0.4%).

Patch testing (de Groot 2008) reflects anyway the difficulties encountered in practice. Several options had been proposed: 5–10% water; 5–10% pet.; 0.5% alcohol. In the above-mentioned study (Lachapelle 2005), the problem has been partially solved.

In recent years, some anaphylactic reactions to povidone-iodine have been reported, and attributed to polyvinylpyrrolidone, not to iodine. They can be considered exceptional, due to the large use of povidone-iodine in clinical practice (Pedrosa et al. 2005; Yoshida et al. 2008; Palobart et al. 2009).

4.3 Hydrogen Peroxide

Hydrogen peroxide has been and is still used as a topical antiseptic (i.e., for the cleansing of wounds) due to its oxidizing properties. The concentration of the hydrogen peroxide solution is expressed in volume or percentage: 10 volumes correspond to 3%. Depending upon its concentration, it is a well-known irritant. Allergic reactions, if any, are exceptional, and, therefore, its implication in occupational dermatology is very limited.

Patch testing: 3% aq.

4.4 Chlorines

4.4.1 Sodium Hypochlorite (Dakin's Solution)

Sodium hypochlorite is an antiseptic which has largely been used in the past. It was introduced by Dakin and some papers refer to the historical aspects of this discovery (Mc Donnell and Sculco 1997; King 2008). Its current popular name is "bleach." It has a large spectrum activity and it is used as antiseptic or disinfectant. Hypochlorites are essentially irritant and, in occupational life, have caused hand, diffuse, or periulcerous dermatitis. Cases of allergic contact dermatitis to sodium hypochlorite have been rarely reported (Osmundsen 1978). Eau de Javel is exclusively used as a disinfectant (see ➋ Sect. 5.2).

Patch testing: 0.5% aq.

4.4.2 Chloramine T (Chloramine, Tosylchloramide Sodium)

Chloramine T (paratoluene-sulfonyl-sodium chloramide) is a potent antiseptic.

It has been described as an occupational hazard for pharmaceutical workers, nurses, butchers, cleaners, and brewers (Key 1961). Immediate reactions are the most frequent side effects: contact urticaria, recurrent attacks of edema around eyelids, rhinitis, dyspnea, asthma (Dooms-Goossens et al. 1983), in particular in industrial settings.

Cases of allergic occupational contact dermatitis are very rare (Lombardi et al. 1989).

Patch testing: 2% aq.

Chloramine-specific IgE serological testing is highly recommended in immediate-type reactions.

4.5 Chlorhexidine

Chlorhexidine is a broad-spectrum antimicrobial agent, a synthetic biguanide used as antiseptic and disinfectant, available under different forms (diacetate, dihydrochloride, and digluconate). The use of chlorhexidine as an antiseptic has increased in recent years at the expense of quaternary ammonium compounds. Chlorhexidine is used clinically for disinfection of hands and operation sites, in the treatment of burns and scalds, in urology and gynecology, and by dentists in the treatment of caries and periodontitis.

Although chlorhexidine is used widely, cases of allergic contact dermatitis are rare, some of them being occupationally related (Muston et al. 1977; Rudzki et al. 1989). Differential diagnosis with irritant reactions is important, in particular when chlorhexidine is used under occlusion.

In recent years, much attention has been paid to immediate IgE-mediated skin reactions, such as urticaria, angioedema, and anaphylaxis. Asthma is another side effect. Many cases have been reported in the literature (Beaudouin et al. 2004; Krautheim et al. 2004; Sharma and Chopra 2009).

Furthermore, chlorhexidine is considered nowadays a new occupational hazard. Urticaria, angioedema, and anaphylaxis have been reported in health care workers (Nagendran et al. 2009). Increased awareness and easier access to chlorhexidine-specific IgE serological testing should facilitate early diagnosis of affected health care workers, avoiding appropriate measures to be investigated, thus reducing the risk of potentially severe allergic reactions in the future.

Patch testing: 0.5% aq.

Chlorhexidine-specific IgE serological testing is highly recommended.

4.6 Quaternary Ammonium Compounds

Quaternary ammonium compounds are a vast family of cationic detergents and are mainly used as disinfectants (and therefore described in ➋ Sect. 5.4).

Their use as antiseptics is rather limited, e.g., topical antiseptics for burns, ointments, and mouth- and hand washes.

4.7 Hexamidine Diisethionate

This antiseptic has been (and it is still) used extensively in some countries, such as France or Belgium. It is well tolerated in most cases, but its antiseptic spectrum (➋ *Table 36.2*) is considered nowadays limited, as compared to other antiseptics, such as povidone-iodine. It is not irritant, but well-documented cases of allergic contact dermatitis have been reported, usually severe in their clinical expression (Revuz et al. 1984; Dooms-Goossens et al. 1989). Some characteristics deserve attention: the long duration of the lesions, after disuse of the allergen; the histopathological features – spongiosis is rare and leukocytoclastic vasculitis is not uncommon (Arthus' phenomenon).

Patch testing: 0.15% aq.

4.8 Hexetidine

Its use is very limited nowadays (mainly as a collutory). Exceptional cases of allergic contact dermatitis have been reported (Merk et al. 1982). Many years ago (but not now), it has also been used as a fungicide.

Patch testing: 0.1 aq.

4.9 Triclosan

Triclosan (Irgasan DP300®) is a lipophilic chlorophenol antiseptic agent, used mainly in soap bars, deodorants, and antiperspirants. It has been shown (Lachapelle and Tennstedt 1979) that the allergenic properties of triclosan were very low, using the maximization test in guinea pigs and in humans. This was confirmed recently by a study conducted in 275 eczema patients. The prevalence of positive patch tests to triclosan was 0.7% (Schena et al. 2008). Nevertheless, allergic contact dermatitis from triclosan used in antibacterial hand washes has been reported (Wong and Beck 2001) and is a potential occupational problem in nursing staff.

Patch testing: 2% pet.

4.10 Potassium Permanganate

Diluted solutions (1/10 000) have been used as wet dressings on weeping dermatitis or leg ulcers.

This use has declined considerably nowadays. A skin side effect was irritation (van der Valk and Maibach 1996) but no case of occupational dermatitis has been described.

4.11 Nitrofurazone (Or Nitrofural)

Nitrofurazone was once a popular antiseptic remedy for the treatment of burns and stasis ulcers.

So many instances of allergic contact dermatitis to this remedy occurred that its use has largely been abandoned. In particular, as nitrofurazone was also used as an antibacterial agent in animal feeds, occupational dermatitis was reported in cattle breeders or farmers (Vilaplana et al. 1990; Condé-Salazar et al. 1995).

Patch testing: 1% pet.

4.12 Chloroxylenol

Chloroxylenol is widely used as a topical antiseptic and/or disinfectant with low irritant potential. It has been a substitute for hexachlorophene in a large number of products. Sensitization has been reported, but it is very rare (Myatt and Beck 1985; Ranchoff et al. 1986).

Patch testing: 1% pet.

4.13 Silver Compounds

4.13.1 Silver Nitrate

Silver nitrate has been used extensively in dermatology in the past, but very much less nowadays.

It was kept in an amber bottle because on exposure to air and light, it decomposes, forming small amounts of nitric acid, silver nitrite, and colloidal silver, which liberate silver ions. The ionized silver is considered allergenic. Some cases of allergic contact dermatitis have been reported (Gaul and Underwood 1948), some of them being of occupational origin. It has also been mentioned that the prolonged use of topical silver nitrate can lead to systemic argyria.

Recently, a new formulation of silver nitrate has been proposed, based upon the "nanoparticles technology." It is developed as a gel, without preliminary side effects (Jain et al. 2009).

Patch testing: 2% aq.

4.13.2 Silver Sulfadiazine

Silver sulfadiazine (often under the trade name Flammazine®) has been (and is still) extensively used in the treatment of burns, and, more recently, of epidermolysis bullosa. A complete review of the literature indicates that allergic contact dermatitis to silver sulfadiazine is quite uncommon, but this has been potentially underestimated (Degreef and Dooms-Goossens 1985; Fuller 2009). Argyria may – exceptionally – be consecutive to its application on large areas of ulcerated skin, as observed in burns or epidermolysis bullosa (Browning and Levy 2008).

Patch testing: 5% pet.

4.13.3 Silver-Based Wound and Burn Dressings

Silver dressings, introduced a few years ago, vary widely according to their matrix, since almost all existing modern dressings (alginates, foams, hydrofibers, interfaces, etc.) are now combined with silver. The shapes, ions (salt, ions exchanger) metallic or organic, as well as the concentrations of silver vary greatly from one dressing to another. No standard has been applied in this field and it is not only the quantity present in the dressing that is important, but above all, the quantity of silver that is left behind by the dressing in the wound. Silver sulfadiazine has been more recently introduced on the market in some dressings.

The efficacy of silver dressings, compared to non-silver dressings, has not been assessed convincingly (Chaby et al. 2007; Trial et al. 2010).

No occupational allergic and/or irritant contact dermatitis to silver dressings has been described so far.

4.14 New Antiseptics Used in Wound Care

Two antiseptics have been introduced recently for cleaning of wounds and/or burns.

4.14.1 Octenidine

Octenidine is a cationic antibacterial of the bispyramidine class, present in Octenilin® Solution and Octenilin® gel, at a concentration of 0.05%. It is also available at a higher concentration (0.10%) as Octenisept®. The areas of application are: the moistening of chronic wounds and burns, facilitation of the mechanical debridement of wounds and burns, and the prevention of bacterial infections.

The efficacy of octenidine in methicillin-resistant *Staphylococcus aureus* decolonization seems evident (Krishna and Gibb 2010).

Skin side effects include irritation and allergic contact dermatitis (Calow et al. 2009). Health care personnel has to be aware nowadays of this potential hazard, if preventive measures are not taken when treating wounds and burns.

Patch testing: 0.1% aq.

4.14.2 Polyhexamethylene Biguanide (PHMB)

PHMB is available as a solution, a gel, and in certain dressings. It belongs to the family of cationic biguanides and has a broad spectrum of activity. The range of antimicrobial dressings offers dressings containing PHMB with a low concentration of 0.2%.

For instance, Suprasorb® X + PHMB is a swab of large cellulose fibers arranged in a broad-woven matrix impregnated with 0.3% PHMB.

A chemical composition close to that of PHMB is found in Prontosan® which is available as a gel or a solution. It contains polyhexamide (polyaminopropyl biguanide) at a concentration of 0.1% used as a preservative.

As far as skin side effects are concerned, polyhexanide and its variants are considered uncommon contact allergens. Nevertheless, in the future, health care personnel has to be aware of a potential risk of occupational disease (Schnuch et al. 2007; Goertz et al. 2010).

A severe case of anaphylaxis has been reported (Olivieri et al. 1998).

Patch testing: 5% aq.

4.15 Mercuric Compounds (Mercurials)

Mercuric compounds have been implicated in the occurrence of innumerable cases of allergic contact dermatitis, already confirmed by patch testing in the last years of the nineteenth century. Cross-reactions between mercury and inorganic and organic mercurials have always been advocated, optional or not.

4.15.1 Mercury

Sensitization to mercury itself is mainly reported when breaking a thermometer and is therefore responsible for occupational allergic contact dermatitis among members of the medical staff. Cases of "baboon syndrome" have been described in this occurrence (Lerch and Bircher 2004; Wen et al. 2007).

Patch testing: 0.5% pet.

4.15.2 Inorganic Mercuric Compounds

Mercuric salts have been broadly used in the past as antiseptics. Ammoniated mercury, yellow mercuric oxide, and cinnabar were considered rightly efficacious antiseptics, before the advent of new molecules. But they were also potent and frequent allergens, occupational and non-occupational. Therefore, their disuse was programmed inexorably. A page of dermato-allergology has been turned, for the sake of everyone. Nevertheless, it is always possible that isolated cases of allergic contact dermatitis occur, and vigilance is needed.

Patch testing: Refer to de Groot's recommendations (2008). Note that when patch testing with mercuric compounds' solutions (aq.) there is an incompatibility between aluminum Finn Chambers®, which are corroded by the mercurials. The use of plastic chambers is therefore compulsory (Lachapelle and Douka 1985).

4.15.3 Mercuric Organic Compounds

Here again, organic mercuric compounds were once popular as skin antiseptics (Rietschel and Fowler 2008), but they also carried the risk of sensitization and they have fallen into disuse (except thiomersal, see later). These compounds likely still appear in many over-the-counter products.

Merbromin (or mercurochrome) is of course the oldest known organic mercurial antiseptic.

Patch testing: 2% aq. or pet.

Thiomersal (thimerosal, merthiolate) is a very particular mercuric organic compound. Its use is still important, when compared to other mercurials. It is used as a disinfectant and a preservative, but less commonly than previously, especially in contact lens fluids, eyedrops, and vaccines. It is prepared by reacting ethylmercuric chloride with thiosalicylic acid. The ethylmercuric moiety is the major allergenic determinant, sometimes associated with mercury sensitivity.

Thiomersal is an indicator of photosensitivity to piroxicam, through its thiosalicylic moiety.

Many publications have been dedicated to thiomersal, and have been broadly reported in most textbooks of environmental dermatology. Patch testing: Thiomersal 0.1% pet.; Thiosalicylic acid 0.1% alcohol.

4.16 Triphenylmethane Dyes

The triphenylmethane dyes, such as gentian violet, methyl violet, rosaniline, malachite green, brilliant green, chrysoidine, and eosine, have been used extensively in dermatological practice; their use has declined due to three factors:

- A rather limited spectrum activity as antimicrobial and/or antifungal agents
- The limitations of the "coloring effect" in terms of antiseptic effectiveness
- The launching of new antiseptics, more efficacious for the treatment of wounds and burns

In retrospect, the dyes were considered mild irritants and weak allergens (Rietschel and Fowler 2008).

Eosine deserves special attention: It has been used extensively in the past and created some allergic reactions. Dermato-allergologists were confronted with patch testing problems. As eosine did not penetrate the skin easily, late reactions did occur and had to be taken into account.

Patch testing: For most dyes: 2% aq.; eosine: 50% pet.

5 The Repertoire of Skin Side Effects of Disinfectants

5.1 Preliminary Remarks

Many chemicals that have disinfectant properties have been quoted in the former sections, due to the fact that they have also been used as antiseptics, either in the past or at present.

Such examples include: alcohols, chlorines such as sodium hypochlorite and chloramine T, hexamidine, hexetidine, etc.

5.2 Eau De Javel (Bleach)

"Eau de Javel" (liquid bleach) is a disinfectant largely used in some countries (France, Belgium, Spain, Italy, Maghreb countries). It has a yellowish color, due to the addition of sodium dichromate used not as a preservative, but as a dye. Many cases of allergic contact dermatitis to chromates have been reported in the past (Lachapelle et al. 1980). Chromates have been removed from the formulation in France in 1978, and this was a good example of prevention in the field of contact dermato-allergology.

Occupational allergic contact dermatitis to "Eau de Javel" still occurs in other countries.

Irritant contact dermatitis of the hands is another skin side effect, depending upon the concentration used and the lack of preventive measures.

Patch testing: Sodium hypochlorite 0.5% aq.; Potassium dichromate 0.5% pet.

5.3 Aldehydes

Aldehydes represent an important class of disinfectants, broadly used throughout the world for various purposes. They are well known for their irritant and/or allergenic properties, and are of daily concern in occupational and/or environmental dermatology.

5.3.1 Formaldehyde

Innumerable publications have been dedicated to formaldehyde, the undisputed "leader" of aldehydes. Its use is so ubiquitous (as well as its skin side effects) that it has always been present in the baseline series of patch tests (Lachapelle and Maibach 2009).

Formaldehyde is an excellent disinfectant. Members of the medical and allied professions may be exposed to formaldehyde when it is used for sterilizing purposes, as a disinfectant, or a fixing solution for tissues. Cleaners, painters, metalworkers, and to a less extent photographers (color developers) and carbonless copy paper users are also at risk.

Depending upon individual situations, many skin side effects have been reported.

- First of all, formaldehyde is a potent primary irritant. Irritant contact dermatitis is therefore common. In fact, a strong solution of formaldehyde (formalin) can coagulate the proteins of the skin and produce necrosis and scarring. Prolonged contact may cause extreme dryness of the skin with fissuring. The nails can become discolored, soft, or brittle. Paronychia and even suppuration of the matrix may follow exposure to the chemical (Rietschel and Fowler 2008).
- Allergic contact dermatitis to formaldehyde is very common. When an allergic sensitization solution

does occur, the dermatitis may become widespread. In sensitive individuals, a minute amount of formaldehyde on thermometers, instruments, slides, and biopsy containers is also sufficient to produce allergic contact dermatitis (Flyvholm and Menné 1992).

- Formaldehyde can induce, in rare cases, immunological contact urticaria (Tupasela and Kanerva 1997).

Patch testing: 1% aq. but it is suggested in recent publications that a 2% concentration is more appropriate (Hauksson et al. 2010).

5.3.2 Glutaraldehyde

Glutaraldehyde (1,5 pentanedial) is available most frequently as a 50% aqueous solution. It is used in a 2% water solution as a cold disinfectant, especially in hospital–medical work for sterilizing instruments, bronchoscopes, cytoscopes, anesthetic equipment and in renal dialysis units for sterilizing forceps. Health care workers are more eight times more likely to be allergic to glutaraldehyde than non-health care workers (Rietschel and Fowler 2008).

Allergic contact dermatitis to glutaraldehyde is considered a common occupational skin disease, as emphasized by recent publications (Takigawa and Endo 2006; Nayebzadeh 2007; Maier et al. 2009).

Patch testing: 0.2–0.3% pet.

5.3.3 Glyoxal

Glyoxal (ethanedial) is a dialdehyde used in medical and dental offices as a disinfectant for surfaces and instruments. It is considered a contact allergen and cross-reactions to formaldehyde and glutaraldehyde have been reported. Occupational hand dermatitis among hospital workers is not uncommon (Uter et al. 2001; Aalto-Korte et al. 2005).

Patch testing: 2% aq.

5.4 Quaternary Ammonium Compounds

These compounds are the active ingredient in disinfectants and sanitizers for homes, farms, offices, and public transportation vehicles. They are also used as algaecides and slimicides for swimming pools, industrial water reservoirs, and farm ponds. They are included in the last rinse in laundering by some hospitals, diaper services, and various institutions (Rietschel and Fowler 2008).

Quaternary ammonium compounds are irritant, for instance even as dilute as 0.1% under occlusion and their allergenic properties do exist, are not so frequent and are masqueraded by their strong irritancy. All of them have been incriminated in the occurrence of occupational dermatitis (irritant and/or allergic) in people at risk.

5.4.1 Benzalkonium Chloride

Benzalkonium chloride is the most widely used quaternary ammonium compound. Its irritation potential is mentioned extensively in all textbooks of environmental dermatology. Allergic contact dermatitis of the hands has been reported in many occupations, particularly in medical personnel from exposure to instruments soaked in it. It has also provoked airborne reactions (Corazza and Virgili 1993).

Patch testing with benzalkonium chloride is a difficult issue (0.1% aq.) (Basketter et al. 2004). When positive, skin reactions are often weak or questionable. As emphasized by the North American Contact Dermatitis Group, caution should be used when interpreting results, and a ROAT test is very often advisable (Warshaw et al. 2010).

Patch testing: 0.1% aq. ROAT test is advised.

5.4.2 Others

Other quaternary ammonium compounds have been incriminated in the occurrence of occupational or non-occupational contact dermatitis, either irritant or allergenic. Their profile of skin side effects can be compared to that of benzalkonium chloride. The most frequently quoted are cetrimonium bromide (Cetrimide®), cetalkonium chloride, and dequalinium chloride.

References

Aalto-Korte K, Mäkelä EA, Huttunen M et al (2005) Occupational contact allergy to glyoxal. Contact Dermatitis 52:276–281

Basketter DA, Marriott M, Gilmoor NJ et al (2004) Strong irritants masquerading as skin allergens: the case of benzalkonium chloride. Contact Dermatitis 50:213–217

Beaudouin E, Kanny G, Morisset M et al (2004) Immediate hypersensitivity to chlorhexidine: literature review. Eur Ann Allergy Clin Immunol 36:123–126

Bloch B (1911) Experimentelle Studien über des Wesen der Iodoformidiosynkrasie. Z Exp Pathol Ther 9:509–538

Browning JC, Levy ML (2008) Argyria attributed to silvadene application in a patient with dystrophic epidermolysis bullosa. Dermatol Online J 15:9

Calow T et al (2009) Contact dermatitis due to the use of Octenisept in wound care. J Dtsch Dermatol Ges 9:759–765

Chaby G, Senet P, Vaneau M et al (2007) Dressings for acute and chronic wounds: a systematic review. Arch Dermatol 143:1297–1304

Condé-Salazar L, Guimaraens D, Gonzales MA et al (1995) Occupational allergic contact dermatitis from nitrofurazone. Contact Dermatitis 32:307–308

Corazza M, Virgili A (1993) Airborne allergic contact dermatitis from benzalkonium chloride. Contact Dermatitis 28:195–196

de Groot AC (2008) Patch testing. Test concentrations and vehicles for 4350 chemicals, 3rd edn. Acdegroot, Wapserveen, p 455 p

Degreef H, Dooms-Goossens A (1985) Patch testing with silver sulfadiazine cream. Contact Dermatitis 12:33–37

Dooms-Goossens A, Gevers D, Mertens A et al (1983) Allergic contact urticaria to chloramine. Contact Dermatitis 9:319–320

Dooms-Goossens A, Van Daele R, Bedert R et al (1989) Hexamidine isethionate: a sensitizer in pharmaceutical products and cosmetics. Contact Dermatitis 21:270

Erdmann S, Herti M, Merk HF (1999) Allergic contact dermatitis from povidone iodine. Contact Dermatitis 40:331–332

Flyvholm MA, Menné T (1992) Allergic contact dermatitis from formaldehyde. A case study focussing on sources of formaldehyde exposure. Contact Dermatitis 27:27–36

Fregert S, Groth O, Hjorth N et al (1963) Dermatitis from alcohol. J Allergy 34:904

Frosch PJ, John SM (2006) Clinical aspects of irritant contact dermatitis. In: Frosch PJ, Menné T, Lepoittevin JP (eds) Contact dermatitis, 4th edn. Springer, Berlin, pp 255–294

Fuller FW (2009) The side effects of silver sulfadiazine. J Burn Care Res 30:464–470

Gaul LE, Underwood GB (1948) The effect of aging a solution of silver nitrate on its cutaneous reaction. J Invest Dermatol 11:7

Goertz O, Abels C, Knive V et al (2010) Clinical safety and efficacy of a novel thermoreversible polyhexanide-preserved wound covering gel. Eur Surg Res 44:96–101

Gosbell IB (2004) Methicillin-resistant *Staphylococcus aureus*: impact on dermatology practice. Am J Clin Dermatol 5:239–259

Hannuksela M, Salo H (1986) The repeated open application test (ROAT). Contact Dermatitis 14:221–227

Hauksson I, Pontén A, Gruvberger B et al (2010) Routine diagnostic patch-testing with formaldehyde 2.0% (0.6 mg/cm^2) may be an advantage compared to 1.0%. Acta Derm Venereol 90:480–484

Jain J, Arora S, Rajwade JM et al (2009) Silver nanoparticles in therapeutics: development of an antimicrobial gel formulation for topical use. Mol Pharm 6:1388–1401

Key M (1961) Some unusual allergic reactions in industry. Arch Dermatol 83:57–60

King M (2008) Our historical roots: Dr Richard Drysdale Dakin, DSc, and his solution. J Wound Ostomy Continence Nurs 35:289–292

Krautheim AB, Jermann THM, Bircher AJ (2004) Chlorhexidine anaphylaxis: case report and review of the literature. Contact Dermatitis 50:113–116

Krishna BV, Gibb AP (2010) Use of octenidine dihydrochloride in methicillin-resistant *Staphylococcus aureus* decolonisation regimens: a literature review. J Hosp Infect 74:199–203

Lachapelle JM (1984) Occupational allergic contact dermatitis to povidone-iodine. Contact Dermatitis 11:189–190

Lachapelle JM (2005) Allergic contact dermatitis from povidone-iodine: a reevaluation study. Contact Dermatitis 52:9–10

Lachapelle JM, de Prost Y (2007) Place de la povidone iodée en dermatologie. Editions Ektopic, Paris, p 84p

Lachapelle JM, Douka MA (1985) An evaluation of the compatibility between aluminium Finn Chambers and various mercurials dissolved in water or dispersed in petrolatum. Derm Beruf Umwelt 33:12–14

Lachapelle JM, Maibach HI (2009) Patch testing and prick testing. A practical guide, 2nd edn. Springer, Berlin, p 195p

Lachapelle JM, Tennstedt D (1979) Low allergenicity of triclosan. Prediction testing in guinea pigs and in humans. Dermatologica 158: 379–383

Lachapelle JM, Lauwerys R, Tennstedt D et al (1980) Eau de Javel and prevention of chromate allergy in France. Contact Dermatitis 6: 107–110

Lee S, Zhai H, Maibach HI (2005) Allergic contact dermatitis from iodine preparations: a conundrum. Contact Dermatitis 52:184–187

Lerch M, Bircher AJ (2004) Systemically induced allergic exanthem from mercury. Contact Dermatitis 50:349–353

Lombardi P, Gola M, Acciai MC et al (1989) Unusual occupational allergic contact dermatitis in a nurse. Contact Dermatitis 20:302–303

Lorette G, Beaulieu P, Allaert FA et al (2009) Superficial community-acquired skin infections: prevalence of bacteria and antibiotic susceptibility in France. J Eur Acad Dermatol Venereol 23:1423–1426

Maier LE, Lampel HP, Bhutani T et al (2009) Hand dermatitis: a focus on allergic contact dermatitis to biocides. Dermatol Clin 27:251–264

Mathelier-Fusade P (1994) L'allergie à l'iode existe-t'elle? Revue du Praticien 8:62

Mc Donnell G, Russell AD (1999) Antiseptics and disinfectants: activity, action and resistance. Clin Microbiol Rev 12:147–179

Mc Donnell KJ, Sculco TP (1997) Dakin's solution revisited. Am J Orthop (Belle Mead NJ) 26:471–473

Merk H, Ebert L, Goerz G (1982) Allergic contact dermatitis due to the fungicide hexetidine. Contact Dermatitis 8:216

Muston HL, Boss JM, Summerly R (1977) Dermatitis from Ammonyx 1.0, a constituent of Hibiscrub. Contact Dermatitis 3:347–348

Myatt AE, Beck MH (1985) Contact sensitivity to parachlorometaxylenol. Clin Exp Dermatol 10:491–494

Nagendran V, Wickin J, Ekbote A et al (2009) IgE-mediated chlorhexidine allergy: a new occupational hazard? Occup Med (Lond) 59:270–272

Nayebzadeh A (2007) The effect of work practices on personal exposure to glutaraldehyde among health care workers. Ind Health 45:289–295

Olivieri J, Eigenmann PA, Hauser C (1998) Severe anaphylaxis to a new disinfectant: polyhexanide, a chlorhexidine polymer. Schweiz Med Wochenschr 128:1508–1511

Ophaswongse S, Maibach HI (1994) Alcohol dermatitis: allergic contact dermatitis and contact urticaria syndrome. Contact Dermatitis 30:1–6

Osmundsen P (1978) Contact dermatitis due to sodium hypochlorite. Contact Dermatitis 4:177–178

Osterlund A, Kahlmeter G, Haeggman S et al (2006) *Staphylococcus aureus* resistant to fusidic acid among Swedish children: a follow-up study. Scand J Infect Dis 38:332–334

Palobart C, Cros J, Orsel I et al (2009) Anaphylactic shock to iodinated povidone. Ann Fr Anesth Reanim 28:168–170

Patruno C, Suppa F, Sarraco G et al (1994) Allergic contact dermatitis due to ethyl alcohol. Contact Dermatitis 31:124

Pecquet C (2003) Allergy to iodine. Ann Dermatol Venereol 130:795–798

Pedrosa C, Costa H, Oliveira G et al (2005) Anaphylaxis to povidone in a child. Pediatr Allergy Immunol 16:361–362

Ranchoff RE, Steck WD, Taylor JS et al (1986) Electrocardiography electrode and hand dermatitis from parachlorometaxylenol. J Am Acad Dermatol 15:348–350

Revuz J, Poli F, Wechsler J et al (1984) Dermatites de contact à l'hexamidine. Ann Dermatol Venereol 111:805–810

Rietschel RL, Fowler JF (2008) Fisher's contact dermatitis, 6th edn. BC Decker, Hamilton, p 862p

Rudzki E, Rebandel P, Grzywa Z (1989) Patch tests with occupational contactants in nurses, doctors and dentists. Contact Dermatitis 20:247–250

Schena D, Papagrigoraki A, Girolomoni G (2008) Sensitizing potential of triclosan and triclosan-based skin care products in patients with chronic eczema. Dermatol Ther 21(suppl 2):S35–S38

Schnuch A, Geier J, Uter W et al (2007) The biocide polyhexamethylene biguanide remains an uncommon contact allergen. Contact Dermatitis 56:235–239

Sharma A, Chopra H (2009) Chlorhexidine urticaria; a rare occurrence with a common mouthwash. Indian J Dent Res 20:377–379

Takigawa T, Endo Y (2006) Effects of glutaraldehyde exposure on human health. J Occup Health 48:75–87

Teot L, Coessens B, Cooper R et al (2004) Wound management. Changing ideas on antiseptics. De Coker, Antwerpen, 77 p

Tosti A, Vincenzi C, Bardazzi F et al (1990) Allergic contact dermatitis due to povidone iodine. Contact Dermatitis 23:197–198

Trial C, Darbas H, Lavigne JP et al (2010) Assessment of the antimicrobial effectiveness of a new silver alginate wound dressing: RCT. J Wound Care 19:20–26

Tupasela O, Kanerva L (1997) Skin tests and specific IgE urticaria caused by low-molecular weight chemicals. In: Amin S, Lahti A, Maibach HI (eds) Textbook of the contact urticaria syndrome. CRC Press, Boca Raton, pp 33–44

Tupker RA, Schuur J, Coenraads PJ (1997) Irritancy of antiseptics tested by repeated open exposures on the human skin, evaluated by noninvasive methods. Contact Dermatitis 37:213–217

Upton A, Lang S, Heffeman H et al (2003) Mupirocin and *Staphylococcus aureus*: a recent paradigm of emerging antibiotic resistance. J Antimicrob Chemother 51:613–617

Uter W, Schwanitz HJ, Lessmann H et al (2001) Glyoxal is an important allergen for (medical care) cleaning staff. Int J Hyg Environ Health 204:251–253

van der Valk GM, Maibach HI (eds) (1996) The irritant contact dermatitis syndrome. CRC Press, Boca Raton, 393 p

Vilaplana J, Grimalt F, Romaguera C (1990) Contact dermatitis from furaltadone in animal feed. Contact Dermatitis 22:232–233

Warshaw EM, Nelsen DD, Sasseville D et al (2010) Positivity ratio and reaction index: patch-test-quality-control metrics applied to the North American contact dermatitis group database. Dermatitis 21:91–97

Wen L, Yin J, Ma DL et al (2007) Baboon syndrome induced by mercury – first case report in China. Contact Dermatitis 56:356–357

Wong CS, Beck MH (2001) Allergic contact dermatitis from triclosan in antibacterial handwashes. Contact Dermatitis 45:307

Yoshida K et al (2008) Anaphylaxis to polyvinylpyrrolidone in povidone-iodine for impetigo contagiosum in a boy with atopic dermatitis. Int Arch Allergy Immunol 146:169–173

37 Formaldehyde and Formaldehyde-Releasers

Anton C. de Groot[1] · *Mari-Ann Flyvholm*[2]
[1]Acdegroot publishing, Wapserveen, The Netherlands
[2]National Research Centre for the Working Environment, Copenhagen, Denmark

Core Messages

- Formaldehyde is a ubiquitous and important allergen. Contact allergy to formaldehyde occurs frequently in women with hand dermatitis. Sensitization may also be caused by occupational exposure to formaldehyde, especially in metalworkers, nurses, other (para)medical professionals, and cosmetologists.
- Formaldehyde is widely distributed in the environment and is difficult to avoid completely. Thus, even in patients actively trying to avoid products containing formaldehyde, the dermatitis will infrequently heal completely and permanently.
- Formaldehyde-releasers are chemicals, which release formaldehyde as a result of decomposition and/or chemicals synthesized from formaldehyde that may still contain residues of free formaldehyde.
- There are over 30 formaldehyde-releasers with a wide array of applications; most are used as preservatives in cosmetics; as antimicrobials in metalworking fluids, paint, lacquers, and varnishes; or as durable press chemical finishes in textiles.
- Positive patch tests to formaldehyde-releasers are often accompanied by concomitant reactions to formaldehyde; in these cases, the patch test to the releaser may be the result of an allergic reaction to the formaldehyde which is present in or released by the donor test material. For most releasers, co-reactivity to formaldehyde is >50%.
- There is very little published information on the relevance of observed positive patch test reactions to formaldehyde-releasers. Most reactions to releasers used in metalworking fluids appear not to be relevant with the exception of *N,N'*-Methylenebis(5-methyloxazolidine). The lack of relevance of reactions to the Bioban ® range of antimicrobials may partly be due to irritancy, leading to false-positive reactions.
- None of the formaldehyde-releasers are important causes of occupational allergic contact dermatitis. The presence of formaldehyde-releasers as durable press chemical finishes in clothes appears to be safe for consumers.

1 Introduction

Formaldehyde is a common cause of contact allergy. Allergic contact dermatitis from this chemical is often chronic, presumably because it is difficult to avoid exposure to the allergen completely. Indeed, formaldehyde may be found in cosmetics, toiletries, household products, and in a great number of industrial applications including adhesives, paints, lacquers, and metalworking fluids. Often, the products are not preserved with formaldehyde itself, but with agents that release formaldehyde under usage conditions, the so-called formaldehyde-releasers (or formaldehyde-donors) (➋ *Table 37.1*). In this chapter, (occupational) contact allergy to formaldehyde and -releasers is discussed. Details of the data presented here can be found in our recent *in-depth* review articles on the subject (de Groot et al. 2009, 2010a, b, c, d, e, f).

2 Formaldehyde

Formaldehyde (methanal) is a colorless gas (HCHO) with a characteristic pungent odor. Formalin is a 37–40% aqueous solution of formaldehyde, to which 10–15% methyl alcohol has been added to inhibit polymerization. This simple aldehyde is ubiquitous in the environment, and is generated in and released from the smoke of burning wood, coal, charcoal, tobacco, natural gas, and kerosene. Formaldehyde also occurs naturally in certain foods such as coffee (especially instant coffee), dried bean curd, cod fish, caviar, maple syrup, shiitake mushrooms, and smoked ham. It is an irritant as well as an allergen and a potential respiratory carcinogen (Scheman et al. 2008).

Formaldehyde can be used as a disinfectant as it kills most bacteria and fungi. It was first commercially used in embalming fluid and as a preservative for laboratory specimens. The chemical is incorporated into a large variety of products and reactants in many chemical processes, including formaldehyde-releasers, polymerized plastics, metalworking fluids, paints and lacquers, topical medicaments, fabrics, cosmetics, and detergents (➋ *Table 37.2*). In finished

T. Rustemeyer, P. Elsner, S.M. John & H.I. Maibach (eds.), *Kanerva's Occupational Dermatology*,
DOI 10.1007/978-3-642-02035-3_37, © Springer-Verlag Berlin Heidelberg 2012

Table 37.1
Formaldehyde-releasers (Adapted from de Groot et al. 2009)

Commonly used name	IUPAC name	Other synonyms	Current trade names	CAS
Formaldehyde-releasers used in cosmetics				
Benzylhemiformal (INCI)	Phenylmethoxymethanol	(Benzyloxy)methanol	Akyposept B [Preventol D2. see there]	14548-60-8
2-Bromo-2-nitropropane-1,3-diol (INCI)	As in column 1	Bromonitropropanediol; Bronopol	Bronopol; Chemynol BP; Myacide Pharma BP; Onyxide 500	52-51-7
Diazolidinyl urea (INCI)	1-[1,3-bis(Hydroxymethyl)-2,5-dioxo-imidazolidin-4-yl]-1,3-bis(hydroxy-methyl)urea	*N,N´*-bis(Hydroxymethyl)urea	Abiol Forte; Germall II; Liposerve DU; Nipa Biopure 200	78491-02-8
DMDM hydantoin (INCI)	1,3-bis(Hydroxymethyl)-5,5-dimethyl-imidazolidine-2,4-dione	Dimethyloldimethylhydantoin; 1,3-dimethylol-5,5-dimethyl-hydantoin; DMDMH	Cosept DM; Dekafald; Glydant (2000, XL-1000); Lanodant DM; Mackstat DM; Microcare DH	6440-58-0
Imidazolidinyl urea (INCI, MI)	3-[3-(Hydroxymethyl)-2,5-dioxo-imidazolidin-4-yl]-1-[[[3-(hydroxy-methyl)-2,5-dioxo-imidazolidin-4-yl] carbamoylamino]methyl]urea	bis(Methylolhydantoin urea) methane; Imidurea (MI)	Germall 115; Liposerve IU; Nipa Biopure 100; Protacide U-13; Unicide U-13	39236-46-9
Quaternium-15 (INCI, MI)	Not available	*N*-(3-Chloroallyl)hexaminium chloride; chloroallylhexaminium chloride; 1-(3-chloroallyl)-3,5,7-triaza-1-azonia-adamantane chloride; hexamethylene tetramine chloro-allyl chloride	Cosept 200; Dowicide Q; Dowicil (75,200);	4080-31-3
Sodium hydroxymethyl-glycinate (INCI)	Not available	Glycine, *N*-(hydroxymethyl)-, sodium salt (1:1); *N*-hydroxymethylglycine (mono)sodium salt; sodium (hydroxymethyl) glycinate	Suttocide A	70161-44-3
Formaldehyde-releasers used in metalworking fluids				
Bioban CS-1135®	4,4-Dimethyloxazolidine; 3,4,4-trimethyl-oxazolidine		Bioban CS-1135	81099-36-7 (Ingred.75673-43-7 and 51200-87-4)
Bioban CS-1246®	5-Ethyl-3,7-dioxa-1-azabicyclo[3.3.0] octane	7-Ethylbicyclooxazolidine	Bioban CS-1246; Chemtan A60; Oxazolidine-E; Zoldine ZE	7747-35-5

Bioban P-1487®	4-[2-(Morpholin-4-ylmethyl)-2-nitro-butyl]morpholine; 4-(2-nitrobutyl) morpholine	Mixture of nitrobutylmorpholine and ethylnitrotrimethylenedimorpholine	Bioban P-1487	37304-88-4 (Ingred.1854-23-5 and 2224-44-4)
Forcide 78® I[a]	(Z)-3-(bis(2-Hydroxyethyl)amino)-2-(2-hydroxyethyl-(hydroxymethyl)amino) prop-2-en-1-ol	2-Hydroxymethylaminoethanol- tri-*N*-ethylhydroxy-2-amino- methylene	Forcide 78[b]	77044-78-1
Forcide 78® II[c]	1,3,5-Triethyl-1,3,5-triazinane (a)	(a) Hexahydro-1,3,5-triethyl-s- triazine;	(a) Vancide-TH Forcide 78[b]	7779-27-3 (a)
		(a) Triethyl-trimethylenetriamine mixture of (1) Triazinetriethanol (see there) and (2) Hexahydro-1,3,5-triethyl-1,3,5-triazine		
N,N′-Methylenebis(5-methyloxazolidine)	5-Methyl-3-[(5-methyloxazolidin-3-yl) methyl]oxazolidine		Grotan OX	66204-44-2
4,4′-Methylenedimorpholine	4-(Morpholin-4-ylmethyl)morpholine	Bismorpholinomethane; dimorpholinomethane; 4,4′-methylenebis-morpholine		5625-90-1
Preventol D2®	Phenylmethoxymethoxymethylbenzene	bis(Benzyloxy)methane; mixture of hydroxymethylene and polyhydroxymethylene monobenzylether; 1,1′-(methylenebis (oxymethylene)) bis-benzene	Preventol D2 This trade name is also often used for benzylhemiformal[d]	2749-70-4
Tris(*N*-hydroxyethyl) hexahydrotriazine	2-[4,6-bis(2-Hydroxyethyl)1,3,5-triazinan-2-yl]ethanol	Hexahydro-1,3,5-tris(hydroxy-ethyl)triazine; triazinetriethanol; trihydroxyethylhexahydro s- triazine; 1,3,5-trihydroxyethylhexahydro-triazine	Forcide 78 (see there); Grotan (B, BK, HD); Onyxide 200; Roksol T 1-7	4719-04-4
Tris(hydroxymethyl)-nitromethane (INCI,MI)	2-(Hydroxymethyl)-2-nitropropane-1,3-diol	Nitromethylidynemethanol; trimethylolnitromethane; tris nitro	Tris Nitro	126-11-4
Formaldehyde-releasers used as durable press chemical finishes				
Dihydroxydimethylol-ethyleneurea, methylated	4,5-Dihydroxy-1,3-bis(hydroxymethyl)-imidazolidin-2-one, methylated	Dimethylolglyoxalurea, methylated	Fixapret (various); Freerez PKF; Knittex LE; Permafresh (various); Sumitex (various)	68411-81-4
Dimethylol dihydroxy-ethyleneurea	4,5-Dihydroxy-1,3-bis(hydroxymethyl)-imidazolidin-2-one	1,3-bis(Hydroxymethyl)-4,5-dihydroxy-2-imidazolidinone	Fixapret (various); Permafresh (various)	1854-26-8
Dimethylolethyleneurea	1,3-bis(Hydroxymethyl)imidazolidin-2-one		Fixapret AH	136-84-5
Dimethylolpropyleneurea	1,3-bis(Hydroxymethyl)-1,3-diazinan- 2-one	DMPU; tetrahydro-1,3-bis(hydroxymethyl)- 1H-pyrimidin-2-one	Fixapret PH; Knittex PRS	3270-74-4

Table 37.1 (Continued)

Commonly used name	IUPAC name	Other synonyms	Current trade names	CAS
Dimethylol urea (INCI)	1,3-bis(Hydroxymethyl)urea	*N,N′*-bis(Hydroxymethyl)urea; carbamol; dihydroxymethylurea; *N,N′*-dimethylolurea; dimethylurea; oxymethurea (MI); urea formaldehyde	Kaurit S; Methural; Permafresh 477; Urofix	140-95-4
Glyoxalurea	4,5-Dihydroxyimidazolidin-2-one	Dihydroxyethyleneurea; glyoxalmonoureine		3720-97-6
Methylol urea	Hydroxymethylurea	*N*-(Hydroxymethyl)urea; methyl hydroxyurea; mono (hydroxymethyl)urea; monomethylolurea		1000-82-4
Polyoxymethylene melamine (INCI)	Not available	Melamine, polymer with formaldehyde; melamine/ formaldehyde resin; nanoplast		9003-08-1
Polyoxymethylene urea (INCI)	Formaldehyde; urea	Polynoxylin; urea-formaldehyde resin; urea, polymer with formaldehyde	Karbamol (B/M); Kaurit (285FL, 240); Uformite	9011-05-6
Propyleneglycolhemiformal	No further data available			
Tetramethylol acetylenediurea	2,4,6,8-Tetrakis(hydroxymethyl)-2,4,6,8-tetraazabicyclo[3.3.0]octane-3,7-dione	Tetrakis(hydroxymethyl)glycoluril; tetramethylolglycoluril	Fixapret 140	5395-50-6
Miscellaneous formaldehyde-releasers				
Dimethyl hydantoin formaldehyde resin	5,5-Dimethylimidazolidine-2,4-dione; formaldehyde	Formaldehyde, polymer with 5,5-dimethyl-2,4-imidazolidinedione; DMHF		26811-08-5
Ethylene urea	Imidazolidin-2-one	2-Imidazolidinone (MI); 2-oxoimidazolidine		120-93-4
MDM hydantoin (INCI)	1-(Hydroxymethyl)-5,5-dimethyl-imidazolidine-2,4-dione	1-Hydroxymethyl-5,5-dimethyl hydantoin (MI); MDMH; methylol dimethyl hydantoin; monomethylol dimethyl hydantoin	Glycoserve	116-25-6
Methenamine (INCI, MI)	Not available	Aminoform; formamine; hexamethylene tetramine; hexamine; methenamide	Cystamine; urotropine; vulkacit H30	100-97-0
N-Methylolchloracetamide	2-chloro-*N*-(hydroxymethyl)acetamide	Chloracetamide-*N*-methylol	Grotan DF-35	2832-19-1
Paraformaldehyde	Formaldehyde	Paraform; poly(oxymethylene)	Aldacide; formagene	30525-89-4

[a]Description of Forcide 78 as by (Hamann 1980)

[b]Forcide 78 is also used as a trade name by Redox Pty Ltd. (www.redox.com/msds/data/TRIAZI80.html) for a preservative containing 75–80% tris(*N*-hydroxyethyl)hexahydrotriazine

[c]Description of Forcide 78 as by (Andersen et al. 1984)

[d]Preventol D2 also is used as a trade name for benzylhemiformal by Lanxess Energizing Chemistry (www.protectedbypreventol.com)

INCI = INCI name (The Cosmetic, Toiletry and Fragrance Association 2006)

MI = Merck Index name (Merck and Co. 2006)

Table 37.2
Examples of applications of and products that may contain formaldehyde[a] (de Groot et al. 2009)

Application/product
Adhesives (glues, pastes, cements)
Agricultural chemicals (seed disinfectants)
Antifreeze agents
Antiperspirants
Asphalt shingles
Binders (polymers)
Castings
Cellulose esters
Chipboard production
Cleaning products
Clothing (wash and wear, crease-resistant)
Coloring agents
Construction materials
Corrosion inhibitors
Cosmetics
Cutting fluids
Dental preparations and dentifrices
Deodorizers
Disinfectants
Dry cleaning materials
Embalming fluids
Explosives manufacture
Filling agents (stopping, putty, etc)
Fish meal industry
Flame retardant
Flooring materials
Footwear (resins and plastics)
Fumigants
Hardeners
Hydrocarbons (e.g., oil)
Impregnating agents
Laboratory chemicals
Latex rubber
Medications: wart remedies, anhydrotics
Metal coatings (not paints)
Metal and tire cleaners
Metalworking fluids
Mildew preventatives (fruits, vegetables)
Mineral wool production
Orthopedic casts
Paints, lacquers, coatings
Paint removers
Paper industry
Phenolic resins in adhesives and footwear
Photographic paper and solutions
Plywood
Polishes and finishes
Printing inks
Starch (spray and powdered)
Surface active agents
Tanning agents
Textiles
Tissue fixatives
Toiletries
Urea plastics in adhesives and footwear

[a]These applications and products have been reported in literature, but it cannot be excluded that some information may be outdated. Additional products that may contain formaldehyde or specific formaldehyde-releasers may be found in de Groot et al. 2009, *Table 37.6*

products, there may be several sources of formaldehyde, for example, active ingredient for preservation or formaldehyde released from a donor. Some sources, however, are "hidden" or "occult" (and indeed sometimes unknown to the manufacturer), such as formaldehyde used for preservation of raw materials used to prepare the product, formaldehyde used to sterilize vessels for storage of raw materials or products, or formaldehyde released by package materials such as formaldehyde resins coating cosmetic and pharmaceutical tubes (Flyvholm 1997).

Exposure to formaldehyde in the EU is subject to restrictions because of its toxicological properties. The maximum allowed concentration in finished cosmetic products is 0.2%. All finished products containing formaldehyde or substances which release formaldehyde must be labeled with the warning "contains formaldehyde" where the concentration of free formaldehyde in the finished product exceeds 0.05 wt% (500 ppm).

Qualitative and quantitative tests for analyzing formaldehyde in products have been discussed recently (de Groot et al. 2009).

2.1 Contact Allergy to Formaldehyde

Patch testing with formaldehyde is not very reliable. Currently, 1% aqua is the standard for patch testing. However, this concentration may result in false-positive and in – up to 40% – false-negative reactions. Irritant, doubtful and follicular reactions also occur (Trattner et al.

1998). The former use of formaldehyde *per se* as a preservative in cosmetics, as a disinfectant, as an antiperspirant and in textile finish resins releasing large amounts of formaldehyde resulted in high sensitization rates into the 1980s. However, its use in cosmetics has largely been abandoned and replaced with formaldehyde-releasers and, as a disinfectant, it was partly replaced by other compounds like glutaraldehyde and glyoxal. Also, low formaldehyde textile resins were introduced. Thus, since the 1980s, there has been a decline in the frequency of sensitization in most countries. Currently, it remains at a stable and relatively low level of around 2–3% in most (European) countries in the general population of patch tested eczema patients (Uter 2008; Uter et al. 2009). In the USA however, where patients undergo stricter selection for patch testing, rates of 8–9% are rule rather than exception (Davis et al. 2008). Women are affected 1.2–1.5 times more frequently than men.

Patients allergic to formaldehyde are often women with hand eczema, presumably from exposure to household cleaning agents (e.g., washing-up liquids), frequently combined with facial dermatitis from contact with formaldehyde in cosmetics (Flyvholm and Menné 1992; Trattner et al. 1998). Sensitization may also be caused by occupational exposure to formaldehyde, especially in metalworkers, nurses, other (para)medical professionals, and cosmetologists (Cronin 1991; Fransway and Schmitz 1991; Schnuch et al. 1998), which usually presents as hand eczema.

As formaldehyde is so widely distributed in the environment, it is difficult to avoid. Thus, even in patients actively trying to avoid products containing formaldehyde, the dermatitis will infrequently heal completely. Most patients will still suffer from exacerbations of dermatitis (Cronin 1991; Kang et al. 1995; Agner et al. 1999).

3 Formaldehyde-Releasers

Formaldehyde-releasers are substances, which release formaldehyde as a result of decomposition and/or chemicals synthesized from formaldehyde that may still contain residues of free formaldehyde (➋ *Table 37.1*). Many patients reacting to formaldehyde also have positive patch tests to one or more formaldehyde-releasers. It is often assumed that this is due to "cross-allergy" to formaldehyde (more correctly termed "pseudo-cross-allergy"), that is, that the patch test reaction to the formaldehyde-releaser is caused by the formaldehyde present in or released by the donor patch test material. In favor of this assumption is the fact that often more than one releaser reacts in formaldehyde-allergic individuals, even when they are not structurally related (which makes cross-reactions unlikely). There is also a significant patch test association between the releasers themselves, including those that are structurally dissimilar; this also suggests an important role for formaldehyde.

The degree of co-reactivity to formaldehyde in eczema patients reacting to formaldehyde-releasers is summarized in ➋ *Table 37.3*. 2-Bromo-2-nitropropane-1,3-diol (15%), Bioban P-1487 ® (8%) and *N*, *N*′-Methylenebis(5-methyloxazolidine) (42%) have less than 50% co-reactivity to formaldehyde. The other 15 (83%) have a co-reactivity score of >50% and the majority of >70% (especially in releasers used as durable press chemical finishes). This means that the (great) majority of positive patch test reactions to these releasers may in fact be caused by formaldehyde sensitivity.

Formaldehyde-releasers are presented here in four groups: releasers mainly used in cosmetics, releasers for antimicrobial activity in metalworking fluids, chemicals used in textiles and clothes as durable press chemical finishes, and a rest group. For most releasers, the application is not limited to one such class of products: Possible applications for individual formaldehyde-releasers are summarized in ➋ *Table 37.4*.

4 Cosmetics

An important source of human skin contact with formaldehyde is the use of cosmetics containing formaldehyde-releasers as preservatives. They are added to water-containing cosmetics (which include personal care products/toiletries) to prevent the growth of microorganisms that may enter during manufacture or during their usage. Microbial contamination may cause discoloration, malodors, and physical and chemical degradation of products, in addition to the potential adverse events of pathogens on consumers. Formaldehyde-releasers used in cosmetics and permitted in the EU are shown in ➋ *Table 37.5*. In the USA, there is no relevant legislation, neither on the ingredients used in cosmetics nor on their permitted concentration in the final product.

4.1 Contact Allergy

The results of (routine) testing of eczema patients with formaldehyde-releasers used in cosmetics are summarized in ➋ *Table 37.3*. In Europe, low frequencies of sensitization have been observed to all releasers used in cosmetics (➋ *Table 37.3*): 2-bromo-2-nitropropane-1,

Table 37.3

Frequency of sensitization to formaldehyde-releasers and co-reactivity to formaldehyde (de Groot et al. 2010a, b, c, d, e, f)[a]

Formaldehyde-releaser	Frequency of sensitization (range %)				Percentages co-reactivity to formaldehyde (mean, adjusted for sample size)
	Unselected patient population[b]		Selected patient population[c]		
	Europe	USA	Europe	USA	
Formaldehyde-releasers used in cosmetics					
Benzylhemiformal			1–2.9		76
2-Bromo-2-nitropropane-1,3-diol	0.4–1.2	2.1–3.3	0–1.8	2.0	15
Diazolidinyl urea	0.5–1.4	2.4–3.7	0.9–1.3	4.9	59
DMDM hydantoin		0.5–3.4	0.5–1.1	1.2	71
Imidazolidinyl urea	0.3–1.4	1.3–3.3	0.6–1.1		51
Quaternium-15	0.6–1.9	7.1–9.6	0.5–0.6		56
Formaldehyde-releasers used in metalworking fluids					
Bioban CS-1135®		6.2	1.1–5.0		72
Bioban CS-1246®		6.2	0.8–3.0		68
Bioban P-1487®	1.5	0.5		0–2.2	8
Forcide®78 (II)	0.6				100 (in 4 patients)
N,N′-Methylenebis(5-methyloxazolidine)			2.9–6.7		42
4,4′-Methylenedimorpholine			4.9		29 (in 7 patients)
Propyleneglycolhemiformal			0.7–0.8		100
Tris(*N*-hydroxyethyl)hexahydrotriazine		4.5	0–8.1	3.4	60
Tris(hydroxymethyl)nitromethane			0–0.3		33 (in 6 patients)
Formaldehyde-releasers used as durable press chemical finishes					
Dihydroxydimethylolethyleneurea, methylated					100 (1 patient only)
Dimethylol dihydroxyethyleneurea	0.7–1.2[d,e]	0.6–2.3		1.9	82
Dimethylol dihydroxyethyleneurea, modified	2.2[d]				
Dimethylolpropyleneurea	2.1[e]		5.5[f]	0.4–1,1[g]	56
Dimethylol urea					100 (in 6 patients)
Ethylene urea, melamine/formaldehyde[h]	2.6–3.1[d,e]	2.1–7.2		1.5	86
Glyoxalurea					100 (in 6 patients)
Polyoxymethylene melamine	2.4–2.6[d,e]		1.7	0.4–1.1[g]	85
Polyoxymethylene urea	2.3–2.4[d,e]			1–2.2[g]	72
Tetramethylol acetylenediurea	2.4[e]		1.8[f]	0.2–0.8[g]	80
Miscellaneous formaldehyde-releasers					
Methenamine			0		
N-Methylolchloracetamide	0.4		0.1–0.4		

[a]Literature reviewed back to 1990

[b]Patients suspected of contact dermatitis

[c]Selection procedures were sometimes specified (e.g., suspected of metalworking fluid dermatitis), but more often not adequately described. The frequency of sensitization obviously depends on the degree of selection

[d]Study from Israel (Lazarov 2004)

[e]Study from Israel (Lazarov et al. 2002)

[f]Study from Israel (Lazarov et al. 2000)

[g]Frequency in an unselected test population, in which an unknown number of patients had been patch tested with these allergens

[h]This is a commercial patch test preparation, not a durable press chemical finished used *per se*

3-diol 0.4–1.2%, diazolidinyl urea 0.5–1.4%, imidazolidinyl urea 0.3–1.4%, and quaternium-15 0.6–1.9%. (For DMDM hydantoin, no recent data are available.) Comparison between Europe and the USA shows that there are (far) higher frequencies in the USA in patients suspected of contact dermatitis. This may partly be explained by stricter selection in the tertiary referral centers where the data come from (NACDG: North American Contact Dermatitis Group [Marks et al. 1998, 2003] and the Mayo Clinic [Davis et al. 2008]) and a far higher frequency of formaldehyde contact allergy in the USA. Whether differences in composition of cosmetics and/or the use pattern of these products (US individuals might for example be heavier users of cosmetics) also play a role, is unknown (de Groot and Veenstra 2010).

4.2 Relevance of Positive Reactions

Only in a small minority of studies, in which selected or unselected patient groups have been tested, has data on relevance been provided. Many such investigations were performed by the North American Contact Dermatitis Group or the Mayo Clinic. Relevance was usually divided into "definite," "probable," and "possible" and expressed as a percentage of the patients tested (Marks et al. 1998, 2003; Davis et al. 2008). Their percentages have ranged widely. In these "prevalence studies," the alleged causative products were never specified and such data actually have little value.

In a detailed study, the great majority of 60 relevant reactions to quaternium-15 were caused by cosmetic products: moisturizers (n = 46), hair preparations (non-coloring, n = 19), and makeup (n = 4). Three occupational cases were caused by similar products (Parker and Taylor 1991). Most reactions to other releasers used in cosmetics such as diazolidinyl urea and imidazolidinyl urea are probably also due to cosmetic products. In a German study, relevance was found in 31% of positive patch test reactions to DMDM hydantoin. Causative products were mainly cosmetics (30%) and topical drugs (22%); the other products were not mentioned (Uter and Frosch 2002).

4.3 Risk of Formaldehyde-Releaser-Containing Products for Patients Allergic to Formaldehyde

Whether cosmetic products containing formaldehyde-releasers will cause allergic contact dermatitis in patients who are sensitive to formaldehyde depends on various factors (➋ *Table 37.6*). The amount of free and releasable formaldehyde in a product is determined – inter alia – by the nature of the releaser, its concentration, the product composition, and the storage conditions. However, the pH of the product, its age, and presence of other ingredients may heavily influence the concentration of free formaldehyde (Rosen and McFarland 1984; Emeis et al. 2007). Although it is unknown what level of formaldehyde in products is safe, levels >200 ppm probably are not (at least for some formaldehyde-allergic subjects) (de Groot et al. 2009). All releasers used in cosmetic products (with the exception of 2-bromo-2-nitropropane-1,3-diol, for which adequate data are lacking) can – in the right circumstances of concentration and product composition – release >200 ppm formaldehyde, which may result in a number of patients in allergic contact dermatitis. Whether this is actually the case in any particular product cannot be decided on the basis of ingredient labeling. It is thus prudent that patients allergic to formaldehyde avoid stay-on cosmetics preserved with quaternium-15, diazolidinyl urea, DMDM hydantoin, or imidazolidinyl urea, especially when to be used regularly and/or on "sensitive" or damaged skin (de Groot et al. 2010b). Rinse-off products in general will have a low risk of causing allergic contact dermatitis.

4.4 Occupational Contact Dermatitis

Among 60 positive patch tests to quaternium-15 considered to be relevant, there were three cases of occupational contact dermatitis, caused by hair products and a barrier cream (Parker and Taylor 1991). Health care workers are more often contact allergic to quaternium-15, which is ascribed to the more frequent use of hand washing preparations and moisturizers (Suneja and Belsito 2008; Cahill and Nixon 2005). Other occupations with overrepresentation of contact allergy to quaternium-15 include the food industry (food preparation), hairdressers and cosmetologists, presumably from similar preparations and cosmetics (Warshaw et al. 2007). Miscellaneous occupational causes have included an electroencephalography skin preparation in a neurophysiology technician (Finch et al. 2001), photocopier toner (Zina et al. 2000), and an industrial cleaner, leading to hand dermatitis and occupational nail dystrophy (Marren et al. 1991). 2-Bromo-2-nitropropane-1,3-diol was an occupational allergen in nylon spin finish (Podmore 2000), in milk recorders (Grattan et al. 1986), and in a veterinary surgeon by its presence in a veterinary lubricant (Wilson and Powel 1990).

Table 37.4

Uses and applications of formaldehyde-releasers[a] (de Groot et al. 2010a, b, c, d, e, f)

Formaldehyde-releaser	Uses
Formaldehyde-releasers used in cosmetics	
Benzylhemiformal	Preservative in rinse-off cosmetics. Biocide in metalworking fluids, slurries, filler suspensions, adhesives, various emulsions and dispersions, paints and lacquers, the paper industry, spinning baths in the textile industry, polishes, waxes, and cleaning products
2-bromo-2-nitropropane- 1,3-diol	Cosmetics, adhesives/glues, cleaning agents, binding agents, coloring agents, construction materials, filling agents, flooring agents, humidifiers, impregnating agents, metalworking fluids, milk processing plants, paints/lacquers, paper mills, water circulating systems, pharmaceutical products, polishes, printing inks, slurries, surface treatment for paper, cardboard and other non-metals, viscosity adjustors, and washing detergents
Quaternium-15	Cosmetics, metalworking fluids, detergents and soaps, floor waxes and polishes, inks, latex-based paints, laundry starch, paper and pulp products, textile finishing solutions, spinning emulsions, printing pastes, joint cements, and photocopier toner
Sodium hydroxymethylglycinate	Cosmetics, neutralizing agent for acids/acrylics polymers, in cleaning/washing agents, in rinsing agents
Formaldehyde-releasers used in metalworking fluids	
Bioban CS-1135®	Bactericide in metalworking fluids, fluids for oil and gas production, and mineral slurries. Also used as an in-can preservative for paints, inks, emulsions, nonfood contact adhesives, surfactants, and in consumer, household and institutional products such as dishwashing and laundry detergents, fabric softeners, household and industrial cleaners, and polishes. Also provides quick cleanup for contaminated process water, and finished formulations
Bioban CS-1246®	Bactericide in metalworking fluids, adhesives, consumer and household products (including dishwashing and laundry liquids, surface cleaners and polishes), industrial products, wax and resin emulsions, inks, nonfood contact adhesives, mineral slurries, paints, and surfactants. Also used for leather tanning
Bioban P-1487®	Bactericidal and fungicidal agent used in metalworking fluids, paints, inks, emulsions, slurries, nonfood contact adhesives, die cast lubricants, mold-release agents and also in consumer, household and institutional products
N,N′-methylenebis(5-methyloxazolidine)	Biocide in metalworking fluids, in nylon spin finish, technical emulsions, and system cleansers
Tris(*N*-hydroxyethyl) hexahydrotriazine	Bactericide and fungicide in adhesives, industrial cleaning systems, polymer emulsions, latex emulsions, soluble lubricants, paints and metalworking fluids, in oilfield water systems, drilling muds, and in workover and completion fluids. In-can preservation of water-based products like paints, glues, emulsions, inks, pigment dispersions, cutting oils and water-soluble cleaners. Fuel protection during storage
Tris(hydroxymethyl) nitromethane	Antimicrobial agent in industrial applications such as household and institutional products, oil field water systems and drilling muds, recirculating water systems, chemical toilets, and metalworking fluids
Formaldehyde-releasers used as durable press chemical finishes	
Dimethylol urea	Production of urea-formaldehyde resins as an unisolated intermediate; also used as textile finish
Glyoxalurea	In paper coating compositions and as a textile finish
Methylol urea	Used to treat textiles and woods and is mixed with fillers for use in molding adhesives. In disinfectants and other biocidal products, methylol urea is used for disinfection of air, surfaces, materials, and equipment. It is a preservative for liquid-cooling and processing systems and is also used as slimicide, e.g., on wood and paper pulp. Present in urea-formaldehyde resins as residual starting material or breakdown product

Table 37.4 (Continued)

Formaldehyde-releaser	Uses
Polyoxymethylene melamine	Surface coating and glues in the furniture and wood industry, bonding agents in plywood and particle board (MDF), plastic composites manufacturing, printing, dyeing, or finishing of textiles, pulp and paper processing, in water-resistant orthopedic plaster, surface coatings, baking enamels, and treatment of leather. Polyoxymethylene melamine increases the wet and folding strength of paper essential for the manufacture of currency, maps, shipping bags, towels, facial tissue, etc
Polyoxymethylene urea	Textile finishes, in cosmetics as bulking agent and to form the outer shell of microcapsules, adhesives, in polymers having incidental contact with food
Miscellaneous formaldehyde-releasers	
MDM hydantoin	Preservative in paints, room deodorizers, and dishwashing detergents. Used as "antimicrobial" in cosmetics according to the EU CosIng database, but is not included in the annex of allowed preservatives
Methenamine	Used in the rubber industry to prevent vulcanized rubber from blocking, as an accelerator and together with resorcinol and silica as adhesion promoter; as a curing agent for thermosetting resins (particularly phenol-formaldehyde and urea-formaldehyde resins); in foundry mold casting as part of binder resins; in the production of nitrilotriacetic acid; for use in the manufacture of adhesives and coatings; as an anticorrosive agent in steel; in the absorption of poisonous gases; in the synthesis of explosives; in flame-retardant materials, paints and lacquers, rubber textile adhesives, the photographic industry; in the production of deodorants and hair fixers, in methenamine solid fuel tablets; as a protein modifier and as a reagent in chemical analysis. Pharmaceutical for intestinal infection and preservative in the food (especially fish) industry. Permitted in cosmetics in the EU in a maximum concentration of 0.15%
N-methylolchloracetamide	Preservative in glues, in metalworking fluids, and spin-finishes applied to nylon
Paraformaldehyde	Used as a fumigant, disinfectant, and fungicide, in root-canal therapy and as a curing agent for phenol-formaldehyde resins. Higher molecule homopolymer is a hard engineering plastic (polyoxymethylene plastic), As paraformaldehyde is essentially a solid form of formaldehyde, it therefore has the same uses as formaldehyde. Permitted in cosmetics in the EU in a maximum concentration of 0.2% (0.1% for products for oral hygiene)

[a]Formaldehyde-rel easers mentioned in *Table 37.1* but *not* here are used mainly in the class of products under which they are classified (cosmetics, metalworking fluids, durable press chemical finishes)

5 Metalworking Fluids

The functions of metalworking fluids (MWF) are primarily those of cooling and lubrication. For these purposes, MWF are directed at the interface of the metal workpiece and the cutting edge of the machine tool. Traditionally, MWF may be classified as insoluble (neat) oils or soluble oils. Soluble oils are usually oil in water emulsions, but sometimes true aqueous solutions. Biocides such as the formaldehyde-releasers are mixed into water-soluble oils to inhibit the overgrowth of bacterial and fungal populations. Such overgrowth, which occurs particularly at oil–water interfaces, is responsible for problems of foul odor ("monday morning stink") and results in decreased tool life (metal corrosion), loss of cutting oil function, increased frictional heat, increased power consumption, and rust. Bacterial growth in these fluids can also cause emulsion breakdown, poor surface finish, excessive solid loads on filters and clarifiers (i.e., slimes and deposits), and discolorations (de Groot et al. 2010e).

5.1 Contact Allergy

The results of (routine) testing with formaldehyde-releasers used in MWF are summarized in *Table 37.3*. The frequency of sensitization in unselected contact dermatitis patients remains largely unknown. The high percentages of positive reactions to Bioban ® CS-1135 and Bioban ® CS-1246 (Anderson et al. 2007) and to tris(*N*-hydroxyethyl)hexahydrotriazine (Davis et al. 2008) in two tertiary US referral centers should not be

Table 37.5
Formaldehyde-releasers permitted in cosmetics in the EU with their maximum concentration

Preservative	Maximum allowed conc.	Comments
Benzylhemiformal	0.15%	Permitted in rinse-off products only
2-Bromo-2-nitropropane-1,3-diol	0.1%	Formation of nitrosamines must be avoided
Diazolidinyl urea	0.5%	
4,4-Dimethyloxazolidine	0.1%	Present in Bioban CS 1135 ®, a preservative mainly used in metalworking fluids
DMDM hydantoin	0.6%	
5-Ethyl-1-aza-3,7-dioxabicyclo-[3.3.0] octane	0.3%	Prohibited in oral hygiene products and products intended to come into contact with mucous membranes. Present in Bioban CS-1246 ®, a preservative in metalworking fluids
Formaldehyde	0.2%	Maximum 0.1% for products for oral hygiene
Imidazolidinyl urea	0.6%	
Methenamine	0.15%	
Paraformaldehyde	0.2%	Maximum 0.1% for products for oral hygiene
Quaternium-15	0.2%	
Sodium methylhydroxyglycinate	0.5%	

taken as representative. They may be due to stricter selection before being patch tested, formaldehyde sensitivity as a cause of positive patch tests and possibly false-positive reactions.

Most studies have been performed in selected patients in contact with MWF suspected of occupational contact dermatitis. In these groups, mean prevalences were 2.8% for Bioban ® CS-1135, 1.9% for Bioban ® CS-1246, 1.9% for Bioban ® P-1487, 4.0% for *N,N'*-methylenebis(5-methyloxazolidine), 4.9% for 4,4'-methylenedimorpholine (one small

Table 37.6
Factors that determine the risk for patients hypersensitive to formaldehyde to develop allergic contact dermatitis from contact with products containing formaldehyde-releasers

Strength of the allergy to formaldehyde in the individual patient
Amount and concentration of free and (upon passage through the skin) releasable formaldehyde in the particular product
Nature of the product (e.g., stay-on versus rinse-off products)
Frequency and duration of skin contact with the products
Localization of skin contact (e.g., thin skin of eyelids or thick skin of the trunk)
Skin status (normal, dry with impaired barrier function, dermatitis)
Concomitant or successive contact with other products containing formaldehyde or -releasers)

study with 144 patients), 1.6% for tris(*N*-hydroxyethyl) hexahydrotriazine and 0.2% for tris(hydroxymethyl) nitromethane. In larger groups of selected patients (selection procedure usually unknown, but *not* patients suspected of MWF dermatitis) generally the same or lower prevalences were observed. It thus appears that most formaldehyde-releasers in MWF cannot be considered frequent and important contact allergens. Even in highly selected patients groups – that is, metalworkers in contact with MWF suspected of occupational contact dermatitis – generally modest prevalence rates have been observed. In the case of the Biobans, it should further be noted that most patch test reactions are only weakly positive (+) and that they are often not reproducible, which suggests that many may be irritant (false-positive) (Brinkmeier et al. 2002). The most frequent contact sensitizer appears to be *N, N'*-methylenebis(5-methyloxazolidine).

5.2 Relevance of Positive Reactions

Relevance data on positive patch tests to Bioban ® CS-1135, Bioban ® CS-1246, and tris(hydroxymethyl)nitromethane are not available; positive patch test reactions to Bioban ® P-1487 and 4,4'-methylenedimorpholine appear to be rarely relevant. In the case of *N,N'*-methylenebis (5-methyloxazolidine), the relevance of positive patch reactions has been stated in one study only and was found to be 47% (7/15 patients) (Madan and Beck 2006). There is extensive literature on contact allergy to tris

(*N*-hydroxyethyl)hexahydrotriazine, but relevance has been addressed in a mere two studies. Of 24 patients with positive reactions to tris(*N*-hydroxyethyl)hexahydrotriazine seen at the Finnish Institute of Occupational Health, only two were exposed to a MWF containing tris (*N*-hydroxyethyl)hexahydrotriazine (Aalto-Korte et al. 2008).

The lack of data on the clinical relevance of contact allergy to formaldehyde-releasers in MWF may partly be explained by the difficulty of establishing exposure. Also, in the safety data sheets (SDS) of other chemicals, the information on the sensitizing substances has sometimes found to be deficient (Henricks-Eckerman et al. 2008). In the case of the Biobans, another explanation for the lack of established relevance may be that a number of the patch test reactions were actually false-positive (Brinkmeier et al. 2002).

5.3 Risk of Formaldehyde-Releaser-Containing Products for Patients Allergic to Formaldehyde

Most metalworking fluid concentrates contain formaldehyde in concentrations ranging from 0.002–1.3% (free and easily released formaldehyde) (Henricks-Eckerman et al. 2008). There appear to be no data on the free and releasable formaldehyde content in fresh and used MWF *in dilutions of actual use*. As a consequence, there is insufficient information to estimate the risk of sensitization in workers exposed to MWF and of elicitation of dermatitis in individuals previously sensitized to formaldehyde. However, it is well known that sensitization to formaldehyde from these sources does occur and is by no means rare. In a recent Finnish study, for example, 40% of new occupational sensitizations to formaldehyde were seen in metalworkers (Aalto-Korte et al. 2008). In a German/Austrian/Swiss study, metalworkers with occupational dermatitis exposed to water-based MWF had a significantly increased risk of sensitization to formaldehyde (odds ratio 4.1) compared to men not working in the metal industry (Geier et al. 2004b).

5.4 Occupational Contact Dermatitis

Occupational hand dermatitis is common in metalworkers exposed to MWF. In one study, current skin symptoms were reported by 10% of metalworkers (Mirabelli et al. 2009); the prevalence or 3-year incidence of hand eczema has also been found to be 20–25% (Berndt et al. 2000). Irritant contact dermatitis is more frequently observed than allergic contact dermatitis. Skin irritation by MWF is not only caused by wet work, but also by the alkaline pH usually ranging from 8.5 to 9.6, and by emulsifiers and biocides in the fluids. Irritant dermatitis promotes and may precede contact sensitization, often caused by biocides, particularly formaldehyde-releasers (Geier et al. 2004a, b; Suuronen et al. 2007).

In several studies, patients suspected of occupational contact dermatitis and/or metalworkers in contact with metalworking fluids have been patch tested with formaldehyde-releasers. In only a few of these studies were positive patch tests often related to occupational contact with metalworking fluids, notably with *N,N'*-methylenebis(5-methyloxazolidine) (Madan and Beck 2006). This formaldehyde-releaser has also caused occupational contact dermatitis in nylon spin finish (Batta et al. 1999).

Hand eczema in an engine fitter was (not quite convincingly) ascribed to Forcide ® 78 I (see ➲ *Table 37.1* for details) (Hamann 1980). Two machinists with hand eczema, who had contact with products containing tris (hydroxymethyl)nitromethane, reacted to this releaser 1% pet. (Robertson and Storrs 1982).

6 Textiles and Clothes: Durable Press Chemical Finishes

Durable press chemical finishes (DPCF) have been used on fabrics since the mid-1920s to impart wrinkle resistance during wear and laundering. Their application primarily concerns cotton, viscose, linen, and their blends with synthetic fibers. DPCF can also facilitate bleaching and dyeing, make fabrics waterproof, non-shrinkable and moth-proof, they can ameliorate nylon and make it electrically antistatic. They give textile body, and improve their quality, touch, and appearance. The early DPCF based on polyoxymethylene urea (urea-formaldehyde resin) and polyoxymethylene melamine (melamine/formaldehyde resin) released large amounts of formaldehyde in clothes; levels of 5,000–12,000 ppm (0.5–1.2%) of formaldehyde were found in rayon and cotton. Consequently, allergic contact dermatitis due to formaldehyde present in textiles was commonly reported in the 1950s and 1960s, especially in Europe (Hatch and Maibach 1986). Presensitization to formaldehyde deodorants and repeated exposure to fabrics treated with DPCF served as the primary sensitizer in many of the cases.

6.1 Contact Allergy

As a result of the many cases of allergic contact dermatitis caused by formaldehyde released from durable press chemical finishes in clothes in the 1950s, the textile industry in the 1960s started using finishes releasing less formaldehyde, notably dimethylol dihydroxyethyleneurea. By 1981 the US textile industry claimed that levels of formaldehyde release had decreased so that 100–200 ppm was the standard; these levels would appear to be safe (Fisher et al. 1962). In spite of this, there has been a resurrection of reports of allergic contact dermatitis to clothes from 1990 on in the USA (Sherertz 1992; Fowler et al. 1992; Scheman et al. 1998; Metzler-Brenckle and Rietschel 2002) and in Israel (Lazarov et al. 2000, 2002; Lazarov 2004). The availability of DPCF for patch testing, including the test mix ethylene urea, melamine/formaldehyde, facilitated the investigation of patients suspected of textile dermatitis.

In the USA, most cases of allergic contact dermatitis were attributed to formaldehyde released from the DPCF; in Israel, however, only about one third of the patients with positive patch test reactions to DPCF co-reacted to formaldehyde. This lead to the conclusion that the DPCF *per se* must be sensitizers as well. However, all studies had one or more (serious) flaws in design and/or interpretation. Recent testing of clothes for formaldehyde in the USA, Europe, New Zealand, and other countries demonstrated low levels of formaldehyde. Such amounts (nearly always <200 ppm) are considered too low to cause sensitization to formaldehyde and also too low to elicit allergic contact dermatitis in individuals already allergic to formaldehyde (with the possible exception of a few patients exquisitely sensitive to formaldehyde). The concept of formaldehyde in clothes as the cause of recent cases of dermatitis has not been proven in a single case and the same applies to DPCF as a putative allergen. Thus, the current use of durable press chemical finishes in clothes is considered to be safe (de Groot and Maibach 2010; de Groot et al. 2010d). The results of (routine) testing with DPCF are summarized in ➋ *Table 37.3.*

6.2 Relevance of Positive Reactions

In the recent studies from the USA and Israel, many reactions to DPCF were considered to be relevant and indicate contact allergy to formaldehyde or DPCF *per se* (in case of a negative reaction to formaldehyde and a positive reaction to DPCF) in clothes (Sherertz 1992; Fowler et al. 1992; Scheman et al. 1998; Metzler-Brenckle and Rietschel 2002; Lazarov et al. 2000, 2002; Lazarov 2004). However, as argued above, the validity of these reports may be questioned (de Groot and Maibach 2010; de Groot et al. 2010d). Most positive reactions observed in routine testing of ethylene urea, melamine/formaldehyde, and dimethylol dihydroxyethyleneurea in the NACDG studies (Marks et al. 1998, 2003) are probably caused by formaldehyde allergy. This leaves the low co-reactivity to formaldehyde in the Israeli studies, however, unexplained (Lazarov et al. 2002; Lazarov 2004).

6.3 Occupational Contact Dermatitis

Reports of occupational allergic contact dermatitis to DPCF in the textile industry and to clothes in an occupational setting are infrequent in the past 30 years. A US pediatrician developed dermatitis attributed to a hospital gown and a face mask, unconvincingly attributed to formaldehyde (Donovan and Skoynicki-Grant 2006). Of 17 patients allergic to ethylene urea, melamine/formaldehyde resin (EUMF) investigated in the USA, there were six occupational cases: three male retirees (one may wonder how can this be occupational) and three women, an office worker, a dialysis technician, and a machinist (Carlson et al. 2004). Among 83 Israeli patients reacting to either a DPCF or a color used in clothes, there were four occupational cases (occupation not specified) (Lazarov 2004). A man handling new readymade clothes in a warehouse had eczema on the hands that improved during weekends and holidays. Patch tests were positive to formaldehyde, quaternium-15 and ethylene urea, melamine/formaldehyde (Cockayne et al. 2001). From Spain, one (atopic) patient was reported with hand eczema that got worse when replacing clothes in a store (Bracamonte et al. 1995). She reacted to formaldehyde and several (high-formaldehyde) DPCF. In the USA, between 1989 and 1994, 19 patients were investigated with dermatitis who were occupationally involved with finished textile products. Six were diagnosed as suffering from allergic contact dermatitis to DPCF on the basis of a positive patch test to formaldehyde or a DPCF (Soni and Sherertz 1996). Between 1975 and 1993, the average annual incidence of formaldehyde-related occupational contact dermatitis in the Finnish Textile and Clothing industries was 0.66/10.000 (Priha 1995). In a US case series (Fowler et al. 1992), there were four cases of occupational contact dermatitis (two garment workers, one printer, and one chemical worker) among 16 patients sensitized to DPCF. From

Table 37.7
Occupational allergic contact dermatitis to melamine/formaldehyde resin

No pat.	No allergic to formaldehyde	Occupation/work activities	Responsible products	References
1	0	Melamine paper impregnating line	Melamine/formaldehyde	Gavin et al. (2008)
3	0	Compositor in chipboard factory	Melamine/formaldehyde resin coating	Aalto-Korte et al. (2003)
		Laboratory technician	Melamine/formaldehyde glue	Aalto-Korte et al. (2003)
		Plywood worker	Melamine/formaldehyde glue	Aalto-Korte et al. (2003)
5	0	Workers in plant producing resin-fiber composites	Melamine/formaldehyde resin	Isaksson et al. (1999)
1	?	?	?	Holness and Nethercott (1997)
1	0	Orthopedic plaster technician	Orthopedic plaster	Ross et al. (1992)
1	1	Production of clay pots	Gypsum molds for clay pots	Fregert (1981)

Italy came a report on 62 textile and garment industry workers with allergic contact dermatitis; not a single case was caused by either formaldehyde or a DPCF (Gasperini et al. 1989). Investigators in Spain ascribed petechial facial dermatitis in a patient working in a textile plant to contact with wool on the basis of a positive patch test reaction to formaldehyde and two high-formaldehyde DPCF (Romaguera et al. 1981). There have been several reports of occupational contact dermatitis from melamine/formaldehyde resin, but all *outside* the textile industry; their details are summarized in ➋ *Table 37.7.*

7 Miscellaneous Formaldehyde-Releasers

7.1 Contact Allergy

A rest group of formaldehyde-releasers (➋ *Table 37.1*) has various applications and functions (➋ *Table 37.4*). None of these are important causes of allergic contact dermatitis (➋ *Table 37.3*). Methenamine has structural similarities to quaternium-15 and about one in three patients allergic to quaternium-15 will also have positive patch tests to methenamine. This is presumably unrelated to formaldehyde sensitivity (Aalto-Korte 2000). Patients allergic to *N*-methylolchloracetamide may co-react to formaldehyde and/or chloracetamide, from which *N*-methylolchloracetamide is synthesized.

7.2 Occupational Contact Dermatitis

7.2.1 Methenamine

A Japanese foundry worker had hand eczema caused by occupational contact with methenamine in a core molding process. He reacted to a patch test with methenamine 1% pet., but was negative to formaldehyde (Hayakawa et al. 1988). In 1998, all 17 employees of a German methenamine production plant were investigated for health effects of methenamine. Patch tests were performed with fresh batches of methenamine 1% and 2% in both water and petrolatum. No sensitizations were found. However, two out of four ex-workers previously considered to be “allergic” had positive patch tests to methenamine. They did not react to formaldehyde. These two patients reported eczema (located at exposed skin areas in one subject and generalized in the other) and conjunctivitis during exposure but were free of symptoms after removal of exposure. All highly exposed individuals showed irritant dermatitis of the hands. The workers were aware of this effect and protected themselves by the frequent use of creams. Because none of these reacted upon patch tests, it was concluded that methenamine is not a potent skin sensitizer (Merget et al. 1999).

7.2.2 *N*-methylolchloracetamide

In a series of 175 Israeli patients suspected of occupational contact dermatitis and working with oils and cooling liquids, one positive patch test was observed to *N*-methylolChloracetamide; the relevance was not stated (Trattner et al. 2009). Dermatitis of the hands was investigated in seven employees in a plant manufacturing nylon yarn in the UK. A "spin finish" was applied to the nylon thread containing Grotan ® HD (active ingredient: *N*-methylolchloracetamide) at a concentration of 0.075%. Patch tests were performed with the chemical at the usage concentration in water. All gave a positive reaction. None reacted to formaldehyde 2% aqua. Chloracetamide was not tested. It was (not explicitly) suggested that the workers had been sensitized to chloracetamide (Savage 1978).

An Italian worker producing modeling plasticine became sensitized to Preventol ® D5, containing 24% *N*-methylolchloracetamide. Patch tests were positive to Preventol ® D5 1%, 0.2%, and 0.04% pet (0.25%, 0.05% and 0.01% *N*-methylolchloracetamide) but not to formaldehyde. He did, however, react to chloracetamide 0.2% pet. Of seven controls known to be allergic to formaldehyde, three reacted to all three concentrations of Preventol ® D5 (Farli et al. 1987).

A man working in a Swedish chemical company developed eczema on his face which he attributed to a preservative that he worked with once a week since 6 months. The preservative, containing *N*-methylolchloracetamide and benzyl alcohol, was patch test positive at 0.1% aqua. Further patch testing showed a positive reaction to *N*-methylolchloracetamide down to 0.01% in alcohol but negative to benzyl alcohol and chloracetamide. Subsequently, 261 patients were routinely tested with *N*-methylolchloracetamide and one 15-year-old boy reacted (negative to formaldehyde and chloracetamide). He had worked with glues, but it was not ascertained whether these contained *N*-methylolchloracetamide (Ågren et al. 1980). The two patients in this report did not react to chloracetamide (0.1%) or to formaldehyde, suggesting the entire molecule can act as hapten. Maximization tests were performed and 6/8 guinea pigs were sensitized to *N*-methylolchloracetamide 1% acetone. Four of these eight also reacted to chloracetamide 1% acetone, which was considered to be a cross-reaction. The *N*-methylolchloracetamide contained less than 0.5% chloracetamide (Ågren et al. 1980).

A 19-year-old Norwegian engine fitter's apprentice with hand eczema tested positively to formaldehyde. It was suspected that he might react to a formaldehyde-releaser in the coolant oil, Parmetol ® K50, containing *N*-methylolchloracetamide + o-formal of benzyl alcohol. Patch tests were positive to Parmetol ® K50 10% pet, chloracetamide 5% pet, and formaldehyde 2% aqua. Parmetol ® K50 was tested on 74 consecutive patients with negative results after 3–5 days. However, seven patients developed late reactions after 17–50 days. Two of these were further analyzed. Both reacted to chloracetamide and one to formaldehyde, which had given a negative reaction previously. Two of the controls were allergic to formaldehyde but did not react to Parmetol ® K 50. A further 66 controls were tested with Parmetol ® K 50 2% pet and one patient reacted to it and to formaldehyde (Hjorth 1979).

A carpenter in Portugal became occupationally sensitized to a glue containing isothiazolinones and *N*-methylolchloracetamide. He also reacted to chloracetamide and formaldehyde (Pereira et al. 1999).

References

Aalto-Korte K (2000) Simultaneous allergic reactions to quaternium-15 and methenamine. Contact Dermatitis 42:365

Aalto-Korte K, Jolanki R, Estlander T (2003) Formaldehyde-negative allergic contact dermatitis from melamine-formaldehyde resin. Contact Dermatitis 49:194–196

Aalto-Korte K, Kuuliala O, Suuronen K et al (2008) Occupational contact allergy to formaldehyde and formaldehyde releasers. Contact Dermatitis 59:280–289

Agner T, Flyvholm M-A, Menné T (1999) Formaldehyde allergy: a follow-up study. Am J Contact Dermatitis 10:12–17

Ågren S, Dahlquist I, Fregert S et al (1980) Allergic contact dermatitis from the preservative *N*-methylol-chloracetamide. Contact Dermatitis 6:202–203

Andersen KE, Boman A, Hamann K et al (1984) Guinea pig maximization tests with formaldehyde releasers. Results of two laboratories. Contact Dermatitis 10:257–266

Anderson BE, Tan TC, Marks JG Jr (2007) Patch-test reactions to formaldehyde, Biobans, and other formaldehyde releasers. Dermatitis 18:92–95

Batta K, McVittie S, Foulds IS (1999) Occupational allergic contact dermatitis from *N*, *N*-methylene-bis-3-methyl-oxazolidine in a nylon spin finish. Contact Dermatitis 41:165

Berndt U, Hinnen U, Iliev D et al (2000) Hand eczema in metalworker trainees – an analysis of risk factors. Contact Dermatitis 43:327–332

Bracamonte BG, Ortiz de Frutos FJ, Iglesias Diez L (1995) Occupational allergic contact dermatitis due to formaldehyde and textile finish resins. Contact Dermatitis 33:139–140

Brinkmeier T, Geier J, Lepoittevin J-P et al (2002) Patch test reactions to Biobans in metalworkers are often weak and not reproducible. Contact Dermatitis 47:27–31

Cahill J, Nixon R (2005) Allergic contact dermatitis to quaternium-15 in a moisturizing lotion. Australas J Dermatol 46:284–285

Carlson RM, Smith MC, Nedorost ST (2004) Diagnosis and treatment of dermatitis due to formaldehyde resins in clothing. Dermatitis 15:169–175

Cockayne SE, McDonagh AJ, Gawdrodger DJ (2001) Occupational allergic contact dermatitis from formaldehyde resin in clothing. Contact Dermatitis 44:109–110

Cronin E (1991) Formaldehyde is a significant allergen in women with hand eczema. Contact Dermatitis 25:276–282

Davis MD, Scalf LA, Yiannias JA et al (2008) Changing trends and allergens in the patch test standard series. A Mayo Clinic 5-year retrospective review, January 1, 2001, through December 31, 2005. Arch Dermatol 144:67–72

de Groot AC, Maibach HI (2010) Does allergic contact dermatitis from formaldehyde in clothes treated with durable-press chemical finishes exist in the USA? Contact Dermatitis 62:127–136

de Groot AC, Veenstra M (2010) Formaldehyde-releasers in cosmetics in the USA and in Europe. Contact Dermatitis 62:221–224

de Groot AC, Flyvholm M-A, Lensen G et al (2009) Formaldehyde-releasers: relationship to formaldehyde contact allergy. I. Contact allergy to formaldehyde and inventory of formaldehyde-releasers. Contact Dermatitis 61:63–85

de Groot AC, White IR, Flyvholm M-A et al (2010a) Formaldehyde-releasers: relationship to formaldehyde contact allergy. II. Formaldehyde-releasers used in cosmetics. Part 1. Characterization, frequency and relevance of sensitization, and frequency of use in cosmetics. Contact Dermatitis 62:2–17

de Groot AC, White IR, Flyvholm M-A et al (2010b) Formaldehyde-releasers: relationship to formaldehyde contact allergy. II. Formaldehyde-releasers used in cosmetics. Part 2. Patch test relationship to formaldehyde contact allergy, experimental provocation tests, amount of formaldehyde released and assessment of risk to consumers allergic to formaldehyde. Contact Dermatitis 62:18–31

de Groot A, Le Coz C, Lensen G et al (2010c) Formaldehyde-releasers: relationship to formaldehyde contact allergy. III. Formaldehyde-releasers in clothes: durable press chemical finishes. Part 1. Contact Dermatitis 62:1–9

de Groot AC, Le Coz C, Lensen G et al (2010d) Formaldehyde-releasers: relationship to formaldehyde contact allergy. III. Formaldehyde-releasers in clothes: durable press chemical finishes. Part 2. Contact Dermatitis 63:1–9

de Groot AC, Geier J, Flyvholm M-A et al (2010e) Formaldehyde-releasers: relationship to formaldehyde contact allergy. IV. Metalworking fluids and remainder. Part 1. Contact Dermatitis 63:117–128

de Groot AC, Geier J, Flyvholm M-A et al (2010f) Formaldehyde-releasers: relationship to formaldehyde contact allergy. IV. Metalworking fluids and remainder. Part 2. Contact Dermatitis 63:129–139

Donovan J, Skoynicki-Grant S (2006) Allergic contact dermatitis from formaldehyde textile resins in surgical uniforms and nonwoven textile masks. Dermatitis 18:40–44

Emeis D, Anker W, Wittern K-P (2007) Quantitative ^{13}C NMR spectroscopic studies on the equilibrium of formaldehyde with its releasing preservatives. Anal Chem 79:2096–2100

Farli M, Ginanneschi M, Francalanci S et al (1987) Occupational contact dermatitis to *N*-methylol-chloroacetamide. Contact Dermatitis 17:182–184

Finch TM, Prais L, Foulds IS (2001) Occupational allergic contact dermatitis in an electroencephalography skin preparation. Contact Dermatitis 44:44–45

Fisher AA, Kanof NB, Biondi EM (1962) Free formaldehyde in textiles and paper. Clinical significance. Arch Dermatol 86:753–756

Flyvholm M-A (1997) Formaldehyde exposure at the workplace and in the environment. Allergologie 20:225–231

Flyvholm M-A, Menné T (1992) Allergic contact dermatitis from formaldehyde. A case study focusing on sources of formaldehyde exposure. Contact Dermatitis 27:227–236

Fowler JF Jr, Skinner SM, Belsito DV (1992) Allergic contact dermatitis from formaldehyde resins in permanent press clothing: an underdiagnosed cause of generalized dermatitis. J Am Acad Dermatol 27:962–968

Fransway AF, Schmitz NA (1991) The problem of preservation in the 1990s: II. Formaldehyde and formaldehyde-releasing biocides: incidences of cross-reactivity and the significance of the positive reponse to formaldehyde. Am J Contact Dermatitis 2:78–88

Fregert S (1981) Formaldehyde dermatitis from a gypsum-melamine resin mixture. Contact Dermatitis 7:56

Gasperini M, Farli M, Lombardi P et al (1989) Contact dermatitis in the textile and garment industry. In: Frosch PJ (ed) Current topics in contact dermatitis. Springer, Berlin, pp 326–329

Gavin JG, Martinez ML, Fernandez-Redondo V et al (2008) Contact allergic dermatitis from melamine formaldehyde resins in a patient with a negative patch-test reaction to formaldehyde. Dermatitis 19:5–6

Geier J, Lessmann H, Dickel H et al (2004a) Patch test results with the metalworking fluid series of the German Contact Dermatitis Research Group (DKG). Contact Dermatitis 51:118–130

Geier J, Lessmann H, Schnuch A et al (2004b) Contact sensitizations in metalworkers with occupational dermatitis exposed to water-based metalworking fluids: results of the research project "FaSt". Int Arch Occup Environ Health 77:543–551

Grattan CE, Harman RR, Tan RS (1986) Milk recorder dermatitis. Contact Dermatitis 14:217–220

Hamann K (1980) Forcide 78 ® – another formaldehyde releaser in coolant oils. Contact Dermatitis 6:446

Hatch KL, Maibach HI (1986) Textile chemical finish dermatitis. Contact Dermatitis 14:1–13

Hayakawa R, Arima Y, Hirose O et al (1988) Allergic contact dermatitis due to hexamethylenetetramine in core molding. Contact Dermatitis 18:226–228

Henricks-Eckerman M-L, Suuronen K, Jolanki R (2008) Analysis of allergens in metalworking fluids. Contact Dermatitis 59:261–267

Hjorth N (1979) N-methylol-chloracetamide, a sensitizer in coolant oils and cosmetics. Contact Dermatitis 5:330–331

Holness DL, Nethercott JR (1997) Results of patch testing with a specialized collection of plastic and glue allergens. Am J Contact Dermatitis 8:121–124

Isaksson M, Zimerson E, Bruze M (1999) Occupational dermatoses in composite production. J Occup Environ Med 41:261–266

Kang KM, Corey G, Storrs FJ (1995) Follow-up study of patients allergic to formaldehyde and formaldehyde releasers: retention of information, compliance, course, and persistence of allergy. Am J Contact Dermatitis 6:209–215

Lazarov A (2004) Textile dermatitis in patients with contact sensitization in Israel: a 4-year prospective study. J Eur Acad Dermatol Venereol 18:531–537

Lazarov A, Trattner A, David M et al (2000) Textile dermatitis in Israel: a retrospective study. Am J Contact Dermatitis 11:26–29

Lazarov A, Trattner A, Abraham D et al (2002) Frequency of textile dye and resin sensitization in patients with contact dermatitis in Israel. Contact Dermatitis 46:119–120

Madan V, Beck MH (2006) Occupational allergic contact dermatitis from *N*, *N*-methylene-bis-5-methyl-oxazolidine in coolant oils. Contact Dermatitis 55:39–41

Marks JG jr, Belsito DV, DeLeo VA et al (1998) North American Contact Dermatitis Group patch test results for the detection of delayed-type hypersensitivity to topical allergens. J Am Acad Dermatol 38:911–918

Marks JG jr, Belsito DV, DeLeo VA et al (2003) North American Contact Dermatitis Group Patch-Test Results, 1998 to 2000. Am J Contact Dermatitis 14:59–62

Marren P, de Berker D, Dawber RPT et al (1991) Occupational contact dermatitis due to quaternium 15 presenting as nail dystrophy. Contact Dermatitis 25:253–255

Merck & Co. (2006) The Merck index, 14th edn. Merck & Co., Whitehouse Station, www.merck.com.html

Merget R, Topcu M, Friese K et al (1999) A cross-sectional study of workers in the chemical industry with occupational exposure to hexamethylenetetramine. Int Arch Occup Environ Health 72:533–538

Metzler-Brenckle L, Rietschel RL (2002) Patch testing for permanent-press allergic contact dermatitis. Contact Dermatitis 46:33–37

Mirabelli MC, Zock J-P, Bircher AJ et al (2009) Metalworkers exposures and persistent skin symptoms in the ECRHS II and SAPALDIA 2 cohorts. Contact Dermatitis 60:256–263

Parker LU, Taylor JS (1991) A 5-year study of contact allergy to quaternium-15. Am J Contact Dermatitis 2:231–234

Pereira F, Rafael M, Pereira MA (1999) Occupational allergic contact dermatitis from a glue, containing isothiazolinones and *N*-methylol-chloroacetamide, in a carpenter. Contact Dermatitis 40:283

Podmore P (2000) Occupational allergic contact dermatitis from both 2-bromo-2-nitropropane-1,3-diol and methylchloroisothiazolinone plus methylisothiazolinone in spin finish. Contact Dermatitis 43:45

Priha E (1995) Are textile formaldehyde regulations reasonable? Experiences from the Finnish textile and clothing industries. Regul Toxicol Pharmacol 22:243–249

Robertson M, Storrs FJ (1982) Allergic contact dermatitis in two machinists. Arch Dermatol 118:997–2002

Romaguera C, Grimalt F, Lecha M (1981) Occupational purpuric textile dermatitis from formaldehyde resins. Contact Dermatitis 7:152–153

Rosen M, McFarland A (1984) Free formaldehyde in anionic shampoos. J Soc Cosmet Chem 35:157–169

Ross JS, Rycroft RJG, Cronin E (1992) Melamine-formaldehyde contact dermatitis in orthopaedic practice. Contact Dermatitis 26:203–204

Savage J (1978) Chloracetamide in nylon spin finish. Contact Dermatitis 4:179

Scheman AJ, Carroll PA, Brown KH et al (1998) Formaldehyde-related textile allergy: an update. Contact Dermatitis 38:332–336

Scheman A, Jacon S, Zirwas M et al (2008) Contact allergy: alternatives for the 2007 North American Dermatitis Group (NACDG) standard screening tray. Dis Mon 54:7–156

Schnuch A, Geier J, Uter W et al (1998) Patch testing with preservatives, antimicrobials and industrial biocides. Results from a multicentre study. Br J Dermatol 138:467–476

Sherertz EF (1992) Clothing dermatitis: practical aspects for the clinician. Am J Contact Dermatitis 3:55–64

Soni BP, Sherertz EF (1996) Contact dermatitis in the textile industry: a review of 72 patients. Am J Contact Dermatitis 7:226–230

Suneja T, Belsito DV (2008) Occupational dermatoses in health care workers evaluated for suspected allergic contact dermatitis. Contact Dermatitis 58:285–290

Suuronen K, Aalto-Korte K, Piipari R et al (2007) Occupational dermatitis and allergic respiratory diseases in Finnish metal working machinists. Occup Med 57:277–287

The Cosmetic, Toiletry and Fragrance Association, Inc (2006) CTFA cosmetic ingredient dictionary and handbook, 11th edn. The Cosmetic, Toiletry and Fragrance Association, Washington, DC, www.personalcarecouncil.org.html

Trattner A, Johansen JD, Menné T (1998) Formaldehyde concentration in diagnostic patch testing: comparison of 1% with 2%. Contact Dermatitis 38:9–13

Trattner A, Freireich-Astman M, David M et al (2009) Patch-test results of chemotechnique oil and cooling fluid series in patients with suspected occupational contact dermatitis in Israel. Dermatitis 20:39–43

Uter W, on behalf of the ESSCA writing group (2008) The European Surveillance System of Contact Allergies (ESSCA): results of patch testing the standard series, 2004. J Eur Acad Dermatol Venereol 22:174–181

Uter W, Frosch PJ (2002) Contact allergy from DMDM hydantoin, 1994–2000. Contact Dermatitis 47:57–58

Uter W, Rämsch C, Aberer W et al (2009) The European baseline series of 10 European countries, 2005/2006 – results of the European surveillance system on contact allergies (ESSCA). Contact Dermatitis 61:31–38

Warshaw EM, Ahmed RL, Belsito DV et al (2007) Contact dermatitis of the hands. Cross-sectional analyses of North American Contact Dermatitis Group Data, 1994–2004. J Am Acad Dermatol 57: 301–315

Wilson CL, Powel SM (1990) An unusual case of allergic contact dermatitis in a veterinary surgeon. Contact Dermatitis 23:42–43

Zina AM, Fanan E, Bundino S (2000) Allergic contact dermatitis from formaldehyde and quaternium-15 in a photocopier toner. Contact Dermatitis 43:241–242

38 Fiberglass, Dusts

Daniel J. Hogan · Megan Morrison
Bay Pines VA Healthcare System, Bay Pines, FL, USA

Core Messages

- Production of fiberglass is increasing.
- Airborne dermatitis may be caused by fiberglass.
- Irritant contact dermatitis is usually caused by fibers greater in diameter.
- Hardening is not prominent and may be less likely development atopics
- Histopathology of dermatitis is nonspecific unless the fiberglass is itself visualized in the skin biopsy or skin tape stripping.
- Treatment is nonspecific except for taking measures to curtail exposure to fiberglass where possible to identify sources of exposure.

1 Introduction

Fiberglass is a type of man-made vitreous fiber (MMVF). There are four general groups of MMVF (➋ *Table 38.1*): glass filament, mineral wool (glass wool, rock wool, and slag wool), refractory ceramic fibers, and fibers for special purposes (Jolanki et al. 2002).

We will be focusing on glass filament MMVF, also known as fiberglass. Fiberglass is the most commonly used mineral fiber because of its wide variety of uses. It has slowly replaced asbestos as the insulation of choice because the health risk involved is less. As opposed to asbestos which breaks longitudinally to make many finer thin fibers, the fiberglass breaks transversely to give rise to many smaller fibers of the same diameter (Sertoli et al. 1992). Also, compared to asbestos, which is a natural mineral, fiberglass can be produced in various dimensions and is best suited to meet the required use.

Since 2002, the demand for fiberglass has been rapidly growing. Between 2002 and 2006 the production capacity increased dramatically at an annual growth rate of 33%. China is the main supplier of fiberglass, and provided 38.1% of the global fiberglass output in 2007. Despite this steady increase in production, the overall demand still exceeds the worldwide supply. In 2007 the global output of fiberglass was 4.2 t, while the demand was 4.5 million tons. By 2010 the fiberglass demand was estimated to be 5.68 million tons (China 2008).

Fiberglass is made from thin strands of glass, the basis of which is silica, SiO_2. These strands are produced through fusion at temperatures ranging from 1,000°C to 1,500°C, after which point they are filtered of the siliceous-based mixtures which contain earthy alkaline additives to improve their workability (Sertoli et al. 2000). Glass fibers and other MMVP products have a variety of uses (➋ *Tables 38.2* and ➋ *38.3*). Depending on their function, they can be made into wool or fibers. Glass wool is commonly used to reinforce polymer products and make heat and sound insulation. Glass fibers are used in the textile industry to make curtains and draperies. These thin fibers are friable and easily break into microscopic particles. Dust is made up of fragmented glass fibers and plastic particles, which are easily carried in the air due to their microscopic size, causing airborne diseases or dust mechanical irritation of the skin and lungs. Contact with the dust can lead to mild respiratory symptoms, itching, and eczema (Minamoto et al. 2002; Cusano and Mariano 2007).

Fiberglass is also used to make casts and dentures. Fiberglass casts require less maintenance than the plastic casts, so are the preferred material, and are excellent additives for dentures because it solidifies dental implants.

A variety of resins are added to assist in the various 'functions of the fiberglass, which can induce allergic contact dermatitis. Commonly used additives are listed in ➋ *Table 38.4.*

Fiberglass dermatitis occurs primarily in the workplace, and was first described in the 1940s by Sulzberger and Baer (1942). Exposure is almost impossible to avoid in the building industry and glass wool factories.

2 Production

As mentioned earlier, glass fibers are produced at extremely high temperatures ranging from 1,000°C to 1,500°C. Three methods are currently still in use

T. Rustemeyer, P. Elsner, S.M. John & H.I. Maibach (eds.), *Kanerva's Occupational Dermatology*,
DOI 10.1007/978-3-642-02035-3_38, © Springer-Verlag Berlin Heidelberg 2012

Table 38.1
Classification and mean diameter of MMVF (Modified from Stam-Westerveld 1995)

Classification	Material	Mean diameter (μm)
Glass filament	Glass fibers	6–25
Mineral wool	Glass wool	4–9
	Rock wool	4–6
	Slag wool	4–6
Refractory ceramic fibers	Ceramic fibers	2.5–4
Fibers for special purposes	Glass fibers	0.2–1.5

Table 38.2
Uses of MMVF (Adapted from Stam-Westerveld 1995)

Classification	Uses
Glass filament	Textiles
	Reinforcement of plastics, cement, papers, and roofing materials
Mineral wool	Thermal insulation
	Acoustic insulation
	Fire protection
	Horticultural growing media
Refractory ceramic fibers	High temperature insulation
Fibers for special purposes (textile fibers)	Aircraft insulation
	Spacecraft insulation
	Filtration applications
	Curtains

Table 38.3
Uses of fiberglass (Adapted from Sertoli et al. 2000)

Use	Type	Product
Acoustic insulators	Glass wool	Used for the internal setting of public buildings, usually in the form of panels
Thermal insulators	Glass wool	Mattresses
		Felts
		Fiberglass tissues
		Insulation for water pipes, stoves, under-roof coverings in houses with wave-form ceiling boards
		Aircraft industry
		Printed circuit boards (PRCB)
Electrical insulators	Glass fibers	Insulation of motors
		Insulation of wires
		Insulation of electric cables
Reinforcing material	Glass fibers/wools with polyester, epoxy and melaminic resins	Reinforced plastic
		Used in the aircraft, automotive, naval and railway industries to make doors, hulls, boards etc.
		Sportswear
		Printed material
Filtering material	Glass fibers	Shaping tissues for air filters, gas filters and liquid filters for chemistry labs, food and drunk industries
		Air filters for private and public air circulating systems

for the production of glass fibers: centrifugation, blowing with hot gasses, and thinning by flame (Sertoli et al. 2000).

2.1 Centrifugation

Special rotating drums are utilized to churn the vitreous mixture. As the mixture exits the furnace, it is melted at high temperatures and percolates through small holes in the shape of the primary filaments, which are then thinned by a high-pressure fluid flux. This enables fibers to maintain a diameter between 6 and 7 μm (Sertoli et al. 2000) (➋ *Fig. 38.1*).

2.2 Blowing Through Hot Gases

This technique is similar to centrifugation, but instead of exiting through a rotating drum, the melted magma exits by gravity out of the special crucible. In this method a gaseous jet is used, instead of a fluid jet, to thin the fibers to a diameter of 15 μm (Sertoli et al. 2000). This method produces more fiberglass dusts due to the blowing process, which can lead to respiratory problems. These effects are discussed later.

Table 38.4
Resins used with fiberglass leading to ACD (Adapted from Björnberg 1985)

Resin
Epoxy resin
Phenyl-formaldehyde resin
Polyvinyl acetate
Silicones
Urea
Starch
Ammonium hydroxide
Mineral oil
Dyes

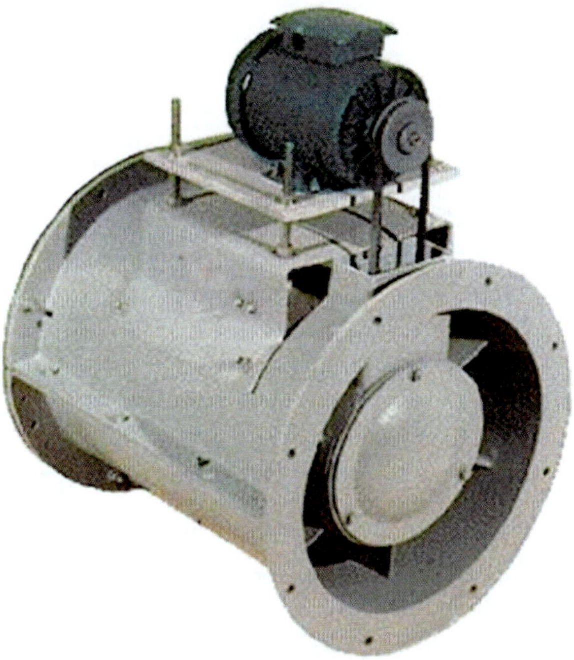

Fig. 38.1
Fiberglass inline centrifugal blower (http://www.troymfg.com/fans/blow_inline.html)

2.3 Thinning by Flame

In this technique, after the vitreous substance is thinned into the primary filaments, it is transferred to an inner combustible chamber where high-speed gas jets thin the filaments to 1 μm or less in diameter using high temperatures. The length of this continuous filament is 10 cm at most. After this process of thinning the glass, the fibers are treated with different resins to bind, protect, and lubricate the fiberglass, especially if it is to be used for reinforced plastics (Sertoli et al. 2000).

After this process is complete, the fiberglass is reinforced with resins. Glass wool is produced by spinning a vitreous mixture into wool and is used in acoustic and heat insulation (*Tables 38.2* and *38.3*) with a maximum operating temperature of 450°C (Sertoli et al. 1992).

3 Pathogenesis

The fiberglass is not only a primary irritant, but may also contain a sensitizer. Because of this it can induce either an irritant contact dermatitis (ICD) or an allergic contact dermatitis (ACD). It is mainly transmitted directly, but because of its small size and ease of breakage, it often travels airborne to lead to cutaneous and respiratory problems. Atopic patients have been specified as easier targets for the effects of fiberglass.

3.1 Irritant Contact Dermatitis (ICD)

Since glass itself is chemically inert, the dermatitis is actually due to the fiberglass fragments breaking through the epidermis, leading to direct microtrauma. The severity of the irritant is inversely proportional to length and directly proportional to the diameter of the fiber. It has been reported that irritation is mainly caused with fibers exceeding 4.5 μm (Stam-Westerveld 1995; Hogan 2008). These microscopic fibers penetrate through the stratum corneum, leading to epidermal cellular changes and cytokine release (Hogan 2008). The particles can be transferred to the worker by direct contact with the fiberglass, contact with contaminated surfaces, contact with garment embedded with fibers, indirect contact with fiber dust on the skin, and inhalation of the fiber dust. The clinical appearance of ICD resembles other eczematous reactions and is almost indistinguishable from ACD (Frosch and John 2006).

3.1.1 Acute

Acute ICD elicits keratinocytic changes that vary based on the irritating substance.

3.1.2 Chronic

Chronic ICD is also referred to as "cumulative insult dermatitis" and by definition persists for a considerable time period with a minimum of 6 weeks (Frosch and John 2006). Histologically the keratinocytic changes have been described as one of hyperkeratosis with areas of parakeratosis, moderate to marked acanthosis and elongation of the rete ridges, with increased numbers of Langerhans cells in the epidermis and dermis (Willis 1996). The ICD is usually aggravated by hand washing with water, which directly disrupts the stratum corneum lipid lamellar bilayers (Frosch and John 2006). Fiberglass rarely causes a chronic ICD due to hardening of the skin.

3.2 Allergic Contact Dermatitis (ACD)

Sensitization causes an ACD reaction, which is not directly caused by the fiberglass trauma, but is a response to the body's sensitization to resins and additives in the fiberglass (➋ *Table 38.4*). The most common causes of ACD are cobalt, peroxides, para-tertiary butyl catechol (PTBC) and unsaturated polyester (UP) base resin which are commonly used in the production of fiberglass-reinforced plastic (Minamoto et al. 2002). As opposed to ICD, ACD may not present with symptoms until at least the second exposure, after the Langerhans cells have migrated and matured. The initial sensitization takes 10–14 days, after which a subsequent exposure can produce a response in several hours or days (Hogan and May 2007; Hogan 2008). Trace amounts of contaminants such as arsenic, mercury, lead, or cadmium can be found in fiberglass and rock wool insulation (Adams 1999).

3.2.1 Patch Testing

Patch testing has shown that the irritation caused by fiber glass and glass wool is transient in nature and is directly related to the diameter of the fiber (Stam-Westerveld 1995). The histology of the patch test shows nonspecific changes due to minor trauma and features of eczema. In a study of 410 patients with chronic eczematous dermatitis reported by Rietschel, it was established that atopic patients were just as likely to have allergic contact dermatitis as nonatopic patients and that they would also benefit from patch testing. Also, atopic dermatitis patients had significantly more positive patch tests (2.7 vs. 2.0) than nonatopic dermatitis patients.

Patch testing done on 66 fiberglass spinners in Germany showed epoxy resin to be the most common allergen in 54% of the workers (Cronin 1980). A negative patch test to epoxy resin does not exclude the resin product as the cause of the allergic dermatitis. There may be a different epoxy resin in the product, or another compound in the resin such as dyes, fillers, plasticizers, or the hardener that could be causing the allergy. In a PRCB factory, 19 workers were tested, and 6 were positive in a patch test for epoxy resin (Sertoli et al. 2000). Also, in a ski factory where the plastics were fiberglass reinforced, 6 out of 22 workers presented with sensitization to epoxy, and all had dermatitis on the back of their hands (Jolanki 1996). Conversely, many patients test positively to epoxy resin in patch testing without having a history of contact (Andersen et al. 1992). This can be due to exposure to uncured resin in common plastic products on a daily basis. Another resin to produce a positive patch test was discovered in a case by Kalimo et al. A 46-year-old glass wool delivery truck driver in Finland had a positive patch test to p-tert-butylphenol-formaldehyde resin after presenting with loss of voice (1980).

3.2.2 Rubbing Tests

This test has been used to establish the diameters and lengths at which the MMVF is most irritating. Assessment of the reaction can be analyzed using laser Doppler flowmetry and erythema scores. Studies using this test have established that the smaller diameter fibers (less than 4.5 μm) are less irritating to the skin (Stam-Westerveld et al. 1993).

3.2.3 Resins

Epoxy Resin

Epoxy resins are used daily as additives in various materials to act as an adhesive. Epoxy resins are not alone in the materials they harden. They are combined with fillers, pigments, plasticizers, reactive diluents, and solvents, which are all mixed together with a hardening agent to cure the resin. The higher the molecular weight of the epoxy resin, the less sensitizing the compound is. After hardening, the cured resins are less sensitizing, but hardened resins are known to contain some uncured molecules which lead to sensitization (Andersen et al. 1992).

One of the most common routes of epoxy resin sensitization is the epoxy resin used in fiberglass. This combination produces strong sheets with many uses, such as hulls for boats and ships and electrical insulation (Andersen et al. 1992). Another common use for the combination of epoxy resin and fiberglass is in the production of printed circuit boards (PRCB). In this, the

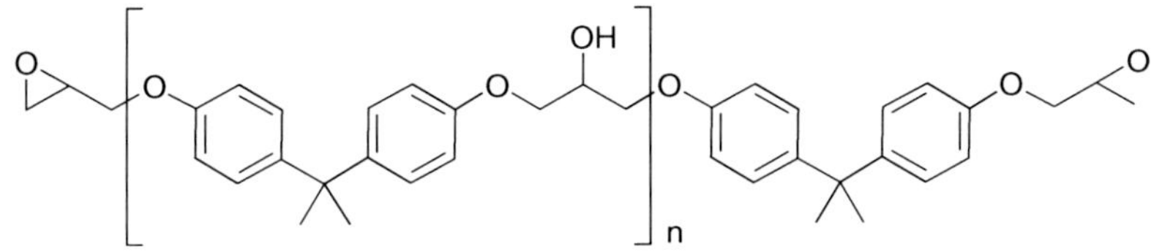

◘ Fig. 38.2
Epoxy resin

fire-proof core made up of fiberglass is soaked in brominated epoxy resin and wrapped in an outer layer of copper sheets (Wang et al. 1993). In the production of skis, plastic sheets that are reinforced with glass fibers are laminated with sheets in epoxy resins (Jolanki et al. 1996) (➋ *Fig. 38.2*).

p-tert-Butylphenol-formaldehyde Resin (PTBP)
PTBP is a very adhesive substance which is durable and pliable, and has good strength and high temperatures. Because of its pliability it is mainly utilized as an adhesive or glue in the manufacturing of rubber shoes and leather goods, neoprene adhesives and glues for furniture and auto upholstery. It is also used for construction materials, such as laminated floors, and in the production of fiberglass and mineral fiber insulation. It acts as a modifier in resin manufacturing (Andersen et al. 1992).

In the case mentioned earlier studied by Kalimo et al., a 46-year-old truck driver had been loading and delivering glass wool rolls used for thermal insulation and air filters since 1972. He developed aphonia without any cutaneous symptoms and tested positive for both a type 1 and delayed type 4 hypersensitivity reactions to PTBP resin. Sixty minutes after patch test application, an urticarial reaction was seen, and after 3 days a delayed type 4 reaction also developed (Rietschel and Fowler 2008) (➋ *Fig. 38.3*).

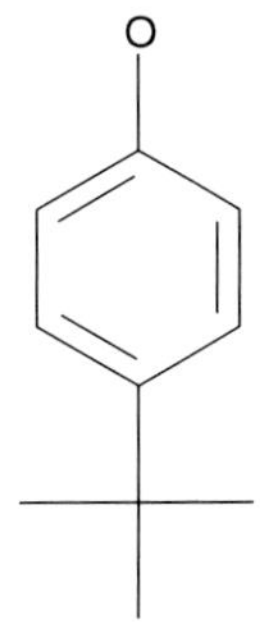

◘ Fig. 38.3
PTBP

3.3 Airborne Contact Dermatitis

Any fibrous material can give rise to an airborne contact dermatitis when it is circulated in the work place. Glass fiber, rock wool, and grain dust are examples of some fibrous materials that can lead to mechanical dermatitis. These dusts impregnate themselves in the fabric of clothing and accumulate in skin folds (Veien 1992). These areas, for example, the eyelids and neck (beside the shirt line), are irritated by friction and can sometimes mimic photo contact dermatitis.

Airborne contact dermatitis that affects the lung has been correlated with the length and diameter of the glass fiber. The hazard is inversely proportional to the diameter and length. Fibers with a length between 5 pm and 80 μm with a diameter less than 3 μm can reach the peripheral areas of the lung to create a potential bronchopneumopathy hazard (Sertoli et al. 2000).

3.4 Atopic Dermatitis

The cause of atopic dermatitis (AD) has yet to be firmly established. The "hygiene hypothesis" attributes the sensitivity to reduced microbial exposure in childhood, which helps to explain why people from well-developed countries are more prone to AD. The allergens that are most important to AD patients are aeroallergens and food allergens in children (Darsow and Ring 2003). The airborne spread of fiberglass dusts particles puts AD patients at a heightened risk. The estimated prevalence of AD is 10–30%, which is imprecise due to the disagreement between physicians about criteria to make a firm diagnosis. A set of criteria that can be agreed upon is the presence of atopy, pruritus, eczema, and altered vascular reactivity (Beltrani and Boguneiwicz 2003). It can also be loosely defined as a susceptibility to start an itch and occurs when usually harmless substances in the stratum corneum meet and react with specific circulating antibodies, presumably

IgE (Rietschel and Fowler 2008). It has been established that some patients with AD have elevated levels of IgE in their serum which may correlate with the disease severity. One proposed hypothesis reported by Darsow and Ring states that Langerhans cells bind to and present "immediate-type" allergens, which then penetrate the impaired epidermal barrier in AD patients (2003). Antigen-presenting cells in both epidermis and dermis express IgE on their surface significantly more than patients with irritant contact dermatitis or allergic contact dermatitis. There is some evidence that substances from the horny layer of skin may induce reactions in people with atopic skin. Such substances include skin's own constituents, soil, and products of microorganisms that colonize the skin (e.g., staphylococci) (Rietschel and Fowler 2008). It has been observed that there is an inverse relationship related to the clinical severity of atopic dermatitis and contact sensitization in atopic dermatitis (Rietschel and Fowler 2008). A female predominance has been reported in atopic patients. In a study reported by Rietschel and Fowler, out of 74 atopic dermatitis patients with persistent facial dermatitis, 39.2% had one or more positive patch test, while 31 out of the 40 positive tests were females (2008).

Atopic patients have been advised in the past to not work with glass fibers because of a low threshold for itch, and an increased risk of being affected by the fiberglass (Adams 1999). Atopic eczema renders skin vulnerable to nonspecific irritants such as dust and dander, so when faced with an abrasive irritant such as fiberglass, it is understandable as to why an atopic individual would have a heightened reaction. This decreased pruritic threshold is attributed to the innate perception of mild mechanical stimulation as itch instead of as touch. Once the scratch has been itched, the surrounding skin has increased liability to react to light stimuli with an itch sensation – a phenomenon called allokinesis (Beltrani and Boguneiwicz 2003). A study done by Björnberg showed that rubbing tests may be a reliable way to determine which workers are more sensitive to glass fiber–induced itching. Despite this, a history of itching from synthetic textile fibers, wool, and hot baths was of no value to predicting itching from fiberglass (1985).

Studies reported by Cronin have shown that patients with a history of irritant contact dermatitis have a high chance of reoccurrence from a new irritant. This has led to the understanding that some people are predisposed to irritant contact dermatitis, or AD, and despite job changes and different chemical exposures, the dermatitis is likely to recur. Because of this, not all irritant hand eczemas heal when the precipitating factor is removed (1992).

4 Clinical Picture

Initial symptoms are most commonly intense pruritus and tingling at the site of exposure and skin folds. Skin lesions are not always initially present, but can appear within hours or days. The characteristic dermatitis appears as pinpoint-sized erythematous papules, which are often follicular (Björnberg 1985; Stam-Westerveld 1995). It appears like papular urticaria without papules. Irritation is most common on the hands, forearms, face, neck, and flexural areas where clothing rubs. Other skin lesions can appear as purpura, urticaria, petechiae, erosions, nummular eczema, and rarely paronychia due to penetration of glass spicules beneath the nail fold (Björnberg 1985; Stam-Westerveld 1995). The fragments and dust can penetrate clothing, so it is not uncommon for the dermatitis to be in a covered area. With continued irritation, secondary changes may occur. These consist of lichenification, bacterial infections, and excoriations (Björnberg 1985; Stam-Westerveld 1995). When present, an excoriated folliculitis is most commonly located on the arms, face, neck, and sometimes legs (Sertoli et al. 1992). Glass fibers and resins may less commonly penetrate leather footwear leading to maceration and dermatitis of the feet (Rietschel and Fowler 2008).

Different environmental changes can aggravate the symptoms of the dermatitis. High temperatures and humidity in the summer or relative low humidity in the winter can make diagnosis more difficult. The humidity is protective in the fact that it prevents the airborne mechanism from being started up, while also supporting the spontaneous elimination of fibers by gravity (Sertoli et al. 2000).

The irritant dermatitis may appear "contagious," as the fibers can be transferred to family members by mixing laundry. This dermatitis is most likely due to large glass fibers. This has been reported as a familial fiberglass microepidemic and appears clinically as scabies when the workers' clothes are mixed with underwear (Stam-Westerveld 1995).

In one case, a 36-year-old woman and her husband had been treated for scabies for 3 months without results. The woman had a mild presentation with a pruritus follicular eruption, while the husband presented more similarly to scabies with marked folliculitis, popular urticaria, and linear erosions in the creases. It was soon established that the husband had recently started a job at a fiberglass factory, and had been washing his work clothes at home with his wife's. To determine if this was the culprit, the husband was instructed to apply talcum powder to his body every day before he put on his work clothes, and to wash his clothing separately from his wife's. One week after these changes were made, the eruption on both the husband and wife completely subsided (Rietschel and Fowler 2008). Scabies is caused by *Sarcoptes scabiei*, var. hominis, and is distributed bilaterally on the wrists, elbows, ankles, and feet. The lesion is indentified by the primary burrow dug where the female mite breaks through the skin and tunnels through the corneum, leaving a gray straight line. The mite usually moves toward the extremities and ends the tunnel with a blister (Sertoli et al. 2000). Itching is the most common symptom, which is more intense at night, as opposed to fiberglass dermatitis which is pruritic throughout the day. Main differentiating features between scabies and fiberglass dermatitis is the distribution of the lesions, the observation of the mite under the microscope after scrapping the skin, and the type of itching that it induces. Also with scabies pruritus, once the itch is treated, it rarely relapses. In fiberglass dermatitis, the pruritus may improve when the irritant is removed, but quickly relapses when reintroduced.

Clothing purpura has been reported and presented as petechial and prupuric eruptions caused by woolen garments such as underwear and from the water-soluble formaldehyde urea finish applied to the woolen khaki skirts worn by British soldiers (Rietschel and Fowler 2008). Many other problems can present similarly to fiberglass dermatitis and are listed in ➋ *Table 38.5.*

◘ Table 38.5

Differential diagnosis with fiberglass dermatitis (Modified from Sertoli et al. 2000)

By external cause
Pediculosis
Swimmers prurigo
Phytodermatitis by thorns
Prurigo by irritant solid airborne particles
Actinic prurigo
Eczema prurigo
Improper or excessive use of detergents
Side effects of drugs
By internal cause
Pruritus senilis
Psychosomatic pruritus
Biliary stasis
Diabetes mellitus
Uremia
Pregnancy (PUPP)
Dysthyroidisms
Cancers
Hodgkin's disease or chronic leukemias
Myeloma

PUPP "pruritic urticarial papules and plaques of pregnancy." This is an uncommon cause of third trimester itching with a polymorphous rash

The transmission of fiberglass in the laundry is not limited to workers' clothing. There have been reports of family outbreaks of fiberglass dermatitis when fiberglass curtains were washed with the clothes (Cronin 1980). Laundry mats are often utilized by the public to wash fiberglass curtains, so caution must be exercised when using one for family clothing. Because of this problem, the Department of National Health and Welfare recommended for curtains containing fiberglass to not be washed in the same laundry machine as clothing (National Institute of Occupational Safety and Health 1977). The proper way to wash fiberglass curtains or fiberglass-laden clothing is with rubber gloves separately in a tub or basin that can be rinsed thoroughly after use (Rietschel and Fowler 2008).

Other rare cases of fiberglass dermatitis have been reported, and a few examples are listed:

- An 8-year-old girl experienced chronic ICD on the posterior thighs from sitting in fiberglass reinforced plastic chairs at school (Cronin 1980).
- A 6-year-old girl came into contact with glass fiber when playing in a barn, leading to the formation of nodules (Sertoli et al. 1992).
- A 37-year-old man experienced an intense pruritic eruption on his forearms after crawling through an insulated attic (Chen et al. 2000).
- Two waitresses in contact with serving trays in a restaurant (Cusano and Mariano 2007).
- A 22-year-old man working in a scrap yard removing heating pipes (Bordel-Gómez and Miranda-Romero 2008).
- A fiberglass epidemic occurred in Italy and was reported by Cusano and Mariano. Ten 8- to 9-year-old children and two female teachers experienced an acute skin itching eruption with excoriated follicular papules and mild respiratory symptoms after being exposed for 10 months to fiberglass felt from a hole kicked in the wall of the classroom. History of atopy was only present in one child (2007).
- The penetration of glass fragments into the hands of employees causing glass-hand syndrome which was first reported by Grzegorczyk in 1982. In this syndrome, there is a painful sensation in the hands,

without any skin lesions. These glass fragments can be visualized by x-rays and computed axial tomography. The fragments were shown to have penetrated into the hands reaching the subcutis among the tendons and the interossei (Sertoli et al. 2000).

Exposure to fiberglass has been associated with various cancers. Asbestos is a well-established occupational carcinogen, and because of the similarities, a relationship of MMVF and cancer has been suspected. In the 1950s a timeline of lung cancer and mesothelioma caused by asbestos was determined. It was established that the average latency interval for lung cancer caused by chronic asbestos exposure was 20 years, and 25–50 years for mesothelioma (Warheit et al. 2001). It was thought in the past that MMVFs were nonrespirable because they are generally manufactured as a continuous filament and the diameters usually exceeded 3 μm. They were thought to be too large to penetrate the distal lung, and if inhaled they would be trapped in the upper lung (Warheit et al. 2001). \It has since been determined that in the production of fiberglass, small fractions of airborne fibers and dusts can be generated during the blowing or extruding process. These particles can travel into the alveoli to induce an airborne bronchopneumopathy. Toxicological research done on synthetic vitreous fibers (fiberglass, mineral wool and refractory fiber) has shown that the pulmonary effects of these dusts are directly related to the fiber dose in the lung over time and have been generally grouped into the three "Ds": (a) Dose – the number of fibers deposited in the distal lung over time. (b) Dimension – the thinner fibers are more respirable, while the longer fibers are more toxic to the pulmonary cells. The thinner the fibers are, the more efficiently they deposit in the lower lungs. (c) Durability – the severity is related to the biopersistance, which is related to the fiber length and inversely related to the dissolution and fragmentation rates (Warheit et al. 2001). The dusts that can irritate the lung are too small to cause any dermatologic symptoms. As stated earlier, cutaneous manifestations of fiberglass irritation are not apparent until the fiberglass is 4.5 μm or larger.

A study done on rats and hamsters by McConnell showed that all vitreous fibers stimulate an inflammatory response, which is characterized by the increase in the number of pulmonary macrophages at the level of the terminal bronchioles and proximal alveoli (1994). The only vitreous fiber in this study to show carcinogenic activity was refractory ceramic fibers, which produced a dose-related increase in primary lung neoplasms and mesotheliomas (McConnell 1994).

Table 38.6
Mortality by selective causes for plant workers, 1955–1997 (Adapted from Shannon et al. 2005)

	SMR
All cancers	115
Lung cancer	163[a]
Respiratory diseases	119
Kidney cancer	146
Ischemic heart disease	81

SMR = (observed number of deaths/expected number of deaths) × 100

[a]$P < 0.05$

A follow-up cohort study done in Ontario of 2557 fiberglass workers between 1955 and 1997 showed a significant increase in lung cancer deaths, with a nonsignificant increase in chronic obstructive pulmonary disease and bronchitis. The study focused on three groups of workers: workers only in the plant (*Table 38.6*), workers only in the office, and workers with mixed exposures. There were slightly more respiratory disease deaths than expected, and the standardized mortality ratio (SMR) was lower for office workers for all selective causes. The study also focused on establishing a relationship between the duration of employment and the time since first employment (TSFE). Although it seems there would be correlation, there was no clear pattern for mortality and incidence in relation to duration of employment and TSFE (Shannon et al 2005). Buchanich et al. established in a study that the males and females working in fiberglass factories had higher rates of ever smoking than the corresponding general populations of the USA (2001). This differentiating factor could further explain the reasoning behind the elevated levels of respiratory system cancers that are found in these workers.

Shannon et al. also found that the number of kidney cancers was nearly double than expected. Literature reviewed by Goldsmith and Goldsmith (1993) concluded that silica was likely to be the cause of the excess renal diseases in fiberglass workers. Fiberglass can be silica based, which gives it more dexterity in production. Silica has no real melting point, but has a softening point at 2,000°C at which point the silica-based fiberglass can be extruded out into thin strands suitable for textile processing (Loewenstein 1973). Thus the finding of increased renal cancer is unlikely to be related directly to the glass fibers (Shannon et al. 2005). Despite these findings, in 2002 the International Agency for Research on

Cancer classified glass and mineral fibers as class 3, which is not classifiable as to carcinogenicity to humans. They established this based on insufficient evidence in humans and limited evidence in experimental animals (Pintos et al. 2008). Two subsequent studies published in 2008 from Canada and 2009 from Italy showed no evidence that continuous glass filament workers experience a significant increased risk of cancer (Pintos et al. 2008; Pira et al. 2009).

A strong relationship between asbestos and mesothelioma has been well established. Because of this relationship, and the similarities between asbestos and MMVFs, the mortality rate from mesothelioma has been studied by Marsh et al. in a group of MMVF factory workers. After reviewing data from a 1992 follow-up study of 32,110 fiberglass workers it was concluded that the overall mortality risk for malignant mesothelioma was not elevated in this cohort (2001).

Some other symptoms of fiberglass exposure are dry hacking cough, sore throat or blood in the sputum, bloody nose, persistent sinusitis and rhinitis, persistent respiratory infections; headaches; nausea; dizziness; insomnia; irritability; depression; asthma-like breathing attacks or constant wheezing; allergy-like symptoms that do not respond to allergy treatment; reactive airway disease; swollen, red, watery infected eyes; and extreme sensitivity to everyday amounts of ambient pollutants. Many of these symptoms overlap with symptoms of allergies, common cold, asthma, and conjunctivitis, making the diagnosis difficult.

5 Hardening

In most cases, after 1–4 weeks of exposure, workers may become unaffected by the irritant, or hardened, allowing individuals to continue with their work. The term "hardening" is mainly in regards to the itching, not the visible dermatitis, and has been defined by some as an adaptation of the skin to the cause of the ICD (Björnberg 1985; Watkins and Maibach 2009). After hardening, the skin is less vulnerable to the secondary effects of the dermatitis and less prone to secondary infection. Because of this, most workers do not request to be transferred after experiencing an acute ICD since the symptoms disappear without any consequences (Sertoli et al. 2000). The gross appearance of hardened skin has been described in some experimental models as having a slight sheen and glossy appearance with a mild scale. Upon manipulation it has been documented to show a decrease in skin elasticity (Watkins and Maibach 2009). This adaptive measure is not permanent though, as a break in exposure for more than 4 weeks will result in the same irritant response on reintroduction of the fiberglass (Stam-Westerveld 1995; van der Valk 1996).

The mechanism of hardening is not completely understood, most likely because research usually does not focus on mechanisms of nondisease or illnesses that self-resolve. Hardening was first described in 1982 by Samuel, who showed that repeated exposure of rabbit ears to croton oil resulted in decreased levels of inflammatory response (Watkins and Maibach 2009). Since then the adaptive effects of hardening have been studied on humans. Theories have been formulated to determine the cause of the hardening. One theory pertains to altered barrier function, which holds that morphological changes in skin structure and composition decreases irritant access to skin (Watkins and Maibach 2009). On histological exam of accommodated skin, it is shown to have a thicker layer of stratum granulosum. It was reported by Van der Valk and Maibach that the thickening of the horny layer was directly proportional to a decrease in transepidermal water loss (TEWL), which is a method of estimating skin water barrier function. TEWL fluctuates throughout the evolution of hardening. Upon initial exposure to the irritant, the TEWL increases. With chronic irritation, the TEWL subsequently decreases with emergence of hardening (Watkins and Maibach 2009). There have also been reports of altered lipid composition in the stratum corneum layer, which could be a contributing factor to the accommodation effect of hardening (Watkins and Maibach 2009).

Hardening has also been described to produce global effects of cutaneous adaptation. In this process, an individual can be exposed to the irritant, or fiberglass, on their hands and become "hardened." When the fiberglass is introduced after the initial hardening to another area of their body, i.e., their feet, there is no irritant reaction because of the global adaptation. The studies done on this provide evidence that chronic exposure to an irritant in low doses can induce a globally hyporeactive state (Watkins and Maibach 2009). A summary of the alterations in hardened skin is provided in ➋ *Table 38.7.*

Less commonly a worker may not adapt to the irritant, leading to chronic ICD. This can lead to emotional, physical, and financial distress for affected individuals (Watkins and Maibach 2009). Chronic ICD can appear as erythematous or dry, scaly, and fissured skin, usually on the hands, and is difficult to treat. The only cure is to withdraw exposure to the irritating substance.

Table 38.7
Alterations in hardened skin (Modified table from Watkins and Maibach 2009)

Alteration	Experimental findings
Physical changes	Thicker stratum granulosum; hyperkeratotic stratum corneum
Skin permeability changes	Adapted skin is more permeable to irritants; accommodated skin is more erythematous after irritant exposure versus non-accommodated skin
Systemic changes	Locally induced hardening can alter skin's response on re-exposure to irritant systemically in previously unexposed areas
Immunologic changes	Localized hardening is accompanied by changes in the expression of various inflammatory mediators and markers

6 Histopathology

6.1 Biopsy

If fiberglass dermatitis is suspected, a biopsy of the irritated skin can aide in the diagnosis. The fragments produce microtrauma and perforate the skin. Under the microscope, the fiberglass particles show up as birefringent fragments in the cornified layer of the skin (Bordel-Gómez and Miranda-Romero 2008). The histopathology induced by glass fiber dermatitis is indistinguishable to that of rock wool dermatitis. This has been described by Björnberg to display the following features: subcorneal vesicles containing neutrophils, sometimes developing into superficial erosions; spongiosis with mononuclear-polynuclear infiltrate in the epidermis; and a perivascular lymphocytic infiltration in the dermis (Björnberg 1985).

The lesions are almost equal to those produced by contact eczema, which present with spongiosis, sometimes diastasis at the basal layer, and lymphocytic perivascular and perifollicular infiltrate. The lesions can sometimes persist into a foreign body granuloma due to the continuous stimulation from the penetration (Sertoli et al. 2000).

6.2 Alternative Methods

Alternatively, particles may be observed through skin stripping or skin scraping. In skin stripping, which can also be used as a treatment, tape is applied to the irritated area and peeled away. It is then mounted on a glass slide, and visualized under polarized light microscopy. If fiberglass is the cause of the dermatitis, the tape would show transparent fine fragments of glass. The tape stripping method can also be used to demonstrate the presence of fiberglass fragments on clothing.

With skin scraping, the sample is prepared with one or two drops of potassium hydroxide at 20% and visualized microscopically to look for the presence of fibers in the horny layer of the epidermis (Stam-Westerveld 1995). Also when the presence of fibers is suspected in tissue, an x-ray should be taken to confirm the results of the biopsy (Sertoli et al. 1992).

7 Treatment

Treatment of acute fiberglass dermatitis is primarily symptomatic. Oral antihistamines or low-power corticosteroids can be applied, along with antibiotics to eradicate any overlapping bacterial infection. Fibers can be removed from the skin to relieve irritation by using scotch tape or plumbers' duct tape and peeling it away (Sertoli et al. 2000).

The only way to successfully treat chronic ICD is to adhere to a strict avoidance of the irritating substance, in this case, fiberglass. This is not a practical treatment in most cases, as this is how the workers earn their livelihood. Because of this, the best treatment is to avoid excessive contact with water, aggressive cleaning materials and abrasives, and use topical emollients until the skin heals. This in combination with protective skin practices will help in the alleviation and avoidance of any future ICD outbreaks (van der Valk 1996). Topical emollients should contain no irritating ingredients, and must contain enough fatty substances to hydrate the skin. Topical corticosteroid therapy is controversial, as it is known to thin the epidermis and make it more vulnerable to trauma. Tar is often known for its anti-eczematous effect on the hands, but is undesirable due to the appearance and smell. This can be masked by wearing cotton gloves (van der Valk 1996).

8 Prevention

Workers in direct contact with fiberglass and the resins should wear gloves, long sleeves, and loose-fitting clothes. Any clothing that is exposed to fiberglass should be washed separately to avoid transferring the fibers to other clothes. To avoid transfer to family members, the washing machine should be wiped out after each washing, or run through an extra cycle to clean out all the fibers. Also, workers should shower right after work to prevent the fibers from being rubbed in (Stam-Westerveld 1995).

Preventative measures can be taken by the workplace to minimize exposure to fiberglass by frequent cleaning of the floor and work surfaces to decrease the amount of indirect dust exposure. Direct contact can be minimized by decreasing the amount of hands on exposure that workers have with the fiberglass. This can be done by making some of the machines a closed cycle, so that the transfers are done automatically. Also, when felts are cut, hand tools would be more ergonomic than power-driven tools, because they would release less fibers and powders (Sertoli et al. 2000). Air quality can be improved by increasing ventilation and adding filters and providing masks. Latent dermatitis can be avoided by providing protective clothing that can be left at work and washed, which would also help in avoiding fiberglass exposure to the family, and providing a shower room to allow the worker to rinse off the fiber dust as soon as possible. Washable leather gloves could also be provided, which are less permeable to the fibers (Schwartz et al. 1947). When spraying insulation containing fiberglass, the wet method would produce less airborne contact than the dry method (Sertoli et al. 2000). The removal of non-resined materials is especially risky and should be done with the material in humidified conditions with adequate ventilation of the rooms.

Exposure in noncommercial buildings can be kept under control by ensuring that there are no holes in the walls and by making sure to wear appropriate clothing while crawling in a fiberglass attic.

These are just a few suggestions that may be costly to implement, but will effectively save money due to less sick days and medical expenses. A study about workers compensation in Washington State showed that 9.1% of skin disorder claims, mainly contact dermatitis, resulted in more than 3 missed work days (Kaufman et al. 1998). The incidence of fiberglass dermatitis should not be underestimated, as an evaluation of 700 workers in the construction industry showed that 65% had skin lesions and/or subjective symptoms from contact with insulation wool (Björnberg 1985). Another study by Sertoli et al. surveyed employees directly exposed to fiberglass and concluded that 20.3% of employees directly exposed and 19.9% of employees indirectly exposed were affected by the fiberglass (2000).

Various protective creams and powders have been used in an attempt to protect against the irritant effect of fiberglass, but none have been of a measureable protective value. The ACD induced by resins can be prevented by barrier creams, mainly due to the fact that it reminds the patient to wash their hands before eating. Because of this, the allergens on the skin are removed (Chen et al. 2000).

References

Adams RM (1999) Appendix: job descriptions with their irritants and allergens: insulation workers. In: Occupational skin disease, 3rd edn. W.B. Saunders, Philadelphia

Andersen KE et al (1992) Allergens from the standard series: epoxy resin. In: Rycroft RJG et al (eds) Textbook of contact dermatitis. Springer, New York

Beltrani VS, Boguneiwicz M (2003) Atopic dermatitis. Dermatol Online J 9(2):1

Björnberg A (1985) Glass fiber dermatitis. In: The chronic effect of repeated mechanical trauma to the skin. Alan R. Liss, New York. Am J Ind Med 8: 395–400

Bordel-Gómez MT, Miranda-Romero A (2008) Fiberglass dermatitis: a report of 2 cases. Contact Dermatitis 59:120–122

Buchanich JM et al (2001) Historical cohort study of US man made citreous fiber production workers: V. Tobacco-smoking habits. J Occup Environ Med 43(9):793–802

Chen JY et al (2000) Irritant contact dermatitis secondary to fiberglass: an unusual presentation. Int J Dermatol 39:372–274

China Fiberglass Industry Report, Research in China. 2008. http://www.researchandmarkets.com/reports/662053/china_fiberglass_industry_report_2008#. Accessed 22 Nov 2011

Cronin E (1980) Clothing and textiles. In: Contact dermatitis. Churchill Livingstone, New York

Cronin E (1992) Hand eczema: contact dermatitis. In: Rycroft RJG et al (eds) Textbook of contact dermatitis. Springer, New York

Cusano F, Mariano M (2007) Fiberglass dermatitis microepidemic in a primary school. Contact Dermatitis 57:351–352

Darsow U, Ring J (2003) The atopy patch test in atopic dermatitis. In: Lachapelle JM, Maibach HI (eds) Patch testing prick testing – a practical guide. Springer, New York

Frosch PJ, John SM (2006) Clinical aspects of irritant contact dermatitis. In: Frosch PJ et al (eds) Contact dermatitis, 4th edn. Springer, New York

Goldsmith JR, Goldsmith DR (1993) Fiberglass or silica exposure and increased nephritis or ESRD (end-stage renal disease). Am J Ind Med 28:873–881

Hogan DJ (2008) Contact dermatitis, Irritant. eMedicine

Hogan DJ, May JM (2007) Contact dermatitis, Allergic. eMedicine http://emedicine.medscape.com/article/1049353-overview. Accessed 22 Nov 2011

Jolanki R et al (1996) Occupational dermatosis from exposure to epoxy resin compounds in a ski factory. Contact Dermatitis 34:390–394

Jolanki R et al (2002) Occupational irritant contact dermatitis from synthetic mineral fibers according to Finnish statistics. Contact Dermatitis 47:329–333

Kalimo K et al (1980) Immediate and delayed type reactions to formaldehyde resin in glass wool. Contact Dermatitis 6(7):496

Kaufman JD et al (1998) Occupational skin diseases in Washington State, 1989 Through 1993: using workers' compensation data to identify cutaneous hazards. Am J Public Health 88(7):1047–1051

Loewenstein KL (1973) The manufacturing technology of continuous glass fibers. Elsevier, New York, pp 2–94

Marsh GM et al (2001) Historical cohort study of US man-made vitreous fiber production workers: II. Mortality from mesothelioma. J Occup Environ Med 43(9):757–766

McConnell EE (1994) Synthetic vitreous fibers—inhalation studies. Regul Toxicol Pharmacol 20(3 Pt. 2):S22–S34

Minamoto K et al (2002) Occupational dermatoses among fiberglass-reinforced plastics factory workers. Contact Dermatitis 46:339–347

Pintos J et al (2008) Occupational exposure to asbestos and man-made vitreous fibers, and risk of lung cancer: evidence from two case–control studies in Montreal, Canada. J Occup Environ Med 50(11):1273–1281

Pira E et al (2009) Cancer mortality in a cohort of continuous glass filament workers. J Occup Environ Med 51(2):239–242

Rietschel RL, Fowler JF (2008a) Noneczematous contact dermatitis. In: Fisher's contact dermatitis, 6th edn. BC Decker, Hamilton

Rietschel RL, Fowler JF (2008b) Plastics, adhesives, and synthetic resins. In: Fisher's contact dermatitis, 6th edn. BC Decker, Hamilton

Rietschel RL, Fowler JF (2008c) Role of age, sex, color of skin, and atopic status. In: Fisher's contact dermatitis, 6th edn. BC Decker, Hamilton

Schwartz L et al (1947) Dermatoses caused by resins and waxes. In: Occupational diseases of the skin, 2nd edn. Lea & Febiger, Philadelphia

Sertoli A et al (1992) Fiberglass dermatitis. Clin Dermatol 10(2):167–174

Sertoli A et al (2000) Fiberglass dermatitis. In: Kanerva L et al (eds) Handbook of occupational dermatology, 1st edn. Springer, Berlin

Shannon H et al (2005) Mortality and cancer incidence in Ontario glass fiber workers. Occup Med 55:528–534

Stam-Westerveld EB (1995) Man-made vitreous fibers: glass fiber and Rockwool dermatitis. In: van der Valk PGM, Maibach HI (eds) The irritant contact dermatitis syndrome. CRC Press, New York

Stam-Westerveld EB et al (1993) Rubbing test responses of the skin to man-made mineral fibers of different diameters. Contact Dermatitis 31(1):1–4

Sulzberger MB, Baer BL (1942) The effects of fiberglass on animal and human skin. Int Med 11:482–484

van der Valk PGM (1996) The treatment of irritant contact dermatitis. In: van der Valk PGM, Maibach HI (eds) The irritant contact dermatitis syndrome. CRC Press, New York

Veien NK (1992) Clinical features: airborne contact dermatitis. In: Rycroft RJG et al (eds) Textbook of contact dermatitis. Springer, New York

Wang BJ et al (1993) Fiberglass dermatitis: report of two cases. J Formos Med Assoc 92:755–758

Warheit DB et al (2001) Potential pulmonary effects of man-made organic fiber (MMOF) dusts. Crit Rev Toxicol 31(6):697–736

Watkins SA, Maibach HI (2009) The hardening phenomenon in irritant contact dermatitis: an interpretative update. Contact Dermatitis 60:123–130

Willis C (1996) The histopathology of irritant contact dermatitis. In: van der Valk PGM, Maibach HI (eds) The irritant contact dermatitis syndrome. CRC Press, New York

39 Drug Allergens

Andreas J. Bircher
Allergy Unit, Department of Dermatology, University Hospital, Basel, Switzerland

Core Messages

- Many drugs from very different drug classes and categories have been reported to elicit allergic contact dermatitis by direct or airborne exposure.
- Rarely, allergic-type reactions with urticaria or anaphylaxis have been observed.
- Employees in the development, production, and maintenance in the pharmaceutical industry and workers in health care are typically affected.
- Most drugs are haptens and therefore need to become reactive to be able to bind to protein to from a complete antigen.
- Some prodrugs and intermediate substances in the synthetisization process are highly reactive and more prone to become allergenic.

1 Introduction

With few exceptions, such as peptides and hormones, drugs and their precursors are typically low-molecular-weight compounds and, therefore, haptens. Some drugs, called prohaptens have to be metabolized to become reactive and therefore sensitizing. To build a complete antigen, they must bind to macromolecules, e.g., to human tissue or serum proteins. Some drugs are primarily reactive, while in others, reactive metabolites are only generated in vivo. Recently, the concept of prehaptens has been proposed, where a molecule, e.g., oxidizes to become a hapten (Lepoittevin 2006). For drugs, however, this is unusual and only feasible if they are inappropriately stored.

Oral administration of a drug is usually better tolerated and is typically associated with tolerance. However, particularly intermittent exposure or application by the epidermal, intradermal, subcutaneous, or by the inhalatory route, as it typically occurs in occupational settings, carries a higher risk of sensitization (Bircher 1996; Merk et al. 2007).

Occupationally related allergic reactions to drugs mainly occur in two groups of employees exposed in different settings. The first group involves workers of pharmaceutical and chemical companies occupied in the production of drugs; the second group consists of professionals using the final drugs in a therapeutic setting. The former includes chemists and laboratory technicians involved in the development of new agents, workers exposed during the manufacturing and synthetisization processes, technicians or cleaning staff employed in the maintenance of equipment, and employees involved in handling and packing the final products. This group may be exposed – directly or by airborne contact – to precursor substances, highly reactive intermediates, and the final drugs, as well as to other agents used in the synthesis, such as accelerators, catalysts, enzymes, etc., which may also act as allergens (Altomare et al. 1992; Sherertz 1994). The second group encompasses health-care workers, such as nurses, physiotherapists, physicians, dentists, pharmacists, masseurs, herbal therapists, veterinarians, animal caretakers, and farmers preparing or applying medicaments for animals. These particular occupations are discussed in depth in other respective chapters of this book.

Apart from drugs for topical use, where contact is possible during treatment of a patient, exposure to systemically applied agents, e.g., powdered substances from vials, may happen by negligence or accident and involves direct or airborne contact with the skin or the mucosae or takes place by inhalation or, rarely, by ingestion. Typical situations involving dust or nebulization exposure occur during the manufacturing of hand-compounded medications by pharmacists, during the preparation of animal feed in farmers, or in nurses crushing tablets or preparing lyophilized drugs for injection (Barbaud 2002). Some health professionals, such as dentists, physiotherapists, or masseurs directly apply the drug to the patient by hand, thus facilitating sensitization by repeated unprotected skin contact. Sometimes, a member of such an occupation needs pharmacotherapy himself and suffers from an adverse drug reaction, e.g., to carbamazepine, which, however, is not necessarily linked to his occupation (Altomare et al. 1992). Another occasionally overlooked way of exposure may happen by connubial contact (Newton and White 1987).

Typical clinical manifestations include allergic and irritant contact dermatitis, airborne dermatoses, photo-induced reactions (Bjorkner 1994), immunologic and non-immunologic contact urticaria, rhinoconjunctivitis,

T. Rustemeyer, P. Elsner, S.M. John & H.I. Maibach (eds.), *Kanerva's Occupational Dermatology*,
DOI 10.1007/978-3-642-02035-3_39,

Table 39.1
Selected drug allergens eliciting immediate-type skin symptoms on contact

Allergen	Symptom	References
Benzalkonium chloride	Urticaria, asthma	Bernstein et al. 1994
Cefotiam	Anaphylaxis	Miyahara et al. 1993; Tadokoro et al. 1994
Chloramine-T	Urticaria	Dooms-Goossens et al. 1983; Kanerva et al. 1997
Cisplatin	Urticaria	Schena et al. 1996
Labetalol	Anaphylaxis	Bause and Kugelman 1990
Levomepromazine	Urticaria	Johansson 1988
Mezlocillin	Urticaria	Keller and Schwanitz 1992
Penicillin	Urticaria	Rudzki and Rebandel 1985; Stejskal et al. 1986
Pentamidine isethionate	Urticaria	Belsito 1993
Piperacillin sodium	Urticaria, asthma	Moscato et al. 1995

asthma and, rarely, anaphylaxis (Bause and Kugelman 1990), or severe skin disorders, such as toxic epidermal necrolysis (Valsecchi et al. 1987). Irritant agents are numerous and may cause symptoms on the skin or the mucosal surfaces (Testud et al. 1994). Examples are potassium salts, chloroquine phosphate, ethylene oxide and, particularly, the cytostatic drugs. Usually, the exposed workers know the hazards of these substances, and preventive measures are used. Accidental contact, however, causes rapidly irritant or toxic skin damage in most or all exposed individuals. The causal relationship is easily recognized, and an extensive diagnostic work-up is often not necessary; therefore, such cases may be under-reported in the literature. However, patients with sensitization to a particular unusual compound are often published as single case reports and dominate the literature.

As a practical consequence of sensitization, an allergic individual must therefore meticulously avoid contact with the allergen or, in a more severe case, change the workplace or even his profession. In cases of drug allergens, a further problem may arise. Occupationally sensitized individuals may encounter their allergen in drug therapy (Bircher 1996). Topical treatment with the occupational allergen or with cross-reacting substances, e.g., the "caine group," may elicit contact dermatitis. Systemic exposure to an allergen, e.g., antibiotics to which the patient has been sensitized by epidermal contact may result in a flare-up of formerly affected sites; it may also result in systemic (hematogenous) contact dermatitis or the so-called Baboon syndrome (Menne et al. 1989) or SDRIFE (Häusermann et al. 2004). Therefore, the exact identification of a presumed occupational allergy and the offending allergens has implications beyond the scope of occupational safety. In this chapter, an overview on drugs and intermediate substances reported as occupational allergens is given (*Tables 39.1* and *39.2*).

1.1 Immediate-Type Reactions

These types of reactions include rhinoconjunctivitis, asthma, contact urticaria, and rarely, anaphylaxis (Belsito 1993). In some patients, urticaria and later eczema may be present, in analogy to protein contact dermatitis (Keller and Schwanitz 1992); patients may also have concomitant skin and respiratory symptoms (Stejskal et al. 1986; Moscato et al. 1995). Pharmaceutical workers and farmers exposed to airborne dust, nurses and veterinarians crushing tablets or preparing vials for injection, farmers exposed to animal feed, and individuals exposed to the dust of medicines derived from plants are typically affected. Common allergens include particularly penicillins and cephalosporins. Chloramine-T is known to induce immunoglobulin E (IgE) antibodies (Piirilä et al. 2002; Kanerva et al. 1997). A list of selected allergens having elicited urticaria or anaphylaxis by contact, with or without respiratory symptoms, is shown in *Tables 39.1*. In such patients, suspected allergens should be first tested in high dilutions on intact skin and only later by prick and, if necessary, intradermal tests. The patients should be carefully monitored during these diagnostic procedures since severe anaphylactic reactions may be elicited by skin tests alone (Bause and Kugelman 1990; Tadokoro et al. 1994).

2 Contact Allergens

2.1 Additives

Some examples of common additives are given which may be used as drugs themselves (such as benzoyl peroxide for acne), in the synthesis of drugs (dicyclohexyl carbodiimide) or as antioxidants in final products. Ethylene diamine is present in topical drugs and in

Table 39.2
Drug and intermediate allergens eliciting occupational contact dermatitis

Allergen	References
Additives	
Benzoyl peroxide	Quirce et al. 1993
Ethoxyquin (CAS 91-53-2)	Savini et al. 1989; Mancuso et al. 1990
Ethylene diamine	Rudzki et al. 1989b; Rudzki 1990; Corazza et al. 1994
Dicyclohexylcarbodiimide (CAS 538-75-0)	Davies 1983; Poesen et al. 1995
Tosyl chloride	Watsky et al. 1993
Analgesics and nonsteroidal anti-inflammatory drugs	
Benzydamine hydrochloride (CAS 132-69-4)	Foti et al. 1992; Rademaker 1994
Piroxicam	Arevalo et al. 1995
Propacetamol	Szczurko et al. 1996; Mathelier-Fusade et al. 1997
Pyrazinobutazone	Dorado Bris et al. 1992
Pyrazolone	Vanuytrecht-Henderickx et al. 1986
Anesthetics	
Isoflurane (1-chloro-2,2,2-trifluoroethyl difluoromethyl ether)	Finch et al. 2000
Pantocaine	Rudzki 1990
Procaine	Rudzki et al. 1989a, b; Bruijn et al. 2009
Proxymetacaine	Riddell et al. 2000
Propanidid	Castelain and Piriou 1980
Tetracaine (amethocaine)	Conde-Salazar et al. 1988, 1989; Rudzki et al. 1989a; Rudzki 1990
Antacids	
Famotidine	Monteseirin and Conde 1990
Lansoprazole	Villaplane et al. 2001
Omeprazole	Meding 1986; Altomare et al. 1992
Ranitidine	Alomar et al. 1987; Romaguera et al. 1988, 1990
Antiasthmatic drugs	
Aminophylline	Tas and Weissberg 1958; Rudzki et al. 1989a; Rudzki 1990
Budesonide	Baeck and Goossens 2009
Metaproterenol	Fung et al. 1996
Antibiotics and tuberculostatics	
Aminopenicillins	Moller et al. 1986, 1990; Stejskal et al. 1986; Moller and Jeppesen 1987; Rudzki et al. 1989b; Rudzki and Rebandel 1991; Moller and Von Wiirden 1992; Gamboa et al. 1995
Cefazolin	Straube et al. 2000
Cefradine	Rudzki et al. 1989b
Ceftiofur	Garcia-Bravo et al. 1995
Cephalosporins	Conde-Salazar et al. 1986; Foti et al. 1994,1997; Filipe et al. 1996
Chloramphenicol	Schwank and Jirasek 1963; Rudzki et al. 1989b; Rudzki 1990
Colistin	Rudzki et al. 1989b
Doxycycline	Rudzki et al. 1989b
Ethambutol	Holdiness 1986a
Gentamicin	Altomare et al. 1992

Table 39.2 (Continued)

Allergen	References
Isoniazid	Holdiness 1986b; Rudzki et al. 1989a
Kitasamycin (leucomycin)	Dooms-Goossens et al. 1990
Mezlocillin	Keller and Schwanitz 1992
Midecamycin	Dooms-Goossens et al. 1990
Oxytetracycline	Rudzki 1990
Penicillin	Stejskal et al. 1986; Rudzki et al. 1989a, b; Pecegueiro 1990
Streptomycin	Holdiness 1986b; Rudzki et al. 1989b; Altomare et al. 1992
Sulfathiazol	Rudzki et al. 1989a; Rudzki 1990
Tetracyclines	Rudzki et al. 1989a, b
Vibramycin	Rudzki 1990
Other anti-infectious agents	
Albendazol	Macedo et al. 1991
Benzalkonium chloride	Kanerva et al.
Chloramine T (CAS 127-65-1)	Lombardi et al. 1989
Chlorhexidine	Sato et al. 2004
Chloroquine	Kellett and Beck 1984
Fentichlor[a]	Norris et al. 1988
Foscarnet	Testud et al. 1994
Griseofulvin	Testud et al. 1994
Metronidazole	Madsen et al. 2009
N-benzyl-*N*,*N*-dihydroxyethyl-*N*-cocosalkyl-ammonium chloride	Placucci et al. 1996
Nifuroxazide	Kieć-Swierczyńska 1998
Piperazine	Calnan 1975; Rudzki and Grzywa 1977; Rudzki et al. 1989b
Quinine[a]	Hardie et al. 1978
Quinidine[a]	Wahlberg and Boman 1981
Cardiovascular and vasoactive drugs	
Alprenolol	Ekenvall and Forsbeck 1978; Stejskal et al. 1986
Captopril	Dziuk et al. 1994
Carbocromen	Martin et al. 1973; Rudzki et al. 1989b
Homatropine	Marcos et al. 1997
Nicergoline (CAS 27848-84-6)	Fumagalli et al. 1992
Oxprenolol	Rebandel and Rudzki 1990
Phenoxybenzamine hydrochloride	Mitchell and Maibach 1975
Phenylephrine	Marcos et al. 1997
Propanolol	Rebandel and Rudzki 1990; Rudzki 1990
Quinidine sulfate[a]	Wahlberg and Boman 1981; Stejskal et al. 1986
Spironolactone	Klijn 1984
Central nervous system drugs	
Apomorphine	Dahlquist 1977
Chloropromazine[a]	Foussereau et al. 1982; Rudzki 1990; Bjorkner 1994
Chlorprothixen	Schwenck et al. 1994

Table 39.2 (Continued)

Allergen	References
Codeine	Romaguera and Grimalt 1983; Conde-Salazar et al. 1991; Waclawski and Aldridge 1995; Coenraads et al. 2001
Cyanamide (CAS 420-04-2)	Goday Bujdn et al. 1994
Diamorphine (heroine)	Coenraads et al. 2001
Meclofenoxate	Foussereau et al. 1982
Morphine	Conde-Salazar et al. 1991
Oxolamine (CAS 959-14-8)	Conde-Salazar et al. 1989; Coenraads et al. 2001
Perazine	Rudzki et al. 1989a
Pyritinol	Dooms-Goossens et al. 1986b; Wigger-Alberti and Elsner 1997
Tetrazepam	Ortiz-Frutos et al. 1995; Ferran et al. 2005
Thebaine	Waclawski and Aldridge 1995
Herbal drugs and plant derivatives	
Arnica	Hausen 1980
Essential oils	Selvaag et al. 1995; Cockayne and Gawkrodger 1997
Eugenol	Rudzki et al. 1989a; Kanerva et al. 1994
Lavender	Rademaker 1994
Pyrethrum	Schmidt 1986
Vincamine tartrate	Van Hecke 1981
Immune modulating drugs	
Azathioprine	Burden and Beck 1992; Soni and Sherertz 1996
Dinitrochlorobenzene	Garcia-Perez 1978; Lubbe 1993
Dinitrofluorobenzene	Garcia-Perez 1978
Diphencyprone	Sansom et al. 1995; Bircher et al. 1999
Squaric acid dibutyl ester	Noster et al. 1976; Frattasio et al. 1997
Intermediate and precursor products	
2-Aminothiophenol	Bonamonte et al. 2002
2,6-Dichloropurine	Rycroft 1981
Allopurinol (ethyl ethoxymethylene cyanoacetate)	Hsu et al. 1992
Azaerythromycin	Milković-Kraus et al. 2007
Azathioprine (5-chloro-1-methyl-4-nitroimidazole)	Jolanki et al. 1997
Bumetanide (sulfonyl benzoic acids)	Moller and Kromann 1989
Chlordiazepoxide (2-chloromethyl-4-phenyl-6-chlorquinazoline-3-oxide)	Rebandel and Rudzki 1986a, b
Chloroquine (4,7-dichloroquinoline)	Pickering and Ive 1982
Clenbuterol (4-amino-(x-bromo-3,5-dichloroacetophenone))	Romaguera et al. 1990
Cytosine arabinoside	Conde-Salazar et al. 1984
Diethyl-*p*-chloroethylamine	Deschamps et al. 1988
Dichlorobenzoyl chloride	De Boer and Van Joost 1988
Erythromycin A oxim hydrochloride	Milković-Kraus et al. 2007
Erythromycin A iminoether	Milković-Kraus et al. 2007
Famotidine	Guimaraens et al. 1994

Table 39.2 (Continued)

Allergen	References
H_2 antagonist (2-(4(5)-methyl-5(4)-imidazolyl-methyl-thio)-C13)	Camarasa and Alomar 1980
Histamine antagonist (heterocyclic chloromethyl compounds)	Sonnex and Rycroft 1986
Methotrexate (2,4-di-amino-6-6-chloromethylpteridine)	Lahti et al. 1990
N-(3-trifluoromethyl-4-nitrophenyl) phthalimide	Jungewelter and Aalto-Korte 2008
Nitrosourea (3-taurinyl-1-(2-chloroethyl)-1-nitrosourea, carbamates)	Niklasson et al. 1990
Oxprenolol (epichlorhydrin)	Rebandel and Rudzki 1990
p-Aminophenol	Walker et al. 2005
Procaine (*p*-nitrobenzoyl chloride)	Foussereau 1989
Propanolol (epichlorhydrin)	Rebandel and Rudzki 1990
Pyridoxine (2-methyl-3-nitro-4-methoxymethyl-5-cyano-6-chloropyridine)	Wigger-Alberti and Elsner 1997
Radiocontrast medium (3,4-dicarbethoxyhexane-2,5-dione)	Niklasson and Bjorkner 1990
Ranitidine (cistoran)	Valsecchi et al. 1989
Cistofur (2-[([(1-Dimethylaminomethyl)] furan-5-1methyl)thio] ß-amino ethane)	Romaguera et al. 1990
1-(Methylamino)-1-(methylthio)-2-nitroethylene	Romaguera et al. 1990
5-1-(2-Aminoethyl)-thiomethyl-*N,N*-dimethyl-2-furanmethanamine	Rycroft 1983; Goh and Ng 1984
Tetramisol (3rd intermediate)	Valsecchi et al. 1987
Virostatic 6-aza-uracil (3,4,6-trichloropyridazine)	Doorns-Goossens et al. 1986a
Veterinary drugs	
Avoparcin	Barriga et al. 1991
Bacitracin	Mancuso et al. 1990
Furaltadone	Vilaplana et al. 1990
Furazolidone	De Groot and Conemans 1990
Lincomycin	Vilaplana et al. 1991
Methylchlorpindol	Mancuso et al. 1990
Monensin (CAS 17090-79-8)	Mancuso et al. 1990
Morantel tartrate (CAS 26155-31-7)	Newton and White 1987
Neomycin	Mancuso et al. 1990
Nitrofurazone	Ancona 1985; Lo et al. 1990
Olaquindox[a]	Francalanci et al. 1986; Schauder et al. 1996
Oxytetracycline	Guerra et al. 1991
Penethamate	Hjorth and Weisman 1973
Penicillin	Hjorth and Weisman 1973; Guerra et al. 1991
Phenothiazines	Schauder et al. 1996
Spectinomycin	Vilaplana et al. 1991; Dal Monte et al. 1994

Table 39.2 (Continued)

Allergen	References
Spiramycin	Veien et al. 1980; Guerra et al. 1991
Streptomycin	Gauchia et al. 1996
Thiabendazole	Mancuso et al. 1990
Tylosin	Veien et al. 1980; Baberda and De la Cuadra 1989; Guerra et al. 1991; Caraffini et al. 1994; Tuomi and Rasanen 1995
Virginiamycin	Tennstedt et al. 1978
Vitamins	
Cyanocobalamin (vitamin B_{12})	Rudzki et al. 1989b; Rodriguez et al. 1994
Menadione sodium bisulfite (vitamin K_3)	Romaguera et al. 1980; Camarasa and Barnadas 1982; Dinis et al. 1988
Pyridoxine	Wigger-Alberti and Elsner 1997
Retinyl acetate (vitamin A acetate)	Heidenheim and Jemec 1995
Thiamine (vitamin B_1)	Ingemann-Larsen et al. 1989
Miscellaneous	
Benzoin	Klein et al. 2009
Carbimazole[a] (CAS 22232-54-8)	Goh and Ng 1985
Disulfiram (CAS 97-77-8)	Rudzki et al. 1989b; Mathelier-Fusade and Leynadier 1994
Ethylene oxide (CAS 75-21-8)	Haddar et al. 1993; Lerman et al. 1995
Meglumine diatrizoate (CAS 131-49-7)	Verschaeve et al. 1984
Mesna (CAS 19767-45-4)	Benyoussef et al. 1996
Minoxidil	Veraldi et al. 1992
Mitomycin C	Fisher 1991
Simvastatin	Peramiquel et al. 2005; Mascaro 2005
Thiomersal	De Groot et al. 1990
Tubocurarine	Rudzki 1990

[a]Photosensitivity

aminophylline and is the allergen in the latter compound. Several cases of occupational contact dermatitis have been reported (Corazza et al. 1994).

2.2 Analgesics and Nonsteroidal Anti-inflammatory Drugs

With the exception of photoallergy, nonsteroidal anti-inflammatory drugs rarely induce immunologically mediated adverse reactions; more commonly, a pseudoallergic pathogenesis is involved, reflected by non-immunologic urticaria, asthma, or anaphylactoid reactions. Nurses have been reported who have developed contact dermatitis and, in one case, an airborne contact dermatitis (Mathelier-Fusade et al. 1997) to propacetamol (Barbaud et al. 1995, 1997), an injectable prodrug which is rapidly hydrolyzed by esterases to paracetamol and diethylglycine. Paracetamol and diethylglycine were patch-test negative, and oral administration was tolerated (Szczurko et al. 1996). Later, diethylglycine has been identified as eliciting moiety, explaining why propacetamol-sensitized individuals tolerate paracetamol (Berl et al. 1998).

However, a patient sensitized to another prodrug, pyrazinobutazone, a piperazine salt of phenylbutazone, reacted with a flare-up to oral provocation (Dorado Bris et al. 1992). Benzydamine, a topical and systemic nonsteroidal anti-inflammatory drug, has caused two cases of occupational sensitization (Foti et al. 1992). An unusual case of a multilocular-fixed drug eruption upon inhalation of pyrazolones with positive oral provocation has also been described (Vanuytrecht-Henderickx et al. 1986).

2.3 Anesthetics

Occupational problems with topically applied local anesthetics, particularly ester derivatives, have been known for many years (Altomare et al. 1992). Contact allergy to procaine used to be a typical professional disease of dentists due to direct handling (Kanerva et al. 1994). Other affected professions include ophthalmologists and veterinary surgeons. An extensive disseminated contact allergy from procaine has been seen in a veterinarian (Bruijn et al. 2009). Allergic contact fingertip dermatitis secondary to proxymetacaine has been reported in an ophthalmologist (Riddell et al. 2000).

There is an extensive cross-reactivity between all *p*-aminobenzoic acid derivatives, such as procaine, benzocaine, and tetracaine, but not to amide derivatives, such as lidocaine. Since the less allergenic amide local anesthetics are used today, the number of occupational cases has declined. The intravenous anesthetic propanidid, a derivative of eugenol (Castelain and Piriou 1980), has caused sensitization in anesthetists by direct and probably also airborne contact (Altomare et al. 1992).

2.4 Antacids

Two pharmaceutical employees with contact allergy to the proton-pump inhibitor omeprazole have been reported (Meding 1986). Another employee with contact dermatitis from lansoprazole and cross-reactivity to omeprazole has also been observed (Vilaplana and Romaguera 2001). More often, pharmaceutical workers with skin problems from the production of the H_2 antagonists (famotidine, ranitidine) have been described. Typically, the patients are not only sensitized to the final products but also to intermediate products from the synthesis process (see ➋ Sect. 2.12).

2.5 Antiasthmatic Drugs

Compared to the widespread and long-term use of β-mimetic drugs, typically by nebulization, the few reports involving antiasthmatic drugs indicate that they are weak allergens (Fung et al. 1996). Aminophylline is of importance since it consists of ethylenediamine and theophylline; therefore, positive patch tests to ethylenediamine are present in patients sensitized to aminophylline (see ➋ Sect. 2.1) (Rudzki et al. 1989a; Rudzki 1990). Corticosteroids and particularly budesonide have resulted in 15 subjects, not themselves treated by budesonide-containing aerosols but taking care of or living together with patients who used them, have been sensitized by airborne exposure, and presented with airborne allergic contact dermatitis (Baeck and Goossens 2009).

2.6 Antibiotics and Tuberculostatics

By far, the largest number of affected workers has symptoms due to antimicrobials for human or animal use (see ➋ Sect. 2.13). Among the antibiotics, the natural and the semisynthetic penicillins are the most common drug allergens causing symptoms, particularly in pharmaceutical workers, followed by cephalosporins and tuberculostatic agents in pharmaceutical industry workers and medical employees. Contact urticaria and anaphylaxis has also been reported (see ➋ Sect. 1.1). In the penicillin group, aminopenicillins have elicited occupational skin problems; cross-reactivity to natural penicillins (penicillin G and V) was not always present, indicating an antigenic determinant on the side chain and not on the β-lactam ring (Rudzki and Rebandel 1991; Moller and Von Wiirden 1992; Gamboa et al. 1995). Contact allergy to cephalosporins has been particularly observed in nurses. The problem of cross-reactivity is more complex, since the antigenic determinants for cephalosporins in IgE- and T cell–mediated reactions are not known. Cases of contact allergy to ceftiofur (Garcia-Bravo et al. 1995) and several structurally different cephalosporins and also a case from cefazolin (Straube et al. 2000) have been described. Occupational contact allergy to tuberculostatics and tetracyclines is of minor relevance today; however, in some countries it was a common problem. Several workers with contact dermatitis from azithromycine and some also from intermediate products such as erythromycin A oxim hydrochloride 5% in pet., erythromycin A iminoether 5% in pet., and azaerythromycin A 5% in pet. were reported (Milković-Kraus et al. 2007).

2.7 Anti-infectious Agents

Common occupational allergens are quinine (an antimalarial) and its D-stereoisomer, quinidine sulfate salt, used as an anti-arrhythmic drug. Both substances have elicited contact allergy without cross-reactivity between the two compounds (Wahlberg and Boman 1981; Stejskal et al. 1986), indicating stereoselectivity for contact allergy (Isaaksson et al. 1994). However, photocontact allergy cross-reactivity between the two isomeric substances is present (Ljunggren et al. 1992), due to practically identical photoproducts after ultraviolet irradiation (Isaaksson et al. 1994).

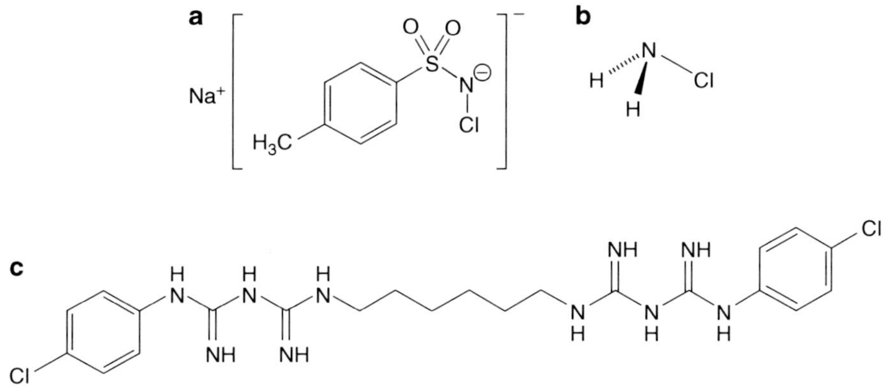

Fig. 39.1
Chemical formulas of chloramine T, monochloramine, and chlorhexidine

An outbreak of irritant quinine dermatitis has been observed in a factory (Hardie et al. 1978), whereas allergic reactions to quinine have declined in recent years. Contact allergy to chloroquine sulfate, another chemically closely related antimalarial, has been observed in a maintenance apprentice in a drug-packing firm; cross-reactivity to quinine was not present. Quinidine was not tested (Kellett and Beck 1984). Also, cases of sensitization to a precursor of chloroquine (4,7-dichloroquinoline) have been published (Pickering and Ive 1982). Nifuroxazide, a compound used in diarrhea, elicited a prurigo-like eruption in an employee filling bottles with the drug (Kieć-Swierczyńska 1998).

Chloramine-T, which should not be confused with (mono)chloramine (NH_2Cl) or chlorhexidine (Krautheim et al. 2004) (*Fig. 39.1*), is a recognized IgE-antibody-inducing immediate-type allergen, which causes contact urticaria and asthma (Kanerva et al. 1997). However, allergic contact dermatitis to chloramine-T was identified in a nurse who was also sensitized to quaternary ammonium compounds and mercury derivatives (Lombardi et al. 1989). Chlorhexidine was a common contact allergen among physicians in one study (Sato et al. 2004). Another quaternary ammonium compound caused contact dermatitis in a dental nurse (Placucci et al. 1996). Also, benzalkonium chloride, a disinfectant with irritant potential, has been identified as occupational contact allergen (Kanerva et al. 2000). Other anti-infectious drugs include albendazole (which induced contact urticaria and dermatitis), fentichlor (eliciting a photoallergic reaction with positive patch and photo patch tests) (Norris et al. 1988), piperazine (another anthelmintic), foscarnet (an antiviral), and griseofulvin (an old antifungal drug) (Testud et al. 1994). Also, topical metronidazole has rarely elicited contact allergy. In two nurses, therapeutic use for rosacea elicited within 1 day severe contact dermatitis of the face (Madsen et al. 2009). Sensitization has likely taken place during occupational exposure.

2.8 Cardiovascular and Vasoactive Drugs

Antihypertensive drugs, which have elicited occupational dermatitis in pharmaceutical workers, include the β-blocking agents, e.g., alprenolol, propanolol, and oxprenolol, and their precursors (Rebandel and Rudzki 1990). Cross-reactivity between alprenolol and metoprolol was present (Ekenvall and Forsbeck 1978). In a patient with contact sensitization to the α-blocker phenoxybenzamine, cross-reactivity to chemically related haloalkylamines was demonstrated (Mitchell and Maibach 1975). Contact dermatitis has been observed to nicergoline and spironolactone in pharmaceutical employees and to carbocromene (a vasodilator), captopril (an angiotensin-converting enzyme inhibitor), and the ophthalmologic agents homatropine and phenylephrine in nurses. Quinidine sulfate has elicited contact allergy in production workers, and patch tests with quinine were negative (Wahlberg and Boman 1981) (see Sect. 2.7).

2.9 Central Nervous System Drugs

Among the drugs acting on the central nervous system, the opium alkaloids and the phenothiazine derivatives have caused most occupation-related cases. Apart from contact dermatitis in pharmaceutical employees and nurses, the opiates have also caused respiratory symptoms. In an IgE-mediated reaction to papaveretum, the allergenic determinant has been located at the *N*-methyl-cyclohexenyl ring in combination with a hydroxyl group on the C atom in position 6 (Harle et al. 1989). For contact allergy, the antigenic determinant is not clear, since cross-reactivity between the opiates is present; thebaine has an $-OCH_3$ group and hydromorphone, an oxygen at this position (Waclawski and Aldridge 1995). It also remains unexplained why most of the patients allergic to opioids were also sensitized to *p*-group substances, since there are no apparent cross-reacting structures (Conde-Salazar et al. 1991). Workers preparing heroin from capsules developed contact sensitivity to heroine (diamorphine), morphine, and codeine (Coenraads et al. 2001).

The phenothiazines may elicit contact dermatitis, airborne dermatitis (Schwenck et al. 1994), and photoallergic dermatitis. In particular, chlorpromazine was a potent contact and photocontact allergen on direct skin contact (Rudzki 1990; Bjorkner 1994). There have also been cases of occupational contact dermatitis to other centrally active compounds, such as tetrazepam (Ferran et al. 2005) and cyanamide. In another benzodiazepine chlordiazepoxide, its precursor quinazoline oxide has caused sensitization (Rudzki and Rebandel 2001). A rare case of airborne allergy from isoflurane (1-chloro-2,2,2-trifluoroethyl difluoromethyl ether) was identified in an anesthetist. A ROAT only identified the culprit; patch tests were negative possibly due to its volatile nature (Finch et al. 2000).

2.10 Herbal Drugs and Plant Derivatives

Plant derivatives are used as fragrances and as drugs in aromatherapy and phytotherapy. Contact allergy and exanthematous reactions to herbal remedies have been observed (Bircher 1996); airborne contact dermatitis and photosensitivity are well-known reactions to members of the Asteraceae (Compositae) family. Occupational allergies have been observed to *Arnica montana* (Hausen 1980); to essential oils in aroma- and phytotherapists; to pyrethrum, which is still used as acaricide, in factory workers; and to the alkaloid vincamine tartrate from *Vinca minor* L. (used for cerebral perfusion problems) (Van Hecke 1981). Eugenol, the essential constituent of clove oil, which is present in impression pastes and cements, may be an allergen for dentists (Kanerva et al. 1994).

2.11 Immune Modulators

Highly reactive chemicals (and, therefore, potent contact sensitizers) include dinitrofluorobenzene, dinitrochlorobenzene (DNCB), diphenylcyprone, and squaric acid dibutyl ester. These sensitize practically all exposed individuals and, therefore, probably only unusual cases are published. The three latter agents have been used in the treatment of alopecia areata, but DNCB has become obsolete due to its mutagenic potential (Happle et al. 1980). The main exposed professions are accidentally exposed chemical workers, dermatologists, and pharmacy employees (Bircher et al. 1999).

Azathioprine, an immunosuppressant, is widely used in transplantation and autoimmune diseases; cutaneous reactions to it are rare (Soni and Sherertz 1996). Two pharmaceutical workers have been described who had a contact allergy to azathioprine; the role of impurities, such as mercaptopurine and chloromethyl-nitroimidazole, could not be elucidated (Burden and Beck 1992).

2.12 Intermediates and Precursors

Intermediate products are often highly reactive chemicals and bind readily to proteins, a prerequisite for sensitization. Contact allergy to intermediates is not uncommon and occurs practically exclusively in individuals involved in the development and production of drugs or in maintenance employees in chemical or pharmaceutical plants. Allergic reactions to intermediates of H_2-antagonists are well established, e.g., for ranitidine (Romaguera et al. 1990), famotidine, and others. Also, synthesis of cytostatic drugs apparently produces allergenic intermediates, as demonstrated for cytosine arabinoside, methotrexate, nitrosoureas, and the immunosuppressant azathioprine. The intermediates of a number of other drugs have been reported as contact allergens (➋ *Tables 39.2*). An unusual case of toxic epidermal necrolysis upon skin contact with an intermediate of tetramisole, an anthelmintic and immunostimulatory agent, has been described. Patch tests were not performed (Valsecchi et al. 1987). Recently, p-aminophenol, a breakdown product of paracetamol (acetaminophen), has been identified as contact allergen in two employees of a production plant (Walker et al. 2005). After accidental exposure without protection to 2-aminothiophenol, an intermediate pharmaceutical substance, a technician developed recurrent contact dermatitis at his working place, even when exposed to minute amounts (Bonamonte et al. 2002). An intermediate (*N*-(3-trifluoromethyl-4-nitrophenyl) phthalimide) of flutamide, an antiandrogen, elicited a disseminated erythema despite extensive protective measures. Patch tests were positive in very high dilutions to this substance only (Jungewelter and Aalto-Korte 2008).

2.13 Veterinary Drugs

Farmers, animal caretakers, and veterinarians are particularly at risk. The majority of the eliciting agents are anti-infectious and antibiotic drugs, which are used as growth promoters or for therapy.

Contact takes place by skin contact while treating or vaccinating (Vilaplana et al. 1991) animals or through dust during feeding or the production of feed. Important allergens are tylosin, a macrolide antibiotic (Veien et al. 1980) that sometimes induced airborne contact dermatitis, and olaquindox, a growth promoter for pigs, which induced severe photoallergic contact dermatitis, and, in some patients, a persistent light reaction (Schauder et al. 1996).

2.14 Vitamins

Thiamine (vitamin B_1) (Ingemann-Larsen et al. 1989) is a typical occupational sensitizer, whereas, e.g., cyanocobalamin has rarely caused occupational problems. In some patients, oral administration of thiamine resulted in a flare of contact dermatitis. Few cases of occupational contact dermatitis have been reported to pyritinol, a compound of two pyridoxine (vitamin B_6) molecules; pyritinol and two bases containing pyridoxine induced airborne occupational contact allergy (Wigger-Alberti and Elsner 1997). The retinols (vitamin A) elicit irritant reactions in higher concentrations more often; a case of allergy to vitamin A acetate has been reported. However, occupational contact allergy (in several pharmaceutical workers and a pig feeder) to the synthetic, water-soluble form of vitamin K_3 (menadione sodium bisulfite) has been observed, with cross-reactivity to vitamin K_4 (menadiol sodium diphosphate) (Dinis et al. 1988).

2.15 Miscellaneous Drugs

Several drugs have caused single cases of occupational contact dermatitis. Carbimazole, a thiourea used as an antithyroid drug, has induced photoallergic reactions in a pharmaceutical laboratory worker. Disulfiram (tetraethylthiuram disulfide) used for adjunctive therapy in alcoholism has elicited contact dermatitis in a nurse handling tablets. A clinically relevant cross-reactivity to other thiurams (eczema under rubber gloves) has been reported (Mathelier-Fusade and Leynadier 1994). A nurse was affected with contact dermatitis from meglumine diatrizoate, an ionic radio-contrast medium; another nurse had a reaction to mesna, a mucolytic also used to prevent cyclophosphamide urotoxicity. A third nurse had a reaction to mitomycin C, a cytostatic drug, and a fourth had a reaction to tubocurarine, a myorelaxant. Finally, a hairdresser became sensitized to minoxidil he applied to a customer, and an ophthalmologic assistant became sensitized to thiomersal from contact lens fluids while instructing customers. Ethylene oxide, a sterilizing agent known to elicit immediate-type hypersensitivity, has caused an epidemic of irritant contact dermatitis due to ethylene oxide-sterilized overalls (Lerman et al. 1995). Two patients, a male and a female with an airborne contact dermatitis on the face from simvastatin with positive patch tests, have been observed; patch tests were positive, and ten controls were negative (Peramiquel et al. 2005).

A male anesthesiologist used a tincture of benzoin aerosol spray to improve adhesion of a small bandage immediately before performing a spinal anesthesia. He experienced severe pruritus and dermatitis in the affected hand 48 h after benzoin exposure (Klein et al. 2009).

3 Summary

A considerable number of drugs have been reported as occupational allergens. Drugs are not the most common occupational allergens but, for several reasons, they may be of considerable importance. Cutaneous and/or respiratory symptoms (and, rarely, systemic reactions) may be elicited. Of particular importance is the possibility of re-exposure to a particular drug for medical purposes in an occupationally sensitized individual. Diagnosis of an occupational allergy and allergen recognition can lead to appropriate control and prevention in many situations (Sherertz 1994).

References

Alomar A, Puig L, Vilaltella I (1987) Allergic contact dermatitis due to ranitidine. Contact Dermatitis 17:154–155

Altomare GF, Capella GL, Veraldi S (1992) Occupational drug dermatitis. Clin Dermatol 10:141–147

Ancona A (1985) Allergic contact dermatitis to nitrofurazone. Contact Dermatitis 13:35

Arevalo A, Blancas R, Ancona A (1995) Occupational contact dermatitis from piroxicam. Am J Contact Dermat 6:113–114

Baberda E, De la Cuadra J (1989) Occupational airborne allergic contact dermatitis from tylosin. Contact Dermatitis 20:308

Baeck M, Goossens AN (2009) Patients with airborne sensitization/contact dermatitis from budesonide-containing aerosols 'by proxy'. Contact Dermatitis 61:1–8

Barbaud A (2002) Occupational dermatitis in health care personnel. La Revue du praticien 52:1425–1432

Barbaud A, Trechot P, Bertrand O, Schmutz JL (1995) Occupational allergy to propacetamol. Lancet 346:902

Barbaud A, Reichert-Penetrat S, Trechot P, Cuny JF, Weber M, Schmutz JL (1997) Occupational contact dermatitis to propacetamol. Allergological and chemical investigations in two new cases. Dermatology 195:329–331

Barriga A, Romaguera C, Vilaplana J (1991) Contact dermatitis from avoparcin. Contact Dermatitis 27:115

Bause GS, Kugelman LC (1990) Contact anaphylactoid response to labetalol. Contact Dermatitis 23:51

Belsito DV (1993) Contact urticaria from pentamidine isethionate. Contact Dermatitis 29:158

Benyoussef K, Bottlaender A, Pfister HR, Caussade P, Heid E, Grosshans E (1996) Allergic contact dermatitis from MESNA. Contact Dermatitis 34:228–229

Berl V, Barbaud A, Lepoittevin JP (1998) Mechanism of allergic contact dermatitis from propacetamol: sensitization to activated N, *N*-diethylglycine. Contact Dermatitis 38:185–188

Bernstein JA, Stauder T, Bernstein DI, Bernstein IL (1994) A combined respiratory and cutaneous hypersensitivity syndrome induced by work exposure to quaternary amines. J Allergy Clin Immunol 94:257–259

Bircher AJ (1996) Arzneimittelallergie und Haut. Georg Thieme, Stuttgart

Bircher AJ, Bigliardi P, Langauer Messmer S, Surber C (1999) Occupational airborne contact dermatitis from diphencyprone in a pharmacy employee. Contact Dermatitis 41:52

Bjorkner BE (1994) Industrial airborne dermatoses. Dermatol Clin 12:501–509

Bonamonte D, Carino M, Mundo L, Foti C (2002) Occupational airborne allergic contact dermatitis from 2-aminothiophenol. Eur J Dermatol 12:592–593

Bruijn MS, Lavrijsen AP, van Zuuren EJ (2009) An unusual case of contact dermatitis to procaine. Contact Dermatitis 60:182–183

Burden AD, Beck MH (1992) Contact hypersensitivity to azathioprine. Contact Dermatitis 27:329–330

Calnan CD (1975) Occupational piperazine dermatitis. Contact Dermatitis 1:126

Camarasa G, Alomar A (1980) Contact dermatitis to an H_2 antagonist. Contact Dermatitis 6:152–153

Camarasa JG, Barnadas M (1982) Occupational dermatosis by vitamin K_3 sodium bisulphite. Contact Dermatitis 8:268

Caraffini S, Assalve D, Stingeni L, Lisi P (1994) Tylosin, an airborne contact allergen in veterinarians. Contact Dermatitis 31:327–328

Castelain PY, Piriou A (1980) Contact dermatitis due to propanidid in an anesthesist. Contact Dermatitis 6:360

Cockayne SE, Gawkrodger W (1997) Occupational contact dermatitis in an aromatherapist. Contact Dermatitis 37:306–307

Coenraads PJ, Hogen Esch AJ, Prevoo RL (2001) Occupational contact dermatitis from diacetylmorphine (heroin). Contact Dermatitis 45:114

Conde-Salazar L, Guimaraens D, Romero L (1984) Occupational contact dermatitis from cytosine arabinoside synthesis. Contact Dermatitis 10:44–45

Conde-Salazar L, Guimaraens D, Romero LV, Gonzalez MA (1986) Occupational dermatitis from cephalosporins. Contact Dermatitis 14:70–71

Conde-Salazar L, Llinas MG, Guimaraens D, Romero L (1988) Occupational allergic contact dermatitis from amethocaine. Contact Dermatitis 19:69–70

Conde-Salazar L, Guimaraens D, Llinas G, Romero L, Gonzalez MA (1989) Occupational allergic contact dermatitis from oxolamine. Contact Dermatitis 21:206

Conde-Salazar L, Guimaraens D, Gonzalez M, Fuente C (1991) Occupational allergic contact dermatitis from opium alkaloids. Contact Dermatitis 25:202–203

Corazza M, Mantovani L, Trimurti S, Virgili A (1994) Occupational contact sensitization to ethylenediamine in a nurse. Contact Dermatitis 31:328–329

Dahlquist I (1977) Allergic reactions to apomorphine. Contact Dermatitis 3:349–350

Dal Monte A, Laffi G, Mancini G (1994) Occupational contact dermatitis due to spectinomycin. Contact Dermatitis 31:204–205

Davies MG (1983) Contact allergy to dicyclohexyl-carbodiimide. Contact Dermatitis 9:318

De Boer J, Van Joost T (1988) Sensitisation to dichlorobenzoyl chloride. Contact Dermatitis 18:116–117

De Groot AC, Conemans JMH (1990) Contact allergy to furazolidone. Contact Dermatitis 22:202–205

De Groot AC, Van Wijnen WG, Van Wijnen-Vos M (1990) Occupational contact dermatitis of the eyelids, without ocular involvement, from thimerosal in contact lens fluid. Contact Dermatitis 23:195

Deschamps D, Gamier R, Savoye J, Chabaux C, Efthymiou ML, Fournier E (1988) Allergic and irritant contact dermatitis from diethyl-b-chloroethylamine. Contact Dermatitis 18:103–105

Dinis A, Branddo M, Faria A (1988) Occupational contact dermatitis from vitamin K_3 sodium bisulphate. Contact Dermatitis 78:170–171

Dooms-Goossens A, Gevers D, Mertens A, Vanderheyden D (1983) Allergic contact urticaria due to chloramines. Contact Dermatitis 9:319–320

Dooms-Goossens A, De Boulle K, Snauwaert J, Degreef H (1986a) Sensitization to 3,4,6-trichloropyridazine. Contact Dermatitis 14:64–65

Dooms-Goossens AE, Debusschere KM, Gevers DM, Dupre KM, Degreef HJ, Loncke JP, Snauwaert JE (1986b) Contact dermatitis caused by airborne agents. A review and case reports. J Am Acad Dermatol 15:1–10

Dooms-Goossens A, Bedert R, Degreef H, Vandaele M (1990) Airborne allergic contact dermatitis from kitasamycin and midecamycin. Contact Dermatitis 23:118–119

Dorado Bris JM, Aragues Montailes M, Sols Candela M, Garcia Diez A (1992) Contact sensitivity to pyrazinobutazone (Carudol) with positive oral provocation test. Contact Dermatitis 26:355–356

Dziuk M, Gall H, Sterry W (1994) Contact dermatitis from the ACE-inhibitor captopril. Dermatosen Beruf Umwelt 42:159–161

Ekenvall L, Forsbeck M (1978) Contact eczema produced by a β-adrenergic blocking agent (alprenolol). Contact Dermatitis 4:190–194

Ferran M, Gimenez-Arnau A, Luque S, Berenguer N, Iglesias M, Pujol R (2005) Occupational airborne contact dermatitis from sporadic exposure to tetrazepam during machine maintenance. Contact Dermatitis 52:173–174

Filipe P, Soares Almeida RSL, Guerra Rodrigo FG (1996) Occupational allergic contact dermatitis from cephalosporins. Contact Dermatitis 34:226

Finch TM, Muncaster A, Prais L, Foulds IS (2000) Occupational airborne allergic contact dermatitis from isoflurane vapour. Contact Dermatitis 42:46

Fisher AA (1991) Allergic contact dermatitis to mitomycine C. Cutis 47:225–227

Foti C, Vena GA, Angelini G (1992) Occupational contact allergy to benzydamine hydrochloride. Contact Dermatitis 27:328–329

Foti C, Vena GA, Cucurachi MR, Angelini G (1994) Occupational contact allergy from cephalosporins. Contact Dermatitis 31:129–130

Foti C, Bonamonte D, Trenti R, Vena GA, Angelini G (1997) Occupational contact allergy to cephalosporins. Contact Dermatitis 36:104–105

Foussereau J (1989) Accidental occupational sensitization to *p*-nitrobenzoyl chloride in a chemistry student synthesizing procaine. Contact Dermatitis 20:397–398

Foussereau J, Benezra C, Maibach HI (1982) Occupational contact dermatitis. Munksgaard, Kopenhagen

Francalanci S, Gola M, Giorgini S, Muccinelli A, Sertoli A (1986) Occupational photocontact dermatitis from olaquindox. Contact Dermatitis 15:112–114

Frattasio A, Germino M, Cargnello S, Patrone P (1997) Side-effects during treatment with SADBE. Contact Dermatitis 36:118–119

Fumagalli M, Bigardi AS, Legori A, Pigatto PD (1992) Occupational contact dermatitis from airborne nicergoline. Contact Dermatitis 27:256

Fung MA, Geisse JK, Maibach HI (1996) Airborne contact dermatitis from metaproterenol in a respiratory therapist. Contact Dermatitis 35:317–318

Gamboa P, Muregui I, Urrutia I (1995) Occupational sensitization to aminopenicillins with oral tolerance to penicillin V. Contact Dermatitis 32:48–49

Garcia-Bravo B, Gines E, Russo F (1995) Occupational contact dermatitis from ceftiofur sodium. Contact Dermatitis 33:62–63

Garcia-Perez A (1978) Occupational dermatitis from DNFB with cross sensitivity to DWB. Contact Dermatitis 4:125–127

Gauchia R, Rodriguez-Serna M, Silvestre JF, Linana JJ, Aliaga A (1996) Allergic contact dermatitis from streptomycin in a cattle breed. Contact Dermatitis 35:374–375

Goday-Bujan JJ, Yanguas-Bayona I, Soloeta-Arechavala R (1994) Allergic contact dermatitis from cyanamide: report of 3 cases. Contact Dermatitis 31:331–332

Goh CL, Ng SK (1984) Allergic contact dermatitis to ranitidine. Contact Dermatitis 11:252

Goh CL, Ng SK (1985) Photoallergic contact dermatitis to carbimazole. Contact Dermatitis 12:58–59

Guerra L, Venturo N, Tardio M, Tosti A (1991) Airborne contact dermatitis from animal feed antibiotics. Contact Dermatitis 25:333–334

Guimaraens D, Gonzales MA, Conde-Salazar L (1994) Occupational allergic contact dermatitis from intermediate products in famotidine synthesis. Contact Dermatitis 31:259–260

Haddar M, Araibia A, Laibldder C, Mekki R, Benmami F (1993) Contact dermatitis due to ethylene oxide. Arch Mal Prof Med Trav Secur Soc 54:358–359

Happle R, Kalveram KJ, Buchner U, Echtemacht-Happle K, Goggelmann W, Summer KH (1980) Contact allergy as a therapeutic tool for alopecia areata: application of squaric acid dibutylester. Dermatologica 161:289–297

Hardie RA, Savin JA, White DA, Pumford S (1978) Quinine dermatitis: investigation of a factory outbreak. Contact Dermatitis 4:121–124

Harle DG, Baldo BA, Coroneos NJ, Fisher MM (1989) Anaphylaxis following administration of papaveretum. Case report: implication of IgE antibodies that react with morphine and codeine, and identification of an allergenic determinant. Anesthesiology 71:489–494

Hausen BM (1980) Arnikaallergie. Hautarzt 31:10–17

Häusermann P, Harr T, Bircher AJ (2004) Baboon syndrome resulting from systemic drugs: is there strife between SDRIFE and allergic contact dermatitis syndrome? Contact Dermatitis 51:297–310

Heidenheim M, Jemec GBE (1995) Occupational allergic contact dermatitis from vitamin A acetate. Contact Dermatitis 33:439

Hjorth N, Weisman K (1973) Occupational dermatitis among veterinary surgeons caused by spiramycin, tylosin and penethamate. Contact Dermatitis 53:229–232

Holdiness MR (1986a) Contact dermatitis to ethambutol. Contact Dermatitis 15:96–97

Holdiness MR (1986b) Contact dermatitis to antituberculosis drugs. Contact Dermatitis 15:282

Hsu CK, Sun CC, Su MS, Kuo EF, Wu YC (1992) Systemic contact allergy from occupational contact with ethyl ethoxymethylene cyanoacetate. Contact Dermatitis 27:58–59

Ingemann-Larsen A, Jepsen JR, Thulin H (1989) Allergic contact dermatitis from thiamine. Contact Dermatitis 20:387–388

Isaaksson M, Bruze M, Gruvberger B, Ljunggren B (1994) Quinine and quinidine photoproducts can be identical. Acta Derm Venereol 74:286–288

Johansson G (1988) Contact urticaria from levomepromazine. Contact Dermatitis 19:304

Jolanki R, Alanko K, Pfaffli P, Estlander T, Kanerva L (1997) Occupational allergic contact dermatitis from 5-chloro-1-methyl-4-nitroimidazole. Contact Dermatitis 36:53–54

Jungewelter S, Aalto-Korte K (2008) A new allergen in the pharmaceutical industry. Contact Dermatitis 59:314

Kanerva L, Estlander T, Jolanki R (1994) Occupational skin allergy in the dental profession. Dermatol Clin 12:517–532

Kanerva L, Alanko K, Estlander T, Sihvonen T, Jolanki R (1997) Occupational allergic contact urticaria from chloramine-T solution. Contact Dermatitis 37:180–181

Kanerva L, Jolanki R, Estlander T (2000) Occupational allergic contact dermatitis from benzalkonium chloride. Contact Dermatitis 42:357–358

Keller K, Schwanitz HJ (1992) Combined immediate and delayed hypersensitivity to mezlocillin. Contact Dermatitis 27:348–349

Kellett JK, Beck MH (1984) Contact sensitivity to chloroquine sulphate. Contact Dermatitis 11:47

Kieć-Swierczyńska M, Krecisz B (1998) Occupational contact allergy to nifuroxazide simulating prurigo nodularis. Contact Dermatitis 39:93–94

Klein T, Woehlck H, Pagel P (2009) Severe allergic contact dermatitis resulting from occupational exposure to tincture of benzoin aerosol spray in an anesthesiologist. J Anesth 23:292–294

Klijn J (1984) Contact dermatitis from spironolactone. Contact Dermatitis 10:105

Krautheim AB, Jermann TH, Bircher AJ (2004) Chlorhexidine anaphylaxis: case report and review of the literature. Contact Dermatitis 50:113–116

Lahti A, Puurunen J, Hannuksela M (1990) Occupational contact allergy to 2,4-di-amino-6-chloromethylpteridine hydrochloride: an intermediate in methotrexate synthesis. Contact Dermatitis 22:294

Lepoittevin JP (2006) Metabolism versus chemical transformation or pro- versus prehaptens? Contact Dermatitis 54:73–74

Lerman Y, Ribak J, Skulsky M, Ingber A (1995) An outbreak of irritant contact dermatitis from ethylene oxide among pharmaceutical workers. Contact Dermatitis 33:280–281

Ljunggren B, Hindsen M, Isaaksson M (1992) Systemic quinine photosensitivity with photoepicutaneous cross-reactivity to quinidine. Contact Dermatitis 26:14

Lo JS, Taylor JS, Oriba H (1990) Occupational allergic contact dermatitis to airborne nitrofurazone. Dermatol Clin 8:165–168

Lombardi P, Gola M, Acciai MC, Sertoli A (1989) Unusual occupational allergic contact dermatitis in a nurse. Contact Dermatitis 20:302–303

Lubbe D (1993) Professional dinitrochlorobenzene contact dermatitis. Eleven cases in the nitration facility of a chemical plant. Derm Beruf Umwelt 41:19–24

Macedo NA, Pineyro I, Carmona C (1991) Contact urticaria and contact dermatitis from albendazole. Contact Dermatitis 25:73–75

Madsen J, Lorentzen H, Paulsen E (2009) Contact sensitization to metronidazole from possible occupational exposure. Contact Dermatitis 60:117–118

Mancuso G, Staffa M, Errani A, Berdondini RM, Fabbri P (1990) Occupational dermatitis in animal feed mill workers. Contact Dermatitis 22:37–41

Marcos NIL, Garces MM, Alonso L, Juste S, Carretero P, Blanco J, Garcia F, Perez R, Herrero D (1997) Occupational allergic contact dermatitis from homatropine and phenylephrine eyedrops. Contact Dermatitis 37:189

Martin P, Bétourné M, Martin JJ, Huriez C (1973) Allergie au carbocromène. Bull Soc Fr Dermatol Syphil 80:620

Mascaro AA (2005) Occupational contact dermatitis from simvastatin. Contact Dermatitis 52:286–287

Mathelier-Fusade P, Leynadier F (1994) Occupational allergic contact reaction to disulfiram. Contact Dermatitis 31:121–122

Mathelier-Fusade P, Mansouri S, Aissaoui M, Chabane MH, Aractingi S, Leynadier F (1997) Airborne contact dermatitis from propacetamol. Contact Dermatitis 36:267–268

Meding B (1986) Contact allergy to omeprazole. Contact Dermatitis 15:36

Menne T, Veien NK, Maibach HI (1989) Systemic contact-type dermatitis to drugs. Semin Dermatol 8:144–148

Merk H, Baron J, Neis M, Obrigkeit D, Karlberg A-T (2007) Skin: major target organ of allergic reactions to small molecular weight compounds. Toxicol Appl Pharmacol 224:313–317

Milković-Kraus S, Macan J, Kanceljak-Macan B (2007) Occupational allergic contact dermatitis from azithromycin in pharmaceutical workers: a case series. Contact Dermatitis 56:99–102

Mitchell JC, Maibach HI (1975) Allergic contact dermatitis from phenoxybenzamine hydrochloride. Contact Dermatitis 1:363–366

Miyahara H, Koga T, Imayama S, Hori Y (1993) Occupational contact urticaria syndrome from cefotiam hydrochloride. Contact Dermatitis 29:210–211

Moller NE, Jeppesen K (1987) Patch testing with semisynthetic penicillins. Contact Dermatitis 16:227–228

Moller NE, Kromann N (1989) Bumetanide allergy in factory workers. Contact Dermatitis 20:393–394

Moller NE, Von Wiirden K (1992) Hypersensitivity to semisynthetic penicillins and cross-reactivity with penicillin. Contact Dermatitis 26:351–352

Moller NE, Nielsen B, Von Wiirden K (1986) Contact dermatitis to semisynthetic penicillins in factory workers. Contact Dermatitis 14:307–311

Moller NE, Nielsen B, Von Wiirden K (1990) Changes in penicillin contamination and allergy in factory workers. Contact Dermatitis 22:106–107

Monteseirin J, Conde J (1990) Contact eczema from famotidine. Contact Dermatitis 22:290

Moscato G, Galdi E, Scibilia J, Dellabianca A, Omodeo P, Vittadini G, Biscaldi GP (1995) Occupational asthma, rhinitis and urticaria due to piperacillin sodium in a pharmaceutical worker. Eur Respir J 8:467–469

Newton JA, White I (1987) Connubial dermatitis from morantel. Contact Dermatitis 16:38–39

Niklasson B, Bjorkner B (1990) Contact allergy to 3,4-dicarbethoxyhexane-2,5-dione. Contact Dermatitis 23:46–47

Niklasson B, Bjorkner B, Hansen L (1990) Occupational contact dermatitis from antitumor agent intermediates. Contact Dermatitis 22:233–235

Norris PG, Hawk JL, White IR (1988) Photoallergic contact dermatitis from fentichlor. Contact Dermatitis 18:318–320

Noster U, Hausen BM, Krische B, Schulz KH (1976) Squaric acid diethyl ester – a strong sensitizer. Contact Dermatitis 2:99–104

Ortiz-Frutos FJ, Alonso J, Hergueta JP, Quintana I, Iglesias L (1995) Tetrazepam an allergen with several clinical expressions. Contact Dermatitis 33:63–65

Pecegueiro M (1990) Occupational contact dermatitis from penicillin. Contact Dermatitis 23:190–191

Peramiquel L, Serra E, Dalmau J, Vila AT, Mascaró JM, Alomar A (2005) Occupational contact dermatitis from simvastatin. Contact Dermatitis 52(5):286–287

Pickering FC, Ive FA (1982) Allergic contact dermatitis from 4,7-dichloroquinoline. Contact Dermatitis 8:269–270

Piirilä P, Hodgson U, Estlander T, Keskinen H, Saalo A, Voutilainen R, Kanerva L (2002) Occupational respiratory hypersensitivity in dental personnel. Int Arch Occup Environ Health 75:209–216

Placucci F, Benini A, Guerra L, Tosti A (1996) Occupational allergic contact dermatitis from disinfectant wipes used in dentistry. Contact Dermatitis 35:306

Poesen N, De Moor A, Busschots A, Dooms-Goossens A (1995) Contact allergy to dicyclohexyl carbodiimide and diisopropyl carbodiimide. Contact Dermatitis 32:368–369

Quirce S, Olaguibel JM, Garcia BE, Tabar AI (1993) Occupational airborne contact dermatitis due to benzoyl peroxide. Contact Dermatitis 29:165–166

Rademaker M (1994) Allergic contact dermatitis from lavender fragrance in Difflam gel. Contact Dermatitis 31:58–59

Rebandel P, Rudzki E (1986a) Dermatitis from quinazoline oxide. Contact Dermatitis 15:63–65

Rebandel P, Rudzki E (1986b) Occupational contact sensitivity in oculists. Contact Dermatitis 15:92

Rebandel P, Rudzki E (1990) Dermatitis caused by epichlorohydrin, oxprenolol hydrochloride and propranolol hydrochloride. Contact Dermatitis 23:199

Riddell CE, Reed J, Shaw S, Duvall-Young J (2000) Allergic contact fingertip dermatitis secondary to proxymetacaine in an ophthalmologist. Eye 14:907–908

Rodriguez A, Echechipia S, Alvarez M, Muro MD (1994) Occupational contact dermatitis from vitamin B_{12}. Contact Dermatitis 31:271

Romaguera C, Grimalt F (1983) Occupational dermatitis from codeine. Contact Dermatitis 9:170

Romaguera C, Grimalt F, Conde-Salazar L (1980) Occupational dermatitis from vitamin K_3 sodium bisulfite. Contact Dermatitis 6:355–356

Romaguera C, Grimalt F, Vilaplana J (1988) Epidemic of occupational contact dermatitis from ranitidine. Contact Dermatitis 18:177–178

Romaguera C, Grimalt F, Vilaplana F (1990) Contact dermatitis caused by intermediate products in the manufacture of clenbutol, ranitidine base, and ranitidine hydrochloride. Dermatol Clin 8:115–117

Rudzki E (1990) Contact sensitivity to systemically administered drugs. Dermatol Clin 8:177

Rudzki E, Grzywa Z (1977) Occupational piperazine dermatitis. Contact Dermatitis 3:216

Rudzki E, Rebandel P (1985) Occupational contact urticaria from penicillin. Contact Dermatitis 13:192

Rudzki E, Rebandel P (1991) Hypersensitivity to semisynthetic penicillins but not to natural penicillin. Contact Dermatitis 25:192

Rudzki E, Rebandel P (2001) Contact sensitivity to quinazoline oxide. Contact Dermatitis 44:56–57

Rudzki E, Rebandel P, Grzywa Z (1989a) Patch tests with occupational contactants in nurses, doctors and dentists. Contact Dermatitis 20:247–250

Rudzki E, Rebandel P, Grzywa Z (1989b) Contact allergy in the pharmaceutical industry. Contact Dermatitis 21:121–122

Rycroft RJG (1981) Occupational contact sensitization to 2,6-dichloropurine. Contact Dermatitis 7:349–350

Rycroft RJG (1983) Allergic contact dermatitis from a novel diamino intermediate, 5-[(2-aminoethyl)-thiomethyl]-*N*, *N*-di-methyl-2-furanmethanamine, in laboratory synthesis. Contact Dermatitis 9:456–458

Sansom JE, Molloy KC, Lovell CR (1995) Occupational sensitization to diphencyprone in a chemist. Contact Dermatitis 32:363

Sato K, Kusaka Y, Suganuma N, Nagasawa S, Deguchi Y (2004) Occupational allergy in medical doctors. J Occup Health 46:165–170

Savini C, Morelli R, Piancastelli E, Restani S (1989) Contact dermatitis due to ethoxyquin. Contact Dermatitis 21:342–343

Schauder S, Schröder W, Geier J (1996) Olaquindox-induced airborne photoallergic contact dermatitis followed by transient or persistent light reactions in 15 pig breeders. Contact Dermatitis 35:344–354

Schena D, Barba A, Costa G (1996) Occupational contact urticaria due to cisplatin. Contact Dermatitis 34:220–221

Schmidt RJ (1986) Compositae. Clin Dermatol 4:46

Schwank R, Jirásek L (1963) Kontaktallergie gegen Chloramphenicol mit besonderer Berücksichtigung der Gruppensensibilisierung. Hautarzt 14:24–30

Schwenck K, Gall H, Sterry W (1994) Aerogene Kontaktdermatitis auf das Neuroleptikum Chlorprothixen. Allergologie 17:467–469

Selvaag E, Holm JO, Thune P (1995) Allergic contact dermatitis in an aroma therapist with multiple sensitizations to essential oils. Contact Dermatitis 33:354–355

Sherertz EF (1994) Occupational skin disease in the pharmaceutical industry. Dermatol Clin 12:533–536

Soni BP, Sherertz EF (1996) Allergic contact dermatitis from azathioprine. Am J Contact Dermat 7:116–117

Sonnex TS, Rycroft RJ (1986) Allergic contact dermatitis from chloromethyl heterocyclic intermediates in the synthesis of a histamine antagonist. Contact Dermatitis 14:265–267

Stejskal VDM, Olin RG, Forsbeck M (1986) The lymphocyte transformation test for diagnosis of drug-induced occupational allergy. J Allergy Clin Immunol 77:411–426

Straube MD, Freitag M, Altmeyer P, Szliska C (2000) Occupational airborne contact dermatitis from cefazolin. Contact Dermatitis 42:44

Szczurko C, Dompmartin A, Michel M, Castel B, Leroy D (1996) Occupational contact dermatitis from propacetamol. Contact Dermatitis 35:299–301

Tadokoro K, Niimi N, Ohtoshi T, Nakajima K, Takafuji S, Onodera K, Suzuki S, Murunaka M (1994) Cefotiam-induced IgE-mediated occupational contact anaphylaxis of nurses; case reports, RAST analysis, and a review of the literature. Clin Exp Allergy 24:127–133

Tas J, Weissberg D (1958) Allergy to aminophylline. Allergy 12:39–42

Tennstedt D, Dumont-Fruytier M, Lachapelle JM (1978) Occupational allergic contact dermatitis to virginiamycin, an antibiotic used as a food additive for pigs and poultry. Contact Dermatitis 4:133–134

Testud F, Descotes J, Evreux JC (1994) Pathologie professionnelle due aux medicaments. Arch Mal Prof 55:279–286

Tuomi ML, Rasanen L (1995) Contact allergy to tylosin and cobalt in a pig-farmer. Contact Dermatitis 33:285

Valsecchi R, Cassina P, Cainelli T (1987) Contact toxic epidermal necrolysis. Contact Dermatitis 16:277

Valsecchi R, Rohrich O, Cainelli T (1989) Contact allergy to cistoran, an intermediate in ranitidine synthesis. Contact Dermatitis 20:396–397

Van Hecke E (1981) Contact sensitivity to vincamine tartrate. Contact Dermatitis 7:53

Vanuytrecht-Henderickx D, Bourgeois M, Mariën K, Dooms-Goossens A (1986) Occupational fixed eruption by inhalation of pyrazolones. Contact Dermatitis 14:115

Veien NK, Hattel T, Justesen O, Norholm A (1980) Occupational contact dermatitis due to spiramycin and/or tylosin among farmers. Contact Dermatitis 6:410–413

Veraldi S, Benelli C, Pigatto PD (1992) Occupational allergic contact dermatitis from minoxidil. Contact Dermatitis 26:211–212

Verschaeve A, Loncke J, Dooms-Goossens A (1984) Occupational contrast media dermatitis: meglumine diatrizoate. Contact Dermatitis 11:318–319

Vilaplana J, Romaguera C (2001) Allergic contact dermatitis due to lansoprazole, a proton pump inhibitor. Contact Dermatitis 44:48

Vilaplana J, Grimalt F, Romaguera C (1990) Contact dermatitis from furaltadone in animal feed. Contact Dermatitis 22:232–233

Vilaplana J, Romaguera C, Grimalt F (1991) Contact dermatitis from lincomycin and spectinomycin in chicken vaccinators. Contact Dermatitis 24:225–226

Waclawski ER, Aldridge R (1995) Occupational dermatitis from thebaine and codeine. Contact Dermatitis 33:51

Wahlberg JE, Boman A (1981) Contact sensitivity to quinidine sulfate from occupational exposure. Contact Dermatitis 7:27–31

Walker SL, Ead RD, Shackleton DB, Beck MH (2005) Two cases of occupational allergic contact dermatitis to p-aminophenol in pharmaceutical workers manufacturing paracetamol. Contact Dermatitis 52:290–291

Watsky KL, Reynolds K, Berube D, Bayer FJ (1993) Occupational contact dermatitis from tosyl chloride in a chemist. Contact Dermatitis 29:211–212

Wigger-Alberti W, Elsner P (1997) Occupational contact dermatitis due to pyritinol. Contact Dermatitis 37:91–92

40 Fragrances and Essential Oils

Anton C. de Groot
Acdegroot publishing, Wapserveen, The Netherlands

Core Messages

- Fragrances are ubiquitous and are present in cosmetics, household products, industrial products and many other applications; they are also used as flavors in foods and drinks.
- Contact allergy to fragrance materials is frequent, both in the general population (2–3.5%) and in patients seen by dermatologists for suspected allergic contact dermatitis (10–12%).
- Only about half of the patients with positive patch tests to fragrances have allergic contact dermatitis from these materials or have a history of a rash from scented products (notably deodorants and fine fragrances).
- Frequent fragrance sensitizers include *Evernia prunastri* (oak moss), *Evernia furfuracea* (tree moss), hydroxyisohexyl 3-cyclohexene carboxaldehyde, hydroxycitronellal, isoeugenol, cinnamal, and farnesol.
- Linalool and limonene may well be frequent sensitizers, but contact allergy is detected only when oxidized patch test materials are used (which is currently not the case).
- Fragrances are not important occupational sensitizers; in the case of eczema of the hands, fragrance allergy may complicate previous irritant or atopic hand dermatitis from their presence in cleansers, hand lotions, etc.
- Essential oils are not important occupational sensitizers, but contact allergy may increasingly be detected in aromatherapists and physiotherapists. Occupational allergic contact dermatitis from oil of cinnamon has been reported in bakers, candy makers, cooks, grocers, confectioners, and housewives.

1 Introduction

Perfumes are so much a part of our culture that we take them for granted, but if they were suddenly taken from us, our culture would suffer immeasurably. We do pay a price for their service, part of which are dermatologic and other medical reactions. This chapter discusses occupational and nonoccupational side effects of fragrance materials and essential oils. For a full review of this subject up to 1997, including adverse reactions to *Myroxylon pereirae* (balsam of Peru, which is used as a marker for fragrance sensitivity) the reader is referred to de Groot and Frosch (1997). Many older literature references for the data in this chapter can be found in the chapter "Fragrances" in the previous edition of the *Handbook of Occupational Dermatology* (de Groot 2000). A book on beneficial and adverse effects of fragrances also provides valuable information (Frosch et al. 1998), as does Dr. Johansen's recent thesis (Johansen 2002). The history of fragrances has been well described by Guin (1982), Scheinman (1996), and Johansen (2002).

2 The Composition of Perfumes

Perfumery is the art of making individuals and products attractive to the olfactory sense. Of the thousands of chemical substances that have an odor, about 3,000 (of which 300–400 are of natural origin), are used in the fragrance industry. A perfume is a creative composition of a few to over 300 fragrance materials. "Proper" perfumes contain approximately 15–30% of the fragrance compound. They are expensive and highly concentrated. The more diluted products (eau de parfum, eau de toilette, colognes) are therefore much more popular. Approximate concentrations of fragrance materials in cosmetics and other products are given in ➋ *Table 40.1*.

Details of the composition of a particular fragrance are closely guarded by industry, which maintains that secrecy of the formulae is fully commensurate with investment in the development and marketing of a product. In several studies, the nature of fragrance materials used in perfumes, deodorants, other cosmetics, and household products (including liquid soap and soap bars, soft/hard surface cleaners, fabric conditioners, laundry detergents, and dish-wash) has been examined (Fenn 1989; Weijland JW, cited by de Groot et al. 1994; Rastogi et al. 1998, 2001); the results are shown in ➋ *Table 40.2* (for synonyms see ➋ *Tables 40.5* and ➋ *40.6*). The results of these studies are difficult to compare because of the

T. Rustemeyer, P. Elsner, S.M. John & H.I. Maibach (eds.), *Kanerva's Occupational Dermatology*,
DOI 10.1007/978-3-642-02035-3_40, © Springer-Verlag Berlin Heidelberg 2012

Table 40.1
Concentrations of perfume in various products (De Groot and Frosch 1997; Johansen 2002)

Aerosol freshener	0.5–2%
Bathroom cleaners	≤5%
Body lotion	0.4%
Compressed powder	0.5%
Deodorant/antiperspirant	1–3%
Dishwashing liquid	0.1–0.5%
Eau de cologne	3–5%
Eau de parfum	8–15%
Eau de toilette	4–8%
Facial make-up	1.0%
Hair pomade	0.5%
Hair spray	0.1–0.3%
Laundry powder	0.1–0.3%
Lipstick	1.0%
Liquid detergents	0.1–1%
Masking perfume	≤0.1%
Perfume (proper)	15–30%
Shampoo (undiluted)	0.5%
Skin care products (emulsions)	0.3–0.5%
Soap (undiluted)	0.5–2%

differences in products investigated, analytical methods, fragrances analyzed (in one study only 20 target fragrances were investigated), geographical differences (Europe versus USA), and period of investigation (usage trends for individual fragrances may vary over time) (Rastogi et al. 2003). Of the 20 fragrances that were investigated in all studies, 10 were found to be in the "Top-25" in each study. These were (in order of decreasing average percentages of being present in the products investigated in the four studies) linalool (85%), linalyl acetate (61%), citronellol (59%), geraniol (53%), hexyl cinnamal (51%), coumarin (49%), benzyl salicylate (44%), butylphenyl methylpropional (Lilial®) (44%), hydroxyisohexyl 3-cyclohexene carboxaldehyde (Lyral®) (36%), and hydroxycitronellal (33%). Fragrances found in three of the four studies were benzyl acetate, methyldihydrojasmonate (Hedione®), heliotropine (piperonal), and amyl cinnamal and benzyl benzoate.

Quantitative data on the fragrances are available from two studies (Rastogi et al. 1998, 2001). The highest fragrance concentrations in deodorants in ppm (10,000 ppm = 1%) were found for benzyl acetate (26,960 ppm), benzyl salicylate (18,758 ppm), and methyldihydrojasmonate (Hedione®) (17,587 ppm). Thirteen of the 20 fragrances investigated had maximum concentrations between 0.1% and 0.56% (1,023–5,585 ppm) (Rastogi et al. 1998). The maximum concentrations found for cinnamal and isoeugenol were high enough to be able to elicit allergic contact dermatitis in patients previously sensitized to these fragrance materials (Bruze et al. 2003). The same applies to hydroxyisohexyl 3-cyclohexene carboxaldehyde (Lyral®). The concentrations of this fragrance ranged from 1 to 1,874 ppm; a concentration as low as 200 ppm in a deodorant use test has been shown to elicit allergic contact dermatitis in the great majority of patients sensitized to this fragrance (Jørgensen et al. 2007).

As can be expected, the concentrations in domestic products were lower with a highest concentration of 9,443 ppm (0.94%) for limonene (this fragrance was present in nearly 4/5 of all products) and 4,060 ppm for hexyl salicylate. The other 17 fragrances were in the concentration range of 3–1,758 ppm, most of them below 500 ppm (0.05%) (Rastogi et al. 2001).

Since 2005, in the EU cosmetic products and detergent products are required to be labeled for the presence of 26 individual fragrance chemicals (➲ *Table 40.5*; these fragrances are identified by the symbol [c]), if present at >10 parts per million (ppm, 0.001%) in leave-on products and >100 ppm (0.01%) in rinse-off products (EU 2003) (http://eur-lex.europa.eu/LexUriServ/LexUriServ.do?uri=OJ:L:2003:066:0026:0035:en:PDF).

In 2006, in the UK 300 products were surveyed and any of the 26 listed fragrances named on the label were recorded (Buckley 2007). Two hundred and sixty-six (89%) contained at least one of the listed fragrances. The top ten most frequently labeled fragrances were linalool (63%), limonene (63%), citronellol (48%), geraniol (42%), butyl phenyl methyl propional (Lilial®) (42%), hexyl cinnamal (42%), benzyl salicylate (38%), α-isomethyl ionone (35%), coumarin (30%), and hydroxyisohexyl 3-cyclohexene carboxaldehyde (29%). Linalool was the most frequently found fragrance in 70 personal care products (soap, shampoo, shower gel) and linalool and limonene the most frequent in 59 products for men (e.g., aftershave). Limonene predominated in household products (washing-up liquid, detergent) and limonene and linalool were found in nearly all perfumes for women. Alpha-isomethyl ionone was the most frequent in cosmetics (foundation, lipstick, etc.) and citronellol predominated in 17 deodorants (88%). The mean number of listed fragrances in a product was 5.9 (mean for perfumes 12, deodorants 7.8, products for men 6.5, household products 3, in dental products 1) (Buckley 2007).

Table 40.2
Most commonly found fragrances in cosmetics, toiletries, and household products

Rank order	Fragrances found in 400 cosmetics and household products in the USA (Fenn 1989)	Fragrances found in 300 cosmetic products in The Netherlands (Weijland, cited by De Groot et al. 1994)	(Targeted) fragrances found in 73 deodorants in Denmark, Sweden, Germany, UK and France (Rastogi et al. 1998)	Fragrances found in 57 domestic and 2 occupational products in Denmark, UK, Germany and Italy (Rastogi et al. 2001)
1	Linalool (90%)	Linalool (91%)	Linalool (97%)	Limonene (78%)
2	Phenethyl alcohol (82%)	Phenethyl alcohol (79%)	Benzyl acetate (84%)	Linalool (61%)
3	Linalyl acetate (78%)	Benzyl acetate (78%)	Citronellol (81%)	Citronellol (47%)
4	Benzyl acetate (74%)	Limonene (71%)	Methyldihydrojasmonate (79%)	Eucalyptol (41%)
5	Benzyl salicylate (74%)	Citronellol (71%)	Geraniol (76%)	Geraniol (41%)
6	Coumarin (68%)	Linalyl acetate (67%)	Linalyl acetate (73%)	α-Pinene (39%)
7	Terpineol (66%)	α-Isomethyl ionone (63%)	Benzyl benzoate (71%)	Hexamethylindanopyran (36%)
8	Methyldihydrojasmonate (56%)	Terpineol (52%)	Hexyl cinnamal (71%)	Isoamyl salicylate (34%)
9	Hexyl cinnamal (51%)	β-Pinene (51%)	α-Isomethyl ionone (61%)	Hexyl cinnamal (32%)
10	α-Isomethyl ionone (51%)	Geraniol (50%)	Coumarin (57%)	Isobornyl acetate (32%)
11	Terpinyl acetate (50%)	Hydroxycitronellal (49%)	Eugenol (57%)	4-*tert*-Butylcyclohexyl acetate (31%)
12	Butylphenyl methylpropional (49%)	Benzyl benzoate (49%)	Hydroxyisohexyl 3-cyclohexene carboxaldehyde (53%)	Nerol (29%)
13	Hydroxyisohexyl 3-cyclohexene carboxaldehyde (46%)	Hexyl cinnamal (48%)	Butylphenyl methylpropional (51%)	Eugenol (27%)
14	Geraniol (43%)	Butylphenyl methylpropional (48%)	Hydroxycitronellal (50%)	Butylphenyl methylpropional (27%)
15	Heliotropine (43%)	Coumarin (44%)	Benzyl salicylate (49%)	Linalyl acetate (27%)
16	Hexamethylindanopyran (41%)	Benzyl salicylate (43%)	Heliotropine (40%)	Coumarin (25%)
17	Acetyl cedrene (41%)	Benzyl alcohol (42%)	Cinnamyl alcohol (39%)	Citral (25%)
18	Musk ketone (38%)	Eugenol (36%)	Amyl cinnamal (31%)	Borneol/isoborneol (25%)
19	Citronellol (38%)	α-Pinene (35%)	Isoeugenol (29%)	Methyl dihydrojasmonate (24%)
20	Amyl salicylate (32%)	Geranyl acetate (35%)	Cinnamal (17%)	Heliotropine (22%)
21	Eugenol (26%)	Amyl cinnamal (35%)		Hexyl salicylate (19%)
22	4-*tert*-Butylcyclohexyl acetate (25%)	Musk ketone (34%)		Hydroxycitronellal (12%)
23	Isobornyl acetate (23%)	β-Caryophyllene (33%)		Hydroxyisohexyl 3-cyclohexene carboxaldehyde (10%)
24	Amyl cinnamal (21%)	Hydroxyisohexyl 3-cyclohexene carboxaldehyde (33%)		Benzyl benzoate (10%)
25	Hydroxycitronellal (21%)	Camphor (31%)		Benzyl salicylate (8%)

3 Contact with Fragrances and Fragranced Products

The use of fragrances is ubiquitous and not limited to those cosmetic products that are used primarily for their scent (such as perfumes, eau de cologne, eau de toilette, deodorant, and aftershave). Virtually all cosmetics and toiletries contain fragrance materials; even "unscented" or "fragrance-free" products may contain a masking perfume or an essential oil (Nardelli et al. 2009b). Flavors used in oral hygiene products – toothpaste, mouthwash, and dental floss are fragrance chemicals. Scented household products include detergents, cleaners, softeners, fabric conditioners, deodorizing sprays, polishes, solvents, and waxes (Magnano et al. 2009). In industry, cutting fluids, electroplating fluids, paints, rubber, plastics, insecticides, herbicides, and additives used in air-conditioning water may all be scented. Eugenol is occasionally used by dentists. Paper and paper products – including diapers, facial tissues, moist toilet paper, and sanitary napkins – may cause a reaction. Fabrics and clothes may contain fragrance materials, especially after they are laundered or treated with a fabric softener (although this never results in sensitization or elicitation of allergic contact dermatitis; Corea et al. 2006). Topical drugs often contain perfumes or essential oils (Nardelli et al. 2009a), and ventilating systems may spread fragrances. The distinction between fragrances and spices is often vague. Many synthetic fragrances are used as spices and flavors. Natural fragrances like cinnamon, clove, vanilla and cardamom are added to foods, soft drinks, lozenges, chewing gum, candies, ice cream, and tobacco. Thus, it can be stated that virtually everyone is in daily contact with fragrance materials.

Contact with fragrances may be from direct product application to the skin or mucous membranes, by occasional contact with an allergen-contaminated product such as towels and pillows; contact with products used by partners, friends, or coworkers (consort or connubial contact dermatitis); airborne contact; and systemic exposure by inhalation and ingestion (fragrances, flavors and spices in foods and drinks). Any part of the body may come in contact with fragranced cosmetics.

4 Contact Allergy to Fragrances

Contact allergy to fragrances is very common. In the general Danish and Norwegian population aged 18–69 years, 1.6% and 1.8% reacted to a patch test with the fragrance mix I (FM I), a diagnostic marker for fragrance sensitivity (Dotterud and Smith-Sivertsen 2007; Thyssen et al. 2009a). The positive reactions were associated with self-reported recent cosmetic dermatitis and use of health care related to cosmetic dermatitis (Thyssen et al. 2009a). Based on 13 studies performed in adults, the weighted average prevalence of FM I sensitization was calculated to be 3.7% (Thyssen et al. 2009b). However, other fragrance compounds not detected by this mix can also cause contact allergy, so the percentage is likely to be higher. It should be appreciated that many such individuals, although sensitized to certain fragrance materials, can tolerate perfumes and scented products and do not suffer from, nor have a history of allergic reactions. Even continuous exposure to fragrances to which contact allergy has been established will not necessarily lead to allergic contact dermatitis (Schubert 2006). Nevertheless, of contact dermatitis patients with a positive reaction to the FM I, many continue to suffer from (periodic) dermatitis, 17% reported sick-leave due to fragrance allergy, and 45% found that fragrance allergy significantly affects their daily living (Hovmand Lysdal and Johansen 2009). Fragrances account for 30–45% of all reactions in patients suffering from allergic contact dermatitis to cosmetics (Adams and Maibach 1985; De Groot et al. 1988).

5 Detecting Fragrance Allergy

A perfume may contain as many as 200 or more individual ingredients. This makes the diagnosis of perfume allergy by patch test procedures complicated. Formerly, *M. pereirae* resin (balsam of Peru) and – to a lesser extent – colophonium (rosin) in the European baseline series (at that moment named European standard series) acted as sole diagnostic markers ("indicators") for fragrance contact allergy: positive patch test reactions raised the possibility of fragrance allergy (they both contain a large number of substances used in fragrances) (Downs and Sansom 1999; Hausen 2001). In the late 1970s, the fragrance mix (now called fragrance mix I) was introduced as a screening tool for fragrance sensitivity (➋ *Table 40.3*).

It is estimated that this mix detects 50–80% of fragrance sensitivity cases (Johansen 2003). The response rate in dermatological patients to the fragrance mix and its ingredients ranges worldwide from 6% to 17.9% (Landeck et al. 2009), and the fragrance mix is (outside the USA, where *M. pereirae* is second) usually the second most frequent allergen after nickel sulfate (ESSCA Writing Group 2008). The rates peaked in the mid- to late 1990s (9.7% in Europe, Bruynzeel et al. 2005) but since then, the frequency of reactions to the mix appears to be decreasing in several European countries (Schnuch et al.

Table 40.3
Fragrances, fragrance mixes and indicators of fragrance contact allergy in the European baseline series

Chemical	Concentration% (w/w) and vehicle
Colophonium (rosin)	20% pet.
Fragrance mix I (including 5% sorbitan sesquioleate)	8% pet.
Amyl cinnamal (α-amylcinnamic aldehyde) (1%) Cinnamal (cinnamic aldehyde) (1%) Cinnamyl alcohol (1%) Eugenol (1%) *Evernia prunastri* (oak moss absolute) (1%) Geraniol (1%) Hydroxycitronellal (1%) Isoeugenol (1%)	
Fragrance mix II	14% pet.
Citral (1%) Citronellol (0.5%) Coumarin (2.5%) Farnesol (2.5%) Hexyl cinnamal (α-hexylcinnamic aldehyde) (5%) Hydroxyisohexyl 3-cyclohexene carboxaldehyde (Lyral ®) (2.5%)	
Hydroxyisohexyl 3-cyclohexene carboxaldehyde (Lyral ®)	5% pet.
Myroxylon pereirae (balsam of Peru)	25% pet.

2004a; Thyssen et al. 2008; Nardelli et al. 2008; Europe 7%, Uter et al. 2009). This may be related to changes in the composition of perfumes (Rastogi et al. 2003), contact allergy to which ingredients may not be detected by the FM I. In the USA rates are still 11.5%, which may partly be related to stricter selection of patients for patch testing (Zug et al. 2009).

Of the ingredients in the mix (➋ *Table 40.3*), most reactions are caused by *Evernia prunastri* (oak moss), isoeugenol, cinnamal, and hydroxycitronellal (Schnuch et al. 2004a; Buckley et al. 2006). Among the >100 constituents identified in oak moss, atranol and chloroatranol (degradation products of atranorin and chloroatranorin) figure as the most potent allergens (Johansen et al. 2006). These substances are found in many perfumes in considerable concentrations (Rastogi et al. 2004). Other lichen acids present in *E. prunastri* that cause reactions in allergic patients include usnic acid, evernic acid, fumarprotocetraric acid, stictic acid, physodes/physodalic acid, and diffractaic acid. Contact allergy to lichen acids may also be acquired from woods and plants.

The FM I, although very useful, is far from ideal. It causes irritant reactions, false-negative reactions (positive reaction to one or more of the ingredients but negative reaction to the mix), and leaves 20–50% of fragrance sensitivities undetected. In addition, it is rather common for patients with positive reactions to the fragrance mix to have a negative break-down, i.e., no positive reactions to one or more of its ingredients (Buckley et al. 2000). This phenomenon (assuming that the reaction to the mix was not false-positive) remains unexplained. In addition, it is likely that testing with the fragrance mix I may occasionally cause active sensitization (White et al. 2008). Also, sorbitan sesquioleate present in the mix may induce an allergic response. Therefore, this emulsifier should always be routinely tested to avoid misinterpreting a positive reaction to sorbitan sesquioleate in the mix as fragrance allergy.

Routine testing with additional fragrances (and essential oils) reveals many cases of fragrance contact allergy not detected by the FM I (Frosch et al. 2002, 2005a). A group of European dermatologists recently developed a new mix of six fragrances, the FM II (➋ *Table 40.3*) (Frosch et al. 2005b). Its constituents are citral, citronellol, coumarin, farnesol, hexyl cinnamal, and hydroxyisohexyl 3-cyclohexene carboxaldehyde (Lyral®). Reaction rates to this mix, which was introduced in the European baseline series in 2008 (Bruze et al. 2008) vary from 2.1% to 4.7% (Frosch et al. 2005b; Nardelli et al. 2008; Uter et al. 2009). In 35–50% of the patients, the FM I was negative. In testing the ingredients separately, by far the most common allergen was hydroxyisohexyl 3-cyclohexene carboxaldehyde, followed by citral, farnesol, and citronellol. There were very few reactions to amyl cinnamal and coumarin. It should be noted that one third of the patients reacting to the FM II had no positive reactions to its ingredients (similar to FM I), which may indicate that some reactions are actually false positive (irritant) (Frosch et al. 2005b).

At the same time, hydroxyisohexyl 3-cyclohexene carboxaldehyde (Lyral ®), the predominant sensitizing constituent of the FM II, was added as single allergen to the baseline series in the higher concentration of 5% (Bruze et al. 2008). The rate of sensitization to this fragrance, which is strongly associated with contact allergy to deodorants, is 1.5–3% throughout Europe, which makes it one of the most frequent allergens in the baseline series (Braendstrup and Johansen 2008).

Sixty fragrance allergens (including mixes and indicators) and 25 essential oils (which are frequently used in fragrances) are commercially available for patch testing (➋ *Table 40.4*). In case of suspected allergic contact dermatitis to perfumes, deodorants, and shaving lotions, it is advisable to test these products also (undiluted), as in about half the cases of positive reactions to the patients' own products the fragrance allergens in the baseline series are negative, and positive reactions to the products strongly suggest relevancy (Uter et al. 2007).

6 Important Fragrance Sensitizers

In a German study, the frequency of sensitization to the 26 fragrance allergens that need to be labeled in the EU (2003) was investigated in 1,658–21,325 patients. Leading allergens were *Evernia prunastri* (oak moss) (2% reactions), *Evernia furfuracea* (tree moss) (2.4%), hydroxyisohexyl 3-cyclohexene carboxaldehyde (2.3%), hydroxycitronellal (1.3%), isoeugenol (1.1%), cinnamal (1.0%), and farnesol (0.9%). A second group with a sensitization rate between 1.0% and >0.5% comprises cinnamyl alcohol, citral, citronellol, geraniol, eugenol, coumarin, butylphenyl methylpropional, amyl cinnamic alcohol, and benzyl cinnamate. The other 10, including the very commonly used linalool and limonene, had scores of 0.3% or lower (Schnuch et al. 2007b). Similar results were obtained in a smaller Dutch investigation (Van Oosten et al. 2009). There are relatively few positive reactions to linalool and limonene, although these fragrances are very often present in fragrances in perfumes, cosmetics, and household products (Buckley 2007). This may well be caused by the fact that these fragrances become (far more) allergenic after auto-oxidation (Matura et al. 2005, 2006; Bråred Christensson et al. 2010). This means that current patch tests may be false negative and should be performed with oxidized patch test material of linalool and limonene.

7 Clinical Picture of Allergic Contact Dermatitis from Fragrances

In general, fragrance allergy (as diagnosed by positive patch tests) occurs predominantly in women with facial and hand eczema. They will typically give a history of previous rash to a fine fragrance or scented deodorant (Johansen 2003). Literature on the clinical picture of perfume dermatitis is rather scant and a good description is lacking. It can be expected, however, that the neck, skin

Table 40.4
Fragrances and essential oils commercially available for patch testing

Patch test allergen	Suppliers		
	Almirall	Chemo	Brial
FRAGRANCES			
Abietic acid	10%	10%	10%
Alantolactone		0.33%	
Amyl cinnamal (α-amylcinnamic aldehyde)	1%	2%	1%
α-Amylcinnamic alcohol	1%	5%	
Anethole		5%	
Anisyl alcohol	1%	10% Softisan	
Atranorin		0.1%	
Benzaldehyde	5%		5%
Benzyl alcohol	1%	10% Softisan	1%
Benzyl benzoate	1%	10%	5%
Benzyl cinnamate	5%	10%	5%
Benzyl salicylate	1%	10%	1%
Butylphenyl methylpropional (Lilial®, *p-tert*-butyl-α-methyl-hydrocinnamic aldehyde)	10%	10%	
Carvone		5%	5%
Cinnamal (cinnamic aldehyde)	1%	1%	1%
Cinnamyl alcohol	1%	2%	1%
Citral	2%	2%	
Citronellal			2%
Citronellol	1%	1%	
Colophonium (rosin)[a]	20%	20%	20%
Coumarin	5%	5%	1%
Dipentene (d,l- (R-S-)-limonene)	2%	1%	
Eugenol	1%	2%	1%
Evernia furfuracea (tree moss)	1%	1%	
Evernia prunastri (oak moss absolute)	1%	2%	1%
Evernic acid		0.1%	
Farnesol	5%	5%	
Fragrance mix I (cinnamyl alcohol, cinnamal, hydroxycitronellal, amyl cinnamal, geraniol, eugenol, isoeugenol, *Evernia prunastri*)[a]	8%	8%	8%
Fragrance mix II (citral, citronellol, coumarin, farnesol, hexyl cinnamal, hydroxyisohexyl 3-cyclohexene carboxaldehyde (Lyral))[a]	14%	14%	14%

Table 40.4 (Continued)

Patch test allergen	Suppliers		
	Almirall	Chemo	Brial
Geraniol	1%	2%	1%
Hexyl cinnamal (α-hexylcinnamic aldehyde)	10%	10%	
Hydroabietyl alcohol (Abitol®)	10%	10%	
Hydroxycitronellal	1%	2%	1%
Hydroxyisohexyl 3-cyclohexene carboxaldehyde (Lyral®)	5%	5%	
Isoeugenol	1%	2%	1%
α-Isomethyl ionone (γ-methylionone)	1%	10%	
Lichen acid mix (atranorin, evernic acid, usnic acid)[a]		0.3%	
d-Limonene		10%	2%
Linalool	10%	10%	
Menthol	1%	2%	1%
Methyl anthranilate		5%	
Methylcoumarin		1%	
Methyl-2-octynoate (methyl heptine carbonate)	1%	0.2%	
Methyl salicylate			2%
Musk ambrette			5%
Musk ketone		1%	
Musk mix (xylene, moskene, ketone)[a]		3%	
Musk moskene		1%	
Musk xylene		1%	
Myroxylon pereirae (Balsam of Peru)[a]	25%	25%	25%
Perfume mix (cinnamyl alcohol, cinnamal, hydroxycitronellal, eugenol, isoeugenol, geraniol)[a]		6%	
Phenyl salicylate		1%	1%
α-Pinene			15%
Propolis[a]	10%	10%	10%
Salicylaldehyde	2%		2%
Sesquiterpene lactone mix (alantolactone, costunolide, dehydrocostus lactone)[a]	0.1%	0.1%	0.1%
Trimethyl benzene propanol (Majantol®)	5%		5%
Usnic acid	0.1%	0.1%	0.1%
Vanillin	10%	10%	10%
ESSENTIAL OILS			
Bergamot oil (*Citrus bergamia*)			2%

Table 40.4 (Continued)

Patch test allergen	Suppliers		
	Almirall	Chemo	Brial
Cananga oil (*Cananga genuina*)		2%	
Cedarwood oil (*Cedrus atlantica*)	10%		10%
Chamomile oil (*Anthemis nobilis*)		1%	
Cinnamon oil (*Cinnamonum cassia*)			0.5%
Clove oil (*Eugenia caryophyllus*)	2%		2%
Eucalyptus oil (*Eucalyptus globulus*)	2%		2%
Geranium oil, Bourbon (*Pelargonium roseum*)		2%	
Hypericum oil (*Hypericum perforatum*)			0.5%
Jasmine absolute, synthetic (*Jasminum officinale*)	5%	2%	2%
Laurel oil (*Laurus nobilis*)	2%		2%
Lavender, absolute (*Lavandula angustifolia*)		2%	2%
Lemongrass oil (*Cymbopogon Schoenanthus*)	2%		2%
Lemon oil (*Citrus limonum*)	2%		2%
Narcissus absolute (*Narcissus jonquilla*)	2%	2%	
Neroli oil (*Citrus aurantium dulcis*)	2%		2%
Orange oil (*Citrus dulcis*)	2%		
Patchouli oil (*Pogostemon cablin*)	10%		
Peppermint oil (*Mentha piperita*)	2%		2%
Rose oil (*Rosa*)			0.5%
Rose oil, Bulgarian (*Rosa centifolia*)		2%	
Rosemary oil (*Rosmarinus officinalis*)			0.5%
Sandalwood oil (*Santalum album*)	10%	2%	
Tea tree oil (*Melaleuca alternifolia*)		5%	5%
Ylang-ylang oil (*Cananga odorata*)	10%	2%	2%

Almirall www.almirall.de; Chemotechnique www.chemotechnique.se; Brial www.brial.com

All test substances are in petrolatum unless otherwise indicated

[a]Not a fragrance ingredient per se, but an indicator of fragrance allergy

behind the ear, and axillae are often implicated, given that they are exposed to products with high concentrations of fragrances (perfume, deodorant). Indeed, the fragrances used in deodorants are an important cause of induction and elicitation of fragrance allergy (Johansen 2003). Also, the sensitive skin of the face and the eyelids should be particularly susceptible to developing allergic contact dermatitis to fragrances in skin-care products, decorative cosmetics, and cleansing preparations, and from airborne contact dermatitis. Micro-traumata from shaving facilitates (photo) contact allergy to aftershave fragrances. Most reactions are erythematous, and some cases may resemble nummular eczema, seborrheic dermatitis, sycosis barbae, or lupus erythematosus (Meynadier et al. 1986). More acute lesions with papules, vesicles, and oozing may sometimes be observed. Lesions in the skin folds may be mistaken for atopic dermatitis. Dermatitis due to perfumes or toilet water tends to be "streaky." Facial psoriasis may be induced/aggravated by allergic contact dermatitis from fragrances. Hand eczema is common in fragrance-sensitive patients and there is a possible but not certain (Nardelli et al. 2008) association between the dermatitis and fragrance sensitization (Heydorn et al. 2003a). Patients may first have irritant dermatitis or atopic dermatitis, which is later complicated by contact allergy to products used for treatment or prevention (hand creams and lotions) of hand dermatitis, or to other perfumed products in the household, hobby, or work environment. Dyshidrotic eruptions are ascribed to ingestion of spices. Atopic dermatitis located at other body sites, perianal dermatitis, and vulvar dermatitis may also be complicated by fragrance allergy. Fragrances present in topical pharmaceutical preparations (corticosteroids, anti-inflammatory drugs, wound healing, antiseptic-disinfectant, antihemorrhoids) can cause iatrogenic allergic contact dermatitis (Nardelli et al. 2009a).

8 Clinical Relevance of Positive Reactions to the Fragrance Mixes

As with any contact allergen, the finding of a positive reaction to the fragrance mixes should be followed by a search for its relevance. Often, however, correlation with the clinical picture is lacking and many patients can tolerate perfumes and fragrance products without problems. About half of those with a positive patch test to a fragrance mix have no history of any cosmetic reaction. This may sometimes be explained by irritant patch test reactions to the fragrance mix. Alternative explanations include the absence of relevant allergens in products used or a concentration too low to elicit clinically visible allergic contact reactions.

In various studies, the relevance of positive patch test reactions to the FM mix I has been investigated. However, criteria were often not provided. In cases with concomitant positive reactions to perfumes or fragranced products used by the patient, interpretation of the reaction as relevant may be quite easy (Uter et al. 2007). In the presence of more than one fragrance reaction and/or co-reactivity to other markers of fragrance sensitivity (*M. pereirae*, colophonium), relevance becomes more likely. Strongly positive patch test reactions are also more likely associated with relevancy than a weak or doubtful reaction (? + 25%, + 40%, ++/+++ >70%; Devos et al. 2008). A repeated FM I positive patch test strongly increases the possibility for a relevant reaction (Devos et al. 2008). Clinical relevance of a positive patch test reaction was estimated to be 45-65% of positive results (de Groot and Frosch 1997). In a recent more detailed study, 61% of positive patch test reactions to one or more fragrances (fragrance mixes I and II, 26 fragrances labeled in the EU) were "definitely" relevant, and 12% "probably" relevant. However, these patients were selected on the basis of certain criteria, among which suspicion of contact allergy to fragrances or cosmetics (van Oosten et al. 2009). A positive ROAT (repeated open application test, twice daily application on the antecubital fossa for at least 2 weeks) with fragrance ingredients makes relevance of the reaction more likely.

9 Other Allergens

In ➔ *Table 40.5*, published fragrance allergens are tabulated with their CAS number, test concentration, vehicle (De Groot 2008), and references. Over 140 fragrances have been reported as sensitizers. It should be noted, however, that for a substantial number of them, only positive patch tests were observed (often with routine testing), without verification of their relevance. There is no consensus in literature on the nomenclature and many different names are used, including trade names. ➔ *Table 40.6* provides a list of synonyms. We have used INCI names and – if not available – names used in the European CosIng data base (http://ec.europa.eu/enterprise/cosmetics/cosing).

10 Occupational Allergic Contact Dermatitis to Fragrances

It may be expected that fragrances will cause dermatological problems for workers in the cosmetics industry (cosmetic chemists, workers handling the raw materials and the final products, salespeople) beauticians, hairdressers, and aromatherapists (see the ➔ Sect. 40.16). In a German study, massage therapists and physiotherapists had the highest occupational risk of fragrance contact allergy (Uter et al. 2001). Housewives, health personnel, and

Table 40.5
Fragrances reported as contact allergens (de Groot and Frosch 1997; de Groot 2000)

Name of fragrance	Chemical abstract service (CAS)	Test concentration and vehicle (de Groot 2008)	Additional references
Abietic acid[a]	514-10-3	See *Table 40.4*	
Acetylcedrene (Vertofix®)	32388-55-9	1–5% pet	
5-Acetyl-1,1,2,3,3,6-hexamethylindan (Phantolide®)	15323-35-0	3% pet	
6-Acetyl-1,1,2,4,4,7-hexamethyltetralin (Fixolide®)	1506-02-1	3% pet	
Alantolactone[a,b]	546-43-0	See *Table 40.4*	
Amyl cinnamal (α-amylcinnamic aldehyde)[a,c]	122-40-7	See *Table 40.4*	Schnuch et al. 2007b; van Oosten et al. 2009
Amyl cinnamate	3487-99-8	8% pet	
Amyl cinnamic alcohol[c]	101-85-9	See *Table 40.4*	Schnuch et al. 2007b; van Oosten et al. 2009
Amyl salicylate	2050-08-0	5% pet	
Anethole	104 46-1	See *Table 40.4*	
Anisyl alcohol[a,c]	105-13-5	See *Table 40.4*	Schnuch et al. 2007b; van Oosten et al. 2009
Anisylidene acetone	943-88-4	2% pet	
Aromadendrene (in tea tree oil)	489-39-4	5% DEP	Hausen 2004
Ascaridol (in tea tree oil)	512-85-6	10% DEP	Hausen 2004
Atranorin (in oak moss)[b]	479-20-9	See *Table 40.4*	
Benzaldehyde[a]	100-52-7	See *Table 40.4*	Schubert 2006
Benzyl acetate	140-11-4; 101-41-7	5% pet	
Benzyl alcohol[a,c,d]	100-51-6	See *Table 40.4*	Curry and Warshaw 2005; Schnuch et al. 2007b; Nardelli et al. 2009a; van Oosten et al. 2009
Benzyl benzoate[a,c]	120-51-4	See *Table 40.4*	Schnuch et al. 2007b; van Oosten et al. 2009
Benzyl cinnamate[c]	103-41-3	See *Table 40.4*	Schnuch et al. 2007b; van Oosten et al. 2009
Benzylidene acetone	122-57-6	0.5% pet	
Benzyl salicylate[c,d]	118-58-1	See *Table 40.4*	Schnuch et al. 2007b; van Oosten et al. 2009
Butylphenyl methylpropional (Lilial®)[c]	80-54-6	See *Table 40.4*	Schnuch et al. 2007b; van Oosten et al. 2009
Camphor	76-22-2	10% pet	Schubert 2006
Carvacrol (isothymol)	499-75-2	5% pet	
d- and l-Carvone	218-827-2 (d-); 6485-40-1 (l-)	See *Table 40.4*	Hausen 2004
β-Caryophyllene	87-44-5	5% pet	Frosch et al. 2002; Matura et al. 2005
Cedrol methyl ether (cedramber)	19870-74-7	5% pet	
Cinnamal (cinnamic aldehyde, cinnamaldehyde)[a,b,c]	104-55-2	See *Table 40.4*	Buckley et al. 2006; Schnuch et al. 2007b; van Oosten et al. 2009
Cinnamyl alcohol (cinnamic alcohol)[a,c,d]	203-212-3	See *Table 40.4*	Buckley et al. 2006; Schnuch et al. 2007b; van Oosten et al. 2009
Cinnamyl benzoate	5320-75-2	5% pet	
Cinnamyl cinnamate[a]	122-69-0	5% pet	

Table 40.5 (Continued)

Name of fragrance	Chemical abstract service (CAS)	Test concentration and vehicle (de Groot 2008)	Additional references
Citral[c]	5392-40-5	See Table 40.4	Heydorn et al. 2003b; Schnuch et al. 2007b; van Oosten et al. 2009
Citronellal	106-23-0	See Table 40.4	
Citronellol[c]	106-22-9	See Table 40.4	Schnuch et al. 2007b; van Oosten et al. 2009
Coumarin[a,b,c]	91-64-5	See Table 40.4	Schnuch et al. 2007b; van Oosten et al. 2009
Cuminaldehyde	122-03-2	5% pet	
Cyclohexyl acetate	622-45-7	5% pet	Larsen et al. 2002
Cyclopentadecanone	502-72-7	5% pet	Larsen et al. 2001
α- and β-Damascone	23726-94-5; 43052-87-5 (α)	2 × 0.1% pet	Frosch et al. 2002; Giménez-Arnau et al. 2002
Dehydroisoeugenol		Test ylang-ylang oil	
Diethyl maleate	141-05-9	2% pet	
Diffractaic acid (in oak moss)		0.1–1% pet	
Dihydrocoumarin	119-84-6	5% pet	
Dihydro pentamethylindanone (Cashmeran®)	33704-61-9	5% pet	
Dimethyl citraconate	617-54-9	10% pet	
3,7-Dimethyl-7-methoxyoctan-2-ol (Osyrol®)	41890-92-0	?	Larsen et al. 2002
Dimethyltetrahydrobenzaldehyde (isomer mixture)	68737-61-1	5% pet	Larsen et al. 2001
DMBCA (dimethylbenzyl carbinyl acetate)	151-05-3	3% pet	
Ebanol (3-Methyl-5-(2,2,3-trimethyl-3-cyclopenten-1-yl)-4-penten-2-ol)	67801-20-1	5% pet	An et al. 2005
Ethyl anisate	94-30-4	4% pet	
Ethylene dodecanedioate	54982-83-1	5% pet	Larsen et al. 2002
Eucalyptol (1,8-cineole, cajeputol)	470-82-6	5% pet	
Eugenol[a,b,c]	97-53-0	See Table 40.4	Buckley et al. 2006; Schnuch et al. 2007b; van Oosten et al. 2009;
Evernia furfuracea (tree moss)[c]	90028-67-4	See Table 40.4	Schnuch et al. 2007b; van Oosten et al. 2009
Evernia prunastri (oak moss)[a,b,c]	90028-68-5	See Table 40.4	Schnuch et al. 2007b; van Oosten et al. 2009
Evernic acid (in oak moss)[b]	537-09-7	See Table 40.4	
Farnesol[c]	4602-84-0	See Table 40.4	Schnuch et al. 2004b, 2007b; van Oosten et al. 2009
Fumarprotocetraric acid (in oak moss)		0.1% pet	
Galbanum resin (*Ferula galbaniflua* gum)	93165-40-3	2% pet	
Geranial	141-27-5	1–5% pet	
Geraniol[a,c,d]	106-24-1	See Table 40.4	Schnuch et al. 2007b; van Oosten et al. 2009

Table 40.5 (Continued)

Name of fragrance	Chemical abstract service (CAS)	Test concentration and vehicle (de Groot 2008)	Additional references
Heliotropine (piperonal)	120-57-0	5% pet	Frosch et al. 2002
Hexadecanolactone (hexadecanolide)	109-29-5	5% pet	An et al. 2005; Larsen et al. 2001
Ω-6-hexadecenlactone	7779-50-2	5% pet	Larsen et al. 2001
Hexamethylindanopyran (Galaxolide®)	1222-05-5	5–15% pet	An et al. 2005
cis-3-Hexenyl salicylate	65405-77-8	3% pet	Shaw 2006
Hexyl cinnamal (α-Hexylcinnamic aldehyde)[c]	101-86-0	See ➋ *Table 40.4*	Schnuch et al. 2007b; van Oosten et al. 2009
Hexyl salicylate	6259-76-3	12% pet	
Hydroabietyl alcohol (Abitol®, dihydroabietyl alcohol)	13393-93-6	See ➋ *Table 40.4*	
Hydroxycitronellal[a,b,c,d]	107-74-4	See ➋ *Table 40.4*	Schnuch et al. 2007b; van Oosten et al. 2009
Hydroxyisohexyl 3-cyclohexene carboxaldehyde (Lyral®)[c]	31906-04-4; 51414-25-6	See ➋ *Table 40.4*	Militello and James 2005; Jørgensen et al. 2007; Schnuch et al. 2007b; Braendstrup and Johansen 2008; van Oosten et al. 2009
Ionone (irisone)	8013-90-9; 79-77-6	8% pet	Nardelli et al. 2009a
Isobornyl cyclohexanol (synthetic sandalwood)[d]	68877-29-2	2% pet	
Isoeugenol[c]	97-54-1	See ➋ *Table 40.4*	Buckley et al. 2006; White et al. 2007; Schnuch et al. 2007b; van Oosten et al. 2009
trans-Isoeugenol	97-54-1	1% pet	Tanaka et al. 2004a
Isoeugenyl acetate	93-29-8	1.3% pet	Tanaka et al. 2004a
Isoeugenyl benzoate		1.6% pet	Tanaka et al. 2004a
Isoeugenyl benzyl ether (benzyl isoeugenol)	120-11-6	1.5% pet	Tanaka et al. 2004a
Isoeugenyl methyl ether (methyl isoeugenol)	93-16-3	1.1–5% pet	Larsen et al. 2002; Tanaka et al. 2004a
Isoeugenyl phenylacetate	120-24-1	1.7% pet	Tanaka et al. 2004a
Isolongifolene ketone	33407-62-4	5% pet	Larsen et al. 2001
α-Isomethyl ionone (γ-methylionone)[a,c]	127-51-5	See ➋ *Table 40.4*	An et al. 2005; Schnuch et al. 2007b; van Oosten et al. 2009
Isopulegol	7786-67-6; 89-79-2	5% pet	
Ledene (viridoflorene) in tea tree oil	21747-46-6	10% DEP/5% pet	Hausen 2004
Ligustral ((methyl-(2,4(3,5)-dimethyl-3-cyclohexen-1-yl)-methylene anthranilate)	68039-49-6	5% pet	
Limonene[c] d-, d,l- (dipentene)	5989-27-5 (d-); 138-86-3 (d,l-)	See ➋ *Table 40.4* (limonene, dipentene)	Matura et al. 2006; Schnuch et al. 2007b; van Oosten et al. 2009
Linalool[c]	78-70-6	See ➋ *Table 40.4*	Matura et al. 2005; Schnuch et al. 2007b; Hagvall et al. 2008; van Oosten et al. 2009; Bråred Christensson et al. 2010
Linalyl acetate	115-95-7	4% pet	Hagvall et al. 2008

Table 40.5 (Continued)

Name of fragrance	Chemical abstract service (CAS)	Test concentration and vehicle (de Groot 2008)	Additional references
Menthol[a]	1490-04-6; 2216-51-5; 89-78-1; 15356-70-4	See *Table 40.4*	Nardelli et al. 2009a
o-Methoxycinnamic aldehyde	1504-74-1	4% pet	
Methoxycitronellal[d]	3613-30-7	10% pet	
Methyl anisate	121-98-2	4% pet	
Methyl anthranilate[b]	134-20-3	See *Table 40.4*	
α-Methyl-1,3-benzodioxole-5-propanal (Helional®)	1205-17-0	5% pet	
Methylcoumarin	92-48-8 (6-); 2445-83-2 (7-)	See *Table 40.4*	
Methyldihydrojasmonate (Hedione®)	2630-39-9	5% pet	Frosch et al. 2002
Methyleugenol	93-15-2	5% pet	Larsen et al. 2002
Methylionantheme		0.04% alc	
6-Methyl-α-ionone (α-Irone)	79-69-6	10% pet	Frosch et al. 2002
Methyl octine carbonate	111-80-8	l% MEK	
Methyl-2-octynoate (methyl heptine carbonate)[c]	111-12-6	See *Table 40.4*	Schnuch et al. 2007b; van Oosten et al. 2009
Methyl salicylate[a]	119-36-8	See *Table 40.4*	
3-Methyl-5-(2,2,3-trimethyl-3-cyclopenten-1-yl)pent-4-en-2-ol	67801-20-1	5% pet	Larsen et al. 2001
Musk ambrette[b,d]	201-493-7	See *Table 40.4*	
Musk ketone	81-14-1	See *Table 40.4*	
Musk moskene (moskene)[b]	116-66-5	See *Table 40.4*	
Musk tibetene	145-39-1	2–5% pet	
Musk xylene[b]	81-15-2	See *Table 40.4*	
Myrcene (in tea tree oil)	123-35-3	5% DEP	Hausen 2004
Neral	106-26-3	2% pet	
Nerol (*cis*-3,7-dimethyl-2,6-octadien-1-ol)	106-25-2	5% pet	Larsen et al. 2002
Nopyl acetate	128-51-8	10% pet	
1-(1,2,3,4,5,6,7,8-Octahydro-2,3,8,8-tetramethyl-2-naphthalenyl)ethanone	54464-57-2	5% pet	Larsen et al. 2001
α-Phellandrene (in tea tree oil)	99-83-2	5% DEP	Hausen 2004
Phenethyl alcohol (phenylethyl alcohol)	60-12-8	5% pet	
Phenylacetaldehyde	122-78-1	0.5–2% pet	Sanchez-Politta et al. 2007
3-Phenyl 1-propanol	122-97-4	5% pet	Larsen et al. 2002
Phenyl salicylate	118-55-8	See *Table 40.4*	
Physodic/physodalic acid (in oak moss)		0.1% pet	
α-Pinene	80-56-8	See *Table 40.4*	
β-Pinene	127-91-3	15% pet	
Propylidene phthalide	17369-59-4	2% pet	

Table 40.5 (Continued)

Name of fragrance	Chemical abstract service (CAS)	Test concentration and vehicle (de Groot 2008)	Additional references
Rhodinol (mixture of 1-citronellol and geraniol)	6812-78-8	3% pet	
Sabinene (in tea tree oil)	3387-41-5	5% DEP	Hausen 2004
Salicylaldehyde	90-02-8	See *Table 40.4*	
Sandalore (5-(-2,2,3-trimethyl-3-cyclopentenyl)-3-methylpentan-2-ol)	65113-99-7	5% pet	
Sandela (isobornyl cyclohexanol + 3-*trans*-isocamphyl cyclohexanol)	70955-71-4	5% pet	
Santalol[d]	11031-45-1; 115-71-9 (α-); 77-42-9 (β-)	2–5% pet	Larsen et al. 2001
Stictic acid (in oak moss)[b]		0.1% pet	
Styryl acetate (in publication "styrol acetate," unknown compound)	10521-96-7	1% pet	Schubert 2006
α-Terpinene (in tea tree oil)	99-86-5	5% DEP	Hausen 2004
Terpinen-4-ol (in tea tree oil)	562-74-3	10% DEP	Hausen 2004
α-Terpineol	10482-56-1; 98-55-5	5% pet	
Terpinolene (in tea tree oil)	586-62-9	10% DEP/pet	Hausen 2004
1,1,6,7-Tetramethyl-6-acetyl decalene (isomers) (Iso E Super®)	54464-57-2; 68155-66-8; 68155-67-9	1–5% pet	
Thymol	89-83-8	1% pet	
1,2,4-Trihydroxy menthane (in tea tree oil)		5% pet	Hausen 2004
Trimethyl benzene propanol (Majantol®, 2,2-dimethyl-3-(3-ethylphenyl)propanol)	103694-68-4	See *Table 40.4*	Larsen et al. 2002; Schnuch et al. 2007a
2,4,6-Trimethyl-4-phenyl-1,3-dioxane (Floropal®)	5182-36-5	5% pet	
Usnic acid (in oak moss)	125-46-2	See *Table 40.4*	
Vanillin[a]	121-33-5	See *Table 40.4*	
Verdyl acetate (tricyclodecen-4-yl 8-acetate, Cyclacet®)	2500-83-6; 5413-60-5	5% pet	

alc alcohol, *DEP* diethyl phthalate, *pet* petrolatum, *MEK* methyl ethyl ketone
[a]Has caused immediate contact reactions
[b]Has caused phototoxicity/photoallergy
[c]Presence labeled in the EU on cosmetics and detergent products, if present at >10 parts per million (ppm) (0.001%) in leave-on products and > 100 ppm (0.01%) in rinse-off products
[d]Has caused pigmented cosmetic/contact dermatitis

cleaning personnel may also be endangered by frequent contact with soap, cleansers, dishwashing liquids and other fragranced products. In spite of this, surprisingly little information on occupational allergic contact dermatitis from fragrances can be found in the literature. This may be because in the majority of people at risk, a definite relationship between dermatitis and fragrances is hard to prove. In many occupations (hairdressers,

Table 40.6
Synonyms/trade names for fragrances

Synonym/trade name	INCI name or other preferred name in Table 40.5
Abitol®	Hydroabietyl alcohol
α-Amylcinnamic aldehyde	Amyl cinnamal
Cajeputol	Eucalyptol
Cashmeran®	Dihydro pentamethylindanone
Cedramber	Cedrol methyl ether
1,8-Cineole	Eucalyptol
Cinnamaldehyde	Cinnamal
Cinnamic alcohol	Cinnamyl alcohol
Cinnamic aldehyde	Cinnamal
Cyclacet®	Verdyl acetate
Dihydroabietyl alcohol	Hydroabietyl alcohol
Dimethylbenzyl carbinyl acetate	DMBCA
2,2-Dimethyl-3-(3-ethylphenyl)propanol	Trimethyl benzene propanol
cis-3,7-Dimethyl-2,6-octadien-1-ol	Nerol
Dipentene	D,L-Limonene
Fixolide®	6-Acetyl-1,1,2,4,4,7-hexamethyltetralin
Floropal®	2,4,6-Trimethyl-4-phenyl-1,3-dioxane
Galaxolide®	Hexamethylindanopyran
Hedione®	Methyldihydrojasmonate
Helional®	α-Methyl-1,3-benzodioxole-5-propanal
Hexadecanolide	Hexadecanolactone
α-Hexylcinnamic aldehyde	Hexyl cinnamal
Irisone	Ionone
α-Irone	6-Methyl-α-ionone
Isobornyl cyclohexanol + 3-trans-Isocamphyl cyclohexanol	Sandela
Iso E Super®	1,1,6,7-Tetramethyl-6-acetyl decalene (isomers)
Isothymol	Carvacrol
Lilial®	Butylphenyl methylpropional
Lyral®	Hydroxyisohexyl 3-cyclohexene carboxaldehyde
Majantol®	Trimethyl benzene propanol
(Methyl-(2,4(3,5)-dimethyl-3-cyclohexen-1-yl)-methylene anthranilate	Ligustral
Methyl heptine carbonate	Methyl-2-octynoate
γ-Methylionone	α-Isomethyl ionone
Methyl isoeugenol	Isoeugenyl methyl ether
3-Methyl-5-(2,2,3-trimethyl-3-cyclopenten-1-yl)-4-penten-2-ol	Ebanol
Moskene	Musk moskene
Oak moss	*Evernia prunastri*
Osyrol®	3,7-Dimethyl-7-methoxyoctan-2-ol
Phantolide®	5-Acetyl-l,1,2,3,3,6-hexamethylindan
Piperonal	Heliotropine
Synthetic sandalwood	Isobornyl cyclohexanol
Tree moss	*Evernia furfuracea*
Tricyclodecen-4-yl 8-acetate	Verdyl acetate
5-(-2,2,3-Trimethyl-3-cyclopentenyl)-3-methylpentan-2-ol	Sandalore
Vertenex®	4-*tert*-Butylcyclohexyl acetate
Vertofix®	Acetylcedrene
Viridoflorene	Ledene

beauticians, housewives, health personnel, cleaning personnel) irritant factors may also be relevant in the etiology of dermatitis, and sometimes other allergens are also considered of paramount importance. In addition, nonoccupational exposure to fragrances occurs in virtually everybody.

In an early study, all workers in a factory became sensitized to cinnamal (Bonnevie 1948). In Germany, 26 female workers in a perfume factory were investigated, who were filling 10 different perfumes into small glass bottles, setting in spray devices, and testing their valves. Six bottlers had dermatitis of the hands, forearms, and the face. All 26 were tested with four perfumes from the factory and 30 of their ingredients, both individual fragrance compounds and essential oils. A total of 97 positive reactions were recorded in 18 out of 26 persons with the majority (50 reactions) in the six eczema patients. The other 12, although sensitized to fragrances, never developed allergic contact dermatitis from working in the factory. Most reactions were caused by the perfumes and their ingredients geraniol, benzaldehyde, cinnamal, and camphor. In 10/18 cases with positive reactions the FM I was also positive. The high prevalence of fragrance allergy in this investigation in a small perfume factory (18/26, 69%) was the result of poor work hygiene and permanent direct and airborne skin contact. The degree of automation was very low, even the bottle-filling machines had to be operated by hand. In all rooms in the perfume factory, there was an intensive smell of perfumes. For the six patients with allergic contact dermatitis, job change to other rooms without exposition to fragrances led to a complete clearing of the dermatitis (Schubert 2006).

Although there should be individual cases of allergic contact dermatitis from fragrances in hairdressers, frequencies of positive patch tests are usually no higher than in the general patch test population (Heydorn et al. 2003a).

Goodfield and Saihan (1988) found a 44% prevalence of sensitivity to one or more fragrances in 35 coal miners, compared with 22% in male and 17% in female non-miner controls. The high frequency was attributed to the use of a highly perfumed body lotion provided at the pit-head bath, and to the facilitation of contact sensitization due to the frequent occurrence of irritant dermatitis from working in the coal mines (Goodfield and Saihan 1988).

There have been case reports of occupational contact dermatitis from oak moss in aftershave lotion in a geriatric nurse (Dahlquist and Fregert 1981); lavender oil in shampoo in a hairdresser (Brandão 1986); pure methyl heptine carbonate in a laboratory technician (English and Rycroft 1988); oak moss in a coolant oil in an engineer (Owen et al. 2000); pure phenylacetaldehyde in a perfume factory worker (Sanchez-Politta et al. 2007); cinnamal in odor-masking powder in a car engineer (Decapite and Anderson 2004); eugenol in restorative material in a dental nurse (Kanerva et al. 1998); dl-limonene (dipentene) in a solvent in a laboratory technician (Wakelin et al. 1998); dipentene and pine oil in waxpolish in a car mechanic (Martins et al. 1995); dipentene in honing oil in three honing machinists (Rycroft 1980); oxidized d-limonene in fruits, flavors, vegetables, and cleaning products (Karlberg and Dooms-Goossens 1997); d-limonene in hand cleanser in a painter/decorator (Topham and Wakelin 2003); fragrances in room-fresheners and an insecticide (Freeman 1990); oak moss in permanent waving solution in a hairdresser (Kanerva et al. 1999); d-limonene in a hand cleanser in a mechanic; and cinnamal in a man making air freshener with perfumes (Nethercott et al. 1983).

On the basis of this data, it is concluded that fragrances may play a role in some cases of occupational contact dermatitis, but in no single profession are they a major cause of occupational allergic contact dermatitis, and rarely are they the sole etiological factor. However, fragrances may play an important role in aggravating hand eczema of other origin (atopic hand eczema, irritant dermatitis, allergic contact dermatitis) by contact with hand cleansers, barrier creams, moisturizing preparations, etc. In addition, flavors and spices may be involved in occupational contact dermatitis in bakers, cooks, caterers, and others working in the food industry (Kanerva et al. 1996).

11 Irritant Dermatitis

Few well-documented cases of irritant dermatitis from fragrance materials can be found in the literature (Rothenborg et al. 1977). A large number of people broke out after the introduction of a lemon-scented detergent in a hospital. The temperature-dependent, primary irritant reaction from the lemon perfume was due to the chemical citral (Rothenborg et al. 1977). Although some authors state that irritant reactions occur frequently and are caused especially by products with high concentrations of perfume (notably deodorants and antiperspirants) no clinical data or literature references are provided to substantiate these statements. Of course, deodorants and antiperspirants are an important cause of irritation, due to the humidity and anatomical occlusion of the axillae. However, this may well be caused by the alcohol or other ingredients rather than by the fragrance materials.

12 Photocontact Dermatitis

Compared with contact allergic reactions, photocontact dermatitis from fragrances is unusual. Only musk ambrette, a fragrance fixative used in both the food and cosmetics industry, has – in the past – caused a considerable number of photocontact allergic reactions. Pigmented photoallergic contact dermatitis, airborne pigmented contact dermatitis, and lichenoid photocontact dermatitis have all been described. Persistent light reactions were not rare, and sometimes lead to erythroderma. Photocross reactions have been observed to musk moskene and musk xylene. Occasionally, positive photopatch tests are observed to the fragrance mix

(Pigatto et al. 2008) and some phototoxic reactions have been noted. Reactions to *E. prunastri* (oak moss) and its ingredients (lichen acids) are usually of the contact allergic type, but photosensitivity may occur to oak moss, atranorin, and evernic acid. In patients with persistent light reactions in chronic actinic dermatitis, a higher incidence of contact sensitivity reactions to certain fragrance materials was found (Chew et al. 2010). Immediate and delayed photopatch test reactions have also been observed, notably to oak moss, musk ambrette, eugenol, cinnamic aldehyde, 6-methylcoumarin, costus root oil, and hydroxycitronellal. Fragrances having caused photosensitivity are identified in ➋ *Table 40.5* by the symbol [b].

13 Immediate Contact Reactions (Contact Urticaria)

Contact urticaria to fragrances is usually nonallergic (nonimmune immediate contact reactions), caused by a nonallergic histamine-liberating effect. Well-known causes are the fragrance mix I, *M. pereirae* (from its ingredient cinnamal), cinnamal (Tanaka et al. 2004b), cinnamic acid, cinnamyl cinnamate, benzyl benzoate, and benzyl alcohol; such immediate reactions have also been caused by cinnamyl alcohol, eugenol and oak moss (*E. prunastri*), α-isomethyl ionone, and terpinyl acetate. Immediate contact reactions can also affect the respiratory tract, as some individuals suffering from chronic respiratory problems experience worsening or precipitation of their symptoms upon exposure to some fragrance materials. Occupational asthma from fragrances has also been reported.

14 Other Adverse Reactions

Pigmented cosmetic dermatitis used to be frequent in Japan. Other cutaneous reactions ascribed to fragrances include depigmented airborne contact dermatitis, a pemphigoid-like allergic reaction, and erythema multiforme-like contact dermatitis.

15 Essential Oils

Essential oils are volatile fragrant organic constituents obtained from plants. Oils may be extracted from different parts of plants such as the leaves (e.g., eucalyptus, peppermint), flowers (e.g., lavender, rose), twigs (e.g., juniper), wood (e.g., sandalwood), roots (e.g., vetivert, calamus), sap (e.g., benzoin, frankincense), and grasses (e.g., palmarosa grass, lemongrass). Essential oils are extracted from the plant often using fresh dried plant materials. The process of steam distillation is used most often to separate the essential oil from the plant. For certain types of oils, such as those extracted from the rinds of citrus fruit, a process of cold expression is used. The oils contain a mixture of many organic compounds which include alcohols, aldehydes, esters, ketones, terpenes, oxides, coumarins, lactones, acids, aromatic aldehydes, and phenols.

Essential oils are used in the food, cosmetic, and perfume industry, which are presently the largest users of essential oils in the world. As essential oils are used extensively in perfumes, their applications parallel those of fragrances. To a lesser extent, but growing steadily, they are used in aromatherapy, which is the therapeutic use of essential oils. Aromatherapists attribute certain therapeutic properties to each organic compound present in essential oils. The relative amount of each compound contained in the various oils denotes its therapeutic value. Oils high in ketones, for example, are considered to have wound healing properties, whereas oils high in alcohols such as tea tree oil (*Melaleuca alternifolia*) are renowned among aromatherapists for their antimicrobial and anti-infectious properties. Lavender oil is high in alcohols, terpenes, and oxides and is noted for its effects in the rapid healing of burns, without scarring or infections. Aromatherapy is used for a wide range of physical, mental, and emotional conditions. Oils may be applied externally via therapeutic massage (mixed with a plain vegetable oil; this is the most common method of application), a compress, as a topical wound dressing (mixed in a gel or paste), as a spray, in a bath, or as an inhalation. The internal use of essential oils may be offered orally, rectally, or vaginally according to the condition. It should be appreciated that the term aromatherapy is very loose and many people associate essential oils purely with the beauty and cosmetics industry (Stevensen 1998).

15.1 Allergic Contact Dermatitis

Contact allergy has been reported to over 80 essential oils (➋ *Table 40.7*). In a (considerable) number of the reports, only positive patch tests were observed, without assessing relevance (i.e., the presence of allergic contact dermatitis was not verified). Rates of >1% positive reactions in patients routinely tested for suspected contact dermatitis have been observed with several oils including lavender oil, geranium oil, ylang-ylang oil, tea tree oil, lemongrass oil, narcissus absolute, and jasmine oil (Sugiura et al. 2000; Frosch et al. 2002; Hausen 2004; Zug et al. 2009). Recently, especially tea tree oil has caused many cases of

Table 40.7

Essential oils reported as contact allergens (De Groot et al. 1994; De Groot and Frosch 1997)

Common name	INCI name[a]	Test concentration and vehicle[b]	Additional references
Abies alba oil	*Abies alba* cone/leaf/needle oil	2% pet	
Angelica root oil[c]	*Angelica archangelica* root oil	2% MEK	
Angelica seed oil	*Angelica archangelica* seed oil	2% pet	Dharmagunawardena et al. 2002
Anise oil	*Pimpinella anisum* fruit oil	0.5% pet	
Avocado oil	*Persea gratissima* oil	Pure	
Basil oil	*Ocimum basalicum* herb oil	5% pet	
Bay oil	*Pimenta acris* fruit oil	2% pet	
Benzoin oil	*Styrax tonkinensis* resin oil	2% pet	
Bergamot oil[c]	*Citrus bergamia* peel oil expressed	See *Table 40.4*	
Black cumin oil[c]	*Nigella sativa* seed oil	0.5% and 1% oo	Zedlitz et al. 2002
Black pepper oil	*Piper nigrum* fruit/seed oil	2% pet	Dharmagunawardena et al. 2002
Bitter orange oil[c]	*Citrus aurantium* peel oil expressed	2% pet	
Cajuput oil	*Melaleuca leucadendron cajuputi* leaf oil	2% pet	Dharmagunawardena et al. 2002
Calamus oil	*Acorus calamus* root oil	2–4% pet	
Cananga oil	*Cananga genuine* oil	See *Table 40.4*	Cockayne and Gawkrodger 1997
Cassia (cinnamon) oil[c,d]	*Cinnamomum cassia* leaf oil	See *Table 40.4*	
Cedarwood oil[c]	*Cedrus atlantica* wood oil	See *Table 40.4*	Frosch et al. 2002
Chamomile oil	*Anthemis nobilis* flower oil	See *Table 40.4*	
Chamomile oil German	*Anthemis nobilis* flower oil	See *Table 40.4*	
Chamomile oil Roman	*Anthemis nobilis* flower oil	See *Table 40.4*	Giordano-Labadie et al. 2000
Cherry pit oil	*Prunus avium* seed oil	2% pet	
Citronella oil	*Cymbopogon nardus* herb oil	1–2% pet	
Clary sage oil	*Salvia sclarea* (flower) oil	2% pet	
Clove oil	*Eugenia caryophyllus* bud oil	See *Table 40.4*	
Coriander oil	*Coriandrum sativum* fruit/herb/seed oil	2% pet	
Costus oil	Costus root oil (*Saussurea lappa*)	0.1–0.5% pet	
Cypress oil	*Cupressus sempervirens* leaf oil	5% pet	
Elemi oil	*Canarium luzonicum* gum oil	2% pet	Dharmagunawardena et al. 2002
Eucalyptus oil	*Eucalyptus* species (*citriodorata, globulus, radiata*) (flower/leaf/stem) oil	See *Table 40.4*	
French marigold oil[c]	*Tagetes* species (*erecta, patula*) flower oil	2% pet	
Geranium oil[e]	*Pelargonium roseum* leaf oil	See *Table 40.4*	
Ginger oil	*Zingiber officinale* root oil	2% pet	Dharmagunawardena et al. 2002
Grapefruit oil	*Citrus* species (*grandis, paradisi*) peel/seed oil (expressed)	2% pet	Dharmagunawardena et al. 2002
Grapeseed oil	*Vitis vinifera* seed oil	2% pet	Trattner et al. 2008
Green grass oil		10% oo	
Guaiac wood oil		2% pet	
Hyssop oil	*Hyssopus officinalis* herb/leaf oil	2% pet	Dharmagunawardena et al. 2002
Jasmine oil	*Jasminum officinale* (flower) oil	See *Table 40.4*	Frosch et al. 2002

Table 40.7 (Continued)

Common name	INCI name[a]	Test concentration and vehicle[b]	Additional references
Juniper berries oil	*Juniperus communis* fruit oil *Juniperus oxycedrus* fruit oil	2% pet	
Juniper oil	*Juniperus* species (*communis, Mexicana, oxycedrus, phoenicea, scopulorum, virginiana*) (wood) oil	1% pet	
Laurel oil	*Laurus nobilis* oil	See *Table 40.4*	Adişen and Önder 2007
Lavandin oil	*Lavandula hybrida* herb oil	2% pet	
Lavender oil[c,e]	*Lavandula officinalis* flower oil	See *Table 40.4*	Hagvall et al. 2008
Lemongrass oil	*Cymbopogon Schoenanthus* oil	See *Table 40.4*	Frosch et al. 2002
Lemon oil[c]	*Citrus limonum* peel oil expressed	See *Table 40.4*	
Litsea cubeba oil	*Litsea cubeba* fruit oil	2% pet	
Lovage oil	*Levisticum officinale* (leaf/root) oil	2% pet	
Mandarin oil	*Citrus* species (*nobilis, reticulata, unshiu*) leaf/peel/fruit oil (expressed)	2% pet	Dharmagunawardena et al. 2002
Marjoram oil	*Origanum* species (*cretium, majorana,vulgare*) (herb/flower/leaf) oil	2–5% pet	
Melissa oil	*Cymbopogon citrates* leaf oil	2% pet	Dharmagunawardena et al. 2002
Mint oil	*Mentha spicata* herb oil	2% pet	Boonchai et al. 2007
Myrrh oil	*Commiphora* species (*abyssinica, myrrha, schimperi*) gum oil	2% pet	
Narcissus oil	*Narcissus jonquilla* flower oil	See *Table 40.4*	Frosch et al. 2002
Neem oil (oil of margosa)	*Melia azadirachta* seed oil	Pure	Reutemann and Ehrlich 2008
Neroli oil[c]	*Citrus aurantium* flower oil	See *Table 40.4*	
Niaouli oil	*Melaleuca quinquenervia* oil	1% alc.	
Nutmeg oil (myristica oil)	*Myristica fragrans* kernel oil		Nardelli et al. 2009a
Olibanum oil (frankincense oil)	*Boswellia carterii* gum oil	2% MEK	Dharmagunawardena et al. 2002
Orange oil[c]	*Citrus* species (*aurantium* [*dulcis*], *bergamia, sinensis*) peel oil expressed	See *Table 40.4*	
Origanum oil	*Origanum vulgare* oil	2% pet	Nardelli et al. 2009a
Patchouli oil[e]	*Pogostemon cablin* leaf oil	See *Table 40.4*	Frosch et al. 2002
Peppermint oil[d]	*Mentha piperita* oil	See *Table 40.4*	Frosch et al. 2002
Petitgrain bigarade oil[c]	*Citrus nobilis* seed oil	2% pet	
Pine needle oil[d] (pine oil)	*Pinus* species needle oil	2% pet	Frosch et al. 2002
Pinus pumilio oil	*Pinus mugo pumilio* twig leaf oil	2% pet	
Pinus sylvestris oil	*Pinus sylvestris* (twig leaf) oil	2% pet	
Ravensara oil	*Ravensara aromatica* leaf/twig oil	2% pet	Dharmagunawardena et al. 2002
Rosemary oil	*Rosmarinus officinalis* flower oil	See *Table 40.4*	
Rose oil (Bulgarian)	*Rosa* species (many) flower oil	See *Table 40.4*	
Rosewood oil		5% pet	

Table 40.7 (Continued)

Common name	INCI name[a]	Test concentration and vehicle[b]	Additional references
Sage oil	*Salvia* species (e.g., *officinalis, sclarea, hispanica, lavandulifolia*) (herb/seed/flower) oil	2% pet	
Sandalwood oil[c,e]	*Santalum album* (wood/seed) oil	See *Table 40.4*	Frosch et al. 2002
Spearmint oil	*Mentha spicata* herb oil	1–2% pet	Frosch et al. 2002; An et al. 2005
Spike oil	*Lavandula* species (*latifolia, spica*) herb oil	2% pet	
Star anise oil	*Illicium verum* fruit/seed oil	0.5% pet	
Suxiaoye-baojianxiang-jin oil		Use test with the oil pure	
Sweet orange oil	*Citrus* species (*aurantium, sinensis*) flower/peel/seed oil (expressed)	2% pet	
Tamanu oil	*Calophyllum inophyllum* (INCI Europe) *Calophyllum tacamahaca* (INCI USA)	1% oo and pure	Le Coz 2004
Tangerine oil	*Citrus tangerina*	2% and 10%	Vilaplana and Romaguera 2002
Tea tree oil	*Melaleuca alternifolia* leaf oil	See *Table 40.4*	Carson and Riley 2001; Hausen 2004; Crawford et al. 2004b
Thuja oil	*Thuja* species (*occidentalis, plicata*) leaf/stem oil	2% pet	
Thyme oil	*Thymus* species (*vulgaris, zygis*) herb oil	2% pet	
Valerian oil	*Valeriana officinalis* root oil	2% pet	Dharmagunawardena et al. 2002
Vetiver oil	*Vetiveria zizanoides* root oil	2–5% pet	
Violet leaves absolute	*Viola odorata oil*	2% pet	Callejo et al. 2007 (synthetic violet oil)
Ylang-ylang oil[e]	*Cananga odorata macrophylla* flower oil	See *Table 40.4*	Frosch et al. 2002
Zdrawetz oil		2% pet	
Zhenghonghua oil		Pure	

INCI international nomenclature cosmetic ingredient, *alc* alcohol, *MEK* methyl ethyl ketone, *oo* olive oil, *pet* petrolatum
[a]Many are not officially INCI names, but Perfuming names
[b]Based on de Groot (2008) and original publications
[c]Has caused (or may cause, according to the International Fragrance Association IFRA) phototoxic and/or photoallergic reactions
[d]Has caused immediate contact reactions
[e]Has caused pigmented contact/cosmetic dermatitis

sensitization (Carson and Riley 2001; Hausen 2004; Crawford et al. 2004b).

Patients have been sensitized to essential oils from many sources, including perfumes (Vilaplana and Romaguera 2002), cosmetics (Hausen 2004), aromatherapy (Adişen and Önder 2007), aromatherapy self-treatment (Schaller and Korting 1995; Le Coz 2004), dried flowers (lavender, Sugiura et al. 2000), and homeopathic preparations (Giordano-Labadie et al. 2000). Essential oils in toothpastes, mouthwashes, and foods and drinks may cause allergic contact cheilitis and stomatitis (anise oil, spearmint oil). Systemic exposure in sensitized individuals (e.g., drinking chamomile tea) has resulted in anaphylactic reactions and systemic contact dermatitis (Giordano-Labadie et al. 2000). Due to the volatile nature of these oils, airborne allergic contact dermatitis occurs (Schaller and Korting 1995; Hausen 2004).

Not infrequently, allergic patients react to various oils, presumably from common ingredients or multiple sensitizations. Often there is co-reactivity with the fragrance-mix, *M. pereirae* and/or colophonium. All oils have many constituents, which may vary according to their origin, time of harvest, manufacturing process, their age, and use (due to volatility). Some oils are allergenic only after photooxidation due to light, oxygen, warmth, and moisture, through creation of degradation products that are moderate or strong sensitizers, e.g., tea tree oil and lavender oil (Hausen 2004; Hagvall et al. 2008). Identification of the specific sensitizer is often difficult. Currently, 25 essential oils are commercially available for patch testing (➋ *Table 40.4*). The literature on adverse reactions to essential oils up to 1997 has been reviewed (de Groot and Frosch 1997). Further information on this subject can also be found in ➋ Chap. 118, "Aromatherapists".

15.2 Occupational Contact Dermatitis

Aromatherapists, when utilizing essential oils for massaging, often have unprotected bare hands, which results in frequent skin contact with the oils. Thus, occupational allergic contact dermatitis from essential oils in aromatherapists and others massaging with products containing essential oils is increasingly recognized (Rademaker 1994; Selvaag et al. 1995; Sánchez-Pérez and García-Díez 1999; Keane et al. 2000; Dharmagunawardena et al. 2002; Boonchai et al. 2007; Trattner et al. 2008). A 12-month prevalence of hand dermatitis in massage therapists was found to be 15% by self-reported criteria and 22% by a symptom-based method. Risk factors were having a history of atopic dermatitis and having frequently used aromatherapy products in oils, creams, and lotions (Crawford et al. 2004a). Allergic contact dermatitis from essential oils has also been documented in bar workers, citrus fruit pickers, hairdressers, and beauticians (Crawford et al. 2004a). Occupational allergic contact dermatitis from oil of cinnamon has been reported in bakers, candy makers, cooks, grocers, confectioners, and housewives (Sánchez-Pérez and García-Díez 1999), and from ylang-ylang oil in a woman packing cosmetics (Kanerva et al. 1995).

15.3 Other Adverse Reactions

Other adverse reactions to (individual) essential oils include irritant dermatitis (*Nigella sativa* black cumin oil) and immediate contact reactions (caraway seed oil, cassia oil, clove oil, peppermint oil; see oils in ➋ *Table 40.7* indicated with the symbol [d]). Photosensitivity reactions (➋ *Table 40.7*, indicated with the symbol [c]) are usually phototoxic, sometimes photoallergic (sandalwood oil); aromatherapy with bergamot oil may lead to bullous phototoxic reactions caused by the furocoumarins contained therein, notably 5-methoxyposoralen, in combination with UV-A radiation (sun, sunbed) (Kaddu et al. 2001). Exposure to lavender and tea tree oils has been linked to prepubertal gynecomastia (Henley et al. 2007).

References

Adams RM, Maibach HI (1985) A five-year study of cosmetic reactions. J Am Acad Dermatol 13:1062–1069

Adişen E, Önder M (2007) Allergic contact dermatitis from *Laurus nobilis* oil induced by massage. Contact Dermatitis 56:360–361

An S, Lee A-Y, Lee CH et al (2005) Fragrance contact dermatitis in Korea: a joint study. Contact Dermatitis 53:320–323

Bonnevie P (1948) Some experiences of war-time industrial dermatoses. Acta Derm Venereol 28:231–237

Boonchai W, Iamtharachai P, Sunthonpalin P (2007) Occupational allergic contact dermatitis from essential oils in aromatherapists. Contact Dermatitis 56:181–182

Braendstrup P, Johansen JB (2008) Hydroxyisohexyl 3-cyclohexene carboxaldehyde (Lyral®) is still a frequent allergen. Contact Dermatitis 59:187–188

Brandão FM (1986) Occupational allergy to lavender oil. Contact Dermatitis 15:249–250

Bråred Christensson J, Matura M, Gruvberger B, Bruze M, Karlberg A-T (2010) Linalool – a significant contact sensitizer after air exposure. Contact Dermatitis 62:32–41

Bruynzeel DP, Diepgen TL, Andersen KE et al, on behalf of the European Environmental and Contact Dermatitis Research Group (EECDRG) (2005) Monitoring the European standard series in 10 centres 1996–2000. Contact Dermatitis 53:146–152

Bruze M, Johansen JD, Andersen KE et al (2003) Deodorants: an experimental provocation study with cinnamic aldehyde. J Am Acad Dermatol 48:194–200

Bruze M, Andersen KE, Goossens A, on behalf of the ESCD and EECDRG (2008) Recommendation to include fragrance mix 2 and hydroxyisohexyl 3-cyclohexene carboxaldehyde (Lyral ®) in the European baseline patch test series. Contact Dermatitis 58: 129–133

Buckley DA (2007) Fragrance ingredient labelling in products on sale in the UK. Br J Dermatol 157:295–300

Buckley DA, Wakelin SH, Seed PT et al (2000) The frequency of fragrance allergy in a patch-test population over a 17-year period. Br J Dermatol 142:203–204

Buckley DA, Basketter DA, Smith Pease CK et al (2006) Simultaneous sensitivity to fragrances. Br J Dermatol 154:885–888

Callejo A, Martínez JC, Martín G, Martín C, Armentia A (2007) Contact dermatitis from a violet fragrance in a florist. Contact Dermatitis 57:191

Carson CF, Riley TV (2001) Safety, efficacy and provenance of tea tree (*Melaleuca alternifolia*) oil. Contact Dermatitis 45:65–67

Chew A-L, Bashir SJ, Hawk JLM et al (2010) Contact and photocontact sensitization in chronic actinic dermatitis: a changing picture. Contact Dermatitis 62:42–46

Cockayne SE, Gawkrodger DJ (1997) Occupational contact dermatitis in an aromatherapist. Contact Dermatitis 37:306–307

Corea NV, Basketter DA, Clapp C et al (2006) Fragrance allergy: assessing the risk from washed fabrics. Contact Dermatitis 55:48–53

Crawford GH, Katz KA, Ellis E, James WD (2004a) Use of aromatherapy products and increased risk of hand dermatitis in massage therapists. Arch Dermatol 140:991–996

Crawford GH, Sciacca JR, James WD (2004b) Tea tree oil: cutaneous effects of the extracted oil of *Melaleuca alternifolia*. Dermatitis 15:59–66

Curry EJ, Warshaw EM (2005) Benzyl alcohol allergy: importance of patch testing with personal products. Dermatitis 16:203–208

Dahlquist I, Fregert S (1981) Atranorin and oak moss contact allergy. Contact Dermatitis 7:168–169

De Groot AC (2000) Fragrances. In: Kanerva L, Elsner P, Wahlberg JE, Maibach HI (eds) Handbook of occupational dermatology. Springer, Berlin/Heidelberg, pp 497–508

De Groot AC (2008) Patch testing, 3rd edn. Acdegroot publishing, Wapserveen, The Netherlands

De Groot AC, Frosch PJ (1997) Adverse reactions to fragrances. A clinical review. Contact Dermatitis 36:57–86

De Groot AC, Bruynzeel DP, Bos JD et al (1988) The allergens in cosmetics. Arch Dermatol 124:1525–1529

De Groot AC, Weyland JW, Nater JP (1994) Unwanted effects of cosmetics and drugs used in dermatology, 3rd edn. Elsevier, Amsterdam

Decapite TJ, Anderson BE (2004) Allergic contact dermatitis from cinnamic aldehyde found in an industrial odour-masking agent. Contact Dermatitis 51:312–313

Devos SA, Constandt L, Tupker RA et al (2008) Relevance of positive patch-test reactions to fragrance mix. Am J Contact Dermat 19: 43–47

Dharmagunawardena B, Takwale A, Sanders KJ et al (2002) Gas chromatography: an investigative tool in multiple allergies to essential oils. Contact Dermatitis 47:288–292

Dotterud LK, Smith-Sivertsen T (2007) Allergic contact sensitization in the general adult population: a population-based study from Northern Norway. Contact Dermatitis 56:10–15

Downs AMR, Sansom JE (1999) Colophony allergy: a review. Contact Dermatitis 41:305–310

English JSC, Rycroft RJG (1988) Allergic contact dermatitis from methyl heptine and methyl octine carbonate. Contact Dermatitis 18:174–175

ESSCA Writing Group (2008) The European surveillance system of contact allergies (ESSCA): results of patch testing the standard series, 2004. J Eur Acad Dermatol Venereol 22:174–181

EU (2003) Directive 2003/15/EC of the European parliament and of the council of 27 February 2003 amending council directive 76/768/EEC on the approximation of the laws of the member states relating to cosmetic products. Off J Eur Union L66:26–35

Fenn RS (1989) Aroma chemical usage trends in modern perfumery. Perfum Flavor 14:3–10

Freeman S (1990) Fragrance and nickel: old allergens in new guises. Am J Contact Dermat 1:47–52

Frosch PJ, Johansen JD, White IR (eds) (1998) Fragrances. Beneficial and adverse effects. Springer, Berlin/Heidelberg/New York

Frosch PJ, Johansen JD, Menné T et al (2002) Further important sensitizers in patients sensitive to fragrances. I. Reactivity to frequently used chemicals. Contact Dermatitis 47:78–85

Frosch PJ, Pirker C, Rastogi SC et al (2005a) Patch testing with a new fragrance mix detects additional patients sensitive to perfumes and missed by the current fragrance mix. Contact Dermatitis 52:207–215

Frosch PJ, Rastogi SC, Pirker C et al (2005b) Patch testing with a new fragrance mix – reactivity to the individual constituents and chemical detection in relevant cosmetic products. Contact Dermatitis 52:216–225

Giménez-Arnau A, Giménez-Arnau E, Serra-Baldrich E et al (2002) Principles and methodology for identification of fragrance allergens in consumer products. Contact Dermatitis 47:345–352

Giordano-Labadie F, Schwarze HP, Bazex J (2000) Allergic contact dermatitis from chamomile used in phytotherapy. Contact Dermatitis 42:247

Goodfield MJD, Saihan EM (1988) Fragrance sensitivity in coal miners. Contact Dermatitis 18:81–83

Guin JD (1982) History, manufacture, and cutaneous reactions to perfumes. In: Frost P, Horwitz SW (eds) Principles of cosmetics for the dermatologist. The CV Mosby, St. Louis, pp 111–129

Hagvall L, Sköld M, Bråred-Christensson J, Börje A, Karlberg A-T (2008) Lavender oil lacks natural protection against autoxidation, forming strong contact allergens on air exposure. Contact Dermatitis 59:143–150

Hausen BM (2001) Contact allergy to Balsam of Peru. II. Patch test results in 102 patients with selected Balsam of Peru constituents. Am J Contact Dermat 12:98–102

Hausen B (2004) Evaluation of the main contact allergens in tea tree oil. Dermatitis 15:213–215

Henley DV, Lipson N, Korach KS, Bloch CA (2007) Prepubertal gynecomastia linked to lavender and tea tree oils. N Engl J Med 356:479–485

Heydorn S, Menné T, Johansen JD (2003a) Fragrance allergy and hand eczema – a review. Contact Dermatitis 48:59–66

Heydorn S, Menné T, Andersen KE et al (2003b) Citral a fragrance allergen and irritant. Contact Dermatitis 49:32–36

Hovmand Lysdal S, Johansen JD (2009) Fragrance contact allergic patients: strategies for use of cosmetic products and perceived impact on life situation. Contact Dermatitis 61:320–324

Johansen JD (2002) Contact allergy to fragrances: clinical and experimental investigations of the fragrance mix and its ingredients. Contact Dermatitis 46(suppl 3):1–31

Johansen JD (2003) Fragrance contact allergy: a clinical review. Am J Clin Dermatol 4:789–798

Johansen JD, Bernard G, Giménez-Arnau E, Lepoittevin JP, Bruze M, Andersen KE (2006) Comparison of elicitation potential of chloroatranol and atranol – 2 allergens in oak moss absolute. Contact Dermatitis 54:192–195

Jørgensen PH, Jensen CD, Rastogi S, Andersen KE, Johansen JD (2007) Experimental elicitation with hydroxyisohexyl-3-cyclohexene carboxaldehyde-containing deodorants. Contact Dermatitis 56: 146–150

Kaddu S, Kerl H, Wolf P (2001) Accidental bullous phototoxic reactions to bergamot aromatherapy oil. J Am Acad Dermatol 45:458–461

Kanerva L, Estlander T, Jolanki R (1995) Occupational allergic contact dermatitis caused by ylang-ylang oil. Contact Dermatitis 33:198–199

Kanerva L, Estlander T, Jolanki R (1996) Occupational allergic contact dermatitis from spices. Contact Dermatitis 35:157–162

Kanerva L, Estlander T, Jolanki R (1998) Dental nurse's occupational allergic contact dermatitis from eugenol used as a restorative dental material with polymethylmethacrylate. Contact Dermatitis 38:339–340

Kanerva L, Jolanki R, Estlander T (1999) Hairdresser's dermatitis caused by oak moss in permanent waving solution. Contact Dermatitis 41:55

Karlberg A-T, Dooms-Goossens A (1997) Contact allergy to oxidised d-limonene among dermatitis patients. Contact Dermatitis 36: 201–206

Keane FM, Smith HR, White IR, Rycroft RJG (2000) Occupational allergic contact dermatitis in two aromatherapists. Contact Dermatitis 43:49–51

Landeck L, Gonzalez E, Baden LA, Neumann K, Schalock PC (2009) Contact sensitization by age group in adults: patch-test data from the Massachusetts General Hospital, 1996 to 2006. Dermatitis 20:287–291

Larsen W, Nakayama H, Fischer T et al (2001) Fragrance contact dermatitis: a worldwide multicenter investigation (part II). Contact Dermatitis 44:344–346

Larsen W, Nakayama H, Fischer T et al (2002) Fragrance contact dermatitis – a worldwide investigation (part III). Contact Dermatitis 46:141–144

Le Coz C-J (2004) Allergic contact dermatitis from tamanu oil (*Calophyllum inophyllum, Calophyllum tacamahaca*). Contact Dermatitis 51:216–217

Magnano M, Silvani S, Vincenzi C, Nino M, Tosti A (2009) Contact allergens and irritants in household washing and cleaning products. Contact Dermatitis 61:337–341

Martins C, Gonçalo M, Gonçalo S (1995) Allergic contact dermatitis from dipentene in wax polish. Contact Dermatitis 33:126

Matura M, Sköld M, Börje A et al (2005) Selected oxidized fragrance terpenes are common contact allergens. Contact Dermatitis 52: 320–328

Matura M, Sköld M, Börje A et al (2006) Not only oxidized R-(+)- but also S-(−)-limonene is a common cause of contact allergy in dermatitis patients in Europe. Contact Dermatitis 55:274–279

Meynadier J-M, Meynadier J, Peyron J-L, Peyron L (1986) Formes cliniques des manifestations cutanées d'allergie aux parfums. Ann Dermatol Venereol 113:31–39

Militello G, James W (2005) Lyral: a fragrance allergen. Dermatitis 16:41–44

NardelliA,CarbonezA,OttoyWetal(2008)Frequencyofandtrendsinfragrance allergyovera15-yearperiod.ContactDermatitis58:134–141

Nardelli A, D'Hooge E, Drieghe J, Dooms M, Goossens A (2009a) Allergic contact dermatitis from fragrance components in specific topical pharmaceutical products in Belgium. Contact Dermatitis 60:303–313

Nardelli A, Thijs L, Janssen K, Goossens A (2009b) *Rosa centifolia* in a "non-scented" body lotion as cause of allergic contact dermatitis. Contact Dermatitis 61:306–309

Nethercott JR, Pilger C, O'Blenis L, Roy A-M (1983) Contact dermatitis due to cinnamic aldehyde induced in a deodorant manufacturing process. Contact Dermatitis 9:241–242

Owen CM, August PJ, Beck MH (2000) Contact allergy to oak moss resin in a soluble oil. Contact Dermatitis 43:112

Pigatto PD, Guzzi G, Schena D et al (2008) Photopatch tests: an Italian multicentre study from 2004 to 2006. Contact Dermatitis 59:103–108

Rademaker M (1994) Allergic contact dermatitis from lavender fragrance in Difflam gel. Contact Dermatitis 31:58–59

Rastogi SC, Johansen JD, Frosch P et al (1998) Deodorants on the European market: quantitative chemical analysis of 21 fragrances. Contact Dermatitis 38:29–35

Rastogi SC, Heydorn S, Johansen JD, Basketter DA (2001) Fragrance chemicals in domestic and occupational products. Contact Dermatitis 45:221–225

Rastogi SC, Menné T, Johansen JD (2003) The composition of fine fragrances is changing. Contact Dermatitis 48:130–132

Rastogi SC, Bossi R, Johansen JD et al (2004) Content of oak moss allergens atranol and chloroatranol in perfumes and similar products. Contact Dermatitis 50:367–370

Reutemann P, Ehrlich A (2008) Neem oil: an herbal therapy for alopecia causes dermatitis. Dermatitis 19:12–15

Rothenborg HW, Menné T, Sjølin K-E (1977) Temperature dependent primary irritant dermatitis from lemon perfume. Contact Dermatitis 3:37–48

Rycroft RJG (1980) Allergic contact dermatitis from dipentene in honing oil. Contact Dermatitis 6:325–329

Sánchez-Pérez J, García-Díez A (1999) Occupational allergic contact dermatitis from eugenol, oil of cinnamon and oil of cloves in a physiotherapist. Contact Dermatitis 41:346–347

Sanchez-Politta S, Campanelli A, Pashe-Koo F, Saurat J-H, Piletta P (2007) Allergic contact dermatitis to phenylacetaldehyde: a forgotten allergen? Contact Dermatitis 56:171–172

Schaller M, Korting HC (1995) Allergic airborne contact dermatitis from essential oils used in aromatherapy. Clin Exp Dermatol 20:143–145

Scheinman PL (1996) Allergic contact dermatitis to fragrance: a review. Am J Contact Dermat 7:65–76

Schnuch A, Lessmann H, Geier J, Frosch PJ, Uter W (2004a) Contact allergy to fragrances: frequencies of sensitization from 1996 to 2002. Results of the IVDK. Contact Dermatitis 50:65–76

Schnuch A, Uter W, Geier J, Lessmann H, Frosch PJ (2004b) Contact allergy to farnesol in 2021 consecutively patch tested patients. Results of the IVDK. Contact Dermatitis 50:117–121

Schnuch A, Geier J, Uter W, Frosch PJ (2007a) Majantol® – a new important fragrance allergen. Contact Dermatitis 57:48–50

Schnuch A, Uter W, Geier J, Lessmann H, Frosch PJ (2007b) Sensitization to 26 fragrances to be labelled according to current European regulation. Contact Dermatitis 57:1–10

Schubert H-J (2006) Skin diseases in workers at a perfume factory. Contact Dermatitis 55:81–83

Selvaag E, Holm J, Thune P (1995) Allergic contact dermatitis in an aromatherapist with multiple sensitization to essential oils. Contact Dermatitis 33:354–355

Shaw DW (2006) Allergic contact dermatitis from octisalate and *cis*-3-hexenyl salicylate. Dermatitis 17:152–155

Stevensen CJ (1998) Aromatherapy in dermatology. Clin Dermatol 16:689–694

Sugiura M, Hayakawa R, Kato Y, Sugiura K, Hashimoto R (2000) Results of patch testing with lavender oil in Japan. Contact Dermatitis 43:157–160

Tanaka S, Royds C, Buckley D et al (2004a) Contact allergy to isoeugenol and its derivatives: problems with allergen substitution. Contact Dermatitis 51:288–291

Tanaka S, Matsumoto Y, Dlova N et al (2004b) Immediate contact reactions to fragrance mix constituents and *Myroxylon pereirae* resin. Contact Dermatitis 51:20–21

Thyssen JP, Carlsen BC, Menné T, Johansen JD (2008) Trends of contact allergy to fragrance mix I and *Myroxylon pereirae* among Danish eczema patients tested between 1985 and 2007. Contact Dermatitis 59:238–244

Thyssen JP, Linneberg A, Menné T, Nielsen NH, Johansen JD (2009a) The prevalence and morbidity of sensitization to fragrance mix I in the general population. Br J Dermatol 161:95–101

Thyssen JP, Menné T, Linneberg A, Johansen JD (2009b) Contact sensitization to fragrances in the general population: a Koch's approach may reveal the burden of disease. Br J Dermatol 160:729–735

Topham EJ, Wakelin SH (2003) d-Limonene contact dermatitis from hand cleansers. Contact Dermatitis 49:108

Trattner A, David M, Lazarov A (2008) Occupational contact dermatitis due to essential oils. Contact Dermatitis 58:282–284

Uter W, Schnuch A, Geier J, Pfahlberg A, Gefeller O (2001) Association between occupation and contact allergy to the fragrance mix: a multifactorial analysis of national surveillance data. Occup Environ Med 58:392–398

Uter W, Geier J, Schnuch A, Frosch PJ (2007) Patch test results with patients' own perfumes, deodorants and shaving lotions: results of the IVDK 1998–2002. J Eur Acad Dermatol Venereol 21:374–379

Uter W, Rämsch C, Aberer W et al (2009) The European baseline series in 10 European countries, 2005/2006; results of the European surveillance system on contact allergies (ESSCA). Contact Dermatitis 61:31–38

Van Oosten E, Schuttelaar M-L, Coenraads PJ (2009) Clinical relevance of positive patch test reactions to the 26 EU-labelled fragrances. Contact Dermatitis 61:217–223

Vilaplana J, Romaguera C (2002) Contact dermatitis from the essential oil of tangerine in fragrance. Contact Dermatitis 46:108

Wakelin SH, McFadden JP, Leonard JN, Rycroft RJG (1998) Allergic contact dermatitis from d,l-limonene in a laboratory technician. Contact Dermatitis 38:164–165

White JML, White IR, Glendinning A et al (2007) Frequency of allergic contact dermatitis to isoeugenol is increasing: a review of 3636 patients tested from 2001 to 2005. Br J Dermatol 157:580–582

White JML, McFadden JP, White IR (2008) A review of 241 subjects who were patch tested twice: could fragrance mix I cause active sensitization? Br J Dermatol 158:518–521

Zedlitz S, Kaufman R, Boehncke W-H (2002) Allergic contact dermatitis from black cumin (*Nigella sativa*) oil-containing ointment. Contact Dermatitis 46:188

Zug KA, Warshaw EM, Fowler JF Jr et al (2009) Patch-test results of the North American contact dermatitis group 2005–2006. Dermatitis 20:149–160

41 Colophony: Rosin in Unmodified and Modified Form

Ann-Therese Karlberg
Dermatochemistry and Skin Allergy, Department of Chemistry and Molecular Biology, University of Gothenburg, Gothenburg, Sweden

Core Messages

- Colophony (rosin) is a common cause of contact allergy and allergic contact dermatitis (ACD).
- Rosin is present in unmodified and modified form in many products with various usages and is ubiquitous in our daily life. Due to this, contact with rosin or rosin derivatives in commercial products is difficult to detect.
- Main usages are printing ink, adhesives, and sealants as well as paper size (2008).
- Rosin/colophony has an EU harmonised classification as skin sensitizing according to Annex VI of the CLP regulation (Regulation (EC) No 1272/2008). This means that the hazard statement H317 « May cause an allergic skin reaction » or the risk phrase R43 "May cause sensitisation by skin contact" shall apply for products containing rosin in a concentration of at least 1%.
- The allergenicity of modified rosins can be caused by new allergenic derivatives, specifically maleopimaric acid, but also due to unmodified rosin still present after modification.
- More investigations with regard to the presence of various modified rosins in different products are needed.
- Studies on the prevalence of ACD in dermatitis patients and in the population caused by modified rosins should be performed.

1 Introduction

Colophony (rosin) obtained from pine trees has been used since ancient times due to its technical (tackifying) and medicinal (antimicrobial) effects. Also, the skin sensitizing effects of rosin are well known since a long time, and it is still one of the most common causes of contact allergy in the Western society. As most natural products, rosin has a complex chemical composition. A majority of rosin is modified in various ways to improve the technical properties. However, the modifications are only performed until desirable technical properties are obtained. This means that in most cases, unmodified rosin is still present in the final product. New allergens are created in the modification processes; thus, technical products can contain allergens from unmodified rosin together with new allergens from modification. Contact allergy to these allergens is not detected in standardized screening using unmodified rosin of the gum rosin–type for patch testing.

2 Production

Colophony (rosin) is the nonvolatile fraction of the fluid oleoresins from coniferous trees mainly pine trees. As it is a natural product, the composition varies depending on the source but also on the way it is produced. There are three types of rosin depending on the way of recovery: gum rosin, wood rosin, and tall oil rosin. Gum rosin is obtained from various species of standing pine trees. The trees are tapped for oleoresin, which is then processed by evaporating the volatile mono- and sesquiterpenoid components, that is, turpentine, leaving the gum rosin as the residue. Wood rosin is extracted with solvent from pine stumps. Tall oil rosin is obtained as one of the major fractions by distillation of crude tall oil, a coproduct of the sulfate (kraft) pulping process of coniferous trees. Today, the major types of rosin are gum rosin and tall oil rosin. In 2008, the total rosin production was estimated to be 1,190, 000 metric tons of which 763,000 t were gum rosin, 415,000 t tall oil rosin, and 12,000 t wood rosin. Seventy-five percent of gum rosin is produced in China. Other big producers of gum rosin are Brazil, Indonesia, and India, while small amounts of gum rosin are produced in Mexico, Argentina, Nepal, Russia, and Portugal. The major producers of tall oil rosin are the United States and the Nordic countries.

In technical literature, the term "colophony" corresponds to gum rosin. In dermatological literature, also wood rosin and tall oil rosin are included in the term colophony as the resins contain the same major chemical components and allergens, and most often, no declaration of the source is found for technical products. In American literature, the term "rosin" is more frequently used. In the following, "rosin" will be used as the general term

T. Rustemeyer, P. Elsner, S.M. John & H.I. Maibach (eds.), *Kanerva's Occupational Dermatology*,
DOI 10.1007/978-3-642-02035-3_41,

including the three major types. Gum rosin is used in the baseline series for patch testing. It should be observed that an important part of the rosin on the market is chemically modified in order to improve its technical properties.

3 Chemical Composition of Unmodified Rosin

Although there are variations in the chemical composition between the different types of rosin, the major components are the same. The composition is complex including about 90% resin acids and 10% neutral components. The acids are monocarboxylic diterpenoid acids of which the abietane- and pimarane-type structures are the most abundant. Tall oil rosin contains less abietane-type acids and more dehydroabietic acid compared to gum rosin. This is due to oxidation-dehydration of abietane-type acids in the pine chips during pulping and tall oil processing and to the high production temperature. The production process also results in some artifacts which are not found in the other types of rosin. The neutral compounds in rosin are mainly diterpenoid alcohols and aldehydes and also hydrocarbons. Tall oil rosin also contains small amounts of fatty acids and alcohols (Holmbom et al. 1974; Zinkel 1975; Soltes and Zinkel 1989). The major resin acid is abietic acid. Dehydroabietic acid and less stable acids of the abietane-type (e.g., levopimaric acid and palustric acid) are present in varying concentrations depending on the production and storage. Pimaric acid is of the pimarane-type acids and isopimaric acid and sandarcopimaric acid of the isopimarane-type (➋ *Table 41.1*, ➋ *Fig. 41.1*).

Unmodified rosin contains varying amounts of oxidized material mainly due to the oxidation of abietic acid which is known to oxidize at exposure to air. The oxidation of abietic acid has been shown to proceed via a free radical chain reaction. Hydrogens in benzylic, allylic, and tertiary positions are preferably abstracted as they yield particularly stable radicals. For abietic acid, the carbon radical in the tertiary position in the isopropyl group is especially stable as it also is allylic to the two conjugated double bonds (➋ *Fig. 41.1*). Hydroperoxides are formed as primary oxidation products, and the first oxidation product identified was 15-hydroperoxyabietic acid (Karlberg et al. 1988a). Also, peroxides, epoxides, ketones, and alcohols of abietic acid and dehydroabietic acid have been identified. The major oxidation products were identified both in gum rosin and tall oil rosin (Karlberg 1991). Oxidation products identified as contact allergens are shown in ➋ *Fig. 41.2*.

Table 41.1
Gas chromatographic analysis of resin acids in Chinese gum rosin, Portuguese gum rosin, and Swedish tall oil rosin from China and Portugal

Resin acids	Resin acids present in the acid fraction (%)		
	Chinese gum rosin	Portuguese gum rosin	Swedish tall oil rosin
Abietic acid	56	48	43
Neoabietic acid	12	15	3
Palustric acid	14	15	8
Dehydroabietic acid	6	5	28
Pimaric acid	9	9	4
Isopimaric acid	1	5	5
Sandarcopimaric acid	2	2	2
Other free resin acids	0	1	7

4 Chemical Modifications of Rosin

Rosin is modified to a large extent. The major component abietic acid, and its isomers are the main targets for the modifications and derivatizations of rosin which are performed to improve its technical properties (Soltes and Zinkel 1989; Illing et al. 2009). Abietic acid contains two reactive sites: the carboxylic acid group and the double bonds. The rosin derivatives all result from chemical reactions on one or both of these sites. The reactions on the carboxylic group that are of commercial importance are esterifications (ester gums) and salt formations. Most important modifications regarding reactions on the conjugated double bonds include hydrogenation, disproportionation, Diels-Alder-type reactions, dimerization/polymerization, and reactions with formaldehyde (polymerization) (Soltes and Zinkel 1989; Gafvert 1994). Different modification processes are often combined. Generally, the resins obtained are characterized by nonspecific and approximate methods such as color grade, acid number, saponification number, etc. It should be noted that in most cases, the modification is interrupted when certain technical properties are achieved. This means that also nonmodified rosin could be present in the final products (Gafvert et al. 1996). Recently, more than 200 derivatives of rosin (named modified rosin resins) were reviewed by a task group within the Hydrocarbon Resins, Rosin Resins and Pine Chemicals

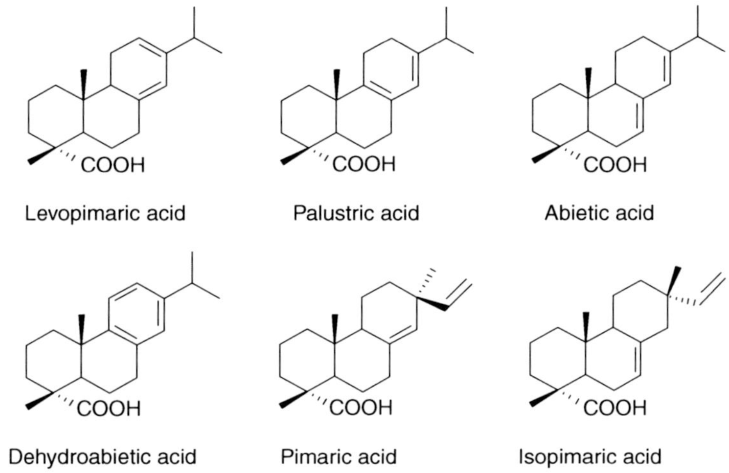

Fig. 41.1
Structures of the different types of major resin acids identified in rosin. Levopimaric, palustric, and abietic acid are all of the abietane-type acids

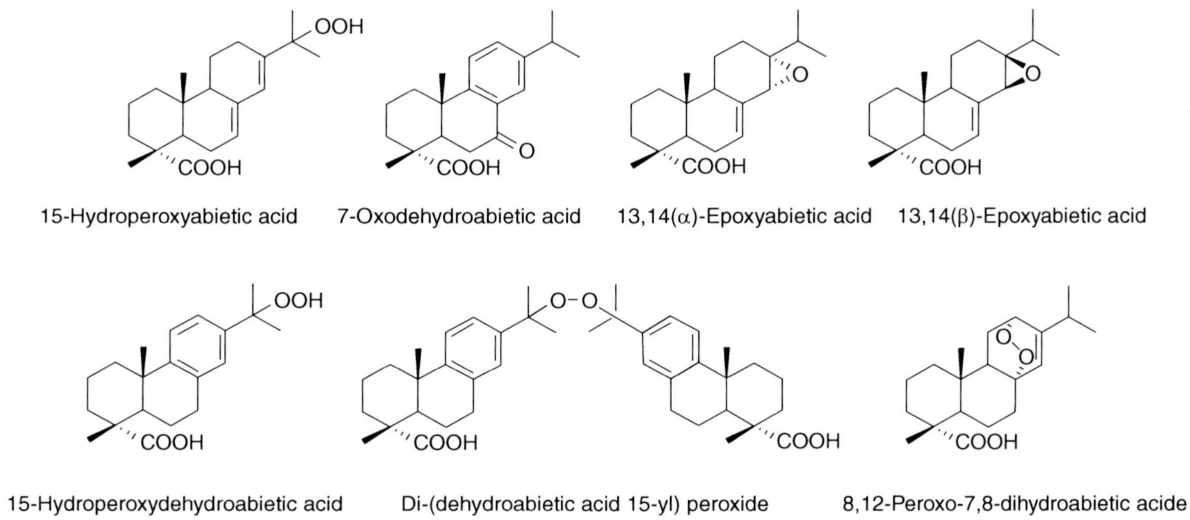

Fig. 41.2
Major oxidation products in rosin identified as contact allergens

Producers Association (HARPA) of which 80 were found to be commercially significant (Illing et al. 2009). These 80 derivatives were allocated into different groupings. The groupings fit well with the modifications of the active sites of abietic acid and its isomers described below.

4.1 Esters

Esterification of the carboxylic acid group with polyalcohols is most often performed with glycerol or pentaerythritol. The esters produced in this reaction are referred to as ester gums. Esterification with glycerol was introduced at the end of the nineteenth century as one of the first commercial modifications used (Soltes and Zinkel 1989). Esterification with polyalcohols can give a mixture of esters when the resin acids react with 1-3 (glycerol) or 1-5 (pentaerythritol) alcohol groups. The esterification process between abietic acid and glycerol has been studied in detail and evaluated with regard to sensitizing capacity (Shao et al. 1993; Gafvert et al. 1994a) (➋ *Fig. 41.3*).

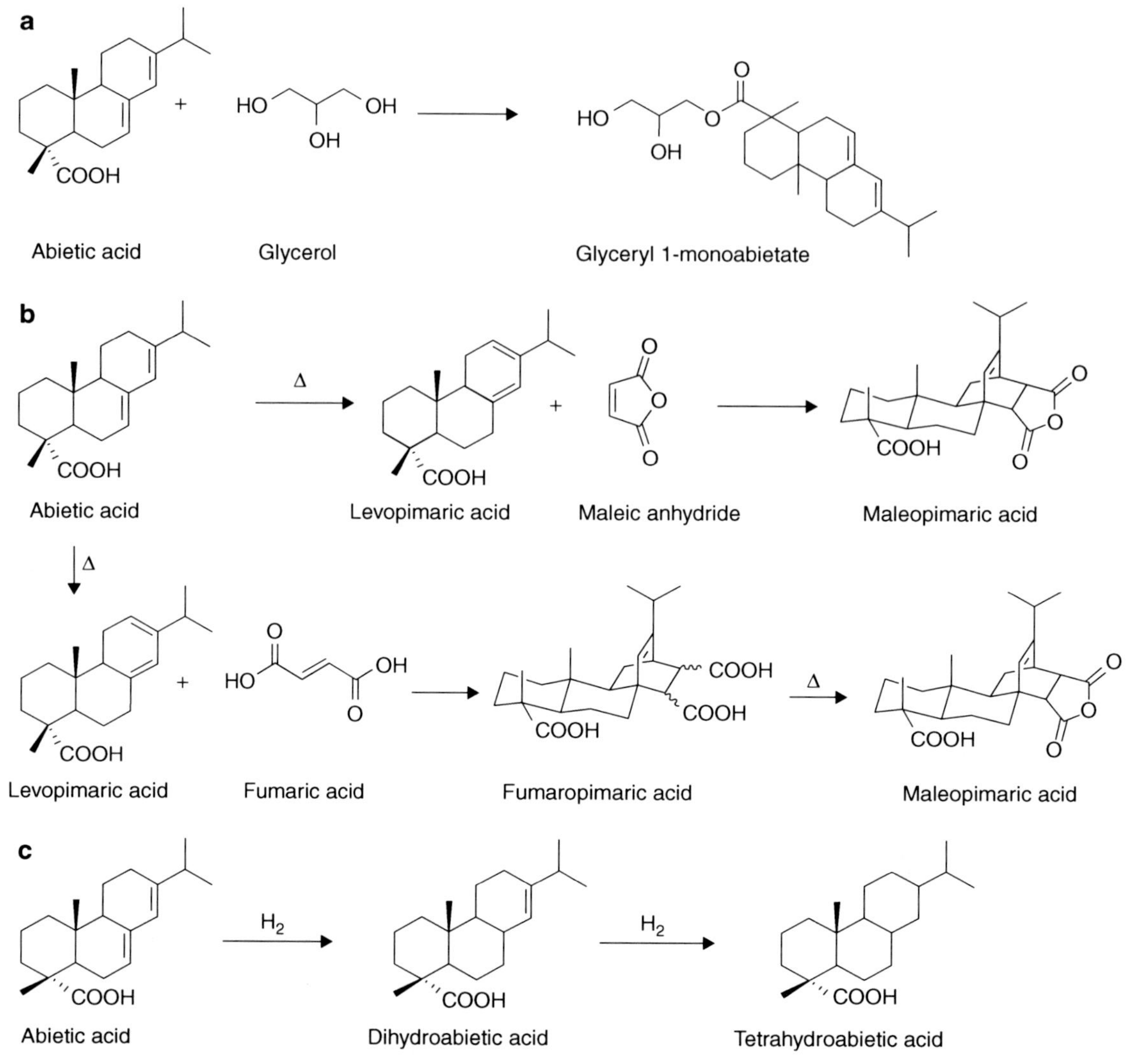

Fig. 41.3

Schemes of important modifications of rosin (using the major component abietic acid as model) which change their technical and skin sensitizing properties. (a) Esterification of abietic acid with glycerol forming monoabietate (weak allergen). (b) Formation of maleopimaric acid (strong allergen) and fumaropimaric acid (weak allergen) by Diels-Alder reactions with maleic anhydride and fumaric acid, respectively. (c) Hydrogenation of abietic acid which reduces the sensitizing capacity of the acid

4.2 Diels-Alder Derivatives

Diels-Alder addition is one of the most common modifications of rosin. In this reaction, an α,β-unsaturated carbonyl compound, referred to as a dienophile, reacts with a conjugated diene such as the ones found in the abietic-type acids. Maleic anhydride or fumaric acid is the dienophile and levopimaric acid is the conjugated diene in the commercial processes. Abietic acid is the major acid in unmodified rosin since it is the more stable, but the equilibrium is changed by heating in the modification process. Maleopimaric acid is formed in the reaction with maleic anhydride, while fumaropimaric acid is formed in the reaction with fumaric acid (Karlberg et al. 1990; Gafvert et al. 1995). However, minor amounts of maleopimaric acid are formed also in the latter process

(➋ *Fig. 41.3*). From a skin sensitizing perspective, this is very important as maleopimaric acid in contrast to fumaropimaric acid is a strong sensitizer not cross-reacting with the sensitizers in unmodified rosin (Gafvert 1994; Gafvert et al. 1996; Illing et al. 2009). Maleopimaric acid is an anhydride and thus very reactive which can explain its sensitizing capacity. Fumaropimaric acid on the other hand is a tricarboxylic acid and as acids are rather unreactive they are also known to be weak allergens.

4.3 Hydrogenated, Dehydrogenated, and Disproportionated Rosin

Hydrogenation, dehydrogenation, and disproportionation are reactions that involve the double bonds and are performed to stabilize and prevent from autoxidation. By hydrogenation, one or both of the easily autoxidized conjugated double bonds could be reduced giving di- or tetraabietic acid (➋ *Fig. 41.3*). Dehydrogenation is the removal of two hydrogen atoms from the abietic-type acids and rearrangement of the double bonds to form dehydroabietic acid. This leads to a reduction of the abietic-type acids to the more stable dehydroabietic acid (➋ *Fig. 41.1*). The disproportionation process can be described as a dehydrogenation-hydrogenation transfer reaction which gives mainly dehydrobietic acid but also a mixture of di- and tetraabietic acids (Soltes and Zinkel 1989).

4.4 Formaldehyde-Modified Rosin

Formaldehyde modifications involve several different reactions performed under various conditions to form addition products. This type of reactions does not necessarily make the abietane-type acids less prone to autoxidation as the conjugated system of double bonds is still present (Soltes and Zinkel 1989).

4.5 Resinates

Salts formed by reacting the resin acids with metal salts are called resinates. These salts can be prepared in mainly two different ways. In the precipitation method, a solution of heavy metal salt is added to a soluble sodium resinate. This will produce a water-insoluble heavy metal resinate. In the fusion method, rosin is fused with a metal hydroxide or oxide. Hydroxides, oxides, and various metal compounds react with the carboxyl group of the resin acids to form soaps and resinates. The alkali metals (e.g., sodium and potassium) form water-soluble salts, while the salts of the alkaline earth metals (e.g., magnesium and calcium) are soluble in organic solvents. The reactive conjugated system of double bonds is still present also for the resinates, but the effect could vary depending on the solubility (Soltes and Zinkel 1989).

5 Usage and Legislation

In the early seventeenth century, extracting resin from living pines became the first widespread industry in America. The business was more famous under the name "naval stores," and the product was used by sailors to seal leaking hulls. Rosin has three main properties: it has good tackifying qualities, it can be used as an emulsifier, and it has acid properties without causing corrosion. The technical properties are modified using chemical reactions as described above. In many cases, modifications are undertaken on both reactive sites (carboxylic acid and double bonds) in different proportions to get the desired technical properties (Soltes and Zinkel 1989; Illing et al. 2009).

Different modifications are important in the various industries. The paper industry uses large amounts of rosin for paper size, that is, to give the paper a smooth and hydrophobic surface. For this purpose, mainly Diels-Alder adducts are used but also formaldehyde-modified rosin. Also, sodium salt is used in the paper industry, while ammonium salt is used in detergents due to their properties as amphiphiles, containing both a hydrophilic and a lipophilic region (Soltes and Zinkel 1989).

Disproportionated rosin is present as polymerization emulsifiers in the production of synthetic rubber and also, e.g., as insulating materials in the electronics industry. Adhesives are primarily composed of a polymeric component and a tackifying resin. Rosin used in tackifying resins is mainly disproportionated, hydrogenated, or polymerized, as well as their esters with glycerol or pentaerythritol. The rosin derivatives are important components both in pressure-sensitive adhesives and hot-melt adhesives. The rosin derivatives are used in large amounts also in paints, coatings, and road markers.

Many of the modified rosin products are not possible to connect to rosin by the name. Thus, trying to find any statistics of the usage of rosin in different industries and products is difficult. The world consumption in 2008 of rosin in unmodified and modified form allocated to market application is seen in ➋ *Fig. 41.4*.

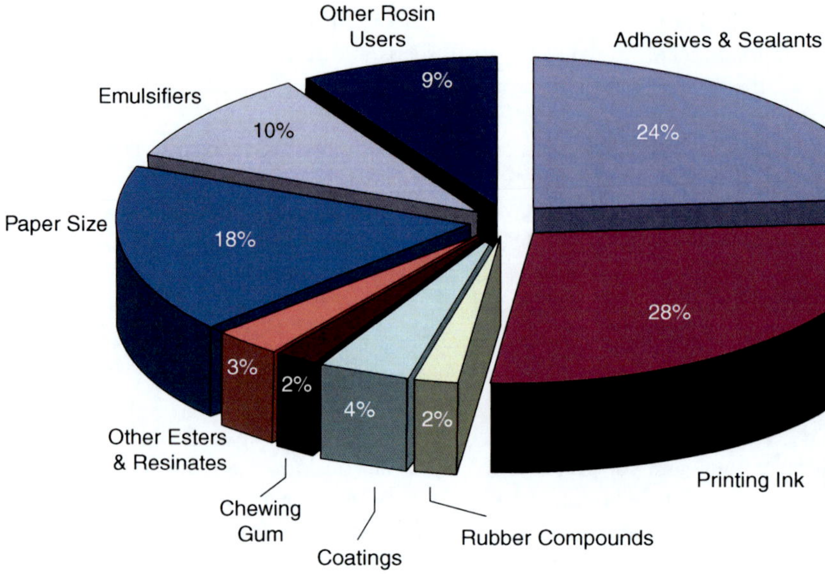

Fig. 41.4
The world consumption in 2008 of rosin in unmodified and modified form allocated to market application (Turner 2010)

According to the EU legislation mixtures containing skin sensitizers in a concentration of at least 1% should be classified for skin sensitization. If classification is conducted according to the preparations directive (Directive 1999/45 EC; valid until 1 June 2015) the risk phrase R43 "May cause sensitisation by skin contact" shall apply (Reference: DIRECTIVE 1999/45/EC OF THE EUROPEAN PARLIAMENT AND OF THE COUNCIL of 31 May 1999 concerning the approximation of the laws, regulations and administrative provisions of the Member States relating to the classification, packaging and labelling of dangerous preparations). If classification is conducted according to the CLP regulation (Regulation (EC) No 1272/2008) the hazard statement H317 « May cause an allergic skin reaction » shall apply (Reference: REGULATION (EC) No 1272/2008 OF THE EUROPEAN PARLIAMENT AND OF THE COUNCIL of 16 December 2008 on classification, labelling and packaging of substances and mixtures, amending and repealing Directives 67/548/EEC and 1999/45/EC, and amending Regulation (EC) No 1907/2006).

Rosin/colophony (CAS numbers 8050-09-7 (preferred name rosin), 8052-10-6 (preferred name tall oil rosin), 73138-82-6 (preferred names resin acids and rosin acids)) has an EU harmonised classification as skin sensitising according to Annex VI of the CLP regulation (Regulation (EC) No 1272/2008). This means that the hazard statement H317 « May cause an allergic skin reaction » or the risk phrase R43 "May cause sensitisation by skin contact" shall apply for products containing rosin in a concentration of at least 1%. The classification and labelling shall be declared in the safety data sheet.

According to the Cosmetics Directive (76/768/EÖF), the component is listed on the INCI list (Index of Cosmetic Ingredients) under the name "colophonium" (EF. Nr. 232-475-7) without any restrictions for its application.

6 Analysis of Content of Unmodified Rosin in Technical Products

The content of rosin in commercial products as demanded from the regulation (see above) is not possible to quantify with a simple chemical analysis. Rosin is a natural product consisting of a mixture of hundreds of components. Quantifying a mixture used as an ingredient of another mixture cannot be achieved by any analytical means. To overcome this impossibility, the quantification must be based on an approximation from the quantification of specific tracers, that is, the major components and calculations from their percentage in rosin. As the content of resin acids varies depending on variations in source, manufacturing, handling, and storage, it is not possible to determine the exact concentration of rosin in a product. A thorough review with regard to analytical methods used for rosin was recently published by the Danish Ministry of the Environment (Nilsson et al. 2009). Two major types of analyses for rosin components are described in literature. Traditionally in the pulp industry, the major resin acids are quantified using gas chromatography with a flame ionization detector (GC/FID). Later on, methods based on liquid chromatography (LC) using UV, fluorescence, and mass spectrometry have been developed, most often for the analyses of specific products (Nilsson et al. 2009).

In all the described methods, the quantification is based on content of the nonoxidized resin acids. Based on this, a low level of abietic acid indicates a low level of rosin; however, it is important to check that a low level is not caused by an oxidative degradation resulting in highly allergenic compounds such as 15-hydroperoxyabietic acid. To avoid such a misinterpretation, a new LC/UV method was developed that besides the two major acids of unmodified rosin, abietic acid and dehydroabietic acid, uses a stable oxidation product, 7-oxodehydroabietic acid as a tracer for oxidative degradation (Nilsson et al. 2008). The necessity of methods and rules for quantification of specific rosin components as tracers for content of rosin in products high enough to be declared according to the EU legislation was demonstrated in a paper on metalworking fluids (Henricks-Eckerman et al. 2008).

7 Allergenic Activity

Unmodified rosin is known to cause contact allergy. The main allergenic components are oxidized resin acids of the abietane-type which are formed on air exposure (➋ *Fig. 41.2*). 15-Hydroperoxyabietic acid was the first oxidation product identified as a contact allergen in unmodified gum rosin and is still considered to be the major sensitizer (Karlberg et al. 1988a). Later, several articles regarding isolation and identification of oxidized resin acids as contact allergens were published (Karlberg et al. 1988b; Hausen and Hessling 1990; Hausen et al. 1990; Gafvert et al. 1992; Hausen and Loll 1993; Khan and Saeed 1994; Gafvert et al. 1994b; Shao et al. 1995; Sadhra et al. 1996). In the pioneer work of rosin allergy, the allergenic resin acids were isolated as their methylates. In a later study, a synthesized 15-hydroperoxyabietic acid was tested in individuals with known contact allergy to gum rosin (Karlberg et al. 2007). The study showed that a similar proportion of individuals (46%) reacted to the acid compared with the percentage (57%) of reactions to its methyl ester used in previous investigations. Corresponding oxidation of the neutral components can also yield allergenic compounds and patch test studies with neutrals have revealed additional cases of rosin allergy (Karlberg et al. 1986; Sadhra and Foulds 1995).

When ranking the sensitizing capacity of the oxidation products in gum rosin according to the original classification by Magnusson and Kligman based on guinea pig studies, most of the compounds were classified as extreme allergens with a ranking grade of V (81–100% sensitized animals) (Karlberg and Gafvert 1996).

The chemical modifications as described above change the reactivity and thus also the allergenic activity of rosin. Modification including hydrogenation of the double bonds will reduce the sensitizing capacity (Karlberg et al. 1988c; Gafvert et al. 1994). Esterifications with polyalcohols forming gum rosins can also reduce the sensitizing capacity depending on how far the process is driven. Studies of esterification of abietic acid with glycerol showed that mono-, di-, and triabietates can be formed. Of these, monoabietate (➋ *Fig. 41.3*) was found to be a sensitizer in guinea pigs, while triabietate was a nonsensitizer (Shao et al. 1993; Gafvert et al. 1994a). The Diels-Alder reaction using maleic anhydride or fumaric acid results in maleopimaric acid which is an anhydride with reactive sites that differ from those in nonmodified rosin (➋ *Fig. 41.3*). Maleopimaric acid is a strong sensitizer, and both maleated and fumarated rosins are sensitizers in animal experiments (Gafvert et al. 1995). A sensitizing capacity of maleated or fumarated rosins is observed also after esterification (Illing et al. 2009). It must be observed that most often, unmodified rosin is still present in a product after modifications have been performed (Gafvert et al. 1996). This has been shown even after double modifications, e.g., analysis of an esterified and maleated rosin showed a content of both unmodified resin acids and maleopimaric acid in addition to the maleated rosin ester which was used in an adhesive for shoe linings (Lyon et al. 1999).

8 Allergic Contact Dermatitis

8.1 Screening and Patch Testing

Gum rosin in petrolatum at a concentration of 20% is used for patch testing under the INCI name colophonium (Karlberg and Liden 1988). In the True Test, a mixture of eight different types of gum rosin is applied in a gel at a concentration 850 μg/cm^2.

The baseline series including gum rosin is also used in screening studies of contact allergy to the most common allergens in cohorts from the general population in different countries. In these studies, prevalence levels of 0.7% positive patch test reactions to gum rosin in 567 tested individuals, 1.2% in 1,141 individuals, and 1.6% in 1,236 individuals, respectively, are reported (Nielsen and Menne 1992; Schafer et al. 2001; Dotterud and Smith-Sivertsen 2007). A 10-year prevalence (1992–2002) of contact allergy to gum rosin in the population in Germany based on the positive reactions to the baseline series in 78,067 dermatitis patients was estimated to 1.4–0.6% (Schnuch et al. 2002). Using the same setup, a prevalence of 0.84–0.62% of rosin allergy was estimated in the Danish population (Thyssen et al. 2007).

Clinical aspects of rosin allergy have been extensively reviewed by Färm (1997). When patch testing consecutive dermatitis patients with the baseline series, gum rosin is among the most common causes of contact allergy with a relative frequency of positive reactions varying from 2% to 7% (Farm 1997; Downs and Sansom 1999; Schnuch et al. 2002; Uter et al. 2010). A dominance of positive reactions in women is observed. Results from testing with the baseline series in about 25,000 consecutive patients in 10 European test centers during the years 1996–2000 were published in 2005 (Bruynzeel et al. 2005). A relative frequency of positive reactions to gum rosin ranging from 2.2% to 5.2% with a mean of 4.0% (3.2% men and 4.5% female) was found. In a Swedish study (Lindberg et al. 2007), a certain decrease in the prevalence of reactions to gum rosin was observed when comparing data from 1992 with those from 2000. More than 3,000 consecutive patients were tested in different clinics at these two occasions. Furthermore, this study showed a clear decrease in the prevalence in the ages <40 years compared to that seen in the older ages for men (2.0% compared with 3.4%) and also for women (2.0% compared with 5.4%). As the use of rosin-containing products for treatment of leg ulcers has been an important source for contact allergy to gum rosin, it might be one of the explanations behind the higher prevalence of allergy in the older group (Lindberg et al. 2007).

Individuals in whom contact allergy to gum rosin had been diagnosed at an occupational clinic were followed up after 9–13 years. At least 30% of the 83 persons investigated had current hand eczema on the follow-up examination. Among those in whom the dermatitis had started on the hands, proportionally more individuals with current hand eczema were observed than among those in whom the onset had been on other parts of the body. At the time of the investigation, 72% of the participants were still patch test positive to gum rosin, and more than half had additional positive reactions to other allergens (Farm 1996).

Various types of rosin are used interchangeably; it is mainly the price that is decisive. When patch testing with various gum rosins and with tall oil rosin, fewer positive reactions were found to the tall oil rosin, but most persons reacted to both gum rosin and tall oil rosin (Karlberg and Liden 1985; Karlberg et al. 1986; Hausen and Loll 1993; Karlberg and Gafvert 1996). The slightly lower allergenic activity of tall oil rosin could be due to a difference in composition, but as the allergenic activity is mainly due to oxidation products, the handling and storage times always affect the allergenic properties (Karlberg 1988; Sadhra et al. 1998). The major oxidation products are identified also in tall oil rosin (Karlberg 1991); thus, it is acceptable to use gum rosin in a well-defined form as the first screening material.

In general, the baseline series for patch testing consists of pure and identified substances, except for some complex natural products among which gum rosin is one. As stated above, the main allergens are found among the oxidation products formed at autoxidation of the resin acids of abietane-type acids, while the pure acids have a very low allergenic activity (Karlberg 1988). The patch test preparations of gum rosin should be as well defined as possible. It is important that the content of oxidation products is kept at a constant and rather high level in the test preparations as they are the main allergens. Investigations have shown that there is a considerable decrease in the content of abietane-type acids in the patch test preparations (21% in the first 6 months after preparation) which was considered to be due to further oxidation followed by formation of less allergenic secondary oxidation products in the preparation process (grinding and heating) as well as at storage; an additional decrease of 6% was seen between 6 and 12 months of storage (Sadhra et al. 1998).

Different rosin components and fractions of unmodified rosin have been suggested for more effective patch test diagnosis (Hausen and Loll 1993; Sadhra and Foulds 1995). However, the problems with the rosin allergens have not been taken into consideration. Testing with the identified allergens will not detect as many cases as testing with gum rosin itself. Simultaneous testing with the major allergens, 15-HPA (the hydroperoxide of abietic acid) and gum rosin, showed that 50%–70% of those reacting to gum rosin reacted to the isolated allergen (Karlberg and Gafvert 1996; Karlberg et al. 2007). In gum rosin, oxidation products are formed continuously due to autoxidation, while pure, isolated, and unstable oxidation products are degradated. In some cases, testing with a major allergen in a newly prepared patch test preparation could detect additional cases of allergy as the concentration of the allergen in the mixture might be too low in the screening of the actual individual. It could therefore be of interest to test with some of the individual sensitizers in addition to the baseline testing in these patients. At present, patch test preparations of the individual sensitizers are not commercially available and, e.g., 15-HPA is unstable and cumbersome to synthesize (Karlberg et al. 2007).

Cross-reactions between rosin, Balsam of Peru (myroxylon pereirae), oil of turpentine, wood tar, and spruce resin were described by Hjorth in 1961 (Hjorth 1961). Today, concomitant reactions to gum rosin, Balsam of Peru, and/or fragrances are frequently seen when testing with the baseline series in consecutive patients. A clear correlation is observed between positive patch test reactions to gum rosin and to oxidized fragrance compounds, that is, oxidized limonene and oxidized linalool in consecutive dermatitis patients (Karlberg and Dooms-Goossens 1997; Matura et al. 2003, 2005). Besides concomitant sensitization, this could be caused by the allergenic hydroperoxides forming nonspecific antigens. As hydroperoxides and peroxides are oxidizing agents, they may oxidize functional groups in the proteins and thereby form nonspecific agents. Thus, cross-reactions between hydroperoxides with significantly different structures would be observed. However, cross-reactivity studies in animals as well as patch test studies show that hydroperoxides have a specific reactivity (Christensson et al. 2006, 2008).

Patch testing with modified rosins and allergens formed by modifications will detect additional cases of contact allergy (Hausen and Mohnert 1989; Gafvert et al. 1996). In an international patch test study, positive reactions were observed to the modified rosin components maleopimaric acid and glyceryl-1-monoabietate (Gafvert et al. 1996). Of the patients who reacted to modified rosin components, some did not react to unmodified gum rosin in the baseline series. This was expected as no cross-reactivity between the modified rosin components and the allergens in gum rosin is observed. Reactions to both gum rosin and the allergens formed after modification could be caused by concomitant sensitization as unmodified rosin is still present in the modified material (Gafvert 1994; Gafvert et al. 1996). It is desirable that at least the potent allergen maleopimaric acid present in commonly used modified rosins could be used as a screening material, but it is presently not commercially available. An alternative is to test with well-defined maleated rosin derivatives with and without esterification (Illing et al. 2009).

8.2 Exposure from Products in Close Contact with the Skin

Several case reports deal with the clinical problems caused by rosin in products that are in close contact with the skin. Intolerance to *adhesive plasters* has been discussed since the beginning of the 1920s (Karlberg 1988). Efforts have been made over the years to make adhesives nonallergenic using acrylate polymers. However, rosin is needed to get a maximum of adhesion effect and therefore it is still used, most often as ester gums. Chemical analysis shows a content of the major resin acids in these types of products (Ehrin and Karlberg 1990). In leg ulcer patients, a high incidence of contact allergy to gum rosin is observed. A recent multicenter study in patients with chronic leg ulcers revealed contact allergy to gum rosin in 7.6% of the tested individuals (Barbaud et al. 2009). A clear correlation was found between rosin allergy and reactions to a *rosin-containing dressing* tested simultaneously. Although the rosin used in these products most often is esterified gum rosin which might be further derivatized, the amount of unmodified rosin still present is high enough to cause allergic contact dermatitis from gum rosin. Contact allergy to the modified rosins was also demonstrated, although no reactions to unmodified rosin in the baseline series were seen (Salim and Shaw 2001; Pereira et al. 2007). Reduction of the allergenic effect of rosin in adhesives and bandages used for treatment of ulcers by addition of zinc oxide could not be confirmed in a specific investigation (Gafvert and Farm 1995).

Epilating waxes and tissues used for removal of hair on the lower legs have caused an epidemic of allergic contact dermatitis due to their content of modified rosin (Goossens et al. 2002). In many cases, a severe systemic eruption led to hospitalization and administration of systemic corticosteroids. Primary sensitization occurred in one-third of the patients. The majority of patients with positive reactions to the modified rosin in the products did not react to the gum rosin in the baseline series. This is in accordance with previous findings when screening with allergens from modified rosin (Gafvert et al. 1996). As specific allergens have been identified in glycerol-modified rosin, this is not surprising. However, recently published chemical analyses show that the modifications are not performed to completeness in epilating waxes but leaving unmodified rosin to ensure the stickiness of the product (Nilsson et al. 2008).

Glycerol esterified rosin is used as a skin conditioner and surfactant-emulsifying agent in eye makeup, hair coloring preparations, blushers, foundations, and lipsticks (Goossens et al. 2002). Allergic contact dermatitis from rosin in unmodified or modified form in various types of *cosmetics* has been reported during the years (Farm 1997). Also, the adhesive of Indian bindi has been reported to cause ACD due to rosin derivatives (Koh et al. 1995).

Rosin in *adhesives for shoe linings* is an important cause of contact allergy. Esterified gum rosins alone or in combination with Diels-Alder derivatization are used, and thus allergic contact dermatitis can be caused by strong allergens formed by modification, especially maleopimaric acid but also due to unmodified rosin still present in the adhesive (Gafvert 1994; Gafvert et al. 1996). A case report describes ACD on the feet caused by rosin in shoe linings in a 5-year-old girl. Although the used adhesive was both maleated and esterified rosin, it contained enough unmodified rosin to cause dermatitis which healed when the girl was wearing unlined shoes. The content of unmodified rosin and maleopimaric acid in the adhesive was confirmed with chemical analysis (Lyon et al. 1999). In an Indian study, patients with footwear dermatitis were tested with the Indian Standard Battery for screening of contact allergy. Contact allergy to gum rosin was detected in 11.6% of the tested patients (Chowdhuri and Ghosh 2007). In cases of ACD caused by the adhesive in shoe linings, it is recommended that individuals allergic to rosin should wear either unlined shoes or leather-lined shoes with the lining stitched, not glued in place, and no heel or toe supports. In comparison with its use and close contact with the skin, contact allergy to modified and unmodified rosin in shoes is very little investigated.

Pharmaceutical uses of oils and pitch from pines were noted by physicians 2,000 years ago (Zinkel 1975), but nowadays, it is mainly used in folk medicine. However, gum rosin is still used in dental materials, e.g., in periodontal dressings, cavity varnishes, and fluoridising dental varnishes. Some reports of stomatitis and lichen planus in the mouth from dental materials containing rosin have been published (Sharma 2006).

Exposure to rosin components in paper products has mainly been a matter of occupational exposure, but rosin components have also been indentified in diapers and sanitary pads (Karlberg and Magnusson 1996; Kanerva et al. 2001).

8.3 Occupational Exposure

Individuals exposed to unmodified rosin in pine wood, sawdust, and wood wool may develop hand dermatitis and dermatitis due to airborne exposure (Burry 1976; Daly and Stevenson 1984; Meding et al. 1996; Watsky 1997). Despite a significant production of gum rosin, no reports of occupational allergic contact dermatitis in gum rosin extractors are found in literature except for a recent report from Brazil (Scherrer and Junqueira 2010). In this case report, a female rosin extractor presented eczematous lesions on her hands, forearms, neck, face, and legs. No protection was used. She reacted to the gum rosin obtained and to gum rosin in the patch test baseline series. Her eczema improved when she left her job. In Brazil, the gum rosin industry employs 15,000 workers (data from the Resin Association in Brazil (ARESB)). The conclusions from the authors are that cases in gum rosin extractors very seldom are reported and diagnosed (Scherrer and Junqueira 2010). The prevalence of contact allergy to gum rosin and tall oil rosin among the employees in a factory for production of tall oil rosin was found to be in accordance with that of dermatitis patients and thus higher than in the general population (Farm et al. 1994). However, the clinical symptoms were rare. A healthy worker effect cannot be excluded among people working with extraction and production of rosin. In the local areas, it is well known that you might get skin problems from working with rosin, and you either continue to work or if possible, leave for another job without involving a dermatologist.

Skin problems among performing *artists* have been reported through the years (Helm et al. 1993; Farm et al. 1995). Artists are often extensively exposed to cosmetics in their occupation. Theatrical cosmetics do not differ essentially from corresponding products for everyday usage, apart from higher pigment content. The frequency of cosmetics intolerance and contact allergy to gum rosin in the baseline series was investigated among artists in an opera house (Farm et al. 1995). Contact allergy to gum rosin was not causing frequent problems among the artists. Among the *dancers* in the opera house, only one subject had an allergic contact dermatitis caused by gum rosin. The dancers use rosin on the floor, on their shoes, and even on the female dresses, as an antislipping agent. Also in this case, a healthy worker effect could be distinguished as it takes many years of training before you become a professional dancer. However, rosin allergy among the dancers' masseurs can be observed (Farm et al. 1995).

The most prevalent skin disorders of instrumental *musicians*, particularly among string instrumentalists, include contact allergy to gum rosin. Several reviews on occupational diseases include this problem (Gambichler et al. 2004). It is well known that gum rosin is used by string players to wax the bow in order to increase the attrition between the bow and the strings. The use of rosin by percussionists to tighten their grip of the sticks is less well known and not discussed in the dermatological literature. It could be concluded that although a member of an orchestra does not use rosin himself, the air exposure caused by other members is significant. The use of rosin in ballet will increase the airborne exposure in the opera orchestra (Farm et al. 1995). It should be remembered that instrumental rosin could cause ACD not only in professional instrumentalists but also in musicians of all ages and ability (Gambichler et al. 2004).

Rosin in *soldering fluxes* for electronic assemblies is a well-known cause of ACD (Widstrom 1983; Liden 1984). As the allergens can be airborne, facial dermatitis is not uncommon in addition to hand eczema. In the late 1980s, the production of electronic equipment was moved from Europe to Asia and so did the reports on occupational problems (Koh et al. 2001). Chemical analysis of a soldering flux revealed a content of abietic acid corresponding to 20% gum rosin in the product (Ehrin and Karlberg 1990).

The content of rosin in *paper and paper products* has been investigated. It was found that so-called environmentally friendly paper of mechanical pulp from coniferous wood contains more components from unmodified rosin than paper based on chemical pulp (Ehrin and Karlberg 1990; Karlberg et al. 1995). As the extractive material containing the rosin components is not separated from the mechanical pulp, a higher response was seen to unprinted paper of mechanical pulps than to paper based on chemical pulps in persons with known contact allergy to gum rosin (Karlberg et al. 1995). When patch testing patients who suspected that their dermatitis was caused by contact with paper, only those with positive patch test reactions to gum rosin or maleopimaric acid reacted to the paper extracts (maleopimaric acid is the main component in maleated rosin used for paper size). The presence of rosin in paper can contribute to hand dermatitis in sensitized subjects, and the use of cotton gloves when in contact with paper might alleviate the dermatitis (Karlberg and Liden 1992). In a study on the prevalence of hand dermatitis and contact allergy in Sweden, it was found that rosin allergy was overrepresented among women in administrative work (Meding and Swanbeck 1990). However, this group showed a low prevalence of hand eczema. Cases of rosin allergy among workers in a paper mill are rare (Meding et al. 1993). Compared with office work the handling of paper in a paper mill is not as intensive as very little work is performed manually.

Metalworking machinists are exposed to diverse skin irritants and sensitizers. Rosin components in metalworking fluids are a common cause of ACD which has been reported throughout the years (Fregert 1979; Matos et al. 1988; Grattan et al. 1989). Recent publications demonstrate that rosin from metalworking fluids still causes contact allergy in the machinists using them (Geier et al. 2004; Suuronen et al. 2007). The source of rosin components in metalworking fluids originates mainly from distilled tall oil which contains typically10–30% tall oil rosin. Chemical analyses detect rosin components in the fluids in amounts high enough to demand a declaration of the content of rosin according to the EU legislation (see above). However, this is not the case (Ehrin and Karlberg 1990; Henricks-Eckerman et al. 2008).

9 Other Health Effects

The potential of rosin fumes to induce occupational asthma has been recognized since the 1970s and is primarily found in employees soldering conductive connections in the electrical or electronic industry. This work caused about 5% of all new cases of occupational asthma according to the UK Surveillance of Work-related Occupational Disease in 1994. The respiratory symptoms have been considered to be due to hypersensitivity. However, specific IgE antibodies were detected in serum from rosin-exposed workers with a likely diagnosis of occupational asthma (Elms et al. 2005).

References

Barbaud A, Collet E, Le Coz CJ et al (2009) Contact allergy in chronic leg ulcers: results of a multicentre study carried out in 423 patients and proposal for an updated series of patch tests. Contact Dermatitis 60:279–287

Bruynzeel DP, Diepgen TL, Andersen KE et al (2005) Monitoring the European standard series in 10 centres 1996–2000. Contact Dermatitis 53:146–149

Burry JN (1976) Contact dermatitis from radiata pine. Contact Dermatitis 2:262–263

Chowdhuri S, Ghosh S (2007) Epidemio-allergological study in 155 cases of footwear dermatitis. Indian J Dermatol Venereol Leprol 73:319–322

Christensson JB, Matura M, Backtorp C et al (2006) Hydroperoxides form specific antigens in contact allergy. Contact Dermatitis 55:230–237

Christensson JB, Johansson S, Hagvall L et al (2008) Limonene hydroperoxide analogues differ in allergenic activity. Contact Dermatitis 59:344–352

Council Directive 67/548/EEC (2004) Annex 1: index of dangerous substances for which harmonized classification and labelling have been agreed at community level, 29th adaption to technical progress. Off J Eur Union L: 152: 30/04/2004. Available from http://ecb.jrc.it/DOCUMENTS/Classification-Labelling/DIRECTIVE_67-548-EEC/ANNEX_1_OF_DIRECTIVE_67-548-EEC/Annex_I_of_Directive_67548EEC.doc

Daly BM, Stevenson CJ (1984) Contact dermatitis to wood wool. Contact Dermatitis 11:123

Directive 1999/45 EC (1999) Directive 1999/45 EC of the European Parliament and of the Council of 31 May 1999, concerning the approximation of the laws, regulations and administrative provisions of the Member States relating to the classification, packaging and labelling of preparations. Off J Eur Union L 200: 1–168

Dotterud LK, Smith-Sivertsen T (2007) Allergic contact sensitization in the general adult population: a population-based study from Northern Norway. Contact Dermatitis 56:10–15

Downs AM, Sansom JE (1999) Colophony allergy: a review. Contact Dermatitis 41:305–310

Ehrin E, Karlberg AT (1990) Detection of rosin (colophony) components in technical products using an HPLC technique. Contact Dermatitis 23:359–366

Elms J, Fishwick D, Robinson E et al (2005) Specific IgE to colophony? Occup Med (Lond) 55:234–237

Farm G (1996) Contact allergy to colophony and hand eczema. A follow-up study of patients with previously diagnosed contact allergy to colophony. Contact Dermatitis 34:93–100

Farm G (1997) Contact allergy to colophony. Clinical and experimental studies with emphasis on clinical relevance. Acta Derm Venereol Suppl (Stockh) 201:1–44

Farm G, Liden C, Karlberg AT (1994) A clinical and patch test study in a tall-oil rosin factory. Contact Dermatitis 31:102–107

Farm G, Karlberg AT, Liden C (1995) Are opera-house artistes afflicted with contact allergy to colophony and cosmetics? Contact Dermatitis 32:273–280

Fregert S (1979) Colophony in cutting oil and in soap water used as cutting fluid. Contact Dermatitis 5:52

Gafvert E (1994) Allergenic components in modified and unmodified rosin. Chemical characterization and studies of allergenic activity. Acta Derm Venereol Suppl (Stockh) 184:1–36

Gafvert E, Farm G (1995) Rosin (colophony) and zinc oxide in adhesive bandages. An appropriate combination for rosin-sensitive patients? Contact Dermatitis 33:396–400

Gafvert E, Nilsson U, Karlberg AT et al (1992) Rosin allergy: identification of a dehydroabietic acid peroxide with allergenic properties. Arch Dermatol Res 284:409–413

Gafvert E, Shao LP, Karlberg AT et al (1994a) Allergenicity of rosin (colophony) esters (II). Glyceryl monoabietate identified as contact allergen. Contact Dermatitis 31:11–17

Gafvert E, Shao LP, Karlberg AT et al (1994b) Contact allergy to resin acid hydroperoxides. Hapten binding via free radicals and epoxides. Chem Res Toxicol 7:260–266

Gafvert E, Shao LP, Karlberg AT et al (1995) Maleopimaric acid – a contact allergen in rosin modified with fumaric acid. Nordic Pulp Paper Res 10:139–144

Gafvert E, Bordalo O, Karlberg AT (1996) Patch testing with allergens from modified rosin (colophony) discloses additional cases of contact allergy. Contact Dermatitis 35:290–298

Gambichler T, Boms S, Freitag M (2004) Contact dermatitis and other skin conditions in instrumental musicians. BMC Dermatol 4:3

Geier J, Lessmann H, Schnuch A et al (2004) Contact sensitizations in metalworkers with occupational dermatitis exposed to water-based metalworking fluids: results of the research project "FaSt". Int Arch Occup Environ Health 77:543–551

Goossens A, Armingaud P, Avenel-Audran M et al (2002) An epidemic of allergic contact dermatitis due to epilating products. Contact Dermatitis 47:67–70

Grattan CE, English JS, Foulds IS et al (1989) Cutting fluid dermatitis. Contact Dermatitis 20:372–376

Hausen BM, Hessling C (1990) Contact allergy due to colophony (VI). The sensitizing capacity of minor resin acids and 7 commercial modified-colophony products. Contact Dermatitis 23:90–95

Hausen BM, Loll M (1993) Contact allergy due to colophony (VIII). The sensitizing potency of commercial products: an investigation of French and German modified-colophony derivatives. Contact Dermatitis 29:189–191

Hausen BM, Mohnert J (1989) Contact allergy due to colophony. (V). Patch test results with different types of colophony and modified-colophony products. Contact Dermatitis 20:295–301

Hausen BM, Krohn K, Budianto E (1990) Contact allergy due to colophony (VII). Sensitizing studies with oxidation products of abietic and related acids. Contact Dermatitis 23:352–358

Helm TN, Taylor JS, Adams RM et al (1993) Skin problems of performing artists. Am J Contact Dermat 4:27–32

Henricks-Eckerman M-L, Suuronen K, Jolanki R (2008) Analysis of allergens in metalworking fluids. Contact Dermatitis 59:261–267

Hjorth N (1961) Eczematous allergy to balsams allied perfumes and flavouring agents. Munksgaard, Copenhagen

Holmbom B, Avela E, Pekkala S (1974) Capillary gas chromatography–mass spectrometry of resin acids in tall oil rosin. J Am Oil Chem Soc 51:397–400

Illing HP, Malmfors T, Rodenburg L (2009) Skin sensitization and possible groupings for "read across" for rosin based substances. Regul Toxicol Pharmacol 54:234–241

Kanerva L, Rintala H, Henriks-Eckerman K et al (2001) Colophonium in sanitary pads. Contact Dermatitis 44:59–60

Karlberg AT (1988) Contact allergy to colophony. Chemical identifications of allergens, sensitization experiments and clinical experiences. Acta Derm Venereol Suppl (Stockh) 139:1–43

Karlberg AT (1991) Air oxidation increases the allergenic potential of tall oil rosin. Gum rosin contact allergens also identified in tall oil rosin. Am J Contact Dermat 2:43–49

Karlberg AT, Dooms-Goossens A (1997) Contact allergy to oxidized d-limonene among dermatitis patients. Contact Dermatitis 36:201–206

Karlberg AT, Gafvert E (1996) Isolated colophony allergens as screening substances for contact allergy. Contact Dermatitis 35:201–207

Karlberg AT, Liden C (1985) Clinical experience and patch testing using colophony (rosin) from different sources. Br J Dermatol 113:475–481

Karlberg AT, Liden C (1988) Comparison of colophony patch test preparations. Contact Dermatitis 18:158–165

Karlberg AT, Liden C (1992) Colophony (rosin) in newspapers may contribute to hand eczema. Br J Dermatol 126:161–165

Karlberg AT, Magnusson K (1996) Rosin components identified in diapers. Contact Dermatitis 34:176–180

Karlberg AT, Boman A, Holmbom B et al (1986) Contact allergy to acid and neutral fractions of rosins. Sensitization experiments in guinea pigs and patch testing in patients. Derm Beruf Umwelt 34:31–36

Karlberg AT, Bohlinder K, Boman A et al (1988a) Identification of 15-hydroperoxyabietic acid as a contact allergen in Portuguese colophony. J Pharm Pharmacol 40:42–47

Karlberg AT, Boman A, Hacksell U et al (1988b) Contact allergy to dehydroabietic acid derivatives isolated from Portuguese colophony. Contact Dermatitis 19:166–174

Karlberg AT, Boman A, Nilsson JL (1988c) Hydrogenation reduces the allergenicity of colophony (rosin). Contact Dermatitis 19:22–29

Karlberg AT, Gafvert E, Hagelthorn G et al (1990) Maleopimaric acid–a potent sensitizer in modified rosin. Contact Dermatitis 22:193–201

Karlberg AT, Gafvert E, Liden C (1995) Environmentally friendly paper may increase risk of hand eczema in rosin-sensitive persons. J Am Acad Dermatol 33:427–432

Karlberg AT, Brared-Christensson J, Borje A et al (2007) Methyl esterification of 15-hydroperoxyabietic acid does not affect the patch-test result in colophonium allergic patients. Contact Dermatitis 56:355–356

Khan L, Saeed MA (1994) 13beta,14beta-dihydroxy-13alpha-isopropylabietic acid, an elicitor of contact allergy. J Pharm Sci 83:909–910

Koh D, Lee BL, Ong HY et al (1995) Colophony in bindi adhesive. Contact Dermatitis 32:186

Koh D, Leow YH, Goh CL (2001) Occupational allergic contact dermatits in Singapore. Sci Total Environ 270:97–101

Liden C (1984) Patch testing with soldering fluxes. Contact Dermatitis 10:119–120

Lindberg M, Edman B, Fischer T et al (2007) Time trends in Swedish patch test data from 1992 to 2000. A multi-centre study based on age- and sex-adjusted results of the Swedish standard series. Contact Dermatitis 56:205–210

Lyon CC, Tucker SC, Gafvert E et al (1999) Contact dermatitis from modified rosin in footwear. Contact Dermatitis 41:102–103

Matos J, Mariano A, Goncalo S et al (1988) Occupational dermatitis from colophony. Contact Dermatitis 18:53–54

Matura M, Goossens A, Bordalo O et al (2003) Patch testing with oxidized R-(+)-limonene and its hydroperoxide fraction. Contact Dermatitis 49:15–21

Matura M, Skold M, Borje A et al (2005) Selected oxidized fragrance terpenes are common contact allergens. Contact Dermatitis 52:320–328

Meding B, Swanbeck G (1990) Predictive factors for hand eczema. Contact Dermatitis 23:154–161

Meding B, Toren K, Karlberg AT et al (1993) Evaluation of skin symptoms among workers at a Swedish paper mill. Am J Ind Med 23:721–728

Meding B, Ahman M, Karlberg AT (1996) Skin symptoms and contact allergy in woodwork teachers. Contact Dermatitis 34:185–190

Nielsen NH, Menne T (1992) Allergic contact sensitization in an unselected Danish population. The Glostrup Allergy Study, Denmark. Acta Derm Venereol 72:456–460

Nilsson U, Berglund N, Lindahl F et al (2008) SPE and HPLC/UV of resin acids in colophonium-containing products. J Sep Sci 31:2784–2790

Nilsson U, Karlberg AT, Lassen P (2009) Development of an analysis method for quantification of colophonium components in cosmetic products. Danish Ministry of the Environment, Environmental Protection Agency, Denmark

Pereira TM, Flour M, Goossens A (2007) Allergic contact dermatitis from modified colophonium in wound dressings. Contact Dermatitis 56:5–9

Sadhra S, Foulds IS (1995) Allergic potential of neutrals in unmodified colophony, and a method for their separation from resin acids. Br J Dermatol 132:69–73

Sadhra S, Foulds IS, Gray CN (1996) Identification of contact allergens in unmodified rosin using a combination of patch testing and analytical chemistry techniques. Br J Dermatol 134:662–668

Sadhra S, Foulds IS, Gray CN (1998) Oxidation of resin acids in colophony (rosin) and its implications for patch testing. Contact Dermatitis 39:58–63

Salim A, Shaw S (2001) Recommendation to include ester gum resin when patch testing patients with leg ulcers. Contact Dermatitis 44:34

Schafer T, Bohler E, Ruhdorfer S et al (2001) Epidemiology of contact allergy in adults. Allergy 56:1192–1196

Scherrer M, Junqueira AF (2010) Allergic contact dermatitis to natural resin rare among gum rosin extractors? Contact Dermatitis 62:64–65

Schnuch A, Uter W, Geier J et al (2002) Epidemiology of contact allergy: an estimation of morbidity employing the clinical epidemiology and drug-utilization research (CE-DUR) approach. Contact Dermatitis 47:32–39

Shao LP, Gafvert E, Karlberg AT et al (1993) The allergenicity of glycerol esters and other esters of rosin (colophony). Contact Dermatitis 28:229–234

Shao LP, Gafvert E, Nilsson U et al (1995) 15-hydroperoxydehydroabietic acid–a contact allergen in colophony from pinus species. Phytochemistry 38:853–857

Sharma PR (2006) Allergic contact stomatitis from colophony. Dent Update 33:440–442

Soltes EJ, Zinkel DF (1989) Chemistry of rosin. In: Zinkel DF, Russel J (eds) Naval stores. Production-chemistry-utilization. Pulp Chemicals Association, New York, pp 261–345

Suuronen K, Aalto-Korte K, Piipari R et al (2007) Occupational dermatitis and allergic respiratory diseases in Finnish metalworking machinists. Occup Med (Lond) 57:277–283

Thyssen JP, Linneberg A, Menne T et al (2007) The epidemiology of contact allergy in the general population–prevalence and main findings. Contact Dermatitis 57:287–299

Turner JM (2010) 2008 international yearbook. Forest Chemicals Review. Kriedt Enterprises, New Orleans, LA:7

Uter W, Geier J, Frosch P et al (2010) Contact allergy to fragrances: current patch test results (2005–2008) from the Information Network of Departments of Dermatology(*). Contact Dermatitis 63: 254–261

Watsky KL (1997) Airborne allergic contact dermatitis from pine dust. Am J Contact Dermat 8:118–120

Widstrom L (1983) Contact allergy to colophony in soldering flux. Contact Dermatitis 9:205–207

Zinkel DF (1975) Chemicals from tree. Chem Technol 4:235–241

42 Industrial Enzymes

David A. Basketter
DABMEB Consultancy Ltd, Sharnbrook, Bedfordshire, UK

Core Messages

- A wide range of enzymes is used in many industrial environments.
- The primary risk that they present to human health is sensitization of the respiratory tract.
- Proteolytic enzymes can give risk to skin irritation.
- All enzymes have the potential to cause immunologic contact urticaria, although this is not common.

1 Introduction

Industrial enzymes are in widespread use, but the major focus for many years has been proteolytic enzymes deployed in fabric washing products (e.g., Peters et al. 2001). These enzymes are very largely of bacterial or fungal origin and are thus foreign to the human immune system. As a consequence, they should all be assumed to be potential respiratory allergens. This property translated into a fairly dramatic outbreak of occupational asthma when proteolytic enzymes were first introduced into detergents (Flindt 1969; Pepys et al. 1969; Schweigert et al. 2000). However, even in this situation, immunologic contact urticaria was not reported, only a limited degree of irritant contact dermatitis (Zachariae et al. 1973). Since then a number of reports of occupational contact urticaria have arisen, but it remains uncommon, perhaps because the often very strict exposure limits related to respiratory sensitization risk tend to ensure that skin contact is also very low.

2 Regulatory Classification of Enzymes

Although it is likely that not all enzymes have been reviewed by regulatory authorities, all those that have in Europe have been judged to be respiratory sensitizers and thus have the annotation "R42: May cause sensitization by inhalation", and such wording must therefore appear on the safety data sheet. Under the new GHS regulations, it should also be indicated by the following symbol:

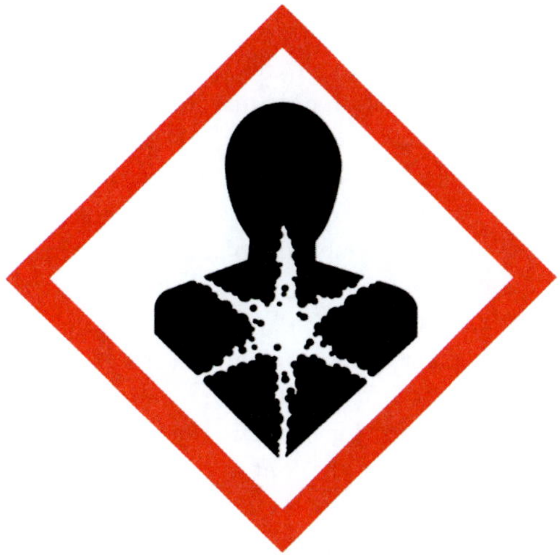

In addition, proteolytic enzymes are likely to be irritant to skin and will be labeled "Causes (mild) skin irritation" and show the following symbol:

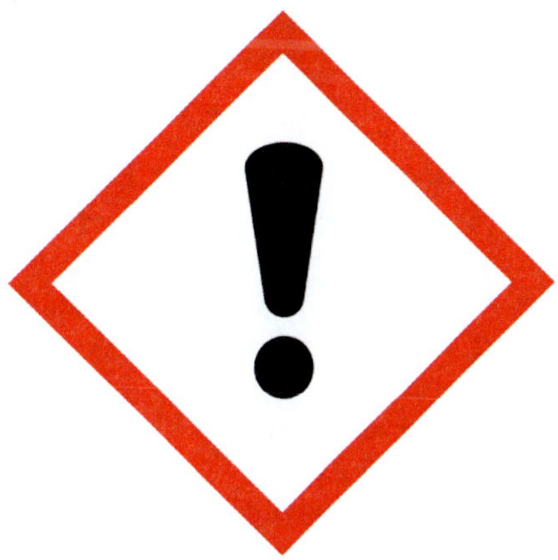

No other hazard classification relevant to skin effects is normally applied to enzymes. In theory, enzymes could be classified as "R43: May cause sensitization by skin contact" if they were to show a sufficient propensity to cause immunologic contact urticaria to a significant extent, but the clinical evidence for this is so sparse (see below) that such an action would not be merited.

T. Rustemeyer, P. Elsner, S.M. John & H.I. Maibach (eds.), *Kanerva's Occupational Dermatology*,
DOI 10.1007/978-3-642-02035-3_42, © Springer-Verlag Berlin Heidelberg 2012

3 Predictive Assays for Enzyme Hazards

Since this is handbook on occupational dermatitis, it is not appropriate to go into details of predictive tests for respiratory sensitization. However, it is worth mentioning that for skin irritation, the traditional toxicology test involved 4 h semi-occluded application of undiluted test material to the shaved skin of three rabbits (Draize et al. 1944). It is well recognized that this is a poor predictor of acute skin irritation potential (Basketter et al. 2004; Jirova et al. 2010) and of course it clearly provides no more than a minimal insight concerning the cumulative irritant potential of a substance. What is evident from testing of enzymes diluted to product and to in use concentrations is that at these exposure levels skin irritation is essentially undetectable (reviewed in Basketter et al. 2009).

However, a key question concerns the possibility of skin-sensitizing activity of enzymes! The experience to date is that all bacterial and fungal enzymes presented to mice and guinea pigs in the context of standard predictive assays for skin sensitization (OECD 1992, 2002) lead to positive results. However, there is no evidence that delayed hypersensitivity reactions occur in human subjects, either under experimental, occupational, or consumer exposure conditions and thus the positive predictive test data from animal models is rightly regarded as an irrelevant consequence of a normal immune reaction to a foreign protein (HERA 2009a, 2009b; Basketter et al. 2009).

4 Immunologic Contact Urticaria

Exposure to enzyme proteins which can generate an IgE antibody response can, in theory, also produce immunologic contact urticaria. After all, this is the basis of the skin prick test for diagnosis of IgE allergy, with the cutaneous weal and flare representing the urticarial response to local mast cell degranulation (Pepys 1972). However, it is well known that proteins struggle to pass the skin barrier, hence the "prick" (Pease et al. 2003). Nevertheless, where the skin barrier is compromised, the proteins, including enzymes, can cause an immunologically mediated dermatitis and this was first identified a quarter of a century ago as "protein contact dermatitis" (Hjorth and Roed-Petersen 1976). The whole subject of contact urticaria/protein contact dermatitis is reviewed in standard textbooks of contact dermatitis (Amin et al. 2008a, b; Levin and Warshaw 2008; Basketter et al. 2010) and there is a recent specific review of immunologic contact urticaria to proteins (Amaro and Goossens 2008). This last mentioned reference notes that there is some suggestion of a delayed (Type IV) hypersensitivity component to protein contact dermatitis (since it is eczematous rather than urticarial), but that this is uncertain and diagnostic testing is best focused on the presence of specific IgE.

A range of enzymes have been reported in the literature as a cause of immunologic contact urticaria and/or protein contact dermatitis. These are summarized with references in *Table 42.1.*

Diagnostic testing for possible immunologic contact urticaria is well covered elsewhere (Amin et al. 2008b). In principle, a skin prick test or an assay for serum IgE such as the radioallergosorbent test (RAST) will give a fairly reliable indication of whether an individual has become sensitized to a particular enzyme, but caution must be exercised. The presence of sensitization does not mean that urticaria and dermatitis must follow. Consider the detergent enzyme industry. Despite stringent exposure controls, such that airborne enzyme is in the very low ng/m^s region, there is still a more than 10% prevalence of sensitization (Nicholson et al. 2001; Sarlo 2003; Basketter et al. 2010). Where factories have not been in control, this level is even higher, such that asthma symptoms begin to appear (Cullinan et al. 2000). However, occupational skin disease due to enzymes in these factory situations is almost unknown. So, the presence of IgE will be a requirement for immunologic contact urticaria but it is probably far from an inevitable consequence. Keep in mind too that skin prick testing with proteolytic enzymes in particular carries an additional risk of false positives, so careful use of controls is necessary (Simesen et al. 1976).

Table 42.1
Enzymes reported to cause immunologic contact urticaria

Enzyme type	References
α-Amylase	Tarvainen et al. (1991); Morren et al. (1993); Wuthrich (1996); Kanerva et al. (1997); Medeiros et al. (2006)
Cellulase	Kanerva and Tarvainen (1990); Kanerva et al. (1998)
Glucoamylase	Kanerva and Vanhanen (1999)
Lactase	Laukkanen et al. (2007)
Papain	Soto-Mera et al. (2000)
Protease	Kanerva and Vanhanen (2001)
Xylanase	Kanerva and Tarvainen (1990)

5 Skin Irritation

There is little to say about this endpoint. Historically, proteolytic enzymes have been reported to cause an occupational irritant contact dermatitis (Zachariae et al. 1973), but this occurred under exceptional conditions of exposure where over half the workforce became sensitized and a substantial minority, perhaps one third, experience bronchoconstriction and/or asthma. At this time, protein contact dermatitis was not recognized as an entity and it must be possible that no differential diagnosis was undertaken, such that the true cause of the skin reactions seen at that time may carry some element of uncertainty concerning the mechanism. However, the proteolytic enzyme was responsible and the skin reactions disappeared as airborne exposure was controlled to eliminate the other clinical symptoms of respiratory sensitization. The diagnosis of irritancy due to proteolytic enzymes remains one of exclusion.

6 Summary

Enzymes are a potential cause of immunologic contact urticaria and, at least for proteolytic enzymes, also of skin irritation. The extent to which either of these types of skin reaction occurs is likely to be extremely low where airborne exposure is properly controlled to minimize the risk of respiratory sensitization. Higher concentration contact, particularly on damaged skin is more likely to produce immunologic contact urticaria/protein contact dermatitis. At very high exposure levels, proteolytic enzymes may well give rise to some degree of skin irritation.

References

Amaro C, Goossens A (2008) Immunological occupational contact urticaria and contact dermatitis from proteins: a review. Contact Dermatitis 58:67–75

Amin S, Lahti A, Maibach HI (2008a) Contact urticaria and Contact urticaria syndrome (immediate contact reactions). In: Zhai H, Wilhelm K-P, Maibach HI (eds) Dermatotoxicology, 7th edn. CRC Press, Boca Raton, pp 525–536

Amin S, Lauerma A, Maibach HI (2008b) Diagnostic tests in dermatology: patch and photopatch testing and contact urticaria. In: Zhai H, Wilhelm K-P, Maibach HI (eds) Dermatotoxicology, 7th edn. CRC Press, Boca Raton, pp 581–586

Basketter DA, Broekhuizen C, Fieldsend M et al (2010) Defining occupational and consumer exposure limits for enzyme protein respiratory allergens under REACH. Toxicol 268:165–170

Basketter DA, English J, Wakelin S et al (2008) Enzymes, detergents and skin: facts and fantasies. Br J Dermatol 158:1177–1181

Basketter DA, York M, McFadden JP et al (2004) Determination of skin irritation potential in the human 4-h patch test. Contact Dermatitis 51:1–4

Commission of the European Communities. Regulation (2006) (EC) No 1907/2006 of the European Parliament and of the Council of 18 December 2006 concerning the Registration, Evaluation, Authorisation and Restriction of Chemicals (REACH), establishing a European Chemicals Agency, amending Directive 1999/45/EC and repealing Council Regulation (EEC) No 793/93 and Commission Regulation (EC) No 1488/94 as well as Council Directive 76/769/EEC and Commission Directives 91/155/EEC, 93/67/EEC,93/105/EC and 2000/21/EC. Off. J. Eur. Union, L 396/1 of 30.12.2006. (http://europa.eu.int/comm/enterprise/reach/index_en.htm)

Cullinan P, Harris JM, Newman Taylor AJ et al (2000) An outbreak of asthma in a modern detergent factory. Lancet 356:1899–1900

Draize JH, Woodard G, Calvery HO (1944) Methods for the study of imitation and toxicity of substances applied topically to the skin and mucous membranes. J Pharmacol Exp Ther 82:377–390

ECHA (2008) Guidance on information requirements and chemical safety assessment. Chapter R.7a: endpoint specific guidance. European Chemicals Agency, Helsinki, pp 256–288

Flindt ML (1969) Pulmonary disease due to inhalation of derivatives of Bacillus subtilis containing proteolytic enzyme. Lancet 1: 1177–1181

HERA. Human and Environmental Risk Assessment 2005 α-Amylases, Cellulases and Lipases, 1st edn. http://www.heraproject.com/files/38-F-Hera_Bridging_document_28.10.05.pdf. Accessed 9 June 2009

HERA. Human and Environmental Risk Assessment 2007 Subtilisins, 2nd edn. http://www.heraproject.com/files/22-F-07_PROTEASE_-HERA_Final%20Edition%20(unsecured%20-%20PDFA-1b).pdf. Accessed 9 June 2009

Hjorth N, Roed-Petersen J (1976) Occupational protein contact dermatitis in food handlers. Contact Dermatitis 2:28–42

Jirova D, Basketter D, Liebsch M et al (2010) Comparison of human skin irritation patch test data with in vitro skin irritation assays and animal data. Contact Dermatitis 62:109–116

Kanerva L, Tarvainen K (1990) Allergic contact dermatitis and contact urticaria from cellulolytic enzymes. Am J Contact Dermat 1:244–245

Kanerva L, Vanhanen M (1999) Occupational protein contact dermatitis from glucoamylase. Contact Dermatitis 41:171–173

Kanerva L, Vanhanen M (2001) Occupational allergic contact urticaria and rhinoconjunctivitis from a detergent protease. Contact Dermatitis 45:49–51

Kanerva L, Vanhanen M, Tupasela O (1997) Occupational allergic contact urticaria from fungal but not bacterial alpha-amylase. Contact Dermatitis 36:306–307

Kanerva L, Vanhanen M, Tupasela O (1998) Occupational contact urticaria from cellulase enzyme. Contact Dermatitis 38:176–177

Laukkanen A, Ruoppi P, Semes S (2007) Lactase-induced occupational protein contact dermatitis and allergic rhinoconjunctivitis. Contact Dermatitis 57:89–93

Levin C, Warshaw E (2008) Protein contact dermatitis: allergens, pathogenesis and management. Dermatitis 19:241–251

Medeiros S, Alves R, Santo R et al (2006) Bakers eczema and occupational asthma. Contact Dermatitis 55:49

Morren M, Janssens V, Doom-Goossens A et al (1993) α-Amylase, a flour additive: an important cause of protein contact dermatitis in bakers. J Am Acad Dermatol 29:723–728

Nicholson PJ, Newman-Taylor AJ, Oliver P et al (2001) Current best practice for the health surveillance of enzyme workers in the soap and detergent industry. Occup Med (Lond) 51:81–92

OECD (1992) Organisation for Economic Cooperation and Development. Guidelines for testing of chemicals no 406. Skin sensitization. Organisation for Economic Cooperation and Development, paris

OECD (2002) Organisation for Economic Cooperation and Development. Test guideline 429: the local lymph node assay. OECD, Paris

Pepys J (1972) Laboratory methods in clinical allergy – skin tests for immediate, type I, allergic reactions. Proc R Soc Med 65:271–272

Pepys J, Longbottom JL, Hargreave FE et al (1969) Allergic reactions of the lungs to enzymes of Bacillus subtilis. Lancet 1:1181–1184

Peters G, Johnson GQ, Golembiewski A (2001) Safe use of detergent enzymes in the workplace. Appl Occup Environ Hyg 16:389–396

Sarlo K (2003) Control of occupational asthma and allergy in the detergent industry. Ann Allergy Asthma Immunol 90:32–34

Schweigert MK, Mackenzie DP, Sarlo K (2000) Occupational asthma and allergy associated with the use of enzymes in the detergent industry – a review of the epidemiology, toxicology and methods of prevention. Clin Exp Allergy 30:1511–1518

Simesen B, Wide L, Zachariae H (1976) Prick and radioallergosorbent tests (RAST) to Alcalase in a population not exposed to enzyme detergents. Acta Allergol 31:71–77

Smith Pease CK, White IR, Basketter DA (2002) Skin as a route of exposure to protein allergens. Clin Exp Dermatol 27:296–300

Soto-Mera MT, Lopez-Rico MR, Filgueira JF et al (2000) Occupational allergy to papain. Allergy 55:983–984

Tarvainen K, Kanerva L, Tupasela O et al (1991) Allergy from cellulase and xylanase enzymes. Clin Exp Allergy 21:609–615

United Nations (2009) Globally harmonized system of classification and labelling of chemicals (GHS). Part 3: health hazards. http://www.unece.org/trans/danger/publi/ghs/ghs_rev03/English/03e_part3.pdf

Wuthrich B (1996) Protein contact dermatitis. Br J Dermatol 135: 332–333

Zachariae H, Thomsen K, Rasmussen OG (1973) Occupational enzyme dermatitis. Results of patch testing with Alcalase. Acta Derm Venereol 53:145–148

43 Nickel

Carola Lidén
Institute of Environmental Medicine, Karolinska Institutet, Stockholm, Sweden

Core Messages

- Nickel is the most frequent cause of contact allergy, affecting up to 17% of women and 3% of men. Certain occupational groups are much more affected.
- Hand eczema is reported by 30–40% of nickel-allergic persons. Occupational exposure to nickel is an important risk factor for hand eczema.
- Occupational nickel dermatitis usually presents as hand eczema. Exposure reduction is essential for the prognosis.
- Pure nickel metal, nickel-containing alloys, coatings, and compounds have different ability to release nickel ions at skin contact, and to cause sensitization and dermatitis.
- The dimethylglyoxime test for nickel ions is very useful in assessment of nickel exposure and exposure reduction in the workplace and elsewhere.
- Skin exposure to nickel can now be quantified. Knowledge on exposure levels in different occupations and in patients will contribute to improved risk assessment and prevention.
- Nickel release from certain consumer items in contact with the skin is limited by the EU Nickel Directive. Regulation of occupational exposure should also be considered.

1 Introduction

Nickel allergy is the most frequent contact allergy in the industrialized world and an important cause of hand eczema. Nickel allergy predominantly affects young girls and women sensitized by jewelry and other personal items. A hundred years ago, however, nickel dermatitis was an occupational disease affecting men. Occupational exposure to this metal is still of great importance for sensitization and elicitation, and for maintaining hand eczema.

2 Prevalence, Use, and Properties

2.1 In Nature and Production

Nickel is present in the earth's crust, occurs naturally in drinking water and in food, and is probably an essential nutrient for humans. Health problems are however not caused primarily by the nickel in the natural environment but are related to industrial activity and manufactured items. Nickel (Ni) is a transitional metal with the atomic number 28. Ni (0) in metal nickel and its alloys, and Ni (II) in nickel salts and stable inorganic compounds, are the most prevalent oxidation states. Numerous nickel salts and sulfides with different properties and uses are known. Nickel ions are formed when metallic nickel is in contact with, e.g., sweat.

Nickel is today the fourth most-used metal after iron, chromium, and lead. During the nineteenth century, white nickel-containing alloys were produced in Europe as substitutes for silver, and around 1870, the use of nickel in steels and platings started. Nickel production has increased considerably since 1940, and today, two thirds the production is used in stainless steels. Nickel is used in numerous alloys and coatings and in chemical compounds. It is also found in products for occupational and private use, many of which may come into contact with the skin (Sunderman 1989; Grandjean et al. 1989; Flint 1998; Lidén et al. 1995, 2011).

2.2 Plating, Alloys, and Corrosion

Metallurgical aspects of nickel and the corrosion of nickel-containing materials in contact with sweat have been reviewed (Flint 1998), and some of the most relevant information is summarized below.

Skin contact with *homogeneous nickel*, other than with some coins, is not common. Many items that are *electroplated* with nickel come into contact with skin. Bright nickel plate contains sulfur which facilitates the release of nickel ions. Nickel plate is often covered with a *top coat* of, e.g., chromium, silver, gold, tin/nickel, or different lacquers which, although reducing formation of nickel ions, may not be adequate to prevent contact dermatitis. Top coats often have pores or cracks, and they are subject to wear. Nickel used as an *interliner* under plating of gold, silver, or chromium causes dermatitis (Lidén et al. 1996).

A broad spectrum of nickel-containing *alloys* is produced. Common examples are stainless steels (iron/nickel/chromium), copper/nickel and nickel–silver (nickel/copper/zinc). Brass (copper/zinc) and red gold

T. Rustemeyer, P. Elsner, S.M. John & H.I. Maibach (eds.), *Kanerva's Occupational Dermatology*,
DOI 10.1007/978-3-642-02035-3_43, © Springer-Verlag Berlin Heidelberg 2012

(gold/silver/copper) are examples of nickel-free alloys. Alloys are compounds or solid solutions of more than one element in metallic form but cannot be considered as mixtures of the metals. Resistance to *corrosion on skin contact* varies widely between different nickel-containing alloys depending on their composition.

Nickel-containing alloys may be placed, regarding their behavior when in *contact with sweat*, in different categories reflecting their probability of causing contact allergy (Flint 1998). Many stainless steels are unlikely to cause allergic contact dermatitis. Sulfur-rich stainless steels, however, may react with sweat, causing contact dermatitis (Haudrechy et al. 1994, 1997). Copper/nickel and nickel–silver (nickel/copper/zinc) are examples of nickel-containing alloys with very high rate of nickel release in sweat (Lidén and Carter 2001; Lidén et al. 2008b).

There is no relationship between the content of nickel in an alloy and its ability to cause an allergic reaction, while there is a close relationship between the rate at which ions form from nickel in contact with sweat and the potential to cause a reaction. This fact may be difficult to understand and has caused demands for "nickel-free" items instead of the generally more relevant demand for "low nickel release."

3 Health Effects

3.1 Toxicology

The major health effect of nickel and its compounds is contact allergy and allergic contact dermatitis as a result of skin exposure to nickel ions, Ni (II). Inhalation exposure to soluble nickel and nickel oxides/sulfides has caused nasal and pulmonary cancer in workers in nickel refineries. Exposure to nickel or nickel compounds via routes other than inhalation has not been shown to increase the cancer risk in humans. The overall evaluation by IARC is that some nickel compounds are carcinogenic to humans (Group 1), and metallic nickel is possibly carcinogenic to humans (Group 2B) (World Health Organization IARC 1997). Inhalation of nickel compounds may induce asthma. Nickel-induced asthma, however, is rare.

3.2 Sensitizing Capacity and Cross-Reactivity in Animals

Nickel sulfate is a moderate or weak sensitizer, according to predictive studies in guinea pigs and in mice (Wahlberg 1989; Basketter et al. 1994). To better understand the simultaneous patch-test reactivity and possible cross-reactivity often recorded in humans (to nickel sulfate–cobalt chloride, to nickel sulfate–potassium dichromate, and to nickel sulfate–palladium chloride, respectively), a series of cross-challenge experiments have been carried out in guinea pigs (Wahlberg and Boman 1992; Lidén and Wahlberg 1994; Lidén et al. 1995). It appears that the reactivity to nickel sulfate–palladium chloride is due to cross-reactivity, while cross-reactivity is not probable for nickel sulfate–cobalt chloride and nickel sulfate–potassium dichromate.

3.3 Sensitization and Prevalence of Allergy

Sensitization to nickel is caused by soluble nickel deposited onto the skin, often by direct, prolonged, or repeated skin contact with items that release nickel ions. The causes of primary sensitization vary depending on fashion and other factors which influence exposure. Suspenders for stockings and jeans buttons have previously been frequent sensitizers. Today, cheap jewelry and piercing are often focused, but nickel allergy is also common among people without piercings. Precious-metal jewelry, watches, spectacle frames, buckets, zips, etc., are other important causes of sensitization and elicitation of dermatitis. The role of occupational exposure in sensitization and elicitation of nickel dermatitis is discussed below.

The prevalence of nickel allergy varies between genders, age groups, countries, and over time (Lidén et al. 2011). Epidemiological studies by patch testing of the *general population* in Europe and North America have shown that up to 17% of women and 3% of men are allergic to nickel and that nickel allergy has increased significantly between the 1960s and the 1990s (Thyssen et al. 2007). Examples are given in ➋ *Table 43.1*. Nickel allergy has generally been more frequent in younger women compared to older women. A decrease in nickel allergy is now being indicated among women in Denmark, in both the population and among patients, which probably is an effect of the EU Nickel Directive and the preceding Danish regulation limiting nickel release from certain items (see below) (Johansen et al. 2000). The prevalence of nickel allergy in patch-tested *dermatitis patients* varies widely. A selection of publications from different parts of the world and different time is listed in ➋ *Table 43.1* showing figures of 10–30% in female patients and 2–8% in male patients.

Table 43.1

Prevalence of nickel allergy in the general population and in dermatitis patients, some examples to illustrate differences over time and between countries

Study population	Nickel allergy Men (%)	Women (%)	References
General population, Finland (n = 980)	0.8	8.0	Peltonen 1979
General population, Germany (n = 1,141)	5.8	20.4	Schäfer et al. 2001
Schoolchildren, Denmark (n = 1,146)	2.5	13.7	Mortz et al. 2002
General population, Thailand (n = 1,397)	3.9	33.8	White et al. 2007
General population, Denmark (n = 3,460)	1.0	9.9	Thyssen et al. 2009
Dermatitis patients, Europe (n = 4,825)	1.8	10.2	Fregert et al. 1969
Dermatitis patients, Germany (n = 36,720)	4.8	18.3	Schnuch et al. 1997
Dermatitis patients, Sweden (n = 3,790)	7.4	24.2	Lindberg et al. 2007
Dermatitis patients, North America (n = 4,425)	Total:	19.0[a]	Zug et al. 2009
Dermatitis patients, Lithuania (n = 816)	4.0	24.1	Beliauskiene et al. 2011

[a]Results not divided by gender

3.4 Hand Eczema

Nickel-sensitive people run a considerably increased risk of developing hand eczema (Lidén et al. 2011). Approximately 30–40% of nickel-sensitive persons report that they ever have experienced hand eczema, versus approximately 15–20% among non-nickel-sensitive controls (Menné 1978; Peltonen 1979; Menné et al. 1982; Meding et al. 2001). Figures from dermatology departments on hand eczema in nickel-sensitive patients vary between 20% and 60%. The relationship between nickel allergy, hand eczema, and atopic dermatitis has been extensively reviewed (Wilkinson and Wilkinson 1989).

Most people, in daily life and in many jobs, have repeated contact with handles, keys, coins, scissors, tools, and other items that may release nickel. Wet work and other irritant factors impair the skin barrier function and facilitate the penetration of nickel and other allergens into the skin. These factors contribute to the development of hand eczema. Dietary intake of nickel has by some authors been proposed to be of significant importance for hand eczema, but this issue is controversial.

4 Exposure Assessment

4.1 The Dimethylglyoxime Test

The dimethylglyoxime (DMG) test is a simple spot test for nickel (Feigl 1972). The test is based on DMG (0.8–1% in alcohol) and ammonia (10%). A cotton-wool-tipped stick with 1–2 drops of each solution is rubbed for up to 20 s against the surface to be tested. A pink-red color indicates presence of nickel ions. In many countries, the DMG test is commercially available, and alternative preparations exist. The DMG test has been validated against nickel release in artificial sweat (see below). The specificity was high, but the sensitivity modest in the range of the limit values of the EU Nickel Directive (0.2 and 0.5 μg/cm^2/week) (Thyssen et al. 2010). A modified DMG test with increased sensitivity by pretreatment of the surface with artificial sweat and heat has been developed (European Committee for Standardization (CEN) 2002).

The DMG test is a very useful tool for screening purposes, but sometimes discoloration or false-negative results may occur. It is used by dermatologists, occupational hygienists, and occupational health services, and it is recommended to nickel-allergic patients for identification of nickel and exposure reduction. The DMG test has also been used in several surveys of nickel release from handheld tools and consumer items (Lidén et al. 1998; Lidén and Norberg 2005; Thyssen and Maibach 2008).

4.2 Nickel Release in Artificial Sweat

Nickel release may be quantitatively determined by immersing items in artificial sweat at 30°C for 1 week and analyzing nickel in the solution at the end of the period (European Committee for Standardization (CEN) 2011). Analysis may be carried out with atomic absorption spectrometry or with inductively coupled plasma detection (ICP). Nickel release of 0.2 and 0.5 μg/cm^2 and week, respectively, are the limits of the Nickel Directive (➋ *Table 43.2*). The CEN standard, EN 1811, was developed to meet the needs of controlling compliance with the EU Nickel Directive. By shorter duration of immersion in artificial sweat, it has been shown that some alloys release substantial amounts of nickel within minutes or hours

Table 43.2
Summary of the EU Nickel Directive and the reference test methods for control of compliance. The Nickel Directive was adopted in 1994, entered into force in 2000, was revised in 2005, and is from 2009 part of REACH, the EU chemicals regulation (European Committee for Standardization 1998, 2002, 2011; Lidén et al. 2011)

Part	Nickel may not be used	CEN standard
1.	In items inserted into pierced parts of the body (not only during epithelialization after piercing) if nickel release is greater than 0.2 μg/cm²/week	EN 1811 (nickel release in artificial sweat)
2.	In products intended to come into direct and prolonged contact with the skin, such as earrings, necklaces, wristwatch cases, watch straps, buttons, zips, and mobile phones, if nickel release is greater than 0.5 μg nickel/cm² per week	EN 1811 (nickel release in artificial sweat)
3.	In coated products in part 2, unless the coating is sufficient to ensure that the nickel release will not exceed 0.5 μg nickel/cm² per week after 2 years of normal use	EN 12472 (wear and corrosion test)

(Lidén and Carter 2001; Lidén et al. 2008b). This is important for understanding that also *brief and repeated skin contact* with coins, tools, and other items may result in sufficient nickel exposure to cause dermatitis, while the Nickel Directive covers items intended for direct and prolonged contact.

4.3 Skin Exposure Assessment

Increasing attention has been given development of methods for skin exposure assessment. Methods for sampling by different removal techniques (wipe sampling, rinsing, and tape stripping) have been developed and used in studies of occupational exposure to nickel (Lidén et al. 2011; Gruvberger et al. 2011).

Acid wipe sampling was developed for assessment of nickel, chromium, and cobalt deposited onto skin (Lidén et al. 2006). Sampling is performed by wiping demarked areas with dilute nitric acid (1%) before and after the work session for exposure, and analysis is performed with ICP-MS. The method has very high sampling efficiency and recovery

Table 43.3
Amount of nickel deposited on hands (index finger dominant hand) in 42 workers and six nickel dermatitis patients. Assessed by acid wipe sampling after 1–2 h of regular work. The amount deposited in 8 h was calculated

Group	Nickel deposited in 8 h, mean (μg/cm²)	References
Carpenters (*n* = 4)	0.7	Lidén et al. 2008a
Locksmiths (*n* = 3)	3.4	Lidén et al. 2008a
Cashiers (*n* = 7)	2.4	Lidén et al. 2008a
Secretaries (*n* = 4)	0.2	Lidén et al. 2008a
Metalworkers (*n* = 24)	3.2	Julander et al. 2010
Nickel-allergic patients with work-related hand eczema (*n* = 6)	0.5	Jensen et al. 2011

(>90%), and the mass per area unit (e.g., μg/cm²) may be calculated. Acid wipe sampling has been used to assess skin exposure to nickel in cashiers, locksmiths, carpenters, metals workers and secretaries, and in patients with nickel allergy and work-related hand eczema (Lidén et al. 2008a, b; Julander et al. 2010; Jensen et al. 2011). Substantial amounts of nickel are deposited onto the hands of these groups (Table 43.3).

Immersion of fingers in water for extraction and analysis of nickel has been used for assessment of exposure to nickel in some occupations (Staton et al. 2006). The recovery of the method has not been stated but is obviously much lower than with acid wipe sampling. *Tape stripping* has been used for studies of how nickel is adsorbed in the skin (Hostýnek et al. 2001). It has recently been shown that nickel on the skin surface can be visualized by the *DMG test* (Julander et al. 2011).

5 Occupational Exposure

Some of the most important jobs and exposures with risk of occupational contact dermatitis due to nickel, and probably primary sensitization, are described below and in *Table 43.4*. Recent publications on occupational nickel dermatitis are added to the extensive reviews by Fischer (1989) and Cavelier and Foussereau (1995).

Table 43.4
Prevalence of nickel allergy in selected occupational groups according to epidemiological studies and among dermatitis patients, examples

Study population	Nickel allergy			References
	Men (%)	Women (%)	Total (%)	
Electroforming plant workers, UK (*n* = 27)	48	–	–	Wall and Calnan 1980
Electroplaters, Finland (*n* = 103)	4	15	–	Kanerva et al. 1997
Electronics industry workers, patients, Singapore (*n* = 149, 57% male)	–	–	32.8	Tan et al. 1997
Hairdressers, patients, Canada (*n* = 53, 87% female)	–	–	17	Holness and Nethercott 1990
Hairdressers, patients, Spain (*n* = 379, 92% female)	–	–	41.4	Condé-Salazar et al. 1995a
Hairdressers, patients, UK (*n* = 725, 91.1% female)	–	–	32.1	O'Connell et al. 2010
Car mechanics, Sweden (*n* = 801)	8	–	–	Meding et al. 1994
Construction workers, patients, Spain (*n* = 408)	10	–	–	Condé-Salazar et al. 1995b
Construction workers, patients, Germany (*n* = 322)	7.5	–	–	Geier and Schnuch 1998
Hospital wet workers, Finland (*n* = 536)	–	–	9.1	Lammintausta et al. 1982
Hospital wet workers, Sweden (*n* = 1,857)	–	26.3	–	Nilsson and Bäck 1986

5.1 Platers

Dermatitis due to nickel exposure was reported among platers in 1889, and up to 1930, nickel dermatitis was a frequent male occupational disease in the plating industry (Blaschko 1889; Schwarz et al. 1957). Since then, improved industrial hygiene and technical development have decreased the risk. Much of the work may today be automated, but handling of hot nickel salt solutions, and heavy contamination of the work environment, skin, working clothes, and protective gloves are still prevalent. While this constitutes a significant risk of sensitization, reports of nickel sensitivity in the electroplating industry since 1960 have been sparse.

An outbreak of occupational dermatitis in an electroforming plant in the UK was due to heavy nickel exposure (Wall and Calnan 1980). Almost half the workers were allergic to nickel (*Table 43.4*). Improvement in industrial hygiene led to an immediate decrease in the incidence of dermatitis.

A worksite survey was carried out in all 38 Finnish electroplating plants (Kanerva et al. 1997). Nickel allergy was found at the same frequency as in Finnish dermatitis patients (*Table 43.4*). Seventy percent of those with nickel allergy reported past or present hand eczema. Sensitized workers were often able to continue their work in the electroplating industry.

5.2 Electronics Industry

Workers in the electronics industry are exposed to skin irritants and contact allergens, among them nickel, colophony (rosin) in soldering flux, rubber chemicals, epoxy, and acrylates (Koh et al. 1990). In Singapore, 24% of occupational dermatology patients were from the electronics industry, and one third of the patients were patch-test positive to nickel (*Table 43.4*) (Tan et al. 1997). Sources of contact included nickel-plated earthing straps, nickel-plated tools, and coolants.

5.3 Metalworkers

Metalworkers are often heavily exposed to cutting fluids and cutting oils, and they are at high risk of developing irritant and allergic contact dermatitis due to additives in the fluids (biocides, antioxidants, fragrances, tall-oil rosin) (Suuronen 20), and to nickel and other sensitizing metals in the materials and equipment they are handling. The role of contamination of recirculating fluids by metals, including nickel, has been discussed and may be of some importance. Skin exposure to metals was assessed among metalworkers. The exposure to nickel was high compared to other studied occupations, and it varied between departments, tasks, and individuals (*Table 43.3*) (Julander et al. 2010).

5.4 Hairdressers

Hairdressers are exposed to several factors that may cause and contribute to hand eczema: wet work, nickel, fragrances, preservatives, hair dyes, and other specific occupational allergens. These factors are responsible for the high prevalence of hand eczema among hairdressers. According to a German workplace regulation aiming at protection of hairdressers' health, their tools (scissors, clips etc.) shall not release nickel.

Nickel allergy among hairdressers was focused by Wahlberg (1975), who reported 40% nickel allergy among hairdresser patients with hand eczema. Results from patch testing of hairdressers referred to dermatology departments and from epidemiological studies have since been published, some shown in ➋ *Table 43.4*. The prevalence of nickel allergy has varied considerably but generally been much higher in hairdressers than in other dermatitis patients or in the general population. It has sometimes been suggested that the high prevalence of nickel allergy among hairdressers is due to other factors than occupational exposure. In an individual case, it must, however, be recognized that occupational nickel exposure might be an important factor contributing to or causing the hairdressers' hand eczema.

5.5 Car Mechanics

Car mechanics have a high prevalence of hand eczema, often related to irritants such as organic solvents and oils. In an epidemiological study of hand eczema, a high prevalence of nickel allergy was found (Meding et al. 1994). Eight percent of the car mechanics were patch-test positive to nickel, which is high for males (➋ *Table 43.4*). Handling of tools with nickel release was suggested as a contributing factor.

5.6 Construction Workers

Construction workers risk occupational contact dermatitis from exposure to irritants, chromate, cobalt, rubber, and epoxy. Nickel allergy, however, is not often discussed in relation to construction work (Coenraads et al. 1984).

Nickel allergy is often more frequent among dermatitis patients who were construction workers than among many other male dermatitis patients (➋ *Table 43.4*). Sources of nickel exposure in plumbers, carpenters, locksmiths, or electricians, shown by a positive DMG test, include tools, pipes, locks, and other items (Lidén 1994a; Lidén et al. 1998). Architectural aluminum, such as doors and window frames, may cause nickel dermatitis due to a method for anodizing aluminum, leaving easily available nickel sulfate on the surface (Lidén 1994b). It has been shown that large amounts of nickel are deposited onto the skin in locksmiths and carpenters performing their normal tasks (Lidén et al. 2008a) (➋ *Table 43.3*).

5.7 Tools

Handheld tools are used in many male- and in some female-dominated occupations. Metal parts may come into repeated contact with the skin, often under friction and wet conditions. The Swedish tool market was surveyed to study the prevalence of tools that release nickel (Lidén et al. 1998). Twenty-seven percent of 565 handheld tools with metal parts that come into contact with the skin were DMG-test positive. It was concluded that such tools may elicit allergic contact dermatitis in already nickel-sensitive people, and present a risk factor for induction of nickel allergy. No relevant information concerning nickel release or composition of the materials is available for workers, consumers, or retailers. It was suggested that tool producers should consider nickel allergy and avoid nickel-releasing materials in parts in contact with the skin, which may be also other parts than the handle. It has been shown that nickel is deposited onto the skin at levels known to elicit nickel dermatitis in workers using tools (Lidén et al. 2008a; Jensen et al. 2011) (➋ *Table 43.3*).

5.8 Coins

Hand eczema in nickel-sensitive cashiers is a problem in clinical occupational dermatology. Coins may cause or aggravate hand eczema among cashiers with nickel allergy, but it is not known to what extent handling of coins induces nickel allergy in cashiers (Gollhausen and Ring 1991).

Cashiers handle coins throughout the workday. The majority of coins worldwide are made of the traditional copper/nickel coin alloy that gives high nickel release in artificial sweat (Lidén and Carter 2001; Lidén et al. 2008b) (➋ *Table 43.3*). The Euro coinage consists of six nickel-free cent coins, and two euro coins made of nickel-containing alloys (copper/nickel combined with nickel/brass). Copper/nickel and similar alloys are much used in the few remaining European national coinage.

Nickel ions are readily available on the surface of coins, and several μg of nickel may be transferred daily to hands by intense handling of high-nickel-releasing coins, as shown by controlled exposure and also in cashiers performing their normal tasks (Bang Pedersen et al. 1974; Staton et al. 2006; Lidén et al. 2008a, b). Provocation studies by coin handling have been performed, with different outcomes.

5.9 Cleaning, Domestic and Hospital Wet Work

Hand eczema is common among people in wet work in hospitals, cleaning and homework, especially among nickel-sensitive individuals. Water and detergents are important skin irritants, and nickel release from frequently handled equipment, tools, handles, and keys may contribute to the hand eczema. Hand eczema and nickel allergy have been studied in hospital employees (➋ *Table 43.4*).

5.10 Miscellaneous Occupations and Exposures

There are numerous reports on occupational nickel dermatitis among workers in different occupations (examples are given by Cronin 1980; Fischer 1989; Lidén et al. 2011). In the individual case, there has often been a convincing relationship between occupational nickel exposure and dermatitis, and sometimes also between the exposure and primary sensitization.

It is important to consider that brief and repeated contact with items, not only contact of long duration, may contribute significantly to nickel exposure (Lidén et al. 2008a, b). It is also important to consider common contacts, and not only contact with occupation-specific items and materials. The list of examples may be extensive. Few examples are given below to display the broad spectrum of potential hazards which may not be shown by epidemiological studies.

Keys, handles, scissors, pens, coins, and mobile phones are just few examples of items that are handled frequently in many occupations and that may cause nickel dermatitis. In restaurants, kitchen, and bars, the employees may be exposed to nickel from kitchen utensils, cutlery, measuring cups, openers, water taps, coins, and handles. Musicians may be intensely exposed to nickel by parts of string instruments, wind and brass instruments, which also may cause lip dermatitis (Gambichler et al. 2004). Tailors and dressmakers are exposed to needles and scissors, some of which release much nickel. Guards, nursing personnel, and many office workers often handle keys, some of which are special keys that may be difficult to substitute.

It is important to identify the causes of exposure and dermatitis and to substitute them with alternatives without nickel release. The DMG test is of great help in this. It is likewise considered important to perform skin exposure assessments in individual cases, to support conclusions on cause-relationships between dermatitis and occupational exposure in nickel allergy.

6 Systemic Exposure

The role of nickel in diet, surgical implants, and dental materials remains controversial and is reviewed elsewhere (Lidén et al. 2011; Veien et al. 2011; Isaksson 2011).

7 Diagnosis

Nickel sulfate 5% in petrolatum is the test material in the European baseline series. Nickel sulfate 2.5% is used in the USA. The ready-to-use patch-test system TRUE Test (Mekos) does also contain a nickel patch.

Patch testing with serial dilution of nickel sulfate or with nickel chloride is sometimes used to gain more information on the degree of sensitivity and to discriminate between allergic reactions and irritant ones (Lidén et al. 2011). Open tests to study the elicitation threshold have been carried out with nickel sulfate or chloride as single or repeated applications (Fischer et al. 2007).

Patch testing with metal discs of different nickel-containing materials may be used as a supplement to the analysis of metal release in artificial sweat. This will give information about the ability of the materials to cause allergic contact dermatitis (Menné et al. 1987; Lidén et al. 1996; Haudrechy et al. 1997).

8 Prevention

8.1 The EU Nickel Directive

The European Union decided in 1994 on a regulation aiming at the prevention of nickel allergy, *the Nickel Directive.* It entered into force in 2000 and has since been slightly revised (➋ *Table 43.2*) (Lidén et al. 2011). The Nickel Directive limits nickel release from certain consumer products intended for direct and prolonged contact with the skin. The aim was to prevent both sensitization and elicitation. Until now, several studies indicate that the legislation has started to give positive effects by reduction of exposure and disease. New cases of nickel allergy are less frequent than before the regulation, and the relationship between nickel allergy and hand eczema may have weakened. It is known that nickel on the market has decreased in Sweden, where it has been followed.

The need to further revise the EU Nickel Directive is obvious, and to include also other type of items and exposures. Items used in the workplace, and items in repeated contact with the skin are not yet covered. Nickel allergy is still the most frequent contact allergy worldwide, causing hand eczema and suffering in large parts of the population. Hopefully, countries outside the EU will implement similar legislation for prevention of nickel allergy.

8.2 Elimination

The DMG test presents a cheap, simple, and powerful tool for prevention of nickel dermatitis by exposure reduction. People with contact dermatitis due to nickel allergy should minimize exposure to nickel, including personal items and exposure in the workplace and during leisure. Nickel-sensitive people and occupational health care may identify objects in the workplace with which skin contact should be avoided and which should possibly be exchanged for other materials.

8.3 Protection

Protective gloves and clothing may be heavily contaminated by soluble nickel salts, especially in platers and battery workers. Good occupational hygiene is of great importance in these kinds of job, as shown by the history of nickel dermatitis. Workers handling metallic items may use protective gloves of fabric, leather, rubber, or plastic, but contamination as well as possible penetration of nickel ions must not be forgotten. *Barrier creams* have until now been of limited value in preventing nickel dermatitis. Possibly useful preparations, with a specific protective effect against nickel, will be presented in the future.

9 Prognosis

Many mild cases of nickel dermatitis will clear, when exposure to the causative object(s) is avoided and by topical treatment. Hand eczema in nickel-sensitive patients is however considered to have a poor prognosis and may in some cases be resistant to treatment and persist for years (Fregert 1975; Lidén et al. 2011). Nickel dermatitis has in Denmark been the second most common dermatological disease, after irritant contact dermatitis, giving rise to compensation for occupational skin disease.

Recent studies in Denmark indicate that the prognosis now is more favorable and that the relationship between nickel allergy and hand eczema has weakened (Nielsen et al. 2002; Lidén et al. 2011). In a 20-year follow-up of patch-tested schoolgirls in Sweden, the prognosis of hand eczema in relation to nickel allergy was also more favorable than previously (Josefson et al. 2009). Severe hand eczema, however, still occurs in nickel-allergic patients.

References

Bang Pedersen N, Fregert S, Brodelius P, Gruvberger B (1974) Release of nickel from silver coins. Acta Derm Venereol (Stockh) 54:231–234

Basketter DA, Scholes EW, Kimber I (1994) The performance of the local lymph node assay with chemicals identified as contact allergens in the human maximization test. Food Chem Toxicol 32:543–547

Beliauskiene A, Valiukeviciene S, Uter W, Schnuch A (2011) The European baseline series in Lithuania: results of patch testing in consecutive adult patients. J Eur Acad Dermatol Venereol 25:59–63

Blaschko A (1889) Berufsdermatosen der Arbeiter. Ein Beitrag zur Gewerbehygiene (I). Das Galvaniseur-Ekzem. Dtsch Med Wochenschr 15:925–927

Cavelier C, Foussereau J (1995) Kontaktallergie gegen Metalle und deren Salze. Teil II: Nickel, Kobalt, Quecksilber und Palladium. Dermatosen 43:152–162

Coenraads PJ, Nater JP, Jansen HA, Latinga H (1984) Prevalence of eczema and other dermatoses of the hands and forearms in construction workers in the Netherlands. Clin Exp Dermatol 9:149–158

Condé-Salazar L, Baz M, Guimaraens D, Cannavo A (1995a) Contact dermatitis in hairdressers: patch test results in 379 hairdressers (1980–1993). Am J Contact Dermat 6:19–23

Condé-Salazar L, Guimaraens D, Villegas C et al (1995b) Occupational allergic contact dermatitis in construction workers. Contact Dermatitis 33:226–230

Cronin E (1980) Metals, nickel. In: Contact dermatitis. Churchill Livingstone, Edinburgh/London/New York

European Committee for Standardization (CEN) (1998) Method for the simulation of wear and corrosion for the detection of nickel release from coated items. EN 12472

European Committee for Standardization (CEN) (2002) Screening tests for nickel release from alloys and coatings in items that come into direct and prolonged contact with the skin. CR 12471

European Committee for Standardization (CEN) (2011) Reference test method for release of nickel from products intended to some into direct and prolonged contact with the skin. EN 1811:2011

Feigl F (1972) Spot tests in inorganic analysis, 6th edn. Elsevier, Amsterdam, pp 325–331

Fischer T (1989) Occupational nickel dermatitis. In: Maibach HI, Menné T (eds) Nickel and the skin: immunology and toxicology. CRC Press, Boca Raton

Fischer LA, Johansen JD, Menné T (2007) Nickel allergy: relationship between patch test and repeated open application test thresholds. Br J Dermatol 157:723–729

Flint GN (1998) A metallurgical approach to metal contact dermatitis. Contact Dermatitis 39:213–221

Fregert S (1975) Occupational dermatitis in a 10-year material. Contact Dermatitis 1:96–107

Fregert S, Hjorth N, Magnusson B et al (1969) Epidemiology of contact dermatitis. Trans St Johns Hosp Dermatol Soc 55:17

Gambichler T, Boms S, Freitag M, 4 (2004) Contact dermatitis and other skin conditions in instrumental musicians. BMC Dermatol 16:3

Geier J, Schnuch A (1998) Kontaktallergien im Bau-Hauptgewerbe. Eine Auswertung der Daten des Informationsverbunds Dermatologischer Kliniken (IVDK) 1994–1996. Dermatosen 46:109–114

Gollhausen R, Ring J (1991) Allergy to coined money. J Am Acad Dermatol 25:365–369

Grandjean P, Nielsen GD, Andersen O (1989) Human nickel exposure and chemobiokinetics. In: Maibach HI, Menné T (eds) Nickel and the skin: immunology and toxicology. CRC Press, Boca Raton

Gruvberger B, Bruze M, Fregert S, Lidén C (2011) Allergens exposure assessment. In: Johansen JD, Frosch PJ, Lepoittevin JP (eds) Contact dermatitis, 5th edn. Springer, Heidelberg

Haudrechy P, Foussereau J, Mantout B, Baroux B (1994) Nickel release from nickel-plated metals and stainless steels. Contact Dermatitis 31:249–255

Haudrechy P, Mantout B, Frappaz A et al (1997) Nickel release from stainless steels. Contact Dermatitis 37:113–117

Holness DL, Nethercott JR (1990) Epicutaneous testing results in hairdressers. Am J Contact Dermat 1:224–234

Hostýnek JJ, Dreher F, Nakada T, Schwindt D, Anigbogu A, Maibach HI (2001) Human stratum corneum adsorption of nickel salts. Investigation of depth profiles by tape stripping in vivo. Acta Derm Venereol 212:11–18

Isaksson M (2011) Dental materials. In: Johansen JD, Frosch P, Lepoittevin J-P (eds) Contact Dermatitis. 5th edn. Springer, Berlin Heidelberg

Jensen P, Thyssen JP, Johansen JD, Skare L, Menné T, Lidén C (2011) Occupational hand eczema caused by nickel and evaluated by quantitative exposure assessment. Contact Dermatitis 64:32–36

Johansen JD, Menné T, Christophersen J, Kaaber K, Veien N (2000) Changes in the pattern of sensitization to common contact allergens in Denmark between 1985–86 and 1997–98, with a special view to the effect of preventive strategies. Br J Dermatol 142:490–495

Josefson A, Färm G, Magnuson A, Meding B (2009) Nickel allergy as risk factor for hand eczema: a population-based study. Br J Dermatol 160:828–834

Julander A, Skare L, Mulder M, Grandér M, Vahter M, Lidén C (2010) Skin deposition of nickel, cobalt, and chromium in production of gas turbines and space propulsion components. Ann Occup Hyg 54:340–350

Julander A, Skare L, Vahter M, Lidén C (2011) Nickel deposited on the skin - visualization by DMG test. Contact Dermatitis 64:151–157

Kanerva L, Kiilunen M, Jolanki R et al (1997) Hand dermatitis and allergic patch test reactions caused by nickel in electroplaters. Contact Dermatitis 36:137–140

Koh D, Foulds IS, Aw TC (1990) Dermatological hazards in the electronics industry. Contact Dermatitis 22:1–7

Lammintausta K, Kalimo K, Havu VK (1982) Occurrence of contact allergy and hand eczemas in hospital wet work. Contact Dermatitis 8:84–90

Lidén C (1994a) Occupational contact dermatitis due to nickel allergy. Sci Total Environ 148:283–285

Lidén C (1994b) Cold-impregnated aluminium. A new source of nickel exposure. Contact Dermatitis 31:22–24

Lidén C, Carter S (2001) Nickel release from coins. Contact Dermatitis 44:160–165

Lidén C, Norberg K (2005) Nickel on the Swedish market. Follow-up after implementation of the nickel directive. Contact Dermatitis 52:29–35

Lidén C, Wahlberg JE (1994) Cross-reactivity to metal compounds studied in guinea pigs induced with chromate or cobalt. Acta Derm Venereol (Stockh) 74:341–343

Lidén C, Wahlberg JE, Maibach HI (1995) Skin. In: Goyer RA, Klaassen CD, Waalkes MP (eds) Metal toxicology. Academic, San Diego/New York/Boston/London/Sydney/Tokyo/Toronto

Lidén C, Menné T, Burrows D (1996) Nickel-containing alloys and platings and their ability to cause dermatitis. Br J Dermatol 134:193–198

Lidén C, Röndell E, Skare L, Nalbanti A (1998) Nickel release from tools on the Swedish market. Contact Dermatitis 39:127–131

Lidén C, Skare L, Lind B, Nise G, Vahter M (2006) Assessment of skin exposure to nickel, chromium and cobalt by acid wipe sampling and ICP-MS. Contact Dermatitis 54:233–238

Lidén C, Skare L, Nise G, Vahter M (2008a) Deposition of nickel, chromium, and cobalt on the skin in some occupations – assessment by acid wipe sampling. Contact Dermatitis 58:347–354

Lidén C, Skare L, Vahter M (2008b) Release of nickel from coins and deposition onto skin from coin handling–comparing euro coins and SEK. Contact Dermatitis 59:31–37

Lidén C, Bruze M, Thyssen JP, Menné T (2011) Nickel. In: Johansen JD, Frosch PJ, Lepoittevin JP (eds) Contact dermatitis, 5th edn. Springer, Berlin, Heidelberg

Lindberg M, Edman B, Fischer T, Stenberg B (2007) Time trends in Swedish patch test data from 1992 to 2000. A multi-centre study based on age- and sex-adjusted results of the Swedish standard series. Contact Dermatitis 56:205–210

Meding B, Barregård L, Marcus K (1994) Hand eczema in car mechanics. Contact Dermatitis 30:129–134

Meding B, Lidén C, Berglind N (2001) Self-diagnosed dermatitis in adults. Results from a population survey in Stockholm. Contact Dermatitis 45:341–345

Menné T (1978) The prevalence of nickel allergy among women. Dermatosen 26:123–125

Menné T, Borgan Ø, Green A (1982) Nickel allergy and hand dermatitis in a stratified sample of the Danish female population: an epidemiological study including a statistic appendix. Acta Derm Venereol (Stockh) 62:35–41

Menné T, Bandrup F, Thestrup-Pedersen K et al (1987) Patch test reactivity to nickel alloys. Contact Dermatitis 16:255–259

Nielsen NH, Linneberg A, Menné T, Madsen F, Frølund L, Dirksen A, Jørgensen T (2002) The association between contact allergy and hand eczema in 2 cross-sectional surveys 8 years apart. Contact Dermatitis 47:71–77

Nilsson E, Bäck O (1986) The importance of anamnestic information of atopy, metal dermatitis and earlier hand eczema for the development of hand dermatitis in women in wet hospital work. Acta Derm Venereol (Stockh) 66:45–50

O'Connell RL, White IR, Mc Fadden JP, White JM (2010) Hairdressers with dermatitis should always be patch tested regardless of atopy status. Contact Dermatitis 62:177–181

Peltonen L (1979) Nickel sensitivity in the general population. Contact Dermatitis 5:27–32

Schäfer T, Böhler E, Ruhdorfer S, Weigl L, Wessner D, Filipiak B, Wichmann HE, Ring J (2001) Epidemiology of contact allergy in adults. Allergy 56:1192–1196

Schnuch A, Geier J, Uter W et al (1997) National rates and regional differences in sensitization to allergens of the standard series.

Population-adjusted frequencies of sensitization (PAFS) in 40,000 patients from a multicenter study (IVDK). Contact Dermatitis 37: 200–209

Schwarz L, Tulipan L, Birmingham DJ (1957) Occupational skin diseases of the skin, 3rd edn. Lea & Febiger, Philadelphia

Staton I, Ma R, Evans N, Hutchinson RW, McLeod CW, Gawkrodger DJ (2006) Dermal nickel exposure associated with coin handling and in various occupational settings: assessment using a newly developed finger immersion method. Br J Dermatol 154:658–664

Sunderman FW Jr (1989) Chemistry, analysis, and monitoring. In: Maibach HI, Menné T (eds) Nickel and the skin: immunology and toxicology. CRC Press, Boca Raton

Tan H-H, Chan MT-L, Goh C-L (1997) Occupational skin disease in workers from the electronics industry in Singapore. Am J Contact Dermat 8:210–214

Thyssen JP, Maibach HI (2008) Nickel release from earrings purchased in the United States: the San Francisco earring study. J Am Acad Dermatol 58:1000–1005

Thyssen JP, Linneberg A, Menné T, Johansen JD (2007) The epidemiology of contact allergy in the general population–prevalence and main findings. Contact Dermatitis 57:287–299

Thyssen JP, Linneberg A, Menné T, Nielsen NH, Johansen JD (2009) Contact allergy to allergens of the TRUE-test (panels 1 and 2) has decreased modestly in the general population. Br J Dermatol 161:1124–1129

Thyssen JP, Skare L, Lundgren L, Menné T, Johansen JD, Maibach HI, Lidén C (2010) Sensitivity and specificity of the nickel spot (dimethylglyoxime) test. Contact Dermatitis 62:279–288

Veien NK, Menné T (2011) Systemic contact dermatitis. In: Johansen JD, Frosch P, Lepoittevin J-P (eds) Contact Dermatitis. 5th edn. Springer, Berlin Heidelberg

Wahlberg JE (1975) Nickel allergy and atopy in hairdressers. Contact Dermatitis 1:161–165

Wahlberg JE (1989) Nickel: Animal sensitization assays. In: Maibach HI, Menné T (eds) Nickel and the skin: immunology and toxicology. CRC Press, Boca Raton

Wahlberg JE, Boman AS (1992) Cross-reactivity to palladium and nickel studied in the guinea pig. Acta Derm Venereol (Stockh) 72:95–97

Wall LM, Calnan CD (1980) Occupational nickel dermatitis in the electroforming industry. Contact Dermatitis 6:414–420

White JM, Gilmour NJ, Jeffries D, Duangdeeden I, Kullavanijaya P, Basketter DA, McFadden JP (2007) A general population from Thailand: incidence of common allergens with emphasis on para-phenylenediamine. Clin Exp Allergy 37:1848–1853

Wilkinson DS, Wilkinson JD (1989) Nickel allergy and hand eczema. In: Maibach HI, Menné T (eds) Nickel and the skin: immunology and toxicology. CRC Press, Boca Raton

World Health Organization. International Agency for Research on Cancer IARC (1997) Monographs on the evaluation of carcinogenic risks to humans, vol 49 Chromium, nickel and welding, 5 Nov 1997

Zug KA, Warshaw EM, Fowler JF Jr, Maibach HI, Belsito DL, Pratt MD, Sasseville D, Storrs FJ, Taylor JS, Mathias CG, Deleo VA, Rietschel RL, Marks J (2009) Patch-test results of the North American contact dermatitis group 2005–2006. Dermatitis 20:149–160

44 Chromium

Geetanjali Sethi[1] · *Viswanath Reddy Belum*[1] · *Desmond Burrows*[2] · *Howard I. Maibach*[3] · *Jurij J. Hostynek*[3]
[1]Wexner Medical Center at The Ohio State University, Columbus, OH, USA
[2]Queens University, Belfast, UK
[3]Department of Dermatology, University of California, San Francisco, CA, USA

Core Messages

- Hexavalent chromium (salt) is a form of chromium responsible for sensitization and contact dermatitis in chromate allergy.
- Exposure to chromium is often occupational and is commonly seen among building workers handling cement, leather workers, electroplaters, welders, and painters.
- Addition of ferrous sulfate has reduced the incidence of chromate allergy in the Scandinavian countries, since it decreases the concentration of hexavalent chromate in cement.
- Simple office-based tests are helpful in detecting chromium in objects.
- Patch testing with chromate (in chromium-sensitive subjects) to detect the minimum elicitation threshold (MET) is best done by using serial dilutions of Cr(III) and Cr(VI).
- Chromium can cause lipid peroxidation, nephrotoxicity and affect the immune system.
- Reduction or elimination of exposure is the best method of prevention of chromium-induced contact allergy.

1 Introduction

Chromium is a metallic element that is commonly found in the environment. Cement was one of the earliest agents incriminated in the causation of chromate dermatitis, with a high incidence among construction workers (handling wet cement). Exposure to chromium may be occupational or household with the skin and mucus membranes both being affected. The risk of exposure to chromium is high among other industries/professions such as leather tanning, chrome plating, welding, carpentry (handling of chromated metal products – screws and fittings), painting (also water coolants), and printing. In susceptible individuals, bleaches and detergents and stainless steel utensils containing chromium may also be potential causes of chromate sensitization.

Chromium is derived from the Greek word *chroma* meaning color due to the brightness of many of its salts. It can occur in every one of the oxidation states from −2 to +6, but the ground states 0, +2, +3, and +6 are common (Love 1983). The metal chromium in itself does not act as an allergen, but does so, in combination with a protein. Only the trivalent and hexavalent salts are able to act as haptens and form potentially antigenic bonds with proteins. It is highly resistant to corrosion in the atmosphere and many aqueous solutions, and is an unlikely cause of contact allergy.

2 Toxicity

While trivalent chromate is not considered toxic, hexavalent chromate has significant toxic effects. In sufficient concentrations it can cause respiratory symptoms such as bronchitis (Langard 1983) and asthma (Fernandez-Nieto et al. 2006), irritant dermatitis and chrome ulcers of the skin and mucous membranes, affect the immune system (Snyder et al. 1996) and also induce cancer, particularly of the lung (Bidstrup 1983).

Its effects on the immune system are demonstrated by the significantly lower levels of IL-6 in workers exposed to chromium, as compared to the normal population (Snyder et al. 1996). However, it was found that exposure to Cr(VI) in early stages can stimulate IL-6 and IL-8 and cause a fall in the percentage of B-cells (Kuo and Wu 2002).

2.1 Chrome Ulcers

The commonest symptoms associated with the irritant effect of chromates are chrome ulcers/holes occurring either on the skin (cement workers) or nasal septum (electroplaters and lithographers). The ulcers occur as 2–5 mm punched out lesions that heal with scarring, when the patient is removed from the source. Necrosis of cartilage (but not bone) can ensue but malignant change does not occur (Williams 1997).

T. Rustemeyer, P. Elsner, S.M. John & H.I. Maibach (eds.), *Kanerva's Occupational Dermatology*,
DOI 10.1007/978-3-642-02035-3_44,

In 1978, there were about 100 reported cases of chrome ulcers occurring in the UK (Burrows 1978).

The ulcer is formed due to the toxic necrotizing action of chromium on tissue. A recent report demonstrated that Cr(VI) causes mitochondrial-dependent apoptosis of the dermal fibroblasts by disrupting their actin cytoskeleton (Rudolf et al. 2005), contributing to the formation of an ulcer. In addition, workers prone to ulcer formation seem to have a lower incidence of allergic contact dermatitis (Walsh 1953). This is probably because the ulcer impairs the ability of the skin to mount an immune response.

An active program of reducing chromate contamination at workplaces can significantly reduce the incidence of chrome ulcers (Dornan 1981; Williams 1997).

3 Contact Dermatitis

3.1 Irritant Contact Dermatitis

Irritant dermatitis is seen particularly in workers exposed to chrome, where the exposure to chromium is high.

3.2 Allergic Contact Dermatitis

Dermatitis occurs more commonly with Cr(VI) than Cr(III) chromate. Cr(III) binds very readily to protein, and thus penetrates the skin poorly; little trivalent chromate gets past the stratum corneum. On the other hand, Cr(VI) penetrates easily and deeply into the dermis where it is transformed to Cr(III), which results in the formation of hapten-protein complex capable of being processed as an allergen. Guinea pig sensitization with Cr(III) is difficult; however, once sensitized, they react to patch testing in a similar fashion to those sensitized with Cr(VI) (Polak 1983).

3.3 Patch Testing

The standard test material is potassium dichromate in petrolatum (0.5%, Europe; 0.25%, USA). At these concentrations contact allergy can be elicited, besides being close to the concentration at which irritant reactions can occur (Burrows 1987). Patch testing with 0.5% and 0.375% potassium dichromate will produce a number of irritant reactions, whereas patch testing with lower percentages, while producing fewer irritant reactions, will miss some allergic reactions (Burrows et al. 1989). Consequently, 0.25% is probably a safer percentage in the hands of those lacking experience in patch testing.

A population-based, serial dilutions patch testing method (➲ *Fig. 44.1*), demonstrating the wide range in patient/worker sensitivity has been published (Nethercott et al. 1994). This method implements the delivery of a controlled amount of *allergen per surface area* of skin, for determination of the *minimum elicitation threshold* (MET). The high water solubility of compounds $K_2Cr_2O_7$ [Cr(VI)] and $CrCl_3$ [Cr(III)] is exploited for their application as T.R.U.E. test patches. The serial dilutions of Cr(III) and Cr(VI) used are given in ➲ *Table 44.1*.

4 Incidence of Chromate Allergy

The incidence of positive patch tests to chromate depends on the subset of workers being studied and illustrates the risk of getting sensitized. In a study of healthy volunteers, the patch test positivity to chromium was 0.5% in those without apparent contact with chromate, as compared to 1.8% in those who had contacted chromate (Peltonen and Fraki 1983). A similar incidence of 1.7% in chromate-pigment workers (Decaestecker et al. 1990), and 2.9% in prefabrication-construction factory workers (Goh et al. 1986b) with normal skin, has been noted. In a review of world literature, the incidence of chromate sensitivity in a routine patch testing clinic was found to be 7.9% (Nethercott 1982). Patch test positivity to dichromate was noted in 6.8% of 1,159 men and 2.8% of 1,823 women, elsewhere (Peltonen and Fraki 1983). Of these, 16.1% of the men and 18.1% of the women had a present or past history of atopic dermatitis; however of the 390 patients with atopic dermatitis as a primary diagnosis, only 1.3% showed a positive reaction to dichromate. These high figures of apparent allergy to dichromate must be accepted with a certain amount of reserve, bearing in mind the potentially irritant nature of 0.5% potassium dichromate, which could give irritant reactions in those with active skin disease. Indeed, Fischer and Rystedt (1985) found that only 40% of their positive chromium patch tests were relevant.

In a skin clinic, the incidence of chromate sensitivity is close to 1–2% and, if the figures are higher, then some special reason should be sought. The data from two British occupational surveillance schemes found 22,184 cases of occupational contact dermatitis over a period of 11 years (1993–2004), of which chromium accounted for 6% of the cases with a male:female ratio of 5:1(Athavale et al. 2007). The Finnish register of occupational diseases observed a 5.6% incidence of ACD due to chromium over a 7 year period (1991–1997). The incidence of chromium allergy per 10,000 working years in different occupations has also been elaborated in ➲ *Table 44.2* (Kanerva et al. 2000).

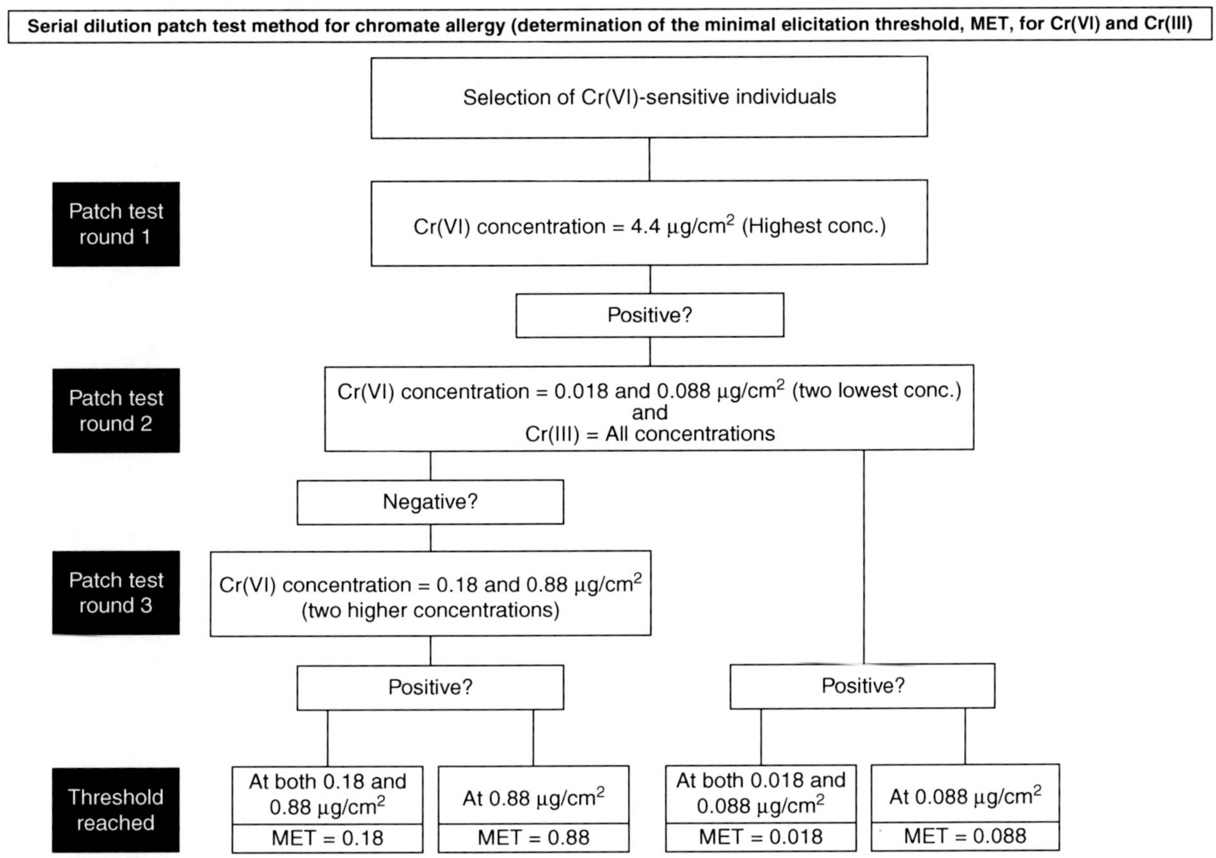

Fig. 44.1
Serial dilution patch test method for determination of minimum elicitation threshold in chromate allergic individuals (Nethercott et al.)

Table 44.1
Serial concentrations (µg/cm²) of Cr(III) and Cr(VI) used

Cr(III)	0.66	3.3	6.6	33	–
Cr(VI)	0.018	0.088	0.18	0.88	4.4

The prevalence of chromate allergy in Denmark decreased significantly from 3.6% (in 1985) to 1% (in 1995), and then increased again to 3.3% in 2007 (Thyssen et al. 2009).

5 Exposure to Chromium

Contact exposure is possible with the following compounds (Burrows and Adams 1990):

- Metals
- Analytic standards/reagents
- Anticorrosion agents
- Batteries
- Catalysts (for hydrogenation, oxidation, polymerization)
- Ceramics
- Cement
- Drilling muds
- Chromium lignosulfonates (from sodium dichromate using lignosulfate waste)
- Electroplating, anodizing agents
- Engraving
- Explosives
- Fire retardant
- Galvanized sheeting
- Hardeners, resins (aircraft industry)
- Leather
- Magnetic tapes
- Metallic chromium
- Milk preservatives
- Paints and varnishes

Table 44.2

Occupational exposure to chromate per 10,000 working years

Occupations	Incidence
Tanners, fellmongers, pelt dressers	12.20
Cast concrete product workers	6.94
Leather goods workers	4.71
Metal plating and coating workers	3.66
Bricklayers	3.44
Reinforcement concreters	2.79
Building workers	1.32

- Paper
- *Chrome cake* (sodium sulfate/dichromate)
- Photography
- Roofing
- Stainless steel
- Sutures
- Tanning leather
- Textile mordants and dyes
- Television screens
- Welding
- Wood preservatives

Chromium is used in the industry as follows:

1. *Metallurgical industries* (85%): primarily stainless steel. It is added to harden the metal and provide high-temperature strength and corrosion resistance. It is also used in combination with aluminum, zirconium, and zinc alloys.
2. *Chemical applications* (8%): predominantly used in leather tanning followed by timber preservation and in paints, inks, textiles, and as pigments in plastics. Zinc and strontium chromates are used as corrosion inhibitors in priming paints. Chromium is used as a catalyst in drilling muds, water treatment, electroplating, passivation treatments of metal, and as a preservative in milk testing.
3. *Refractory bricks* (7%): useful in refractory linings for furnaces and the kilns of the cement industry, and in molding sands in foundries because of its high melting point and relatively low cost.

5.1 Cement

Cement, of course, is by far the most common and best-recognized cause of chromate allergy. Cement contains varying amounts of chromate; for instance, it was found that the chromate content of water-soluble cement in Australia varied from less than 1 ppm to 124 ppm, with the majority tested showing less than 10 ppm (Ellis and Freeman 1986). Cement, upon addition of water, becomes alkaline (pH,12) and is probably a factor in facilitating sensitization to the chromate in cement. This probably explains the rarity of allergic contact dermatitis to chromate in cement-manufacturing workers or in those handling dry, powdered cement. The percentage of patients with cement dermatitis who have positive patch tests to chromate is probably 80–85%, but some (Conde-Salazar et al. 1995) have found lower levels (42%; 20% had positive patch tests to cobalt). Chromate in cement derives from the ingredients (clinker), the machinery used in processing (grinders, etc.), and from refractory bricks. Most of the chromate that goes into the cement is trivalent, but a varying proportion of this is changed to hexavalent chromate during manufacture.

This is important, because in future it is likely that the amount of chromate in cement will decrease due to the following factors: (1) a number of magnesium chrome refractories are currently beginning to use magnesium aluminate (spinal refractories) (Tandon and Aarts 1993); (2) slag from iron blast furnaces, which contains little or no chromate (Goh and Gan 1996), is likely to be increasingly used as a clinker substance; (3) with increased mechanization, cement is being decreasingly handled, leading to a reduction in cement dermatitis (see Chap. 48, "Cement"); and (4) addition of ferrous sulfate to cement (originally reported by Fregert et al.) decreases the concentration of hexavalent chromate in cement (Fregert et al. 1979). This has been substantiated by the findings of significant decreases in the urinary chromium of workers with hand dermatitis after the addition of ferrous sulfate in cement (Chou et al. 2008), and chromium allergy due to cement from 12.7% in 1989–1994 to 3% in 1995–2007 (Thyssen et al. 2009).

5.2 Anticorrosion Agents

Chromates are still being exploited as anticorrosion agents in water-cooling systems and paints. Their use persists despite their toxicity, as they are very effective, persistent, relatively inexpensive agents, and moreover, they do not form insoluble complexes as some other anticorrosion agents do.

5.3 Welding

Chromium may be present in electrorods used in electric arc welding, together with the metals which are being welded. During welding, chromium is oxidized to hexavalent chrome (present in fumes), which causes dermatitis (Fregert and Ovrum 1963; Shelley 1964).

5.4 Leather

The incidence of chromate allergy in footwear dermatitis varies in different studies. Trivalent chromate is used; hence, the sensitization potential is low. Nevertheless, chromate allergy should always be considered in shoe dermatitis, and possibly even as a factor in hand dermatitis due to wearing of leather gloves. Chromate is used in leather tanning, as a water-repellent [Cr(III) stearate chloride], stain-repellent [Cr(III) and fluorinated carboxylic acids], and as a dye. In those carrying out tanning, the sensitization risk is increased because of contact with other irritants, oxidation of small amounts of Cr(III) to Cr(VI) (Hansen et al. 2002) and wetness in the process of tanning. In Denmark, 35% of leather products had Cr(VI) content exceeding the detection limits of 3 ppm (Hansen et al. 2002), and an increase in the prevalence of chromate allergy due to leather exposure from 24.1% during 1989–1994 to 45% during 1995–2007, ($p < 0.02$) has been noted (Thyssen et al. 2009), further proving the role of chromate in leather allergy. The histocompatibility antigens (HLA-B8 and DR-3 alleles) have been incriminated in the susceptibility of patients to immunotoxicity with Cr(VI) (Mignini et al. 2004).

5.5 Chrome Plating

Chrome plating, in which chromic acid and sulfuric acid are used, provides a significant risk for exposure to chromate (Lee and Goh 1988).

5.6 Galvanizing

Galvanizing iron with zinc, either by electroplating or dipping in molten zinc, protects it from rusting. Coating with chromate enhances the protective effect. However, this has led to its recognition as a cause of dermatitis to chromate (Rycroft and Calnan 1977).

5.7 Pigments

Chromates are used as:

1. Dye substances (e.g., lead chromate): They are used in an insoluble hexavalent form and, thus, not relevant as a skin hazard. Chromium oxide, a trivalent form, is used in artists' paints and ceramics.
2. Soluble sodium dichromate: Used as a chelating agent in the presence of acid to yield an insoluble dyestuff. This is particularly used in wool processing.
3. Dyestuffs: This occasional addition prevents wool from reducing the dye.

5.8 Printing

Printing was a relatively common source of allergy to chromate (Burrows 1983); however, with the use of acrylates, this has become infrequent.

5.9 Stainless Steel

Most stainless steel contains about 18% chromate, but this can be as high as 30%. A thin layer of chromium oxide is formed under conditions of acidity and high chloride content. The oxide film may break down and permit corrosion to occur. Corrosion products are trivalent, but with an oxidizing agent present, hexavalent chromium could be produced. The literature on leaching of chromium from various cooking utensils has been reviewed (Kanerva 1997). It has been concluded that chromium is leached only in small amounts, from stainless steel in contact with marked acidity and high temperature. It is unlikely, that the amount leached from stainless steel utensils – even with acidic food – would exceed 50 μg/day, the amount considered to be beneficial to health. A similar observation was made when the difference in nickel and chromium content was studied in 11 habitual menus cooked in different grades of stainless steel utensils (Accominotti et al. 1998).

5.10 Bleaches and Detergents

A large percentage of female patients tested positive to chromate on routine patch testing, without any obvious cause. A case of a person previously sensitized to dichromate, developing inflammation of the sweat ducts by dipping the forearm in a solution containing 25 μg/mL of chromate for 30 min, has been reported (Nethercott et al. 1996). Allenby and Goodwin (1983) found one patient who reacted to as little as 1 ppm and could not rule out detergents as a factor in chromate dermatitis. A study done on various commonly used detergents in India showed chromate levels (by diphenyl carbazide spot test) to be less than 10 ppm, indicating that chromium may not be an important cause of dermatitis (Krupashankar et al. 2009). Note that the spot test may, because of its detection limits, have missed small amounts of chromate. In Israel, it was found that

90% of detergents and bleaches contained chromium levels higher than 1 ppm, thus resulting in a high incidence of chromium allergy (Ingber et al. 1998). Therefore, to prevent the development of chromium allergy and to decrease the incidence of chromium dermatitis in already sensitized individuals, it is now recommended that the chromium content of household products should not normally exceed 1 ppm (Basketter et al. 2003).

It has been suggested that contact with ashes in cigarette trays could be an explanation of some cases of chromate allergy in females (Clemmensen et al. 1981). The ashes contain a relatively high amount of chromate, and the cloth used to wipe these (by cleaners) would contain increasing concentrations of chromate as the day went on.

5.11 Other Sources of Contact Dermatitis

- Magnetic tapes (Krook et al. 1977)
- Paper pulp manufacture (Pirila and Kilpi 1954; Conner 1972; Fregert et al. 1972)
- Cutting fluids (Calnan 1978a)
- Tire fitters (Burrows 1981)
- Milk testers (Huriez et al. 1975; Rogers and Burrows 1975)
- Food laboratories (Pedersen 1977)
- Machine oils (Oleffe et al. 1971; Einarsson et al. 1975; Calnan 1978b)
- Pigment in soap (Mathias 1982)
- Resin hardeners containing high amounts of chromate (this is especially seen in aircraft workers) (Handley and Burrows 1994)
- Antifreeze (Freeman 1995)

6 Detection of Chromate

Chromate is often a hidden allergen, and in any situation where a patient has a positive patch test to chromate and has contact dermatitis, one should always suspect the possibility of contact with chromate; spot testing for chromate can be helpful.

6.1 Spot Test for Detection of Hexavalent Chromium (Chromate)

Reagents:

(a) Reagent I: 1,5–diphenylcarbazide (1% wt./vol. in ethanol)
(b) Concentrated sulfuric acid

Investigative procedures:

- *Chromate on the surface of a solid object*: A few drops of each reagent are applied on a cotton swab. The cotton swab is thereafter rubbed against the surface of the object for 1 min. If chromate is present, a red-violet color appears.
- *Chromate in solutions*: To a sample of approximately 10 mL a few drops of each reagent is added. If chromate is present, a red-violet color appears.
- *Chromate in powders insoluble in water (cement)*: Cement is mixed with 10 mL water for some minutes. The mixture is then filtered and the filtrate is handled in the same way as described for chromate in solutions.

Reagent I must be prepared immediately before the investigation. Spot testing is not so accurate or easily carried out as the dimethylglyoxime test for nickel.

6.2 Acid Wipe Sampling

This technique detects the presence/amount of nickel, chromium, and cobalt in the skin of workers at their workplace. It is performed by an inductively coupled plasma mass spectrometer and has a high sampling efficiency (Liden et al. 2008).

7 Photosensitivity and Chrome Allergy

Photosensitivity has been suggested as a factor in chrome allergy, since many patients develop dermatitis on the exposed areas. This might be expected in a substance that is a potential airborne allergen (El Sayed and Bazex 1994). However, negligible amounts of chromate were found, in the atmosphere of a Singapore cement construction factory and a busy city center (Goh et al. 1986a). Patients have developed a more intense reaction when sites were irradiated with short-wavelength ultraviolet light (Wahlberg and Wennersten 1977), and recently, both immediate and delayed reactions on patch testing were noted, when subsequently irradiated with ultraviolet light (Manciet et al. 1995). However, White and Rycroft (personal communication) were unable to find an increased incidence of chromate sensitivity in patients with photosensitivity. Even though one can find a certain element of photosensitivity, this is unusual and rare.

8 Effect of Systemic Chromium

Chromium is an essential element, especially in glucose metabolism; and the daily addition of 200 mcg chromium to diet improved the metabolism of glucose in diabetics. It was found that 63% of patients with type 2 diabetes mellitus responded to treatment with chromium as compared to 30% with placebo (Wang et al. 2007). This was substantiated by Ghosh et al. who stipulated that the effect of chromium may be due to an increase in insulin action, rather than stimulation of insulin secretion (Ghosh et al. 2002).

However, a randomized double-blind placebo-controlled study in Netherlands did not find any relation between chromium administration and glycemic control (Kleefstra et al. 2007).

There have been several open studies on the systemic effects of chromate in patients with chromate dermatitis (Schleiff 1968) suggesting an association. Joensen et al. (1979) found that 11 out of 31 patients experienced a flare with 2.5 mg potassium dichromate. Veien et al. (1994), in a placebo-controlled oral challenge of 2.5 mg, found a significant number of flares. McMillen (1990), however, found no connection.

Chromium has been found to induce lipid peroxidation in humans, the precise mechanism of which is not known (Bagchi et al. 1995; Kasprzak 1995). Increased concentrations of chromium and malondialdehyde (product of lipid peroxidation) have been observed, in chromium-exposed workers. Therefore, malondialdehyde may be used as a biomarker for occupational chromium exposure (Huang et al. 1999).

Excessive chromium intake or contact has also been associated with nephrotoxicity (Zhang and Jin 2006).

The daily human chromium intake varies in different geographical areas, and is usually between 20 μg and 85 μg per day, although values up to "130 μg" per day have been reported (Kanerva 1997). In other studies from the USA, the daily dietary intake of chromium was estimated to be 5 μg and 100 μg per day (Kumpulainen et al. 1979; Anderson and Kozlovsky 1985). The doses used in these trials of oral aggravation of chromate dermatitis, therefore, bear no resemblance to anything one might meet in everyday life (even in exceptional circumstances), and do not offer any evidence that chromate dermatitis is aggravated by oral intake. While it is well recognized that nickel and cobalt implants can aggravate dermatitis, particularly in the vicinity of the implant, this does not appear to be a problem with chromium.

9 Prognosis

It is well documented that the prognosis in chromium dermatitis is probably worse than in any other form of dermatitis. A very small percentage was found to be clear after 10–15 years (Burrows 1972). This was later confirmed (Halbert et al. 1992), and a review of the prognosis of occupational hand dermatitis further highlighted the finding (Hogan et al. 1990). Outcome studies were performed before current understanding of exposure, protection, and therapeutics. In the authors' experience, at least in San Francisco, many workers have a good outcome.

10 Change of Occupation

Data pertaining to the benefits of a change in occupation are unclear, but common wisdom and clinical experience suggest that it would be beneficial. In a review of chromate allergy in 122 patients, followed up for 6–9 years, it was found that 62 (52%) continued in the same occupation and, of these, 55 (89%) had ongoing dermatitis and 7 (11%) had completely cleared despite continuing chromate exposure. The remaining 58 (48%) had completely changed their type of work since initial presentation and, despite this change dermatitis persisted in 40 (69%) workers. The period an individual continued in employment (with dermatitis) prior to change of occupation appeared to be a significant factor in improvement (Halbert et al. 1992).

11 Management

11.1 Prevention

Reduction of exposure is clearly the best method of prevention. Mechanization in the construction industry and allergen replacement, for instance, change to trivalent chromate for plating results in significant improvement (Burrows and Cooke 1980). A survey of the chrome industry reflected the need and scope for further considerable improvement, and efforts to improve hygiene have been worthwhile (Dornan 1981). In a study conducted at an electroplating facility, significant neglect of preventive measures was noted; workers wore internally contaminated gloves, de-gloved themselves in a manner which led to contamination of skin, did not wear personal protective equipment, and displayed unsafe habits (nose-picking) (Cohen et al. 1974).

Hence, employee education regarding high standards of personal hygiene accompanied by the presence of a "responsible person" trained in identifying and reporting any abnormal signs and symptoms among workers are important steps in preventing morbidity (Williams 1998). In addition, proper environmental control of chromic acid mists also needs to be taken into consideration.

Replacing Cr(III) with Cr(VI) in cement is underway in four countries (Norway, Sweden, Finland, and Denmark), which has led to a significant reduction in chromate dermatitis in the cement industry (Bock et al. 2003).

The universal adoption of this practice is hindered by:

1. The decreasing incidence of chromate allergy in the cement industry worldwide (irrespective of the addition of ferrous sulfate).
2. The cost of this preventative measures, which may be considered prohibitive by some. The cost of ferrous sulfate is £150/t/works for bag material; taking into account transport costs and possible price reduction for bulk orders, one could assume a delivered price of £150. The maximum effective level is likely to be 0.5% and, in some circumstances, would need to be 1%. For an annual cement production of 14 million tons in Britain, the additional cost would thus be between £10.5 million and £21 million. There would also be a capital cost of approximately £150,000 for each works. In the UK, there are 19 works, with a capital cost of three million pounds.
3. The change in refractory materials (Tandon and Aarts 1993) and raw materials (Goh and Gan 1996) used, which will anyway lead to a decrease in the amount of chromate in cement. Cement dermatitis is also reviewed elsewhere.
4. The use of dedicated rotary machinery for large-scale mixing, in many countries, thus decreasing skin exposure.

11.2 Barrier Creams and Protective Gloves

It is doubtful that ordinary barrier creams will provide any protective effect. Specific barrier creams that change hexavalent chrome into trivalent chrome have been suggested, including ascorbic acid (Valsecchi and Cainelia 1984), ascorbic acid with ethylenediamine tetra-acetic acid (Romaguera et al. 1985), dithionate (Wall 1982), tartaric acid plus glycine (Romaguera et al. 1985), and sodium metabisulfite (Burrows and Calnan 1965). Romaguera has also found a preparation containing silicone, glyceryl lactate, glycine, and tartaric acid to be effective in a clinical trial. A polymer resin with a chelating agent was found effective in suppressing nickel patch tests positivity (Niklasson et al. 1996). This is also effective in chelating chromate (Niklasson, personal communication). The utility of good protective gloves (Boman 2004) made of proper rubber must not be underestimated.

11.3 Treatment

One of the most important steps in improving prognosis is to isolate the patient from the source as soon as possible (Halbert et al. 1992). A discussion must take place with the patient, because improvement of their dermatitis cannot be guaranteed, and many patients will continue to experience discomfort even though they have no obvious further contact with chromate. Although a satisfactory explanation does not exist, the prolonged persistence in skin or the requirement of only minute quantities of chromate (as found in soil, paper, etc.) might account for the continuing dermatitis. Nevertheless, it is ideal, that the patient be relocated to another area of the company, where there is no exposure to chromate-containing compounds. Otherwise, treatment options remain the same, as for any other eczematous condition; emollients and use of topical steroids, when necessary.

References

Accominotti M, Bost M, Haudrechy P et al (1998) Contribution to chromium and nickel enrichment during cooking of foods in stainless steel utensils. Contact Dermat 38(6):305–310

Allenby CF, Goodwin BF (1983) Influence of detergent washing powders on minimal eliciting patch test concentration of nickel and chromium. Contact Dermat 9(6):491–499

Anderson RA, Kozlovsky AS (1985) Chromium intake, absorption and excretion of subjects consuming self-selected diets. Am J Clin Nutr 41:1177–1183

Athavale P, Shum KW, Chen Y, Agius R, Cherry N, Gawkrodger DJ (2007) Occupational dermatitis related to chromium and cobalt: experience of dermatologists (EPIDERM) and occupational physicians (OPRA) in the U.K. over an 11-year period (1993–2004). Br J Dermatol 157:518–522

Bagchi D, Hassoun EA, Bagchi M, Stohs SJ (1995) Chromium-induced excretion of urinary lipid metabolites, DNA damage, nitric oxide production, and generation of reactive oxygen species in Sprague-Dawley rats. Comp Biochem Physiol C Pharmacol Toxicol Endocrinol 110:177–187

Basketter DA, Angelini G, Ingber A, Kern PS, Menne T (2003) Nickel, chromium and cobalt in consumer products: revisiting safe levels in the new millennium. Contact Dermat 49:1–7

Bidstrup PL (1983) Effects of chrome compounds on the respiratory system. In: Burrows D (ed) Chromium: metabolism and toxicity. CRC, Boca Raton, pp 31–51

Bock M, Schmidt A, Bruckner T, Diepgen TL (2003) Developments in chromate allergy in the German construction industry. Hautarzt 55:460–464

Boman A, Estlander T, Wahlberg JE (2004) Protective gloves for occupational use, 2nd edn. CRC, Boca Raton

Burrows D (1972) Prognosis in industrial dermatitis. Br J Dermatol 87:145–148

Burrows D (1978) Chromium and the skin. Br J Dermatol 99:587–595

Burrows D (1981) Chromium dermatitis in a tyre fitter. Contact Dermat 7:55–56

Burrows D (1983) Chromium: metabolism and toxicity. CRC, Boca Raton

Burrows D (1987) Comparison of 0.25 and 0.5% potassium dichromate in patch testing. Bull Dermatol Allerg Prof 2:117–120

Burrows D, Adams RM (1990) In: Adams RM (ed) Occupational skin disease, 2nd edn. W.B. Saunders, Philadelphia, pp 349–386

Burrows D, Calnan CD (1965) Cement dermatitis. Trans St Johns Hosp Dermatol Soc 51:27–39

Burrows D, Cooke MD (1980) Trivalent chrome plating. Contact Dermat 6:222

Burrows D, Andersen KE, Camaras JG et al (1989) Trial of 0.5% versus 0.3750% potassium dichromate. Contact Dermat 21:351

Calnan CD (1978a) Chromate dermatitis from soluble oil. Contact Dermat 4:378

Calnan CD (1978b) Chromate in coolant water of gramophone record presses. Contact Dermat 4:246–247

Chou TC, Chang HY, Chen CJ, Yu HS, Wu JD, Sheu SC, Shih TS (2008) Effect of hand dermatitis on the total body burden of chromium after ferrous sulfate application in cement among cement workers. Contact Dermat 59:151–156

Clemmensen OJ, Jorgensen J, Jons O et al (1981) Exposure to chromium from hospital cleaning. Derm Beruf Umwelt 3:31–54

Cohen SR, Davis DM, Kramkowski PE (1974) Clinical manifestations of chromic acid toxicity: nasal lesions in electroplate workers. Cutis 13:558–568

Conde-Salazar L, Guimaraens D, Villegas C et al (1995) Occupational allergic contact dermatitis in construction workers. Contact Dermat 33:226–230

Conner B (1972) Chromate dermatitis and paper manufacture. Contact Dermat Newsl 11:265

Decaestecker AM, Marez T, Jdaini J et al (1990) Hypersensitivity to dichromate among asymptomatic workers in a chromate pigment factory. Contact Dermat 23:52–53

Dornan JD (1981) Occupational dermatoses amongst chrome platers in the Sheffield area 1977–80. Contact Dermat 7:354–355

Einarsson O, Kylin B, Lindstedt G et al (1975) Chromium and cobalt in nickel in using cutting fluids. Contact Dermat 1:182–183

El Sayed F, Bazex J (1994) Air-borne contact dermatitis from chromate in cement with recall dermatitis on patch testing. Contact Dermat 30:58

Ellis V, Freeman S (1986) Dermatitis due to chromate in cement. Part 1. Chromate content in cement in Australia. Aust J Dermatol 27:86–90

Fernandez-Nieto M, Quirce S, Carnes J et al (2006) Occupational asthma due to chromium and nickel salts. Int Arch Occup Environ Health 79(6):483–486

Fischer T, Rystedt I (1985) False-positive follicular and irritant patch test reactions to metal salts. Contact Dermat 12:93–98

Freeman S (1995) Chromate allergy from 'antifreeze-antiboil'. Australas J Dermatol 36:168

Fregert S, Ovrum P (1963) Chromate in welding fumes with special reference to contact dermatitis. Acta Derm Venereol 43:119–124

Fregert S, Gruvberger B, Heijer A (1972) Sensitization to chromium and cobalt in processing of sulfate pulp. Acta Derm Venereol 52:221–224

Fregert S, Gruvberger B, Sandahl E (1979) Reduction of chromate in cement by iron sulfate. Contact Dermat 5:39–42

Ghosh D, Bhattacharya B, Mukherjee B, Manna B, Sinha M, Chowdhury J, Chowdhury S (2002) Role of chromium supplementation in Indians with type 2 diabetes mellitus. J Nutr Biochem 13:690–697

Goh CL, Gan SL (1996) Changes in cement manufacturing process, a cause for decline in chromate allergy? Contact Dermat 34:51–54

Goh CL, Gan SL, Ngui SJ (1986a) Occupational dermatitis in a prefabrication construction factory. Contact Dermat 15:235–240

Goh CL, Wong PH, Kwok SF et al (1986b) Chromate allergy: total chromium and hexavalent chromium in the air. Derm Beruf Umwelt 34:132–134

Halbert AR, Gebaver KA, Wall LM (1992) Prognosis of occupational chromate dermatitis. Contact Dermat 27:214–219

Handley J, Burrows D (1994) Dermatitis from hexavalent chromate in the accelerator of an epoxy sealant (PT 1422) used in the aircraft industry. Contact Dermat 30:193–196

Hansen MB, Rydin S, Menne T, Duus Johansen J (2002) Quantitative aspects of contact allergy to chromium and exposure to chrome-tanned leather. Contact Dermat 47:127–134

Hogan DJ, Dannaker W, Lal S et al (1990) An international survey of the prognosis of occupational contact dermatitis of the hands. Derm Beruf Umwelt 38:143–147

Huang YL, Chen CY, Sheu JY, Chuang IC, Pan JH, Lin TH (1999) Lipid peroxidation in workers exposed to hexavalent chromium. J Toxicol Environ Health A 56:235–247

Huriez C, Martin P, Lefebvre M (1975) Sensitivity dichromate in a milk analysis laboratory. Contact Dermat 1:247–248

Ingber A, Gammelgaard B, David M (1998) Detergents and bleaches are sources of chromium contact dermatitis in Israel. Contact Dermat 38:101–104

Joensen HD, Thormann J, Jespersen NP et al (1979) Kromallergi medicinsice og sociale aspekter. Ugeskr Laeger 141:1405–1407

Kanerva L (1997) Dermatotoxicological aspects of metallic chromium. Eur J Dermatol 7:79–84

Kanerva L, Jolanki R, Estlander T, Alanko K, Savela A (2000) Incidence rates of occupational allergic contact dermatitis caused by metals. Am J Contact Dermat 11:155–160

Kasprzak KS (1995) Possible role of oxidative damage in metal-induced carcinogenesis. Cancer Invest 13:411–430

Kleefstra N, Houweling ST, Bakker SJ, Verhoeven S, Gans RO, Meyboom-de Jong B, Bilo HJ (2007) Chromium treatment has no effect in patients with type 2 diabetes in a Western population: a randomized, double-blind, placebo-controlled trial. Diab Care 30:1092–1096

Krook G, Fregert S, Gruvberger B (1977) Chromate and cobalt eczema due to magnetic tapes. Contact Dermat 3:60–61

Krupashankar DS, Manjushree D, Rathna MS (2009) Absence of chromates in detergents in India confirmed by diphenyl carbazide spot test. Dermatitis 20:351–352

Kumpulainen JT, Wolf WR, Veillon C, Mertz W (1979) Determination of chromium in selected United States diets. J Agric Food Chem 27:490–494

Kuo HW, Wu ML (2002) Effects of chromic acid exposure on immunological parameters among electroplating workers. Int Arch Occup Environ Health 75(3):186–190

Langard S (1983) The carcinogenicity of chrome compounds in man and animals. In: Burrows D (ed) Chromium: metabolism and toxicity. CRC, Boca Raton, pp 13–31

Lee HS, Goh CL (1988) Occupational dermatitis among chrome platers. Contact Dermat 18:89–93

Liden C, Skare L, Nise G, Vahter M (2008) Deposition of nickel, chromium, and cobalt on the skin in some occupations - assessment by acid wipe sampling. Contact Dermat 58:347–354

Love G (1983) Chromium - biological and analytical considerations. In: Burrows D (ed) Chromium: metabolism and toxicity, edn. CRC, Boca Raton, pp 1–12

Manciet JR, Barrade A, Janssen F, Morel P (1995) Contact allergy with immediate and delayed photoaggravation to chromate and cobalt. Contact Dermat 33:282–284

Mathias CGT (1982) Pigmented cosmetic dermatitis from contact allergy to a toilet soap containing chromium. Contact Dermat 8:29–31

Mignini F, Streccioni V, Baldo M, Vitali M, Indraccolo U, Bernacchia G, Cocchioni M (2004) Individual susceptibility to hexavalent chromium of workers of shoe, hide, and leather industries. Immunological pattern of HLA-B8, DR3-positive subjects. Prev Med 39:767–775

Nethercott JR (1982) Results of routine patch testing of 200 patients in Toronto, Canada. Contact Dermat 8:389–395

Nethercott J, Paustenbach D, Adams R, Fowler J, Marks J, Morton C, Taylor J, Horowitz S, Finley B (1994) A study of chromium induced allergic contact dermatitis with 54 volunteers: implications for environmental risk assessment. Occup Environ Med 51:371–380

Nethercott J, Fowler J, Kauffman L et al (1996) Human response to repetitive hexavalent chromium challenge at 25 flg/ml in water. Jadassohn Centenary Congress, London

Niklasson B, Bjorkner B et al (1996) In vivo evaluation of an active barrier cream in nickel contact allergy. Jadassohn Centenary Congress, London

Oleffe J, Roosels D, Vanderkell J et al (1971) Presence due chrome dans l-environment de travail. Derm Beruf Umwelt 19:57

Pedersen NB (1977) Chromate in a food laboratory. Contact Dermat 3:105

Peltonen L, Fraki J (1983) Prevalence of dichromate sensitivity. Contact Dermat 9:190–194

Pirila V, Kilpi O (1954) On occupational dermatoses in Finland: a report of 1752 cases. Acta Derm Venereol 34:395–402

Polak L (1983) Immunology of chromium. In: Burrows D (ed) Chromium: metabolism and toxicity. CRC, Boca Raton, pp 51–136

Rogers S, Burrows D (1975) Contact dermatitis in milk testers. Contact Dermat 1:387–388

Romaguera C, Grimalt F, Vilaplana J, Carreras E (1985) Formulation of a barrier cream against chromate. Contact Dermat 13:49–52

Rudolf E, Cervinka M, Cerman J, Schroterova L (2005) Hexavalent chromium disrupts the actin cytoskeleton and induces mitochondria-dependent apoptosis in human dermal fibroblasts. Toxicol In Vitro 19:713–723

Rycroft UG, Calnan CD (1977) Relapse of chromate dermatitis from sheet metal. Contact Dermat 3:177–180

Schleiff P (1968) Provokation des Chromatekzems zu Testwecken durch interne Chrornzufubr. Hautarzt 19:209–210

Shelley WB (1964) Chromium in welding fumes as cause of eczematous hand eruption. JAMA 189:772–773

Snyder CA, Udasin I, Waterman SJ et al (1996) Reduced IL-6 levels among individuals in Hudson County, New Jersey, an area contaminated with chromium. Arch Environ Health 51:26–28

Tandon R, Aarts B (1993) Chromium, nickel and cobalt contents of some Australian cements. Contact Dermat 28:201–205

Thyssen JP, Jensen P, Carlsen BC, Engkilde K, Menne T, Johansen JD (2009) The prevalence of chromium allergy in Denmark is currently increasing as a result of leather exposure. Br J Dermatol 161: 1288–1293

Valsecchi R, Cainelia T (1984) Chromium dermatitis and ascorbic acid. Contact Dermat 10:252–253

Veien NK, Hattel T, Laurberg G (1994) Chromate-allergic patients challenged orally with potassium dichromate. Contact Dermat 31:137–139

Wahlberg JE, Wennersten G (1977) Light sensitivity and chromium dermatitis. Br J Dermatol 97:411–416

Wall LM (1982) Chromate dermatitis and sodium dithionite. Contact Dermat 8:291–293

Walsh EN (1953) Chromate hazards in industry. J Am Med Assoc 153:1305–1308

Wang ZQ, Qin J, Martin J, Zhang XH, Sereda O, Anderson RA, Pinsonat P, Cefalu WT (2007) Phenotype of subjects with type 2 diabetes mellitus may determine clinical response to chromium supplementation. Metabolism 56:1652–1655

Williams N (1997) Occupational skin ulceration in chrome platers. Occup Med Lond 47:309–310

Williams N (1998) Nasal septal ulceration and perforation in jiggers. Occup Med Lond 48:135–137

Zhang GS, Jin YL (2006) Studies on the nephrotoxicity of chromium compounds. Wei Sheng Yan Jiu 35:659–662

45 Cobalt

Carola Lidén · Anneli Julander
Institute of Environmental Medicine, Karolinska Institutet, Stockholm, Sweden

Core Messages

- Cobalt is a frequent cause of contact allergy, often seen together with allergy to nickel or chromium. Workers in the hardmetal, construction, and electronics industries and dental technicians, among others, are often allergic to cobalt.
- The clinical relevance of patch test reactivity to cobalt is often difficult to establish. Scarce knowledge about sources of skin exposure contributes to the difficulties.
- Cobalt has broad applications. Cobalt-containing materials such as hardmetals, alloys, coatings, and compounds have different ability to release cobalt ions upon skin contact and to cause dermatitis.
- Quantification of cobalt on the skin by wipe sampling, a new spot test for identifying cobalt release, and assessment of cobalt release from materials immersed in artificial sweat, will increase knowledge and facilitate prevention of cobalt allergy.
- Cobalt and cobalt compounds cause occupational lung disease and they are classified as probably and possibly carcinogenic, and as toxic to the environment.

1 Introduction

Cobalt (Co) is one of the most frequent causes of contact allergy. Cobalt allergy affects women more often than men, but the gender difference is not as large as is the case with nickel allergy. The causes of cobalt allergy in dermatitis patients do often remain unknown, probably largely due to scarce knowledge among dermatologists about how cobalt is used and how exposure occurs.

2 Prevalence and Use

Cobalt is a silvery and magnetic metal. It belongs to the transition metals together with nickel and chromium. Cobalt is present in the earth's crust, and it is mainly a by-product of nickel and copper mining. During recent decades, the price of cobalt has increased, which has resulted in more efficient refining, and, thus, nickel is not contaminated by cobalt to the same extent as formerly. Vitamin B_{12} (cobalamin) contains cobalt, which is an essential trace element.

Cobalt has been used for more than 4,000 years, initially for coloring of glass and pottery. Since the middle of the nineteenth century the use of cobalt has found many new applications, such as electroplating, tungsten carbides (hardmetals), as paint dryer, in magnets, dental alloys and orthopedic implants, as a catalyst, and in batteries (Cobalt Facts 2011). The current main uses of cobalt are given in ➲ *Table 45.1*. Cobalt and cobalt compounds are widely used in different types of industry where skin exposure occurs, and contact allergy to cobalt has been described (Rietschel and Fowler 2008; Lidén et al. 2011; Burrows et al. 1999).

Hardmetal has 90–95% of the hardness of diamond and is used in the cutting edges of tools and drills, for milling and many other industrial applications. Hardmetal is manufactured by mixing tungsten powder with carbon to produce tungsten carbide, which is then mixed with cobalt as a binder. The mixture is milled and processed to produce an ultrafine powder, which is pressed, formed, sintered, and grinded. The typical cobalt content in hardmetals is 3–15%. Titanium (Ti) and other metals are often added. Hardmetal items may also be coated with titanium and aluminum compounds. See (➲ Chap. 159, "Grinders and Brazers of Hard Metal and Stellite").

There is a wide range of *cobalt-containing alloys*, mainly for industrial use. They have different properties based on the composition and different fields of application. Orthopedic implants are often made of Co–Cr steels, with 52–62% cobalt. Cobalt-containing dental alloys are much used. Cobalt is also used in jewelry. Examples are Co–Cr steels used in rings, black cobalt-containing platings, and cobalt-containing gold plating.

Many *cobalt compounds* are used in processes and products of interest in occupational dermatology. Cobalt is widely used as a pigment (cobalt blue) in pottery and glass production. Cobalt compounds are also used as pigments in inks, as dryers in paints, and in putties. Cobalt naphtenate is used in the synthesis of polyester. *Household products and cosmetics* may contain cobalt, chromium, and nickel. Based on risk assessment addressing contact

T. Rustemeyer, P. Elsner, S.M. John & H.I. Maibach (eds.), *Kanerva's Occupational Dermatology*,
DOI 10.1007/978-3-642-02035-3_45,

Table 45.1
Main uses of cobalt (based on Cobalt Facts (2011))

Area	Materials
Metallurgical	Superalloys, wear-resistant coatings, high-speed steels, prosthetic alloys, low-expansion alloys, steels, corrosion-resistant alloys, spring alloys
Magnetic alloys	Hard and soft magnets
Chemicals	Batteries, catalysts, adhesives, cobalt soaps, driers, pigments, colors, electroplating, agriculture and medicine, electromagnetic recording
Cemented carbides (hardmetal, tungsten carbide)	Machining metal (cutting tools), metal forming (drawing of wire, cold rolling, press tools, cutting knives), mining (rock drills), wear resistance (valves, seats, seals), high modulus applications (boring bars, guide tools)
Cobalt-bonded diamonds	
Electronics	Recording material, matched-expansion alloys, leads, batteries
Ceramics and enamels	Colors in glass, enamels, pottery, china

dermatitis, it has been recommended that such products shall not contain more than 5 ppm of each of the metals (Basketter et al. 2003).

Cement products and clay used in pottery may contain cobalt in addition to possible nickel and chromium content (Tandon and Aarts 1993).

3 Health Effects

Cobalt is a well-known skin sensitizer. Other known skin effects are skin irritation, urticaria, granuloma, and photosensitization. Severe health effects by inhalation, particularly hardmetal pneumoconiosis and occupational asthma by inhalation of hardmetal dust, have attracted much concern. Cardiomyopathy has been described among heavy consumers of cobalt-containing beer. Cobalt and several cobalt compounds are classified by the EU as sensitizing by inhalation and skin contact (R42/R43), and as toxic and dangerous to the environment. The International Agency for Research on Cancer (IARC) has classified cobalt and cobalt compounds as probably and possibly carcinogenic to humans (Groups 2A and 2B).

3.1 Sensitizing Capacity and Cross-Reactivity in Animals

The skin sensitizing potential of cobalt chloride has been evaluated in animal experiments. Cobalt chloride is an extreme skin sensitizer (grade V) in the guinea pig maximization test. Animals induced with cobalt chloride did not react to nickel sulfate or potassium dichromate at challenge – the results speaking in favor of multiple sensitization rather than cross-reactivity (Wahlberg and Lidén 2000; Lidén and Wahlberg 1994). Cobalt chloride is a potent skin sensitizer also in the local lymph node assay (LLNA) (Basketter et al. 1999). It is a skin sensitizer as shown by the human maximization test (Kligman 1966).

3.2 Sensitization and Prevalence of Allergy

Cobalt allergy is typically observed in about 1% of adults in the general population (Thyssen et al. 2007). Contact allergy to cobalt has been reported at approximately 5–8% of patch-tested dermatitis patients, and generally at a higher rate in women than in men (*Table 45.2*). Contact allergy to cobalt is often associated with concomitant contact allergy to nickel or chromate. Cobalt allergy has however not decreased in parallel with nickel that has started to decrease as a result of the EU regulation limiting nickel release. Solitary cobalt allergy is seen mainly in hardmetal workers and in the glass and pottery industries. It is often difficult to identify the source of isolated positive cobalt patch tests.

4 Occupational Exposure and Occupational Contact Dermatitis

Cobalt and cobalt compounds are important cause of occupational contact dermatitis, particularly hand eczema. Construction workers, hardmetal workers, metal workers, dental technicians, and electronics workers belong to the occupational groups in which allergic contact dermatitis to cobalt is well known. *Table 45.3* displays the frequency of contact allergy to cobalt in some larger studies.

Table 45.2
Prevalence of cobalt allergy in dermatitis patients, examples from different parts of the world

Study population (no. patch tested)	Cobalt allergy	Reference
Dermatitis patients, 10 European countries (n = 18,440)	Total: 6.7%	(Uter et al. 2009)
Dermatitis patients, Denmark (n = 9,138)	Men: 2.2; women: 4.7%	(Carøe et al. 2011)
Dermatitis patients, Sweden (n = 3,790)	Men: 7.0%; women 9.0%	(Lindberg et al. 2007)
Dermatitis patients, North America (n = 4,454)	Total: 8.4%	(Zug et al. 2009)
Dermatitis patients, Singapore (n = 3,074)	Total: 8.2%	(Goon and Goh 2005)

Table 45.3
Cobalt allergy in some occupational groups according to larger workplace studies and reports on dermatitis patients. Examples

Study population (no. patch tested)	Cobalt allergy	Reference
Hardmetal workers, Sweden (n = 853)	4.6%	(Fischer and Rystedt 1983)
Dental technicians, health examination, Korea (n = 49)	12%	(Lee et al. 2001)
Construction workers, dermatitis patients, Germany and Austria (n = 1,238)	8.6%	(Uter et al. 2004)
Registered cases of occupational skin disease, construction industry, Germany (n = 335)	20%	(Bock et al. 2003)
Cement workers, Taiwan (n = 166)	4.2%	(Guo et al. 1999)
Electronics workers (n = 183) and reference workers (n = 185), Taiwan	9.8% and 2.2%	(Shiao et al. 2004)
Reported cases of occupational contact dermatitis, all occupations, UK (n = 22,184)	4%	(Athavale et al. 2007)

Occupational contact dermatitis from metallic cobalt dust in a factory producing tungsten carbide was first described in 1945 (Schwartz et al. 1945) and in a pottery factory from exposure to wet clay containing cobalt in 1953 (Pirilä 1953). Cobalt is an important occupational

Table 45.4
Causes of work-related cobalt dermatitis. See also *Tables 45.1* and *45.3*. Examples

Cause or tasks	Reference
Clay in pottery industry	(Pirilä 1953)
Cobalt in porcelain dyes	(Pirilä and Geier 1964)
Cement workers, tile setters, terrazzo workers, painters	(Bock et al. 2003)
Metal working fluids	(Geier et al. 2004)
Cobalt naphthenate in polyester resin	(Cahill and Andersen 2010)
Underground workers	(Irvine et al. 1994)
Animal feeds	(Ratcliffe and English 1998)
Cobalt in offset printing	(Malten 1975)

contact allergen in construction workers, and it has often been associated with allergy to chromium. Occupational contact dermatitis is frequent in metal workers exposed to water-based metal working fluids, cobalt being an important cause, together with other metals, biocides, skin irritants, etc.

There are several publications, including case reports, on dermatitis related to occupational exposure to cobalt-containing materials and processes, some of them displayed in *Table 45.4*. The wide applications of cobalt as metal, in alloys and hard metals and in compounds (*Table 45.1*), should be considered.

5 Exposure Assessment

5.1 Cobalt Spot Test

The cobalt spot test is a new and simple spot test for cobalt (Thyssen et al. 2010). It has been shown to detect cobalt release from alloys at levels that approximate the elicitation concentration seen in cobalt-allergic patients. A cotton-wool-tipped stick with drops of the yellow cobalt test solution is rubbed for up to 30 s against the surface to be tested. A color change from yellow to red indicates presence of cobalt ions. The test is based on oxalic acid, nitroso R salt, and sodium acetate in deionized water. The cobalt spot test can be prepared in the laboratory, and it may become commercially available. It has, until now, been applied mainly in research, but may in the near future serve as a useful tool in the clinical setting and in workplaces to identify sources of sensitization and elicitation of cobalt dermatitis, as the dimethylglyoxime test for nickel does (see Chap. 43, "Nickel").

5.2 Cobalt Release in Artificial Sweat

Cobalt release may be quantitatively determined by immersing items and materials in artificial sweat and analyzing cobalt in the solution, according to the European standard EN 1811 (Julander et al. 2009) (see Chap. 43, "Nickel"). The standard was developed to meet the needs of controlling compliance with the EU Nickel Directive. It has been shown that some materials release substantial amounts of cobalt. A broad selection of discs made of cobalt-containing hardmetals were immersed in artificial sweat for 1 min to 1 week (Julander et al. 2009). The cobalt release varied significantly from different materials. The highest cobalt release from the hardmetals was 290 μg/cm^2/week, to be compared with nickel release from two euro coins at 99 μg/cm^2/week (Lidén et al. 2008b), and the limit value of 0.5 μg/cm^2/week by the EU nickel regulation. Little is known about release of cobalt ions from other materials.

5.3 Skin Exposure Assessment

Increasing attention has been given to the development of methods for skin exposure assessment (Gruvberger et al. 2011). *Acid wipe sampling* was developed for assessment of nickel, chromium, and cobalt deposited onto skin (Lidén et al. 2006). Sampling is performed by wiping demarked areas with dilute nitric acid (1%) before (cleaning the skin) and after a normal work session. After extraction of the wipes, analysis is performed with ICP-MS or other suitable equipment. The method has very high sampling efficiency and recovery (>90%) and the mass per area unit (e.g., μg/cm^2) may be calculated.

Acid wipe sampling has been used to assess skin exposure to metals in cashiers, locksmiths, carpenters, metal workers, and secretaries (Julander et al. 2010; Lidén et al. 2008a). Cobalt was detected in all samples, and the largest amounts of cobalt (up to 4.5 μg/cm^2/h) were deposited onto the hands in metal workers sharpening hard metal tools (Julander et al. 2010). Skin exposure has also been described as an important route of uptake of cobalt in workers sharpening hard metal blades (Linnainmaa and Kiilunen 1997). Skin and surface contamination by cobalt, chromium, and nickel was assessed in the production of cemented tungsten carbides by another wipe sampling technique (Day et al. 2009). All sampled skin and work surfaces were contaminated with cobalt and the other metals.

6 Systemic Exposure

The role of systemic exposure from cobalt in diet, surgical implants, and dental materials remains controversial and is reviewed elsewhere (see Chaps. 17, 35 and 39 in Contact Dermatitis 5th edn 2011).

7 Diagnosis

Cobalt chloride 1% in petrolatum is the test material in the European baseline series (Lidén et al. 2011). Cobalt chloride 0.5% has, however, been used in Sweden since the 1980s, as 1% may cause nonallergic, porous reactions (Fischer and Rystedt 1985). The ready-to-use patch test system TRUE Test (Mekos) also contains a cobalt chloride patch.

Patch testing with a serial dilution of cobalt chloride is sometimes used to gain more information on the degree of sensitivity and to discriminate between allergic reactions and irritant ones (Lidén et al. 2011). The minimum concentration of cobalt chloride hexahydrate required to elicit a positive patch test reaction was assessed and was found to be approximately 10,000 ppm on normal skin, while it was 10–100 ppm on skin that had been pretreated with an irritant (Allenby and Basketter 1989).

Patch testing with metal discs of cobalt-containing materials may be used as a supplement to the analysis of metal release in artificial sweat. This will give important information about the ability of materials to cause allergic contact dermatitis. When consecutive dermatitis patients were tested simultaneously with cobalt chloride and a metallic disc of 100% cobalt, 11 of 23 cobalt-allergic patients reacted also to the cobalt disc (de Fine Olivarius and Menné 1992). Patch testing has been performed with discs of cobalt-containing hardmetals and dental alloys in cobalt-allergic subjects and controls (Julander et al. 2009; Thyssen et al. 2010). The hardmetals elicited positive patch test reactions, and the release of cobalt in artificial sweat was very high from many of the materials.

8 Prevention

There is no regulatory limitation in the EU of cobalt for prevention of contact dermatitis, as for nickel and chromium in cement. These regulations may, however, affect exposure and sensitization to cobalt. It has been feared that the use of cobalt might increase, as a substitute for nickel (Lidén et al. 2011). This could result in severe increase in cobalt allergy, since cobalt is a potent skin sensitizer. It has been speculated that the limitation of chromium in cement may decrease the risk of cobalt allergy in construction workers, secondary to the reduction of chromium dermatitis from cement (Uter et al. 2004; Kanerva et al. 2000). Contact allergy has not decreased while nickel allergy has started to decrease in young age groups, indicating that exposure to cobalt is not as closely related to nickel as is often assumed.

To reduce exposure to cobalt within the industrial setting, knowledge about the exposure must exist. The focus has often been on reducing cobalt in the breathing zone, and protection of the skin has generally been overlooked. It is suggested that systematic use of the cobalt spot test (Thyssen et al. 2010) and skin exposure assessments by acid wipe sampling (Lidén et al. 2006; Julander et al. 2010) may be important tools for primary and secondary prevention of cobalt allergy in workplaces.

References

Allenby CF, Basketter DA (1989) Minimum eliciting patch test concentrations of cobalt. Contact Dermatitis 20:185–190

Athavale P, Shum KW, Chen Y et al (2007) Occupational dermatitis related to chromium and cobalt: experience of dermatologists (EPIDERM) and occupational physicians (OPRA) in the U.K. over an 11-year period (1993–2004). Br J Dermatol 157:518–522

Basketter DA, Lea LJ, Cooper KJ et al (1999) Identification of metal allergens in the local lymph node assay. Am J Contact Dermat 10:207–212

Basketter DA, Angelini G, Ingber A et al (2003) Nickel, chromium and cobalt in consumer products: revisiting safe levels in the new millennium. Contact Dermatitis 49:1–7

Bock M, Schmidt A, Bruckner T et al (2003) Occupational skin disease in the construction industry. Br J Dermatol 149:1165–1171

Burrows D, Adams RM, Flint GN (1999) Metals. In: Adams RM (ed) Occupational skin disease. W.B. Saunders, Philadelphia

Cahill JL, Andersen KE (2010) Occupational cobalt-allergic contact dermatitis resulting from polyester resin. Contact Dermatitis 63:292–294

Carøe C, Andersen KE, Mortz CG (2011) Fluctuations in the prevalence of nickel and cobalt allergy in eczema patients patch tested after implementation of the nickel regulation in Denmark. Contact Dermatitis 64:126–131

Cobalt Facts (2011) Cobalt Development Institute, http://www.thecdi.com/cobaltfacts.php. Accessed 28 Aug 2011

Day GA, Virji MA, Stefaniak AB (2009) Characterization of exposures among cemented tungsten carbide workers. Part II: assessment of surface contamination and skin exposures to cobalt, chromium and nickel. J Expo Sci Environ Epidemiol 19:423–434

de Fine Olivarius F, Menné T (1992) Skin reactivity to metallic cobalt in patients with a positive patch test to cobalt chloride. Contact Dermatitis 27:241–243

Fischer T, Rystedt I (1983) Cobalt allergy in hard metal workers. Contact Dermatitis 9:115–121

Fischer T, Rystedt I (1985) False-positive, follicular and irritant patch test reactions to metal salts. Contact Dermatitis 12:93–98

Geier J, Lessmann H, Schnuch A et al (2004) Contact sensitizations in metalworkers with occupational dermatitis exposed to water-based metalworking fluids: results of the research project "FaSt". Int Arch Occup Environ Health 77:543–551

Goon AT, Goh CL (2005) Metal allergy in Singapore. Contact Dermatitis 52:130–132

Gruvberger B, Bruze M, Fregert S et al (2011) Allergens exposure assessment. In: Johansen JD, Frosch P, Lepoittevin J-P (eds) Contact Dermatitis, 5th edn. Springer, Berlin

Guo YL, Wang BJ, Yeh KC et al (1999) Dermatoses in cement workers in southern Taiwan. Contact Dermatitis 40:1–7

Irvine C, Pugh CE, Hansen EJ et al (1994) Cement dermatitis in underground workers during construction of the channel tunnel. Occup Med (Lond) 44:17–23

Julander A, Hindsén M, Skare L et al (2009) Cobalt-containing alloys and their ability to release cobalt and cause dermatitis. Contact Dermatitis 60:165–170

Julander A, Skare L, Mulder M et al (2010) Skin deposition of nickel, cobalt, and chromium in production of gas turbines and space propulsion components. Ann Occup Hyg 54:340–350

Kanerva L, Jolanki R, Estlander T et al (2000) Incidence rates of occupational allergic contact dermatitis caused by metals. Am J Contact Dermat 11:155–160

Kligman AM (1966) The identification of contact allergens by human assay. 3. The maximization test: a procedure for screening and rating contact sensitizers. J Invest Dermatol 47:393–409

Lee JY, Yoo JM, Cho BK et al (2001) Contact dermatitis in Korean dental technicians. Contact Dermatitis 45:13–16

Lidén C, Wahlberg JE (1994) Cross-reactivity to metal compounds studied in guinea pigs induced with chromate or cobalt. Acta Derm Venereol 74:341–343

Lidén C, Skare L, Lind B et al (2006) Assessment of skin exposure to nickel, chromium and cobalt by acid wipe sampling and ICP-MS. Contact Dermatitis 54:233–238

Lidén C, Skare L, Nise G et al (2008a) Deposition of nickel, chromium, and cobalt on the skin in some occupations – assessment by acid wipe sampling. Contact Dermatitis 58:347–354

Lidén C, Skare L, Vahter M (2008b) Release of nickel from coins and deposition onto skin from coin handling–comparing euro coins and SEK. Contact Dermatitis 59:31–37

Lidén C, Bruze M, Thyssen JP et al (2011) Metals. In: Johansen JD, Frosch P, Lepoittevin J-P (eds) Contact dermatitis, 5th edn. Springer, Berlin

Lindberg M, Edman B, Fischer T et al (2007) Time trends in Swedish patch test data from 1992 to 2000. A multi-centre study based on age- and sex-adjusted results of the Swedish standard series. Contact Dermatitis 56:205–210

Linnainmaa M, Kiilunen M (1997) Urinary cobalt as a measure of exposure in the wet sharpening of hard metal and stellite blades. Int Arch Occup Environ Health 69:193–200

Malten KE (1975) Cobalt and chromium in offset printing. Contact Dermatitis 1:120

Pirilä V (1953) Sensitization to cobalt in pottery workers. Acta Derm Venereol 33:193–198

Pirilä V, Geier L (1964) On cobalt allergy among porcelain workers. Hautarzt 15:491–493

Ratcliffe J, English JS (1998) Allergic contact dermatitis from cobalt in animal feed. Contact Dermatitis 39:201–202

Rietschel RL, Fowler JFJ (2008) Metals. In: Rietschel RL, Fowler JFJ (eds) Fisher's contact dermatitis, 6th edn. BC Decker, Hamilton

Schwartz L, Peck SM, Blair KE et al (1945) Allergic dermatitis due to metallic cobalt. J Allergy Clin Immunol 16:51–53

Shiao JS, Sheu HM, Chen CJ et al (2004) Prevalence and risk factors of occupational hand dermatoses in electronics workers. Toxicol Ind Health 20:1–7

Tandon R, Aarts B (1993) Chromium, nickel and cobalt contents of some Australian cements. Contact Dermatitis 28:201–205

Thyssen JP, Linneberg A, Menné T et al (2007) The epidemiology of contact allergy in the general population–prevalence and main findings. Contact Dermatitis 57:287–299

Thyssen JP, Menné T, Johansen JD et al (2010) A spot test for detection of cobalt release – early experience and findings. Contact Dermatitis 63:63–69

Uter W, Ruhl R, Pfahlberg A et al (2004) Contact allergy in construction workers: results of a multifactorial analysis. Ann Occup Hyg 48:21–27

Uter W, Ramsch C, Aberer W et al (2009) The European baseline series in 10 European Countries, 2005/2006–results of the European Surveillance System on Contact Allergies (ESSCA). Contact Dermatitis 61:31–38

Wahlberg JE, Lidén C (2000) Cross-reactivity patterns of cobalt and nickel studied with repeated open applications (ROATS) to the skin of guinea pigs. Am J Contact Dermat 11:42–48

Zug KA, Warshaw EM, Fowler JF Jr et al (2009) Patch-test results of the North American Contact Dermatitis Group 2005–2006. Dermatitis 20:149–160

46 Gold

Marléne Isaksson
Department of Occupational and Environmental Dermatology, Department of Clinical Sciences
Malmö Lund University, Skane University Hospital, Malmö, Sweden

Core Messages

- Patch testing to gold is best performed with gold sodium thiosulfate 2.0% petrolatum. If negative and if there is a strong suspicion that gold allergy is present, 5.0% petrolatum can be used.
- Reading of patch tests to gold is necessary both on day 3 or 4 and on day 7 not to miss contact allergy. Sometimes allergic reactions show up even later, up to 3 weeks after patch testing.
- The frequency of gold allergy in dermatitis patients is high, around 10–15%.
- The clinical relevance of gold allergy in dermatitis patients is rather low.
- Gold allergy is correlated to dental gold.
- The more dental gold, the higher the blood level of gold.

1 Introduction

Gold, Aurum in Latin, is the only metal except copper that is markedly colored. It is abundant in low concentrations almost all over the earth's crust, in sea water, above all in metallic form and also as gold tellurid. Gold is found as grains in the bottom of rivers in California, Australia, Alaska, and Russia, while in South Africa gold ore is won from mines with auriferous leaders. Gold is also won as a by-product from the production of copper, nickel, and lead. The world's yearly production of gold is 1,000 t, of which 150 t is used in the electronics industry.

2 Physical Properties

The purity of gold is measured in carat, one carat being a 24th part and where the carat number indicates the proportion of gold in an alloy. Hence, 24 carat is absolutely pure gold. High-carat gold easily produces black dermografism, which is the most common cause of skin discoloration from metal jewelry. It refers to thin deposits of metallic powder, which is always black because these fine particles do not reflect light, and they are produced by friction of a metallic object on skin that is contaminated by powders or abrasives. Dusty environments or fabrics may contaminate the skin with abrasive particles (Rapson 1985).

Pure gold is very soft but malleable and ductile. To increase its strength, alloys of other metals such as silver, copper, nickel, palladium, and zinc are added. The color of gold is influenced by the alloy addition, where silver gives a greenish-yellow, copper a red, and nickel a light-yellow cast to white gold.

As pure gold is malleable, it can be rolled or beaten to a thickness of less than 1 μm. From 1 g of gold, a thread of 2–3 km in length can be made. Gold has good electrical conductivity and, through its durability, a low and stabile contact resistance is achieved. It has a high reflective power, especially within the infrared spectrum, which makes surfaces covered by gold good for heat reflectors. Thin gold foils that reflect heat radiation and yet are able to let visible light through can be used in windowpanes of trains and airplanes. If these panes are electrically heated, mist and rime can be avoided (Cavelier and Foussereau 1995).

3 Chemical Properties

Gold is resistant to corrosion as it does not combine with oxygen or other substances in the atmosphere, even at elevated temperatures. Gold occurs in oxidation states 0, +I, and +III, the latter being most stable, and the equilibrium between these states can be altered easily (Brown et al. 1982). All halogens attack gold and so do halogen acids mixed with nitric acid or other oxidizers. Aqua regia (kingly water), a mixture of hydrochloric and nitric acids, and cyanide solutions attack gold. Gold can also dissolve in water solutions that contain thiol-substituted amino acids (cysteine, glutathione) and can be absorbed through animal skin (Brown et al. 1982).

T. Rustemeyer, P. Elsner, S.M. John & H.I. Maibach (eds.), *Kanerva's Occupational Dermatology*,
DOI 10.1007/978-3-642-02035-3_46, © Springer-Verlag Berlin Heidelberg 2012

4 Applications

Gold is found in a variety of applications:

1. In jewelry, either as an alloy, as gold plating, or as rolled gold (Cronin 1980). In alloys of 18-carat and 22-carat gold, copper and silver are added; in 14-carat gold, copper, nickel, and zinc are added. White gold is hardened by the addition of palladium and nickel and can also contain copper and zinc. In plating, a base metal such as copper is electrolytically covered with nickel, and then gold of varying thickness is added. Rolled gold can be applied to a metal base by mechanical pressure.
2. As gold leaf, used for lettering, decoration of books and the like.
3. In dentistry, as alloys with silver, copper, palladium, platinum, and zinc to make crowns, bridges, etc.
4. As a colloidal solution of a gold salt in stannic acid (purple of Cassius), to make ruby glass and to color enamel and porcelain. Gold hydroxide, gold oxide, and potassium and sodium gold trichloride are also used in this decorative application. The gold salt is painted on the object and, when heated, the gold salt is reduced to metallic gold.
5. As gold salts, such as gold trichloride, and complex gold salts, such as sodium tetrachloroaurate dihydrate (Cronin 1980), for toning and stabilizing silver images in photography. Gold chloride in neutron-activated form has been used in the intensifying of very weak images formed in some modern photographic applications.
6. In gilding, where two techniques principally occur: methods free of water and wet methods. The former is when gold leaf is placed on objects that are covered with varnish or when gold is applied on glass through vacuum methods by means of a pigmented lacquer or a solution of a gold salt. The object is then heated to a temperature near the glass-softening level. Wet methods imply electrolytic gilding, and this method has been in use since the middle of the nineteenth century. Pretreatment of the base metal (if made of copper alloys) with electrolytically won nickel to stop the copper and other alloy metals from diffusing into the gold surface is a prerequisite. Sometimes the nickel surface needs to be activated in an acid bath to increase the attachment of the gold. In electrolytic gilding, different baths are used: acid cyanide baths are used for decorative purposes as well as within the industry; neutral baths were formerly used as alloy baths, but, nowadays, to get very pure coatings in the electronics industry, alkaline baths are used for decorative purposes to get different colors; gold baths free of cyanide are used for decorative purposes and when thick coatings are wanted; and current-free gold baths are used in the manufacture of electronics. Gold potassium cyanide (potassium dicyanoaurate) ($KAu(CN)_2$) is used in the acid, neutral, alkaline, and current-free baths; whereas gold sodium sulfite ($NaAuSO_3$) and gold chloride ($AuCl_3$) are used in the cyanide-free baths (Asthner 1990). Gilding through electroplating is common in the manufacture of alloys for electrical contacts, when bonding transistors and diodes to wires is needed, and in printed circuit boards in the manufacture of electronics (Adams 1990).
7. As an anti-rheumatic drug since the 1920s (chrysotherapy) (Forestier 1929). Myocrisin [gold sodium (I)thiomalate] [GSTM], intended for intramuscular injections, and Auranofin [2,3,4,6-tetra-O-acetyl-1-thio-ß-D-glucopyranosato-5-triethylphosphine gold (I)], to be given orally, are used.
8. As a topical goldsalt (Auranofin) in the treatment of psoriasis (Helm et al. 1995; Marks et al. 1995).
9. As a deposit of wealth (gold bars).
10. In the medical profession, as Hulka clips for the ligation of the Fallopian tube in sterilization procedures (Trathen and Stanley 1985), as a gold ball inserted into the capsule after enucleation of an eye (Forster and Dickey 1949), as a radioactive isotope in the form of colloidal gold or seeds used either therapeutically or diagnostically (Merck 1983), in gold-plated stents, metallic implants, used in patients with stenosis of the cardiac vessels (Ekqvist et al. 2007).
11. In alcoholic beverages (Russel et al. 1999)
12. As metallic gold in makeup, such as lipstick, mascara, eye shadow (Fisher 1967), and in some leave-on products.

5 Contact Allergy to Gold

In the past, contact allergy to metallic gold and gold salts was considered rare (Cronin 1980), but since the beginning of the 1990s when gold sodium thiosulfate (GSTS) [$Na_3\ Au(S_2\ O_3)_2$] was added to many baseline series, several reports on a high frequency of contact allergy among dermatitis patients have been published.

Figures ranging from 0.78% to 13.0% are presented (Björkner et al. 1994; Mc Kenna et al. 1995; Sabroe et al. 1996; Fleming et al. 1997b; Silva et al. 1997; Leow et al.

1998; Nonaka et al. 2003). In dental patients with gold restorations, the frequency of gold allergy is even higher with figures ranging from 12.4% to GSTS (Räsänen et al. 1996). In a recent study of 134 patch-tested dental patients, gold allergy was noted in 14% (Khamaysi et al. 2006). A multicenter study of patch-test reactions with dental screening series from Finland revealed a contact allergy frequency of 7.7% for gold (Kanerva et al. 2001).

In patients with endovascular coronary gold-plated stents, 37–45.5% gold allergy was found (Svedman et al. 2005; Ekqvist et al. 2007). Gold allergy is more frequent in women (Fowler 1988; Nonaka et al. 2003). This predominance probably reflects increased contact with jewelry rather than increased susceptibility (Elgart and Higdon 1971). Hypersensitivity to gold may be seen together with contact allergy to other metals such as mercury, nickel, and palladium (Koch and Bahmer 1995; Heise et al. 1997). Other investigators found no positive statistical correlation with other allergens in a baseline series (Björkner et al. 1994; Sabroe et al. 1996).

6 Patch-Test Materials

Formerly, several gold salts as well as elemental gold in the form of gold leaf have been utilized in patch testing for gold allergy but, as many gold salts are acidic (Cronin 1980), irritant reactions have followed. Gold trichloride often causes irritant, false-positive, and persistent reactions (Fowler 1990). The test solution, which is $HAuCl_3$, is a solution of gold chloride in hydrochloric acid since it is insoluble in water. Hence, it is a strong primary irritant that causes damage to the horny layer and can elicit a lympho-monocytic reaction with pseudo-lymphomatous features (Monti et al. 1983). This has been noted by others (Bowyer 1967; Comaish 1969) and, clinically, it consists of a papular, non-eczematous reaction sometimes persisting for weeks to months (Fowler 1987). Gold chloride was shown to be a potent sensitizer in the human maximization test (Kligman 1966). Also, gold sodium thiomalate (GSTM) has been used in concentrations from 0.5% to 2.0% in petrolatum (Fox et al. 1961; Bowyer 1967; Elgart 1972; Fowler 1987; Björkner et al. 1994). There are no reports of persistent or severe reactions to this salt (Fowler 1987). Sometimes these low concentrations may give false-negative reactions, and when a high concentration (11.5% aqueous) was tested on 12 gold-allergic individuals, all reacted to GSTM. No irritant patch-test reactions were noted, and controls reacted to the salt neither epicutaneously nor intracutaneously (Bruze et al. 1995a).

Several studies have shown that potassium dicyanoaurate often has caused false-negative reactions. The patch-test concentrations have then been low and probably too low to elicit a positive reaction. In one study, this salt gave concordant positive reactions compared with GSTS when the same volumes of solutions of GSTS and potassium dicyanoaurate at equimolar concentrations were used (Björkner et al. 1994). Gold leaf is unsatisfactory due to the often negative patch-test result (Fox et al. 1961; Bowyer 1967; Comaish 1969), and it is presumed to be due to the insolubility of metallic gold (Fowler 1987). Rarely have gold leaf (Forster and Dickey 1949; Cowan 1960), gold rings (Cowan 1960), gold earrings (Cowan 1960), or a gold ball (Forster and Dickey 1949) given positive patch-test responses when tested as is. GSTS at 0.5% petrolatum has been recommended as a reliable patch-test allergen for gold allergy (Fowler 1987; Koch et al. 1997) and in addition also at 2.0% and 5.0% petrolatum (Bruze and Björkner 1996) (➋ *Fig. 46.1*). Positive reactions to this salt represent true contact allergy rather than an irritant contact reaction (Björkner et al. 1994).

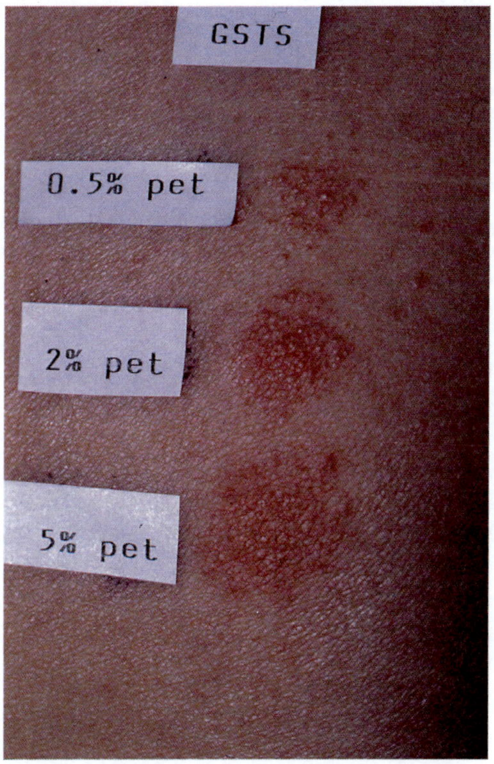

Fig. 46.1

Results of serial dilution test with GSTS with strong allergic test reaction to 5.0% in petrolatum and a weak allergic test reaction to 0.5% petrolatum

This gold salt has been used when high prevalence figures of contact allergy have been reported. Epicutaneous and intracutaneous test reactions to GSTS are long-lasting (Bruze et al. 1995b) and may persist for several months. Intracutaneous positive tests to this salt have a tendency to change from thin infiltrates to deep nodules (Bruze et al. 1995b).

7 Patch-Test Readings

Delayed readings at 96 h and 7 days (168 h) are essential when patch testing with GSTS epicutaneously. Even readings after 1 week are insufficient and should be supplemented by a reading after 3 weeks (Bruze et al. 1995b). If intracutaneously injected GSTS was used, all test reactions appeared within the first week after testing, making only a D7 reading useful, albeit intracutaneous testing might lead to persistent nodules (Bruze et al. 1995a, b).

8 In Vitro Testing

A lymphocyte blast transformation test was positive in a patient patch-tested allergic to GSTS (Silvennoinen-Kassinen and Niinimäki 1984; Aro et al. 1993) and GSTM (Kobayashi et al. 1992). In vitro blast transformation test was suggested to be of significant value in the diagnosis of gold contact dermatitis (Silvennoinen-Kassinen and Niinimäki 1984) and gold allergy (Aro et al. 1993) and might be useful in the diagnosis of drug reactions due to systemic gold therapy used in rheumatic diseases (Silvennoinen-Kassinen and Niinimäki 1984). A positive lymphocyte transformation test in 12 of 13 arthritic patients with skin reactions to systemic gold therapy was reported (Räsänen et al. 1999). Several cytokines, such as IL-1 receptor antagonist and TNF-α in particular, were detected in the elicitation phase of gold allergy in sensitized patients and also in the flare-up reaction after systemic provocation (Möller et al. 1998). The TNF-α and the IL-1 receptor antagonist were released in blood when GSTM was given by intramuscular injection to patients with contact allergy to gold (Larsson et al. 1997). The release was allergen specific (Möller et al. 1999).

9 Allergic Contact Dermatitis from Gold

There are several sporadic cases of allergic contact dermatitis from both metallic gold and gold salts reported in the literature. Elemental gold found in jewelry, such as earrings, rings, and necklaces, seems to make up the majority of causes (Fowler 1987; Wiesner and Pambor 1998) (➋ *Fig. 46.2*). It was shown that gold (0) dissolved in various aqueous amino acid solutions exposed to dioxygen, suggesting that gold jewelry in close skin contact could slowly solubilize to gold complexes in sweat and be absorbed through the skin (Brown et al. 1982), thus leading to an allergic contact dermatitis from gold. The process of dissolution of metallic gold is facilitated by the presence of other metals in the alloy or in the neighborhood (Brown et al. 1982; Holland 1980). The dermatitis under rings is often more severe in summer due to warm (Gaul 1954), humid (Elgart and Higdon 1971) weather, or if the ring is broad and tight (Comaish 1969). One patient stated that in cold weather he could wear gold jewelry for 4 days without problems, but in warm weather it took only 2 days for the dermatitis to appear (Fox et al. 1961). Gold allergy may present solely as eyelid dermatitis (Bruze et al. 1995a), and for two women with eyelid dermatitis and contact allergy to gold, the dermatitis cleared when avoiding gold jewelry (Fowler 1988). It was thought that the allergen was being transferred from the hands to the eyelids. An orbital implant – a 14-carat gold ball – gave an eczematous reaction on the eyelids of a patient 4 years after its insertion (Forster and Dickey 1949). In a study, 60 female patients with pierced ears, tested positive to GSTS, wore earrings coated with gold or titanium nitride for eight weeks. Seventeen of the 60 female patients got a skin reaction, either on the earlobes or distant, 12 of whom had received gold-plated earrings compared to 5 with titanium. The difference was statistically significant and the conclusion was that exposure to gold jewelry can be clinically relevant in persons hypersensitive to gold (Ahnlide et al. 2000). Four patients with paralysis of the

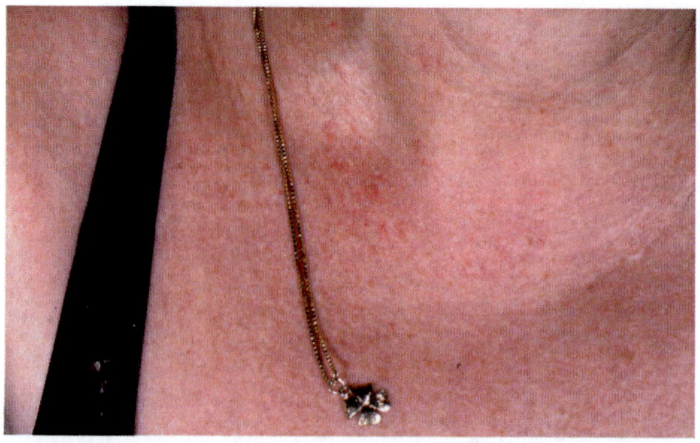

Fig. 46.2
Allergic contact dermatitis from a gold necklace in a gold-allergic individual

orbicularis oculi muscle had a gold weight implanted in the upper eyelid to be able to close the eye. They all got an inflammatory reaction due to gold allergy, but when the implant was removed, the dermatitis resolved completely (Björkner et al. 2008).

Gold rings, but also earrings, are believed to sensitize, and several cases are reported where the piercing of ears (Comaish 1969; Fisher 1974a; Armstrong et al. 1997), followed by wearing of gold earrings, often studs, has resulted in an eczema on the earlobes not long after (Elgart and Higdon 1971; Petros and MacMillan 1973; Iwatsuki et al. 1982), and, at patch testing, allergic reactions to various gold salts were noted (Elgart and Higdon 1971; Petros and MacMillan 1973; Iwatsuki et al. 1982; Nakada et al. 1997). Subsequent development of persistent papular elements on earlobes but without superficial eczematous changes have been seen, where the microscopic specimen showed dense dermal infiltration of lymphocytes and plasma cells (Petros and MacMillan 1973; Fisher 1974c; Iwatsuki et al. 1982; Kobayashi et al. 1992; Fleming et al. 1997a). A lymphomatoid contact reaction to gold earrings due to persistent gold exposure has been suspected, and gold has actually been identified in a skin specimen taken from a dermatitic earlobe in a gold allergic woman who had not used gold studs for 4 months (Suzuki 1998) and also beneath gold rings (Brown et al. 1982). Histological examination of earlobe nodules in another such patient with persistent nodules demonstrated a sarcoidal-type granulomatous reaction (Armstrong et al. 1997). After ear piercing and after the channel is epithelialized, any earrings may be inserted (Fisher 1974a, 1987).

10 Stent Implantation and Gold Allergy

Percutaneous coronary interventions are used to treat atherosclerotic coronary artery disease. The risk of restenosis has been shown to be greatly reduced by intravascular stenting. Among metallic implants, stents, some brands have been coated with gold. A pilot study showed a high prevalence of contact allergy to gold in patients given gold-plated stents (Svedman et al. 2005). In a retrospective study 484 patients, treated with coronary stent implantation, were patch-tested to metals used in the stents to investigate the contact allergy rate, especially to gold and nickel. Results showed that the frequency of contact allergy to gold was higher in the stented patients compared to controls irrespective of stent material. The authors suggested that an induction of gold allergy was possible through a gold-plated stent implanted in the coronary vessel. They also found a statistically significant correlation between the gold-plated stents and contact allergy to gold in a multivariate analysis considering other risk factors for gold allergy, such as dental gold, old age, and ear piercing (Ekqvist et al. 2007).

Restenosis is the recurrence of stenosis at the site of a previously successful intervention. The factors predisposing to in-stent restenosis are still largely unknown. Studies have reported higher restenosis rates with gold-plated stents than with stainless steel stents of the same configuration (Park et al. 2002) but contact allergy was not evaluated. In the aforementioned retrospective study comprising 484 patients treated with percutaneous coronary interventions and stented, the frequency of gold allergy was 39% in the gold-stented group. A correlation between contact allergy to gold, gold-stent, and restenosis was found with a threefold increased risk for restenosis if the patient was gold allergic and stented with a gold-plated stent (Svedman et al. 2009).

11 Allergic Contact Stomatitis and Glossitis

Dental appliances, such as crowns (Wiesenfeld et al. 1984), bridges, and dentures (Fregert et al. 1979), have also been implicated in allergic contact stomatitis and glossitis. The first case of allergic contact stomatitis to metallic gold was reported in 1971, when a patient had irritation and superficial ulceration of the gingival mucosa adjacent to a gold crown and where there already was a history of sensitivity to gold jewelry, such as earrings, rings, and wristwatches. Patch testing with GSTM and gold trichloride (0.5% aqueous) confirmed contact allergy to gold (Elgart and Higdon 1971). After that, several cases were published in which gold crowns have given soreness and erosions of the tongue (Fisher 1974b), mucosal erosions (Klaschka 1975; Wiesenfeld et al. 1984), and oral burning or stinging sensations (Young 1974; Fregert et al. 1979; Aro et al. 1993), and where gold sensitizing was considered to be due to earrings (Fisher 1974b) and a signet ring (Wiesenfeld et al. 1984). After removal of the incriminating gold, the patient has usually recovered fully (Elgart and Higdon 1971; Fisher 1974b; Wiesenfeld et al. 1984). Primarily gold stomatitis seems rare, and only a few cases have been reported (Schöpf et al. 1970; Young 1974; Fregert et al. 1979; Aro et al. 1993) in which gold applications, such as crowns, bridges, and dentures, soon after insertion gave problems in the oral mucosa, and in which tests were positive for gold salts and no history of gold jewelry intolerance was found prior to this event.

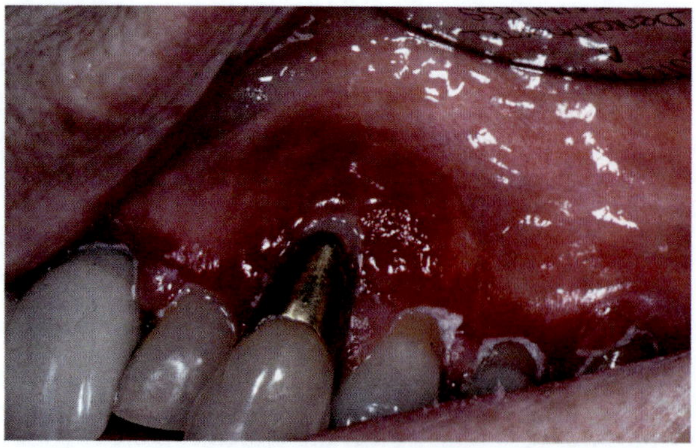

◘ Fig. 46.3
Parodontitis in a gold-allergic individual with a ceramic crown on a gold-alloy post

Oral mucosal reactions ascribed to gold allergy are rare, and the reason for this is thought to be due to the low solubility of metallic gold. Still, the moist oral environment with bacteria, enzymes, and other substances in the saliva may dissolve gold and thus form allergenic gold compounds (Aro et al. 1993; Björkman et al. 1998) (➋ *Fig. 46.3*).

In the last few years it has been shown that gold-based dental restorations seem to be an important risk factor for gold allergy. A significant correlation was found between the amount of gold surfaces in dental gold alloys in examined patients and contact allergy to gold. However, no statistical relationship to oral lesions was found (Ahlgren et al. 2002). Patients with dental gold restorations had a statistically significantly higher blood level of gold than patients without gold restorations. There was also a positive correlation between the blood level of gold and the number of dental gold surfaces, implying that gold is released from dental restorations and taken up into the circulation (Ahnlide et al. 2002).

12 Occupational Exposure and Allergic Contact Dermatitis

Sporadic cases of occupational contact dermatitis to gold salts in gold electroplaters have been reported (Somov and Khaimovsky 1964; Schmollack 1971; Cronin 1980; Adams 1983; Goh 1988; Larsen et al. 1992); nevertheless, gold salts should be considered as significant sensitizers in electroplaters. The reason sensitization seems uncommon is claimed to be due to the infrequent contact with the salts by workers, as factory supervisors only are allowed to handle and prepare the salts. These salts are usually locked away due to their toxicity (Goh 1988). Potassium dicyanoaurate sensitized a Chinese electroplater leading to a subacute dermatitis on exposed skin, beginning 2 weeks after starting work (Goh 1988). Gold cyanide sensitized Russian workers gilding watches, and patch testing was performed using 1.0% gold cyanide (Somov and Khaimovsky 1964). In Germany, gold plating with potassium dicyanoaurate led to a hand and face contact dermatitis in three of ten workers. The eruptions came after 3 weeks to 3 months of starting work The patients were positive to 1.0% gold trichloride at patch testing and two of these also to 0.01% potassium dicyanoaurate aqueous (Schmollack 1971).

A man accidentally rested his bare right forearm on a laboratory bench where crystals of gold trichloride were present, and irritation and subsequent sensitization to gold followed, presenting as pigmented papules and with no eczematous change. A pathological specimen of a papule showed lymphoma-like features, and a patch test to gold trichloride 1.0% appeared as a local, delayed, papular, noneczematous reaction, whereas a patch test to gold potassium chloride 1.0% resulted in an eczematous picture clinically (Shelley and Epstein 1963).

Gold chloride is said to cause dermatitis among photographers who use it in their work (Schwartz et al. 1947). After working 10 years, a female sales clerk in jewelry had dyshidrotic eczema of the fingers and intolerance to wearing gold jewelry, such as necklaces and earrings. She reacted positively to a patch test to GSTS. Cotton gloves improved her hand dermatitis markedly (Felix and Ducombs 1993). Another woman worked in gilding of fountain pens and prepared the gold salt bath. Hand eczema and asthmatic dyspnea soon followed, and patch testing showed her to be allergic to the gold bath (Sidi and Hincky 1965). A machinist in a gold jewelry manufacturing plant had a hand eczema that went away when he was off work and relapsed when at work. Patch testing to GSTS 0.5% was positive (Collet et al. 1994). A merchant jeweler had fingertip dermatitis and experienced great difficulty in handling jewelry. A positive reaction to gold leaf showing as a bright erythema was noted. A generalized purpuric eruption resembling allergic vasculitis flared on three patch-test occasions utilizing gold leaf. The authors state that the cutaneous vasculitis was produced through prolonged cutaneous exposure to elemental gold, although they do not rule out a toxic reaction due to topical absorption from the patient's hands or the gold dental fillings the patient had had for several years (Roenigk and Handel 1974).

In a study from Italy, the incidence of allergic contact dermatitis due to gold in 60 jewelers (13 men, 47 women) was evaluated. Eighteen percent (two men and nine women, 82%) of the individuals had a contact allergy to gold as shown with a positive patch test to gold chloride 0.1% aqueous (Vassilopoulou and Bertazzoni 1997). Japanese students involved in the manufacture of prosthetic materials in a dental clinic were shown to be hypersensitive to gold (Kawahara et al. 1993).

13 Occupational Exposure and Irritancy

When refining and extracting gold from other metals sometimes present in ores, workers are exposed to skin-, eye-, and mucous membrane–irritating chemicals, such as hydrocyanic acid and sulfur monochloride (Adams 1990). In the gold electroplating industry, irritating gold salts such as gold potassium cyanide and gold sodium cyanide are used and they bear a high level of irritancy because of their acidity (Cronin 1980). A man worked with cleaning gold electrode contacts, and in the mixture where these were placed, gold potassium cyanide was formed. After 2 years without mishap, he suddenly developed scattered sterile pustules on the backs of the fingers of the right hand and erosions of the lower lip. When he was off work for 2 weeks, both sets of lesions healed, but a purplish-brown discoloration and partial onycholysis of the free ends of most of his fingernails on the right hand developed. A month later, the nails had returned to normal (Budden and Wilkinson 1978). A woman made up solutions of potassium gold cyanide for 1 year, when she then presented with eczema on the volar surfaces and sides of her fingers. Patch testing with different gold salts gave irritant responses (Cronin 1980). A man cleaning gold clock faces at work presented with an erythematous pruritic dermatitis with papules on the trunk and forearms, where patch testing showed a positive reaction only to gold chloride 0.1%. Eight months later, he was seen with an erythematous circular plaque at the site of the former patch test. The patch test was repeated but with a negative result. The former test was interpreted as false positive (Monti et al. 1983).

14 Chrysotherapy

The most common side effects of gold therapy are mucocutaneous reactions (Svensson and Theander 1992), such as pruritus, lichen planus and pityriasis rosea-like eruptions, erythema nodosum, pemphigus flares, exfoliative dermatitis, and toxic epidermal necrolysis, which is sometimes fatal. Loss of taste, metallic taste, and glossitis are also reported (Thomas 1987). Side effects may prompt up to 45% of patients to discontinue therapy (van Gestel et al. 1994). It was suggested that some of the frequent cutaneous side effects of systemic gold therapy were due to a previous, but unrecognized, contact allergy to gold (Möller et al. 1996). Speaking against this theory is a study involving 55 rheumatoid arthritis (RA) patients, 35 of whom had received gold therapy and 20 who had not; these individuals were patch-tested with GSTS 0.5% and 0.05% petrolatum. All but one, who had never received gold, tested negative (Fleming et al. 1998). Skin testing for contact allergy to gold was also carried out in 77 patients with RA; 10.4% positive skin tests to gold were found. When dividing the 77 into a retrospective group, i.e., treatment with gold previously, and a prospective group (intended for gold therapy), gold allergy was observed in 1 of 57 (1.8%) and in 7 of 20 (35.0%) patients, respectively. The almost nonexisting gold allergy in the rheumatic patients after long-term administration of gold salts was hypothesized to be due to a hyposensitization phenomenon. The authors conclude that RA patients intended for chrysotherapy should probably first be investigated for gold allergy, but that a positive skin test to gold does not necessarily contraindicate further treatment with gold. Starting with a low dose of gold and gradually increasing it seems to work in selected cases (Möller et al. 1997).

15 Treatment and Prevention

Dermatitis caused by metallic gold and gold salts occurring on the skin is treated as other cases of contact dermatitis are treated. As gold salts are strong sensitizers and irritants, the latter mainly due to their acidity, care should be taken to prevent direct skin contact with these chemicals. Proper protective equipment, such as gloves and other protective garments, is sufficient. Dental patients with gold allergy should not be given dental gold restorations. However, if they already have such restorations and have no signs of mucosal lesions, there is no need to remove the gold from the mouth.

References

Adams R (1983) Occupational skin disease. Grune and Stratton, New York

Adams R (1990) Occupational skin disease, 2nd edn. W.B. Saunders, Philadelphia

Ahlgren C, Ahnlide I, Björkner B et al (2002) Contact allergy to gold is correlated to dental gold. Acta Derm Venereol 82:41–44

Ahnlide I, Björkner B, Bruze M et al (2000) Exposure to metallic gold in patients with contact allergy to gold sodium thiosulfate. Contact Dermatitis 43:344–350

Ahnlide I, Ahlgren C, Björkner B et al (2002) Gold concentrations in blood in relation to the number of gold restorations and contact allergy to gold. Acta Odontol Scand 60:301–305

Armstrong DKB, Walsh MY, Dawson JF (1997) Granulomatous contact dermatitis due to gold earrings. Br J Dermatol 136:776–778

Aro T, Kanerva L, Häyrinen-Immonen R, Silvennoinen-Kassinen S, Konttinen YT, Jolanki R, Estlander T (1993) Long-lasting allergic patch test reaction caused by gold. Contact Dermatitis 28:276–281

Asthner B (1990) Textbook of electrolytic and chemical finishing (in Swedish). Ytforum Förlags AB, Linköping

Björkman L, Ekstrand J, Lind BB (1998) Determination of gold released from dental alloys in saliva (abstract). J Dent Res 77:765

Björkner B, Bruze M, Möller H (1994) High frequency of contact allergy to gold sodium thiosulfate. An indication of gold allergy? Contact Dermatitis 30:144–151

Björkner B, Bruze M, Möller H et al (2008) Allergic contact dermatitis as a complication of lid loading with gold implants. Dermatitis 19:148–153

Bowyer A (1967) Epidermal reactions and prolonged dermal reactions to patch testing with gold salts. Acta Derm Venereol 47:9–14

Brown DH, Smith WE, Fox P, Sturrock RD (1982) The reactions of gold (0) with amino acids and the significance of these reactions in the biochemistry of gold. Inorg Chim Acta 67:27–30

Bruze M, Björkner B (1996) Patch testing with gold sodium thio-sulfate. Abstract 49, Jadassohn Centenary Congress, London

Bruze M, Björkner B, Möller H (1995a) Skin testing with gold sodium thiomalate and gold sodium thiosulfate. Contact Dermatitis 32:5–8

Bruze M, Hedman H, Björkner B, Möller H (1995b) The development and course of test reactions to gold sodium thiosulfate. Contact Dermatitis 33:386–391

Budden MG, Wilkinson DS (1978) Skin and nail lesions from gold potassium cyanide. Contact Dermatitis 4:172–173

Cavelier C, Foussereau J (1995) Kontaktallergie gegen Metalle and deren Salze. Dermatosen Occup Environ 43:100–112

Collet E, Lacroix M, Dalac S (1994) Allergie de contact á l'or métal et á ses alliages. Ann Derm Syph 121:21–24

Comaish S (1969) A case of contact hypersensitivity to metallic gold. Arch Dermatol 99:720–723

Cowan MA (1960) Contact dermatitis due to gold. Br J Dermatol 72: 348–349

Cronin E (1980) Contact Dermatitis. Churchill Livingstone, Edinburgh

Ekqvist S, Svedman C, Möller H et al (2007) High frequency of contact allergy to gold in patients with endovascular coronary stents. Br J Dermatol 157:730–738

Elgart M (1972) Allergic contact dermatitis to gold. Arch Dermatol 106:254

Elgart ML, Higdon RS (1971) Allergic contact dermatitis to gold. Arch Dermatol 103:649–653

Felix B, Ducombs G (1993) Allergie professionelle á l'or. Lettre du GERDA 10:44–45

Fisher AA (1967) Contact dermatitis. Lea & Febiger, Philadelphia

Fisher AA (1974a) Ear piercing hazard of nickel-gold sensitization. JAMA 228:1226, letter

Fisher AA (1974b) Allergic reactions due to metals used in dentistry. Cutis 14:797–800

Fisher AA (1974c) Metallic gold: the cause of a persistent allergic "dermal" contact dermatitis. Cutis 14:177–180

Fisher AA (1987) Ear piercing and sensitivity to nickel and gold. J Am Acad Dermatol 17:853

Fleming C, Burden D, Fallowfield M, Lever R (1997a) Lymphomatoid contact reaction to gold earrings. Contact Dermatitis 37:298

Fleming C, Forsyth A, MacKie R (1997b) Prevalence of gold contact hypersensitivity in the West of Scotland. Contact Dermatitis 36:302–304

Fleming C, Porter D, MacKie R (1998) Absence of gold sodium thiosulfate contact hypersensitivity in rheumatoid arthritis. Contact Dermatitis 38:55–56

Forestier JM (1929) L'aurothérapie dans les rheumatismes chroniques. Bull Soc Med Hop Paris 53:323–327

Forster HW Jr, Dickey RF (1949) A case of sensitivity to gold-ball orbital implant. Eczematous contact-type dermatitis due to 14-karat gold. Am J Ophthalmol 32:659–662

Fowler JF Jr (1987) Selection of patch test materials for gold allergy. Contact Dermatitis 17:23–25

Fowler JF Jr (1988) Allergic contact dermatitis to gold. Arch Dermatol 124:181–182

Fowler JF Jr (1990) Allergic contact dermatitis to metals. Am J Contact Dermat 1:212–223

Fox JM, Kennedy R, Rostenberg A Jr (1961) Eczematous contact-sensitivity to gold. Arch Dermatol 83:956–959

Fregert S, Kollander M, Poulsen J (1979) Allergic contact stomatitis from gold dentures. Contact Dermatitis 5:63–64

Gaul LE (1954) Incidence of sensitivity to chromium, nickel, gold, silver, and copper compared to reactions to their aqueous salts including cobalt sulfate. Ann Allergy 12:429–444

Goh CL (1988) Occupational dermatitis from gold plating. Contact Dermatitis 18:122–123

Heise H, Beyer H, Rauschenbach D (1997) Ergebnisse der Epikutantestung auf Goldsalze versus Amalgam. Z Dermatol 183: 68–72

Helm KF, Marks JG Jr, Leyden JJ, Guzzo C, Krueger GG, Griffiths TW, Griffiths CEM (1995) Topical auranofin ointment for the treatment of plaque psoriasis. J Am Acad Dermatol 33:517–519

Holland RI (1980) Galvanic currents between gold and amalgam. Scand J Dent Res 88:269–272

Iwatsuki K, Tagami H, Moriguchi T, Yamada M (1982) Lymphadenoid structure induced by gold hypersensitivity. Arch Dermatol 118: 608–611

Kanerva L, Rantanen T, Aalto-Korte K et al (2001) A multicenter study of patch test reactions with dental screening series. Am J Contact Dermat 12:83–87

Kawahara D, Oshima H, Kosugi H et al (1993) Further epidemiologic study of occupational contact dermatitis in the dental clinic. Contact Dermatitis 28:114

Khamaysi Z, Bergman R, Weltfriend S (2006) Positive patch test reactions to allergens of the dental series and the relation to the clinical presentations. Contact Dermatitis 55:216–218

Klaschka F (1975) Contact allergy to gold. Contact Dermatitis 1:264–265

Kligman AM (1966) The identification of contact allergens by human assay. III. The maximization test, a procedure for screening and rating contact sensitizers. J Invest Dermatol 47:393–409

Kobayashi Y, Nanko H, Nakamura J, Mizoguchi M (1992) Lymphocytoma cutis induced by gold pierced earrings. J Am Acad Dermatol 27: 457–458

Koch P, Bahmer FA (1995) Oral lichenoid lesions, mercury hypersensitivity and combined hypersensitivity to mercury and other metals: histologically-proven reproduction of the reaction by patch testing with metal salts. Contact Dermatitis 33:323–328

Koch P, Kiehn M, Frosch PJ (1997) Epikutane Testung mit Goldsalzen. Hautarzt 48:812–816

Larsen W, Adams RM, Maibach HI (1992) Color text of contact dermatitis. W.B. Saunders, Philadelphia

Larsson Å, Möller H, Björkner B et al (1997) Morphology of endogenous flare-up reactions in contact allergy to gold. Acta Derm Venereol 77:474–479

Leow Y-H, Ng S-K, Goh C-L (1998) A preliminary study of gold sensitization in Singapore. Contact Dermatitis 38:69–170

Marks JG Jr, Helm KF, Kreuger GG, Griffiths CEM, Guzzo CA, Leyden JJ (1995) Contact dermatitis from topical auranofin. J Am Acad Dermatol 32:813–814

Mc Kenna KE, Dolan O, Walsh MY, Burrows D (1995) Contact allergy to gold sodium thiosulfate. Contact Dermatitis 32:143–146

Merck Index (1983) In: Windholz M (ed) Merck index, 10th edn. Merck and Co Inc, Rahway

Möller H, Björkner B, Bruze M (1996) Clinical reactions to systemic provocation with gold sodium thiomalate in patients with contact allergy to gold. Br J Dermatol 135:423–427

Möller H, Svensson Å, Björkner B, Bruze B, Lindroth Y, Manthorpe R, Theander J (1997) Contact allergy to gold and gold therapy in patients with rheumatoid arthritis. Acta Derm Venereol (Stockh) 77:370–373

Möller H, Ohlsson K, Linder C et al (1998) Cytokines and acute phase reactants during flare-up of contact allergy to gold. Am J Contact Dermat 9:15–22

Möller H, Ohlsson K, Linder C et al (1999) The flare-up reactions after systemic provocation in contact allergy to nickel and gold. Contact Dermatitis 40:200

Monti M, Berti E, Cavicchini S, Sala F (1983) Unusual cutaneous reaction after a gold chloride patch test. Contact Dermatitis 9:150–151

Nakada T, Iijima M, Nakayama H, Maibach HI (1997) Rôle of ear piercing in metal allergic contact dermatitis. Contact Dermatitis 36:233–236

Nonaka H, Nakada T, Iijima M (2003) Gold allergy in Japan. Contact Dermatitis 48:112–114

Park SJ, Lee CW, Hong MK et al (2002) Comparison of gold-coated Nir stents with uncoated Nir stents in patients with coronary artery disease. Am J Cardiol 89:872–875

Petros H, Macmillan AL (1973) Allergic contact sensitivity to gold with unusual features. Br J Dermatol 88:505–508

Rapson WS (1985) Skin contact with gold and gold alloys. Contact Dermatitis 13:56–65

Räsänen LR, Kalimo K, Laine J et al (1996) Contact allergy to gold in dental patients. Br J Dermatol 134:673–677

Räsänen L, Kaipiainson-Seppanon O, Thyllykangas-Ludswarvi R et al (1999) Hypersensitivity to gold in gold sodium thiosulfate induced dermatitis. Br J Dermatol 141:683–688

Roenigk HR Jr, Handel D (1974) Gold vasculitis. Arch Dermatol 109: 253–255

Russel MA, Langley M, Truett AP III et al (1999) Lichenoid dermatitis after consumption of gold-containing liquor. J Am Acad Dermatol 36:841–844

Sabroe RA, Sharp LA, Peachey RDG (1996) Contact allergy to gold sodium thiosulfate. Contact Dermatitis 34:345–348

Schmollack E (1971) Berufliche Kontaktekzeme durch Kaliumgoldzyanid. Dermatol Monatsschr 157:821–824

Schöpf E, Wex O, Schulz KH (1970) Allergische Kontaktstomatitis mit spezifischer Lymphocytenstimulation durch Gold. Hautarzt 21: 422–424

Schwartz L, Tulipan L, Peck S (1947) Occupational diseases of the skin, 2nd edn. Lea & Febiger, Philadelphia

Shelley WB, Epstein E (1963) Contact sensitivity to gold as a chronic papular eruption. Arch Dermatol 87:388–391

Sidi E, Hincky M (1965) Problèmes d'actualité concernant les dermatoses professionelles. Rev Fr Allergol 5:198–209

Silva R, Pereira F, Bordalo O, Silva E, Barros A, Gonçalo M, Correia T, Pessoa G, Baptista A, Pecegueiro M (1997) Contact allergy to gold sodium thiosulfate. A comparative study. Contact Dermatitis 37: 78–81

Silvennoinen-Kassinen S, Niinimäki A (1984) Gold sensitivity blast transformation. Contact Dermatitis 11:156–158

Somov BA, Khaimovsky GD (1964) Allergic dermatitis caused by aurum compounds in watch industry. Vestn Dermatol Venerol 10:33

Suzuki H (1998) Nickel and gold in skin lesions of pierced earlobes with contact dermatitis. A study using scanning electron microscopy and x-ray microanalysis. Arch Dermatol Res 290:523–527

Svedman C, Tillman C, Gustavsson CG et al (2005) Contact allergy to gold in patients with gold -plated intracoronary stents. Contact Dermatitis 52:192–196

Svedman C, Ekqvist S, Möller H et al (2009) A correlation found between contact allergy to stent material and restenosis of the coronary arteries. Contact Dermatitis 60:158–164

Svensson Å, Theander J (1992) Skin rashes and stomatitis due to parenteral treatment of rheumatoid arthritis with sodium aurothiomalate. Ann Rheum Dis 51:326–329

Thomas I (1987) Gold therapy and its indications in dermatology. J Am Acad Dermatol 16:845–854

Trathen WT, Stanley RJ (1985) Allergic reaction to Hulka clips. Obstet Gynecol 66:743–744

van Gestel A, Koopman R, Wijnands M, van de Putte L, van Riel P (1994) Mucocutaneous reactions to gold: a prospective study of 74 patients with rheumatoid arthritis. J Rheumatol 21:1814–1819

Vassilopoulou A, Bertazzoni M (1997) Dermatite da contatto negli orafi. Bollettino di Dermatologia Allergologica e Professionale 12: 9–14

Wiesenfeld D, Ferguson MM, Forsyth A, MacDonald DG (1984) Allergy to dental gold. Oral Surg 57:158–160

Wiesner M, Pambor M (1998) Allergic contact dermatitis from gold. Contact Dermatitis 38:52–53

Young E (1974) Contact hypersensitivity to metallic gold. Dermatologica 149:294–298

47 Some Other Metals

Carola Lidén · Anneli Julander
Institute of Environmental Medicine, Karolinska Institutet, Stockholm, Sweden

Core Messages

- Several metals, except the well-known nickel, chromium, and cobalt, are able to cause skin sensitization, dermatitis, and other skin effects.
- Pure metals, alloys, and metal compounds have different ability to cause sensitization and dermatitis.
- Many of the metals and their compounds are known to cause systemic toxicity and cancer.
- The clinical relevance of patch test reactivity to some of the metals is not known.
- The prevalence of contact allergy to many metals in occupationally exposed groups, consumers or dermatitis patients is not known.
- Some of the precious metals are increasingly used in dental alloys and jewelry, and may pose new health risks.

1 Introduction

Several metals besides nickel, chromium, and cobalt may cause adverse skin effects. The most well-known skin effects caused by metals and their compounds are allergic and irritant contact dermatitis, but granuloma and pigmentation also occur (➋ *Table 47.1*). Nickel, chromium, cobalt, and gold are reviewed separately in ➋ Chaps. 46–49, and some other metals are briefly described below.

Very little is known concerning the other metals and the prevalence of contact allergy, allergic and irritant contact dermatitis, and other skin effect in exposed workers, consumers, and dermatitis patients. The knowledge base consists mainly of case reports and few workplace studies. Even less is known about the causes and levels of skin exposure, or the properties of the pure metals and their alloys in contact with skin. There is also limited experience of patch testing with the metals, except palladium. ➋ *Table 47.2* summarizes patch test substances used, but it should be noted that the experience of their use is limited. Considerably more is known concerning systemic exposure by inhalation or oral intake of some of the most toxic metals.

To improve diagnosis and prevention of work-related skin disease caused by metals, it is essential to learn more about skin exposure and properties of metals and their compounds in contact with the skin. This is important also for prevention of systemic toxicity by skin absorption of metals. Acid wipe sampling is a recently developed method for assessment of skin exposure to nickel, chromium, and cobalt, which can be used also for other metals (Julander et al. 2010; Lidén et al. 2008).

Metals are often categorized based on their physical or chemical characteristics or cost. Some of the commonly used and overlapping categories are light, heavy, precious, platinum, transition, toxic, essential, and soluble metals. However, the terminology is not used consistently, and it may sometimes be confusing, but also helpful for understanding.

2 Aluminum

Aluminum (Al) is the most frequently occurring metal in the earth's crust, and it is present as bauxite in nature. Its production requires a lot of energy, and recycling of aluminum has increased significantly during recent decades. Aluminum and aluminum alloys are used in a wide range of materials and products, many of which come in contact with skin of workers and consumers. Examples are construction materials, vehicles, packaging of food and beverages, and cookware.

In an extensive health risk assessment report (Krewski et al. 2007), it was concluded that workers in aluminum production and user industries experience considerable exposure. Asthma-like symptoms (potroom asthma) and neurological symptoms have been extensively investigated. There are still large research needs to assess these risks.

Aluminum is a weak skin sensitizer and contact allergy to elemental aluminum is considered very rare. Aluminum-adsorbed vaccines have caused contact allergy to aluminum and persistent subcutaneous nodules from hyposensitization therapy. Water-soluble aluminum salts are widely used as antiperspirants and may cause axillary dermatitis, generally irritant contact dermatitis, or granulomatous reactions (Böhler-Sommeregger and Lindemayr 1986).

T. Rustemeyer, P. Elsner, S.M. John & H.I. Maibach (eds.), *Kanerva's Occupational Dermatology*,
DOI 10.1007/978-3-642-02035-3_47,

Table 47.1

Potential of metals or metal compounds to cause contact dermatitis or other skin effects (Lidén et al. 2011; Rietschel and Fowler 2008; Lidén et al. 1995; Burrows et al. 1999). Chromium, cobalt, gold, and nickel are described in other chapters of this book

Metal or metal compound	Irritant contact dermatitis	Allergic contact dermatitis	Other skin effect
Aluminum (Al)	x	x	Granuloma
Arsenic (As)	x	–	Folliculitis, ulcerations, pigmentation, keratosis, cancer
Beryllium (Be)	x	x	Granuloma, ulcers
Cadmium (Cd)	x	–	Granuloma, phototoxic reactions
Chromium (Cr)	x	x	Granuloma
Cobalt (Co)	x	x	Urticaria, granuloma
Copper (Cu)	x	x	Pigmentation
Gold (Au)	x	x	Pigmentation, granuloma
Mercury (Hg)	x	x	Pigmentation, de-pigmentation, granuloma
Nickel (Ni)	x	x	
Palladium (Pd)	–	x	Granuloma, urticaria
Platinum (Pt)	–	x	Urticaria
Rhodium (Rh)	–	x	
Silver (Ag)	x	–	Pigmentation (argyria)
Tin (Sn)	x	–	

x confirmed, – less certain or not known

Occupational exposure to aluminum has been reported to cause itch and contact dermatitis in aluminum production, in aircraft manufacture, and in a machine construction plant (Peters et al. 1998; Lidén et al. 2011). Cold sealing of aluminum with nickel fluoride constitutes a risk of contact dermatitis when handling aluminum products, however not from aluminum but from nickel ions on the surface of cold-sealed items (Lidén 1994).

Patch testing is generally performed with an empty Finn Chamber (elemental aluminum) and with aluminum chloride hexahydrate 2% in pet.

3 Arsenic

Arsenic (As) is a widely distributed metalloid. Inorganic arsenic is present in groundwater, salt water, and metal ores. Organic arsenic compounds are primarily found in fish and shell-fish. Arsenic compounds are used as wood preservatives, insecticides, herbicides, and rodenticides. They are added to animal food and have medical use. White arsenic (arsenic trioxide) is a by-product of the smelting of copper and other metals.

Inorganic arsenic is acutely toxic and intake of large quantities may lead to death. Exposure to arsenic is mainly via food and drinking water, and long-term exposure to arsenic in drinking water is related to increased risks of skin cancer, but also some other cancers (Vahter et al. 2007). Occupational exposure to arsenic, primarily by inhalation, is associated with lung cancer (Järup 2003; Wild et al. 2009). International Agency for Research on Cancer (IARC) has classified arsenic and arsenic compounds as carcinogenic to humans (Group 1).

Arsenic dermatitis is seen mainly in smelter workers, and also in mining and glass production. Irritant contact dermatitis and follicular reactions are most frequent. Cases of allergic contact dermatitis have been described (Rietschel and Fowler 2008; Burrows et al. 1999).

Occupational risk for skin cancer by arsenic exposure occurs in the manufacture of insecticides or herbicides, by agricultural exposure to pesticides, and in smelting of copper, lead, zinc, and mining of arsenic. Systemic absorption via ingestion is considered to be the main exposure route rather than skin absorption (Gawkrodger 2004).

One or 10% sodium arsenate in water may be used for patch testing.

Table 47.2
Examples of patch test preparations for other metals and metal compounds than those included in the European baseline series. It should be noted that experience from testing with many of the substances is limited and scientific literature should be consulted before testing (Lidén et al. 1995, 2011; Rietschel and Fowler 2008; Burrows et al. 1999)

Metal	Substance	Concentration in vehicle
Aluminum (Al)	Aluminum chloride hexahydrate, and aluminum metal	2% or 10% pet 100% (patch test chamber)
Arsenic (As)	Sodium arsenate	1% or 10% aq
Beryllium (Be)	Beryllium chloride or sulfate	1% pet
Cadmium (Cd)	Cadmium chloride	0.5% pet
Copper (Cu)	Copper sulfate	2% pet
Mercury (Hg)	Mercuric chloride	0.05% aq
Palladium (Pd)	Palladium chloride	1% pet
Platinum (Pt)	Ammonium tetrachloroplatinate	0.25% pet
Rhodium (Rh)	Rhodium chloride	1% aq
Silver (Ag)	Silver nitrate	1% aq
Tin (Sn)	Tin chloride	1% pet

pet petrolatum, *aq* water

4 Beryllium

Beryllium (Be) is a light metal, which is hard and has a relatively high melting point. It is used as the metal, in alloys, and as its oxide. Mostly it is used as a hardening agent in alloys, particularly in copper-beryllium. Beryllium alloys have wide applications such as in nuclear weapons, aerospace, ceramics, fluorescent lights, medical equipment, dental alloys and orthodontics, electronic equipment, and also in consumer items that come into contact with the skin (golf clubs, fishing rods, jewelry, etc.). The majority of beryllium is produced in the USA.

Beryllium is extremely toxic. Acute exposure may cause acute inflammation of the lungs and pneumonitis. Chronic occupational exposure by inhalation may result in chronic beryllium disease (berylliosis), in which granulomatous lesions in the lungs, reduced lung capacity, and general symptoms are seen. Chronic beryllium disease is a cell-mediated immune response. Sensitization can be measured with a beryllium-specific lymphocyte proliferation test (Kreiss et al. 2007). IARC has classified beryllium and beryllium compounds as carcinogenic to humans (Group 1).

Beryllium may cause irritant contact dermatitis, allergic contact dermatitis, chemical ulcers, ulcerating granulomas, and allergic dermal granulomas (Berlin et al. 2003). It is a skin sensitizer as shown by human maximization test, guinea pig maximization test, and local lymph node assay (Kligman 1966; Wahlberg and Boman 1985; Basketter et al. 1996).

In 1951, contact allergy to beryllium was first diagnosed by patch testing with various beryllium salts in workers at two beryllium plants (Curtis 1951). Since then, cases of contact allergy have been described, among them a dental technician with hand eczema and dental patients with stomatitis from beryllium-containing dental alloys (Berlin et al. 2003; Rietschel and Fowler 2008; Burrows et al. 1999). A worker in beryllium alloy production developed simultaneously granulomatous eruptions on arms and legs and symptoms of chronic beryllium disease (Berlin et al. 2003).

Attempts to prevent chronic beryllium disease by reduction of inhalation of beryllium have often failed. A study of levels of beryllium in workplace air, on work surfaces, and on necks and faces of employees was performed at a beryllium alloy facility. It was concluded that skin may be an important route of exposure for sensitization and chronic beryllium disease, and that it is necessary to minimize also skin exposure to beryllium salts and fine particles (Day et al. 2007). It has recently been shown that beryllium ions are released from particulate beryllium materials, copper-beryllium alloys, and copper-beryllium tools in artificial sweat, suggesting that skin exposure is a pathway for development of sensitization and chronic beryllium disease (Stefaniak et al. 2011).

Patch testing has been performed with beryllium chloride or sulfate 1% in petrolatum.

5 Cadmium

Cadmium (Cd) belongs to the heavy metals. It is one of the most toxic metals and environmental poisons. Cadmium occurs naturally together with zinc, and is a by-product of zinc production. The major part is used in rechargeable nickel-cadmium batteries. Cadmium and cadmium compounds are also used as pigment in paints, for plating, and as stabilizer in plastic materials. The main industrial exposure is to fumes and dust by inhalation, and environmental exposure is via food and smoking (Vahter et al. 2007; Järup 2003). Cadmium red (cadmium selenide) has previously been used for coloration of dentures. Yellow cadmium sulfide is used as a pigment for yellow and red tattoos.

According to the EU chemicals regulation (REACH), cadmium is limited in many products including new plastic materials, paints, and jewelry. According to the EU directive on electric and electronic equipment (RoHS Directive), cadmium is restricted in electrical and electronic equipment, including batteries but with exception for cadmium platings. Acute toxicity may be fatal, and chronic toxicity affects many organs (kidney, lung, bones, hematopoetic system). The itai-itai disease in Japan affected mainly women (Vahter et al. 2007; Järup 2003). IARC has classified cadmium and cadmium compounds as carcinogenic to humans (Group 1).

The skin-sensitizing potential of cadmium chloride was evaluated in a guinea pig maximization test, and no statistically significant reactivity was noted in induced animals compared to controls (Wahlberg and Boman 1979). Cadmium sulfides in tattoos may cause phototoxic reactions and sarcoid-like granulomas.

Three large series of dermatitis patients were patch-tested with different preparations of cadmium chloride. The overall conclusion from testing with cadmium chloride 2% in water (Wahlberg 1977) and cadmium chloride 1% in petrolatum (Gebhart and Geier 1996) was that the observed reactions were irrelevant; 0.5% has been recommended for patch testing (Geier et al. 1996).

6 Copper

Copper (Cu) is an important metal in industry. Pure copper is soft and has high electrical and thermal conductivity. More than half the production is used in electrical equipment, and other high-volume uses are in roofing and plumbing. Copper is widely used in alloys; copper-tin alloys are called bronzes and may contain also other metals, and copper-zink alloy is called brass. Copper-nickel alloys have a wide use in coinage, and copper is used in gold and silver alloys. Copper sulfate and organic copper salts are used in agriculture as fungicide and algicide.

The skin-sensitizing potential of copper sulfate was evaluated in animal experiments; in the guinea pig maximization test it was graded as a weak sensitizer or grade I allergen (Karlberg et al. 1983); in the local lymph node assay (LLNA) it was a sensitizer (Basketter et al. 1996).

Concentrated solutions of copper sulfate are corrosive and cause skin irritation.

Copper has generally been considered a rare skin sensitizer and only few occupationally related cases have been described (Burrows et al. 1999; Rietschel and Fowler 2008; Lidén et al. 2011; Hostynek and Maibach 2004). Cases of systemic eczematous dermatitis have been related to copper-containing intrauterine contraceptive devices (IUCD), and cases of oral lesions have been related to dental fillings and orthodontic materials. When copper sulfate (2% in petrolatum) was used for patch test in two large series of dermatitis patients, 1% and 3.5% of the patients were tested positive, but the reactions were considered to be uncertain or nonrelevant (Karlberg et al. 1983; Wöhrl et al. 2001). Also other patch test concentrations have been suggested.

7 Mercury

Mercury (Hg) belongs to the heavy metals, and it is liquid at room temperature. Mercury is one of the most toxic metals and environmental poisons. Mercury and its compounds are used in many industrial processes and products; in the chlor alkali process, dental amalgam, cosmetics and medicines, as preservative and pesticide, in thermometers, fluorescent lamps and batteries, etc. Mercuric sulfide (cinnabar) is a red pigment used in tattoos.

Due to its toxicity, mercury has been banned or restricted for certain applications in many countries. According to the EU Batteries Directive mercury is banned in batteries, and it is banned in thermometers, barometers, and some other instruments. According to the EU directive on electric and electronic equipment (RoHS Directive), mercury is restricted in electrical and electronic equipment. Mercury and its compounds are highly toxic to the environment and humans. The nervous system, kidneys, and other organs are affected. Methyl mercury poisoning may be very severe and even fatal. Intake of contaminated fish and of mercury-polluted grain resulted in large catastrophes in Minamata, Japan, and in Iraq (Järup 2003).

Systemic mercury poisoning in industry is caused by contamination by mercury from broken thermometers, etc. Occupational exposure to metallic mercury is also caused by dental amalgam in dentist, dental nurses, and dental technicians, who may develop contact allergy (Kanerva et al. 1993; Lee et al. 2001; Burrows et al. 1999). Nonoccupational exposure to mercury-containing antiseptics (merbromin), preservatives (thimerosal) in vaccines and contact lens solution, cosmetics, skin-lightening creams, shampoos and antifungal agents, and mercuric sulfide (cinnabar) in tattoos may cause sensitization and dermatitis (Burrows et al. 1999).

There is no general consensus regarding which mercury compounds to use for patch testing. Mercury compounds may be irritant to the skin and aqueous solutions of mercury salts may react with aluminum in Finn Chambers to produce irritant compounds. Patch test reactivity to thimerosal is considered to indicate mercury allergy.

8 Palladium

Palladium (Pd) is a silvery-white metal, belonging to the platinum group of metals and the precious metals. It has high resistance to corrosion. The main uses are as a catalyst, in electric and electronic equipment as contacts, platings, and solders. It is used in jewelry, mainly as whitener in white gold. Palladium is increasingly used in dental alloys. Occupational asthma and urticaria are known to be caused by the platinum group metals, including palladium in refineries, electroplating, and catalyst and recycling industry (Daenen et al. 1999; Cristaudo et al. 2005).

Palladium chloride has been shown to be a potent skin sensitizer in the guinea pig. Animals induced with palladium chloride do also react to nickel sulfate and vice versa. The results are interpreted as being due to cross-reactivity (Wahlberg and Lidén 1999; Wahlberg and Boman 1992).

Since the 1980s, palladium chloride has been included in routine patch testing in many clinics. The prevalence of contact allergy to palladium in more than 10,000 patients in several countries, patch-tested during the period 1986–2008, has been reviewed (Faurschou et al. 2011). The prevalence was 7.8% in dermatitis patients and 7.4% in dental patients (including dental personnel). The prevalence of allergy to palladium but not to nickel was 0.2% and 0.5% in the two groups, respectively. Thus, in almost every case of patch test reactivity to palladium chloride, simultaneous reactivity to nickel is shown, a finding which is not fully understood, but possibly is due to cross-reactivity as indicated by animal experiments. Palladium has, by some authors, been related to contact stomatitis or oral lichen planus and to granuloma from earrings in pierced ears. The safety for consumers of palladium in these applications has been questioned (Faurschou et al. 2011).

Only single cases of occupational contact dermatitis from palladium have been reported including two analytical chemists working in precious metals analysis (Munro-Ashman et al. 1969; Watsky 2007). They had work-related hand eczema or facial lesions, and were patch-tested positive to palladium chloride. One case was tested positive also to nickel, the other to platinum and gold sodium thiosulfate.

Patch testing is generally performed with palladium chloride 1% in petrolatum. The clinical relevance of routine patch testing with palladium has been questioned because few clinically relevant cases of palladium allergy have been reported, and the significance of the reactions is not fully understood. Patch testing with metallic palladium has been negative (Burrows et al. 1999; Lidén et al. 2011; Faurschou et al. 2011).

9 Platinum

Platinum (Pt) is a gray-white metal, belonging to the platinum group of metals and the precious metals. It has high resistance to corrosion. The main uses are in vehicle emission control, in jewelry and electronics, and as a catalyst. Occupational exposure to platinum occurs in mining, refineries, and in manufacturing catalysts and jewelry.

Exposure to platinum salts is known to cause asthma, rhinitis, eye irritation, contact urticaria, and contact dermatitis. Occupational asthma and urticaria and positive skin-prick tests to platinum salts were shown in studies of precious metals refinery workers (Baker et al. 1990) and workers in catalyst manufacturing (Cristaudo et al. 2005). Single cases of occupational contact allergy to platinum salts have been described in refinery workers, a chemical process worker, and an analytical chemist (Watsky 2007; Lidén et al. 2011). Platinum metal has, however, been questioned as a cause of skin sensitization. When 446 dermatitis patients were patch-tested with ammonium tetrachloroplatinate (0.25% in water) to assess the prevalence of allergy, only two tested positive (Fowler et al. 2008). Ammonium tetrachloroplatinate is a skin sensitizer according to the local lymph node assay (LLNA) (Basketter et al. 1999).

Ammonium tetrachloroplatinate (0.25%) and ammonium hexachloroplatinate (0.1%) have been used for patch testing. The experience is however limited, and they may cause irritant reactions.

10 Rhodium

Rhodium (Rh) is a hard, corrosion-resistant silvery-white metal, belonging to the platinum group of metals and the precious metals. The main uses are as catalyst, in jewelry and electronics, and among other things it is used in high-reflective mirrors and nozzles for glass-fiber spinning. Rhodium is often alloyed with platinum or palladium, and sterling silver and white gold are often plated with a thin layer of rhodium.

Little is known about the toxicology of rhodium. Rhodium chloride is a potent sensitizer in guinea pigs. Animals induced with rhodium chloride also reacted to cobalt chloride indicating cross-reactivity, the clinical relevance of which is not known (Lidén et al. 1995). A range of gold- and rhodium-containing jewelry alloys stored in artificial sweat for 1 and 3 weeks did not release rhodium ions (Lidén et al. 1998). Elemental rhodium has not been described as a sensitizer.

Reports have been published on contact allergy to rhodium salts, in platers, gold- and silversmiths, and a precious metals refinery worker (Goossens et al. 2011; Lidén et al. 2011). Seven hundred and twenty consecutive dermatitis patients in Italy were patch-tested with rhodium chloride. Two were tested positive to rhodium chloride, the significance was, however, unknown (Stingeni et al. 2004). Patch testing has been performed with rhodium chloride 1% in water, but experience is limited.

11 Silver

Silver (Ag) is a white and soft precious metal with the highest electrical and thermal conductivity. Among the main uses of silver are photography, jewelry, and industrial applications. The use of silver in photography is, however, declining, while silver is increasingly used as biocide for surface treatment of products in contact with skin. This is controversial due to the environmental toxicity of silver and also due to known and suspected health risks.

Bluish-gray discoloration of the skin (argyria) or eyes (argyrosis) is an adverse health effect of exposure to soluble silver. The lesions from direct contact are considered to be localized and reversible, but generalized and irreversible from inhalation, ingestion, or injection. Exposure to soluble silver compounds may also cause other toxic effects while metallic silver appears to pose little risk to health (Drake and Hazelwood 2005).

Argyria has been described in the photographic industry, from wound dressings and other applications. Silver-treated textiles are used in the treatment of atopic dermatitis. The increasing use of silver in health care is controversial. The effectiveness has not been proven; silver resistance of antibiotic-resistant bacteria and penetration of silver nanoparticles through wounded skin have been described (Drake and Hazelwood 2005; Lidén et al. 2011; Rietschel and Fowler 2008).

Silver is not a skin sensitizer. It is often used together with nickel in jewelry and other items, which may result in nickel dermatitis. Nickel silver (also called German silver or alpacca) is an alloy of Cu–Ni–Zn which often is silver-coated. Silver nitrate is widely used to mark patch test sites, for wound healing, and cauterizing bleeding. Silver nitrate might be a skin sensitizer, and it may cause local toxic reactions when used as a patch test marker. Silver nitrate 1% in water has been used for patch testing, but it may cause irritant reactions, particularly if the solution is old (Lidén et al. 2011; Rietschel and Fowler 2008).

12 Tin

Tin (Sn) is widely used in solders alloyed with lead, for tin-plating of steel, and in brass and other alloys. Tin is used in dental amalgam alloyed with mercury, silver, copper, and zinc. Organotin compounds are used as biocides and catalysts. Tributyltin (TBT) compounds are highly toxic to the environment.

Tributyltin oxide is severely toxic to humans, and it is a strong skin irritant. Acute foot dermatitis in 70 soldiers was caused by socks disinfected with tributyltin oxide (Molin and Wahlberg 1975). An outbreak of irritant contact dermatitis in painters was caused by exposure to tributyltin oxide containing paints (Goh 1985). Tin chloride is a skin sensitizer according to the local lymph node assay (LLNA) (Basketter et al. 1999). Positive patch test reactions to metallic tin were recorded in nickel allergic individuals, the clinical relevance is, however, not known (Menné et al. 1987; Lidén et al. 2011). Tin chloride (1% in petrolatum) has been used for patch testing in single cases.

References

Baker DB, Gann PH, Brooks SM et al (1990) Cross-sectional study of platinum salts sensitization among precious metals refinery workers. Am J Ind Med 18:653–664

Basketter DA, Gerberick GF, Kimber I et al (1996) The local lymph node assay: a viable alternative to currently accepted skin sensitization tests. Food Chem Toxicol 34:985–997

Basketter DA, Lea LJ, Cooper KJ et al (1999) Identification of metal allergens in the local lymph node assay. Am J Contact Dermat 10:207–212

Berlin JM, Taylor JS, Sigel JE et al (2003) Beryllium dermatitis. J Am Acad Dermatol 49:939–941

Böhler-Sommeregger K, Lindemayr H (1986) Contact sensitivity to aluminium. Contact Dermatitis 15:278–281

Burrows D, Adams RM, Flint GN (1999) Metals. In: Adams RM (ed) Occupational skin disease. W.B. Saunders, Philadelphia

Cristaudo A, Sera F, Severino V et al (2005) Occupational hypersensitivity to metal salts, including platinum, in the secondary industry. Allergy 60:159–164

Curtis GH (1951) Cutaneous hypersensitivity due to beryllium; a study of thirteen cases. AMA Arch Derm Syphilol 64:470–482

Daenen M, Rogiers P, Van de Walle C et al (1999) Occupational asthma caused by palladium. Eur Respir J 13:213–216

Day GA, Dufresne A, Stefaniak AB et al (2007) Exposure pathway assessment at a copper-beryllium alloy facility. Ann Occup Hyg 51:67–80

Drake PL, Hazelwood KJ (2005) Exposure-related health effects of silver and silver compounds: a review. Ann Occup Hyg 49:575–585

Faurschou A, Menné T, Johansen JD et al (2011) Metal allergen of the 21st century–a review on exposure, epidemiology and clinical manifestations of palladium allergy. Contact Dermatitis 64:185–195

Fowler JF Jr, Perryman JH, Quinlan B (2008) Positive patch-test reactions to platinum are rare. Dermatitis 19:146–147

Gawkrodger DJ (2004) Occupational skin cancers. Occup Med (Lond) 54:458–463

Gebhart M, Geier J (1996) Evaluation of patch test results with denture material series. Contact Dermatitis 34:191–195

Geier J, Vieluf D, Fuchs T (1996) Patch testing with cadmium chloride. Contact Dermatitis 34:73–74

Goh CL (1985) Irritant dermatitis from tri-N-butyl tin oxide in paint. Contact Dermatitis 12:161–163

Goossens A, Cattaert N, Nemery B et al (2011) Occupational allergic contact dermatitis caused by rhodium solutions. Contact Dermatitis 64:158–161

Hostynek JJ, Maibach HI (2004) Copper hypersensitivity: dermatologic aspects. Dermatol Ther 17:328–333

Järup L (2003) Hazards of heavy metal contamination. Br Med Bull 68:167–182

Julander A, Skare L, Mulder M et al (2010) Skin deposition of nickel, cobalt, and chromium in production of gas turbines and space propulsion components. Ann Occup Hyg 54:340–350

Kanerva L, Komulainen M, Estlander T et al (1993) Occupational allergic contact dermatitis from mercury. Contact Dermatitis 28:26–28

Karlberg AT, Boman A, Wahlberg JE (1983) Copper–a rare sensitizer. Contact Dermatitis 9:134–139

Kligman AM (1966) The identification of contact allergens by human assay. 3. The maximization test: a procedure for screening and rating contact sensitizers. J Invest Dermatol 47:393–409

Kreiss K, Day GA, Schuler CR (2007) Beryllium: a modern industrial hazard. Annu Rev Public Health 28:259–277

Krewski D, Yokel RA, Nieboer E et al (2007) Human health risk assessment for aluminium, aluminium oxide, and aluminium hydroxide. J Toxicol Environ Health B Crit Rev 10(Suppl 1):1–269

Lee JY, Yoo JM, Cho BK et al (2001) Contact dermatitis in Korean dental technicians. Contact Dermatitis 45:13–16

Lidén C (1994) Cold-impregnated aluminium. A new source of nickel exposure. Contact Dermatitis 31:22–24

Lidén C, Wahlberg JE, Maibach HI (1995) Skin. In: Goyer RA, Klaassen CD, Waalkes MP (eds) Metal toxicology. Academic, San Diego

Lidén C, Nordenadler M, Skare L (1998) Metal release from gold-containing jewelry materials: no gold release detected. Contact Dermatitis 39:281–285

Lidén C, Skare L, Nise G et al (2008) Deposition of nickel, chromium, and cobalt on the skin in some occupations – assessment by acid wipe sampling. Contact Dermatitis 58:347–354

Lidén C, Bruze M, Thyssen JP et al (2011) Metals. In: Johansen JD, Frosch P, Lepoittevin J-P (eds) Contact dermatitis, 5th edn. Springer, Berlin

Menné T, Andersen KE, Kaaber K et al (1987) Tin: an overlooked contact sensitizer? Contact Dermatitis 16:9–10

Molin L, Wahlberg JE (1975) Toxic skin reactions caused by tributyltin oxide (tbto) in socks. Berufsdermatosen 23:138–142

Munro-Ashman D, Munro DD, Hughes TH (1969) Contact dermatitis from palladium. Trans St Johns Hosp Dermatol Soc 55:196–197

Peters T, Hani N, Kirchberg K et al (1998) Occupational contact sensitivity to aluminium in a machine construction plant worker. Contact Dermatitis 39:322–323

Rietschel RL, Fowler JFJ (2008) Metals. In: Fisher's contact dermatitis, 6th edn. BC Decker, Hamilton

Stefaniak AB, Virji MA, Day GA (2011) Release of beryllium from beryllium-containing materials in artificial skin surface film liquids. Ann Occup Hyg 55:57–69

Stingeni L, Brunelli L, Lisi P (2004) Contact sensitivity to rhodium and iridium in consecutively patch tested subjects. Contact Dermatitis 51:316–317

Vahter M, Åkesson A, Lidén C et al (2007) Gender differences in the disposition and toxicity of metals. Environ Res 104:85–95

Wahlberg JE (1977) Routine patch testing with cadmium chloride. Contact Dermatitis 3:293–296

Wahlberg JE, Boman A (1979) Guinea pig maximization test method – cadmium chloride. Contact Dermatitis 5:405

Wahlberg JE, Boman A (1985) Guinea pig maximization test. Curr Probl Dermatol 14:59–106

Wahlberg JE, Boman AS (1992) Cross-reactivity to palladium and nickel studied in the guinea pig. Acta Derm Venereol 72:95–97

Wahlberg JE, Lidén C (1999) Cross-reactivity patterns of palladium and nickel studied by repeated open applications (ROATs) to the skin of guinea pigs. Contact Dermatitis 41:145–149

Watsky KL (2007) Occupational allergic contact dermatitis to platinum, palladium, and gold. Contact Dermatitis 57:382–383

Wild P, Bourgkard E, Paris C (2009) Lung cancer and exposure to metals: the epidemiological evidence. Methods Mol Biol 472: 139–167

Wöhrl S, Hemmer W, Focke M et al (2001) Copper allergy revisited. J Am Acad Dermatol 45:863–870

48 Cement

Christian Avnstorp
Dermatology Clinic, Rødovre, Denmark

Core Messages

- The content of chromium in cement is mostly determined by the presence of chromium compounds in the raw materials.
- Water-soluble hexavalent chromate, Cr(VI), in the cement causes chromium allergy.
- Cement eczema is of an irritant and allergic nature.
- The medical course of allergic cement eczema is often of a chronic nature.
- The development of allergic cement eczema may be prevented by adding ferrous sulfate to the cement.

Cement eczema is of an irritant and allergic nature. Water-soluble hexavalent chromate, Cr(VI), in the cement causes chromium allergy, that may cause the development of allergic cement eczema. The medical course of allergic cement eczema is often of a chronic nature. The development of allergic cement eczema may be prevented by adding ferrous sulfate to the cement. Ferrous sulfate reduces the highly water-soluble allergenic Cr(VI) to Cr(III) with a lower solubility.

1 Introduction

Irritant dermatitis caused by cement was described as early as 1700 (Calnan 1960). In 1908, the first cases of cement eczema since the introduction of modern Portland cement were seen among workers building the Metro in Paris and were described as "la gale du ciment" (Martial 1908). In 1950, Jaeger and Pelloni brought to light the importance of the chromium content of cement as the cause of chromium allergy among workers with cement eczema. In 1970, Høvding published an epidemiological study in which 20 (5.5%) from a group of 366 bricklayers and bricklayers' assistants had cement eczema. Seventeen of these workers with cement eczema (85%) reacted positively to patch tests with chromate (Høvding 1970).

Since then, cement eczema has been found to be one of the most serious occupational health problems in building trades and industries. This has been further illustrated by the high frequency of cement dermatitis in underground workers during construction of the English Channel tunnel between England and France (Irvine et al. 1994), among workers from the construction industry in Taiwan (Sun et al. 1995), construction workers in Spain (Condé-Salazar et al. 1995) and developing countries such as Senagal (Niang et al. 2007). In the United States, the Occupational Health Foundation has been focusing on the problem (Occupational Health Foundation 1996).

In Singapore, being a high active building and construction area, prevalences of chromium allergy decreased from 6.3% in 1984–1985 to 2.7% in 1986–1990. But increased again to 5.6% in the years 2001–2003 (Goon and Goh 2005). Another study from the same area showed increasing numbers of workers from the building and construction trades affected by irritant contact dermatitis to cement and chromium being a constant sensitizer from 1989–1998 to 2003–2004 (Lim and Goon 2007). In a retrospective study from Turkey, occupational contact dermatitis was diagnosed in 77 of the patients with positive reactions (27.5%), most of these being construction workers and house painters who showed relevant sensitizations to potassium dichromate, cobalt chloride, thiuram mix and carba mix. (Akasya-Hillenbrand and Özkaya-Bayazit 2002).

In a survey from Taiwan the most important source of chromate exposure was cement. There are about 846,000 construction workers in Taiwan (about 12% of all laborers), and this was the most common occupation of the individuals who were sensitized to chromate. In fact, 21% of construction workers have experienced occupational dermatitis. The prevalence of chromate-sensitized individuals did not change much over time (4.7% in 1978–1990 to 4.4% in 1991–2003). (Cheng et al. 2008). This study is based on data from the National Taiwan University Hospital. The hospital is a tertiary referral center. Therefore these data are not representative for the conditions on the working places. Taiwan has introduced chromate reduction 2003 (Chia-Yu Chu, 2010, Personal communication).

In Finland incidence rates of occupational allergic dermatitis among men was found highest due to chromium allergy. Among these a high proportion was caused by cement contact (Kanerva et al. 2000). In the UK 22,184 cases of occupational contact dermatitis were reported by dermatologists in the period 1993–2004. This comprised

T. Rustemeyer, P. Elsner, S.M. John & H.I. Maibach (eds.), *Kanerva's Occupational Dermatology*,
DOI 10.1007/978-3-642-02035-3_48,

77% of all types of occupational skin diseases reported. Of these chromium supported to play a role in 1,226 cases (6%). The commonest occupations were within building and construction (Athavale et al. 2007).

In Brazil apparently there have been no changes in allergenic substances, contrary to what is happening in more socially and economically developed countries, where the use of ferrous sulfate has been adopted to decrease sensitization to chromium and precautions have been taken in rubber manufacture. In the period May 2000 to December 2005, workers who were submitted to the Outpatient's Clinic of Skin Allergy and Occupational Dermatoses in Sao Paulo, where patch tested with the standard series of the Brazilian Contact Dermatitis Research Group (GBEDC). In the study period, 596 patients were patch tested. Of these 86 were construction workers. The five most frequent allergens among the construction workers were potassium dichromate (57.0%), carba mix (34.9%), cobalt chloride (30.2%), thiuram mix (27.9), and neomycin (19.8%) (Macedo et al. 2007).

Latest data on chromium allergy related to cement exposure are summarized in *Table 48.1.*

By adding ferrous sulfate to the cement, it is possible to prevent the development of allergic cement eczema. This was illustrated in an epidemiological intervention study from Denmark (Avnstorp 1992) and in a 12 year follow-up study also from Denmark (Johansen et al. 2000).

Same trends have been reported from Finland and Sweden (Roto et al. 1996). The total burden of chromium on the body has shown to decrease after adding ferrous sulfate to cement. Especially among cement workers with severe and continuous hand dermatitis (Chou et al. 2008). This is an essential finding that put further light to the induction and chronicity of allergic cement eczema among workers daily exposed to Cr(VI) in cement-containing products.

Further information about those being affected by cement eczema is detailed in Chap.135, "Cement Workers," and Chap.141, "Construction Workers."

Table 48.1
Latest epidemiological data on chromium allergy related to cement exposure

Prevalences in percentages		
Singapore	5.6	Goon and Goh (2005)
Taiwan	4.4–4.7	Cheng et al. (2008)
UK	6.0	Athavale et al. (2007)

2 The Evolution of Cement

Cement is a material which binds together solid bodies (aggregate) by hardening from a plastic state. The Latin word "cementum" means crushed stone. In 1824 Joseph Aspdin, a British builder, patented a cement produced by firing a mixture of limestone and clay (Bogue 1949). He called his product Portland cement because it was similar in appearance to a building stone quarried on the island of Portland of the south coast of England. In 1845, the first Portland cement, in the modern sense of the term, was produced by firing such a mixture to temperatures from 1200°C to 1400°C (Cement and Concrete Association Publication 1977).

Portland cement is a hydraulic cement. Hydraulic cements are defined as cements that not only harden by reacting with water but also form a water-resistant product. Portland cement is produced by pulverizing clinkers consisting essentially of hydraulic calcium silicates, usually containing one or more of the forms of calcium sulfate as an interground addition. Clinkers are 5–25-mm diameter nodules of a sintered material which is produced when a raw mixture of limestone and clay is heated to high temperatures (Mehta 1986). The chemical reactions taking place in the cement kiln system can be approximately represented as shown in *Fig. 48.1.*

The concrete used today is a mixture of Portland cement, sand, stones, and water. Mortar consists of a mixture of Portland cement, sand, water, and often also hydrated lime. The exact composition depends on the purpose for which the product is to be used.

The potential source of water-soluble hexavalent chromate Cr(VI) in cement is the trivalent Cr(III) compound

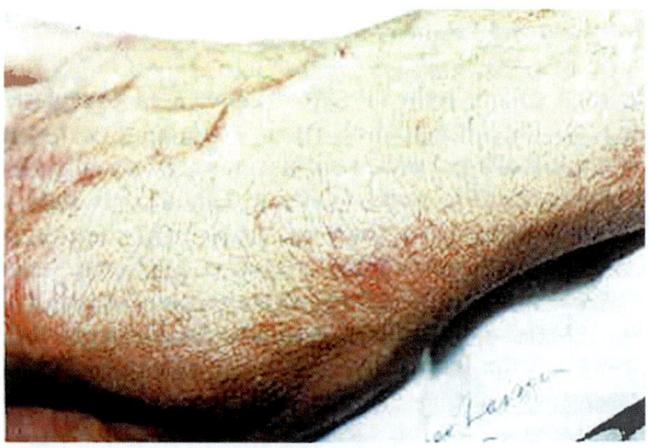

Fig. 48.1
Basic chemical reactions taking place in the cement kiln system

(Cr2O3) in the raw materials from which it is produced. Cr(III) compounds are oxidized to Cr(VI) compounds (CrO2-/4) when heated in the kilns to temperatures of approximately 1,400°C. The content of chromium in cement is determined by the presence of chromium compounds in the raw materials, by the kiln lining and by chromium steel abrasion during the grinding processes (Skomorowski 1985). The Cr(VI) content of cement varies from country to country according to variations in the amount of chromium in the raw materials (Fregert and Gruvberger 1972).

3 Chromate in Cement

The potential source of water-soluble hexavalent chromate Cr(VI) in cement is the trivalent Cr(III) compound (Cr2O3) in the raw materials from which it is produced. Cr(III) compounds are oxidized to Cr(VI) compounds (CrO2-/4) when heated in the kilns to temperatures of approximately 1,400°C. The content of chromium in cement is determined by the presence of chromium compounds in the raw materials, by the kiln lining and by chromium steel abrasion during the grinding processes (Skomorowski 1985). The Cr(VI) content of cement varies from country to country according to variations in the amount of chromium in the raw materials (Fregert and Gruvberger 1972).

3.1 Reduction and Solubility

Ferrous sulfate reduces Cr(VI) in cement to Cr(III) (➋ *Fig. 48.2*). Burckhardt et al. (1971) reported that 62/78 chromium-allergic patients did not react to a solution of 40% cement in water to which 0.3% ferrous sulfate had been added. In a study including eight chromium-hypersensitive individuals, negative reactions were obtained after patch testing with 1.76 ppm of potassium dichromate in water solution. Furthermore, no reactions were found from patch testing with buffered cement after ferrous sulfate was added (Bruze et al. 1990a).

Chromate is highly water soluble (Gammelgaard et al. 1992).

3.2 The Origin of Chromate

In ordinary Danish Portland cement, the chromium content is 40.5 ppm and, of this, 9.6 ppm is water-soluble chromate (Lund 1977). Cr(III) compounds have lower solubility with increasing pH (Gammelgaard et al. 1992). The addition of 0.35% (w/w) ferrous sulfate to cement reduces a Cr(VI) content of 20 ppm to very low concentrations (Fregert et al. 1979). In vitro studies on human skin showed no statistically significant difference in chromium content of skin layers between skin exposed to cement suspensions with the content of 2.1 ppm Cr(VI) and unexposed skin. The content in the dry cement was 3.3 ppm (Fullerton et al. 1993). These findings support the theory that dry cement should not contain more than approximately 2 ppm of water-soluble chromium.

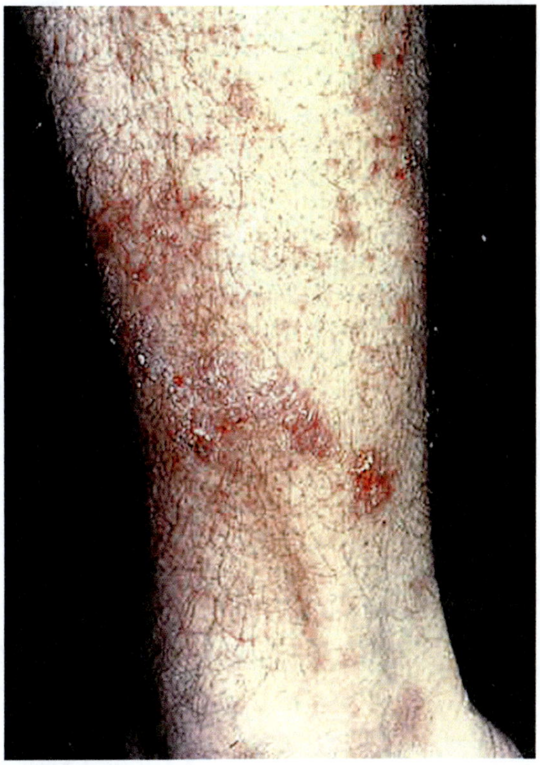

■ Fig. 48.2
The chemical reaction in the reduction of water-soluble chromate by the addition of ferrous sulfate

In 1981, Aalborg Portland A/S (Ltd), the only manufacturer of cement in Denmark, patented a method whereby the amount of chromate in the cement could be reduced using this method, thus reducing the content of water-soluble chromate in cement to not more than 2 ppm at a cost of about 1% of the total value of the cement. Legislation stating that the content of water-soluble chromate in dry cement must not exceed 2 mg/kg (2 ppm) was passed in Denmark in 1983 (Danish Working Environment Service 1983). Since then, both Finland (in 1987) and Sweden (in 1989) have established the same regulation.

Since 1999 the same regulation has been performed in the European Union (EU Directive 1999/45/EF).

The chromate in both bagged cement and bulk cement will remain in a reduced state, as Cr(III) compounds, for 8 weeks. The type of storage conditions used may be essential, especially if bagged cement is stored in open sacks or exposed to moisture because the Cr(VI) will not be reduced when the cement is subsequently mixed with water (Bruze et al. 1990b). These findings were supported in Taiwan where it was noticed that the effects of ferrous sulfate added during production were poor due to the hot and humid environment. Therefore, ferrous sulfate has been provided with the cement and then added on location at the building-places since 2003 (Chia-Yu Chu 2010, Personal communication).

4 Clinical Patterns of Cement Eczema

Cement eczema may be of an irritant nature, allergic or both.

4.1 Irritant Cement Eczema

Depending on exposure, concentration and time, and individual factors, different clinical manifestations of irritant cement eczema are seen (Avnstorp 1995).

4.1.1 Acute Reactions

Cement eczema may initially develop as a result of daily irritation of the skin by contact with cement. The skin of those who have daily contact with wet cement becomes irritated by the hygroscopic and alkaline constitution of the cement. Erythema and dry skin on the dorsal aspects of the hands and fingers are the most frequent findings. Itching of the hand and fingers is the most important symptom (Avnstorp 1983). Acute reactions may develop within weeks. Cement burns are mostly seen in "amateurs," who are not familiar with the handling of cement products. These caustic reactions develop on the lower legs after prolonged contact with wet cement (Vickers and Edwards 1976).

4.1.2 Chronic Reactions

By repetition of the same stimulus or by combinations of varying stimuli, the degree of impairment surpasses a critical level (Malten 1981). Repeated and continual contact with wet cement products in combination with other physical traumas due to the work processes may lead to the development of chronic irritant cement eczema. This may take months or years. The efflorescences may vary with time. These are erythema, lichenification and hyperkeratoses on the dorsal and volar aspects of the hands, fingers and fingertips, and also on the wrists (➲ *Fig. 48.3*). The eczema may be nummular in morphology (➲ *Fig. 48.4*) or include the whole skin on the affected area. Vesicles are seldom found (Calnan 1960; Høvding 1970; Avnstorp 1983).

In general, irritant cement eczema cannot be differentiated from allergic cement eczema clinically. This differentiation should be made after patch testing. If the test reveals a positive reaction to chromate, the eczema must

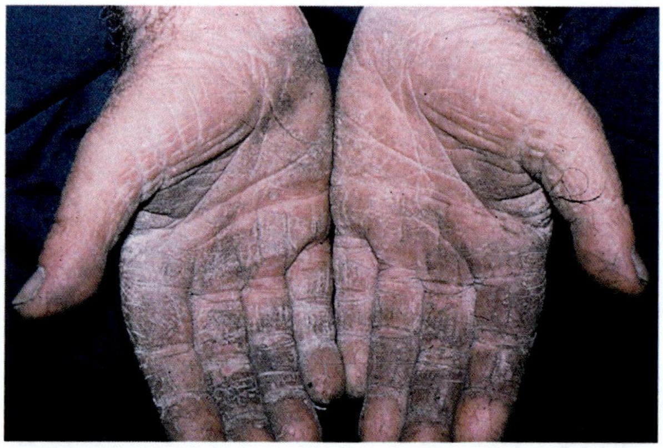

◘ Fig. 48.3
Hyperkeratotic cement eczema

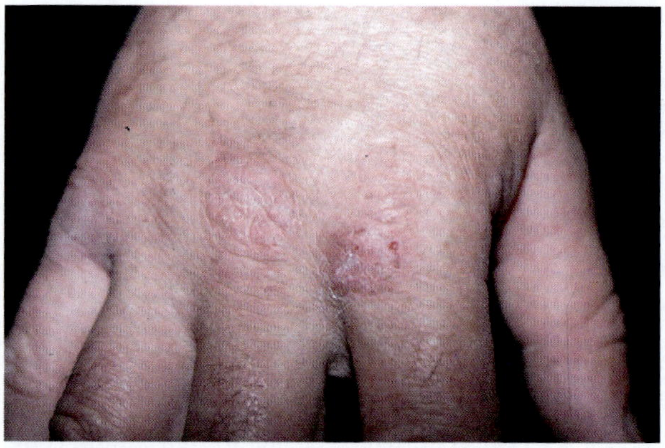

◘ Fig. 48.4
Nummular cement eczema

be classified as allergic cement eczema (Avnstorp 1992). The severity of irritant cement eczema with respect to extension has been found to be mild to moderate, whereas allergic cement eczema has tended to be more severe (Avnstorp 1991).

4.1.3 Noneczematous Skin Changes

Minor skin complaints are accepted as normal among workers who have daily contact with wet cement products (Avnstorp 1983). Mechanical traumas from the handling of bricks, tools, and machines cause occupational stigmata in the form of hyperkeratoses, with fissures on the palmar aspects of the hands and fingers. This phenomenon is particularly seen among individuals working outdoors in cold weather (Avnstorp 1992). In a field study among bricklayers and bricklayers' assistants in Norway, the prevalence of such skin changes was found to be 10% (Høvding 1970).

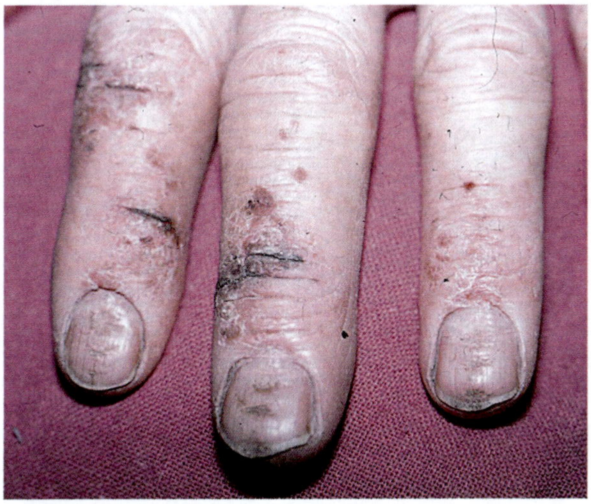

Fig. 48.5
Allergic cement eczema with nail dystrophy

4.2 Allergic Cement Eczema

Allergic cement eczema is primarily located on the hands, fingers, and wrists (Burrows and Calnan 1965; Høvding 1970; Avnstorp 1983). Eczema on the dorsal aspect of the right hand, in particular, has been shown to be associated with chromium hypersensitivity (Avnstorp 1983). Furthermore, allergic cement eczema has been found to have a greater extent of involvement than irritant cement eczema (Avnstorp 1991). Fissures may occur together with nail dystrophy (*Fig. 48.5*). Allergic cement eczema may also spread to the forearms, the feet, and sometimes the face and parts of the trunk (*Fig. 48.6*).

Heat and high humidity exacerbated allergic cement eczema among workers in Kuwait. This phenomenon was explained by the fact that excessive hydration of the skin could lead to increased leaking of chromium through the skin (Kanan 1972). In Singapore, where the climate is hot and humid year round, the number of heat-related dermatoses was, nevertheless, lower than expected, possibly due to the use of air conditioning and good factory ventilation (Goh and Soh 1984).

Although workers with chromium allergy may not be exposed to high levels of chromate in cement, their eczema tends to be chronic. One explanation could be that the exposure to chromium compounds is abundant in daily life, including exposure to leather fabrics (Mälkönen et al. 2009). Leather contains both Cr(III) and Cr(VI) compounds that may elicit eczema (Hansen et al. 2006). Chromated metal products may be another source (Geier et al. 2009).

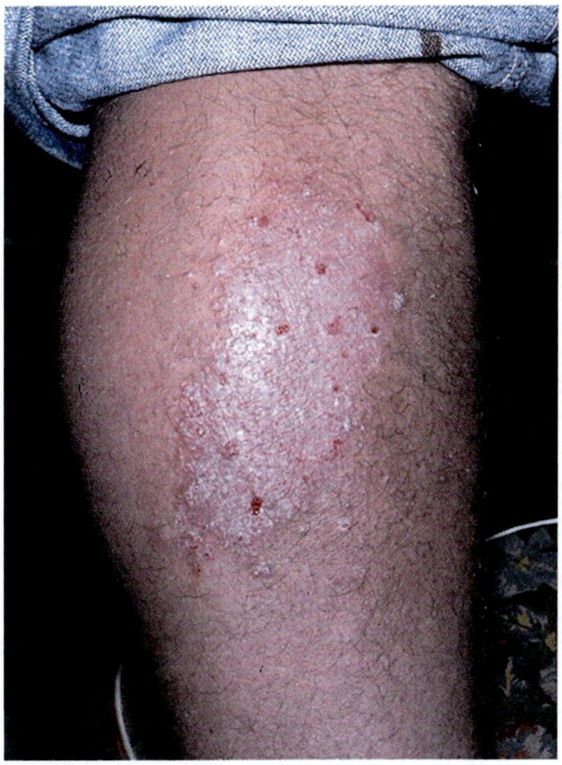

Fig. 48.6
Allergic cement eczema on the leg

4.3 Concomitant Sensitizations

Concomitant sensitivities to cobalt and rubber chemicals have been found significantly more often among chromium-hypersensitive workers than among those not hypersensitive to chromium (Fregert and Rorsman 1966; Høvding 1970; Fregert 1975; Avnstorp 1983; Macedo et al. 2007; Akasya-Hillenbrand and Özkaya-Bayazit 2002; Bock et al. 2003). Among 172 chromium-allergic workers from the Spanish building industry, 82 (47.6%) were sensitized to rubber chemicals. It was suggested that chromium allergy facilitated the rubber sensitization, particularly when gloves were worn in an almost occlusive way for many hours over eczematous skin (Conde-Salazar et al. 1995). A similar correlation has been described among workers from a factory in Singapore manufacturing pre-cast concrete building components (Goh and Gan 1987).

Cobalt could be regarded as a co-sensitization to primary chromium allergy (Goon and Goh 2005).

In a study from Taiwan only one third of cobalt-sensitized individuals were found not co-sensitized to nickel or chromate. Construction workers were found to be the second most common occupation among individuals sensitized to cobalt (Cheng et al. 2008).

Cobalt occurs in cement as water-insoluble oxides, but forms complexes with amino acids in eczematous skin, thereby possibly forming haptens (Fregert and Gruvberger 1978). In cement eczema, cobalt sensitivity is therefore probably secondary to the chromium hypersensitivity.

Nickel is a contaminant of cement in the form of insoluble NiO which, in contrast to the cobalt oxides, is not allergenic (Wahlberg et al. 1977). In a study using multivariate regression analysis, no statistically significant association between nickel allergy and cement eczema was found (Avnstorp 1983, 1989).

Epoxy sensitivity has been observed with relatively high frequency. Bricklayers and workers engaged in pre-cast concrete building component factories are exposed to products containing epoxy resins (van Putten et al. 1984; Avnstorp 1992; Conde-Salazar et al. 1994).

4.4 Hereditary Factors

Combined influences of endogenous and exogenous factors may lead to the development or to aggravation of hand eczema (Nilsson 1985). Atopic eczema in childhood has been found to be a more important predictive factor for hand eczema than occupational exposure (Meding and Swanbeck 1990). In a population of individuals with atopic dermatitis in childhood, 57% developed sporadic or continuous hand eczema during concrete work (Rystedt 1985). When compared with other occupations, such as the metal industry, cleaning, and even office work, equal prevalences were found. Atopic dermatitis and occupational hand eczema has been found to be independent risk factors for sick leave (Cvetkovski et al. 2005).

Mälkönen et al. (2009) found respiratory atopy to be a significant risk factor for the chronicity of occupational contact dermatitis.

In a prevalence study among concrete workers from the building industry, up to 13% of the workers reported previous episodes of eczema other than hand eczema; among those, approximately 50% developed hand eczema (Avnstorp 1983).

Even if in epidemiological terms atopic dermatitis is an effect modifier, it can be argued that irritant contact dermatitis associated with atopy is primarily an exacerbation of underlying atopic dermatitis (Coenraads and Diepgen 2006).

The validity of the information about previous eczema and, therefore, also about atopic heredity may be significantly influenced by the accuracy of recall. It will decrease with time, since those persons who did not have symptoms recently more often will forget their previous eczema episodes.

Age may influence the development of irritant cement eczema. Workers in the age group of 26–30 years are more affected by the irritant properties of cement (Geiser and Girard 1965). The reason may be that younger, inexperienced workers tend to be more careless and, thereby, are more frequently exposed (Goh et al. 1986).

With respect to the development of chronic occupational hand eczema, age more than 45 years has been found to be a risk factor (Mälkönen et al. 2009).

Psoriasis may be triggered by repeated mechanical traumas from handling bricks, tools and machines, and from daily contact with wet cement products.

Filaggrin is a structural protein of the cornified envelope and important for the formation of the epidermal skin barrier. Heterozygosity for nonfunctional mutations in the filaggrin gene may contribute to the manifestation and maintenance of a particular chronic hand eczema subtype that is characterized by the combination of allergic and irritant contact dermatitis (Molin et al. 2009).

Tumor necrotizing factor-alfa promoter and GST-T1 genotype may predict the development of chromium allergy in workers exposed to cement containing high values of chromate (Wang et al. 2007).

5 Prophylaxis

5.1 General Prophylaxis

Irritant cement eczema should, in part, be prevented by automation of work processes whenever possible. The risk of developing allergic cement eczema could be brought to a very low level by the addition of ferrous sulfate to the cement (Avnstorp 1992). Ferrous sulfate reduces the allergenic Cr(VI) to Cr(III) in the cement (see section 3.1; reduction and solubility). In Scandinavian countries, this intervention has shown to be a significantly effective method in the prevention of allergic cement eczema (Avnstorp 1992; Roto et al. 1996; Zachariae et al. 1996). In the period 1996–2000 a decrease in chromium allergy in 10 European centers was found by monitoring the European standard series in 26,210 patients. Although there was a moderate difference in results between the centers, the overall percentage of chromium allergy, 4.6, suggested that the sensitization rate for chromium was decreasing. This could reflect the addition of ferrous sulfate to cement (Bruynzeel et al. 2005). In a prospective study from Germany the incidence of occupational skin disease in the construction industry was calculated from 1990 until 1999. The most important allergen was found to be Cr(VI). In about half of all cases of sensitization, this was the relevant allergen (153 of 335). In Germany cement has partially been Cr(VI) reduced since 1998. Fully reduction was performed in 2002. Therefore, future data will reveal whether the German measure will be effective (Bock et al. 2003).

Changes in the cement manufacturing process by using slag as a substitute for clinker, proportionally, decrease the Cr(VI) concentration of cement. This phenomenon was considered to be one of the reasons for a periodical decline in the prevalence of cement dermatitis among construction workers in Singapore (Goh and Gan 1996). But since then, it has been rising again (Goon and Goh 2005). These results support that prevention of allergic cement eczema needs general prophylaxis in the form of Cr(VI) reduction of cement by the addition of ferrous sulfate.

Reduced numbers of statements and approved claims of cement eczema have been found following the addition of ferrous sulfate to cement in Denmark and Finland (Avnstorp 1992; Roto et al. 1996. Skoet et al. 2004). This economic benefit should be included in the calculation together with spared costs for medical support, lost working days, and personal suffering of the workers developing allergic cement eczema.

5.2 Individual Prophylaxis

The dynamics of the development of occupational hand eczema are not fully understood, but irritation and contact sensitivity, together with individual constitutional factors, influence its development. Theoretically, at least one of the triggering factors could be eliminated if the workers used individual preventive measures. Skin protection creams alone had a small effect on the skin barrier in workers in the building industries compared with skin care alone or in combination with skin protection (Winker et al. 2009). Use of gloves, protective hand creams, and hand washing were not found to influence the propensity for developing irritant cement eczema (Avnstorp 1991). Furthermore, no additional effect was found from individual preventive measures. The absence of influence from individual preventive measures could be explained by the possibility that the work processes are so hazardous that they overwhelm the protective effect. It could also be that the preventive initiatives were not conducted systematically or carefully enough.

In workers with chromium allergy, the use of leather gloves may deteriorate the dermatitis because of the chromium tanning (Fregert and Gruvberger 1979). The use of rubber gloves can cause secondary sensitization to rubber chemicals (Conde-Salazar et al. 1995). Often gloves also contain the remains of cement spills and may be soaked with mould oil (➋ *Fig. 48.7*). The moderate use of gloves may be advisable to protect against trauma from specific work processes, but prolonged occlusion of the skin with gloves should be avoided.

Barrier creams and ointments containing chemicals such as ethylenediaminetetraacetate (EDTA); ascorbic acid; and combinations of sodium pyrosulfite, tartaric

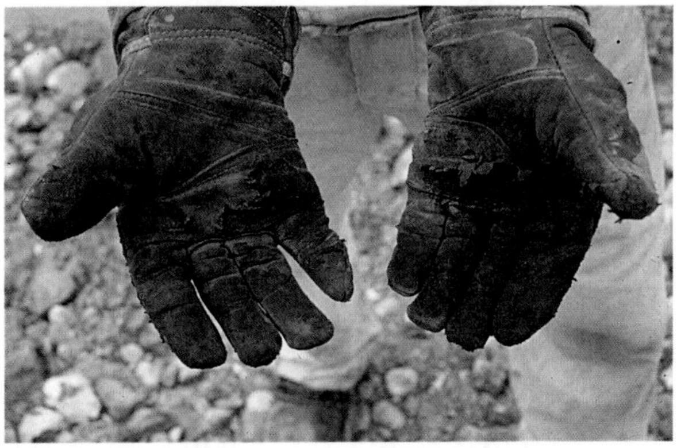

Fig. 48.7
Leather gloves soaked with cement and mould oil

acid, and glycerine have been used in an attempt to reduce Cr(VI) to Cr(III) and to chelate Cr(III) on the skin (Samitz and Pomeranz 1958; Samitz and Gross 1962; Samitz 1970; Shuppli 1970; Amphoux et al. 1975; Romaguera et al. 1985). The effect of these measures under actual working conditions is, however, doubtful. A thin layer of cream can easily be rubbed and washed off, and it can hardly be thought of as an effective barrier for those carrying out manual work. The creams themselves do not inhibit the absorption of chromium (Wahlberg 1971). In general barrier creams cannot replace other protective measures and should be maximally used to inhibit low-grade irritants or in combination with other protectants or in body areas where other protective measures are not applicable (Teichmann et al. 2006).

References

Amphoux M, Woerth P, Grimonnet J, Ha-Hau-Cam J (1975) Doppelblind Versuch mit einer Schutzsalbe (Ivosin) an den Händen von Cementarbeitern. Dermatosen 23:214–226

Akasya-Hillenbrand E, Özkaya-Bayazit E (2002) Patch test results in 542 patients with suspected contact dermatitis in Turkey. Contact Dermatitis 46:17–23

Athavale P, Shum KW, Chen Y et al (2007) Occupational dermatitis related to chromium and cobalt: experience of dermatologists (EPIDERM) and occupational physicians (OPRA) in the U.K. over an 11-year period (1993–2004). Br J Dermatol 157:518–522

Avnstorp C (1983) Cement eczema in Danish workers engaged in the building trades and industries. PhD thesis, University of Copenhagen, Denmark (In Danish with English summary)

Avnstorp C (1989) Prevalence of cement eczema in Denmark before and since addition of ferrous sulfate to Danish cement. Acta Derm Venereol 69:151–155

Avnstorp C (1991) Risk factors for cement eczema. Contact Dermatitis 25:81–88

Avnstorp C (1992) Cement eczema. An epidemiological intervention study. Acta Derm Venereol Suppl (Stockh) 179:14–17

Avnstorp C (1995) Irritant cement eczema. In: van der Valk PGM, Maibach HI (eds) The irritant contact dermatitis syndrome. CRC Press, Boca Raton, pp 111–119

Bock M, Schmidt A, Bruckner T, Diepgen TL (2003) Occupational skin disease in the construction industry. Br J Dermatol 149:1165–1171

Bowles O (1918) Rock Quarrying for Cement Manufacture, U.S dept of the Interior as Bulletin 160, Mineral Technology 22, p 4

Bruze M, Fregert S, Gruvberger B (1990a) Patch testing with cement containing iron sulfate. Dermatol Clin 8:173–176

Bruynzeel DP, Diepgen TL, Andersen KE et al (2005) Monitoring the European standard series in 10 centres 1996–2000. Contact Dermatitis 53:146–149

Bruze M, Gruvberger B, Hradil E (1990b) Chromate sensitization and elicitation from cement with iron sulfate. Acta Derm Venereol Suppl (Stockh) 70:160–162

Burckhardt W, Frenk E, de Sepidus D, Paschoud JM, Szadurski J, Schwartz K (1971) Abwächung der Ekzematogenen Wirkung des Zementes durch Ferrosulfat. Dermatologica 142:271–273

Burrows D, Calnan CD (1965) Cement dermatitis, 2. clinical aspects. Trans St John's Hosp Derm Soc 51:27–39

Calnan CD (1960) Cement dermatitis. J Occup Med 2:15–22

Cement and Concrete Association Publication 98.001 (1977) Portland cement in the making. Wexham Springs, Slough

Cheng TY, Tseng YH, Sun CC et al (2008) Contact sensitization to metals in Taiwan. Contact Dermatitis 59:353–360

Chou TC, Chang HY, Chen CJ et al (2008) Effect of hand dermatitis on the total body burden of chromium after ferrous sulfate application in cement among cement workers. Contact Dermatitis 59:151–156

Cvetkovski RS, Rothman KJ, Olsen J et al (2005) Relation between diagnoses on severity, sick leave and loss of job among patients with occupational hand eczema. Br J Dermatol 152:93–98

Coenraads PJ, Diepgen T (2006) Epidemiology. In: Frosch PJ, Menné T, Lepoittevin JP (eds) Contact dermatitis, 4th edn. Springer, Berlin Heidelberg/New York, pp 147–148

Conde-Salazar L, Gonzalez MA, Guimaraens D (1994) Sensitization to epoxy resin systems in special flooring makers. Contact Dermatitis 31:157–160

Condé-Salazar L, Guimaraens D, Villegas C, Romero A, Gonzalez MA (1995) Occupational allergic contact dermatitis in construction workers. Contact Dermatitis 33:226–230

Danish Working Environment Service (1983) Order on water-soluble chromate in cement. Order no. 661 (in Danish)

Fregert S (1975) Occupational dermatitis in a 10-year material. Contact Dermatitis 1:96–107

Fregert S, Gruvberger B (1972) Chemical properties of cement. Dermatosen 20:238–248

Fregert S, Gruvberger B (1978) Solubility of cobalt in cement. Contact Dermatitis 4:14–18

Fregert S, Gruvberger B (1979) Chromium in industrial leather gloves. Contact Dermatitis 5:189

Fregert S, Rorsman H (1966) Allergy to chromium, nickel and cobalt. Acta Derm Venereol 46:114–118

Fregert S, Gruvberger B, Sandahl E (1979) Reduction of chromate in cement by iron sulfate. Contact Dermatitis 5:39–42

Fullerton A, Gammelgaard B, Avnstorp C, Menné T (1993) Chromium content in human skin after in vitro application of ordinary cement and ferrous-sulfate-reduced cement. Contact Dermatitis 29:133–137

Gammelgaard B, Fullerton A, Avnstorp C, Menné T (1992) Permeation of chromium salts through human skin in vitro. Contact Dermatitis 27:302–310

Geier J, Lessmann H, Hellweg B et al (2009) Chromated metal products may be hazardous to patients with chromate allergy. Contact Dermatitis 60:199–202

Geiser JD, Girard A (1965) Remarques sur les cas déczéma au ciment observés á la clinique de dermato-vénéreologie de Lausanne de 1947–1961. Dermatologica 131:93–102

Goh CL, Gan SL (1987) Rubber allergy among construction workers in a prefabrication construction factory. Clin Exp Dermatol 12:332–334

Goh CL, Gan SL (1996) Change in cement manufacturing process, a cause for decline in chromate allergy? Contact Dermatitis 34:51–54

Goh CL, Soh SD (1984) Occupational dermatoses in Singapore. Contact Dermatitis 11:288–293

Goh CL, Gan SL, Ngui SJ (1986) Occupational dermatitis in a prefabrication construction factory. Contact Dermatitis 15:235–240

Goon ATJ, Goh CL (2005) Metal allergy in Singapore. Contact Dermatitis 52:130–132

Hansen MB, Menné T, Johansen JD (2006) Cr(III) and Cr(VI) in leather and elicitation of eczema. Contact Dermatitis 54:278–282

Høvding G (1970) Cement eczema and chromium allergy, an epidemiologic investigation. Thesis. University of Bergen, Norway

Irvine C, Pugh CE, Hansen EJ, Rycroft RJG (1994) Cement dermatitis in underground workers during construction of the channel tunnel. Occup Med 44:17–23

Jaeger H, Pelloni E (1950) Test épicutanés aux bichromates, positifs dans léczema au ciment. Dermatologica 100:207–215

Johansen JD, Menné T, Christophersen J et al (2000) Changes in the pattern of sensitization to common contact allergens in Denmark between 1985–86 and 1997–98, with a special view to the effect of preventive strategies. Br J Dermatol 142:490–495

Kanan MW (1972) Cement dermatitis and atmospheric parameters in Kuwait. Br J Dermatol 86:155–159

Kanerva L, Jolanki R, Estlander T et al (2000) Incidence rates (IR) of occupational dermatosis. Am J Contact Dermat 11:155–160

Lim YL, Goon ATJ (2007) Occupational skin diseases in Singapore 2003–2004. Contact Dermatitis 56:157–159

Lund MH (1977) Chrom i cement. Nordisk betong 6:28–30

Macedo MS, Alchorne AOA, Costa EB et al (2007) Contact allergy in male construction workers in Sao Paulo, Brazil, 2000–2005. Contact Dermatitis 56:232–234

Malten KE (1981) Thoughts on irritant contact dermatitis. Contact Dermatitis 7:238–247

Martial R (1908) La "Gâle" du ciment. Presse Med 64:507–508

Meding B, Swanbeck G (1990) Occupational hand eczema in an industrial city. Contact Dermatitis 22:13–23

Mehta PK (1986) Concrete. Structure, properties and materials. Prentice-Hall, Englewood Cliffs

Molin S, Vollmer S, Weiss H et al (2009) Filaggrin mutations may confer susceptibility to chronic hand eczema characterized by combined allergic and irritant contact dermatitis. Br J Dermatol 161:801–807

Mälkönen T, Jolanki R, Alanko K et al (2009) A 6-month follow-up study of 1048 patients diagnosed with an occupational skin disease. Contact Dermatitis 61:261–268

Niang SO, Cissé M, Gaye FM et al (2007) Occupational allergic contact dermatitis in Dakar. Mali Med 22:34–37

Nilsson E (1985) Contact sensitivity and urticaria in "wet" work. Contact Dermatitis 13:321–328

Occupational Health Foundation (1996) How to save your skin: preventing skin problems in the construction industry. Symposium findings and recommendations. Occupational Health Foundation, Washington DC

Romaguera C, Grimalt F, Vilaplana J, Carreras E (1985) Formulation of a barrier cream against chromate. Contact Dermatitis 13:49–52

Roto P, Sainio H, Reunala T, Laippala P (1996) Addition of ferrous sulfate to cement and risk of chromium dermatitis among construction workers. Contact Dermatitis 43:43–50

Rystedt I (1985) Work-related hand eczema in atopics. Contact Dermatitis 12:164–171

Samitz MH (1970) Ascorbic acid in the prevention and treatment of toxic effects from chromates. Acta Derm Venereol 50:59–64

Samitz MH, Gross S (1962) Inactivation of chromium ion in allergic eczematous dermatitis. J Invest Dermatol 38:5–12

Samitz MH, Pomeranz H (1958) Studies on the effect on the skin of nickel and chromium salts. Arch Ind Health 18:473–479

Shuppli RF (1970) Über eine neuen Typus von Schutzsalben gegen Chromatekzeme. Dermatosen 18:350–355

Skoet R, Olsen J, Mathiesen B et al (2004) A survey of occupational hand eczema in Denmark. Contact Dermatitis 51:159–166

Skomorowski E (1985) Chromium in Portland cement. Cement Wapno-Gips 1:1–16

Sun CC, Guo YL, Lin RS (1995) Occupational hand dermatitis in a tertiary referral dermatology clinic in Taipei. Contact Dermatitis 33:414–418

Teichmann A, Jacobi U, Waibler E et al (2006) An in vivo model to evaluate the efficacy of barrier creams on the level of skin penetration of chemicals. Contact Dermatitis 54:3–13

van Putten PB, Coenraads PJ, Nater JP (1984) Hand dermatoses and contact allergic reactions in construction workers exposed to epoxy resins. Contact Dermatitis 10:146–150

Vickers HR, Edwards DH (1976) Cement burns. Contact Dermatitis 2:73–78

Wahlberg JE (1971) Absorption-inhibiting effect of barrier creams. Dermatosen 19:197–207

Wahlberg JE, Lindsted G, Einarsson Ö (1977) Chromium, cobalt and nickel in Swedish cement, mould and cutting oils. Dermatosen 25:220–228

Wang BJ, Shiao JS, Chen J et al (2007) Tumour necrotizing factor-alfa promotor and GST-T1 genotype predict skin allergy to chromate in cement workers in Taiwan. Contact Dermatitis 57:309–315

Wexham Springs (1977) Portland cement in the making. Cement and concrete association publication 98.001. Wexham Springs, Slough

Winker R, Salameh B, Stolkovich S et al (2009) Effectiveness of skin protection creams in the prevention of occupational dermatitis: results of a randomized, controlled trial. Int Arch Occup Environ Health 82:653–662

Zachariae COC, Agner T, Menné T (1996) Chromium allergy in consecutive patients in a country where ferrous sulfate has been added to cement since 1981. Contact Dermatitis 35:83–85

49 Adverse Effects of Skin Protective Products, Including Sunscreens

Sibylle Schliemann
Department of Dermatology, University Hospital Jena, Jena, Germany

Core Messages

- The overall incidence of adverse reactions to skin protection products seems to be low.
- Possible types of adverse reactions include aggravation of preexisting irritation, induction of allergic contact dermatitis, photocontact dermatitis, and enhancement of percutaneous absorption of particular chemicals.

1 Introduction

Skin protection products may have unsatisfactory protective action or they may even aggravate the preexisting disease, such as irritant contact dermatitis (ICD). In rare instances, the product ingredients themselves may induce allergic contact dermatitis (ACD). In addition, the potential of some preparations to enhance penetration of certain hazardous substances through the epidermal barrier in the experimental setting caused concern. Altogether, barrier and after-work creams apparently only rarely induce adverse effects, judging by the low number of published case reports on intolerance reactions and experimental studies in the scientific setting.

While many authors reported a satisfactory protective action of PCs, others found no protection (see also ➋ Chap. 112, "Barrier Creams and Emollients") or even aggravation of ICD in the experimental setting. A particular "skin protector" aggravated irritation due to sodium hydroxide and failed to provide action against two other irritants, SLS and toluene, in a guinea pig study (Frosch et al. 1993). Also using a guinea pig model, it was shown that treatment with inappropriate BCs may increase skin irritation induced by cutting oil fluids (Goh 1991). Especially protection against solvents such as toluene appears to be a difficult task (Wigger-Alberti et al. 1998; Schliemann-Willers et al. 2001). Recently, experimental efficacy testing of six skin protection products marketed to protect against "organic solvents" revealed in a human repetitive irritation test that two out of six products aggravated skin irritation induced by *n*-octane and cumene (personal communication) more significantly. These examples illustrate that the protective action of prework creams may be highly specific and depends on the type of irritant chosen. Accordingly, skin protective products should undergo standardized efficacy testing considering the fields of intended use into account by including tests against different relevant types of irritants.

Apart from insufficient efficacy against irritants or even amplification of barrier damage, cream constituents may induce allergic contact dermatitis. Intolerance of skin protection products or after-work creams should be considered in case of worsening of the preexisting hand eczema without other potential explanation. Patch testing should not only include the product as is, but also the ingredients should be ordered from the manufacturer and patch-tested in appropriate concentration(s) and vehicles according to the pertinent literature (de Groot 2006). It is important to identify the single responsible allergen in order to prevent further relapses caused by the same ingredient in other cosmetics used on the impaired skin or by working material. A subsequent confirmatory repeated open application test (ROAT) with the product (➋ *Fig. 49.1*) can be very useful in cases of doubtful reactions, especially in atopics, to differentiate mild irritant reactions (Hannuksela and Salo 1986). Preservatives, emulsifiers, and fragrances are the main potential allergens. Fragrances are ubiquitous and part of many domestic and occupational products intended for hand exposure (see also ➋ Chap. 40, "Fragrances and Essential Oils"). Hands with impaired epidermal barrier function are more prone to secondary contact sensitization. Therefore, the results of a systematic literature research revealing a possible association between fragrance allergy and hand eczema are not surprising (Heydorn et al. 2003). In the EU, 26 fragrances have to be labeled in cosmetics according to current regulation. As a result, a tendency of manufacturers to avoid those fragrances in favor of alternatives that they do not have to declare is observed in Germany (Fartasch 2009). The allergenic potential of those fragrances is unknown in many cases. It is recommended that manufacturers should avoid well-known sensitizers in their products and at best fragrances

T. Rustemeyer, P. Elsner, S.M. John & H.I. Maibach (eds.), *Kanerva's Occupational Dermatology*,
DOI 10.1007/978-3-642-02035-3_49,

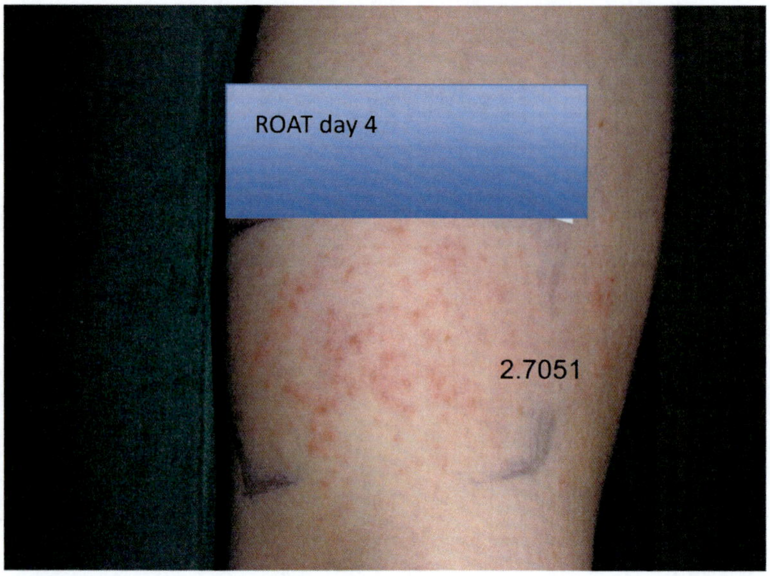

Fig. 49.1

Positive confirmatory repeated open application test (ROAT) to an after-work moisturizer at day 4, after a doubtful patch test result. The contact dermatitis of this hairdresser had worsened in spite of treatment with topical corticosteroids and implementation of personal protective equipment

at all. Potent fragrance allergens such as limonene and geraniol may cause ACD in barrier creams (Tanko et al. 2009) and even when contained in rinse-off products such as hand cleansers (Topham and Wakelin 2003) or washing-up liquids used at the work place (Murphy and White 2003). Methyldibromo glutaronitrile is a preservative that has caused an epidemic of contact allergy in Europe (Schnuch et al. 2011), with creams and lotions accounting for 31% of the identified causative products and liquid soaps for 23% (Johansen et al. 2005). The substance was as well found to be relevant in work creams (Wong and Beck 2001). From 2008 onward, it has been totally banned from all leave-on and rinse-off cosmetic products in the EU and will therefore no longer be found in barrier creams and after-work creams (Commission of the European Communities 2007). Methylisothiazolinone (MI) is another contact allergen of increasing relevance in cosmetics since its introduction as a cosmetic preservative in 2005. Out of 2,536 patients tested in Denmark, 1.5% reacted to MI, and exposure from cosmetic products, such as soaps and moisturizers, accounted for 32% of contact dermatitis caused by MI (Lundov et al. 2010). Contact allergy to MI has not yet been published in the context of being a constituent of barrier or after-work creams. However, the widespread use in industrial products and the potential cross-reactivity to methylchloroisothiazolinone have risen concern and questions about the need for more thorough regulation of this preservative, especially in leave-on products (Garcia-Gavin et al. 2010). Quaternium 15 is one example of a group of formaldehyde donors used as preservatives in cosmetics. It may induce allergic contact dermatitis in persons allergic to formaldehyde, such as health care workers, as has been described after usage of a moisturizing lotion, (Microshield®) (Cahill and Nixon 2005). Chlorocresol is an antiseptic and preservative used not only in topical medications but also rarely in cosmetics. In a single patient from Australia, it was identified as the cause of a severe contact allergy after application of a common moisturizer, Sorbolene®, as a barrier cream (MacKenzie-Wood and Freeman 1997). Coconut diethanolamide (CDEA), manufactured from coconut oil, is used as a surface-active agent in cosmetics and altogether a rare contact allergen. Nevertheless, in Finland, two out of six patients were sensitized from a barrier cream, while three became sensitized from a hand-washing liquid and one from either hand-washing liquid or metalworking fluid (Pinola et al. 1993).

Skin protection products are commonly used together with protective gloves, and some products are explicitly claimed to reduce the unfavorable effects of prolonged occlusion on the epidermal barrier that are caused by gloves. Studies investigating the effects of barrier creams on leaching of allergens from glove material are scarce and produced conflicting results either by showing reduced or enhanced release (Baur et al. 1998; Allmers 2001). Ideally, skin protection products recommended to be used under gloves should be tested in this context.

Topical sunscreens are recommended in outdoor professions as a part of a comprehensive UV protection strategy for outdoor workers to prevent acute sunburns, cumulative actinic skin damage and non-melanoma skin cancer (Glanz et al. 2007; Schmitt et al. 2011). Sunscreen chemicals, in particular UV filters, may as well cause allergic or photoallergic contact dermatitis. The diagnostic method in case of suspected photoallergy is photopatch testing. Photopatch testing should be considered in case a dermatitis predominantly affects UV-light-exposed sites and in patients with chronic actinic dermatitis or obvious photoaggravated eczema. A European consensus statement on methodology, test materials, and interpretation of photopatch testing was given by the European Taskforce for Photopatch Testing (Bruynzeel et al. 2004). Benzophenones ranged among the most common sunscreen photoallergens in several studies (Schauder and Ippen 1997; Bryden et al. 2006; Agin et al. 2008; Victor et al. 2010) (reviewed in Wong and Orton 2011). Other common sensitizers are para-aminonbenzoic acid (PABA), isopropyl dibenzoylmethane (de Groot et al. 1987; Schauder and Ippen 1997), butyl methoxydibenzoylmethane (Bryden et al. 2006), oxybenzone (Cook and Freeman 2001), and octyl dimethyl, 4-tert-butyl-4′-methoxydibenzoylmethane in the USA (Victor et al. 2010). Isoamyl p-methoxycinnamate appears to be a rare photocontact allergen (Darvay et al. 2001; Ghazavi and Johnston 2011). Octocrylene (2-ethylhexyl 2-cyano-3,3-diphenyl-2-propenoate) is a filter covering UVB and short UVA that was recently shown to be both a photocontact allergen and a contact allergen (Avenel-Audran et al. 2010; Karlsson et al. 2011). Other constituents of sun protection products might cause contact allergies as well. Recently, four cases of copolymer allergy to C30–38 olefin/isopropyl maleate/MA copolymer (CAS 75535-27- 2) in a sunscreen were reported. Copolymers are chemical compounds that are used in many consumer products. They can be found in sunscreens, other cosmetic types, and topical medications and have been reported as a cause of contact allergy in cosmetics and adhesives (Kai et al. 2011). Other cases of allergic contact dermatitis were reported from Decyl Glucoside as a component of Tinosorb® (Andrade et al. 2010), from tetrasodium EDTA (Sanchez-Pedreno et al. 2009), and case reports upon further ingredients were reviewed in (Avenel-Audran 2010).

An additional concern regarding PCs is the possibility for enhanced penetration of particular industrial chemicals and carcinogenic substances. Skin protection preparations are aimed at prevention of irritant barrier impairment and not at prevention of systemic absorption. However, they are used also on already damaged skin and should not facilitate epidermal penetration of chemicals. Recent research demonstrated that it cannot be generally assumed that prework creams do reduce percutaneous absorption of chemicals, although there are examples of studies showing diminished dermal penetration, e.g., of N, N-dimethylformamide. Application of a particular barrier cream was indeed as effective as wearing impermeable rubber gloves in this study (Wang et al. 2006). Industrial solvents and aromatic amines are capable to penetrate through intact skin, and the penetration may go ahead without any visible signs of skin irritation, although the penetration rates through a damaged epidermal barrier are significantly higher than through healthy skin (Korinth et al. 2003, 2006, 2007). Using diffusion cells, it was demonstrated that penetration of three chemicals, namely, ethyleneglycol (EG), isopropylalcohol (IA), and 1,2,4-trimethylbenzene (TMB), was enhanced when the excised skin had been pretreated with a protective cream against water-based (EG and IA) and oil-based workplace substances, respectively (Korinth et al. 2003). A field study by the same group examined the influence of several factors on the percutaneous absorption of aromatic amines (AA) in the rubber industry (Korinth et al. 2007). The use of a protective cream and frequent washing were associated with increased systemic exposure to AA. The other protective measures, such as breathing masks, prolonged wearing of gloves and after-work creams, were associated with decreased exposure. The authors suggest that some PCs may facilitate the adhesion of particles from the air to the skin in certain industries; as in the rubber industry the aromatic amines in the air are mainly bound to particles (Korinth et al. 2007). There are other examples, such as experimental studies with diffusion chambers or microdialysis, that generated conflicting results, depending on the PC preparations and chemicals used (Loden 1986; Boman and Mellstrom 1989; Klede et al. 2005). These studies show that a potentially increased systemic toxicity risk of specific hazardous chemicals, due to epidermal penetration facilitated by barrier creams, should be considered in selected industries.

References

Agin PP, Ruble K et al (2008) Rates of allergic sensitization and irritation to oxybenzone-containing sunscreen products: a quantitative meta-analysis of 64 exaggerated use studies. Photodermatol Photoimmunol Photomed 24(4):211–217

Allmers H (2001) Wearing test with 2 different types of latex gloves with and without the use of a skin protection cream. Contact Dermatitis 44(1):30–33

Andrade P, Goncalo M et al (2010) Allergic contact dermatitis to decyl glucoside in Tinosorb M. Contact Dermatitis 62(2):119–120

Avenel-Audran M (2010) Sunscreen products: finding the allergen. Eur J Dermatol 20(2):161–166

Avenel-Audran M, Dutartre H et al (2010) Octocrylene, an emerging photoallergen. Arch Dermatol 146(7):753–757

Baur X, Chen Z et al (1998) Results of wearing test with two different latex gloves with and without the use of skin-protection cream. Allergy 53(4):441–444

Boman A, Mellstrom G (1989) Percutaneous absorption of 3 organic solvents in the guinea pig. (III). Effect of barrier creams. Contact Dermatitis 21(3):134–140

Bruynzeel DP, Ferguson J et al (2004) Photopatch testing: a consensus methodology for Europe. J Eur Acad Dermatol Venereol 18(6):679–682

Bryden AM, Moseley H et al (2006) Photopatch testing of 1155 patients: results of the U.K. multicentre photopatch study group. Br J Dermatol 155(4):737–747

Cahill J, Nixon R (2005) Allergic contact dermatitis to quaternium 15 in a moisturizing lotion. Australas J Dermatol 46(4):284–285

Commission of the European Communities (2007) Commission directive 2007/17/EC of 22 March 2007. Off J Eur Union 82:27–30

Cook N, Freeman S (2001) Report of 19 cases of photoallergic contact dermatitis to sunscreens seen at the Skin and Cancer Foundation. Australas J Dermatol 42(4):257–259

Darvay A, White IR et al (2001) Photoallergic contact dermatitis is uncommon. Br J Dermatol 145(4):597–601

de Groot A (ed) (2006) Patch testing. Acdegroot publishing, Wapserveen

de Groot AC, van der Walle HB et al (1987) Contact allergy to 4-isopropyl-dibenzoylmethane and 3-(4′-methylbenzylidene) camphor in the sunscreen Eusolex 8021. Contact Dermatitis 16(5):249–254

Fartasch M (2009) Skin protection. From TRGS 401 to guidelines on "occupational skin protection products". Hautarzt 60(9): 702–707

Frosch PJ, Schulze-Dirks A et al (1993) Efficacy of skin barrier creams (I). The repetitive irritation test (RIT) in the guinea pig. Contact Dermatitis 28(2):94–100

Garcia-Gavin J, Vansina S et al (2010) Methylisothiazolinone, an emerging allergen in cosmetics? Contact Dermatitis 63(2):96–101

Ghazavi MK, Johnston GA (2011) Photo-allergic contact dermatitis caused by isoamyl p-methoxycinnamate in an 'organic' sunscreen. Contact Dermatitis 64(2):115–116

Glanz K, Buller DB et al (2007) Reducing ultraviolet radiation exposure among outdoor workers: state of the evidence and recommendations. Environ Health 6:22

Goh CL (1991) Cutting oil dermatitis on guinea pig skin (I). Cutting oil dermatitis and barrier cream. Contact Dermatitis 24(1):16–21

Hannuksela M, Salo H (1986) The repeated open application test (ROAT). Contact Dermatitis 14(4):221–227

Heydorn S, Menne T et al (2003) Fragrance allergy and hand eczema – a review. Contact Dermatitis 48(2):59–66

Johansen JD, Veien NK et al (2005) Contact allergy to methyldibromo glutaronitrile–data from a 'front line' network. Contact Dermatitis 52(3):138–141

Kai AC, White JM et al (2011) Contact dermatitis caused by C30-38 olefin/isopropyl maleate/MA copolymer in a sunscreen. Contact Dermatitis 64(6):353–354

Karlsson I, Vanden Broecke K et al (2011) Clinical and experimental studies of octocrylene's allergenic potency. Contact Dermatitis 64(6):343–352

Klede M, Schmitz H et al (2005) Transcutaneous penetration of toluene in rat skin a microdialysis study. Exp Dermatol 14(2):103–108

Korinth G, Geh S et al (2003) In vitro evaluation of the efficacy of skin barrier creams and protective gloves on percutaneous absorption of industrial solvents. Int Arch Occup Environ Health 76(5):382–386

Korinth G, Weiss T et al (2006) Dermal absorption of aromatic amines in workers with different skin lesions: a report on 4 cases. J Occup Med Toxicol 1:17

Korinth G, Weiss T et al (2007) Percutaneous absorption of aromatic amines in rubber industry workers: impact of impaired skin and skin barrier creams. Occup Environ Med 64(6):366–372

Loden M (1986) The effect of 4 barrier creams on the absorption of water, benzene, and formaldehyde into excised human skin. Contact Dermatitis 14(5):292–296

Lundov MD, Thyssen JP et al (2010) Prevalence and cause of methylisothiazolinone contact allergy. Contact Dermatitis 63(3):164–167

MacKenzie-Wood AR, Freeman S (1997) Severe allergy to sorbolene cream. Australas J Dermatol 38(1):33–34

Murphy LA, White IR (2003) Contact dermatitis from geraniol in washing-up liquid. Contact Dermatitis 49(1):52

Pinola A, Estlander T et al (1993) Occupational allergic contact dermatitis due to coconut diethanolamide (cocamide DEA). Contact Dermatitis 29(5):262–265

Sanchez-Pedreno P, Garcia-Bravo B et al (2009) Contact allergy to tetrasodium EDTA in a sunscreen. Contact Dermatitis 61(2):125–126

Schauder S, Ippen H (1997) Contact and photocontact sensitivity to sunscreens. Review of a 15-year experience and of the literature. Contact Dermatitis 37(5):221–232

Schliemann-Willers S, Wigger-Alberti W et al (2001) Efficacy of a new class of perfluoropolyethers in the prevention of irritant contact dermatitis. Acta Derm Venereol 81(6):392–394

Schmitt J, Diepgen T et al (2011) Occupational exposure to non-artificial UV-light and non-melanocytic skin cancer – a systematic review concerning a new occupational disease. J Dtsch Dermatol Ges 8(4):250–263, 250–64

Schnuch A, Lessmann H et al (2011) Contact allergy to preservatives. Analysis of IVDK data 1996–2009. Br J Dermatol 164(6):1316–1325

Tanko Z, Shab A et al (2009) Polyvalent type IV sensitizations to multiple fragrances and a skin protection cream in a metal worker. J Dtsch Dermatol Ges 7(6):541–543

Topham EJ, Wakelin SH (2003) D-Limonene contact dermatitis from hand cleansers. Contact Dermatitis 49(2):108–109

Victor FC, Cohen DE et al (2010) A 20-year analysis of previous and emerging allergens that elicit photoallergic contact dermatitis. J Am Acad Dermatol 62(4):605–610

Wang SM, Shih TS et al (2006) Evaluation of the effectiveness of personal protective equipment against occupational exposure to N, N-dimethylformamide. J Hazard Mater 138(3):518–525

Wigger-Alberti W, Rougier A et al (1998) Efficacy of protective creams in a modified repeated irritation test. Methodological aspects. Acta Derm Venereol 78(4):270–273

Wong CS, Beck MH (2001) Occupational contact allergy to methyldibromo glutaronitrile in abrasive cleansers and work creams. Contact Dermatitis 44(5):311–312

Wong T, Orton D (2011) Sunscreen allergy and its investigation. Clin Dermatol 29(3):306–310

50 Acrylic Resins

Kristiina Aalto-Korte
Health and Work Ability, Control of Hypersensitivity Diseases Team, Finnish Institute of Occupational Health, Helsinki, Finland

Core Messages

- Contact allergy to acrylic resin monomers is most often induced by dental products, artificial nails, and anaerobic glues, which usually contain aliphatic methacrylates. Patients exposed to methacrylate products commonly have allergic reactions to a large number of different methacrylates. 2-Hydroxyethyl methacrylate (2-HEMA), ethyleneglycol dimethacrylate (EGDMA), and 2-hydroxypropyl methacrylate (2-HPMA) are the most commonly positive, due to the strong cross-allergy between them. Other commonly positive methacrylates include ethyl methacrylate (EMA), methyl methacrylate (MMA), triethyleneglycol dimethacrylate (TREGDMA), and tetrahydrofurfuryl methacrylate (THFMA). Patients have not necessarily been exposed to all patch-test-positive methacrylates.
- Some products contain mostly aliphatic acrylates, e.g., UV-cured printing inks, lacquers, paints, varnishes, and glues. Contact allergy to acrylates is relatively rare. The main aliphatic acrylate allergens in these products include tripropyleneglycol diacrylate (TPGDA) and dipropyleneglycol diacrylate (DPGDA). Exposure to acrylates does usually not lead to cross-allergy to methacrylates.
- Dental composite resins, UV-curable printing inks, and some glues contain epoxy acrylates such as bis-GMA and bis-GA. Most of the reactions to epoxy acrylates are cross-allergies to epoxy resin – about 20% of epoxy resin allergic patients react to some epoxy acrylates. Specific allergy to epoxy acrylates is rare, and diagnosis requires testing with the specific compound(s).
- Cyanoacrylates and acrylamide derivatives are also rare independent allergens, which cannot be screened by other acrylic compounds, e.g., 2-HEMA.
- Allergic contact dermatitis from acrylic resins typically affects the fingertips.
- Risk occupations include dentists, dental nurses, dental technicians, nail technicians, assemblers of machines and mechanical devices, printers, painters, and workers in paint factories.

1 Introduction

Acrylic resins are a group of plastic substances derived from acrylic acid, methacrylic acid, and other related compounds. Acrylic acid is a carboxylic acid with a carbon-carbon double bond connected to its acid functionality (➋ *Fig. 50.1*). The carbon-carbon double bond (a vinyl group) is the reactive group responsible for the formation of plastics by polymerization. The monomers include acrylic acid and methacrylic acid and their esters, cyanoacrylic acid and its esters, acrylamides, and acrylonitrile. A large number of different acrylic polymers are formed from the monomers, and can be combined with other types of resins such as epoxies, polyurethanes, polyesters, and polyethers.

2 Chemical Structures and Main Uses

2.1 Acrylic Acid and its Esters (Acrylates)

Acrylic acid and its esters, which are also known as acrylates (➋ *Fig. 50.1*), are flammable, volatile, colorless liquids. They all polymerize very easily. Polymerization is catalyzed by heat, light, and peroxides, and inhibited by stabilizers such as the monomethyl ether of hydroquinone, or hydroquinone itself. These phenolic inhibitors are only effective in the presence of oxygen (Ohara et al. 2010).

The primary role of acrylic acid in the production of acrylates is as an intermediate. Acrylic esters are used exclusively for the production of polymers (polyacrylates). Polymers are used mainly in coatings, paints, adhesives, binders for leather, paper, and textiles. About 80% of the methyl acrylate (MA) produced is used as a copolymer component of acrylic fibers. Ethyl acrylate (EA) is used for both solvent- and water-based paints, and in textiles as a binder in nonwoven fabrics and flocking. Butyl acrylate (BA) is mainly used in water-based paints and adhesives. 2-Ethylhexyl acrylate (2-EHA) is used for almost the same purposes as butyl acrylate, in stick-on labels, and in the caulking of building materials. The above mentioned

T. Rustemeyer, P. Elsner, S.M. John & H.I. Maibach (eds.), *Kanerva's Occupational Dermatology*,
DOI 10.1007/978-3-642-02035-3_50,

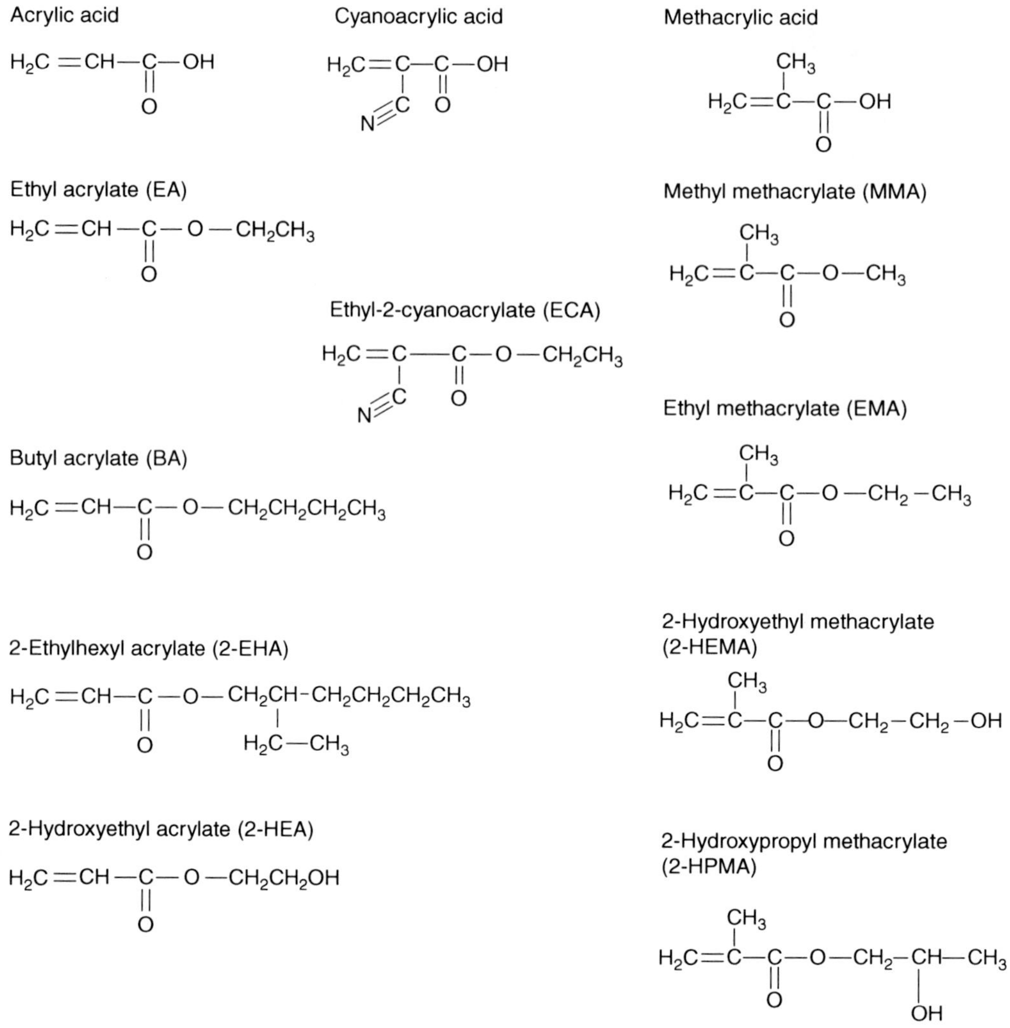

Fig. 50.1
Acrylic acid, cyanoacrylic acid, methacrylic acid, and their monoesters

acrylates have only one reactive acrylic group and are called monoacrylates (*Fig. 50.1*). Compounds with at least two reactive groups are called multifunctional acrylates. Representative multifunctional acrylates comprise trimethylolpropane triacrylate (TMPTA), pentaerythritol triacrylate (PETA), 1,4-butanediol diacrylate (1,4-BUDA), 1,6-hexanediol diacrylate (1,6-HDDA), and poly(ethylene glycol) diacrylates (*Figs. 50.2*, *50.3*, *50.4*). These esters of polyhydric alcohols are used as cross-linking agents and modifiers in rubber and synthetic resins, in adhesives, and as active diluents in photosensitive resins. They are also applied in the coating and ink industries because they can be cured with ultraviolet light or electron-beam radiation. Examples of two industrially significant esters are 2-hydroxyethyl acrylate (2-HEA) and 2-hydroxypropyl acrylate (2-HPA), which are particularly used as cross-linking agents in heat-cured paints, adhesives, and textile preparations, etc. (*Fig. 50.1*) (Ohara et al. 2010) (*Table 50.1*).

2.2 Methacrylic Acid and its Esters (Methacrylates)

Methacrylates are esters of methacrylic acid, which has an additional methyl group compared to acrylic acid (*Fig. 50.1*). Compounds with one methacrylic group are called monomethacrylates (*Fig. 50.1*), and those

Trimethylolpropane triacrylate (TMPTA)

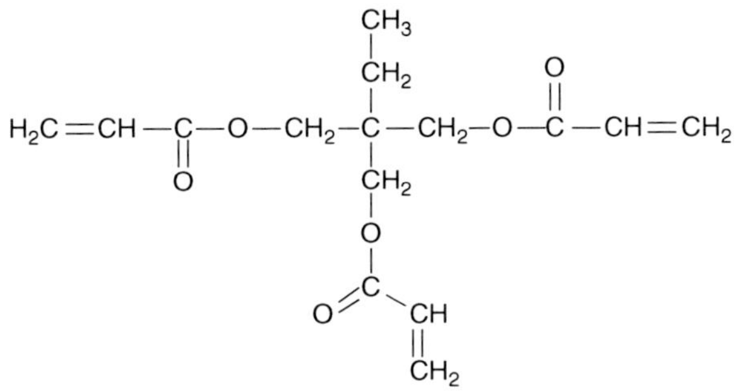

Pentaerythritol triacrylate (PETA)

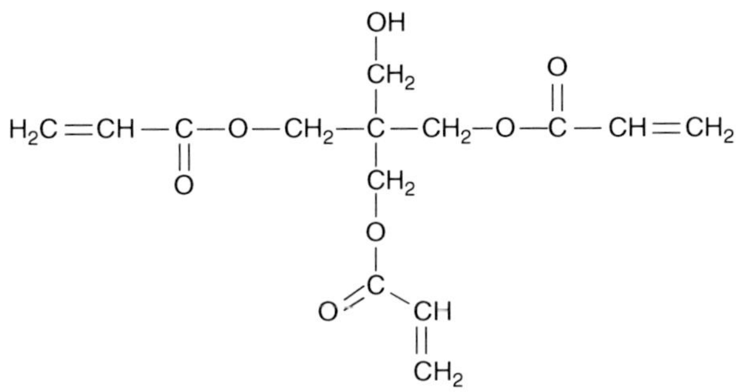

Dipropyleneglycol diacrylate (DPGDA)

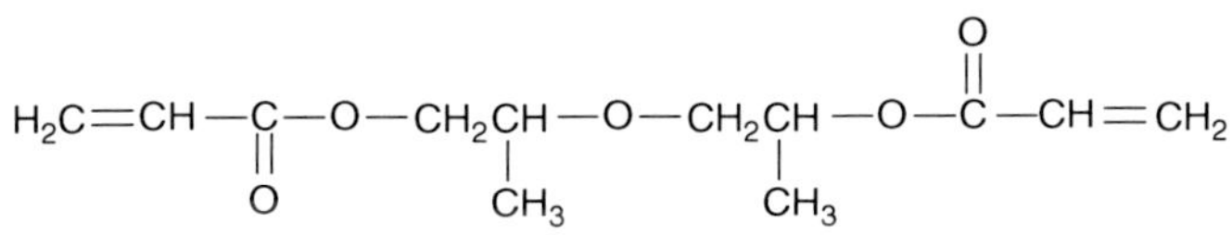

Tripropyleneglycol diacrylate (TPGDA)

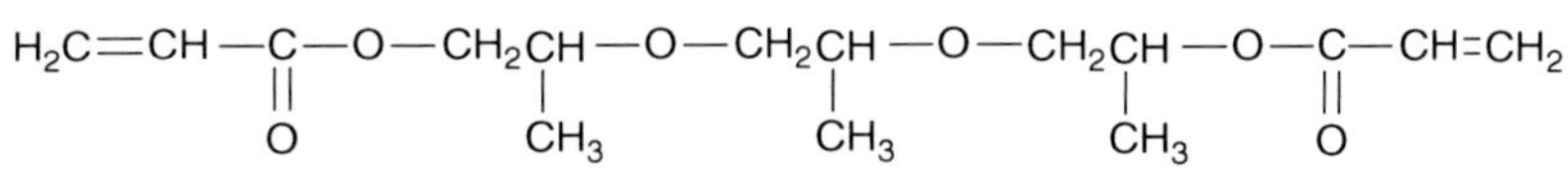

Fig. 50.2
Some multifunctional acrylates

with at least two methacrylic groups are called multifunctional methacrylates (Figs. 50.3, 50.4). Methacrylic acid and methacrylate esters are used to prepare a wide range of polymers. Polymethyl methacrylate (PMMA) is the primary polymer in this category, and provides water-clear, tough plastics that are used in sheet form in glazing, signs, displays, and lighting panels. Automotive lighting lenses and similar products can be prepared from molding pellets. Methyl methacrylate, incorporated into copolymers, forms the basis for durable coatings and inks. Higher methacrylate polymers are useful in the manufacture of oil additives, solvent-free inks and coatings, and binders for xerography. Salts of polymethacrylic acid can serve as the basis for water-soluble thickeners and detergent additives (Bauer 2010). As regards contact allergy, important applications include dental restorative materials, dentures, artificial nails, glues, and orthopedic cements.

2.3 Cyanoacrylates

Cyanoacrylates are based on cyanoacrylic acid (*Fig. 50.1*). 2-cyanoacrylates are utilized almost exclusively as instant adhesives. Methyl, ethyl, butyl, allyl, and methoxyethyl 2-cyanoacrylates are available for a wide

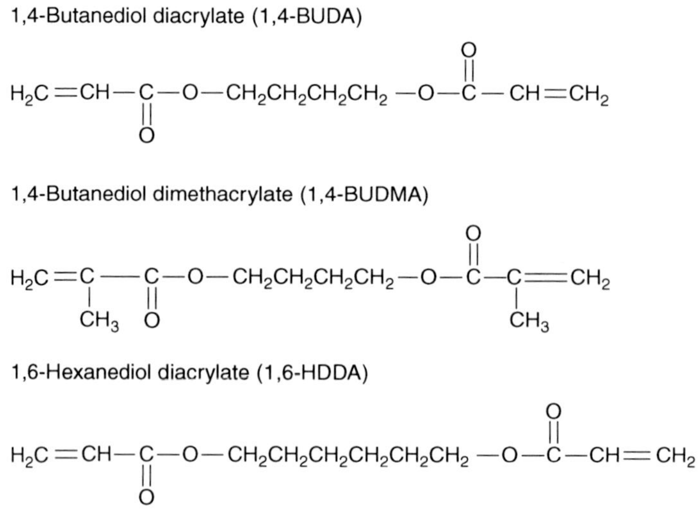

Fig. 50.3
Some multifunctional (meth)acrylates

field of applications. They are used in the electrical and electronics industries, as well as in many areas of mechanical engineering such as automobile, ship, and aircraft construction. In addition to these purely technical applications, 2-cyanoacrylates are used in medicine to close wounds, and in artificial nail glues (Ohara et al. 2010).

2.4 Epoxy Acrylates (Acrylated Epoxy Resins)

Epoxy resins are reacted with acrylic acid to form epoxy acrylates (➋ *Fig. 50.5*), which can be cured by light (most commonly UV lights) or electron beams. Epoxy diacrylate, named also bis-GA, 2,2-Bis[4-(2-hydroxy-3-acryloxypropoxy)phenyl]-propane or epoxy acrylate, is the diacrylate of the diglycidyl ether of bisphenol A (DGEBA) epoxy resin. Major applications include coatings for overprint varnishes, wood substrates, and plastics. Both aromatic and aliphatic epoxy acrylates exist, as well as acrylated epoxidized oils such as soybean oil and linseed oil (Bjorkner 2006; Pham and Marks 2010). In the 1960s, the first epoxy methacrylate, 2,2-bis[4-(2-hydroxy-3-methacryloxypropoxy) phenyl]propane (bis-GMA; also named bisphenol A diglycidyl-methacrylate or epoxy dimethacrylate), was developed for dental composite resins. It is manufactured by reacting DGEBA with methacrylic acid, or bisphenol A with glycidyl methacrylate (Jolanki et al. 2000b). 2,2-Bis[4-(methacryl-oxyethoxy)phenyl] propane (bis-EMA) and 2,2-bis[4-(methacryloxy)phenyl]-propane (bis-MA) have been developed as substitutes for bis-GMA.

2.5 Combinations with Other Plastics

Acrylic resins can be combined with other resins to form, e.g., urethane acrylates, polyester acrylates, polyether acrylates. These compounds are used as prepolymers in dental composites, UV-curable inks, varnishes, and coatings.

2.6 Acrylamide and Derivatives

Acrylamide is used to produce water-soluble polymers or copolymers used for paper manufacturing, waste treatment, mining applications, and enhanced oil recovery (Langvardt 2010). Acrylamide and its derivatives are also used in the production of photopolymer printing plates and polyacrylamide electrophoresis.

2.7 Acrylonitrile

Acrylic textile fibers are by far the largest end-use product for acrylonitrile, which is also used for nitrile rubber and in the production of acrylonitrile-butadiene-styrene and styrene-acrylonitrile resins. These products are used to

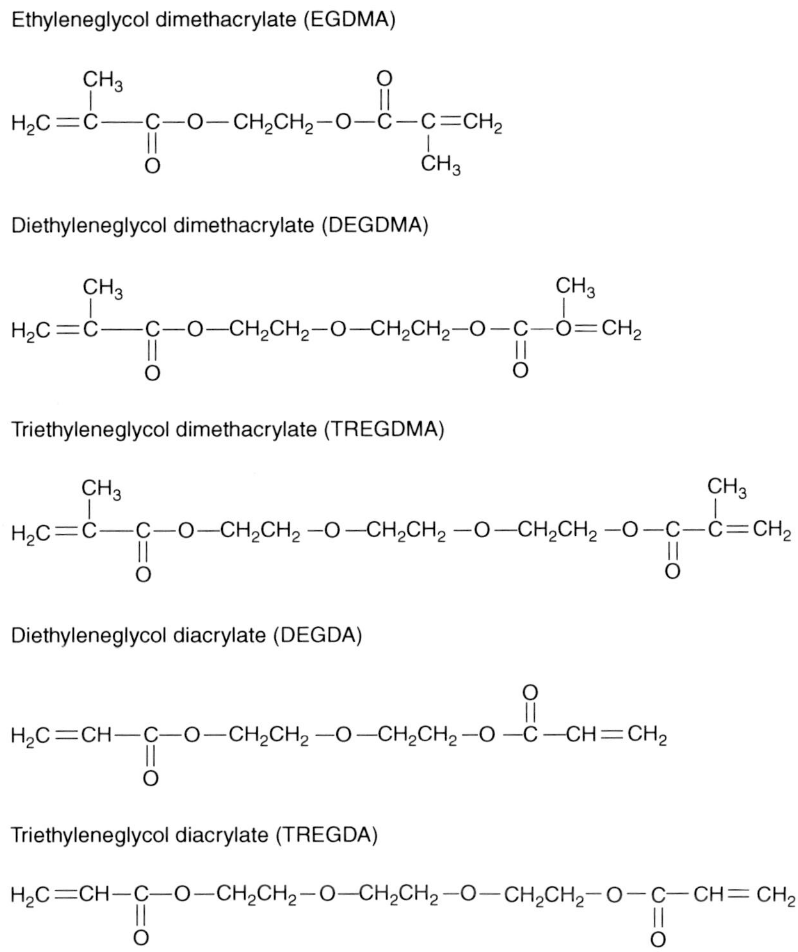

Fig. 50.4
(Poly)ethylene glycol di(meth)acrylates

fabricate components for automotive and recreational vehicles, pipe fittings, house ware, electrical appliances, suitcases, and disposable dishes (Bjorkner 2006; Langvardt 2010).

2.8 Radiation Curing Systems

Radiation curing is a relatively new technology which uses electromagnetic (mainly UV) or ionizing (mainly accelerated electrons) radiation to initiate a chain reaction in which mixtures of polyfunctional compounds are transformed into a cross-linked polymer network. During irradiation with UV light, the reactive species are formed by the chemical decomposition of a photo initiator. Radiation-cured systems can be based on several resin systems. Prepolymers and monomers bearing acrylic functionalities dominate the market. Products with methacrylic groups have special end uses, e.g., in dental products and in the electronics industry. Other resin systems include polyester-styrene mixtures, thiol-thiene mixtures, and epoxy resins (Streitberger et al. 2010).

A UV-curable acrylate system usually contains four main components: prepolymer(s), monomer(s), photo initiator(s), and additives. The most common prepolymers are acrylated epoxy resins. In acrylated urethanes, an isocyanate-functional prepolymer with a polyol backbone can be reacted with a hydroxy-functional monomer (e.g., 2-HEA or 2-HPA). Polyester acrylates are another example of commercially significant prepolymers; they are used in a wide range of applications from

Table 50.1
Abbreviations

Acrylic monomer	Abbreviation
Acrylates	
Methyl acrylate	MA
Ethyl acrylate	EA
Butyl acrylate	BA
2-Ethylhexyl acrylate	2-EHA
2-Hydroxyethyl acrylate	2-HEA
2-Hydroxypropyl acrylate	2-HPA
1,4-Butanediol diacrylate	BUDA
1,6-Hexanediol diacrylate	HDDA
Diethyleneglycol diacrylate	DEGDA
Triethyleneglycol diacrylate	TREGDA
Pentaerythritol triacrylate	PETA
Dipropyleneglycol diacrylate	DPGDA
Tripropyleneglycol diacrylate	TPGDA
Trimethylolpropane triacrylate	TMPTA
Isobornyl acrylate	IBA
Oligotriacrylate 480	OTA480
Urethane diacrylate, aliphatic	al-UDA
Urethane diacrylate, aromatic	ar-UDA
Methacrylates	
Methyl methacrylate	MMA
Ethyl methacrylate	EMA
N-Butyl methacrylate	BMA
2-Hydroxyethyl methacrylate	2-HEMA
2-Hydroxypropyl methacrylate	2-HPMA
Ethyleneglycol dimethacrylate	EGDMA
Diethyleneglycol dimethacrylate	DEGDMA
Triethyleneglycol dimethacrylate	TREGDMA
Tetraethyleneglycol dimethacrylate	TETEGDMA
Pentaethyleneglycol dimethacrylate	PEGDMA
Tetrahydrofurfuryl methacrylate	THFMA
1,4-Butanediol dimethacrylate	BUDMA
N,N-Dimethylaminoethyl methacrylate	DMAEMA
Urethane dimethacrylate	UDMA
Polymethyl methacrylate	PMMA
Others	
Ethyl cyanoacrylate	ECA
N,N-Methylenebisacrylamide	MBAA
Epoxy (meth)acrylates	
Epoxy diacrylate (epoxy acrylate)	bis-GA
2,2-bis[4-(2-Hydroxy-3-methacryl-oxypropoxy)phenyl] propane	bis-GMA
2,2-bis[4-(Methacryl-oxyethoxy) phenyl] propane	bis-EMA
2,2-bis[4-(Methacryloxy) phenyl]propane	bis-MA
Glycidyl methacrylate	GMA
Diglycidyl ether of bisphenol A (epoxy resin)	*DGEBA*

overprinting varnishes to lithographic (offset) inks. In radiation-curable systems, the solvent is replaced by reactive diluents (monomers) which are incorporated into the network during cross-linking. These monomers have two important functions: they reduce the viscosity of the mixture, and they strongly influence the physical and chemical properties of the final coating. Monomers can be divided into three groups: (1) Monofunctional monomers: e.g., isobornyl acrylate (IBA), N-vinylpyrrolidone, (2) difunctional monomers: e.g., 1,6-HDDA, tripropylene glycol diacrylate (TPGDA), and (3) tri- or tetrafunctional monomers: e.g., TMPTA, PETA, and pentaerythritol tetraacrylate (which increase the cross-linking density of the final coating). Compounds such as benzophenone, thioxanthone, and benzoin ethers are used as photo initiators. Additives include, e.g., pigments, fillers, defoamers and wetting agents, flatting agents, surfactants, and slip aids (Streitberger et al. 2010).

Radiation curing is used for protective coatings, inks, adhesives, and in other minor areas. Coatings for paper include clear-coats for laminated paper on pressboard (wood-grain papers to simulate natural wood). Inks and overprint varnishes for the graphic art industry, high-gloss overprint varnishes for magazine covers, record jackets, and various other consumer items are also often radiation-cured, as are plastic coatings for interior and exterior applications. The coating of wood is another important use of radiation curing, and UV-curable coatings are also used for cork in Spain and Portugal. Industrial metal applications also exist: electronics applications, photoresists, solder masks, potting compounds, and conformal coatings are all products based on UV-curable materials. Optical fibers are coated with a protective layer of UV-curable materials. Radiation-curable inks are applied to metal, paper, wood, and plastics. Lithographic (offset) and screen printing inks are the main printing inks, but flexographic inks, intaglio inks, and ink-jet printing are also used. In the printing industry, flexographic printing plates are manufactured from UV-curable materials. UV-cured adhesives on the other hand are often used in lamination,

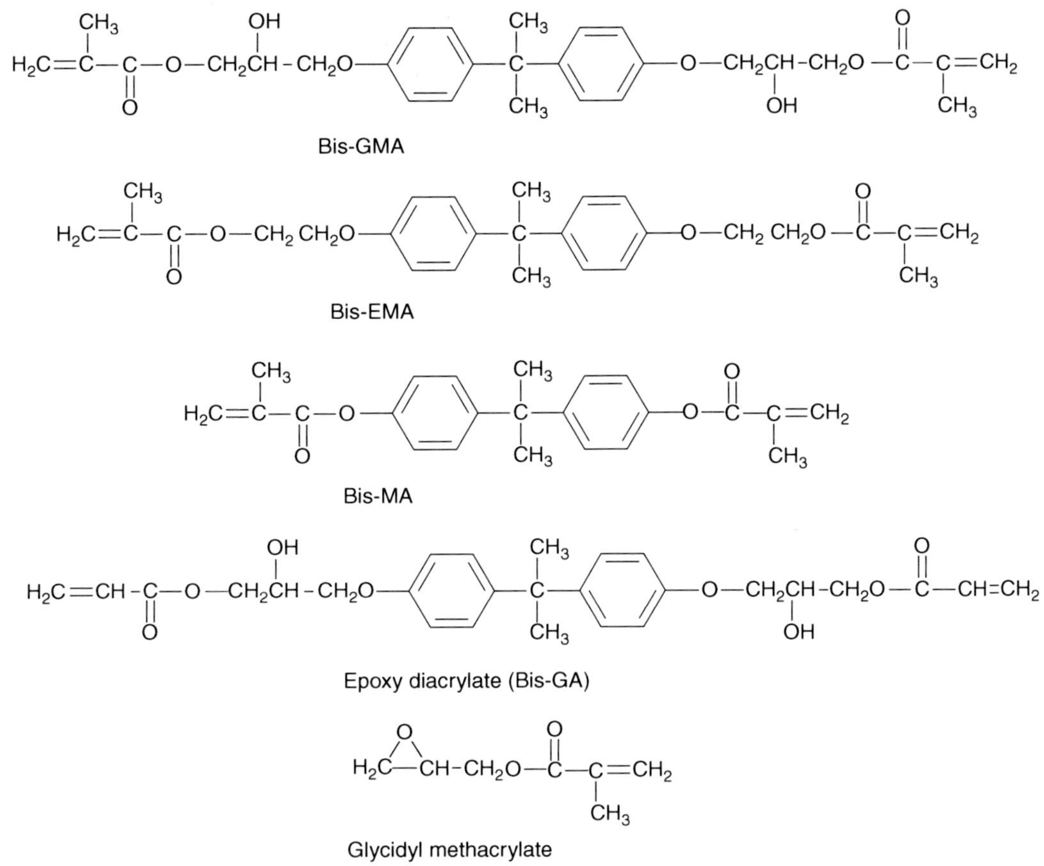

Fig. 50.5
Epoxy (meth)acrylates

and some UV-curable pressure-sensitive adhesives are used in the automotive industry.

An interesting application is three-dimensional modeling (stereo lithography), in which a solid part is made from a vat of UV-curable liquor by the use of UV lasers controlled by computers using CAD/CAM software. Release coatings (casting paper, caul sheet, labels) are manufactured by electron beam curing. Other new applications of radiation curing include binders for magnetic media, leather coatings, and paper upgrading (Streitberger et al. 2010).

3 Allergic Contact Dermatitis from Acrylic Resins

The cured end products of acrylic resin systems do not normally sensitize or cause symptoms in previously sensitized individuals, as they do not contain enough reactive monomers, which represent the actual contact allergens.

Uncured products, in turn, contain sensitizing monomers. Contact allergy to acrylic resin monomers is most often induced by dental products, artificial nails, and glues (Guerra et al. 1993; Tucker and Beck 1999; Geukens and Goossens 2001; Sood and Taylor 2003; Goon et al. 2006; Teik-Jin Goon et al. 2007; Aalto-Korte et al. 2008). These products usually contain methacrylates, to which patients have allergic reactions more commonly than to acrylates. 2-Hydroxyethyl methacrylate (2-HEMA), ethyleneglycol dimethacrylate (EGDMA), and 2-hydroxypropyl methacrylate (2-HPMA) are the most commonly positive allergens. Some products contain mainly acrylates, e.g., UV-cured printing inks and lacquers (Emmett 1977), paints and varnishes (Conde-Salazar et al. 2007), and glues (Fregert 1978; Whittington 1981; Kiec-Swierczynska et al. 2005). In many occupations, dermatitis typically affects the fingertips; sometimes also the hands, the forearms, and the face.

3.1 Dental Acrylates

Dental fillings are now often composed of resin-based composites, various glass-ionomers and combinations of composite resins and glass-ionomers. These essentially consist of an organic methacrylate functional resin matrix, inorganic fillers, and coupling agents. Light-curing systems are popular (Onusseit et al. 2010a). The key chemical in dental restorative resins is bis-GMA (epoxy dimethacrylate). Today, monomer mixtures of bis-GMA and triethylene glycol dimethacrylate (TREGDMA), some other dimethacrylates which act as diluents, and certain urethane dimethacrylates are used. The resins are used together with inorganic filler, usually silica, to form the composite resins. The inorganic filler material is treated with special silanes, e.g., 3-methacryloxypropyltrimethoxysilane, in order to enable a chemical bond between matrix and filler. In a more recent development, glass particles (barium or strontium silicate glass) are mixed with silica. The composites were formerly used as two-paste systems: base paste and catalyst paste. Today, light-cured one-component polymers are more common. They contain a photo initiator system: to cure the composites, visible light is used with camphoroquinone as the initiator, and aliphatic and aromatic amines as polymerization promoters, and only common halogen lamps or blue LED lights are required (Craig et al. 2006). In ormocer-based filling material, the main component of the monomer matrix is an organically modified ceramic. This is a cross-linked silicone oligomer bearing methacrylate groups. Dimethacrylates are used as diluents (Craig et al. 2006).

Carious lesions can potentially arise in the fissures of the posterior teeth. However, when these fissures are sealed with thin layers of bis-GMA or related compounds, the occlusal surfaces can largely be protected from caries. The sealant resins, such as restorative resins, are available as either cold-cured or light-cured systems (Craig et al. 2006).

The acid-etch technique has been used to bond enamel to composite resins. The dental enamel surface is first roughened with an approximately 35% solution of phosphoric acid. A thin layer of resin of the bis-GMA type is then applied to the etched surface, and finally, the restorative resin is applied (Craig et al. 2006).

PMMA has a dominant position in denture base resins. Methacrylates are available as powder and liquid. The polymer powder is mixed with the liquid monomer. Mineral pigments are the principal coloring agents used; organic dyes less so. To avoid formation of stress cracks and to improve mechanical properties, the liquid monomer generally contains up to 10% of a cross-linking agent, usually EGDMA. Depending on the polymerization initiator used, four types of materials can be distinguished: heat-, cold-, light-, and microwave-cured polymers. In heat-cured polymers, dibenzoyl peroxide is generally used. In cold-cured polymers, the polymerization is initiated by a two-component redox system, which is usually composed of tertiary amines, e.g., N,N-dimethyl-p-toluidine, and peroxides, dibenzoyl peroxide in particular. The addition of UV stabilizers is customary to reduce discoloration. Instead of MMA, diesters of methacrylic acid with high molecular mass diols similar to bis-GMA, or high molecular mass urethane dimethacrylates are used as the monomer in light-cured polymers. The reaction of microwave-cured polymers is almost the same as for heat-cured materials. Dental technicians also use similar methacrylates in artificial teeth, crowns and bridges (Craig et al. 2006).

Orthodontic treatment corrects the position of the teeth. For removable orthodontic devices, cold-cured polymers are used. For fixed orthodontic appliances, resins very similar in chemical composition to those used in cold-cured restorative materials are employed as adhesives (Craig et al. 2006).

When commonly used dental restorative materials in the Finnish market were analyzed, bonding materials most often contained 2-HEMA and bis-GMA, the composite resins bis-GMA and TREGDMA, and glass-ionomers 2-HEMA and TMPTA (Henriks-Eckerman et al. 2004).

Dentists and dental nurses are most commonly exposed to 2-HEMA, TREGDMA, and bis-GMA, they most often react to 2-HEMA, sometimes also to TREGDMA, but rarely to bis-GMA (Goon et al. 2006; Aalto-Korte et al. 2007b). Among dental technicians, MMA and EGDMA are the most significant allergens (Aalto-Korte et al. 2007b). Reactions to 2-HPMA, tetrahydrofurfuryl methacrylate (THFMA), ethyl methacrylate (EMA), butanediol dimethacrylate (BUDMA), and urethane dimethacrylate (UDMA) are quite common among dental workers, but these reactions possibly represent cross-allergy to other methacrylates (Aalto-Korte et al. 2007b).

At FIOH in the 1980s, contact allergy to epoxy acrylates was found in five dental professionals, and was always connected with reactions to DGEBA-based epoxy resin (Kanerva et al. 1986; Kanerva et al. 1989; Kanerva and Zwanenburg 2000). These cases, along with the patch tests of other epoxy allergic patients at FIOH, indicated that exposure to DGEBA epoxy resin results in cross-reactivity to epoxy acrylates and vice versa (Kanerva and Zwanenburg 2000; Kanerva 2001). In a 1984 animal study, impurities in commercial products of bis-GMA had a high sensitizing capacity, for which the presence of epoxy resin was a probable explanation (Bjorkner et al. 1984). In 1991, dental restorative materials were analyzed at FIOH, and small amounts (0.01–0.06%) of DGEBA epoxy resin were present in all of the seven dental restorative materials that contained bis-GMA (Aalto-Korte et al. 2007b). In 2001, DGEBA epoxy resin oligomers were no longer detected in analyses of bis-GMA-containing dental materials at FIOH (Aalto-Korte et al. 2009). Although dental composite resins still contain bis-GMA, contact allergy to it was rare in a recent series at FIOH, possibly either because the products no longer contain sensitizing impurities, or because the use of gloves prevents sensitization to this high-molecular-weight compound and its possible impurities.

Patients sensitized to methacrylates may develop symptoms such as stomatitis, cheilitis, or perioral dermatitis after dental care, but these usually disappear in 1–2 weeks. The relevance of contact allergy to symptoms of longer duration and to conditions such as burning mouth syndrome is difficult to ascertain.

3.2 Artificial Nail Products

The use of artificial nails has gained much popularity in recent decades. With the increasing number of nail studios, artificial nails are nowadays among the main causes of (meth)acrylate contact allergy in developed countries (Sood and Taylor 2003; Constandt et al. 2005; Lazarov 2007; Teik-Jin Goon et al. 2007).

There are various types of artificial nails: preformed plastic nail tips (press-on nails), "silk nails," and sculptured nails, which include so-called chemically cured "acrylic nails" and photo-bonded "gel nails." Nail tips and silk nails are usually glued using cyanoacrylate products, but more sensitizing acrylic monomers may also be used. In the "acrylic nail" method, liquid monomer and powdered polymer are mixed and painted onto the nail and extension template. The liquid monomer is typically composed of EMA or another monomethacrylate, and the polymer powder usually contains PMMA or polyethyl methacrylate (PEMA). The liquid monomer is highly sensitizing, but the polymer may also contain traces of monomers, e.g., MMA and EMA (Kanerva et al. 1996). In light-cured sculptured "gel nails," the resins are similar to dental bonding resins: they are serially applied in many layers, first a primer and then the acrylic nail resin, after which the layer is cured in a "photo-bonding box," and the procedure is repeated. A primer can be composed of methacrylic acid or 2-HEMA, but traces of other undeclared monomers can also be found. The resin part is typically based on epoxy acrylates (bis-GMA) or acrylated urethane as matrix monomers in combination with mono- and polyfunctional cross-linking monomers such as TREGDMA, EGDMA, 2-HPMA, TPGDA, and 2-HEA (Kanerva et al. 1996; Sauni et al. 2008). Knowledge of the exact composition of nail acrylics is sparse.

Both nail beauticians and their customers are in danger of being sensitized to acrylic resins. Nail beauticians often wear artificial nails themselves. Allergic contact dermatitis from (meth)acrylates in artificial nails usually affects the hands, especially the fingertips. With nail customers, periungual involvement may lead to onycholysis and deformations of the nail bed, while nail technicians develop symptoms on the face and forearms more commonly than their customers (Constandt et al. 2005; Lazarov 2007). In a Belgian study of 27 nail acrylate patients, nearly all reacted to 2-HEMA, and this allergen was recommended together with ethyl cyanoacrylate (ECA) for screening contact allergy from artificial nail products (Constandt et al. 2005). Although 2-HEMA has also been among the most commonly positive allergens in other nail patient series (Lazarov 2007; Teik-Jin Goon et al. 2007), the results are difficult to compare because patients have not been tested with a similar tray of allergens and there is little information on the chemical composition of the products. In general, the nail patients have allergic reactions to the same methacrylates as the dental cases, but sensitization to cyanoacrylates, epoxyacrylates, and acrylates is also possible.

3.3 Acrylic Glues

Glues, sealants, and adhesives are a relatively common occupational source of sensitization to methacrylates and acrylates, in addition to dental restorative materials and artificial nails (Guerra et al. 1993; Geukens and Goossens 2001; Sood and Taylor 2003). Anaerobic sealants are typical glue products that cause contact allergy (Conde-Salazar et al. 1988; Guerra et al. 1993; Holme and Statham 2000; Sood and Taylor 2003; Aalto-Korte et al. 2008).

Anaerobic adhesives are mixtures of acrylic esters which remain liquid when exposed to air but harden when confined between metal surfaces. These mixtures can be used for a large number of industrial purposes such as locking threaded fasteners; sealing threaded pipe connections; retaining cylindrical machine components; sealing flange joints; bonding structural components; sealing porous metal castings, welds and powdered metal parts; and many other applications (Onusseit et al. 2010b). Anaerobic adhesive compositions usually consist of mixtures of methacrylate esters or methacrylated urethanes, initiators, accelerators, and other additives. Traditionally, methacrylate esters are polyether types based on oligomeric polyethylene or polypropylene glycols (Onusseit et al. 2010a).

In chemical analyses at FIOH, the main components of anaerobic glues were found to be TREGDMA, and diethyleneglycol dimethacrylate (DEGDMA) and 2-HPMA were used as reactive diluents (Kanerva et al. 1997). Further analyses of anaerobic products have also detected methacrylates 2-HEMA, EGDMA, tetraethyleneglycol dimethacrylate (TETEGDMA) and pentaethyleneglycol dimethacrylate (PEGDMA), and MMA (Aalto-Korte et al. 2008) and epoxyacrylate bis-GA (Aalto-Korte et al. 2009). The typical clinical picture of allergic contact dermatitis due to anaerobic glues is dermatitis of the distal fingers (Conde-Salazar et al. 1988). Typical occupations include assemblers of machines and mechanical devices, mechanics, and plumbers. The most commonly positive acrylic monomers in patients exposed to anaerobic glues have been methacrylates 2-HEMA, EGDMA, TREGDMA, and 2-HPMA (Conde-Salazar et al. 1988; Holme and Statham 2000; Aalto-Korte et al. 2008). It is noteworthy that anaerobic glues may contain epoxy acrylates bis-EMA, bis-GMA, glycidyl methacrylate, and bis-GA (Aalto-Korte et al. 2009). In the USA, three glue-related cases were positive to glycidyl methacrylate, and one of them had used an anaerobic sealant that contained glycidyl methacrylate (Dempsey 1982). Bis-GA in an anaerobic sealant had sensitized one worker in Finland (Aalto-Korte et al. 2009). These acrylated epoxies need to be tested separately, as the patients need not have contact allergy to epoxy resin or acrylates.

Two-component acrylate adhesives are cold-setting products which contain methacrylates or acrylates as the monomer, and other polymers (Onusseit et al. 2010b). There are a few reports of sensitization to methacrylates in 2-component acrylic glue products (Kanerva et al. 1995; Aalto-Korte et al. 2008). The patch-test-positive products of these patients contained methacrylates such as 2-HEMA, EGDMA and MMA, and acrylates. The reaction patterns of these patients did not essentially differ from those of other patients who had handled mono-component anaerobic products, i.e., strong allergic reactions to many methacrylates, and milder or fewer reactions to acrylates.

Cyanoacrylate adhesives are one-component polymerization adhesives. Methyl, ethyl, butyl, and methoxyethyl esters of cyanoacrylic acid (methylcyanoacrylate, ethylcyanoacrylate, butylcyanoacrylate, methoxyethylcyanoacrylate) are used for these products; soluble polymers and plasticizers are incorporated to control viscosity, and rubbers for elastification. Cyanoacrylate adhesives rapidly polymerize to form a high molecular mass, but largely uncross-linked polymers. In most cases, atmospheric moisture, or the film of moisture on the substrate is sufficient to initiate polymerization. However, due to this sensitivity to atmospheric moisture, the adhesives must be stored in tightly sealed containers. Cyanoacrylates are used for bonding small items of nearly all substrates. Cyanoacrylate adhesives are also used in surgery and wound management (Onusseit et al. 2010b). Cyanoacrylate glues are rare sensitizers in industrial settings (Bruze et al. 1995; Conde-Salazar et al. 1998) and a few cases have been reported in nail technicians, their customers, and hair dressers (Belsito 1987; Tomb et al. 1993; Constandt et al. 2005; Lazarov 2007). Cyanoacrylates have to be tested separately as there is no cross-allergy between them and other (meth)acrylates.

UV-cured acrylic glues have also caused contact allergy (Whittington 1981; Brooke and Beck 2002; Kiec-Swierczynska et al. 2005; Minamoto and Ueda 2005). These products may contain only acrylates, and the patients may not necessarily react to methacrylates.

Orthopaedic Adhesives (Bone Cements) are used to anchor long-term implantable devices to the neighboring bone. Bone cements consist of separate powder and liquid components which are mixed prior to application. Though many products exist, the powder components always contain methacrylate polymer, a polymerization initiator, and a radiopaque medium. The liquid component contains MMA with small amounts of accelerator for the hardening process (Onusseit et al. 2010a). Contact allergy to bone cements in orthopedic surgeons and nurses is rare.

Window screen repair products are used for repairing small cracks in window screens, and the systems can be UV-cured. A windscreen repairer at FIOH, and three other previously reported cases have reacted to 2-HEMA (Bang Pedersen 1998; Banerjee et al. 2001; Geukens and Goossens 2001).

Non-occupational sources of sensitization include not only nail glues and instant adhesives but also adhesives in electrosurgical grounding plates, skin tapes, and glues in insulin pump infusion sets.

3.4 Paints, Varnishes, and Coatings

Both the workers that manufacture UV-curable paints, varnishes, lacquers, and coatings, and the workers that use these products are at risk of developing contact allergy to acrylates. Significant allergens in these products include dipropyleneglycol diacrylate (DPGDA) (Estlander et al. 1998; Isaksson and Zimerson 2007), TPGDA (Conde-Salazar et al. 2007), and 2-HEA (Geukens and Goossens 2001). Patients often react positively to various acrylates (e.g., DEGDA), but whether the reactions represent cross-allergy or primary sensitization is difficult to assess with the sparse information available on exact exposure. Paints sometimes contain methacrylates, such as 2-HEMA (Geukens and Goossens 2001). As regards wood coatings, nine cases of PETA allergy from UV-curable water-based acrylate lacquer in a furniture factory were reported in Sweden (Saval et al. 2007). The literature contains two cases of acrylate allergy from the coating of optical fibers: one caused by urethane acrylate and TMPTA (Maurice and Rycroft 1986) and another caused by phenoxyethoxy ethylacrylate (Jolanki et al. 2001). Glycidyl methacrylate, an epoxy methacrylate used in the coating of spectacle lenses, caused allergic contact dermatitis in Spain (Sanchez-Perez et al. 2008). In Finland, TMPTA used in the manufacture of printed circuit boards induced dermatitis in one worker (Kanerva et al. 1998).

3.5 Printing Work

Radiation-curable inks are applied to metal, paper, wood, and plastics. Lithographic (offset) and screen printing inks are the main printing inks, while flexographic inks, intaglio inks, and ink-jet printing are also common. In the printing industry, flexographic printing plates are also manufactured from UV-curable materials (Streitberger et al. 2010). In earlier reports of allergic contact dermatitis from UV-cured inks, patients were often exposed and sensitized to TMPTA and PETA (Emmett and Kominsky 1977; Bjorkner et al. 1980; Isaac et al. 1992). In later reports, TPGDA and/or epoxyacrylates bis-GA and bis-GMA have been the primary allergens (Goossens et al. 1998; Scotnicki and Pratt 1998; Kanerva et al. 2000). The main allergens in UV-curable printing inks are thus acrylates and epoxyacrylates, but methacrylates can also be used: 2-HEMA together with diaminodiphenylmethane and triglycidylisocyanurate were the causes of allergic dermatitis in a silk-screen printer in the manufacture of circuit boards (Jolanki et al. 1994). Sensitizing acrylamide derivatives are used in printing plates work (see below ➲ Sect. 3.7), as is 2-HEMA (Pedersen et al. 1983).

3.6 Allergic Contact Dermatitis from Epoxyacrylates

Allergic reactions to bis-GMA, bis-GA, glycidyl methacrylate, and bis-EMA are usually seen in patients with allergic contact dermatitis from DGEBA epoxy resin, who are exposed to only epoxy resin products. About 20% of patients who are allergic to DGEBA epoxy resin react to some of the chemicals, most often to bis-GA and bis-GMA (Lee et al. 2002; Aalto-Korte et al. 2009). The majority of the reactions to epoxyacrylates probably represent cross-allergy, but some patients, however, are sensitized as a result of specific exposure. In particular, allergic reactions to bis-GA without concomitant DGEBA epoxy resin allergy point to specific sensitization. To detect the specific contact allergy, these compounds should be tested separately, because the patients do not necessarily have a concomitant allergy to DGEBA epoxy resin or acrylates.

UV-cured printing inks are a significant source of bis-GA sensitization (Emmett and Kominsky 1977; Bjorkner et al. 1980; Nethercott et al. 1983; Guimaraens et al. 1994; Kanerva et al. 2000; Aalto-Korte et al. 2009), and bis-GA in the production of UV-cured paints has sensitized one patient (Jolanki et al. 1995). In these cases, specific exposure to bis-GA led to specific sensitization without allergy to DGEBA epoxy resin. At FIOH, an assembler of hydraulic devices was investigated. He developed dermatitis while using anaerobic sealants, and in patch tests, he reacted to 2-HPMA and bis-GA, but not to epoxy resin. In the chemical analysis, bis-GA was detected in one of his sealants at an 8% concentration (Aalto-Korte et al. 2009). The literature nevertheless presents many bis-GA-positive cases with no shown specific exposure, but these patients usually have allergic reactions to DGEBA epoxy resin and bis-GMA (Kanerva et al. 2000; Lee et al. 2002; Aalto-Korte et al. 2009). The majority of the reactions probably represent cross-allergy.

Bis-GMA was introduced as a component of dental composite resin in the 1960s. Since then it has been widely found in products used by dentists (Estlander et al. 2006), denture materials (Kanerva et al. 1993; Aalto-Korte et al. 2007b), artificial nail preparations (Hemmer et al. 1996; Geier et al. 2007; Sauni et al. 2008), and in printing work (Goossens et al. 1998). According to the Finnish Product Register, it was also found in some adhesives, in a wind screen repair resin, and in a filler for motor vehicles (Aalto-Korte et al. 2009). Contact allergy to bis-GMA has been reported in dental workers (Kanerva et al. 1986; Kanerva et al. 1989; Rustemeyer and Frosch 1996; Kanerva and Zwanenburg 2000; Geukens and Goossens 2001;

Wrangsjo et al. 2001; Sood and Taylor 2003; Goon et al. 2006), dental patients (Kanerva and Alanko 1998; Lee et al. 2002; Goon et al. 2006), a printer (Bong and English 2000), a silk-screen maker (Goossens et al. 1998), and a mechanic handling coating materials (Kanerva et al. 2000). The allergic reactions to bis-GMA in these studies usually occurred concomitantly with an allergic reaction to the DGEBA epoxy resin. Many of the previously reported dental patients and the mechanic were reported to have been sensitized to DGEBA epoxy resin before developing symptoms from materials containing bis-GMA (Kanerva and Alanko 1998; Kanerva et al. 2000; Lee et al. 2002). In a German study, six (15%) out of 40 bis-GMA positive patients did not react to DGEBA epoxy resin, and the only probable bis-GMA exposure was to artificial nails in one patient (Geier et al. 2007). At FIOH, all bis-GMA-positive patients also reacted to DGEBA epoxy resin. In the literature, 10–18% of the epoxy resin allergic cases had had an allergic reaction to bis-GMA (Lee et al. 2002; Geier et al. 2007; Aalto-Korte et al. 2009). Bis-GMA per se has either low sensitizing capacity or none at all (Bjorkner et al. 1984). The probable explanation for concomitant reactions is a cross-allergy between DGEBA epoxy resin and epoxy (meth)acrylates (bis-GMA and bis-GA) (Kanerva et al. 2000; Lee et al. 2002; Geier et al. 2007; Aalto-Korte et al. 2009).

Glycidyl methacrylate was reported to be the cause of occupational allergic contact dermatitis in a chemist who impregnated paper and textile materials to make them water- and oil-resistant (Matura et al. 1995), and in Sweden an allergic patch test reaction to glycidyl methacrylate was seen in a production worker in a paint binder factory which used the chemical (Gruvberger et al. 1998). In the USA, three glue-related cases were positive to glycidyl methacrylate, and one of them had used an anaerobic sealant that contained glycidyl methacrylate (Dempsey 1982). In Spain, a worker developed occupational allergic contact dermatitis due to glycidyl methacrylate in a liquid that was used in coating spectacle lenses (Sanchez-Perez et al. 2008). None of the six patients were reported as having DGEBA epoxy resin allergy. One case of chemical burn from glycidyl methacrylate has recently been reported (Shimizu et al. 2008). Glycidyl methacrylate is an ester of methacrylic acid and epichlorohydrin; it has a methacrylate structure at one end of the molecule and an epoxy group at the other. At FIOH, in a series of ten patients with allergic reactions to glycidyl methacrylate, the majority of the cases also reacted to DGEBA epoxy resin in the baseline series, and had been occupationally exposed to epoxy products. At FIOH, however, no specific exposure to glycidyl methacrylate was found (Aalto-Korte et al. 2009).

In the Finnish Product Register of Chemicals, bis-EMA appears in numerous glues and in some dental products. In the literature, some cases of allergic reactions to bis-EMA are reported, many of them in dental personnel, often with a simultaneous reaction to the DGEBA epoxy resin and bis-GMA. However, in the literature there are no detailed descriptions of primary sensitization with known exposure to bis-EMA. At FIOH, a manicurist with allergic reactions to bis-EMA and glycidyl methacrylate was investigated, but these compounds were not mentioned in the product declarations, and the products were not analyzed (Aalto-Korte et al. 2009).

Allergic reactions to bis-MA have also been reported in single dental workers. Cross-allergy to epoxy resin does not seem to be common, as 41 epoxy-resin-allergic patients remained negative to this substance in the USA (Lee et al. 2002). In 2008, a search in the Finnish Chemical Register of Chemicals yielded no products containing bis-MA (Aalto-Korte et al. 2009).

3.7 Allergic Contact Dermatitis from Acrylamide Derivatives and Acrylonitrile

Acrylamide used in polyacrylamide gel electrophoresis may cause allergic contact dermatitis in exposed workers (Lambert et al. 1988; Dooms-Goossens et al. 1991; Beyer and Belsito 2000; Aalto-Korte et al. 2002). Piperazine diacrylamide, a cross-linker of acrylamide gel electrophoresis, can also sensitize (Bjorkner 2006). Secondary acrylamides such as N,N'-methylene-bis-acrylamide (MBAA), have been identified as sensitizers in photo polymerizing printing plates (Malten et al. 1978; Pedersen et al. 1982; Pedersen et al. 1983). Patients sensitized to the secondary acrylamides used in Nyloprint® printing plates may react to acrylamide on patch testing (Pedersen et al. 1982). Although printing plates may contain other (meth)acrylic monomers, the patients may have monosensitization to secondary acrylamides and thus do not react to commonly tested acrylic monomers.

A few cases of allergic contact dermatitis from acrylonitrile have been reported (Bjorkner 2006).

4 Patch Testing with Acrylic Resins

It is common that (meth)acrylate-allergic patients have simultaneous allergic reactions to several (meth)acrylate test substances, although they have probably not been exposed to all the positive compounds. Some of the multiple reactions probably derive from cross-allergy between acrylic monomers. However, it is difficult to establish an individual's history of exposure to various acrylic monomers in acrylic products, as he/she will have used various different products during their work life. Acrylic products often contain many undeclared acrylic monomers, and differences probably occur between different batches of the same product (Kanerva 2001; Henriks-Eckerman et al. 2004). When commonly used dental restorative materials in the Finnish market were analyzed, SDSs proved to be unreliable: information regarding methacrylates was provided in only half of the products which, according to the analysis, contained methacrylates. Moreover, some methacrylic compounds given in the safety data sheets could not be detected (Henriks-Eckerman et al. 2004). Impurities in patch test preparations may also have led to false interpretations of patch test results: for instance, in the 1980s technical grade raw materials were sometimes used in commercial test preparations (Kanerva et al. 1989). Many problems with test substances still remain to be solved, e.g., Chemotechnique declares that their aromatic urethane acrylate (ar-UDA) contains some PETA and pentaerythritol tetraacrylate. Sensitization to PETA explains reactions to ar-UDA.

In all larger patient materials, methacrylates 2-HEMA, EGDMA, and 2-HPMA have been among the most commonly positive allergens (Tucker and Beck 1999; Geukens and Goossens 2001; Sood and Taylor 2003; Aalto-Korte et al. 2007b; Teik-Jin Goon et al. 2007). These three allergens are significant for patients exposed to dental products, glues and artificial nails, products which usually contain methacrylates and often epoxyacrylates, but seldom acrylates (Aalto-Korte et al. 2007b; Aalto-Korte et al. 2008). The methacrylate-exposed patients often react not only to the cross-reacting 2-HEMA, EGDMA, and 2-HPMA, but also to other methacrylates, such as MMA, EMA, TREGDMA, and THFMA. Reactions to acrylates occur, but are not very common. Patients with strong allergic reactions to some methacrylate(s) tend to react to large numbers of methacrylates, as well as to some acrylates. The most commonly positive acrylates in methacrylate-exposed patients are EA, TREGDA, and DEGDA.

Contact allergy to acrylates is not as common as allergy to methacrylates. There are no large published materials on acrylate allergy, and in the available small series the relative importance of different acrylate allergens depends on the products the patients have been exposed to. Among the patients investigated at FIOH were several cases in which acrylate contact allergy was limited to the chemical the patients were exposed to, and the patients exposed solely to acrylates did not react to methacrylates. Thus, the results of FIOH imply that although exposure to methacrylates might induce cross-reactivity to acrylates, exposure to acrylates does not usually lead to cross-sensitization to methacrylates. Guin's textbook presents similar cross-reactivity rules concerning monoacrylates and monomethacrylates (Guin and Work 1995). The acrylate-allergic patients at FIOH were mainly exposed and sensitized to diacrylates (TPGDA, DPGDA, DEGDA, and TREGDA), but not to monoacrylates to the same extent. Multiple reactions to several acrylates are also quite common, which imply a cross-allergy between them. When clinical patients are analyzed, it is difficult to draw firm conclusions regarding cross-allergy, because concomitant exposure to several acrylic monomers is always an alternative explanation.

While the pattern of concomitant reactions in methacrylate-exposed patients varies only slightly according to the type of exposure, the diagnosis of contact allergy to acrylates, epoxyacrylates, cyanoacrylates, and acrylamide derivatives often requires testing with the specific allergen.

At FIOH in the 1980s, acrylates EA, 2-HEA, and 2-HPA caused active sensitization in several patients when tested at concentrations of 0.5–1% (Kanerva et al. 1988). The present recommended concentration for acrylates is 0.1% in petrolatum, and most methacrylates are tested at a concentration of 2%. Late reactions appearing after D7 are not necessarily due to active sensitization (Isaksson et al. 2005), and reactions to low concentrations and to cross-reacting secondary allergens in particular tend to appear later.

When testing patients' own products, the concentration of the methacrylate/acrylate product should be adjusted to the concentrations of the monomers in the product so that 2% for any sensitizing methacrylate monomer or 0.1% for any sensitizing acrylate monomer is not exceeded (Jolanki et al. 2000a). At FIOH, no active sensitizations to patients' own products have been observed (Aalto-Korte et al. 2007a). The recommendation for cyanoacrylates is 10% in petrolatum. Testing acetone dilutions of cyanoacrylates in aluminum chambers yields false negative results. Acetone dilutions may be used in plastic-coated aluminum chambers (Bruze et al. 1995). At FIOH cyanoacrylate glues are tested as is, dried in Finn-Chambers due to the simplicity of the procedure (Aalto-Korte et al. 2008).

5 Skin Irritation and Other Effects

Acrylic acid is moderately toxic and very corrosive. The vapor is an irritant to the eyes and respiratory tract, and skin contact may cause burns. Acrylic esters are of moderately acute toxicity, which decreases as the number of carbon atoms in the alkyl group increases. Generally speaking, methacrylates are less toxic than their corresponding acrylates. The mucous membranes of the eyes, nose, and throat are particularly sensitive to irritation. Acrylic monomers can produce eye and skin irritation ranging from slight to corrosive, depending on the monomer and the type of exposure. Liquid methyl and ethyl acrylates severely irritate the skin and mucous membranes, and are corrosive to the eyes, whereas the butyl and 2-ethylhexyl acrylates have less severe effects. Methyl and ethyl acrylate vapors are very lachrymatory, extremely irritating to the respiratory tract, and corrosive to the eyes, causing corneal injury. The lachrymatory effect of the butyl and 2-ethylhexyl esters is weak. Methacrylic acid is more corrosive than its esters (Bauer 2010; Ohara et al. 2010). Handling methacrylate products has caused respiratory problems, rhinitis, and asthma in dental workers and nail technicians.

In humans and laboratory animals, single or repeated exposure to acrylamide caused local irritations on contact with the skin and neurological symptoms. The peripheral neuropathy is a result of long-term accumulation and appears after a latent period. Acrylamide is readily absorbed during oral, inhalation, and dermal exposure. Its genotoxicity, the formation of the genotoxic metabolite glycidamide in humans, and long-term animal studies, indicate that acrylamide has the potential to cause cancer in humans. Accordingly, acrylamide has been classified as probably carcinogenic to humans (Ohara et al. 2010).

6 Prevention

Protection required for the safe handling of acrylic acid and methacrylic acid and their esters includes chemical-resistant gloves and clothing, splash-proof goggles, and effective ventilation of the workplace. Small molecular acrylic compounds permeate common disposable natural rubber and vinyl gloves rapidly. In dental care, at least double gloving with thin vinyl or natural rubber gloves should be used for a 15-min task. For a task lasting 15–30 min, good nitrile rubber gloves should be used, preferably as a double layer with other gloves. A simple polyethylene glove under another glove may improve protection considerably when performing longer work tasks. Double gloving becomes easier if the inner gloves are of a larger size (Mäkelä and Jolanki 2005). The development of so-called no-touch techniques in the application of dental composite resins (e.g., pistols and syringes) has most likely played a significant role in the prevention of sensitization to methacrylates; at least in Finland, methacrylate allergy in dentists and dental nurses is no longer as common as it was in the 1990s. Furthermore, most workers in these two occupations are aware of the rapid permeation of gloves to small methacrylates, and many of them change gloves immediately when they notice glove contact with materials containing methacrylate.

References

Aalto-Korte K, Jolanki R, Suuronen K, Estlander T (2002) Biochemist's occupational allergic contact dermatitis from iodoacetamide and acrylamide. Contact Dermatitis 47:361–362

Aalto-Korte K, Alanko K, Kuuliala O, Jolanki R (2007a) Late reactions in patch tests: a 4-year review from a clinic of occupational dermatology. Contact Dermatitis 56:81–86

Aalto-Korte K, Alanko K, Kuuliala O, Jolanki R (2007b) Methacrylate and acrylate allergy in dental personnel. Contact Dermatitis 57:324–330

Aalto-Korte K, Alanko K, Kuuliala O, Jolanki R (2008) Occupational methacrylate and acrylate allergy from glues. Contact Dermatitis 58:340–346

Aalto-Korte K, Jungewelter S, Henriks-Eckerman ML, Kuuliala O, Jolanki R (2009) Contact allergy to epoxy (meth)acrylates. Contact Dermatitis 61:9–21

Banerjee PP, Banerjee S, Brown TR (2001) Increased androgen receptor expression correlates with development of age-dependent, lobe-specific spontaneous hyperplasia of the brown Norway rat prostate. Endocrinology 142:4066–4075

Bang Pedersen N (1998) Allergic contact dermatitis from acrylic resin repair of windscreens. Contact Dermatitis 39:99

Bauer W (2010) Methacrylic acid and derivatives. In: Ullmann's encyclopedia of industrial chemistry, 7th edn. Wiley, New York

Belsito DV (1987) Contact dermatitis to ethyl-cyanoacrylate-containing glue. Contact Dermatitis 17:234–236

Beyer DJ, Belsito DV (2000) Allergic contact dermatitis from acrylamide in a chemical mixer. Contact Dermatitis 42:181–182

Bjorkner B (2006) Acrylic resins. In: Frosch PJ, Menné T, Lepoittevin J-P (eds) Contact dermatitis, 4th edn. Springer, Berlin, pp 584–594

Bjorkner B, Dahlquist I, Fregert S (1980) Allergic contact dermatitis from acrylates in ultraviolet curing inks. Contact Dermatitis 6:405–409

Bjorkner B, Niklasson B, Persson K (1984) The sensitizing potential of di-(meth)acrylates based on bisphenol A or epoxy resin in the guinea pig. Contact Dermatitis 10:286–304

Bong JL, English JS (2000) Allergic contact dermatitis from airborne exposure to acrylates. Contact Dermatitis 43:242

Brooke RC, Beck MH (2002) A new source of allergic contact dermatitis from UV-cured (meth)acrylate adhesive. Contact Dermatitis 47: 179–180

Bruze M, Bjorkner B, Lepoittevin JP (1995) Occupational allergic contact dermatitis from ethyl cyanoacrylate. Contact Dermatitis 32:156–159

Conde-Salazar L, Guimaraens D, Romero LV (1988) Occupational allergic contact dermatitis from anaerobic acrylic sealants. Contact Dermatitis 18:129–132

Conde-Salazar L, Rojo S, Guimaraens D (1998) Occupational allergic contact dermatitis from cyanoacrylate. Am J Contact Dermat 9:188–189

Conde-Salazar L, Vargas I, Tevar E, Barchino L, Heras F (2007) Sensitization to acrylates in varnishes. Dermatitis 18:45–48

Constandt L, Hecke EV, Naeyaert JM, Goossens A (2005) Screening for contact allergy to artificial nails. Contact Dermatitis 52:73–77

Craig RG, Welker D, Rothaut J, Krumbholz KG, Stefan K-P, Dermann K, Rehberg H-J, Franz G, Lehmann KM, Borchert M (2006) Dental materials. Ullmann's encyclopedia of industrial chemistry. Wiley Online Library

Dempsey KJ (1982) Hypersensitivity to Sta-Lok and Loctite anaerobic sealants. J Am Acad Dermatol 7:779–784

Dooms-Goossens A, Garmyn M, Degreef H (1991) Contact allergy to acrylamide. Contact Dermatitis 24:71–72

Emmett EA (1977) Contact dermatitis from polyfunctional acrylic monomers. Contact Dermatitis 3:245–248

Emmett EA, Kominsky JR (1977) Allergic contact dermatitis from ultraviolet cured inks. Allergic contact sensitization to acrylates. J Occup Med 19:113–115

Estlander T, Jolanki R, Kanerva L (1998) Occupational allergic contact dermatitis from UV-cured lacquer containing dipropylene glycol diacrylate. Contact Dermatitis 39:36

Estlander T, Alanko K, Jolanki R (2006) Dental materials. In: Frosch PJ, Menné T, Lepoittevin J-P (eds) Contact dermatitis, 3rd edn. Springer, Berlin, pp 653–678

Fregert S (1978) Allergic contact dermatitis from ethylacrylate in a window sealant. Contact Dermatitis 4:56

Geier J, Lessmann H, Uter W, Schnuch A (2007) Are concomitant patch test reactions to epoxy resin and BIS-GMA indicative of cross-reactivity? Contact Dermatitis 57:376–380

Geukens S, Goossens A (2001) Occupational contact allergy to (meth) acrylates. Contact Dermatitis 44:153–159

Goon AT, Isaksson M, Zimerson E, Goh CL, Bruze M (2006) Contact allergy to (meth)acrylates in the dental series in southern Sweden: simultaneous positive patch test reaction patterns and possible screening allergens. Contact Dermatitis 55:219–226

Goossens A, Coninx D, Rommens K, Verhamme B (1998) Occupational dermatitis in a silk-screen maker. Contact Dermatitis 39:40–42

Gruvberger B, Bruze M, Almgren G (1998) Occupational dermatoses in a plant producing binders for paints and glues. Contact Dermatitis 38:71–77

Guerra L, Vincenzi C, Peluso AM, Tosti A (1993) Prevalence and sources of occupational contact sensitization to acrylates in Italy. Contact Dermatitis 28:101–103

Guimaraens D, Gonzalez MA, Del Rio E, Conde-Salazar L (1994) Occupational airborne allergic contact dermatitis in the national mint and fiscal-stamp factory. Contact Dermatitis 30:172–173

Guin JD, Work WJ (1995) Other plastics. In: Guin JD (ed) Practical contact dermatitis, a handbook for the practioner. McGraw-Hill, New York, pp 433–475

Hemmer W, Focke M, Wantke F, Gotz M, Jarisch R (1996) Allergic contact dermatitis to artificial fingernails prepared from UV light-cured acrylates. J Am Acad Dermatol 35:377–380

Henriks-Eckerman ML, Suuronen K, Jolanki R, Alanko K (2004) Methacrylates in dental restorative materials. Contact Dermatitis 50:233–237

Holme SA, Statham BN (2000) A cluster of 6 cases of occupational allergic contact dermatitis from (meth)acrylates. Contact Dermatitis 43:179–180

Isaac MA, Thiboutot DM, Vasily DB, Marks JG (1992) Contact dermatitis from printing inks. Am J Contact Dermat 3:142–144

Isaksson M, Zimerson E (2007) Risks and possibilities in patch testing with contaminated personal objects: usefulness of thin-layer chromatograms in a patient with acrylate contact allergy from a chemical burn. Contact Dermatitis 57:84–88

Isaksson M, Lindberg M, Sundberg K, Hallander A, Bruze M (2005) The development and course of patch-test reactions to 2-hydroxyethyl methacrylate and ethyleneglycol dimethacrylate. Contact Dermatitis 53:292–297

Jolanki R, Kanerva L, Estlander T, Tarvainen K (1994) Concomitant sensitization to triglycidyl isocyanurate, diaminodiphenylmethane and 2-hydroxyethyl methacrylate from silk-screen printing coatings in the manufacture of circuit boards. Contact Dermatitis 30:12–15

Jolanki R, Kanerva L, Estlander T (1995) Occupational allergic contact dermatitis caused by epoxy diacrylate in ultraviolet-light-cured paint, and bisphenol A in dental composite resin. Contact Dermatitis 33:94–99

Jolanki R, Estlander T, Alanko K, Kanerva L (2000a) Patch testing with a patient's own materials handled at work. In: Kanerva L, Elsner P, Wahlberg JE, Maibach HI (eds) Handbook of occupational dermatology. Springer, Berlin, pp 375–384

Jolanki R, Kanerva L, Estlander T et al (2000b) Epoxy resins. In: Kanerva LEP, Wahlberg JE, Maibach HI (eds) Handbook of occupational dermatology. Springer, Berlin, pp 570–590

Jolanki R, Kanerva L, Estlander T, Henriks-Eckerman ML, Suhonen R (2001) Allergic contact dermatitis from phenoxyethoxy ethylacrylates in optical fiber coating, and glue in an insulin pump set. Contact Dermatitis 45:36–37

Kanerva L (2001) Cross-reactions of multifunctional methacrylates and acrylates. Acta Odontol Scand 59:320–329

Kanerva L, Alanko K (1998) Stomatitis and perioral dermatitis caused by epoxy diacrylates in dental composite resins. J Am Acad Dermatol 38:116–120

Kanerva L, Zwanenburg R (2000) Allergic contact reactions to poly (oxy-1,2-ethanediyl) alpha, alpha'-[(1-methylethylidene)di-4, 1-phenylene]bis[omega-[(2-methyl-1-oxo-2-propenyl)oxy](BIS-EMA). Contact Dermatitis 43:115–117

Kanerva L, Jolanki R, Estlander T (1986) Occupational dermatitis due to an epoxy acrylate. Contact Dermatitis 14:80–84

Kanerva L, Estlander T, Jolanki R (1988) Sensitization to patch test acrylates. Contact Dermatitis 18:10–15

Kanerva L, Estlander T, Jolanki R (1989) Allergic contact dermatitis from dental composite resins due to aromatic epoxy acrylates and aliphatic acrylates. Contact Dermatitis 20:201–211

Kanerva L, Estlander T, Jolanki R, Tarvainen K (1993) Occupational allergic contact dermatitis caused by exposure to acrylates during work with dental prostheses. Contact Dermatitis 28:268–275

Kanerva L, Jolanki R, Leino T, Estlander T (1995) Occupational allergic contact dermatitis from 2-hydroxyethyl methacrylate and ethylene glycol dimethacrylate in a modified acrylic structural adhesive. Contact Dermatitis 33:84–89

Kanerva L, Lauerma A, Estlander T, Alanko K, Henriks-Eckerman ML, Jolanki R (1996) Occupational allergic contact dermatitis caused by photobonded sculptured nails and a review of (meth) acrylates in nail cosmetics. Am J Contact Dermat 7:109–115

Kanerva L, Henriks-Eckerman ML, Jolanki R, Estlander T (1997) Plastics/acrylics: material safety data sheets need to be improved. Clin Dermatol 15:533–546

Kanerva L, Tarvainen K, Jolanki R, Henriks-Eckerman ML, Estlander T (1998) Airborne occupational allergic contact dermatitis due to trimethylolpropane triacrylate (TMPTA) used in the manufacture of printed circuit boards. Contact Dermatitis 38:292–294

Kanerva L, Estlander T, Jolanki R, Alanko K (2000) Occupational allergic contact dermatitis from 2,2-bis[4-(2-hydroxy-3-acryloxypropoxy) phenyl]-propane (epoxy diacrylate) in ultraviolet-cured inks. Contact Dermatitis 43:56–59

Kiec-Swierczynska M, Krecisz B, Swierczynska-Machura D, Zaremba J (2005) An epidemic of occupational contact dermatitis from an acrylic glue. Contact Dermatitis 52:121–125

Lambert J, Matthieu L, Dockx P (1988) Contact dermatitis from acrylamide. Contact Dermatitis 19:65

Langvardt PW (2010) Acrylonitrile. In: Ullmann's encyclopedia of industrial chemistry, 7th edn. Wiley, New York

Lazarov A (2007) Sensitization to acrylates is a common adverse reaction to artificial fingernails. J Eur Acad Dermatol Venereol 21:169–174

Lee HN, Pokorny CD, Law S, Pratt M, Sasseville D, Storrs FJ (2002) Cross-reactivity among epoxy acrylates and bisphenol F epoxy resins in patients with bisphenol A epoxy resin sensitivity. Am J Contact Dermat 13:108–115

Mäkelä EA, Jolanki J (2005) Chemical permeation through disposable gloves. In: Estlander T, Wahlberg JE, Maibach HI, Boman A (eds) Protective gloves for occupational use. CRC Press, Boca Raton, pp 299–314

Malten KE, van der Meer-Roosen CH, Seutter E (1978) Nyloprint-sensitive patients react to NN' methylene bis acrylamide. Contact Dermatitis 4:214–222

Matura M, Poesen N, de Moor A, Kerre S, Dooms-Goossens A (1995) Glycidyl methacrylate and ethoxyethyl acrylate: new allergens in emulsions used to impregnate paper and textile materials. Contact Dermatitis 33:123–124

Maurice PD, Rycroft RJ (1986) Allergic contact dermatitis from UV-curing acrylate in the manufacture of optical fibres. Contact Dermatitis 15:92–93

Minamoto K, Ueda A (2005) Occupational allergic contact dermatitis due to ultraviolet-cured acrylic glue. J Occup Health 47:340–342

Nethercott JR, Jakubovic HR, Pilger C, Smith JW (1983) Allergic contact dermatitis due to urethane acrylate in ultraviolet cured inks. Br J Ind Med 40:241–250

Ohara T, Sato T, Shimizu N, Prescher G, Schwind H, Weiberg O, Marten K, Greim H (2010) Acrylic acid and derivatives. In: Ullman's encyclopedia of industrial chemistry, 7th edn. Wiley, Weinheim

Onusseit H, Wefringhaus R, Dreezen G, Kneafsey B, Wichelhaus J, Bachon T, Becker K, Chen C, Dausmann D, Gillitzer T, Gossen R, Gupta S, Holloway M, Iida K, Jacobine AF, Kopannia S, Lammerschop O, Lu D, Mayer B, Meckel-Jonas C, Picker S, Pröbster M, Ruytens M, Sattler HP, Schöttmer B, Windhövel U (2010a) Adhesives, 2. Applications. In: Ullmann's encyclopedia of industrial chemistry, 7th edn. Wiley, Hoboken

Onusseit H, Wefringhaus R, Dreezen G, Wichelhaus J, Schall J, Thiele L, van Halteren A (2010b) Adhesives, 1. General. In: Ullmann's encyclopedia of industrial chemistry, 7th edn. Wiley, Hoboken

Pedersen NB, Chevallier MA, Senning A (1982) Secondary acrylamides in Nyloprint printing plate as a source of contact dermatitis. Contact Dermatitis 8:256–262

Pedersen NB, Senning A, Nielsen AO (1983) Different sensitising acrylic monomers in Napp printing plate. Contact Dermatitis 9: 459–464

Pham HQ, Marks MJ (2010) Epoxy resins. In: Ullmann's encyclopedia of industrial chemistry, 7th edn. Wiley, Weinheim

Rustemeyer T, Frosch PJ (1996) Occupational skin diseases in dental laboratory technicians. (I). Clinical picture and causative factors. Contact Dermatitis 34:125–133

Sanchez-Perez J, Gonzalez-Arriba A, Goiriz R, Garcia-Diez A (2008) Occupational allergic contact dermatitis to acrylates and methacrylates. Contact Dermatitis 58:252–254

Sauni R, Kauppi P, Alanko K, Henriks-Eckerman ML, Tuppurainen M, Hannu T (2008) Occupational asthma caused by sculptured nails containing methacrylates. Am J Ind Med 51(12):968–974

Saval P, Kristiansen E, Cramers M, Lander F (2007) Occupational allergic contact dermatitis caused by aerosols of acrylate monomers. Contact Dermatitis 57:276

Scotnicki S, Pratt MD (1998) Occupational dermatitis to ultraviolet-cured acrylic-based inks in computer hard disc manufacturing. Am J Contact Dermat 9:179–181

Shimizu A, Kamada N, Kambe N, Matsue H (2008) Chemical burn caused by glycidyl methacrylate. Contact Dermatitis 59:316–317

Sood A, Taylor JS (2003) Acrylic reactions: a review of 56 cases. Contact Dermatitis 48:346–347

Streitberger HJ, Urbano E, Laible R, Meyer BD, Bagda E, Waite FA, Philips M (2010) Paints and coatings, 3. Paint systems. In: Ullmann's encyclopedia of industrial chemistry, 7th edn. Wiley, Weinheim

Teik-Jin Goon A, Bruze M, Zimerson E, Goh CL, Isaksson M (2007) Contact allergy to acrylates/methacrylates in the acrylate and nail acrylics series in southern Sweden: simultaneous positive patch test reaction patterns and possible screening allergens. Contact Dermatitis 57:21–27

Tomb RR, Lepoittevin JP, Durepaire F, Grosshans E (1993) Ectopic contact dermatitis from ethyl cyanoacrylate instant adhesives. Contact Dermatitis 28:206–208

Tucker SC, Beck MH (1999) A 15-year study of patch testing to (meth) acrylates. Contact Dermatitis 40:278–279

Whittington CV (1981) Dermatitis from UV acrylate in adhesive. Contact Dermatitis 7:203–204

Wrangsjo K, Swartling C, Meding B (2001) Occupational dermatitis in dental personnel: contact dermatitis with special reference to (meth) acrylates in 174 patients. Contact Dermatitis 45:158–163

51 Epoxy Resins

Rosemary Nixon[1] · *Jennifer Cahill*[1] · *Riitta Jolanki*[2]
[1]Occupational Dermatology Research and Education Centre, Skin and Cancer Foundation, Carlton South, Melbourne, VIC, Australia
[2]Control of Hypersensitivity Diseases, Finnish Institute of Occupational Health (FIOH), Helsinki, Finland

Core Messages

- Allergic contact dermatitis to epoxy resin systems may be caused by resins, hardeners, or reactive diluents.
- Patch testing with the standard epoxy resin based on diglycidyl ether of bisphenol A (DGEBA) will miss many cases of epoxy system allergy.
- Patch testing with workers' own samples is necessary.
- Allergic contact dermatitis to epoxy chemicals may present with dermatitis on the hands, arms, neck, and face.
- Rubber gloves offer poor protection against epoxy chemicals.
- If a worker develops allergic contact dermatitis to epoxy chemicals, consider the factors which led to sensitization. It may be that other workers are also at risk.

1 Introduction

It is reported that products now known as epoxy resins were synthesized as early as 1891 with the first patent applications occurring in the 1930s and the first commercial production in the 1940s (Potter 1975; Ellis 1993). Large-scale production of epoxy resins began in the early 1950s. By the end of the 1960s, at least 25 distinct types of epoxy resins were commercially available (Lee and Neville 1967). The first cases of epoxy dermatitis were observed in the 1950s, shortly after epoxy resins were introduced (Calnan 1958; Jolanki 1991).

2 Epoxy Compounds

2.1 Chemistry and Properties

Epoxy resins are normally used in what is called an "epoxy resin system." This consists of the epoxy resin, hardener, and reactive diluent or other additives, such as fillers, modifiers, pigments, and reinforcements. These may all influence the properties of the resulting epoxy resin system.

2.1.1 Epoxy Resins

Epoxy resins contain at least two cyclic three-membered-ring structures containing oxygen, called epoxy groups, oxirane, or epoxide groups, in their molecules. The term "epoxy resin" may refer to the resins in either the uncured thermoplastic or cured thermoset states (Lee and Neville 1967). The uncured resins can be cross-linked through the use of a variety of curing agents or hardeners to form cured plastics with insoluble three-dimensional structures. Epoxy resins are generally prepared by the coupling of epichlorohydrin [CAS 106-89-8] with compounds that possess at least two reactive hydrogen atoms (Muskopf and McCollister 1987). The reaction products of epichlorohydrin and bisphenol A [CAS 80-05-7] resulted in the first commercial epoxy resins, which are generally mixtures of monomeric diglycidyl ether of bisphenol A (DGEBA), with a molecular weight (MW) of 340 Da, and oligomers with a higher MW. The average number of repetitive parts in the oligomers ranges from essentially 0 to approximately 25 (➋ *Fig. 51.1*) (Bauer 1985). The sensitizing capacity decreases with higher MW (Thorgeirsson et al. 1978b). DGEBA epoxy resins account for 75–95% of epoxy resins used worldwide, while 1% is based on diglycidyl ether of bisphenol F (DGEBF) (Pontén et al. 2002). DGEBA epoxy resins with an average MW as high as 8,000 Da are available (Guin and Work 1995). When DGEBA epoxy resins are prepared, apart from DGEBA and higher oligomers, side reactions result in the formation of low levels of impurities that both decrease the epoxide content from the theoretical amount of two per molecule and affect the resin properties, both before and after curing. DGEBA epoxy resins with a low average MW of 350–400 Da are liquids with a relatively high viscosity, and they contain monomeric DGEBA up to more than 90%. Resins with an average MW of more than 900 Da are solids (Muskopf and McCollister 1987), but may contain more than 15% DGEBA (Henriks-Eckerman and Laijoki 1986b). DGEBA epoxy resins are relatively expensive, but have a unique combination of properties,

T. Rustemeyer, P. Elsner, S.M. John & H.I. Maibach (eds.), *Kanerva's Occupational Dermatology*,
DOI 10.1007/978-3-642-02035-3_51, © Springer-Verlag Berlin Heidelberg 2012

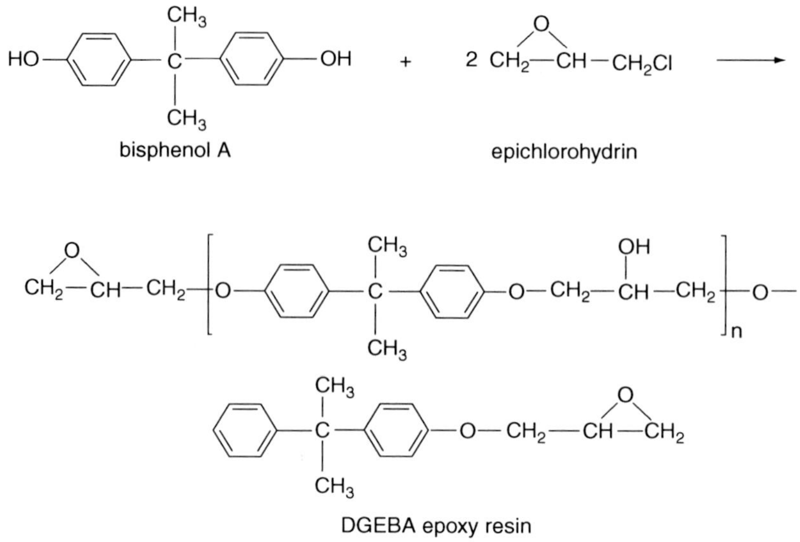

Fig.51.1
Diglycidyl ether of bisphenol A (*DGEBA*) epoxy resin

such as electrical insulation, good chemical and mechanical resistance, and versatility (Jolanki 1994). Non-DGEBA epoxy resins possess special properties that have made them competitive with less expensive DGEBA resins for certain applications. A list of chemical names and CAS numbers of available epoxy resins is given in *Table 51.1.* The chemical structures of some dermatologically interesting non-DGEBA epoxy resins are presented in *Fig. 51.2.* The resin or mixture of resins chosen for a particular application depends on the desired balance of properties. For example, brominated epoxy resins are semisolids and resistant to ignition, while epoxy novolacs exhibit better high-temperature performance and chemical resistance than DGEBA epoxy resins.

2.1.2 Reactive Diluents

Reactive diluents are used to reduce the viscosity of the resin and improve polymerization (Angelini et al. 1996). The reactive diluents are generally glycidyl ethers and sometimes glycidyl esters; structurally, they are aliphatic or aromatic, and they also contain epoxy groups in their molecules. Reactive diluents participate in the curing process by the epoxy groups and become chemically linked to cured epoxy resins (Muskopf and McCollister 1987). A list of chemical names and CAS numbers of representative examples of available reactive diluents is given in *Table 51.2.* The chemical structures of some compounds are also shown in *Fig. 51.3.* Reactive diluents based on diols, such as 1,4-butanediol diglycidyl ether (BDDGE) and 1,6-hexanediol diglycidyl ether (HDDGE), may also be used as low-MW epoxy resins (Muskopf and McCollister 1987). It has been estimated that more than half of epoxy-resin products contained varying (0.1–20%) amounts of reactive diluents (Henriks- Eckerman and Laijoki 1986b; Jolanki et al. 1987a).

2.1.3 Hardeners

A wide variety of hardeners or curing agents is currently available. *Tables 51.3–51.6* list representative examples of available hardeners with their CAS numbers. The chemical structures of some amine hardeners are also presented in *Fig. 51.4.* When epoxy resins are used in two-component products, the hardeners are added to the resins immediately before the application, and the subsequent cross-linking occurs at either an ambient or an elevated temperature. Aliphatic and cycloaliphatic polyamines are low-viscosity liquids which react readily with epoxy resins at ambient temperatures; less reactive aromatic polyamines require an elevated curing temperature (Muskopf and McCollister 1987). 3-Dimethylaminopropylamine (DMAPA) is an aliphatic alkyl polyamine hardener (*Fig. 51.4*) and is also an intermediary in cocamidopropyl betaine synthesis and exists as an impurity of cocamidopropyl betaines

Table 51.1
Epoxy resins (Muskopf and McCollister 1987; Guin and Work 1995)

Diglycidyl ether of bisphenol A based epoxy resins
Diglycidyl ether of bisphenol A (DGEBA) [1675-54-3]
Brominated bisphenol A based epoxy resins
Diglycidyl ether of tetrabromo bisphenol A [68928-70-1, 26265-08-7, 40039-93-8]
Phenol and cresol epoxy novolacs
Cresol epoxy novolacs [37382-79-9]
Diglycidyl ether of bisphenol F [54208-63-8]
2,2′,2″,2‴-[1,2-ethanediylidenetetrabis (4,1-phenyleneoxymethylene)]tetrabisoxiran [7328-97-4]
Phenol epoxy novolacs [9003-36-5]
Resorcinol diglycidyl ether [101-90-6]
Trisphenol novolac epoxy resin [66072-38-6]
Glycidyl ethers of phenol-aldehyde adducts
1,1,2,2-tetrakis[4-(2,3-epoxypropyl)phenyl]ethane [27043-37-4]
T ris[4-(2,3-epoxypropoxy)phenyl]methane [66072-39-7]
Glycidyl ethers of phenol-hydrocarbon novolacs
2,5-bis[(2,3-epoxypropoxy)phenyl]octahydro-4,7-methano-
5 H-indene [13446-85-0]
Glycidyl ethers of aliphatic diols
Ethylene glycol diglycidyl ether [2224-15-9]
Diglycidyl and triglycidyl ether of glycerol
Diglycidyl ether of polypropyleneglycol [16096-30-3]
Diglycidyl ether of hydrogenated bisphenol A [30583-72-3]
Sorbitol polyglycidyl ether [68412-01-1]
Aromatic glycidyl amines
4-glycidyloxy-N,N-diglycidylaniline
N,N′-tetraglycidyl-4,4′-methylenedianiline (TGMDA) [28768-32-3]
Triglycidyl-p-aminophenol (TGPAP) [5026-74-7]
Heterocyclic glycidyl imides
1,3-bis(2,3-epoxypropyl)-5,5-dimethylhydantoin; dimethylhydantoin epoxy resin [15336-81-9]
3-(2-glycidyloxypropy1)-1-glycidyl-5,5-dimethylhydantoin [32568-89-l]
Triglycidyl isocyanurate (TGIC) [2451-62-9]
Glycidyl esters
Diglycidyl ester of hexahydrophthalic acid [5493 -45-8]
Diglycidyl ester of phthalic acid [7 195-45-1]
Glycidyl ester of dimerized linoleic acid and epichlorohydrin

Table 51.1 (Continued)

Fluorinated epoxy resins
Epoxidized cycloaliphatic olefins
3′,4′-epoxycyclohexylmethyl-3,4-epoxycyclohexane-carboxylate (cycloaliphatic epoxy resin) [2386-87-0]
4-epoxyethyl-l,2-epoxycyclohexane (vinyl cyclohexene diepoxide) [25550-49-6]
Naphthalene epoxy resins
1,6-bis(2,3-epoxypropoxy)naphthalene [27610-48-6]

(Angelini et al. 1995). Polyamines are often troublesome to work with because of their reactivity and volatility, and also because of their irritating and sensitizing properties to the skin and respiratory tract. To overcome these problems, less volatile, less reactive, and less irritating and sensitizing polyamides, amine-epoxy adducts have been developed. Polyamides are prepared by combining aliphatic polyamines, e.g., diethylenetriamine (DETA) or triethylenetetramine (TETA), with fatty acids. Amine-epoxy adducts are formed in a reaction between epoxy resin and an excess of polyamine, mostly DETA, TETA, or isophoronediamine (IPDA) (Bauer 1985). The content of free amine is about 5% in the amine-epoxy adduct hardeners used in metal paints, but for those used in floor and concrete coatings the corresponding figure is about 20% (Back and Saarinen 1986). Free DGEBA is not found in amine-epoxy adducts (Henriks-Eckerman and Laijoki 1986b).

When DGEBA epoxy resins are cured by polyamine-bearing hardeners at room temperature, the amounts of unreacted DGEBA and polyamine diminish rapidly within 1–2 days, but thereafter the decrease is slow. Nevertheless, after 1 week's cure, 0.02–12% of free DGEBA and 0.01–1% of free DETA were found when six different epoxy resin products were experimentally cured by DETA (Henriks-Eckerman and Laijoki 1986a). Exposure to uncured resin may be the cause of unexplained epoxy resin sensitization. A patient was reported to react to DGEBA in a mop handle at a concentration of 0.015% and on patch testing to dilutions was positive down to 0.00032% (Kanerva et al. 2000a). The use of an elevated curing temperature is more effective in reducing the DGEBA concentration than simply waiting until the next day (Hansson 1994). One-component products contain curing agents which are inactive at storage temperatures, but which initiate a curing process when heated. Typical latent curing agents include organic acid anhydrides (*Table 51.4*, *Fig. 51.5*), which are used mainly in the electrical industry when good electrical properties are

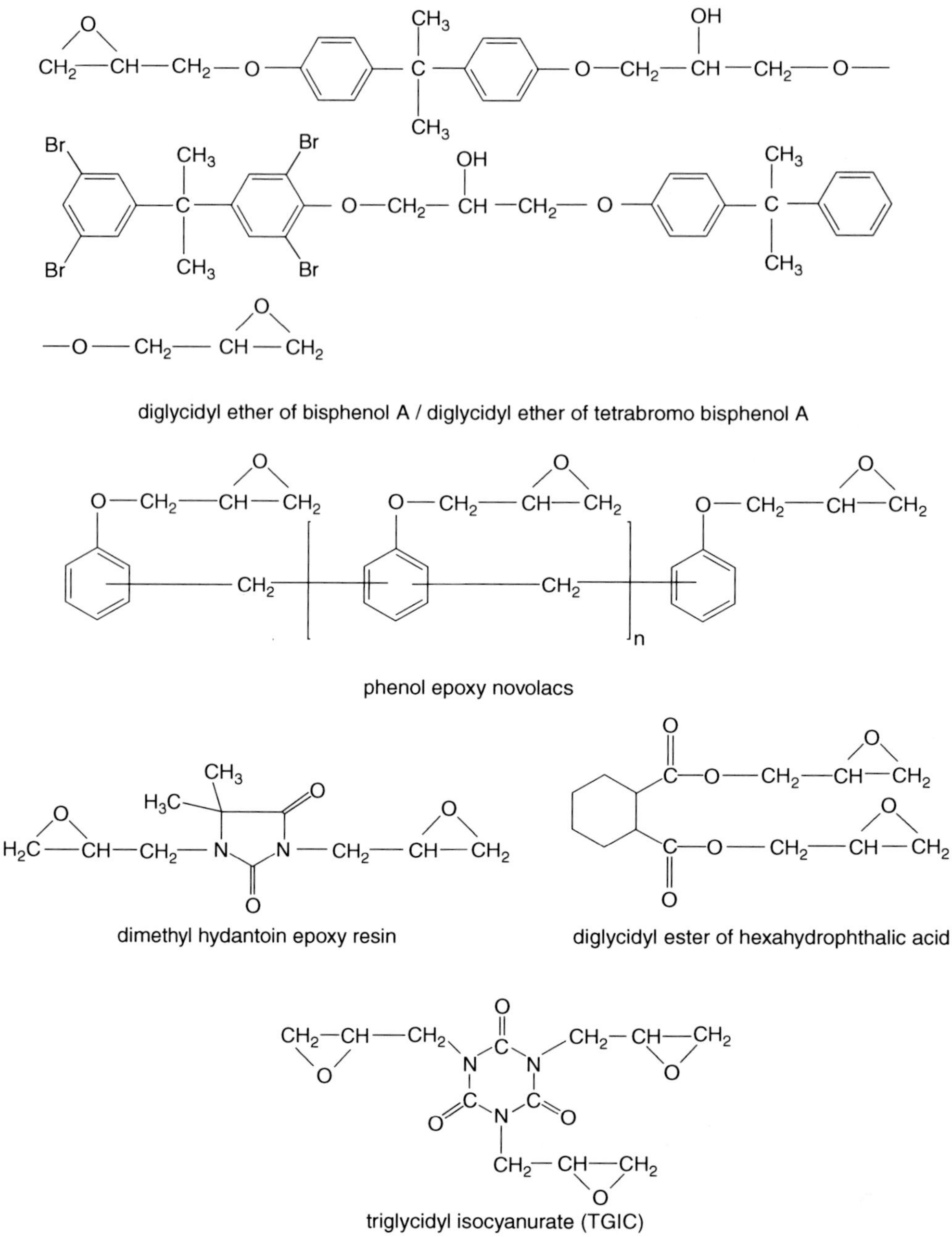

Fig. 51.2
Non-diglycidyl ether of bisphenol A (*DGEBA*) epoxy resin

required. Other examples of one-component epoxy products include powder epoxy or epoxy-polyester paints, polyester paints (Peltonen 1986), one-pack glues (Dahlquist et al. 1979), and prepreg-laminates (Mathias 1987). With the anhydrides, the cross-linking reaction is achieved using tertiary amines (➋ *Table 51.6*) as catalysts and an elevated curing temperature (50–200°C). The anhydrides used as epoxy hardeners include phthalic anhydride (PA) and PA derivatives (Muskopf and McCollister 1987; Jolanki et al. 1997b). The typical latent

Table 51.2
Reactive diluents (Muskopf and McCollister 1987; Angelini et al. 1996; Jolanki 1991)

Aliphatic glycidyl ethers
Allyl glycidyl ether (AGE) [106-92-31]
1,4-butanediol diglycidyl ether (BDDGE) [2425-79-8]
n-Butyl glycidyl ether (*n*-BGE) [2426-08-6]
tert-Butyl glycidyl ether (tert-BGE) [7665-72-7]
Diethyleneglycol diglycidyl ether (DEGDGE)
Diglycidyl ether of pentaerythritol
2-ethyl hexyl glycidyl ether
Glycidyl ether of aliphatic alcohols (Epoxide 8) [68609-97-2]
Glycidyl ether of polypropyleneglycol [9072-62-2]
1,6-hexanediol diglycidyl ether (HDDGE) [16096-31-4]
Neopentyl glycol diglycidyl ether (NPGDGE) [17557-23-2]
Cycloaliphatic glycidyl ethers
Cyclohexanedimethanol diglycidyl ether
Aromatic glycidyJ ethers
tert-Butylphenyl glycidyl ether [3101-60-8]
Cresyl glycidyl ether (CGE) [26447-14-3]
p-Fluorphenyl glycidyl ether
Alpha-naphthyl glycidyl ether
Phenyl glycidyl ether (PGE) [122-60-1]
Glycidyl esters
Castor oil glycidyl ether [74398-71-3]
Glycidyl ester of neodecanoic acids (Cardura E 10) [26761-45-5]
Glycidyl methacrylate [106-91-2]
Glycidyl neodecanoate [26761-45-5]

curing agents in powder epoxy paints are composed of about 4% hardeners, such as dicyandiamide or pyromellitic anhydride. Triglycidyl isocyanurate (TGIC) is used to cure powder polyester paints. Blocked isocyanates are latent curing agents used in waterborne coatings (Muskopf and McCollister 1987). Polysulfides and hexavalent chromate are constituents found especially in the curing agents of epoxy sealants used in the aircraft industry (Handley and Burrows 1994; Bruze et al. 1996). Polyamine and organic acid anhydride hardeners serve as co-reactive hardeners, which become incorporated into the epoxy resin, whereas tertiary amines, such as 2,4,6-tris-(dimethylaminomethyl)phenol (tris-DMP) and N,N-dimethylbenzylamine, imidazoles, and boron trihalide amine complexes are catalyst-type curing agents, which may not be chemically bound to the resin molecules during epoxy curing reactions (Guin and Work 1995; Muskopf and McCollister 1987).

2.1.4 Epoxy Di(meth)acrylates

Epoxy di(meth)acrylates (also called vinyl esters) are another name for β-hydroxyester acrylates, because they are usually obtained by reacting epoxy resins of glycidyl derivatives with (meth)acrylic acid. They can also be manufactured from bisphenol A and glycidyl (meth)acrylates. Although prepared from compounds containing reactive epoxy groups, completed epoxy di(meth)acrylate molecules do not contain these groups. Both aromatic and aliphatic epoxy di(meth)acrylates are available, as well as acrylated epoxydized oils (Jolanki 1991; Jolanki et al. 1995). The first epoxy dimethacrylate, known as bis-GMA (2,2-bis(4-(2-hydroxy-3-methacryloxypropoxy) phenyl)propane) [CAS 1565-94-2] (*Fig. 51.6*), was developed by Bowen in 1956. bis-GMA is manufactured from DGEBA and methacrylic acid or bisphenol A and glycidyl methacrylate (Bowen 1962; Jolanki et al. 1995). Analyses have shown that epoxy di(meth)acrylate products may contain DGEBA as an impurity (Kanerva et al. 1989; Henriks-Eckerman and Kanerva 1997). bis-GA (2,2-bis[4-(2-hydroxy-3-acryloxypropoxy) phenyl]propane) is an example of epoxy diacrylates based on bisphenol A (*Fig. 51.6*). Epoxy di(meth)acrylates can be polymerized, not only by exposure to an electron beam, ultraviolet (UV) light, or even visible light, but also chemically activated by the use of various peroxides and tertiary amines. Chemically cured dental restorative composite material is usually available in two bis-GMA-based components. The tooth-colored base paste contains a tertiary amine (1–2%), and the catalyst paste contains dibenzoyl peroxide (1–1.5%). The light-cured composite material consists of only one component (Anderson and Messick 1985; Janda 1987). Epoxy di(meth)acrylates have the desirable properties of both epoxy resins and poly(meth) acrylates, including relatively low volumetric shrinkage during the curing process (epoxy resins), and an adequate polymerization rate (2–5 min at 37°C) (methacrylates of low MW) (Vanherle and Smith 1985; Janda 1987).

2.1.5 Other Epoxy Compounds

Apart from epoxy resins, reactive diluents and epichlorohydrin, other compounds containing at least one epoxy

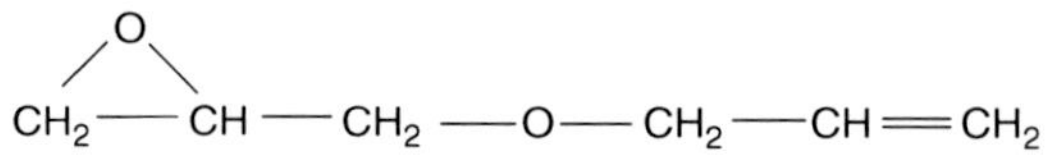

allyl glycidyl ether (AGE)

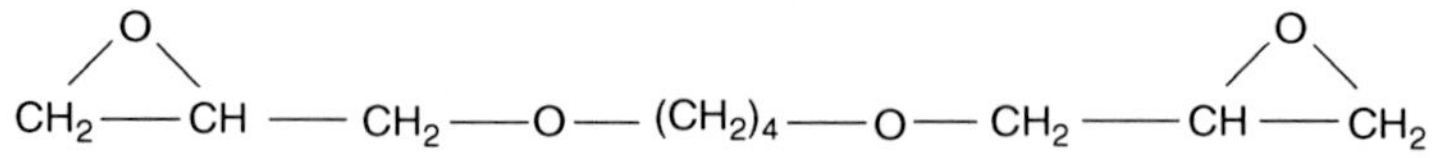

1,4-butanediol diglycidyl ether (BDDGE)

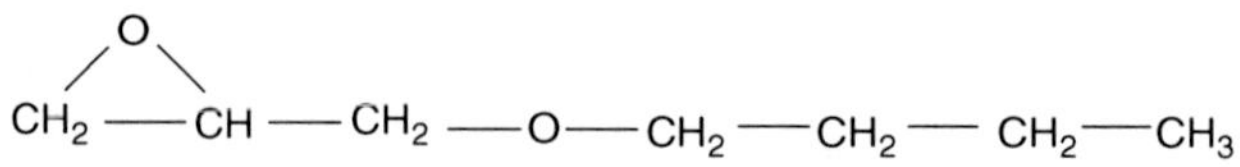

n-butyl glycidyl ether (n-BGE)

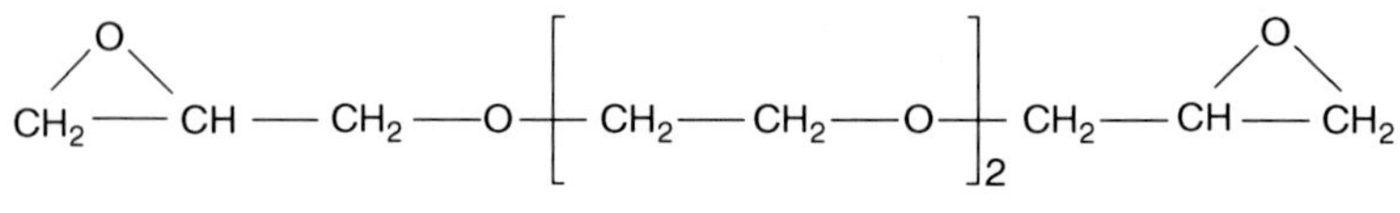

diethyleneglycol diglycidyl ether (DEGDGE)

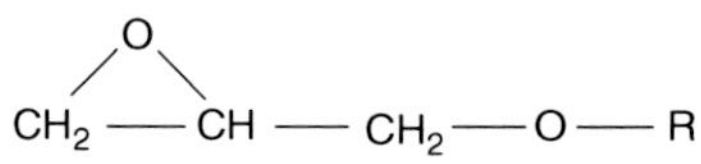

glycidyl ether of aliphatic alcohols (Epoxide 8) (R is predominantly a C12 or C14 alkyl chain)

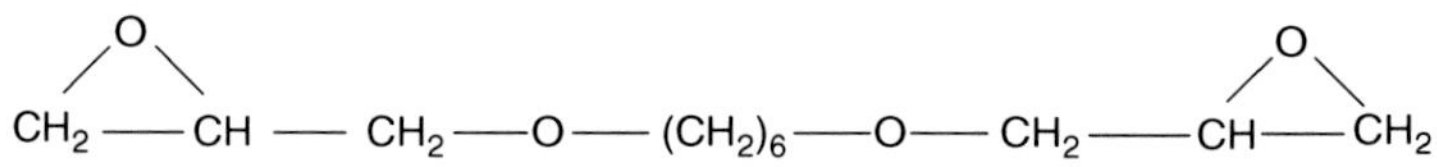

1,6-hexanediol diglycidyl ether (HDDGE)

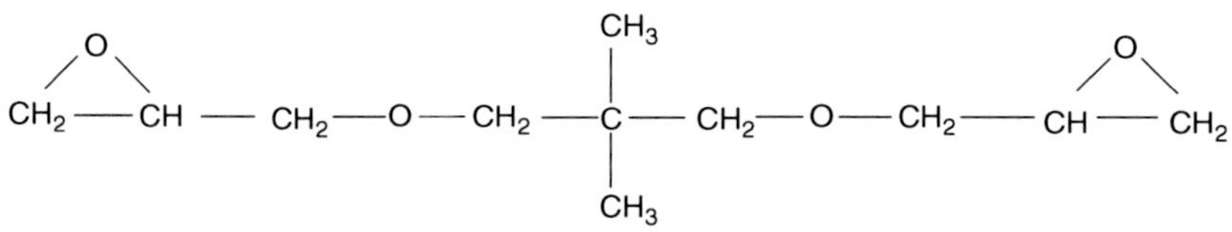

neopentyl glycol diglycidyl ether (NPGDGE)

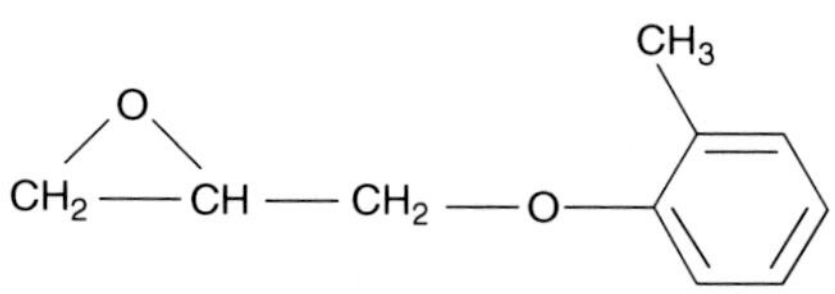

O-cresyl glycidyl ether (CGE)

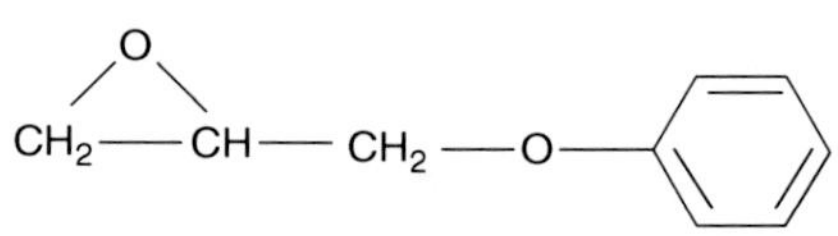

phenyl glycidyl ether (PGE)

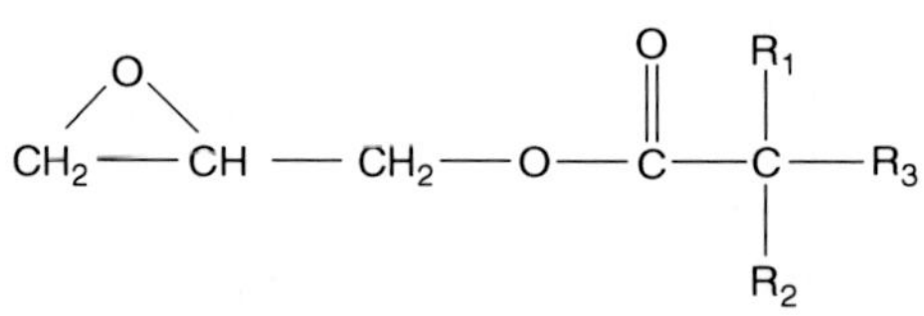

glycidyl ester of neodecanoic acids (Cardura E 10) (R_1, R_2 and R_3 are alkanes)

Fig. 51.3
Reactive diluents

Table 51.3
Polyamine hardeners (Muskopf and McCollister 1987; Guin and Work 1995; Kanerva et al. 1996)

Aliphatic polyamines
N′-(3-aminopropyJ)-N,N-dimethyl-l,3-propanediamine [10563-29-8]
Diethylenetriamine (DETA) [111-40-0]
Diethylamino propylamine (DEAPA) [104-78-9]
3-dimethylaminopropylamine (DMAPA) [109-55-7]
Dipropylene triamine (DPTA) [56-18-8]
Ethylene diamine (EDA) [107-15-3]
p-Menthane-l,8-diamine (80-52-4]
Poly(oxypropylenediamine) [9046-10-0]
Poly(oxypropylenetriamine) [39423-51-3]
Tetraethylene pentamine (TEPA) [112-57-2]
Triethylenetetramine (TETA) [112-24-3]
2,2,4-Trimethylhexamethylene 1,6-diamine [3236-53-1]
2,4,4-Trimethylhexamethylene 1,6-diamine [3236-53-2]
Cycloaliphatic polyamines
1,2-Cyclohexanediamine [694-83-7]
3-Cyclohexylaminopropylamine [3312-60-5]
1,4-Diaminocyclohexane [3114-70-3]
Isophoronediamine (IPDA) [2855 -13-2]
2,2′-Dimethyl-4,4′ –methylene-bis(cyclohexylamine) [6864-37-5]
Aromatic polyamines
4,4′-Diaminodiphenylmethane (DDM) [101-77-9]
4,4′-Diaminodiphenyl sulfone (DDS) [80-08-0]
Diethyltoluenediamine [75389-89-8]
m-Phenylenediamine (MPDA) [108-45-2]
o-Tolyl biguanide [93-69-6]
m-Xylene diamine [1477-55-0]
Polyamide diamines
Polymeric amido-amine alkoxylated triethylene tetramine
Adducts of aliphatic amines with mono- and diepoxides and ketones (i.e., amine-epoxy adducts)
Diethylenetriamine-ethylene oxide adduct
Ethylene diamine adduct to solid epoxy
Triethylenetetramine-propylene oxide adduct

group in their molecules are also potential causes of contact allergy. Examples of these epoxy compounds include glycidyl methacrylate [98104-93-9] (Matura et al. 1995, *Fig. 51.6*), epoxy propane [CAS 75-56-91] (Steinkraus and Hausen 1994; Morris et al. 1998), 2.3-epoxypropyl trimethyl ammonium chloride (EPTMAC) [CAS 3033-77-01] (Estlander et al. 1996), and trans-3-(4-methoxyphenyl) glycidate (Buisson et al. 1991).

Table 51.4
Organic acid anhydride hardeners (Guin and Work 1995; Jolanki et al. 1997b)

Chlorendic anhydride [115-27-5]
cis-Cyclohexane-l,2-dicarboxylic anhydride [13149-00-3]
Dodecenylsuccinic anhydride (DDS) [25377-73-5]
Hexahydrophthalic anhydride (HHPA) [85-42-7]
Maleic anhydride (MA) [108-31-6]
Methyl endo-methylene-tetrahydrophthalic anhydride
Methylhexahydrophthalic anhydride (MHHPA) [19438-60-9]
Methyl nadic anhydride [25134-21-8]
Methyltetrahydrophthalic anhydride (MTHPA) [26590-20-5]
Phthalic anhydride (PA) [85-44-9]
Polyazelaic polyanhydride
Polysebacic polyanhydride [26776-29-4]
Pyromellitic dianhydride (PMDA) [89-32-7]
Succinic anhydride [108-30-5]
Tetrahydrophthalic anhydride (THPA) [85-43-8]
Trimellitic anhydride (TMA) [552-30-7]

2.2 Use

2.2.1 Epoxy-Resin Compounds

The scope of epoxy resin application is broad. Epoxy resins are used mostly in two-component paints and other protective coatings, and two-component adhesives. Epoxy resins are used to provide good resistance against water, many chemicals, corrosion, heat and abrasion, and to form tough, high-strength adhesive bonds on metal and many other surfaces (including plastics, rubber, wood, glass, and ceramics). Epoxy resins are also used to insulate or encapsulate and they are used in the assembly of a wide variety of electrical and electronic devices, in the manufacture of glass fibers as sizing agents (Toffoletto et al. 1994) and in the manufacture of sporting goods or other plastic items. They can also be used as injection resins to repair cracks in concrete, in flooring materials (Conde-Salazar et al. 1994), and stone work (Angelini et al. 1996). Powder paints (Peltonen 1986), and even nail polishes (Jolanki et al. 1996a) may contain epoxy resin compounds. Epoxy resins were introduced in 1956

Table 51.5
Miscellaneous curing agents (Muskopf and McCollister 1987; Guin and Work 1995; Kanerva et al. 1996)

N-Aminoethylpiperazine [140-31-8]
Cyanoethyl modified aliphatic amine
2,4-Diamino-6-(2′-alkylimidazol-l-yl)ethyl-5-triazine
Dicyandiamide [461 -58-5]
Di- and polyisocyanates
Diethylene glycol diaminopropyl ether
Hexavalent chromate
Melamineformaldehyde resins [9003-08-1]
Phenolformaldehyde resins [9003-35-4]
Polycarboxylic acid polyesters
Ureaformaldehyde resins [9011-05-6]

Table 51.6
Catalyst-curing agents (Guin and Work 1995; Kanerva et al. 1996)

Aliphatic thioester
Boron trichloride-amine complex
Boron trifluoride-benzylamine complex [696-99-1]
Boron trifluoride:monomethylamine
l-Cyanoethyl-2-(alkyl or phenyl)imidazoles
l-Cyanoethyl-2-(alkyl or phenyl)imidazole-trimellitates
1-Cyanoethyl-2-phenyl-4,5-di(cyanoethoxymethyl) imidazole
Dimethylaminomethylphenol [25338-55-0]
2,4,6-Tris-(dimethylaminomethyl)phenol (tris-DMP) [CAS 90-72-2]
Tris(dimethylaminomethyl)phenol-tri(2-ethylhexoate)
N,N-Dimethylbenzylamine [CAS-l03-83-3]
Imidazolinealkyl imidazoles
Ketimine
2-(Methyl or phenyl)imidazole-isocyanuric acid adduct
4,4′-Methylene-bis(2-ethyl-5-methylimidazole)
Morpholine salt of p-toluenesulfonic acid
2-Phenylimidazole [670-96-2]
Thioether
Trifunctional mercaptan terminated polymer

in the preparation of samples for electron microscopy (Jolanki et al. 1988; Sommer et al. 1997) and are still widely used. A more recent use has been in the manufacture of wind turbines (Ponten et al. 2004a). In the manufacture of epoxy composite products, for example, by lamination; glass fibers, woven cloth, and matting are impregnated with an epoxy resin/curing agent matrix. Glass fibers usually form composites with a DGEBA epoxy resin/diamine matrix. Epoxy composites are used in the manufacture of pipes and vessels; in sporting goods, such as tennis racquets, skis, ski poles, and fishing rods; in the automotive, boat-building and aircraft industries; in military and aerospace applications; and in electrical applications in articles such as electronic circuit boards (Fregert 1981b; Burrows et al. 1984; Muskopf and McCollister 1987; Tarvainen et al. 1995b). Most epoxy surface coatings are based on DGEBA epoxy resins, but epoxy resins based on DGEBF and phenolic novolac resins have also been increasingly used. Liquid epoxy resins are used in two-component solventless coatings. Waterborne epoxy coatings are prepared by the dispersion of epoxy resins modified with water-soluble functional groups or by the emulsification of DGEBA epoxy resins with surfactants. Both solventless and solvent-borne epoxy coatings have been employed mainly as anticorrosion protection for metals (marine and maintenance coatings), as waterproof protection for concrete, and as chemical-resistant protection for floors and walls (Muskopf and McCollister 1987). Two-component coatings can be cured at ambient temperatures with polyamines, polyamides, and amine-epoxy adducts. Tertiary amines, e.g., tris-DMP are frequently used to accelerate the curing rates (Lee and Neville 1967).

Epoxy adhesives range from those used as two pack, ambient-cure, general adhesives in domestic applications to high-performance, one-component sheet adhesives for aircraft assembly (Gardiner et al. 1992). Araldite™ is a registered trademark of Huntsman Advanced Materials (previously part of Ciba Geigy) used for consumer epoxy adhesives. Liquid DGEBA epoxy resins are used in most of the one- and two-component epoxy adhesives. The curing agent generally consists of polyamides or aliphatic polyamines, e.g., DETA and TETA. Casting resins are liquid and solventless mixtures of low-MW epoxy resin, a curing agent, and additives, e.g., fillers, reinforcements, and catalysts. The mixture is poured into molds and cured to solid structures. The casting resins are used mainly as electrical insulating material in the manufacture of transformers, switching gear, circuit breakers, conductors, and insulators. Anhydride-cured cycloaliphatic epoxy resins are commonly used when durability is required, such as in outdoor electrical insulators (Muskopf and McCollister 1987; Jolanki et al. 1989). Epoxy molding compounds are solid mixtures of epoxy resin (epoxy novolac), a curing agent and catalyst, mold-release

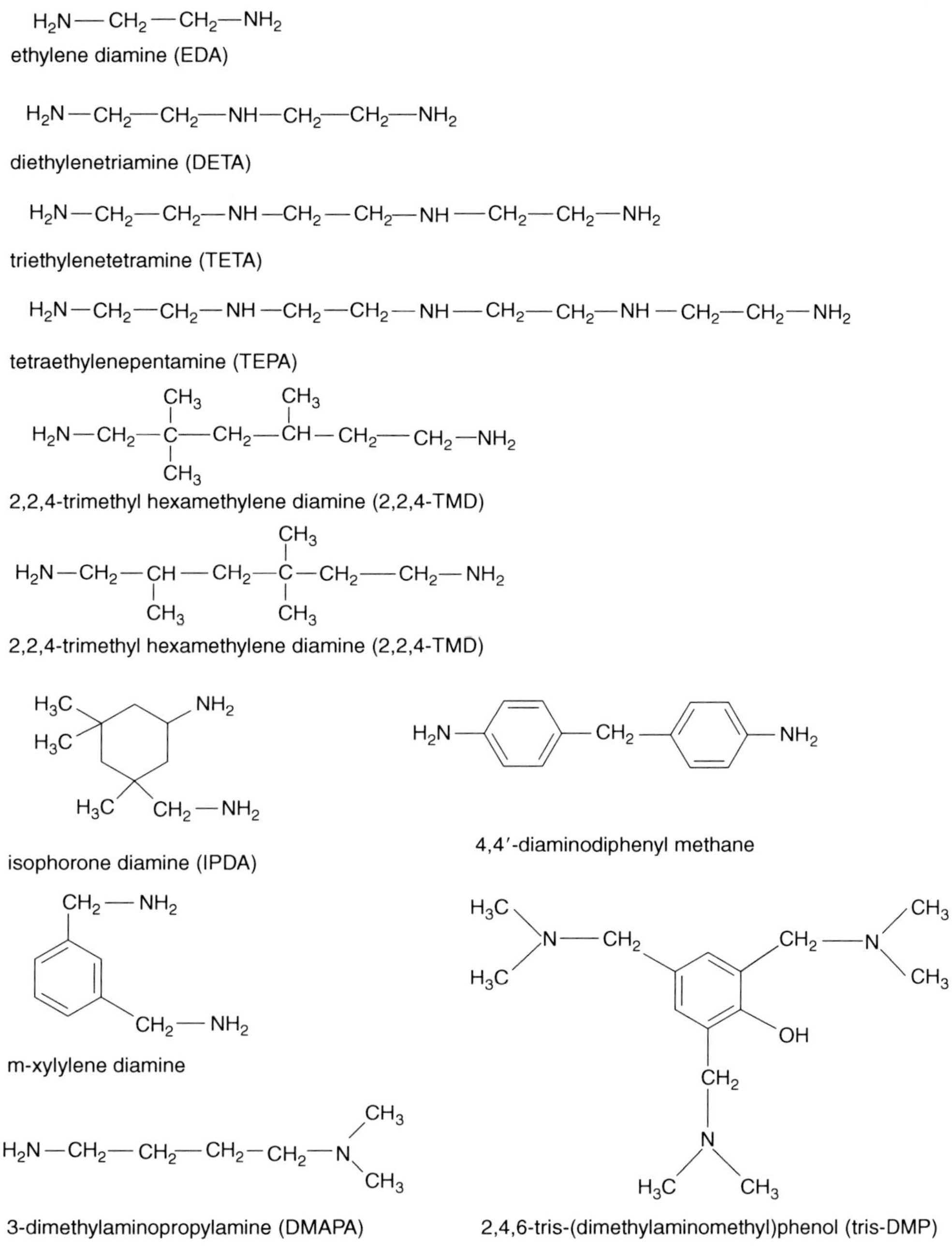

Fig. 51.4
Polyamine hardeners and catalyst-curing agents

compounds, fillers, and other additives. The molding compounds become liquid at relatively low temperatures (200°C) (Muskopf and McCollister 1987). Epoxy molding compounds are used, for example, in the manufacture of models and engine covers and in the encapsulation of electrical components (Fregert 1981b). TGIC is one of the non-DGEBA epoxy resins (*Table 51.1*) and is mainly used in thermosetting one-component powder polyester paints as a hardener (Muskopf and McCollister 1987).

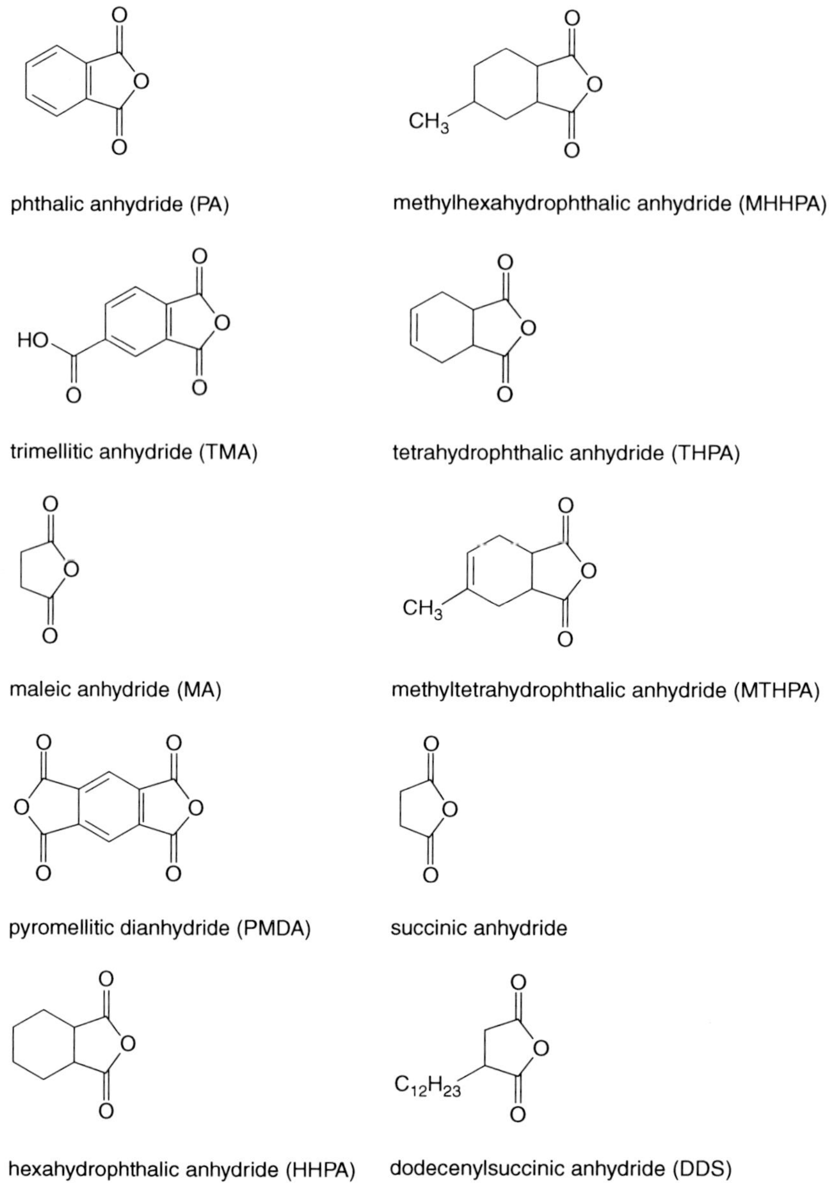

Fig. 51.5
Organic acid anhydride hardeners

2.2.2 Epoxy (Meth)acrylates

bis-GMA is used in dental restoration work, in dental filling and coating materials, in dentin primers, and also when fissures in posterior teeth are sealed to protect them from caries (Vanherle and Smith 1985; Janda 1987). Several similar epoxy dimethacrylate compounds have also appeared as substitutes for bis-GMA or in addition to bis-GMA in dental resins.

Epoxy di(meth)acrylates also have many industrial applications. They are used in UV-curable printing processes (Emmett and Kominsky 1977; Björkner 1984), in corrosion-resistant equipment; land transportation equipment; electrical insulation for heavy electrical equipment, and in marine applications. In the manufacture of composite plastic products, epoxy di(meth)acrylates are used after being dissolved in styrene (Anderson and Messick 1985; Janda 1987).

Solventless epoxy acrylate coatings are cured by initiation with UV light (Bauer 1985). Glycidyl methacrylate, which contains an epoxy group (➋ *Fig. 51.6*), is used in emulsions for impregnating paper and textile materials (Matura et al. 1995).

2.2.3 Other Epoxy Compounds

EPTMAC is used in the manufacture of cationic starch as a cationizing chemical, in the manufacture of ion-exchange resins and in many other applications (Bergquist-Karlsson 1985). Other epoxy compounds are used in drug synthesis (Rudzki and Rebandel 1990) or found among the oxidation products of abietic and related acids (Hausen et al. 1990).

2.3 Allergic Contact Dermatitis to Epoxy Chemicals

2.3.1 Epoxy Resin Compounds

The first reports of sensitization to epoxy chemicals were published in the 1950s in Switzerland, the Netherlands, the United States, and Great Britain, where most of the epoxy resin development had taken place (Calnan 1958; Jolanki 1991). By the beginning of the 1970s, epoxy chemicals began to cause increasing numbers of occupational dermatoses. During 1990–1995, epoxy chemicals were clearly more frequent causes than other plastic chemicals. They caused 11.7–12.5% of the cases of occupational ACD (Jolanki 1991; Holness and Nethercott 1992), and roughly 1% of the exposed workers, annually, developed an occupational dermatosis caused by epoxy chemicals (Jolanki 1991). Patients diagnosed in 1974–1995 at the Finnish Institute of Occupational Health showed that about 80% of 182 patients who had occupational ACD from epoxy chemicals were sensitized to DGEBA epoxy resins. Contact allergy from non-bisphenol A type epoxy resins was found in about 9% of patients, from polyamine hardeners 23%, and from reactive diluents 16%. Six patients had ACD from TGIC. Simultaneous contact allergy to different epoxy chemicals was also found in 29% of the patients (Jolanki et al. 2001).

High rates of contact allergy from exposure to epoxy chemicals have been reported in studies emanating from workplaces, such as 56% in aircraft manufacturing workers (Burrows et al. 1984), 45% in marble workers (Angelini et al. 1996), 27% in ski-factory workers (Jolanki et al. 1996b), and 12.1% in workers exposed to epoxy chemicals from Australia (Nixon and Frowen 1991). In Germany, the frequencies of ACD to epoxy chemicals were reported to be 18.2% in tile setters and terrazzo workers, 9.7% in construction and cement workers, 10.2% in electronics industry workers, and 8.2% in painters (Dickel et al. 2002) The incidence rate of ACD to epoxy chemicals in painters in the Norwegian oil industry was calculated to be 4.5/1,000 person years (Romhyr et al. 2006). Important factors for the development of dermatitis from epoxy chemicals include the type of exposure, frequency of skin contact with the causative agent, the concentration of the epoxy chemical used, the size of the contaminated skin area, and the use of protective gloves (Jolanki 1991).

In some instances, the latent period before onset of ACD to epoxy chemicals may be quite short, ranging from less than 1 month to several years (Suhonen 1983; Holness 1992). Even a single accidental exposure may induce primary sensitization to epoxy resin (Kanerva et al. 1994). Most of the patients contracting dermatitis to epoxy chemicals are men (Fregert 1975; Jolanki 1991; Nethercott et al. 1994). The difference in the frequency of dermatosis between the two genders probably represents differences in exposure.

Epoxy chemicals can induce direct or airborne contact dermatitis, but the skin symptoms are located mainly on the patients' hands or arms, and to a lesser extent, face and neck. The fingers and interdigital spaces, forearms and wrists, and the eyelids are the most typical locations of the skin disorders caused by epoxy chemicals (Jolanki et al. 1990; Geier et al. 2004). In addition, genital involvement may occur because of contamination from hands (Nixon 1997). Reactive diluents and hardeners have been considered the most probable causes of airborne epoxy chemical dermatitis, because these substances are more volatile than DGEBA epoxy resins (Dahlquist and Fregert 1979). In another study, facial dermatitis was found in 60% of patients, but it was not especially common among patients allergic to reactive diluents or hardeners (Jolanki et al. 1990).

2.3.2 Diglycidyl Ether of Bisphenol A (DGEBA) Epoxy Resins

Thorgeirsson and Fregert (1977) confirmed that the main sensitizer in epoxy resin systems was DGEBA, with a MW of 340 Da. In the guinea-pig maximization test, the oligomer with a MW of 624 Da was also a sensitizer, but with minor sensitizing capacity, whereas oligomers with a MW of more than 900 Da did not induce sensitivity (Thorgeirsson et al. 1978). Until 1964, 1.6% of 1,690 patients who were not employed in the epoxy resin

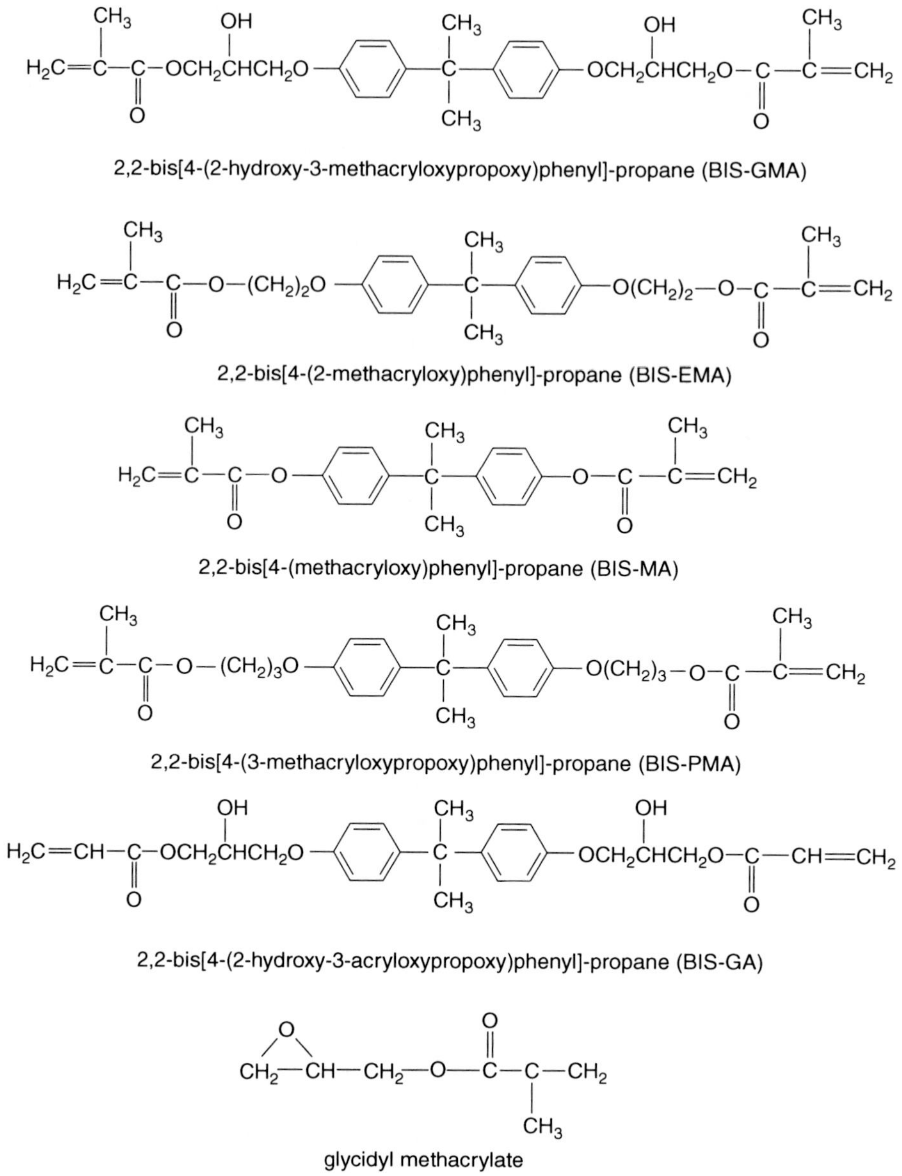

Fig. 51.6
Methacrylated epoxy compounds

industry developed allergic patch test reactions to DGEBA epoxy resin at the Department of Dermatology, University of Lund (Fregert and Rorsman 1964). Thus, the DGEBA epoxy resin, as one of the top 20 contact allergens, was included in the European standard patch-test series in 1966 (Jolanki 1991). In the beginning of the 1990s, the positive rate from the North American Contact Dermatitis Group (NACDG) was 1.8% among 3,500 patients studied (Marks et al. 1995). Edman (1988) found a lower frequency of 1%, among 3,562 patients patch tested during 1982–1987 at the Malmo General Hospital, Sweden. Similarly, in Denmark, 0.8% of 10,423 patients (Veien et al. 1992) and, in China, 0.7% of 1,135 patients were found to be patch test positive to epoxy resin (Liu et al. 1997). However, the positive rates from selective occupational dermatology clinics in Helsinki and Toronto were as high as 3.7% (Jolanki 1991; Holness and Nethercott 1992). The Information Network of Departments of Dermatology (IVDK) in Germany reported rates of 0.9–1.5% (1992–2000) (Geier et al. 2004).

In a recent large multicenter compilation of patch test results in North America, the percentage of positive reactions to epoxy resins have remained relatively stable at 1.8%, with 30.8% of reactions thought to be definitely or probably relevant in 2005–2006 (Zug et al. 2009). In Portugal the rate over 10 years in 2,440 patients was 0.9% (Canelas et al. 2010).

Epoxy resin was the only allergen more often associated with occupational exposure than nonoccupational exposure in North America (Rietschel et al. 2002). Paints, varnishes, and other surface coatings as well as exposure in the electronics industry are common causes of DGEBA epoxy-resin sensitization (Jolanki 1991). Epoxy sensitization is also often caused by exposure to two-component glues and bonding agents (Conde-Salazar et al. 1993; Jolanki et al. 1994b). Several reports describe workers sensitized to epoxy resins used as binders in carbon- or glass-fiber reinforced plastic products (Suhonen 1983; Holness and Nethercott 1989; Tarvainen et al. 1995b).

Epoxy resin used as a sizing agent in glass fibers has also induced contact allergy during the production (Toffoletto et al. 1994). A recent source of exposure to epoxy chemicals has been the production of wind turbines, where 10.9% of 603 workers studied had ACD caused by epoxy chemicals. DGEBA was the causative factor in approximately 50% of cases: the remaining cases were caused by amine hardeners and catalysts (Pontén et al. 2004a). Nonoccupationally induced ACD has been reported from epoxy resin in medical devices, such as hemodialysis needles, polyvinyl ostomy bags, infusion sets of an insulin pump, nasal cannulae, pacemaker, and amputation prosthesis (Mann et al. 1983; Boom and van Driel 1985; Requena et al. 1986; Toome 1989; Skoet et al. 2003; Haussmann et al. 2005).

Furthermore, there are numerous case reports of epoxy ACD from hidden sources of epoxy resin, such as oil painting (Conde-Salazar et al. 1982), lamination of glass products (Heskel 1988), adhesive plaster (Dooms-Goossens et al. 1993), bowls polish (Lyon et al. 1998), a billiard cue (Gonçalo et al. 1992), and microscopy immersion oils (Sommer et al. 1997). Solid, completely polymerized resins rarely cause dermatitis, but traces of unhardened monomeric DGEBA epoxy resin have been identified on sign boards, bottle caps, film cassettes, metal packages, and brass doorknobs (Fregert 1981a). Tooling, including sawing and drilling of epoxy resin in cured state, promotes the release of epoxy allergens (Hansson 1994). ACD has also been induced by unhardened epoxy resin in several finished products (Taylor et al. 1983; Malanin and Kalimo 1985; Fischer et al. 1987; Goulden and Wikinson 1996). In addition, a few cases of ACD from DGEBA epoxy resins with a high average MW have been reported (Jolanki et al. 1987b; Suhonen 1983), even though the amount of DGEBA has been as low as 0.2% in the causative products (Jolanki et al. 1987b). Epoxy resins used as stabilizers and plasticizers for polyvinyl chloride have also been shown to be sensitizers (Ancona-Alayon et al. 1976; Toome 1989).

Both Swedish and Danish groups have reported associations between contact allergy to DGEBA resin and fragrance mix 1, of unclear relevance (Pontén et al. 2004b; Andersen et al. 2009).

2.3.3 Non-Diglycidyl Ether of Bisphenol A

Since the 1980s, ACD has also been reported from non-DGEBA epoxy resins, such as N-N-tetraglycidyl-4,4′-methylene dianiline and o-diglycidyl phthalate (Burrows et al. 1984; Ayala et al. 1990; Tarvainen et al. 1995b; Kanerva et al. 2000b), 4-glycidyloxy-N, N-diglycidylaniline (Burrows et al. 1984; Mathias 1987), vinyl cyclohexene dioxide (Dannaker 1988), triglycidyl derivative of p-aminophenol (TGPAP) (Ayala et al. 1990; Tarvainen et al. 1995b; Bruze et al. 1996; Jappe et al. 2005), and 1,6-bis (2,3-epoxypropoxy) naphthalene (Yokota and Michitsuji 2004). In addition, cycloaliphatic epoxy resins based on diglycidyl ester of hexahydrophthalic acid, heterocyclic dimethylhydantoin epoxy resins, phenol novolac epoxy resins, and brominated epoxy resins have been found to be causes of ACD (Jolanki et al. 1987b, 1989; Kanerva et al. 1991b; Bruze et al. 1996). Many of the patients sensitized to these non-DGEBA epoxy resins do not have contact allergy to DGEBA resin. Cycloaliphatic epoxy resins have been found in jet aviation hydraulic fluid (Maibach and Mathias 2001) and in neat oil when added as a stabilizer (Jensen and Andersen 2003). TGIC is a known skin irritant (Nishioka et al. 1988), but has also been shown to be an allergen. Workers may become sensitized to TGIC from short-term exposure to the chemical during its production, in the manufacture and use of TGIC-containing powder polyester paints, and from silk-screen printing coatings in the manufacture of circuit boards (Nishioka et al. 1988; Munro and Lawrence 1992; Jolanki et al. 1994a).

There have been an increasing number of reports of ACD to diglycidyl ether of bisphenol F (DGEBF) (Pontén and Bruze 2001; Pontén et al. 2004c; Sakata et al. 2005). There is immunological cross-reactivity between DGEBA and isomers of DGEBF, the p,p′-DGEBF and o,p′-DGEBF (Pontén et al. 2002). The addition of DGEBF prevents

DGEBA from crystallizing. Patients reacted to both DGEBA and DGEBF based on both cross-sensitization and co-exposure (Geier et al. 2004).

2.3.4 Reactive Diluents

Fregert and Rorsman (1964) described contact allergy to reactive diluents. Epoxy reactive diluents have been revealed to be strong sensitizers in guinea pigs, especially phenylglycidyl ether (Thorgeirsson 1978a), and in humans, reactive diluents have caused allergy in exposed workers (Jolanki 1991; Tosti et al. 1992; Angelini et al. 1996). Contact allergy to reactive diluents without contact allergy to epoxy resins is also possible (Jolanki et al. 1987a; Jolanki 1991; Angelini et al. 1996). Recently it was shown in guinea pigs that induction of sensitization with DGEBA was associated with allergy to PGE, while induction of sensitization to PGE was not associated with allergy to DGEBA (Pontén et al. 2009). In addition, when considering the allergenicity of PGE analogues, small changes in chemical structure were associated with appreciable differences in sensitizing capacity (Niklasson et al. 2009). Reactive diluents are more volatile than DGEBA epoxy resin, and may cause an airborne dermatitis pattern (Dahlquist and Fregert 1979; Tosti et al. 1988; Angelini et al. 1996). Most patients sensitized to reactive diluents are allergic to PGE, cresyl glycidyl ether, hexanediol diglycidyl ether, butanediol diglycidyl ether, or butyl glycidyl ether, and cross-sensitization between reactive diluents is common (Jolanki et al. 1987a; Jolanki 1991, 1997; Tosti et al. 1992; Conde-Salazar et al. 1994; Angelini et al. 1996). Contamination of epoxy resins with low levels of PGE has also been reported (Pontén et al. 2008). Rare reactive diluent contact allergens include allyl glycidyl ether (Jolanki 1991; Angelini et al. 1996), cyclohexanedimethanol glycidyl ether (Angelini et al. 1996), neopentyl glycol diglycidyl ether (Jolanki 1991), Cardura E10 (Lovell et al. 1984), Epoxide 8 (Björkner et al. 1980), diethyleneglycol diglycidyl ether (Jolanki et al. 1996b), and alphanaphthyl glycidyl ether and p-fluorphenyl glycidyl ether (De Groot 1994). Allyl glycidyl ether has also caused ACD in the plastics industry from the use of epoxy silane in a single-component sealant (Dooms-Goossens et al. 1995).

2.3.5 Hardeners

In the guinea-pig maximization test, polyamine hardeners with a low MW were found to be strong sensitizers (Thorgeirsson 1978b). Most of the patients with contact allergy to epoxy hardeners have reacted to 4,4′-diaminodiphenyl methane (DDM), DETA, and TETA (Jolanki 1991; Tosti et al. 1992). In addition, cases of contact allergy to IPDA (Lachapelle et al. 1978; Kanerva et al. 1998), trimethyl hexamethylene diamine (Kanerva et al. 1991a, 1998), tetraethylenepentamine (TEPA) (Kanerva et al. 1998), m-xylylene diamine (MXDA) (Kanerva et al. 1991a, 1998; Romhyr et al. 2006), diaminocyclohexane (Kirkup et al. 2001), or other cyclohexylamines (Gordon and McLelland 1998) have been reported. More recent reports have emphasized reactions occurring to MXDA, as well as IPDA and DDM (Geier et al. 2004). Cross-reactivity between polyamine hardeners is possible (Rudzki and Krajewska 1976; Kirkup et al. 2001). Isolated contact allergy to epoxy hardeners is uncommon (Tosti et al. 1992; Kanerva et al. 1991a, 1996). tris-DMP has been reported to be probably a more common allergen than expected (Kanerva et al. 1991a, 1996; Brooke and Beck 1998; Romhyr et al. 2006). Positive patch-test reactions to DDM or ethylene diamine (EDA) are not necessarily an indication of sensitivity from exposure to epoxy hardeners. The relevance of DDM allergy is sometimes difficult to detect. For example, a positive patch-test reaction to DDM may represent allergy to para-amino compounds, such as p-phenylene diamine (Gailhofer and Ludvan 1989), or exposure to diphenyl methane diisocyanate (Jolanki et al. 1990). EDA allergy may be caused by exposure, for example, to rubber, synthetic coolants, or topical creams (Rietschel and Fowler 2008). Another aliphatic amine hardener, DMAPA, is an impurity responsible for cocamidopropylbetaine allergy from cosmetics (Speight et al. 1993; Angelini et al. 1995; Kanerva et al. 1996). A few reports of contact allergy to non-amine hardeners have been published in the case of dicyandiamide (Senff et al. 1988), dodecenyl succinic anhydride (Göransson 1977), methylhexahydrophthalic anhydride (Kanerva et al. 1997), hexavalent chromate, an accelerator additive (Handley and Burrows 1994; Bruze et al. 1996), polysulfides (Bruze et al. 1996), and a polymercaptan hardener (Guin 2005).

2.3.6 Bisphenol A and Epichlorohydrin

Occupational contact dermatitis caused by epichlorohydrin and bisphenol A is uncommon (Jolanki 1991). In the finished DGEBA epoxy resin, the proportion of free epichlorohydrin is less than 0.001%. The proportion of bisphenol A is even smaller because, in the manufacturing process, epichlorohydrin is always present in excess to ensure that the molecules terminate in epoxy groups. In epoxy resin plants, despite closed manufacturing systems, workers may have a higher risk of becoming sensitized to epichlorohydrin, but they do not generally become sensitized to bisphenol A (van Joost et al. 1990). Allergy to epichlorohydrin has also been reported from a solvent cement (Beck and King 1983) and from drug synthesis of propranolol hydrochloride and oxprenolol hydrochloride (Rebandel and Rudzki 1990). One patient with ACD from exposure to epoxy propane reacted also to epichlorohydrin and to diglycidyl ester of hexahydrophthalic acid (Morris et al. 1998). Reports of bisphenol A sensitization have been rather controversial (van Joost et al. 1990). Krajewska and Rudzki (1976) described positive patch tests to bisphenol A in 13 of 17 Polish workers sensitized to epoxy resin by patch testing bisphenol A at a concentration of 2% in water, but they did not mention how the positive reactions were scored. Additional data on the high incidence of bisphenol A allergy among those sensitized to epoxy resin are lacking. The group of van Joost (van Joost 1988; van Joost et al. 1990) found very few cases of bisphenol A allergy in workers at epoxy resin manufacturing plants, although several patients had been sensitized to epichlorohydrin. Cases of allergy to bisphenol A have been reported from fiberglass made of epoxy resin (Gaul 1960), bis-GMA-based dental composite resins containing 0.014–0.015% bisphenol A (Jolanki et al. 1995), semisynthetic waxes (Freeman and Warin 1984), plastic footwear (Srinivas et al. 1989), and PVC gloves (Aalto-Korte et al. 2003). Contact allergy to bisphenol A may also be a cross-reaction with compounds responsible for phenolformaldehyde resin allergy, such as dihydroxydiphenyl methanes (bisphenol F) (Bruze and Zimerson 1985; Jolanki 1991).

Epoxy (Meth)acrylates

The guinea-pig maximization test has shown that epoxy di (meth)acrylates range from being weak to extreme sensitizers (Björkner 1984). Despite the increasing use of epoxy di(meth)acrylates in dental care and in industry, relatively few reports of contact allergy caused by these compounds have been published (Emmett and Kominsky 1977; Kanerva and Alanko 1998; Aalto-Korte et al. 2009). The sensitized subjects have mainly been workers in the UV-light printing industry (Emmett and Kominsky 1977; Björkner 1984) or in dental nursing (Kanerva et al. 1989; Aalto-Korte et al. 2009). In addition, work in the manufacture of UV-curable epoxy diacrylate paints (Jolanki et al. 1995), UV-curable coating varnish containing epoxy acrylate oligomers (Guimaraens et al. 1994), and UV-curable inks (Kanerva et al. 2000c; Aalto-Korte et al. 2009) is associated with contact allergy. Patients who acquire their epoxy dimethacrylate allergy from products that contain bis-GMA as the main monomer are, in general, concomitantly allergic to both bis-GMA and the standard epoxy resin (Kanerva et al. 1989; Goossens et al. 1998; Kanerva and Alanko 1998; Aalto-Korte et al. 2009). It has been shown that bis-GMA-borne dental materials may contain minute amounts of DGEBA, enough to induce sensitization (Niinimäki et al. 1983; Kanerva et al. 1989). Contact allergy to epoxy di(meth)acrylates has also been found in patients who had been exposed to DGEBA epoxy resins, but with no known exposure to the epoxy di(meth)acrylates (Jolanki et al. 1990; Kanerva et al. 1991c). Matura et al. (1995) reported on a chemist who had developed ACD to glycidyl methacrylate from compounding emulsions used to impregnate paper and textile materials to make them oil- and water-resistant. The role of glycidyl methacrylates in bis-GMA contact allergy is unknown. Patients with ACD from products containing epoxy dimethacrylate may also have contact allergy to bisphenol A from handling products containing dental composite resin (Jolanki et al. 1995). Cross-reactivity among epoxy acrylates, together with DGEBF and DGEBA allergy was also reported in North America (Lee et al. 2002).

2.3.7 Other Epoxy Compounds

EPTMAC has been shown to be a moderate sensitizer in guinea pigs and to cause ACD in humans (Bergquist-Karlsson 1985; Estlander et al. 1986). An intermediate product in the synthesis of the drug, diltiazem hydrochloride, 2,3-epoxy-3-(4-methoxyphenyl) propionate, has induced contact allergy in two cases (Rudzki and Rebandel 1990; Buisson et al. 1991). Another epoxy compound, 13,14(p)-epoxyabietic acid, is an isolated allergen of unmodified colophony (Hausen et al. 1990; Karlberg and Gafvert 1996). Epoxy propane (propylene oxide) used as a solvent in histology has also been shown to be a contact allergen (Steinkraus and Hausen 1994; Morris et al. 1998).

2.4 Contact Urticaria

Relatively few cases of immediate-type contact urticaria (CU) caused by epoxy chemicals have been reported.

Both epoxy resins (Jolanki et al. 1997a) and organic acid anhydride hardeners (Jolanki et al. 1997b) should be regarded as potential causes of the CU syndrome. In 1974, a patch test with an epoxy resin was reported to induce generalized urticaria and an asthmatic reaction (Woyton et al. 1974). In 1983, Subonen reported on two patients who, in a patch test, showed immediate urticarial reactions, probably caused by an impure DGEBA epoxy resin used in a ski-pole factory. Kanerva et al. (1991c) described two patients with both delayed allergy to DGEBA epoxy resin and specific immunoglobulin E (IgE)-mediated immediate sensitization from DGEBA with a MW of 340 Da. Nixon and Frowen (1991) reported eight cases of CU in 198 workers exposed to epoxy chemicals. Sasseville (1998) reported a case of CU from an aircraft factory. On patch testing after 30 min, the worker experienced urticarial reactions to epoxy resin (1% pet), PGE (0.25% pet), and cresylglycidyl ether (0.25% pet). No delayed reactions were seen. Similarly, Miyamoto and Okumura (1998) reported CU confirmed by a 15 min open test and a 15 min closed patch test for epoxy resin at 1% in petrolatum. Anaphylaxis was reported to epoxy resin in a root canal sealer after a patient became unconscious when visiting the dentist (Stutz et al. 2008).

Occupational asthma was reported by Kanerva et al. (2000c) and Hannu et al. (2009). In another case, the CU test reaction was augmented when the allergen was wiped off with an alcohol swab, presumably because the alcohol enhanced skin penetration of the allergen (Kanerva et al. 2002). Urticarial reactions have been reported in workers involved in the manufacture of phthalic anhydride (Menschik 1955). Other case reports describe patients who developed CU from methylhexahydrophthalic anhydride or methyltetrahydrophthalic anhydride (MTHPA) epoxy hardeners from the manufacture of condensers (Jolanki et al. 1987b, 1990), electrical machines (Tarvainen et al. 1995a; Kanerva et al. 1997), or ski poles (Tarvainen et al. 1995a). Appreciable respiratory symptoms from MTHPA were reported from a plant producing barrels from rocket guns from an epoxy resin (Nielsen et al. 1992). Acid anhydrides have the ability to induce specific IgE-mediated sensitization (Jolanki et al. 1990; Tarvainen et al. 1995a; Kanerva et al. 1997), resulting in CU and allergic respiratory and conjunctival symptoms. The Finnish experience of occupational CU from cyclic acid anhydrides (21 cases) was recently reviewed (Helaskoski et al. 2009). In addition, CU can be caused by aliphatic polyamine hardeners (Rietschel and Fowler 2008) and possibly by other amines (Savonius et al. 1994).

2.5 Irritant Contact Dermatitis from Epoxy Compunds

Irritating, low-MW degradation products may be produced in the tooling of epoxy products and in heating processes (Engstrom and Henriks-Eckerman 1988). Amine and anhydride hardeners and epichlorohydrin irritate the skin and conjunctivae. In addition to causing irritant contact dermatitis, epichlorohydrin, as a highly reactive compound, and aliphatic polyamines, as highly alkaline compounds (pH 13-14), can cause corrosive burns on the skin (Ippen and Mathies 1970; Rietschel and Fowler 2008). Ippen and Mathies (1970) described protracted chemical burns after the exposure of five patients to epichlorohydrin. DGEBA epoxy resins are not strong irritants and their irritancy decreases with the increasing MW of the oligomer (Hine et al. 1958). Lea et al. (1958) found that an epoxy reactive diluent, butyl glycidyl ether, also caused irritation in human volunteers. Curing agents in powder paints, such as dicyandiamide and organic anhydrides are also potentially irritant (Peltonen 1986; Jolanki et al. 1997b). Organic anhydrides, when cold, are not very harmful to dry skin, but hot compounds may cause severe chemical burns. On sweating skin, anhydrides are hydrated to the corresponding acids and can cause caustic dermatitis and burns (Menschik 1955; Malten and Zielhuis 1964). Four patients developed irritant contact dermatitis from paints or paint raw materials containing DGEBA epoxy resins with a high average MW and one patient from a mixture of a DGEBA epoxy resin with a low average MW and its anhydride hardener, used in electrical insulation (Jolanki et al. 1987b, 1990).

2.5.1 Active Sensitization

Patch testing has occasionally produced sensitization to patch test allergens (active sensitization). Active sensitization is especially common when acrylics are tested (Kanerva et al. 1992), but has also complicated testing with epoxy chemicals (Fregert and Rorsman 1964; Calnan 1967, 1975; Lachapelle et al. 1978; Jolanki 1991; Kanerva and Estlander 1998). At the Finnish Institute of Occupational Health, the test concentration of epichlorohydrin was lowered to 0.1% in petrolatum because of active sensitization. (Kanerva et al. 1999). It has not been established whether false negative tests occur. PGE at 0.25% in petrolatum has also been reported to cause active sensitization (Kanerva and Estlander 1998).

2.6 Other Skin Disorders Caused by Epoxy Chemicals

Purpuric ACD, scleroderma-like disorders, atypical psoriasis, and erythema multiforme have all been reported to be caused by exposure to epoxy chemicals (Holness and Nethercott 1989). Bachurzewska and Borucka (1986) reported findings similar to Raynaud's disease. Rycroft (1980) reported on a patient whose epoxy resin sensitization was followed by atypical psoriasis, while Lichter et al. (1992) described a patient whose sensitization to epoxy resin and hardener was followed by lichenoid contact dermatitis. The development of vitiligo in the sites of positive patch tests to TGPAP has been reported (Jappe et al. 2005) together with contact vitiligo following ACD to reactive diluents (Silvestre et al. 2004). Photosensitivity has been reported in relation to the heating of DGEBA epoxy resin and the use of epoxy powder paints (Allen and Kaidbey 1979; Göransson et al. 1984). It is thought to be caused by bisphenol A contained in the resin (Maguire 1988).

2.7 Skin Testing and Chemical Investigations

No single chemical can be used alone to screen for sensitization to the different epoxy chemical contact allergens. Approximately 30% of patients with contact allergy to epoxy chemicals have been found to be sensitive to more than one of the three main epoxy chemical groups: resins, hardeners, and reactive diluents. In addition, individual contact allergies to hardeners, reactive diluents and non-DGEBA epoxy resins without simultaneous contact allergy to the standard epoxy resin are quite common among workers exposed to epoxy chemicals (Jolanki 1991; Tosti et al. 1992). It is therefore recommended that patients suspected of contact dermatitis from epoxy chemicals should also be tested with the individual allergenic compounds, hardeners, reactive diluents, and non-DGEBA epoxy resins to which they have been exposed. They should also be tested with their own specific materials, especially if there is no response to the standard epoxy resin (Holness and Nethercott 1993). It should be borne in mind that testing only with the patients' own materials is not always completely reliable, because the allergens may become too diluted and thus give negative patch-test results (Jolanki 1991).

A patch-test concentration of 0.5% in petrolatum for non-DGEBA epoxy resins is probably preferable to 1% when low-viscosity resins are being tested, because 1% non-DGEBA resins may irritate (Jolanki et al. 1989). Patch testing with the resinous part alone does not exclude contact allergy to reactive diluents if the patient is also sensitive to the resin. The test concentration of 0.25% in petrolatum was found to be suitable for testing reactive diluents (Jolanki 1991; Jolanki et al. 1996b; Geier et al. 2004). On patch testing, cross-reactivity has been found between compounds that are chemically closely related, especially between reactive diluents. Reactive diluents do not produce cross-reactions with DGEBA epoxy resins, and contact allergy to reactive diluents is not revealed by testing with the standard epoxy resin. However patients who are allergic to cycloaliphatic epoxy resins often react to reactive diluents, and vice versa (Jolanki 1991).

Aromatic compounds, especially PGE, have been observed to cause allergic patch test reactions in most of the patients who were allergic to reactive diluents. BDDGE was found to screen contact allergy to aliphatic reactive diluents. Thus PGE and BDDGE are probably enough to also screen contact allergy to other related compounds (Jolanki 1991).

Patch testing with DETA, TETA, DDM, IPDA, and tris-DMP should be performed when allergy to polyamine hardeners is suspected. All but tris-DMP are available from the test substance suppliers. The recommended test concentration for tris-DMP is 0.5–1% in petrolatum (Kanerva et al. 1996; Brooke and Beck 1998). Because of the vast variety of hardeners used, it is highly recommendable to test patients with the hardeners that they have been exposed to; test concentrations of up to 10% should be used for the amine-epoxy adducts. A test concentration of about 1% is the most suitable for polyamine-type hardeners (Jolanki 1991).

bis-GMA and bis-GA should be tested for the detection of contact allergy caused by epoxy di(meth)acrylates. An allergic reaction induced by the standard epoxy resin may indicate contact allergy to epoxy di(meth)acrylates and this possibility should be clarified by additional patch tests (Kanerva et al. 1989; Jolanki 1991).

In general, petrolatum seems to be a good vehicle for testing epoxy chemicals. For solid materials containing uncured epoxy resins, it is preferable to use acetone instead of water for ultrasonic cleaning bath extractions or to soften the material in the patch test chamber (Jolanki et al. 1990; Bruze et al. 1992).

A recent study reported late patch test reactions to epoxy resin, at or after day 7, occurring in 0.3% of 1428 cases (Hillen et al. 2006). It is necessary to combine chemical and dermatological experience for the optimal investigation of occupational skin diseases induced by epoxy chemicals. The methods include clarification of the causative agents through patch testing and planning of preventive measures for both the patient and, especially, unaffected fellow workers. In problematic cases, skin prick testing with epoxy chemicals, consultations with industrial hygienists, visits to the patients' work sites and analyses of the materials handled by the patients are also important (Estlander 1990; Jolanki 1991). It is also important to note that safety data sheets are occasionally incorrect, and epoxy chemicals have sometimes been not listed (Nixon 1997). Thin-layer chromatography and other chromatographic methods (gas chromatography and high-performance liquid chromatography) can be used to demonstrate the presence or absence of particular allergens (Fregert 1988; Jolanki et al. 1988; Ayala et al. 1990; Kanerva et al. 1991a).

2.8 Prevention of Epoxy Chemical Dermatitis

Complete avoidance of contact with the causative allergens is always necessary. In a patient highly sensitive to epoxy compounds, even a minimal amount of an allergen may be enough to evoke the symptoms on the exposed skin. Most patients with occupational dermatitis caused by epoxy chemicals have to leave their work. This may also be beneficial for the prevention of possible respiratory allergy following skin sensitization (Kanerva et al. 1991c). ACD to epoxy chemicals, nevertheless, has been thought to have a good prognosis, predominantly because it is easier to avoid contact with these chemicals than to avoid contact with more ubiquitous allergens, such as nickel or chromate (Rosen and Freeman 1993).

However, recent work suggests that this may not always be the case, and in some cases workers develop persistent skin symptoms. This may relate to the initial severity of the dermatosis (Cahill et al. 2005). It may also result in the development of persistent post-occupational dermatitis (Sajjachareonpong et al. 2004).

Those working with epoxy compounds should be made aware of the risk of sensitization. Gloves made of laminated, multilayered plastic (Silver Shield 4 H Glove, North Safety Products), containing ethylene-vinyl alcohol copolymer, developed especially for the handling of epoxy chemicals give the best protection (Henriksen and Petersen 1986; Roed-Petersen 1989; McClain and Storrs 1992). Unpublished data from glove manufacturers has also suggested that thicker, reusable nitrile gloves may be effective, but not thinner disposable nitrile gloves (Sakata et al. 2005).

Another complicating factor is concurrent solvent use, which may adversely affect glove function. The suitability of gloves with other chemicals may be obtained from websites, such as http://www.ansellpro.com/download/Ansell_7thEditionChemicalResistanceGuide.pdf. The use of less sensitizing products may reduce the possibility of developing allergy to epoxy, as high MW epoxies do not sensitize readily. The use of one-bag epoxies, which mix in the package (Van Putten et al. 1984), may reduce the possibility of skin contact. Recent work suggests that small changes to the structure of PGE are associated with less allergenicity (Niklasson et al. 2009).

The airways should also be protected from exposure to the epoxy compounds, because these compounds may cause asthma. Even use of an automated process does not guarantee protection against skin contact and exposure of the respiratory tract, because of the possibility of exposure during maintenance, machine repair, or sampling (Jolanki 1991).

An "Epoxy Code" was developed for use in the construction industry involving Denmark, Germany, the Netherlands, and the UK (Spee et al. 2006).

Finally, once a case of ACD to epoxy chemicals has been diagnosed, it is worth reflecting on the factors that led to sensitization, and the risks to other workers, who have not (yet) developed dermatitis. As Boris Lushniak said: "By its nature, occupational dermatology is also related to occupational preventive medicine." The ideal role of the medical practitioner involved in occupational dermatology is not only to diagnose and treat patients, but also to determine the etiology of the occupational skin disease and to make recommendations for its prevention" (Lushniak 2004).

References

Aalto-Korte K, Alanko K, Henriks-Eckerman ML et al (2003) Allergic contact dermatitis from bisphenol A in PVC gloves. Contact Dermatitis 49:202–205

Aalto-Korte K, Jungewelter S, Henriks-Eckerman ML et al (2009) Contact allergy to epoxy (meth)acrylates. Contact Dermatitis 61:9–21

Allen H, Kaidbey K (1979) Persistent photosensitivity following occupational exposure to epoxy resin. Arch Dermatol 115:1307–1310

Ancona-Alayon A, Jimenez-Castilla JL, Gomez-Alvarez EM (1976) Dermatitis from epoxy resin and formaldehyde in shampoo packers. Contact Dermatitis 2:356

Andersen KE, Christensen LP, Volund A et al (2009) Association between positive patch tests to epoxy resin and fragrance mix 1 ingredients. Contact Dermatitis 60:155–157

Anderson TF, Messick VB (1985) Vinyl ester resins. In: Pritchard G (ed) Developments in reinforced plastics, vol 1. Elsevier, London, pp 29–58

Angelini G, Foti C, Rigano L, Vena GA (1995) 3-Dimethylaminopropylamine: a key substance in contact allergy to cocamidopropylbetaine? Contact Dermatitis 32:96–99

Angelini G, Rigano L, Foti C, Grandolfo M et al (1996) Occupational sensitization to epoxy resin and reactive diluents in marble workers. Contact Dermatitis 35:11–16

Ayala F, Lembo G, Balato N et al (1990) The use of laboratory methods in contact dermatitis induced by composite materials. Contact Dermatitis 22:262–266, erratum 23:384

Bachurzewska B, Borucka I (1986) Gefässläsionen bei Eisenbahnarbeiterinnen, die mit Epoxidharzen in Berührung kommen. Dermatosen 34:77–79

Back B, Saarinen L (1986) Free amines in epoxy hardeners and in workplace air (in Finnish with English summary). Työterveyslaitoksen tutkimuksia 1:31–36

Bauer RS (1985) Epoxy resins. In: Tess RW, Poehlein GW (eds) Applied polymer science, 2nd edn. American Chemical Society, Washington, DC, pp 931–961

Beck MH, King CM (1983) Allergic contact dermatitis to epichlorhydrin in a solvent cement. Contact Dermatitis 9:315

Bergquist-Karlsson A (1985) Contact allergy to glycidyl trimethyl ammonium chloride. Contact Dermatitis 12:61–62

Björkner B (1984) Sensitizing capacity of ultraviolet curable acrylic compounds. Doctoral dissertation, University of Lund, Sweden

Björkner B, Dahlquist I, Fregert S, Magnusson B (1980) Contact allergy to Epoxide 8, an epoxy reactive diluent. Contact Dermatitis 6:156

Boom BW, van Driel LMJ (1985) Allergic contact dermatitis to epoxy resin in infusion sets of an insulin pump. Contact Dermatitis 12:280

Bowen RL (1962) Dental filling material comprising vinyl silane treated fused silica and a binder consisting of the reaction product of bis phenol and glycidyl acrylate. US Patent 3,066,112

Brooke R, Beck MH (1998) Contact allergy to 2,4,6-tris(dimethylaminomethyl) phenol. Contact Dermatitis 38:284–285

Bruze M, Zimerson E (1985) Contact allergy to dihydroxydiphenyl methanes (bisphenol F). Dermatosen 33:216–220

Bruze M, Trulson L, Bendsoe N (1992) Patch testing with ultrasonic bath extracts. Am J Contact Dermatitis 3:133–137

Bruze M, Edenholm M, Engstrom K, Svensson G (1996) Occupational dermatoses in a Swedish aircraft plant. Contact Dermatitis 34:336–340

Buisson H, Vaillant L, Lasfargues G, Muller C, Lorette G (1991) Occupational contact dermatitis from trans-methyl-3(4-methoxyphenyl) glycidate. Contact Dermatitis 25:262–263

Burrows D, Fregert S, Campbell H, Trulsson L (1984) Contact dermatitis from the epoxy resins tetraglycidyl-4.4′ –methylene dianiline and o-diglycidyl phthalate in composite material. Contact Dermatitis 11:80–82

Cahill J, Keegel T, Dharmage S et al (2005) Prognosis of contact dermatitis in epoxy resin workers. Contact Dermatitis 52:147–153

Calnan CD (1958) Studies in contact dermatitis. Trans St John's Hosp Dermatol Soc 40:12–19

Calnan CD (1967) Studies in contact dermatitis XX. Active sensitization. Trans St John's Hosp Dermatol Soc 53:128–134

Calnan CD (1975) Epoxy resin dermatitis. J Soc Occup Med 25:123–126

Canelas MM, Gonçalo M, Figueiredo A (2010) Contact allergy to epoxy reins- a 10 year study. Contact Dermatitis 62:55

Conde-Salazar L, Romero L, Guimaraens D, Harto A (1982) Contact dermatitis in an oil painter. Contact Dermatitis 8:209–210

Conde-Salazar L, Gorospe M, Guimaraens D (1993) A new source of sensitivity to epoxy resin. Contact Dermatitis 28:292

Conde-Salazar L, Conzalez de Domingo MA, Guimaraens D (1994) Sensitization to epoxy resin system in special flooring workers. Contact Dermatitis 31:157–160

Dahlquist I, Fregert S, Persson K, Trulsson (1979) Exopy resin in a one-pick glue. Contact Dermatitis 5:189–190

Dahlquist I, Fregert S (1979) Allergic contact dermatitis from volatile epoxy hardeners and reactive diluents. Contact Dermatitis 5:406–407

Dannaker CJ (1988) Allergic sensitization to a non-bisphenol A epoxy of the cycloaliphatic class. J Occup Med 30:641–643

De Groot AC (1994) Occupational contact allergy to alphanaphthyl glycidyl ether. Contact Dermatitis 30:253–254

Dickel H, Kuss O, Schmidt A, Diepgen TL (2002) Occupational relevance of positive standard patch-test results in employed persons with an initial report of an occupational skin disease. Int Arch Occup Environ Health 75:423–434

Dooms-Goossens A, Boden G, Auoaix F, Bruze M (1993) Allergic contact dermatitis from adhesive plaster due to colophony and epoxy resin. Contact Dermatitis 28:120–121

Dooms-Goossens A, Bruze M, Buysse L et al (1995) Contact allergy to allyl glycidyl ether present as an impurity in 3-glycidyloxypropoxyltrimethoxysilane. A fixing additive in silicone and polyurethane resins. Contact Dermatitis 33:17–19

Edman B (1988) Computerized patch data in contact allergy. Doctoral dissertation, Lund University. Sweden

Ellis B (ed) (1993) Chemistry and technology of epoxy resins. Blackie Academic and Professional, Glasgow

Emmett EA, Kominsky JR (1977) Allergic contact dermatitis from ultraviolet cured ink. J Occup Med 19:113–115

Engstrom B, Henriks-Eckerman M-L (1988) Welding and paint (in Finnish). Tyoterveyslaitos (Työolot 68.), Helsinki

Estlander T (1990) Occupational skin disease in Finland: observations made during 1974-88 at the Institute of Occupational Health, Helsinki. Doctoral dissertation, Acta Derm Veneral Suppl 155

Estlander T, Jolanki R, Kanerva L (1986) Occupational dermatitis to 2,3-epoxypropyl trimethyl ammonium chloride. Contact Dermatitis 14:49–52

Fischer T, Fregert S, Thulin I, Trulsson L (1987) Unhardened epoxy resin in tool handles. Contact Dermatitis 16:45

Freeman K, Warin AP (1984) Contact dermatitis due to bisphenol A in semi-synthetic waxes. Contact Dermatitis 11:259–260

Fregert S (1975) Occupational dermatitis in a 10-year material. Contact Dermatitis 1:96–107

Fregert S (1981a) Epoxy dermatitis from the non-working environment. Br J Dermatol 105(Suppl 21):63–64

Fregert S (1981b) Manual of contact dermatitis, 2nd edn. Munksgaard, Copenhagen

Fregert S (1988) Physicochemical methods for detection of contact allergens. Dermatol Clin 6:97–104

Fregert S, Rorsman H (1964) Allergens in epoxy resins. Acta Allergol 19:296–299

Gailhofer G, Ludvan M (1989) Zur Wertigkeit positive Epikutantestreaktionen auf 4,4′-Diamino-diphenylmethan. Dermatosen 37:17–22

Gardiner TH, Waechter JM Jr, Wiedow MH, Solomon WA (1992) Glycidyloxy compounds used in epoxy resin systems: a toxicology review. Regul Toxicol Pharmacol 15:S1

Gaul LE (1960) Sensitivity to bisphenol A. Arch Dermatol 82:1003

Geier J, Lessmann H, Hillen U et al (2004) An attempt to improve diagnostics of contact allergy due to epoxy resin systems. First results of the multicentre study EPOX 2002. Contact Dermatitis 51:263–272

Gonçalo S, Gonçalo M, Matos J, Marçues C (1992) Contact dermatitis from a billiard cue. Contact Dermatitis 26:263

Göransson K (1977) Allergic contact dermatitis to an epoxy hardener: dodecenyl-succinic anhydride. Contact Dermatitis 3:277–278

Göransson K, Andersson R, Andersson G, Marklund S, Anderson K, Ostbye P, Zingmark P-A (1984) An outbreak of occupational photodermatosis of the face in a factory in northern Sweden. In: Berglund B, Lindvall T, Sundell J (eds) Indoor air, vol 3. Swedish Council for Building research, Stockholm, pp 367–375

Gordon PM, McLelland J (1998) Contact sensitivity to Ancamine® 2280 (p-aminocyclohexylamine) following a change in work practice. Contact Dermatitis 38:54

Goulden V, Wilkinson SM (1996) Occupational allergic contact dermatitis from epoxy resin on clipboard. Contact Dermatitis 35:62–263

Guimaraens D, Gonzalez MA, Del Rio E, Conde-Salazar L (1994) Occupational airborne allergiC contact dermatitis in the national mint and fiscal-stamp factory. Contact Dermatitis 30:172–173

Guin JD (2005) Airborne contact dermatitis from a polymercaptan hardener in a finished epoxy resin. Contact Dermatitis 52:45

Guin JD, Work W (1995) Plastics: epoxy resins. In: Guin JD (ed) Practical contact dermatitis. A handbook for the practitioner. McGraw-Hill, New York, pp 433–446

Handley J, Burrows D (1994) Dermatitis from hexavalent chromate in the accelerator of an epoxy sealant (PR1422) used in the aircraft industry. Contact Dermatitis 30:193–196

Hannu T, Frilander H, Kauppi P et al (2009) IgE-mediated occupational asthma from epoxy resin. Int Arch Allergy Immunol 148:41–44

Hansson C (1994) Determination of monomers in epoxy resin hardened at elevated temperature. Contact Dermatitis 31:333–334

Hausen BM, Krohn K, Budianto E (1990) Contact allergy due to colophony. VII. Sensitizing studies with oxidation products of abietic and related acids. Contact Dermatitis 23:352–358

Haussmann J, Pratt M, Linett L, Zimmerman D (2005) Allergic contact dermatitis and eosinophilia in association with a hemodialysis cannula. Am J Kidney Dis 45:e23–e26

Helaskoski E, Kuuliala O, Aalto-Korte K (2009) Occupational contact urticaria caused by cyclic acid anhydrides. Contact Dermatitis 60:214–221

Henriks-Eckerman M-L, Kanerva L (1997) Product analysis of acrylic resins compared to information given in material safety data sheets. Contact Dermatitis 36:164–165

Henriks-Eckerman M-L, Laijoki T (1986a) Aliphatic polyamines and epoxy oligomers in cold cured epoxy products (in finnish with english summary). Työterveyslaitoksen tutkimuksia 4:37–40, summary p 69

Henriks-Eckerman M-L, Laijoki T (1986b) Glycidyl ethers in epoxy resin products (in finnish with english summary). Työterveyslaitoksen tutkimuksia 4:41–46, summary p 70

Henriksen HR. Petersen HJS (1986) Better gloves against epoxy products and other chemicals: protective clothing against chemicals (In Danish with English summary). Arbejdsmiljöfondet (Arbejdsmiljöfondets forskningsrapporter), Copenhagen

Heskel NS (1988) Epoxy resin dermatitis in a stained glass window maker. Contact Dermatitis 18:182–183

Hillen U, Jappe U, Frosch PJ et al (2006) Late reactions to the patch-test preparations para-phenylenediamine and epoxy resin: a prospective multicentre investigation of the German Contact Dermatitis Research Group. Br J Dermatol 154:665–670

Hine CH, Kodama JK, Anderson HH et al (1958) The toxicology of epoxy resins. Arch Ind Health 17:129–144

Holness DL (1992) Outbreak of allergic contact dermatitis caused by epoxy resin in a gluing and swaging operation. Am J Contact Dermat 3:150–154

Holness DL, Nethercott JR (1989) Occupational contact dermatitis due to epoxy resin in a fiberglass binder. J Occup Med 31:87–89

Holness DL, Nethercott JR (1992) Results of testing with epoxy resin in an occupational health clinic population. Am J Contact Dermat 3:169–174

Holness DL, Nethercott JR (1993) The performance of specialized collections of bisphenol A epoxy system components in the evaluation of workers in an occupational health clinic population. Contact Dermatitis 28:216–219

Ippen H, Mathies V (1970) Die "protrahierte Verätzung" (unter besonderer Berlücksichtigung der Hautschäden durch Epoxide und Propansulton). Berufsdermatosen 18:144–165

Janda R (1987) Synthetic resins. In: Gerhartz W, Yamamoto YS, Kaudy L, Pfefferkorn R, Rounsaville JF (eds) Ullmann's encyclopedia of industrial chemistry, 5th completely revised edition, vol A8. VCH Verlagsgesellschaft, Weinheim, pp 277–284

Jappe U, Geier J, Hausen BM (2005) Contact vitiligo following a strong patch test to triglycidyl-p-aminphenol in an aircraft industry worker: case report and review of the literature. Contact Dermatitis 53:89–92

Jensen CD, Andersen KE (2003) Two cases of occupational allergic contact dermatitis from a cycloaliphatic epoxy resin in a neat oil: a case report. Environ Health 2:3

Jolanki R (1991) Occupational skin diseases from epoxy compounds. Epoxy resin compounds, epoxy acrylates and 2,3-epoxypropyl trimethyl ammonium chloride (doctoral dissertation). Acta Derm Venerol Suppl 159:1–80

Jolanki R (1994) Epoxy dermatitis. Occup Med 9:97–112

Jolanki R, Estlander T, Kanerva L (1987a) Contact allergy to an epoxy reactive diluent: 1,4-butanediol diglycidyl ether. Contact Dermatitis 16:87–92

Jolanki R, Estlander T, Kanerva L (1987b) Occupational contact dermatitis and contact urticaria caused by epoxy resins. Acta Derm Venereol Suppl (Stockh) 134:90–94

Jolanki R, Estlander T, Henriks-Eckerman M-L et al (1988) Skin protection and sensitizing epoxy compounds in electron microscopy laboratories. In: Mansdorf SZ, Sager R, Nielsen AP (eds) Performance of protective clothing: second symposium. American Society for Testing and Materials (ASTM STP 989), Philadelphia, pp 389–395

Jolanki R, Sysilampi M-L, Kanerva L, Estlander T (1989) Contact allergy to cycloaliphatic epoxy resins. In: Frosch PI, Dooms-Goossens A, Lachapelle J-M, Rycroft RJG, Scheper RJ (eds) Current topics in contact dermatitis. Springer, Berlin/Heidelberg/New York, pp 360–367

Jolanki R, Kanerva L, Estlander T et al (1990) Occupational dermatoses from epoxy resin compounds. Contact Dermatitis 23:172–183

Jolanki R, Kanerva L, Estlander T, Tarvainen K (1994a) Concomitact sensitization to triglycidyl isocyanurate. Diaminodiphenylmethane and 2-hydroxyethyl methacrylates from silk-screen printing coatings in the manufacture of circuit boards. Contact Dermatitis 30:12–15

Jolanki R, Kanerva L, Estlander T, Tarvainen K (1994b) Epoxy dermatitis. In: Nethercott JR (ed) Occupational skin disease, occupational medicine: state of the art reviews, vol 9, part 1. Hanley & Belfus/Medical, Philadelphia, pp 97–112

Jolanki R, Kanerva L, Estlander T (1995) Occupational allergic contact dermatitis caused by epoxy diacrylate in ultraviolet light-cured paint, and bisphenol A in dental composite resin. Contact Dermatitis 33:94–99

Jolanki R, Kanerva L, Estlander T (1996a) Allergic patch test reactions to diglycidyl ether of bisphenol A in hardened nail base and top coat. Contact Dermatitis 35:246–247

Jolanki R, Tarvainen K, Tatar T et al (1996b) Occupational dermatoses from exposure to epoxy resin compounds in a ski factory. Contact Dermatitis 34:390–396

Jolanki R, Kanerva L, Estlander T (1997a) Contact urticaria from epoxy resins. In: Amin S, Lahti A, Maibach HI (eds) Contact urticaria syndrome. CRC Press, Boca Raton, pp 143–147

Jolanki R, Kanerva L, Estlander T, Tarvainen K (1997b) Skin allergy caused by organic acid anhydrides. In: Amin S, Lahti A, Maibach HI (eds) Contact urticaria syndrome. CRC Press, Boca Raton, pp 217–224

Jolanki R, Estlander T, Kanerva L (2001) 182 patients with occupational allergic epoxy contact dermatitis over 22 years. Contact Dermatitis 44:121–123

Kanerva L, Alanko K (1998) Stomatitis and perioral dermatitis caused by epoxy diacrylete in dental composite resins. J Am Acad Dermatol 38:116–120

Kanerva L, Estlander T (1998) Simultaneous active sensitization to multiple chemicals. Contact Dermatitis 38:174–175

Kanerva L, Estlander T, Jolanki R (1989) Allergic contact dermatitis from dental composite resins due to aromatic epoxy acrylates and aliphatic acrylates. Contact Dermatitis 20:201–211

Kanerva L, Jolanki R, Estlander T (1991a) Allergic contact dermatitis from epoxy resin hardeners. Am J Contact Dermatitis 2:88–97

Kanerva L, Jolanki R, Estlander T (1991b) Allergic contact dermatitis from non-diglycidyl ether of bisphenol A epoxy resins. Contact Dermatitis 24:293–300

Kanerva L, Jolanki R, Tupasela O et al (1991c) Immediate and delayed allergy from epoxy resins based on diglycidyl ether of bisphenol A. Scand J Work Environ Health 17:208–215

Kanerva L, Estlander T, Jolanki R (1992) Active sensitization caused by 2-hydroxyethyl methacrylate, 2-hydroxypropyl methacrylate, ethyleneglycol dimethacrylate and N, N-dimethylaminoethyl methacrylate. J Eur Acad Derm Venereol 1:165–169

Kanerva L, Tarvainen K, Pinola A et al (1994) A single accidental exposure may result in a chemical burn, primary sensitization and allergic contact sensitization. Contact Dermatitis 31:229–235

Kanerva L, Estlander T, Jolanki R (1996) Occupational allergic contact dermatitis caused by 2.4,6-tris-(dimethylaminomethyl) phenol, and a review of sensitizing epoxy resin hardeners. Int J Dermatol 35:852–856

Kanerva L, Hyry H, Jolanki R et al (1997) Delayed and immediate allergy caused by methylhexahydrophthalic anhydride. Contact Dermatitis 36:34–38

Kanerva L, Jolanki R, Estlander T (1998) Occupational epoxy dermatitis with patch test reactions to multiple hardeners including tetraethylenepentamine. Contact Dermatitis 38:299–301

Kanerva L, Jolanki R, Alanko K, Estlander T (1999) Patch test reactions with plastic and glue allergens at an occupational dermatology clinic. Acta Derm-Venereol (Stock) 79:296–300

Kanerva L, Jolanki R, Estlander T, Alanko K (2000a) Latent (subclinical) contact dermatitis evolving into occupational allergic contact dermatitis from extremely small amounts of epoxy resin. Contact Dermatitis 43:47–49

Kanerva L, Estlander T, Jolanki R, Alanko K (2000b) Occupational allergic contact dermatitis from 2,2-bis[4-(2-hydroxy-3-acryloxypropoxy) phenyl] propane (epoxy diacrylate) in ultraviolet-cured inks. Contact Dermatitis 43:56–59

Kanerva L, Estlander T, Keskinen H, Jolanki R (2000c) Occupational allergic airborne contact dermatitis and delayed bronchial asthma from epoxy resin revealed by bronchila provocation test. Eur J Dermatol 10:475–477

Kanerva L, Pelttari M, Jolanki R et al (2002) Occupational urticaria from diglycidyl ether of bisphenol A resin. Allergy 57:1205–1207

Karlberg A-T, Gafvert E (1996) Isolated colophony allergens as screening substance for contact allergy. Contact Dermatitis 35:201–207

Kirkup ME, Murphy J, Beck MH, Sansom JE (2001) Occupational sensitization to 1,2-diaminocyclohexane. Contact Dermatitis 45:121–122

Krajewska D, Rudzki E (1976) Sensitivity to epoxy resins and triethylenetetramine. Contact Dermatitis 2:135–138

Lachapelle JM, Tennstedt D, Dumont Fruytier M (1978) Occupational allergic contact dermatitis to isophorone diamine (IPD) used as an epoxy resin hardener. Contact Dermatitis 4:109–112

Lea WA, Block WD, Cornish HH (1958) The irritating and sensitizing capacity of epoxy resins. Arch Dermatol 78:304–308

Lee H, Neville K (1967) Handbook of epoxy resins. McGraw-Hill, New York

Lee HN, Pokorny CD, Law S et al (2002) Cross-reactivity among epoxy acrylates and bisphenol F epoxy resins in patients with bisphenol A epoxy resin sensitivity. Am J Contact Dermat 13:108–115

Lichter M, Drury D, Remlinger K (1992) Lichenoid dermatitis caused by epoxy resin. Contact Dermatitis 26:275

Liu YQ, Zhao S, Zhuang LH, Fan WX (1997) Patch test reactions to the Chinese standard screening allergens in 1,135 patients investigated for allergic contact dermatitis. Am J Contact Dermat 8:141–143

Lovell CR, Rycroft RJG, Matood J (1984) Isolated Cardura EIO sensitivity in an epoxy resin chemical process. Contact Dermatitis 11:190–191

Lushniak B (2004) Occupational contact dermatitis. Dermatol Ther 17:272–277

Lyon CC, O'Driscoll I, Erikstam U et al (1998) Bowlers' grip. Contact Dermatitis 38:223

Maguire HC (1988) Experimental photoallergic contact dermatitis to bisphenol A. Acta Derm Venerol 68:408–412

Maibach HI, Mathias CT (2001) Allergic contact dermatitis from cycloaliphatic epoxide in jet aviation hydraulic fluid. Contact Dermatitis 45:56

Malanin G, Kalimo K (1985) Facial dermatitis from epoxy resin in a helmet. Contact Dermatits 12:221

Malten K, Zielhuis R (1964) Polyester resins. Industrial toxicology and dermatology in the production and processing of plastics. Elsevier, Amterdam, pp 71–84

Mann RI, Stewart E, Peachey RDG (1983) Sensitivity to urostomy pouch plastic. Contact Dermatitis 9:80–81

Marks JG, Belsito DV, DeLeo VA et al (1995) North American Contact Dermatitis Group standard tray patch test results (1992 to 1994). Am J Contact Dermat 6:160–165

Mathias CGT (1987) Allergic contact dermatitis from a nonbisphenol A epoxy in a graphite fiber reinforced epoxy laminate. J Occup Med 29:754–755

Matura M, Poesen N, de Moor A et al (1995) Glycidyl methacrylate and ethoxyethyl acrylate: new allergens in emulsions used to impregnate paper and textile materials. Contact Dermatitis 33:123–134

McClain DC, Storrs FJ (1992) Protective effect of both a barrier cream and a polyethylene lamintate glove against epoxy resin, glyceryl monothioglycolate, frullania, and tancy. Am J Contact Dermat 3:201–205

Menschik H (1955) Gesundheitliche Gefahren bei der Herstellung von Phthalsäureanhydrid. Arch Gewerbepathol Gewerbehyg 183:454–475

Miyamoto T, Okumura M (1998) Occupational contact urticaria due to epoxy resin. Environ Dermatol 5:53–57

Morris AD, Ratcliffe J, Dalziel KL, English JSC (1998) Allergic contact dermatitis from epoxy propane. Contact Dermatitis 38:57

Munro CS, Lawrence CM (1992) Occupational contact dermatitis from triglycidyl isocyanurate in a powder paint factory. Contact Dermatitis 26:59

Muskopf JW, McCollister SB (1987) Epoxy resins. In: Gerhartz W, Yamamoto YS, Kaudy L, Rounsaville JF, Schulx G (eds) Ullmann's encyclopedia of industrial chemistry, 5th completely revised edition, vol A9. VCH Verlagsgesellschaft, Weinheim, pp 547–563

Nethercott JR, Holness DI, Adams RM et al (1994) Multivariate analysis of the effect of selected factors on the elicitation of patch test response to 28 common environmental contactants in North America. Am J Contact Dermatol 5:13–18

Nielsen J, Welinder H, Horstmann V, Skerfving S (1992) Allergy to methyltetrahydrophthalic anhydride in epoxy resin workers. Br J Ind Med 49:769–775

Niinimäki A, Rosberg J, Saari S (1983) Traces of epoxy resin in acrylic dental materials. Contact Dermatitis 9:532

Niklasson IB, Broo K, Jonsson C et al (2009) Reduced sensitizing capacity of epoxy resin systems: a structure-activity realationship study. Chem Res Toxicol 22:1787–1794

Nishioka K, Ogasawara M, Asagami C (1988) Occupational contact allergy to triglycidyl isocyanurate (TGIC, TepicR). Contact Dermatitis 19:379–380

Nixon RL (1997) Material safety data sheets and contact dermatitis: a misleading case. Aust J Dermatol 38:165

Nixon R, Frowen K (1991) Allergic contact dermatitis caused by epoxy resins. J Occup Health Safety-Aust NZ 7:417–424

Peltonen K (1986) Thermal degradation of epoxy powder paints. Doctoral dissertation, University of Kuipo, Kuopio

Pontén A, Bruze M (2001) Contact allergy to epoxy resin based on diglycidyl ether of bisphenol F. Contact Dermatitis 44:98–99

Pontén A, Zimerson E, Sörensen Ö, Bruze M (2002) Sensitizing capacity and cross-reaction pattern of the isomers of diglycidyl ether of bisphenol F in the guinea pig. Contact Drmatitis 47:293–298

Pontén A, Carstensen O, Rasmussen K et al (2004a) Epoxy-based production of wind turbine rotor blades: occupational dernatoses. Contact Dermatitis 50:329–338

Pontén A, Bjork J, Carstensen O et al (2004b) Associations between contact allergy to epoxy resin and fragrance mix. Acta Derm Venereol (Stockh) 84:151–152

Pontén A, Zimerson E, Bruze M (2004c) Contact allergy to the isomers of diglycidyl ether of bisphenol F. Acta Derm Venereol 84:12–17

Pontén A, Zimerson E, Bruze M (2008) Can simultaneous contact allergies to phenyl glycidyl ethers and epoxy resins of the bisphenol A/F-types be explained by contamination of the epoxy resins? Contact Dematitis 59:273–279

Pontén A, Zimerson E, Bruze M (2009) Sensitizing capacity and cross-reactivity of phenyl glycidyl ether studied in the guinea-pig maximization test. Contact Dermatitis 60:79–84

Potter WG (1975) Uses of epoxy resins. Newnes-Butterworths, London

Rebandel P, Rudzki E (1990) Dermatitis caused by epichlorohydrin. oxprenolol hydrochloride and propranolol hydrochloride. Contact Dermatitis 23:199–200

Requena L, Vazquez C, Requena C et al (1986) Epoxy dermatitis of an amputation stump. Contact Dermatitis 14:320

Rietschel RL, Fowler JF Jr (2008) Fisher's contact dermatitis, 6th edn. McGraw-Hill, New York

Rietschel RL, Mathias CGT, Fowler JF Jr et al (2002) Relationship of occupation to contact dermatitis: evaluation in patients tested from 1998 to 2000. Am J Contact Dermat 13:170–176

Roed-Petersen J (1989) A new glove material protective against epoxy and acrylate monomer. In: Lachapelle JM, Frosch PJ, Dooms-Goossens A (eds) Current topics in contact dermatitis. Springer, Berlin/Heidelberg/New York, pp 603–606

Romhyr O, Nyfors A, Leira HL, Smedbold HT (2006) Allergic contact dermatitis caused by epoxy resin systems in industrial painters. Contact Dermatitis 55:167–172

Rosen RH, Freeman S (1993) Prognosis of occupational contact dermatitis in New South Wales, Australia. Contact Dermatitis 29:88–93

Rudzki E, Krajewska D (1976) Cross-reactivity between ethylenediamine, diethylenetriamine and triethylenetetramine. Contact Dermatitis 2:311–313

Rudzki E, Rebandel P (1990) Dermatitis from methyl 2,3 epoxy-3-(4-methoxyphenyl)propionate. Contact Dermatitis 23:382

Rycroft RJG (1980) Atypical psoriasis following epoxy resin sensitization. J Soc Occup Med 30:132–134

Sajjachareonpong P, Cahill J, Saunders H et al (2004) Persistent post-occupational dermatitis. Contact Dermatitis 51:278–283

Sakata S, Cahill J, Barton D, Nixon R (2005) Occupational allergic contact dermatitis to bisphenol F epoxy resin. Australas J Dermatol 46:90–92

Sasseville D (1998) Contact urticaria from epoxy resin and reactive diluents. Contact Dermatitis 38:57–58

Savonius B, Keskinen H, Tuppurainen M, Kanerva L (1994) Occupational asthma caused by ethanolamines. Allergy 49:877–881

Senff H, Kuhlwein A, Hausen BM (1988) Allergisches Kontaktekzem auf Dicyandiamid. Dermatosen 36:99–101

Silvestre JF, Albares MP, Escutia B et al (2004) Contact vitiligo appearing after allergic contact dermatitis in an epoxy resin system. Contact Dermatitis 49:113–114

Skoet R, Tollund C, Bloch-Thomsen PE (2003) Epoxy contact dermatitis due to pacemaker compounds. Cardiology 99:112

Sommer S, Wilkinson SM, Wilson CL (1997) Airborne contact dermatitis caused by microscopy immersion fluid containing epoxy resin. Contact Dermatitis 39:141–142

Spee T, Van Duivenbooden C, Terwoert J (2006) Epoxy resins in the construction industry. Ann N Y Acad Sci (United States), 2006, 1076, p 429–438

Speight EL, Beck MH, Lawrence CM (1993) Occupational allergic contact dermatitis due to 3-dimethylaminopropylamine. Contact Dermatitis 28:49–50

Srinivas CR, Devadiga R, Aroor AR (1989) Footwear dermatitis due to bisphenol A. Contact Dermatitis 20:150–151

Steinkraus V, Hausen BM (1994) Contact allergy to propylene oxide. Contact Dermatitis 31:120

Stutz N, Hertl M, Löffler H (2008) Anaphylaxis caused by contact urticaria because of epoxy resins: an extraordinary emergency. Contact Dermatitis 58:307–309

Suhonen R (1983) Epoxy-dermatitis in a ski-stick factory. Contact Dermatitis 9:131–133

Tarvainen K, Iolanki R, Estlander T et al (1995a) Immunologic contact urticaria due to airborne methylhexahydrophthalic and methyltetrahydrophthalic anhydride. Contact Dermatitis 32:204–209

Tarvainen K, Kanerva L, Jolanki R, Estlander T (1995b) Occupational dermatoses from the manufacture of plastic composite products. Am J Contact Dermatoses 6:95–104

Taylor JS, Bergfeld WF, Guin JD (1983) Contact dermatitis to knee patch adhesive in boy's jeans: a nonoccupational cause of epoxy resin sensitivity. Cleveland Clin Q 50:123–127

Thorgeirsson A (1978a) Sensitization capacity of epoxy reactive diluents in the guinea pig. Acta Derm Venerol 58:329–331

Thorgeirsson A (1978b) Sensitization capacity of epoxy resin hardeners in the guinea pig. Acta Derm Venerol 58:332–336

Thorgeirsson A, Fregert S (1977) Allergenicity of epoxy resins in the guinea pig. Acta Derm Venerol 57:253–256

Thorgeirsson A, Fregert S, Ramnäs O (1978) Sensitization capacity of epoxy resin oligomers in the guinea pig. Acta Derm Venerol 58:17–21

Toffoletto F, Cortona G, Feltrin G et al (1994) Occupational contact dermatitis from aminefunctional methoxysilane in continuous-glass-filament production. Contact Dermatitis 31:320–321

Toome BK (1989) Allergic contact dermatitis to a nasal cannula. Arch Dermatol 125:571

Tosti A, Guerra L, Toni F (1988) Occupational airborne contact dermatitis due to epoxy resin. Contact Dermatitis 19:220–222

Tosti A, Guerra L, Bardazzi F (1992) Occupational contact dermatitis from exposure to epoxy resins and acrylates. Clin Dermatol 10:133–140

Van Joost T (1988) Occupational sensitization to epichlorohydrin and epoxy resin. Contact Dermatitis 19:278–280

Van Joost T, Roesyanto ID, Satyawan I (1990) Occupational sensitization to epichlorohydrin (ECH) and bisphenol-A during the manufacture of epoxy resin. Contact Dermatitis 22:125–126

Van Putten PB, Coenraads PJ, Nater JP (1984) Hand dermatoses and contact allergic reactions in construction workers exposed to epoxy resins. Contact Dermatitis 10:146–150

Vanherle G, Smith DC (eds) (1985) Posterior composite resin dental restorative materials. Minnesota Mining & Mfg, St. Paul

Veien NK, Hattel T, Laurberg G (1992) Patch test results from a private dermatologic practice for two periods of 5 years with a 10-year interval. Am J Contact Dermatol 3:189–192

Woyton A, Wasik F, Bliζanowska A (1974) An uncommon anaphylactic and eczematous reaction after contact with epoxide resins (in Polish). Przegl Dermatol 61:303–308

Yokota K, Michitsuji H (2004) Occupational allergic contact dermatitis from 1,6-bis (2,3-epoxypropoxy) naphthalene in a one-component epoxy coating. Contact Dermatitis 51:154–155

Zug KA, Warshaw EM, Fowler JF et al (2009) Patch-test results of the North American Contact Dermatitis Group 2005-2006. Dermatitis 20:149–160

52 Contact Allergy to Phenol-Formaldehyde Resins

Erik Zimerson[1] · *Magnus Bruze*[2,3]
[1]Department of Occupational and Environmental Dermatology, Malmö University Hospital, Malmö, Sweden
[2]University of California Medical School, San Francisco, CA, USA
[3]Department of Occupational and Environmental Dermatology, Skåne, University Hospital Malmö, Lund University, Malmö, Sweden

Core Messages

- The raw materials, phenols and aldehydes, are not important allergens in phenol-formaldehyde resins.
- The strongest allergens are found among monomers and dimers with reactive hydroxymethyl groups, the hydroxymethyl phenols.
- Resins produced with a deficit of formaldehyde (novolac resins) show low allergenicity because they contain very low concentrations of hydroxymethyl phenols. Addition of formaldehyde needs to be done before curing. Novolac resins should not be used for patch testing.
- The concentrations of allergens usually drop significantly when the resins are cured (e.g., phenol-formaldehyde resin), while some resins more or less retain their levels of allergens regardless of treatment (e.g., *p-tert*-butylphenol-formaldehyde resin).
- Phenol-formaldehyde resins made from different phenols and/or aldehydes will contain different allergens and cross-reactions between different resins should not be expected.
- Patch testing should be performed with the specific phenol-formaldehyde resin the patient is exposed to.
- *p-tert*-butylcatechol is a strong sensitizer used as a stabilizer in plastic monomers (e.g., styrene) and is also found in *p-tert*-butylphenol-formaldehyde resin. In case of a positive patch test reaction to *p-tert*-butylphenol-formaldehyde resin with no clinically relevant exposure to this resin *p-tert*-butylcatechol should be patch tested and exposure to this substance investigated.

1 Introduction

The first successful commercial exploitation of phenol-formaldehyde resin was made in 1909 under the name of Bakelite. This was the first wholly synthetic polymer ever made but in spite of this it is still used in many applications and products. Fillers and other additives are used to improve the product. From the first resins, other varieties have been developed so that phenol-formaldehyde resins now designates a group of resins with varying properties made from different phenols and aldehydes.

2 Chemistry

The most used phenol-formaldehyde resins are based on phenol or *p-tert*-butylphenol and formaldehyde. However, other phenols can be used such as resorcinol, cresols, guayacol (2-methoxy phenol), *p*-phenylphenol, xylenols, amylphenol, octylphenol, nonylphenol, and bisphenol A. In some resins, a mixture of phenols is used. Aldehydes other than formaldehyde are occasionally used, for example furfural.

Modified phenol-formaldehyde resins are, for example, used for surface coatings and impregnation. In these cases, the phenol-formaldehyde resin can be mixed with colophony, terpenes, fatty acids, amines, or epoxy resins.

Formaldehyde reacts with phenols giving methylol-substituted phenols. Another word for methylol phenol is hydroxymethyl phenol. These substances are the monomers in the resin. Formaldehyde also creates chemical bonds between the monomers. This bond can be either of the methylene type ($-CH_2-$) or of the methylene-ether type ($-CH_2-O-CH_2-$) thus forming dimers, trimers, tetramers, and so on. Phenol-formaldehyde resin can be produced in two principal ways, either as resol or novolac resins.

Resol resins are produced by the reaction of phenol with a molecular excess of formaldehyde under alkaline conditions. The monomers form dimers, trimers, and other oligomers in which the monomers are mainly

T. Rustemeyer, P. Elsner, S.M. John & H.I. Maibach (eds.), *Kanerva's Occupational Dermatology*,
DOI 10.1007/978-3-642-02035-3_52, © Springer-Verlag Berlin Heidelberg 2012

connected by methylene groups. The excess of formaldehyde in the reaction makes all the constituents of the resin rich in reactive methylol groups. The methylol groups in o- or *p*-position to the hydroxy group of the phenol make the resol substances reactive by giving them the possibility to split off a water molecule and become extremely reactive quinonmethides. This is the mechanism behind formation of dimers, trimers, and other oligomers. This reactivity also means that the substances can react with proteins in the skin and act as type IV allergens. The resol resins are viscous dark reins, which often are used, dissolved in a solvent (such as methanol) before being applied to different materials such as paper. Stabile products are then created by curing (polymerization) of the resins by application of pressure and heat. Curing transforms the resins into rigid network polymers.

Novolac resins are produced when formaldehyde reacts with a molecular excess of phenol under acidic conditions. Almost all of the added formaldehyde is consumed producing methylene groups which create bonds between the monomers. As there are few or no methylol groups in the molecules, these resins show very low reactivity and more aldehyde must be added in the process before curing. This is often done by the addition of a formaldehyde releaser such as paraformaldehyde or hexamethylenetetramine.

p-tert-butylphenol-formaldehyde resin is produced as a resol resin in a similar way as resins based on phenol but has several different properties. The constituents of the resin are more lipophilic and thus more fat soluble. The bonds between the monomers are mostly of the methylene-ether-type, which are more unstable than the methylene bonds in phenol-formaldehyde resin. The methylene-ether bonds can, for example, be split by reaction with water (hydrolysis) or light-catalyzed reaction with oxygen (oxidation). The resins cannot create a network polymer when cured due to blocking of one position on the aromatic ring of the phenol by the *tert*-butyl group. As a consequence, the resin will often contain relatively high levels of monomers, dimers, and trimers. If the resin is more condensed and thus contains larger molecules, these can still be converted back to smaller ones by spontaneous hydrolysis and/or oxidation. If the resin is heavily condensed at high temperatures, a part of the methylene-ether bonds will be converted into methylene bonds and this will make the polymer more stable to degradation but it will still be a thermoplastic polymer.

All the phenol-formaldehyde resins are produced with different degrees of condensation (curing). In this way, resins with different viscosity or tackiness can be achieved. Resins with a low degree of condensation are rich in low molecular weight compounds such as monomers and dimers. These resins consist of hundreds or thousands of substances of which the vast majority is not chemically identified. However, efforts to identify the main sensitizers in resins based on phenol and *p-tert*-butylphenol have been made.

3 Use

Phenol-formaldehyde resins were earlier much used as casting compounds for products such as knobs, electrical switches, ashtrays, and many others. This use has diminished and, nowadays, the resins are mainly used as binders in different products. Large quantities are used, for example, in building, construction, car, leather, shoe, molding, and electric industries.

Resins based on phenol and formaldehyde or a combination of phenol, resorcinol, and formaldehyde are used in many glues and adhesives. The resins are used for decorative boards, laminated boards for floors, plywood, water-resistant boards, glass and mineral fibers for insulating, brake and clutch linings, abrasive cloth and paper, grinding wheels, and molds for casting metal and plastic. Phenol-formaldehyde resins are developed for new applications which includes being a base for nanoparticles and for use in the production of foaming boards from wastepapers.

p-tert-butylphenol-formaldehyde resin is used in adhesives based on neoprene and other rubbers. These glues are used when flexibility of the joint or when extra water resistance is needed. The resin is frequently used in glues for shoes and other leather products such as watch straps. Other uses include glues for automobile upholstery, furniture, hobbies, artificial fingernails, and adhesive labels. Other products reported to contain the resin include athletic tapes, glue in hearing aid, and ink in marking pens.

Modified resins or resins based on *p-tert*-butylphenol or other alkyl-substituted phenols are used for surface coatings as protective and isolating varnishes for packing due to their water-repellent properties. Modified resins can be used as binders in inks, typewriter correction papers, and different laminates.

4 Contact Dermatitis and Allergy

Phenol-formaldehyde resins can cause several types of damage to the skin. The most frequently reported effects are different types of contact dermatitis such as irritant contact dermatitis and allergic contact dermatitis. Depigmentation and contact urticaria have also been described. Reaction products such as monomers and dimers, or remaining raw material such as phenols and aldehydes are causative agents.

Phenol-formaldehyde resins can cause irritant contact dermatitis (Fregert 1980) and chemical burns (Fisher 1973). Many phenols are known to be irritating and can cause chemical burns and the level of remaining or free phenol can vary in the resins. The reaction products, methylol phenols, generally seem to be less irritating to the skin than the phenols. Low or high pH of the resin can contribute to irritant contact dermatitis. The pH of a resin mainly depends on remaining or added catalyst which can be an acid or a base. In a case report, a life-threatening condition involving necrotic lesions of the skin and renal functional impairment is reported of a patient who had spilled phenol-formaldehyde resin over a large area of the skin (Cohen et al. 1989).

Depigmentation can be caused by certain resins and are likely due to remaining phenols such as *p-tert*-butylphenol (Malten et al. 1971; Stevenson 1981).

Contact urticaria has been ascribed to *p-tert*-butylphenol-formaldehyde resin in a case report due to handling of glass fiber insulation (Kalimo et al. 1980).

Most reports about adverse effects from phenol-formaldehyde resins describe allergic contact dermatitis. Although free formaldehyde can be found in many phenol-formaldehyde resins, it is not a major sensitizer in these resins (Hjort and Fregert 1967; Bruze et al. 1985). Free phenols also seem to be of little or no significance concerning allergic reactions to the resins (Fregert and Hjort 1969; Bruze et al. 1985), although *p-tert*-butylphenol once was considered the main sensitizer in resins based on this phenol (Malten 1958).

There are relatively few reports on contact allergy to resins based on phenol. In some investigations of workers in laminate productions, high frequencies of allergies have been reported (Bruze and Almgren 1988; Isaksson et al. 1999). Reports on occupational sensitization have also concerned a secretary handling typewriter correction paper (Jordan and Bourlas 1975), a newspaper dealer (Castelain et al. 1980), painters (Hjort and Fregert 1967), a worker in a rubber factory (van der Willingen et al. 1987), bricklayers (Sonneck 1964), workers producing abrasive paper (Bompart and Smagge 1959), a worker manufacturing gasoline filters (Gaul 1967), and workers sawing masonite or using grinding wheels (Fregert and Tegner 1972). In one investigation, 17 cases of occupational allergic contact dermatitis due to phenol-formaldehyde resin are reported. Their occupations were friction material production, fiberglass manufacture, foundry work, aircraft construction, joinery, and adhesives processing (Owen and Beck 2001). Occupational allergic contact dermatitis from cured and used casting sand containing phenol formaldehyde has been reported (Isaksson 2002). Also occupational airborne allergic contact dermatitis from medium-density fiberboard (MDF-board) has been reported (Ezughah et al. 2001). Phenol-formaldehyde resin has also been reported to cause palmoplantar dermatitis (Downs and Sansome 1998). One factor that can contribute to the relatively few reported cases is that resins of this type usually are not used in standard patch test series.

It has been shown that resol resins based on phenol contain highly sensitizing substances. Fourteen sensitizers from this type of resin have been isolated and described. Some of the allergens are shown in ➲ *Fig. 52.1.* Both monomers and dimers were shown to be sensitizers. Patch testing with serial dilutions showed that some of the sensitizers, for example, the dimer 4,4′-dihydroxy-3,3′-dimethylol-diphenylmethane, could elicit an allergic reaction down to a concentration of about 0.01 ppm in patients with a high sensitivity. The presence of these sensitizers in resins and products based on phenol and formaldehyde has been investigated. Concentrations of allergens in cured products were reduced by a factor of 100–1,000 when compared to the contents of the uncured resins (Bruze 1985; Bruze et al. 1986).

p-tert-butylphenol-formaldehyde resin is the most frequently reported sensitizer among the phenol-formaldehyde resins. As this resin is used both in industries and in personal products, sensitization can be of occupational origin or caused by contact with the resin in ordinary daily life. In 1958, contact allergy was described among cobblers (Malten 1958). Since then, more patients working with shoe manufacturing or shoe repairing have been reported (Mancuso et al. 1996) as well as patients with shoe dermatitis (Freeman 1997) and still a major problem facing sensitized persons is to find shoes that they can tolerate. Among 140 patients with suspected shoe dermatitis in Israel, 8.7% showed an allergic reaction to *p-tert*-butylphenol-formaldehyde resin (Trattner et al. 2003), while a retrospective study (1998–2004) showed a frequency of 1.3% among dermatitis patients also in Israel (Lazarow 2006). There seems to be a tendency that allergy frequencies to *p-tert*-butylphenol-formaldehyde resin are declining in European countries but are increasing in other countries. In a study in England (1994–2003), 0.5% out of 230 patients with foot dermatitis were allergic to *p-tert*-butylphenol-formaldehyde resin (Holden and Gawcrodger 2005), but in Iran 8.0% of 250 dermatitis

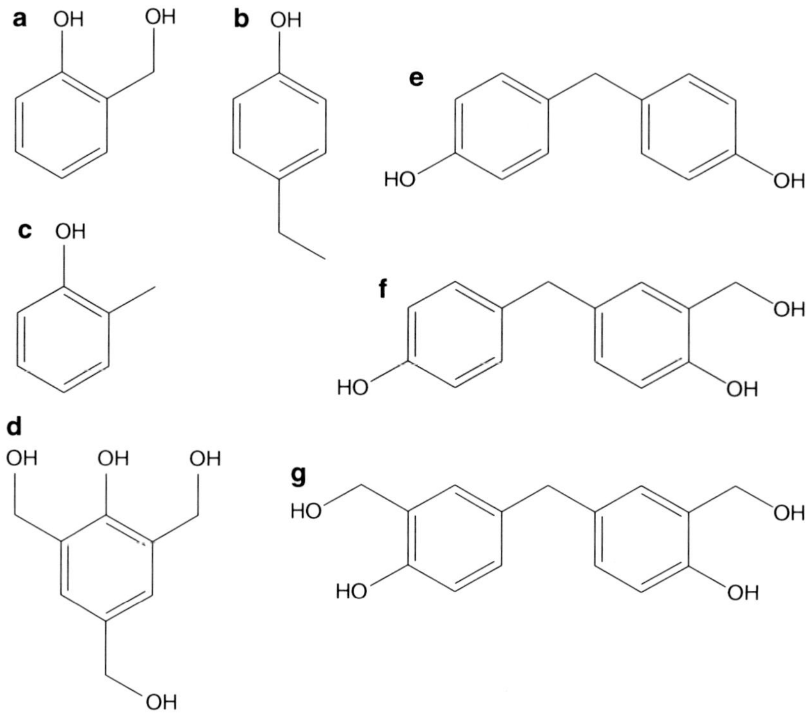

Fig. 52.1

Chemical structures of some of the identified sensitizers in resins based on phenol and formaldehyde. (a) 2-methylol phenol. (b) 4-methylol phenol. (c) o-cresol. (d) 2,4,6-trimethylol phenol. (e) 4,4′-dihydroxy diphenylmethane. (f) 4,4′-dihydroxy-3-hydroxymethyl-diphenylmethane (a main allergen). (g) 4,4′-dihydroxy-3,3′-dihydroxymethyl-diphenylmethane (a main allergen)

patients were shown to be allergic to *p-tert*-butylphenol-formaldehyde resin (Kashani et al. 2005). Also among workers in a car factory (Calnan and Harman 1959; Engel and Calnan 1966), painters (Högberg and Wahlberg 1980), and glue users (Moran and Martin-Pascual 1978; Cronin 1980), contact allergy has been reported. Other causes of mainly nonoccupational sensitization and/or allergic contact dermatitis can be leather watch straps (Foussereau et al. 1968; Mobacken and Hersle 1976), use of certain plastic finger nail adhesives (Rycroft et al. 1980), athletic tape (Shono et al. 1991), an hearing aid (Matrolonardo et al. 1993), a lip liner (Angelini et al. 1993), a knee guard (Vincenzi et al. 1992), detoration brace after an orthopedic operation and a rain coat (Hayakawa et al. 1994), a waist support for treatment of scoliosis and leather glues (Tarvainen 1995), marking pens (Hagdrup et al. 1994), prosthesis (Romaguera et al. 1985), and electrocardiograph-monitoring electrodes (Avenel-Audran et al. 2003).

The first allergen reported in *p-tert*-butylphenol-formaldehyde resin was *p-tert*-butylphenol (Malten 1958). Formaldehyde is a known allergen which is present in the resin. However, most individuals sensitized to *p-tert*-butylphenol-formaldehyde resin are not sensitive to *p-tert*-butylphenol or formaldehyde (Malten 1987). The two monomers, 2-hydroxymethyl-*p-tert*-butylphenol and 2,6-dimethylol-*p-tert*-butylphenol, have been shown to be allergens in the resin, the latter being the stronger sensitizer of the two (Zimerson and Bruze 2002d). Some theoretical constituents and theoretical degradation products have been synthesized and among these a linear tetramer has been reported as an allergen (Agatha and Schubert 1979; Schubert and Agatha 1979). Present investigations in our department regarding isolation of allergens directly from the resin has shown the presence of many other allergens and some of which have a potency comparable to the strongest allergens in resins based on phenol (Zimerson et al. 1999; Zimerson and Bruze 1998, 2000a, b, 2002a, b, c). Chemical structures of some allergens in *p-tert*-butylphenol-formaldehyde resin are shown in *Fig. 52.2.*

p-tert-butylphenol-formaldehyde resin is included in the International Contact Dermatitis Research Group (ICDRG) standard patch test series. Positive patch test reactions have varied between 0.3% and 2.6% among

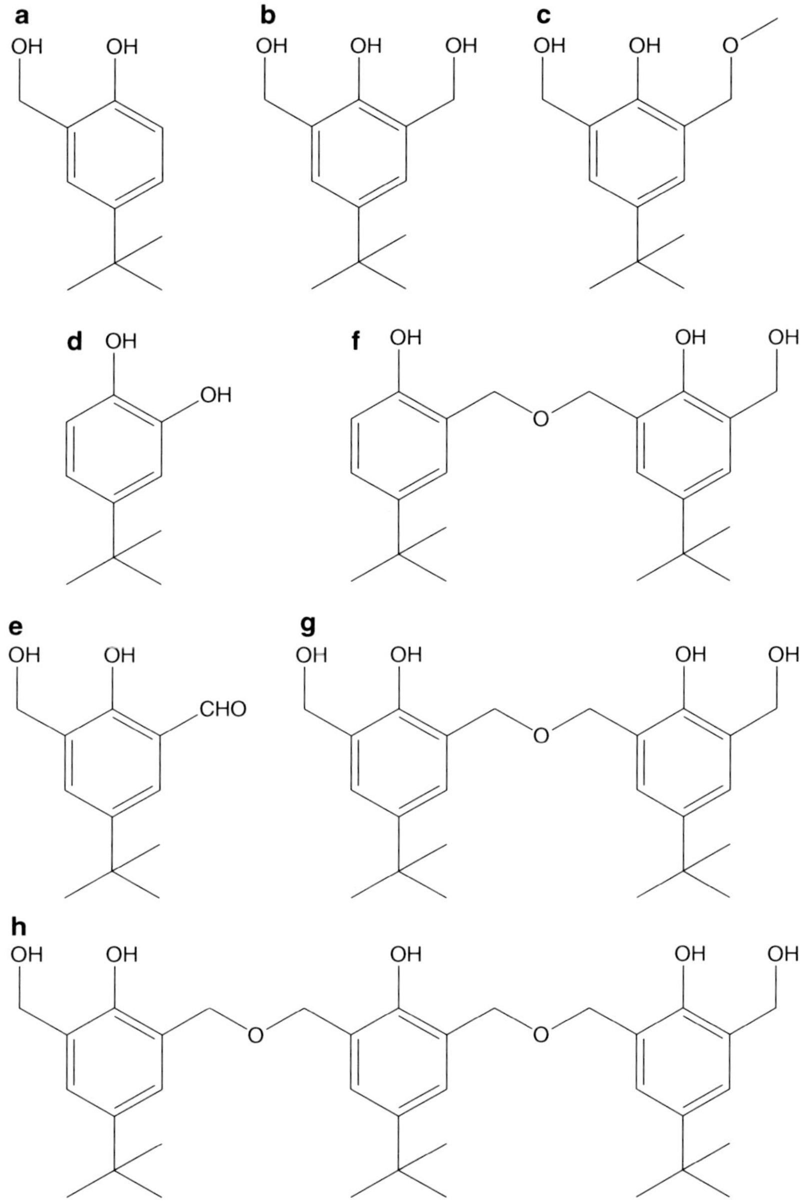

Fig. 52.2

Chemical structures of some of the identified sensitizers in resins based on *p-tert*-butylphenol and formaldehyde. (a) 4-*tert*-butyl-2-hydroxymethyl-phenol. (b) 4-*tert*-butyl-2,6-bis-hydroxymethyl-phenol. (c) 4-*tert*-butyl-2-hydroxymethyl-6-methoxymethyl-phenol. (d) *p-tert*-butylcatechol (PTBC). (e) 5-*tert*-butyl-2-hydroxy-3-hydroxymethyl-benzaldehyde. (f) 4-*tert*-butyl-2-(5-*tert*-butyl-2-hydroxy-benzyloxymethyl)-6-hydroxymethyl-phenol (a main allergen). (g) 4-*tert*-butyl-2-(5-*tert*-butyl-2-hydroxy-3-hydroxymethyl-benzyloxymethyl)-6-hydroxymethyl-phenol (a main allergen). (h) 4-*tert*-butyl-2,6-bis-(5-*tert*-butyl-2-hydroxy-3-hydroxymethyl-benzyloxymethyl)-phenol

dermatological patients (Tarvainen 1995; Handley et al. 1993). In Portugal, positive reactions varied between 1.4% (1984) and 3.8% (1992), with an increasing tendency mainly in woman (Marques et al. 1994). However, patch testing with this resin is not sufficient to detect allergies to phenol-formaldehyde resins based on other phenols and patch testing with the patients' own resin/material can therefore be indicated (Bruze 1985, 1988).

Active sensitization has been reported when patch testing with 1.0% *p-tert*-butylphenol-formaldehyde resin.

However, the authors point out that the benefits of patch testing with this substance, outweighs the risks for sensitization, as this seems to happen very seldom (Arpa et al. 2002).

5 Connections to Other Sensitizers

In 1967, a possible relation between contact allergy to phenol-formaldehyde resin and coal tar was noted (Hjort and Fregert 1967). Some simple phenols have been shown to be probable cross-reacting substances in patients hypersensitive to phenol-formaldehyde resin, for example, o-cresol (Bruze and Zimerson 1997). o-cresol is also a known component in coal and wood tar (Snell and Ettre 1973; Richardson 1993) and it has been identified as an allergen in phenol-formaldehyde resin (Bruze and Zimerson 2002). This could explain the connection to coal tar. It also indicates a possible connection to other sources of o-cresol, for example, tobacco smoke (Jeanty et al. 1984).

In patients hypersensitive to phenol-formaldehyde resin (resol), simultaneous patch test reactions to formaldehyde, colophony, hydroabietyl alcohol, balsam of Peru, perfume mixture, and *p-tert*-butylphenol-formaldehyde resin have been reported. In patients hypersensitive to *p-tert*-butylphenol-formaldehyde resin (resol), simultaneous patch test reactions to hydroabietyl alcohol, balsam of Peru, and phenol-formaldehyde resin have been reported (Bruze 1986).

Simultaneous patch test reactions to *p-tert*-butylphenol-formaldehyde resin and *p-tert*-butylcatechol have been reported (Estlander et al. 1998) and *p-tert*-butylcatechol has been shown to be a component in at least some resins based on *p-tert*-butylphenol-formaldehyde (Zimerson and Bruze 1999). This can indicate a connection to other sources of *p-tert*-butylcatechol which is used as an antioxidant (Gellin et al. 1970) and as a stabilizer in different plastic monomers (Macfarlane et al. 1990).

6 Treatment and Prevention

Dermatitis caused by phenol-formaldehyde resins is treated in the same way as other contact dermatitis. Irritant dermatitis can usually be successfully treated if it is possible to reduce exposure to the irritating resin. In many cases of occupationally related allergic dermatitis caused by phenol-formaldehyde resin, the person cannot continue the job. However, the prognosis is usually good when they can change job. Work including handling of cured products can be tolerated if the sensitivity is not too high.

For patients hypersensitive to *p-tert*-butylphenol-formaldehyde resin and for whom no clinically relevant contact to this resin can be found, patch testing with *p-tert*-butyl catechol can be indicated. Patch testing with *p-tert*-butylphenol-formaldehyde resin is not sufficient to detect hypersensitivity to phenol-formaldehyde resins based on other phenols. A more complete patch testing for allergies to this group of resins should include testing with phenol-formaldehyde resin and the patients' own resins/materials. Extracts of finished products can be useful for patch testing. Resins based on phenol and *p-tert*-butylphenol can be tested as a mix (Bruze 1985, 1988).

Phenol-formaldehyde resin included in standard or supplementary test series should be of the resol type, as this type of resin contains higher levels of potent allergens than novolac resins.

References

Agatha G, Schubert H (1979) Untersuchungen zur Allergen-Identifizierung bei der p-tertiären Butylphenol-Formaldehydharz-Allergie. Dermatol Monatschr 165:337–345

Angelini E, Marinaro C, Carrozzo AM, Bianchi L, Delogu A, Gianello G, Nini G (1993) Allergic contact dermatitis of the lip margins from para-tertiary-butylphenol in a lip liner. Contact Dermatitis 28:146–148

Arpa MG, Ortiz-Frutos FJ, Donoso CG, Pérez SP, Dies LI (2002) Active sensitization to para-tertiary-butylphenol-formaldehyde resin. Contact Dermatitis 47:124–125

Avenel-Audran M, Goossens A, Zimerson E, Bruze M (2003) Contact dermatitis from electrocardiograph-monitoring electrodes: role of *p-tert*-butylphenol-formaldehyde resin. Contact Dermatitis 48:108–111

Bompart PV, Smagge G (1959) Quelques remarques d'ardre pratique á propos d'une application industrielle des résines formo-phénolique. Arch Mal Prof Méd Trav Sécuri Soc 20:64–67

Bruze M (1985) Contact sensitizers in resins based on phenol and formaldehyde. Acta Dermato-venereologica suppl 119:1–83

Bruze M (1986) Simultaneous reactions to phenol-formaldehyde resins colophony/hydroabietyl alcohol and balsam of Peru/perfume mixture. Contact Dermatitis 14:119–120

Bruze M (1988) Patch testing with a mixture of 2 phenol-formaldehyde resins. Contact Dermatitis 19:116–119

Bruze M, Almgren G (1988) Occupational dermatoses in workers exposed to resins based on phenol and formaldehyde. Contact Dermatitis 19:272–277

Bruze M, Zimerson E (1997) Cross-reaction patterns in patients with contact allergy to simple methylol phenols. Contact Dermatitis 37:82–86

Bruze M, Zimerson E (2002) Contact allergy to o-cresol – a sensitizer in phenol-formaldehyde resin. Am J Contact Dermat 13:198–200

Bruze M, Fregert S, Zimerson E (1985) Contact allergy to phenol-formaldehyde resins. Contact Dermatitis 12:81–86

Bruze M, Persson L, Trulsson L, Zimerson E (1986) Demonstration of contact sensitizers in resins and products based on phenol and formaldehyde. Contact Dermatitis 14:146–154

Calnan CD, Harman RRM (1959) Studies in contact dermatitis. X. Sensitivity to para-tertiary butylphenol. Trans St John's Hosp Derm Soc 43:27–32

Castelain PY, Pirious A, Raulot-Lapointe H, Rabaglia JL (1980) Sensitization to abieto-formo-phenolic resin in printing ink. Contact Dermatitis 6:145

Cohen N, Modai D, Khahil A, Golik A (1989) Acute resin phenol-formaldehyde intoxication. A life threatening occupational hazard. Hum Toxicol 8:247–250

Cronin E (1980) Contact dermatitis. Churchill Livingstone, Edinburgh, pp 617–619

Downs AM, Sansome JE (1998) Palmoplantar dermatitis may be due to phenol-formaldehyde resin contact dermatitis. Contact Dermatitis 39:147–148

Engel HO, Calnan CD (1966) Resin dermatitis in a car factory. Br J Ind Med 23:62–66

Estlander T, Kostiainen M, Jolanki R, Kanerva L (1998) Active sensitization and occupational allergic contact dermatitis caused by para-tertiary-butylcatechol. Contact Dermatitis 38:96–100

Fisher AA (1973) Contact dermatitis, 2nd edn. Lea and Febiger, Philadelphia, pp 16–18

Foussereau MJ, Petitjean J, Barré JG (1968) Eczema aux bracelets-montres par allergie a des résines formol-p.t.butylphénol des colles pour cuir (résines du type c.k.r. 1634). Bull Soc Fr Dermatol Syphiligr 75:630–633

Freeman S (1997) Shoe dermatitis. Contact Dermatitis 36:247–251

Fregert S (1980) Irritant dermatitis from phenol-formaldehyde resin powder. Contact Dermatitis 6:493

Fregert S, Hjort N (1969) Results of standard patch tests with substances abandoned. Contact Dermatitis Newslett 5:85–86

Fregert S, Tegner E (1972) Allergic contact dermatitis due to phenolic resin in ready products. Contact Dermatitis Newslett 12:328

Gaul LE (1967) Absence of formaldehyde sensitivity in phenol formaldehyde dermatitis. J Invest Dermatol 48:485–486

Gellin GA, Possick PA, Perone VB (1970) Depigmentation from 4-tertiary butyl catechol: an experimental study. J Invest Dermatol 55:190–197

Hagdrup H, Egsgaard H, Carlsen L, Andersen KE (1994) Contact allergy to 2-hydroxy-5-*tert*-butyl benzylalcohol and 2,6-bis (hydroxymethyl)-4-tert-butylphenol, components of a phenolic resin used in marking pens. Contact Dermatitis 31:154–156

Handley J, Todd D, Bingham A, Corbett R, Burrows D (1993) Allergic contact dermatitis from para-tertiary-butylphenol-formaldehyde resin (PTBP-F-R) in Northern Ireland. Contact Dermatitis 29:144–146

Hayakawa R, Ogino Y, Suzuki M, Kaniwa M (1994) Allergic contact dermatitis from para-tertiary-butylphenol-formaldehyde resin (PTBP-F-R). Contact Dermatitis 30:187–188

Hjort N, Fregert S (1967) Sensitivity to formaldehyde and formaldehyde resins. Contact Dermatitis Newslett 2:18–19

Högberg M, Wahlberg JE (1980) Health screening for occupational dermatoses in house painters. Contact Dermatitis 6:100–106

Holden CR, Gawcrodger DJ (2005) 10 years' experience of patch testing with a shoe series in 230 patients: which allergens are important? Contact Dermatitis 53:37–39

Isaksson M (2002) Occupational allergic contact dermatitis from cured and used casting sand. Contact Dermatitis 46:239–240

Isaksson M, Zimerson E, Bruze M (1999) Occupational dermatoses in composite production. J Occup Environ Med 41:261–266

Jeanty G, Massé J, Bercot P, Coq F (1984) Quantitative analysis of cigarette smoke condensate monophenols by reverse-phase high-performance liquid chromatography. Beiträge zur Tabakforschung Int 12:245–250

Jordan WP, Bourlas M (1975) Contact dermatitis from typewriter correction paper. Cutis 15:594–595

Kalimo K, Saarni H, Kytta J (1980) Immediate and delayed type reactions to formaldehyde resin in glass wool. Contact Dermatitis 6:496

Kashani MN, Gorouhi F, Behnia F, Nazemi MJ, Dowlati Y, Firooz A (2005) Allergic contact dermatitis in Iran. Contact Dermatitis 52:154–158

Lazarow A (2006) European standard series patch test results from a contact dermatitis clinic in Israel during the 7-year period from 1998–2004. Contact Dermatitis 55:73–76

Macfarlane AW, Yu RC, King CM (1990) Contact sensitivity to para-tertiary-butylcatechol in an artificial limb. Contact Dermatitis 22:56–57

Malten KE (1958) Occupational eczema due to para-tertiary butylphenol in a shoe adhesive. Dermatologica 117:103–109

Malten KE (1987) Old and new, mainly occupational dermatological problems in the production and processing of plastics. In: Maibach HI (ed) Occupational and industrial dermatology. Year Book Medical, Chicago, pp 290–340

Malten KE, Seutter E, Hara I et al (1971) Occupational vitiligo due to *p-tert*-butylphenol and homologues. Trans St John's Hosp Dermatol Soc 57:115–134

Malten KE, Rath R, Pastors PMH (1983) *p-tert*-butylphenol formaldehyde and other causes of shue dermatitis. Derm Beruf Umwelt 31:149–153

Mancuso G, Reggiani M, Berdondini RM (1996) Occupational dermatitis in shoemakers. Contact Dermatitis 34:17–22

Marques C, Goncalo M, Goncalo S (1994) Sensitivity to para-tertiary-butylphenol-formaldehyde resin in Portugal. Contact Dermatitis 30:300–301

Matrolonardo M, Loconsole F, Conte A, Rantuccio F (1993) Allergic contact dermatitis due to para-tertiary-butylphenol-formaldehyde resin in a hearing aid. Contact Dermatitis 28:179

Mobacken H, Hersle K (1976) Allergic contact dermatitis caused by paratertiary butylphenol-formaldehyde resin in watch straps. Contact Dermatitis 2:59

Moran M, Martin-Pascual A (1978) Contact dermatitis to para-tertiary-butylphenol formaldehyde. Contact Dermatitis 4:372–373

Owen CM, Beck MH (2001) Occupational allergic contact dermatitis from phenol-formaldehyde resins. Contact Dermatitis 45:294–295

Richardson ML (1993) The dictionary of substances and their effects. The Royal Society of Chemistry, Cambridge, pp 675–678

Romaguera C, Grimalt F, Vilaplana J (1985) Paratertiary butylphenol formaldehyde resin in prosthesis. Contact Dermatitis 12:174

Rycroft RJG, Wilkinson JD, Holmes R, Hay RJ (1980) Contact sensitization to *p*-tertiary-butylphenol (PTBP) resin in plastic nail adhesive. Clin Exp Dermatol 5:411–445

Schubert H, Agatha G (1979) Zur Allergennatur der para-*tert.* Butylphenol-formaldhydharze. Dermatosen 27:49–52

Shono M, Ezoe K, Kaniwa M-A, Ikarashi Y, Kojima S, Nakamura A (1991) Allergic contact dermatitis from para-tertiary-butylphenol-formaldehyde resin (PTBP-FR) in athletic tape and leather adhesive. Contact Dermatitis 24:281–288

Snell FD, Ettre LS (1973) Enzyclopedia of industrial chemical analysis, vol 17. Interscience, New York, pp 9–10

Sonneck HJ (1964) Hautschäden durch Kunstharzäurekitte. Berufsdermatosen 12:42–48

Stevenson CJ (1981) Occupational vitiligo: clinical and epidemiological aspects. Br J Dermatol 105(suppl 21):51–56

Tarvainen K (1995) Analysis of patients with allergic patch test reaction to a plastics and glue series. Contact Dermatitis 32:346–351

Trattner A, Tarachi Y, David M (2003) Shoe contact dermatitis in Israel. Am J Contact Dermat 14:12–14

van der Willingen AH, Stolz E, van Joost T (1987) Sensitization to phenol formaldehyde in rubber glue. Contact Dermatitis 16:291–292

Vincenzi C, Guerra L, Peluso AM, Zucchelli V (1992) Allergic contact dermatitis due to phenol-formaldehyde resin in a knee-guard. Contact Dermatitis 27:54

Zimerson E, Bruze M (1998) Contact allergy to the monomers in *p-tert*-butylphenol formaldehyderesin in the guinea pig. Contact Dermatitis 39:222–226

Zimerson E, Bruze M (1999) Demonstration of the contact sensitizer *p-tert*-butylcatechol in *p-tert*-butylphenol-formaldehyde resin. Am J Contact Dermat 10:2–6

Zimerson E, Bruze M (2000a) Contact allergy to 5,5′-di-*tert*-butyl-2,2′-dihydroxy-(hydroxymethyl)-dibenzyl ethers, sensitizers, in *p-tert*-butylphenol-formaldehyde resin. Contact Dermatitis 43:20–26

Zimerson E, Bruze M (2000b) Sensitizing capacity of 5,5′-di-*tert*-butyl-2,2′-dihydroxy-(hydroxymethyl)-dibenzyl ethers in the guinea pig. Contact Dermatitis 43:72–78

Zimerson E, Bruze M (2002a) Sensitizing capacity of two monomeric aldehyde components in *p-tert*-butylphenol-formaldehyde resin. Acta Derm Venereol 82:418–422

Zimerson E, Bruze M (2002b) Sensitizing capacity of some trimers in *p-tert*-butylphenol-formaldehyde resin. Contact Dermatitis 47:40–46

Zimerson E, Bruze M (2002c) Low-molecular-weight contact allergens in *p-tert*-butylphenol-formaldehyde resin. Am J Contact Dermat 13:190–197

Zimerson E, Bruze M (2002d) Contact allergy to the monomers in *p-tert*-butylphenol-formaldehyde resin. Contact Dermatitis 47:147–153

Zimerson E, Bruze M, Goossens A (1999) Simultaneous *p-tert*-butylphenol- formaldehyde resin and *p-tert*-butylcatechol allergies in man and sensitizing capacities of *p-tert*-butylphenol and *p-tert*-butylcatechol in the guinea pig. J Occup Environ Med 41:23–28

53 Polyurethane Resins

Malin Frick-Engfeldt[1] · *Tuula Estlander*[2] · *Riitta Jolanki*[3]
[1]Department of Occupational and Environmental Dermatology, Skåne University Hospital (SUS), Lund University, Malmö, Sweden
[2]Terveystalo Healthcare Oyj, Helsinki, Finland
[3]Control of Hypersensitivity Diseases, Finnish Institute of Occupational Health (FIOH), Helsinki, Finland

Core Messages

- Polyurethane (PU) products are formed by reacting a di- or polyfunctional isocyanate with a polyol in the presence of suitable catalysts and additives.
- The main occupationally hazard associated with PU chemicals are isocyanates, which have an adverse effect on the respiratory tract including both airway irritation and immunologically mediated outcomes.
- Exposure to isocyanates and auxiliary chemicals may also result in both allergic and irritant contact dermatitis, as well as contact and generalized urticaria, and the typical localization is hands and face.
- When patch-testing workers exposed to polyurethane chemicals it is advisable to test with their own work material in addition to the commercially available patch-test preparations of diisocyanates. A second reading on day 7 is advisable since positive reactions may appear late. Positive reactions to methylenedianiline (MDA) (also known as diaminodiphenylmethane) should be taken into account as it may be an important marker for diphenylmethane diisocyanate (MDI) sensitivity.

1 Introduction

Poluyurethanes (PUs) are used in a wide range of products including paints, glues, castings, surface coatings, adhesives, and soft and rigid foam. The main occupationally hazard associated with PU chemicals are isocyanates, which are known to affect the airways and eyes, and can cause rhinitis, asthma, hypersensitive pneumonitis or alveolitis, conjunctivitis, and chronic obstructive lung disease (Baur et al. 1994; Klees and Ott 1999). Isocyanates are toxic and poisonous chemicals, e.g., an accidental massive exposure to toluene diisocyanate (TDI) has been reported to cause acute intoxication, including severe pulmonary, gastric, and neurological symptoms (Cronin 1980; Adams 1983) and milder symptoms of intoxication were seen in the workers of a glass-bottle factory exposed to dicyclohexylmethane diisocyanate (DMDI) (Israeli et al. 1981). Furthermore, pyrolysis products of PU have been reported to cause fever (Kanerva et al. 1991; Littorin et al. 1994).

Exposure to isocyanates and auxiliary chemicals may also result in both allergic and irritant contact dermatitis, as well as contact and generalized urticaria (Rothe 1976; Malten 1984a; Kanerva et al. 1989, 1991; Estlander et al. 1992; Mancuso et al. 1996; Thompson and Belsito 1997; Schroder et al. 1999; Goossens et al. 2002; Frick et al. 2003a, b; Belsito 2003; Valks et al. 2003; Morgan and Haworth 2003; Liippo and Lammintausta 2008; Stingeni et al. 2008; Donovan et al. 2009).

2 Composition

PUs are formed as a result of a condensation or an adduction reaction between isocyanates and multifunctional alcohols (polyols). Isocyanates can be classified based on the number of –NCO groups in the molecule (i.e., monoisocyanates contain one –NCO, diisocyanate contains two –NCO, and polyisocyanates contain multiple –NCO groups). The chemical structures of the most common diisocyanate monomers and their technical grade counterparts are shown in ➋ *Fig. 53.1*. Di- and polyisocyanates form thermosetting end products when reacting with polyols. Generally the polyols are polyesters or polyethers with terminal hydroxyl groups, or castor oil or tall oil with secondary hydroxyl groups but other compounds containing active hydrogen atoms such as water and amines can also serve as polyols. Isocyanates can also be classified as either aromatic (containing one or more aromatic rings) or aliphatic. The aromatic isocyanates dominate the market. The most commonly used aromatic diisocyanate is diphenylmethane diisocyanate (MDI) followed by TDI. They are frequently used in the production of rigid and flexible foam but also in coatings,

T. Rustemeyer, P. Elsner, S.M. John & H.I. Maibach (eds.), *Kanerva's Occupational Dermatology*,
DOI 10.1007/978-3-642-02035-3_53,

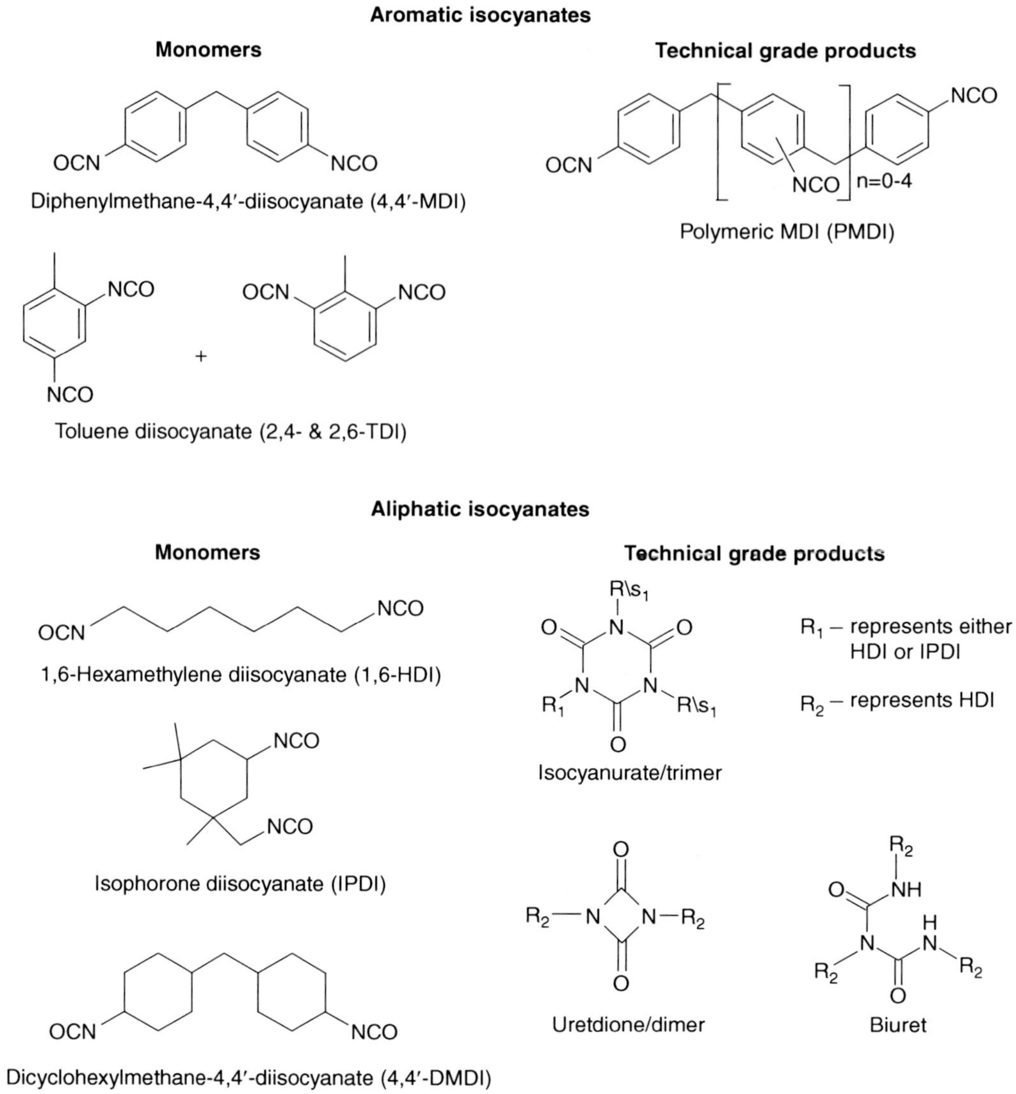

Fig. 53.1
Chemical formulae of various isocyanates used in the production of polyurethane plastics

adhesives, binders, and elastomers. Aliphatic isocyanates such as isophorone diisocyanate (IPDI) and hexamethylene diisocyanate (HDI) are generally more expensive to produce but they are used when the performance of aromatic isocyanates is inadequate, mainly because of their tendency to undergo oxidative discolouration upon exposure to light and moisture (Ulrich 2001). Due to their light and weather resistance, the aliphatic isocyanates are commonly used in lacquers, coatings, and paints. The production of both aromatic and aliphatic diisocyanates is mainly based on synthesizing the corresponding molecular structure with primary amine groups. The amino groups are then transformed into isocyanate groups by treatment with phosgene (Thorpe 2002).

In industry, technical grade isocyanate products are mainly used. They often consist of a mixture of isomers of monomers (i.e., diisocyanates) and oligomers (i.e., higher molecular weight molecules with more than two –NCO groups), and they are often referred to as polyisocyanates of the diisocyanate monomer. TDI is industrially available as mixtures of the 2,4- and 2,6-TDI isomers at ratios of 80:20 or 65:35 (2,4:2,6) or as pure 2,4-TDI (*Fig. 53.1*). Commercial MDI products generally contain a complex mixture of 25–80% monomeric 4,4′-MDI as well as oligomers containing predominately 3–6 aromatic rings, but also smaller amounts of oligomers containing a higher number of rings (➋ *Fig. 53.1*). They also contain low amounts of the monomeric isomers 2,2′- and 2,4′-MDI (Anonymous 2001). These MDI mixtures are usually referred to as polymeric MDI (PMDI), but the synonyms crude MDI and polymethylene polyphenyl isocyanate (PAPI or PMPPI) are sometimes also used. Phenyl isocyanate has been reported as a trace constituent in commercial MDI products (Karol and Kramarik 1996). Technical products of HDI and IPDI are often produced by reacting the monomeric isocyanates either with themselves (di- or trimerization) forming uretdiones, biurets, and isocyanurates, or with urea or urethane compounds to form higher molecular weight polyisocyanates (Thorpe 2002) (➋ *Fig. 53.1*). The monomer content in the technical products of IPDI and HDI is generally low (Marand et al. 2004).

Several auxiliary substances are also used in the manufacturer of PU products. The hardening process can be modified by heat or with a catalyst, usually tertiary amines and/or organometallics (primarily tin compounds) (Zimmerman 2002). Other additives, e.g., fire retardants, fillers, coloring agents, and cross-linking agents can be added to modify the polyurethane reaction as well as the properties of the final product. In the production of foamed plastics, blowing agents, e.g., pentane, carbon dioxide, or water, is also added (Anonymous 1996). When used as activators or hardeners, diisocyanates are often dissolved in aliphatic or aromatic hydrocarbon solvents or a mixture of different organic solvents, e.g., aliphatic hydrocarbon solvents, petroleum, and butyl acetate. Adhesives, varnishes, and paints may also contain solvents.

3 Skin Exposure

Exposure to isocyanates is mainly an occupational problem that occurs in work places where isocyanates or PUR are manufactured and processed. However, there have recently been reports describing isocyanate exposure in domestic settings (Militello et al. 2004; Morgan and Haworth 2003). Occupational exposure has been considered to occur mainly through inhalation, which has led to strict regulations regarding occupational exposure limits for airborne isocyanates in order to avoid adverse health effects on the respiratory tract. Monomeric diisocyanates with high vapor pressures, such as TDI, IPDI, and HDI, cause airborne exposure already at room temperature. MDI and most prepolymers, on the other hand, have low vapor pressures and are only volatile at elevated temperatures. Isocyanate exposure has also been reported in spraying applications, in which exposure to isocyanates with low vapor pressures becomes significant even at room temperature (Crespo and Galan 1999).

Completely hardened polyurethane products usually do not cause skin problems. Unreacted isocyanate monomer may, however, remain in excess inside polyurethane foams even after curing. This can create a health hazard due to isocyanate exposure when polyurethane dust is produced during machining or cutting (Emmett 1976; Kanerva et al. 1997). Additionally, processing of PUR materials at temperatures above 150°C causes thermal degradation, which leads to dissociation of the PUR into a complex mixture of isocyanates, amines, and aminoisocyanates (Karlsson et al. 2001).

Recently, concerns have been raised about the role of skin exposure from isocyanates in the development of occupational asthma (Bello et al. 2008), and animal studies have shown that animals sensitized by dermal contact alone exhibit respiratory response upon inhalation of isocyanates (Rattray et al. 1994).

4 Skin Problems Caused by PU Chemicals

Exposure to isocyanates may result in both allergic and irritant contact dermatitis, as well as contact urticaria (Larsen et al. 2001; Goossens et al. 2002; Valks et al. 2003; Stingeni et al. 2008) and the typical localization is hands and face. According to Liippo et al. facial dermatitis seem more common in patients with positive patch-test reactions to TDI and/or IPDI than in patients with positive reactions to MDI (Liippo and Lammintausta 2008), which is in accordance with the fact that TDI and IPDI are more volatile than MDI.

4.1 Allergic Contact Dermatitis

Diisocyanates are strong contact sensitizers, judged by the results of animal studies (Tanaka et al. 1987; Thorne et al. 1987). Animal experiments have also shown that polyisocyanate prepolymers are capable of causing skin sensitization in guinea pigs (Zissu et al. 1998). However, in spite of this, reports on allergic contact dermatitis are relatively few in number considering the extensive use of these chemicals in manufacturing processes and other applications. The low contact allergy frequency has been explained by the fact that (i) contamination of the skin is minimized by the application of strict regulations to the handling of isocyanates in order to avoid respiratory problems; (ii) that the reactive isocyanates react before penetrating the skin (Malten 1984b); and (iii) that the patch-test diagnostics of isocyanates is inadequate due to instability of patch-test allergens and lack of late readings (i.e., reading after day 7)(Frick-Engfeldt et al. 2007a, b).

Heavy exposure to diisocyanates may result in a rapid sensitization within a week to some months after exposure (Estlander et al. 1992; Frick et al. 2003b; Donovan et al. 2009). It has been proposed that aromatic diisocyanates are strong respiratory sensitizers but weak cutaneous sensitizers (Emmett 1976), and that the opposite could be true for aliphatic diisocyanates (Rietschel and Fowler 2001). Contact allergy to MDI, TDI, IPDI, HDI, DMDI, naphthalene diisocyanate (NDI), and trimethyl hexamethylene diiosocyanate (TMDI) has been reported (Kanerva et al. 1989; Estlander et al. 1992; Rothe 1976; Malten 1984a; Schroder et al. 1999; Frick et al. 2003a, b; Thompson and Belsito 1997; Belsito 2003; Morgan and Haworth 2003; Goossens et al. 2002; Mancuso et al. 1996; Liippo and Lammintausta 2008). Most recorded cases were sensitized to MDI or DMDI. HDI trimers are novel occupational contact allergens (Pesonen et al. 2010).

DMDI has been reported as a very potent dermal sensitizer (Emmett 1976; White et al. 1983; Frick et al. 2003a; Donovan et al. 2009). In a company manufacturing medical equipment 13 out of 100 workers were sensitized to DMDI, which was used in a glue (Frick et al. 2003a). At a factory making car badges two out of seven workers showed positive patch-test reactions to DMDI. It was also believed that irritant contact dermatitis from DMDI was the cause of three of the workers' skin problems (White et al. 1983). Recently, a case describing allergic contact dermatitis to DMDI in an office environment where DMDI-charged cartridges were used was described (Kerre 2008). DMDI exposed patients have been reported to show positive reactions to TDI, HDI, and IPDI without any previously known contact with the substances in question (Frick et al. 2003a; Militello et al. 2004). Militello et al. attributed this to cross-sensitivity, referring to Thorne et al. who investigated MDI, TDI, HDI, and DMDI and showed cross-reactions between all isocyanates, regardless of whether they were aromatic or aliphatic, in animal experiments based on the mouse-ear swelling test (Thorne et al. 1987; Militello et al. 2004). In the same study it was postulated that HDI was the most potent sensitizer, followed by DMDI, MDI, and TDI in declining order of potency (Thorne et al. 1987).

MDI-positive patients may also react to the corresponding amine methylenedianiline (MDA) (also known as diaminodiphenylmethane) (Fregert 1967; Rothe 1976; Estlander et al. 1992; Goossens et al. 2002; Frick et al. 2003b; Liippo and Lammintausta 2008). In 1967, Fregert was the first to report these simultaneous reactions (Fregert 1967). He attributed this to cross-reactivity. In 1976, Rothe suggested that MDA might be the actual allergen and that it is formed from hydrolysis of MDI when MDI comes into contact with the skin (Rothe 1976). Several reports describe workers exposed to MDI with positive patch-test reactions to MDA but negative reactions to MDI (Alomar 1986; Estlander et al. 1992; Tait and Delaney 1999; Goossens et al. 2002; Frick et al. 2003b) and it has been proposed that MDA might be an important marker for MDI hypersensitivity (Estlander et al. 1992; Goossens et al. 2002; Frick et al. 2003b). MDA may also represent cross-allergy to p-phenylenediamine (Rothe 1976; Uter et al. 2002).

Other examples of products and tasks or manufacturing processes which have caused sensitization and allergic eczema to PU chemicals are workers exposed to PU chemicals and prepolymers in laboratories (Rothe 1976; Kanerva et al. 1989; Estlander et al. 1992), in paint industry (Pesonen et al. 2010), and in the manufacture of PUs, e.g., car spray painters, adhesive workers – such as those exposed to two-part glues used by floor layers (Lodi et al. 1993), consolidation of brittle ground (Bertrand et al. 1984) and sealants used to repair cracks in concrete buildings (Rothe 1995), and the making of PU casts (Vaichere et al. 1986). Furthermore, rare sources of sensitization to PU chemicals include a plastic watch strap (Alomar 1986), a PU covering (Synthaderm) used to treat leg ulcers (Helland et al. 1983), spectacle frames (Vilaplana et al. 1987), and a pacemaker lining (Abdallah et al. 1994).

Polyols are not considered to be sensitizers. However, Verdich and Skoven reported that a man, whose job was to mix polyols and different catalysts in open barrels, was patch-test positive to the polyol but not to any other chemicals used in the production (Verdich and Skoven 1979). Although rare, there are also some cases describing allergic contact dermatitis caused by accelerators (Wodiansky 1967; Emmett 1976).

4.2 Irritant Contact Dermatitis

Isocyanates are described as mild to strong skin irritants and are listed in material safety data sheets as skin irritating substances. Liquid monomer coming into contact with the skin has been reported to cause edema and redness if it is not immediately washed away (Fisher 1986). Irritant contact dermatitis seems to be more common than allergic contact dermatitis and small epidemics have occurred in certain plants using isocyanates.

Itchy rash-like eruptions on exposed skin areas in the factory workers who coat car badges with the resin have been reported within 1 week to 6 months of exposure to DMDI (White et al. 1983). The same was reported in workers of a glass-bottle factory, where DMDI was used to coat the bottles (Israeli et al. 1981), as well as in the workers of a PU-molding plant (Emmett 1976). Irritant dermatitis appearing in a laboratory technician within a few hours of contact with TDI and in a repair man have also been described (Rothe 1976).

After heavy exposure to TDI, pulmonary symptoms followed by thrombocytopenia and purpura have been reported (Jennings and Gower 1963). Pruritus and exanthema without proven contact sensitization have also been reported in workers exposed to MDI (Mowe 1980). Irritant dermatitis, in addition to allergic dermatitis from HDI occurred in the workers of two clothing mills handling cloths previously coated with an antipill finish containing HDI. The eruption was located typically on the hands and face (Wilkinson et al. 1991).

Skin irritation can also be caused by amine accelerators, e.g., MDA (Van Joost et al. 1987), triethylenediamine (Adams 1983), and triethylamine (Malten 1964). Concentrated liquids may even be corrosive. The irritant effect of diisocyanates in the hardeners, glues, and paints may also be attributed to the solvents used in these products.

4.3 Urticaria

Generalized or contact urticaria from isocyanate exposure has relatively seldom been reported (Israeli et al. 1981; Kanerva et al. 1991, 1999; Valks et al. 2003; Stingeni et al. 2008). One case of concomitant Type I and Type IV allergy to MDI has been described in a man working with a polyurethane glue and who showed an immediate urticarial-type contact reaction when patch tested and read after 20 min as well as an eczematous reaction when patch tested and read after 2 and 4 days, respectively (Stingeni et al. 2008). Additionally, specific IgE antibodies against MDI were detected in the patient.

Occupational urticaria and fever caused by inhalation of dissociation products of heated PUR has been described in a welder (Kanerva et al. 1991). The causative agent in the PUR fume was not determined and it could not be shown whether the urticaria was nonimmunologic or mediated by immunoglobins.

5 Examination of Dermatoses Caused by PU Chemicals and Their Prevention

Examinations should include clinical follow-up of the symptoms and exploration of the exposing chemicals, as well as patch testing. Patch testing is necessary to distinguish between sensitization and irritation caused by PU chemicals. In commercially available isocyanate series the patch-test preparations of TDI and MDI only contain one isomer of the respective monomers. Therefore, patients are generally tested with the isomers 4,4′-MDI, and 2,4-TDI. Patch-test preparations of DMDI is not commercially available but is normally tested as the 4,4′-DMDI isomer. Most reports found in literature refer to contact allergy to these specific isomers. However, when previously described, the general abbreviations MDI, TDI, and DMDI have often been used. The significance of the various subtypes (i.e., biuret, isocyanurate, and asymmetric) of HDI trimers is still unknown and commercially available test substances are lacking. Allergic reactions to HDI trimers cannot be explained by sensitization to HDI monomer as it has been shown that HDI trimer allergic patients are negative in patch testing to the HDI monomer (Pesonen et al. 2010).

Isocyanates are highly reactive and their stability in patch-test preparations has been discussed. In 1992, Estlander et al. suggested that preparations of TDI and 4,4′-MDI could be used for over a year since preparations that were 5.5 and 15.5 months old had elicited positive reactions in two patients (Estlander et al. 1992). No chemical analyses were done. In 2004 and 2005, Frick et al. and Frick-Engfeldt et al. performed chemical analysis on commercially available patch-test preparations from isocyanate series obtained from four American and nine European patch-testing departments showing that patch-test preparations of 2,4-TDI, 1,6-HDI, and IPDI contained the declared concentrations, but the concentration of 4,4′-MDI was generally so low that patch testing with the same could not be considered reliable (Frick et al. 2004; Frick-Engfeldt et al. 2005). It was concluded that there is a high risk of false-negative reactions when using these preparations of 4,4′-MDI and, therefore, additional patch testing with the patients' own fresh work material was recommended (Frick et al. 2004). The same recommendation was given by Gossens et al. (2002) when reporting 13 patients with positive patch-test reactions to isocyanate-based products and where only one of these patients reacted to any commercially available patch-test preparation of diisocyanates. In the case of MDI it has been suggested that patch-test preparations of PMDI with a monomer content of at least 35% are used instead of preparations of 4,4′-MDI. The recommended patch-test concentration for PMDI was 2% in petrolatum (Frick-Engfeldt et al. 2007b). Additionally, preparations should be stored in a freezer, for no longer than 1 year in order to ensure stability (Frick-Engfeldt et al. 2007b).

Patch-testing workers exposed to polyurethane chemicals should include relatively fresh preparations of the most common diisocyanates MDI, TDI, HDI, and IPDI as well as MDA and the actual chemicals to which the workers have been exposed. It has been proposed that positive reactions to isocyanates appear late and, therefore, it is advisable that isocyanate patch tests are also read on day 7 and that patients should be advised to make contact with the clinic, if any reactions appear after day 7 (Frick-Engfeldt et al. 2007b).

One case of a possible active patch-test sensitization with TDI 1% in pet. has been reported (Le Coz et al. 1999).

In the case of urticaria, prick tests with MDI, TDI, and HDI human serum albumin (HSA) conjugates and the determinations of the same diisocyanate IgE-specific antibodies in the serum should be included in the examinations. An IgE-mediated reaction may also be the cause of diisocyanate-induced urticaria. It is one of the mechanisms of sensitization in occupationally derived asthma, and explained less than half of the immediate reactions in the bronchial provocation test in 35 cases of occupational asthma caused by MDI, TDI, and HDI (Keskinen et al. 1988). However, a challenge test in an exposure chamber (Kanerva et al. 1991) is probably the most reliable method of confirming the diagnosis of generalized diisocyanate-induced urticaria, and open application with an isocyanate product to confirm the diagnosis of contact urticaria. The open test is recommended to be performed in prick-positive patients using either the same diisocyanate HSA conjugate as in the prick test or the isocyanate-containing product from the workplace diluted to the desired concentration. The vehicle, water, petrolatum, or ethanol is used as control (Helaskoski et al. 2009).

In the prevention of dermatoses induced by PU chemicals, it is important to inform all exposed workers about all the health hazards of mainly isocyanates, and to give detailed instructions on how isocyanate products should be handled correctly. This means using appropriate personal protective equipment, such as EC conformity-marked chemical protective gloves, masks, eye and face protectors, and other protective clothing. In countries belonging to the European Union, all gloves used for chemical protection must be certified to fulfill the requirements of Directive *89/686/EEC* category III, and supplied with CE markings. Data on the workplace performance of protective gloves and clothing are limited and, although nitrile gloves (thickness >0.3 mm) have been suggested as preferable to latex, studies have shown that isocyanates can be detected underneath both types of glove (Bello et al. 2007). Thus, Silver Shield®/4H gloves made of a multilayer of polyethylene/ethylene vinyl alcohol/polyethylene probably give the best protection against polyurethane chemicals (Forsberg and Mansdorf 2007). Good ventilation, local exhausts, and general cleanliness are also essential. During patient examination it is heard much too often that no information had been given about the health hazards of PU chemicals or products such as paints, adhesives, sealants, and lacquers.

References

Abdallah HI, Balsara RK, O'Riordan AC (1994) Pacemaker contact sensitivity: clinical recognition and management. Ann Thorac Surg 57(4):1017–1018

Adams RM (1983) Plastics. Occupational skin disease. Grune and Stratton, New York, pp 238–266

Alomar A (1986) Contact dermatitis from a fashion watch. Contact Dermatitis 15:44–45

Anonymous (1996) Thermosetting plastics. Statue Book of the Swedish National Board of Occupational Safety and Health. AFS 1996:4

Anonymous (2001) TA: Concise International Chemical Assessment Document (CICAD) PG:25 p YR:2001 IP: VI:27

Baur X, Marek W, Ammon J et al (1994) Respiratory and other hazards of isocyanates. Int Arch Occup Environ Health 66(3):141–152

Bello D, Herrick CA, Smith TJ et al (2007) Skin exposure to isocyanates: reasons for concern. Environ Health Perspect 115(3):328–335

Bello D, Redlich CA, Stowe MH et al (2008) Skin exposure to aliphatic polyisocyanates in the auto body repair and refinishing industry: II. A quantitative assessment. Ann Occup Hyg 52(2):117–124

Belsito DV (2003) Common shoe allergens undetected by commercial patch-testing kits: dithiodimorpholine and isocyanates. Am J Contact Dermat 14(2):95–96

Bertrand JP, Wantz JM, Heintz P et al (1984) Pathologic lies e l'utilisation des isocyanates dans les mines de charles. Archives des Maladies Professionelles de Medecine de Travail et de Sécurité Soviale 45:3–9

Crespo J, Galan J (1999) Exposure to MDI during the process of insulating buildings with sprayed polyurethane foam. Ann Occup Hyg 43(6):415–419

Cronin E (1980) Contact dermatitis. Churchill Livingstone, Edingburgh

Donovan JC, Kudla I, DeKoven JG (2009) Rapid development of allergic contact dermatitis from dicyclohexylmethane-4,4′-diisocyanate. Dermatitis 20(4):214–217

Emmett EA (1976) Allergic contact dermatitis in polyurethane plastic moulders. J Occup Med 18(12):802–804

Estlander T, Keskinen H, Jolanki R et al (1992) Occupational dermatitis from exposure to polyurethane chemicals. Contact Dermatitis 27(3):161–165

Fisher AA (1986) Contact dermatitis. Lea and Febiger, Philadelphia

Forsberg K, Mansdorf SZ (2007) Quick selection guide to chemical protective clothing. Wiley, New Jersey

Fregert S (1967) Allergic contact reaction to diphenyl-4,4′-diisocyanate. Contact Dermatitis Newsl 2:17

Frick M, Bjorkner B, Hamnerius N et al (2003a) Allergic contact dermatitis from dicyclohexylmethane-4,4′-diisocyanate. Contact Dermatitis 48(6):305–309

Frick M, Isaksson M, Bjorkner B et al (2003b) Occupational allergic contact dermatitis in a company manufacturing boards coated with isocyanate lacquer. Contact Dermatitis 48(5):255–260

Frick M, Zimerson E, Karlsson D et al (2004) Poor correlation between stated and found concentrations of diphenylmethane-4,4′-diisocyanate (4,4′-MDI) in petrolatum patch-test preparations. Contact Dermatitis 51(2):73–78

Frick-Engfeldt M, Zimerson E, Karlsson D et al (2005) Chemical analysis of 2,4-toluene diisocyanate, 1,6-hexamethylene diisocyanate and isophorone diisocyanate in petrolatum patch-test preparations. Dermatitis 16(3):130–135

Frick-Engfeldt M, Isaksson M, Zimerson E et al (2007a) How to optimize patch testing with diphenylmethane diisocyanate. Contact Dermatitis 57(3):138–151

Frick-Engfeldt M, Zimerson E, Karlsson D et al (2007b) Is it possible to improve the patch-test diagnostics for isocyanates? A stability study of petrolatum preparations of diphenylmethane-4,4′-diisocyanate and polymeric diphenylmethane diisocyanate. Contact Dermatitis 56(1):27–34

Goossens A, Detienne T, Bruze M (2002) Occupational allergic contact dermatitis caused by isocyanates. Contact Dermatitis 47(5):304–8

Helaskoski E, Kuuliala O, Aalto-Korte K (2009) Occupational contact urticaria caused by cyclic acid anhydrides. Contact Dermatitis 60(4):214–221

Helland S, Nyfors A, Utne L (1983) Contact dermatitis to Synthaderm. Contact Dermatitis 9(6):504–506

Israeli R, Smirnov V, Sculsky M (1981) Intoxication due to dicyclohexylmethane-4-4′ diisocyanate exposure (author's transl). Int Arch Occup Environ Health 48(2):179–184

Jennings GH, Gower ND (1963) Thrombocytopenic purpura in toluene di-isocyanate workers. Lancet 1(7278):406–408

Kanerva L, Lähteenmäki MT, Estlander T et al (1989) Allergic contact dermatitis from isocyanates. In: Frosch PJ, Dooms-Goossens A, Lachapelle J-M, Rycroft RJG, Scheper RJ (eds) Current topics in contact dermatitis. Springer, Berlin/Heidelberg/New york, pp 368–373

Kanerva L, Estlander T, Jolanki R et al (1991) Occupational urticaria from welding polyurethane. J Am Acad Dermatol 24(5 Pt 2):825–826

Kanerva L, Jolanki R, Estlander T (1997) 10 years of patch testing with the (meth)acrylate series. Contact Dermatitis 37(6):255–258

Kanerva L, Grenquist-Norden B, Piirila P (1999) Occupational IgE-mediated contact urticaria from diphenylmethane-4,4-diisocyanate (MDI). Contact Dermatitis 41(1):50–51

Karlsson D, Dalene M, Skarping G et al (2001) Determination of isocyanic acid in air. J Environ Monit 3(4):432–436

Karol MH, Kramarik JA (1996) Phenyl isocyanate is a potent chemical sensitizer. Toxicol Lett 89(2):139–146

Kerre S (2008) Allergic contact dermatitis to DMDI in an office application. Contact Dermatitis 58(5):313–314

Keskinen H, Tupasela O, Tiikkainen U et al (1988) Experiences of specific IgE in asthma due to diisocyanates. Clin Allergy 18(6):597–604

Klees JE, Ott MG (1999) Diisocyanates in polyurethane plastics applications. Occup Med 14(4):759–776

Larsen TH, Gregersen P, Jemec GB (2001) Skin irritation and exposure to diisocyanates in orthopedic nurses working with soft casts. Am J Contact Dermat 12(4):211–214

Le Coz CJ, El Aboubi S, Ball C (1999) Active sensitization to toluene di-isocyanate. Contact Dermatitis 41(2):104–105

Liippo J, Lammintausta K (2008) Contact sensitization to 4,4′-diaminodiphenylmethane and to isocyanates among general dermatology patients. Contact Dermatitis 59(2):109–114

Littorin M, Truedsson L, Welinder H et al (1994) Acute respiratory disorder, rhinoconjunctivitis and fever associated with the pyrolysis of polyurethane derived from diphenylmethane diisocyanate. Scand J Work Environ Health 20(3):216–222

Lodi A, Mancini LL, Pozzi M et al (1993) Occupational airborne allergic contact dermatitis in parquet layers. Contact Dermatitis 29(5):281–2

Malten KE (1964) Occupational dermatoses in the processing of plastics. Trans St John's Hosp Dermatol Soc 59:78–113

Malten KE (1984a) Dermatological problems with synthetic resins and plastics in glues. Part I. Derm Beruf Umwelt 32(3):81–86

Malten KE (1984b) Dermatological problems with synthetic resins and plastics in glues. Part II. Derm Beruf Umwelt 32(4):118–125

Mancuso G, Reggiani M, Berdondini RM (1996) Occupational dermatitis in shoemakers. Contact Dermatitis 34(1):17–22

Marand A, Dahlin J, Karlsson D et al (2004) Determination of technical grade isocyanates used in the production of polyurethane plastics. J Environ Monit 6(7):606–614

Militello G, Sasseville D, Ditre C et al (2004) Allergic contact dermatitis from isocyanates among sculptors. Dermatitis 15(3):150–153

Morgan CJ, Haworth AE (2003) Allergic contact dermatitis from 1,6-hexamethylene diisocyanate in a domestic setting. Contact Dermatitis 48(4):224

Mowe G (1980) Health risks from isocyanates. Contact Dermatitis 6(1):44–45

Pesonen M, Jolanki R, Kuuliala O (2010) Contact allergy to aliphatic polyisocyanates (hexamethylene-1,6-diisocyanate homopolymers). Contact Dermatitis 63 (Suppl. 1):46-47

Rattray NJ, Botham PA, Hext PM et al (1994) Induction of respiratory hypersensitivity to diphenylmethane-4,4′-diisocyanate (MDI) in guinea pigs. Influence of route of exposure. Toxicology 88(1–3): 15–30

Rietschel RL, Fowler JF (2001) Fisher's contact dermatitis, 5th edn. Lipingcott, Williams & Wilkins, Philadelphia, p 512

Rothe A (1976) Occupational dermatoses due to polyurethane drugs. Berufsdermatosen 24:7–24

Rothe A (1995) Gefahren bei der Injektion von Rissen in Betonbauwerk. Bau 2:72–75

Schroder C, Uter W, Schwanitz HJ (1999) Occupational allergic contact dermatitis, partly airborne, due to isocyanates and epoxy resin. Contact Dermatitis 41(2):117–118

Stingeni L, Bellini V, Lisi P (2008) Occupational airborne contact urticaria and asthma: simultaneous immediate and delayed allergy to diphenylmethane-4,4′-diisocyanate. Contact Dermatitis 58(2): 112–113

Tait CP, Delaney TA (1999) Reactions causing reactions: allergic contact dermatitis to an isocyanate metabolite but not to the parent compound. Australas J Dermatol 40(2):116–117

Tanaka K, Takeoka A, Nishimura F et al (1987) Contact sensitivity induced in mice by methylene bisphenyl diisocyanate. Contact Dermatitis 17(4):199–204

Thompson T, Belsito DV (1997) Allergic contact dermatitis from a diisocyanate in wool processing. Contact Dermatitis 37(5):239

Thorne PS, Hillebrand JA, Lewis GR et al (1987) Contact sensitivity by diisocyanates: potencies and cross-reactivities. Toxicol Appl Pharmacol 87(1):155–165

Thorpe D (2002) Isocyanates. In: Lee S (ed) The Huntsman polyurethanes book, 1st edn. Wiley, UK, pp 63–88

Ulrich H (2001) Diisocyanates. In: Ulrich H (ed) Chemistry and technology of isocyanates. Wiley, Chichester/NewYork/Brisbane/Toronto/Singapore, pp 315–467

Uter W, Lessmann H, Geier J et al (2002) The spectrum of allergic (cross-) sensitivity in clinical patch testing with "para amino" compounds. Allergy 57(4):319–322

Vaichere E, Lefevre A, Choudat D et al (1986) Allergies cutanées et respiratoires liées a la confection de "platres" orthopédiques à base de résines synthétique. Archives des Maladies Professionnelles de Médicine de Travail et de Sécurité Sociale 47:35–36

Valks R, Conde-Salazar L, Barrantes OL (2003) Occupational allergic contact urticaria and asthma from diphenylmethane-4,4′-diisocyanatae. Contact Dermatitis 49(3):166–167

Van Joost T, Heule F, de Boer J (1987) Sensitization to methylenedianiline and para-structures. Contact Dermatitis 16(5):246–248

Verdich J, Skoven I (1979) Allergic contact dermatitis from Desmophen, a polyether alcohol. Contact Dermatitis 5(2):120

Vilaplana J, Romaguera C, Grimalt F (1987) Allergic contact dermatitis from aliphatic isocyanate on spectacle frames. Contact Dermatitis 16(2):113

White IR, Stewart JR, Rycroft RJ (1983) Allergic contact dermatitis from an organic di-isocyanate. Contact Dermatitis 9(4):300–303

Wilkinson SM, Cartwright PH, Armitage J et al (1991) Allergic contact dermatitis from 1,6-diisocyanatohexane in an anti-pill finish. Contact Dermatitis 25(2):94–96

Wodiansky P (1967) Hautschäden beider Erzeugung von Polyurethan-Kunstoffen. Berufsdermatosen 15:81–92

Zimmerman R (2002) Catalysts. In: Lee S (ed) The Huntsman polyurethanes book, 1st edn. Wiley, UK, pp 137–150

Zissu D, Binet S, Limasset JC (1998) Cutaneous sensitization to some polyisocyanate prepolymers in guinea pigs. Contact Dermatitis 39(5):248–251

54 Polyester Resins

Rosemary Nixon[1] · *Jennifer Cahill*[1] · *Riitta Jolanki*[2]
[1]Occupational Dermatology Research and Education Centre, Skin and Cancer Foundation, Carlton South, Melbourne, VIC, Australia
[2]Control of Hypersensitivity Diseases, Finnish Institute of Occupational Health (FIOH), Helsinki, Finland

Core Messages

- Allergic contact dermatitis from polyester resins is rare.
- Allergic reactions are more likely to occur from other components of the resin system, but are still uncommon. Irritant contact dermatitis may occur from peroxides and styrene.
- Contact urticaria may occur from anhydrides.

1 Introduction

Polyester resins are polycondensates prepared in two different forms: saturated and unsaturated. Saturated polyesters, alkyd resins, are produced from polybasic acids and polyalcohols. Polybasic acids, mainly phthalic acid or maleic acid, are used in their anhydride forms. The polyalcohols most often used are glycerol, pentaerythriol, or trimethylolpropane.

The saturated polyesters, synthesized in this way, are also named unmodified alkyd resins, macromolecules commonly used as plasticizers for other plastic materials. Alkyd resins can be modified by oil-containing fatty acids to be used in water-based paints and surface coatings (Kanerva et al. 1996a; Björkner 2006).

Unsaturated polyester (UP) resins are produced through esterification of dicarboxylic acids or their anhydrides, such as maleic anhydride, phthalic anhydride, or fumaric acid, and diols, such as diethylene glycol or 1,2-propylene glycol (➲ *Fig. 54.1*). Styrene is the most commonly used monomer for the cross-linking of UP resins. Vinyl toluene and methyl methacrylate are examples of other cross-linking agents.

An initiator or catalyst is required to start the cross-linking process, and is usually a peroxide such as benzoyl peroxide or methyl ethyl ketone peroxide. Accelerators, such as cobalt naphthenate or octoate, or tertiary amines such as dimethyl aniline, diethyl aniline, and dimethyl-p-toluidine, are also necessary for the curing of plastics at room temperature. The ultraviolet light (UV)-curable polyester system is used in the furniture industry as top coating and for orthopedic casts. The UV-curable polyester system contains vinyl toluene as the cross-linking agent and a benzoin-ether molecule as photoinitiator (Kanerva et al. 1996a; Björkner 2006). UP resins have been used extensively in the reinforced plastics industry in the manufacture of products for transportation, construction, and marine applications. They are also used for coatings, finishes, lacquers, cements, and glues (Kanerva et al. 1996a; Björkner 2006).

2 Skin Problems from Polyester Resins

Saturated polyester resins are generally not considered to be sensitizing. Allergic contact dermatitis (ACD) has, however, been caused by an epoxy compound, triglycidyl isocyanurate (TGIC) used as cross-linker in polyester paints (Mathias 1988). Phthalic anhydrides have been reported to cause ICD (Malten and Zielhuis 1964), immediate IgE-mediated hypersensitivity with asthma, allergic rhinitis, urticaria (Jolanki et al. 1987, 1997; Tarvainen et al. 1995a) and, rarely, ACD (Kanerva et al. 1997). The contact urticaria reaction from methyl hexahydrophthalic anhydride was reported to be enhanced by wiping off the substance with an alcohol disinfectant, which was presumed to enhance penetration of the allergen (Kanerva et al. 1999a).

Most reports of skin problems involve workers in plastics manufacture. In one workplace study (Minamoto et al. 2002a), ACD was most common but irritant contact dermatitis (ICD) was also reported, from both chemicals and mechanical irritants such as glass fiber and dust. As manufacturing processes become increasingly automated, exposure to alkyd resins is generally a result of accidents or maintenance work.

T. Rustemeyer, P. Elsner, S.M. John & H.I. Maibach (eds.), *Kanerva's Occupational Dermatology*,
DOI 10.1007/978-3-642-02035-3_54,

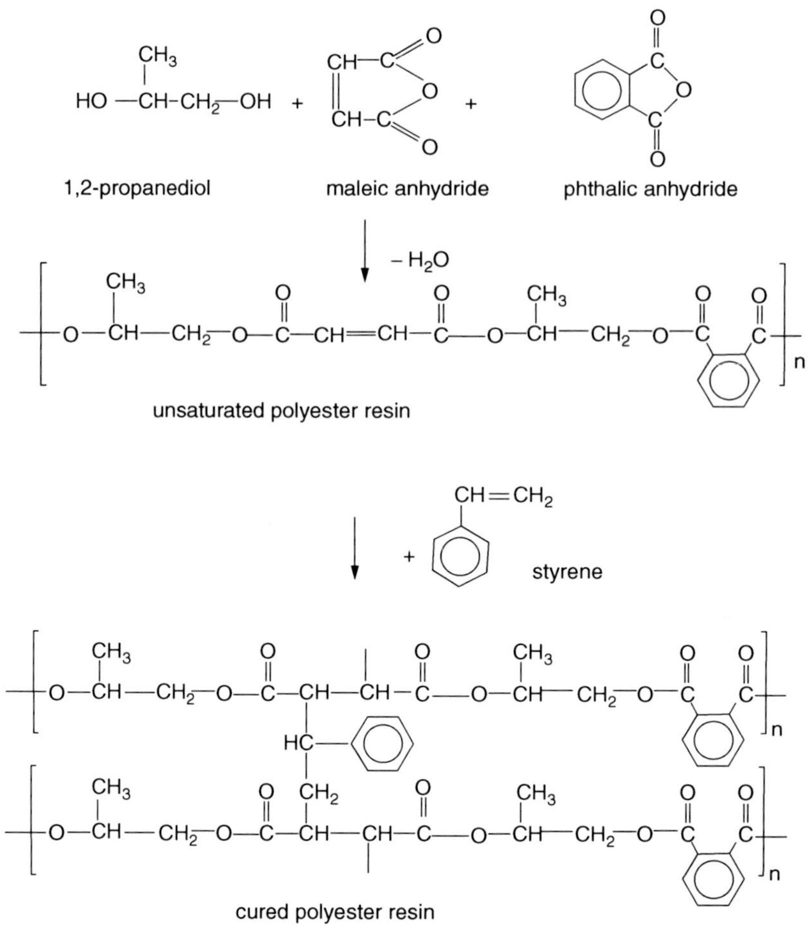

Fig. 54.1
Unsaturated polyester resin is made by condensing 1,2-propanediol, maleic anhdyride, and phthalic anhydrides. Styrene is used as a cross-linking monomer

3 Irritant Contact Dermatitis

ICD from UP resins occurs from cross-linking styrene (Rietschel and Fowler 2008) or, in earlier times, diallylphthalate (Fregert 1971). Styrene is classified as a mild irritant, although it has been reported to cause blisters (Bourne and Milner 1963) and even chemical burns (Bruze et al. 2000).

Prolonged exposure to styrene has caused a case of skin atrophy, neurogenic muscular atrophy, and anxiety reaction (Araki et al. 1971). Levels of styrene vapor exceeding 300 ppm (1,260 mg/m) have been reported to induce erythema of the skin (Stewart et al. 1968). Even at levels of 50 ppm (215 mg/m), styrene vapor may irritate conjunctival and nasal mucous membranes (Gotell et al. 1972). The mucous membrane irritation may be caused by the vinyl group in styrene (Alarie 1973). However, workers may develop a tolerance to the irritation after prolonged exposure (Gotell et al. 1972).

Organic peroxides, used as 3–10% solutions to catalyze the hardening reactions of UP, are weak sensitizers but strong irritants (Haustein et al. 1985). In the plastic composite industry, organic peroxides have caused severe ICD (Bourne and Milner 1963). Reactive organic peroxide molecules in unhardened resin dust may cause stinging on uncovered areas of the skin during spray lamination (Schumes 1990).

Hydrogen peroxide is an irritant but very rarely an allergen (Aguirre et al. 1994; Kanerva et al. 1998). Phthalic anhydride used in the manufacture of alkyd resins can cause ICD, and even caustic blisters especially on moist skin, where the anhydride is transformed into the corresponding acid (Malten and Zielhuis 1964).

In addition to chemicals included in the resin system, mold-releasing chemicals have also caused ICD (Bourne and Milner 1963). Acetone is used to clean equipment in UP resin industries. With repeated contact, acetone may defat the skin and disrupt the epidermal barrier (Fartasch 1997). It has been reported to be a contributing factor for ICD in this industry (Bourne and Milner 1963; Tarvainen et al. 1993b, 1994). Chlorinated hydrocarbon solvents such as methylene chloride and trichloroethane are often used for cleaning purposes and are also skin irritants (Midtgard and Knudsen 1994).

4 Allergic Contact Dermatitis

ACD was first reported from UP resins in 1955 (Lieber 1955). Five patients with ACD and positive patch tests to UP resins were reported from a group of 30 workers in an airplane factory (Malten 1956). Most cases of ACD have been caused by exposure to UP resin in lamination work (Malten 1956; Bourne and Milner 1963; Lidén et al. 1984), in painting (Kadlec et al. 1974), or in the use of UV light-cured inks (Björkner 1982).

UP dust from reinforced plastic products (Bourne and Milner 1963; Tarvainen et al. 1993b, 1995b) or UP automobile-repair putty (Tarvainen et al. 1993a; Kanerva et al. 1999b; Dooms-Goossens and De Jonge 1985) have also caused ACD.Guin (2001) reported a machine repairman who had developed ACD from adipic acid while working in the synthesis of polyester resins.

Adipic polyester, produced from adipic acid and propylene glycol, is a thermoplastic polyester used as a plasticizer in vinyl gloves, and has also caused ACD (Sowa et al. 2005). Nonoccupational ACD from UP resin is infrequent, but has been reported from "hypoallergenic" nail varnish (Shaw 1989), UP glue (Sjoborg et al. 1982), and limb prostheses (MacFarlane et al. 1986; Freeman 1986; Vincenzi et al. 1991; Haddad et al. 1996).

The allergens are often the auxiliary chemicals used, such as cobalt naphthenate (Key et al. 1961; Bourne and Milner 1963; Malten and Zielhuis 1964; Kadlec et al. 1974), cobalt octoate (cobalt-2-ethylhexanoate) (Kanerva et al. 1996b) and more recently in a spa bath laminator (Anavekar and Nixon 2006); dibutyl phthalate, dimethyl phthalate, dioctyl phthalate (Malten and Zielhuis 1964), tricresyl phosphate (Key et al. 1961), or a cross-linking monomer, such as styrene (Key et al. 1961; Bourne and Milner 1963; Sjoborg et al. 1982; Conde-Salazar et al. 1989), or a catalyst such as benzoyl peroxide (Bourne and Milner 1963; Malten and Zielhuis 1964;

Table 54.1
Allergens in unsaturated polyester (UP) resins

Actual allergen in UP resin	
Maleic acid	Malten and Zielhuis (1964)
Fumaric acid	Malten and Zielhuis (1964)
Adipic acid	Malten and Zielhuis (1964), Guin (2001)
Phthalic anhydride	Malten and Zielhuis (1964), Lidén et al. (1984)
Maleic anhydride	Minamoto et al. (2002b)
Maleic esters	Minamoto et al. (2002b), Malten (1984)
Polyester methacrylate	Björkner (1982)
Methyl methacrylate	Wehle (1966)
Diethylene glycol maleate	Tarvainen et al. (1993a), Kanerva et al. (1999b); Pfaffli et al. (2002)
Cross-linking monomers	
Styrene	Key et al. (1961), Bourne and Milner (1963), Sjoborg et al. (1982), Conde-Salazar et al. (1989)
Vinyltoluene	Sjoborg et al. (1982)
Hardening catalysts	
Benzoyl peroxide	Bourne and Milner (1963), Vincenzi et al. (1991)
Cyclohexanone hydroperoxide	Malten (1964)
Methyl ethyl ketone peroxide	Bourne and Milner (1963), Malten and Zielhuis (1964)
Cobalt salts	Kanerva et al. (1996b), Minamoto et al. (2002)
Cobalt naphthenate	Key et al. (1961), Bourne and Milner (1963), Malten and Zielhuis (1964), Kadlec et al. (1974)
Cobalt octoate	Anavekar and Nixon (2006)
Inhibitor	
Hydroquinone	Torres et al. (1993)
p-tert-Butyl catechol (in styrene)	Estlander et al. (1998)
Artificial limbs (made of UP resin)	
p-tert-Butyl catechol	MacFarlane et al. (1986), Freeman (1986)
Benzoyl peroxide	Vincenzi et al. (1991)
Dimethyl-p-toluidine	Haddad et al. (1996)
Others	
Pthalates	Malten and Zielhuis (1964)
Tricresyl phosphate	Key et al. (1961)

Table 54.2
Allergic and nonallergic (negative) patch-test reactions to the components of polyester resin (Kanerva et al. 1999b, Pfaffli et al. 2002)

Allergic patch-test reaction to:	Negative patch-test reaction to:
Patient's own two-component polyester cement (sanding dust)	Hardener component (including benzoyl peroxide) (1%)
Resin component (UP resin in styrene with auxiliary substances and filling materials) (1–10%)	Filling materials (100%)
UP resin in styrene with auxiliary substances (10%)	Styrene (1%)
Pure UP resin in styrene (2.5% in acetone)	Auxiliary substances (1%)
Purification: TLC bands found at Rf-value of 0.24 ± 0.03 ($n = 6$) (100%)	Ingredients of UP resin
Identification: Diethylene glycol maleate (MW 204) (0.1–0.01%)	

TLC thin-layer chromatography, *MW* molecular weight (in kilodaltons), *Rf* retention factor

Vincenzi et al. 1991), cyclohexanone hydroperoxide (Malten 1964), or methyl ethyl ketone hydroperoxide (Bourne and Milner 1963; Malten and Zielhuis 1964). Lymphomatoid-like contact dermatitis in a marble worker was reported from cobalt naphthenate (Schena et al. 1995).

The allergens have been summarized in *Table 54.1.* Eight patients were reported to be allergic to UP resins from car-repair painting and mold manufacturing (Tarvainen et al. 1993a; Kanerva et al. 1999b).

A patch testing strategy was developed by Kanerva's group in order to clarify the allergic components of UP resins and has been summarized in *Table 54.2.* All patients reacted on patch testing to the UP resin component of a cement they had used in their work.

Five patients also reacted to hardened UP resin cements, indicating that the hardened UP resin contains reactive monomers. Grinding the resin can give airborne allergic reactions many years after it has been hardened (Kanerva et al. 1999b). The causative allergen was found to be diethylene glycol maleate (DEGM) (Tarvainen et al. 1993a; Kanerva et al. 1999b; Pfaffli et al. 2002).

In another workplace study, ACD was caused not only by UP resin, but by cobalt, benzoyl peroxide, methyl ethyl ketone peroxide, para-tertiary butyl catechol, styrene, and formaldehyde (Minamoto et al. 2002b).

UP resins have been patch tested at concentrations of 0.5–10% (Tarvainen et al. 1993a; Kanerva et al. 1999b) but also at 20% in acetone (Foussereau et al. 1982). In one patient, a concentration of 1% caused a weak allergic reaction (Tarvainen et al. 1993a), and it was suggested that the test concentration may need to be as high as 5% (Kanerva et al. 1999b). However, it is not clear at what concentration active sensitization may occur.

References

Aguirre A, Zabala R, Sanz de Galdeano C, Landa N, Diaz-Perez JL (1994) Positive patch tests to hydrogen peroxide in 2 cases. Contact Dermatitis 30:113

Alarie Y (1973) Sensory irritation of the upper airways by airborne chemicals. Toxicol Appl Pharmacol 24:279–297

Anavekar A, Nixon R (2006) Occupational allergic contact dermatitis to cobalt octoate included as an accelerator in polyester resin. Australas J Dermatol 47:143–144

Araki S, Abe A, Vshio K, Fujino M (1971) A case of skin atrophy, neurogenic muscular atrophy and anxiety reaction following long exposure to styrene. Jpn J Ind Health 13:427–431

Björkner B (1982) Sensitizing capacity of polyester methacrylate in ultraviolet curing inks tested in the Guinea pig. Acta Derm Venereol 62:153–182

Björkner B (2006) Other Plastics 34.5. In: Frosch PJ, Menné T, Lepoittevin J-P (eds) Contact dermatitis. Springer, Berlin/Heidelberg/New York, pp 607–608

Bourne L, Milner F (1963) Polyester resin hazards. Br J Ind Med 20: 100–109

Bruze M, Fregert S, Gruvberger B (2000) Chemical skin burn. In: Menné T, Maibach HI (eds) Hand eczema. CRC Press, Boca Raton, pp 117–125

Conde-Salazar L, Gonzales M, Guimaraens D, Romero L (1989) Occupational allergic contact dermatitis from styrene. Contact Dermatitis 21:112

Dooms-Goossens A, De Jonge G (1985) Contact allergy to unsaturated polyester in a boat builder. Contact Dermatitis 12:238

Estlander T, Kostiainen M, Jolanki R, Kanerva L (1998) Active sensitization and occupational allergic contact dermatitis caused by para-tertiary-butylcatechol. Contact Dermatitis 38:96–100

Fartasch M (1997) Ultrastructure of the epidermal barrier after irritation. Microsc Res Tech 37:193–199

Foussereau J, Benezra C, Maibach HI, Hjorth N (1982) Occupational contact dermatitis. Clinical and chemical aspects. Munksgaard, Copenhagen

Freeman S (1986) Contact dermatitis of a limb stump caused by p-tertiary butyl catechol in the artificial limb. Contact Dermatitis 14:68–69

Fregert S (1971) Outbreak of irritant contact dermatitis from diallylphthalate in polyester resin. Contact Dermatitis Newslett 10:234

Gotell P, Axelson O, Lindelof B (1972) Field studies on human styrene exposure. Work Environ Health 9:76–83

Guin JD (2001) Sensitivity to adipic acid used in polyester synthesis. Contact Dermatitis 44:256–257

Haddad FS, Cobb AG, Bentley G, Levell NJ, Dowd PM (1996) Hypersensitivity in aseptic loosening of total hip replacements. The role of constituents of bone cement. J Bone Joint Surg Br 78:546–549

Haustein V-F, Tegetmeyer L, Ziegler V (1985) Allergic and irritant potential of benzoyl peroxide. Contact Dermatitis 13:252–257

Jolanki R, Estlander T, Kanerva L (1987) Occupational contact dermatitis and contact urticaria caused by epoxy resins. Acta Derm Venereol Suppl (Stockh) 134:90–94

Jolanki R, Kanerva L, Estlander T, Tarvainen K (1997) Skin allergy caused by organic acid anhydrides. In: Amin S, Lahti A, Maibach HI (eds) Contact urticaria syndrome. CRC Press, Boca Raton, pp 217–224

Kadlec K, Hanslian L, Forprechtová A (1974) Occurrence of skin disease as a result of work with polyester varnishes (in Czech). Cesk Dermatol 49:281–289

Kanerva L, Björkner B, Estlander T, Jolanki R, Tarvainen K (1996a) Plastic materials: occupational exposure, skin irritancy and its prevention. In: van der Valk P, Maibach HI (eds) The irritant contact dermatitis syndrome. CRC Press, Boca Raton, pp 127–155

Kanerva L, Jolanki R, Estlander T (1996b) Offset printer's occupational allergic contact dermatitis caused by cobalt-2-ethylhexoate. Contact Dermatitis 34:67–68

Kanerva L, Hyry H, Jolanki R, Hytonen M, Estlander T (1997) Delayed and immediate occupational allergy caused by methylhexahydrophthalic anhydride. Contact Dermatitis 36:34–38

Kanerva L, Jolanki R, Riihimäki V, Kalimo K (1998) Patch test reactions and occupational dermatoses caused by hydrogen peroxide. Contact Dermatitis 39:146

Kanerva L, Alanko K, Jolanki R, Estlander T (1999a) Airborne allergic contact urticaria from methyl hexahydrophthalic anhydride and hexahydrophthalic anhydride. Contact Dermatitis 41:339–341

Kanerva L, Estlander T, Alanko K, Pfäffli P, Jolanki R (1999b) Occupational allergic contact dermatitis from unsaturated polyester resin an a car repair putty. Int J Dermatol 38:447–452

Key MM, Perone VB, Birmingham DJ (1961) Patch testing in dermatitis from the newer resins. J Occup Med 3:361–364

Lidén C, Löfström A, Storgårds-Hatam K (1984) Contact allergy to unsaturated polyester in a boat builder. Contact Dermatitis 11: 262–264

Lieber EE (1955) Dermatitis – an industrial problem. Br Plastics 28: 428–429

MacFarlane AW, Curley RK, King CM (1986) Contact sensitivity to unsaturated polyester resin in a limb prosthesis. Contact Dermatitis 15:301–303

Malten KE (1956) Occupational eczema in processing plastics (doctoral dissertation in Dutch with English summary). University of Amsterdam, Amsterdam

Malten KE (1964) Einige Bemerkungen zur Hautsensibilisierung durch Aethoxylin (Epoxyd)-Kunstharze und deren Prophylaxe. Derm Beruf Umwelt 2:78–85

Malten KE, Zielhuis R (1964) Polyester resins. In: Malten KE, Zielhuis R (eds) Industrial toxicology and dermatology in the production and processing of plastics. Elsevier, Amsterdam, pp 71–84

Malten KE (1984) Dermatological problems with synthetic resins and plastics in glues. Part 11. Derm Beruf Umwelt 32:81–86

Mathias CGT (1988) Allergic contact dermatitis from triglycidyl isocyanurate in polyester paint pigments. Contact Dermatitis 19: 67–68

Midtgard U, Knudsen LE (1994) Fibre-reinforced plastics and advanced polymer composites. Occupational hazards and toxicity of selected compounds.. Nordic Council of Ministers and National Institute of Occupational Health, Copenhagen, pp 1–73

Minamoto K, Nagano M, Inaoka T, Futatsuka M (2002a) Occupational dermatoses among fiberglass-reinforced plastics factory workers. Contact Dermatitis 46:339–347

Minamoto K, Nagano M, Yonemitsu K, Futatsuka M (2002b) Allergic contact dermatitis from unsaturated polyester resin consisting of maleic anhydride, phthalic anhydride, ethylene glycol and dicyclopentadiene. Contact Dermatitis 46:62–63

Pfaffli P, Jolanki R, Estlander T, Tarvainen K, Kanerva L (2002) Identification of sensitizing diethyleneglycol maleate in a two-component polyester cement. Contact Dermatitis 46:170–173

Rietschel RL, Fowler JF Jr (2008) Fisher's contact dermatitis, 6th edn. McGraw-Hill, New York

Schena D, Rosina P, Chieregato C, Colombari R (1995) Lymphomatoid-like contact dermatitis from cobalt napthenate. Contact Dermatitis 33:197–198

Schumes E (1990) Solvents and plastizers. In: Adams RM (ed) Occupational skin disease, 2nd edn. WB Saunders, Philadelphia

Shaw S (1989) A case of contact dermatitis from "hypoallergenic" nail varnish. Contact Dermatitis 20:385

Sjoborg S, Dahlquist I, Fregert S, Trulson L (1982) Contact allergy to styrene with cross reaction to vinyltoluene. Contact Dermatitis 8:207–208

Sowa J, Kobayashi H, Tsuruta D et al (2005) Allergic contact dermatitis due to adipic polyester in vinyl chloride gloves. Contact Dermatitis 53:243–244

Stewart RD, Dodd HC, Baretta ED, Schaffer AW (1968) Human exposure to styrene vapor. Arch Environ Health 16:656–662

Tarvainen K, Jolanki R, Estlander T (1993a) Occupational contact allergy to unsaturated polyester resin cements. Contact Dermatitis 28: 220–224

Tarvainen K, Jolanki R, Forsman-Gronholm L, Estlander T, Pfaffli P, Juntunen J, Kanerva L (1993b) Exposure, skin protection and occupational skin diseases in the glass-fibre reinforced plastics industry. Contact Dermatitis 29:119–127

Tarvainen K, Estlander T, Jolanki R, Kanerva L (1994) Occupational dermatoses caused by man-made mineral fibers. Am J Contact Dermat 5:22–29

Tarvainen K, Jolanki R, Estlander T, Tupasela O, Pfaffli P, Kanerva L (1995a) Immunologic contact urticaria due to airborne methylhexahydrophthalic and methyl tetrahydrophthalic anhydrides. Contact Dermatitis 32:204–209

Tarvainen K, Kanerva L, Jolanki R, Estlander T (1995b) Occupational dermatoses from the manufacture of plastic composite products. Am J Contact Dermat 6:95–104

Torres V, Mano-Azul AC, Correia T, Soares AP (1993) Allergic contact cheilitis and stomatitis from hydroquinone in an acrylic dental prosthesis. Contact Dermatitis 29:102–193

Vincenzi C, Cameli N, Vassilopoulou A, Tosti A (1991) Allergic contact dermatitis due to benzoyl peroxide in an arm prosthesis. Contact Dermatitis 24:66–67

Wehle U (1966) Arbeitsbedingte Ekzeme durch Polyester. Allerg Asthma (Leipz) 12:184–186

55 Other Plastics

George-Sorin Ţiplica[1] · *Letiţia Bucur*[2] · *Gheorghe Bucur*[3] · *Carmen Maria Sălăvăstru*[1]
[1]Colentina Clinical Hospital, "Carol Davila" University of Medicine and Pharmacy, Bucharest, Romania
[2]Department of Occupational Health, Belsana Grup LLC, Bucharest, Romania
[3]Dermato-venereologist, Morarilor Medical Center, Bucharest, Romania

Core Messages

- Health risks, including dermatoses, are mainly induced by monomers or by-products used or produced during the polymerization process (hardeners, plasticizers, stabilizers, initiators, accelerators, inhibitors, catalyzers, antioxidants, coloring agents).
- The general population uses only on rare occasions incompletely polymerized plastic resins. Polyethylene and polypropylene are the most widely used plastics in the world.
- Amino plastics usually contain formaldehyde, which is both irritating and sensitizing. Contact and airborne dermatitis were described. *Para*-tertiary-butyl-phenol-formaldehyde resin can also produce occupational vitiligo.
- Polycarbonates and polyamide resins rarely induce skin allergies or irritation.
- Polystyrene is obtained from styrene – a mild primary irritant. Styrene acts as sensitizer only in rare situations.
- Polyurethanes contain isocyanates known for their sensitizing actions.
- Polyolefin resins can induce skin irritation and allergy. Sicca syndrome and epidermal necrolysis were described in workers in contact with polyethylene. Exposure to polypropylene can modify color perception.
- Polytetrafluoroethylene is a skin irritant.

1 Introduction

Plastics are organic macromolecular substances made by chains of similar molecules (monomers). Polymers are plastics made from identical monomers (in the process of polymerization) and polycondensated polymers contain different monomers (combined in the reaction of polycondensation). Plastics do not have the tendency to crystallize, are usually nontoxic, and are stable at ambient conditions. Health risks, including dermatoses, are mainly induced by monomers or by-products used or produced during the chemical reactions (hardeners, plasticizers, stabilizers, initiators, accelerators, inhibitors, catalyzers, antioxidants, coloring agents). Thermic disintegration can produce potentially dangerous substances (Rusu 2009).

The rapid development of plastic industry generated an immense number of different types of plastic materials with diverse properties and many applications. By their nature polymers can be naturals, artificials, or synthetics (➋ *Table 55.1*). Natural polymers can be found in this form in nature (rubber, cellulose). Artificial polymers are produced using natural polymers (ebonite, viscose). Synthetic polymers are generated entirely by chemical synthesis and are classified in thermoplastic resins and thermoset

Table 55.1
Polymers

Group of polymers	Examples
1. Natural polymers	Rubber, cellulose
2. Artificial polymers	Rubber derivates: vulcanized rubber, ebonite
	Cellulose derivates: viscose, cellulose acetate (zyl), nitrocellulose (flash paper)
	Proteic derivates: casein (galalith)
3. Synthetic polymers	Thermoplastics: polyolefins, polystyrene, polyacryls and polymethacryls, polyamides, polycarbonates, vinyl derivatives
	Thermostables: amino-plastics, pheno-plastics, epoxy resin, alchidic resins, polyurethane resins

T. Rustemeyer, P. Elsner, S.M. John & H.I. Maibach (eds.), *Kanerva's Occupational Dermatology*,
DOI 10.1007/978-3-642-02035-3_55, © Springer-Verlag Berlin Heidelberg 2012

resins. Thermoplastic resins are malleable if heated and on cooling they become hard and keep their new shape. Thermoplastic resins are made by linear chains of monomers. Thermostable resins are also malleable when heated but overheated they develop a tri-dimensional network generating a rigid material.

The polymerization or polycondensation process involves many types of adjuvants: curing agents, plasticizers, stabilizers, initiators, accelerators and inhibitors, catalysts, antioxidants, coloring agents, flavoring agents, etc. Mainly those adjuvants and not the plastics are responsible for the occurrence of the majority of occupational pathology in the plastics industry. The health risks are generated by exposure during plastics manufacturing (direct contact with monomer molecules and adjuvants). In the case of further processing or alteration of plastics (grinding, melting, burning, etc.), molecules with irritating or allergic potential can be released: phenols, aldehydes, acrylonitrile, vinyl chloride, styrene, etc. For this reason sensitization among persons working in the plastics industry is four times more common than in other industries (Foussereau and Benezra 1970).

The technological processes for producing plastics can be divided into: (a) technological processes highly harmful to the health of exposed workers (e.g., epoxy resins, phenol-formaldehyde resins, carbamid-formaldehyde resins, acrylic resins, polyester resins); (b) technological processes rarely harmful to the health of exposed workers (e.g., polypropylene, polyurethane, polystyrene, siliconic resins, polyvnyl chloride, polycarbonates, polyethylene). Among adjuvants the most notorious noxious are phthalates (e.g., dibutyl-, dioctyl-) and maleates, dimethylaniline, cobalt naphtenate, toluene sulphonic acid, benzoyl peroxide, phenylenediamine group, mercaptobenzothiazole group, epoxy compounds, phenols, and naphthylamines. Plastics in general are involved in 8% of skin allergies of which 45% are due to epoxy and acrylic resins, 9% to methacrylic resins, 8% to phenol-formaldehyde resin, 4% to urea-formaldehyde resins, 3% to polyester resin, and 1% to polyurethane resins (Rudzki 1978). The process of plastic recycling can be also harmful for the exposed workers as involves heating of the plastic materials in the processes of heat compression, thermal depolymerization, or monomer recycling. Recycling codes are used to identify the material from which an item is made, to facilitate easier recycling or other reprocessing. Such symbols for plastics have been developed by the Society of the Plastics Industry in 1988 and are internationally used (➲ *Table 55.2*).

The general population uses only on rare occasions incompletely polymerized/polycondensed resins: nail varnish containing formaldehyde resins or toluene sulphonamidic resin; acrylic artificial nails; dental and orthopedic prostheses from acrylic/methacrylic resins; cement and adhesives containing epoxy or formaldehyde resins.

Patch testing of synthetic resins should be done with caution in order to avoid side effects or errors in results interpretation. Acetone is the preferred vehicle for urethane monomers and pre-polymers, polyester and epoxy resins because it does not react with these substances. Solutions must always be fresh as acetone is very volatile. Other vehicles: petroleum jelly, alcohol, methyl-ethyl-ketone. Patch testing for plastics uses PG-1000 Plastic and glues series (➲ *Table 55.3*).

2 Chemistry, Use, and Skin Problems

2.1 Amino Plastics

Amino plastics are produced by polycondensation of aldehydes (such as formaldehyde) with amines (urea, melamine, thiourea) using heat curing and an inorganic acid as catalyst (hydrochloric acid, phosphoric acid etc.). Urea–formaldehyde resin accounts for more than 80% of amino plastics; melamine–formaldehyde resin accounts for most of the rest (Williams 2002). All amino plastic resins have an excess of formaldehyde that may be gradually eliminated. Today amino plastics release much lower quantities of formaldehyde by comparison with amino plastics produced in the past decades (Belsito 1997). Amino plastics have excellent solvent resistance and resistance to abrasion and heat. Their hardness is much appreciated and they are used in the wood and furniture industry as surface coatings and adhesives to make plywood, chipboard, and sawdust board. Amino plastics are often reinforced with silica, cloth, cotton fabric, and glass (Björkner 2000). Both urea- and melamine-formaldehyde resins are of low toxicity. Melamine-formaldehyde resins may be used in paper that contacts aqueous and fatty foods (Williams 2002).

2.1.1 Phenol-Formaldehyde Resins

Phenol-formaldehyde resins are based on phenols (alkyl phenols, bisphenol-A, cresols, *p*-tertiary-phenyl-phenol, phenol, resorcinol, xylenol, etc.) and formaldehyde (See also: ➲ Chap. 52, "Contact Allergy to Phenol-Formaldehyde Resins"). There are four major forms of these resins: solid

Table 55.2
Plastic identification code (according to the Society of the Plastics Industry and the Plastics and Chemical Industries Association)

Plastic identification code	Type of plastic polymer	Common properties	Applications
01 PET	Polyethylene terephthalate (PET, PETE)	Clarity, strength, toughness, barrier to gas and moisture	Beverage bottles; textile fibers
02 PE-HD	High-density polyethylene (HDPE)	Stiffness, strength, toughness, resistance to moisture, permeability to gas	Shopping bags; water pipes; buckets; milk, juice and water bottles
03 PVC	Polyvinyl chloride (PVC)	Versatility, ease of blending, strength, toughness	Blister packaging for non-food items; cling films for non-food use; blood bags; electrical cable insulation; rigid piping; vinyl records; watch straps
04 PE-LD	Low-density polyethylene (LDPE)	Ease of processing, strength, toughness, flexibility, ease of sealing, barrier to moisture	Frozen food bags; squeezable bottles; cling films; flexible container lids; garbage bags
05 PP	Polypropylene (PP)	Strength, toughness, resistance to heat, chemicals, grease and oil, versatile, barrier to moisture	Reusable microwaveable ware; kitchenware; yogurt containers; margarine tubs; carpet fiber; toys; caps
06 PS	Polystyrene (PS)	Versatility, clarity, easily formed	Egg cartons; packing peanuts; disposable cups, plates, trays and cutlery; disposable take-away containers; refrigerator bins; medical disposables; dairy containers
07 O	Other plastics, including acrylic, acrylonitrile butadiene styrene (ABS), fiberglass, nylon, polycarbonate, polylactic acid	Dependent on polymers or combination of polymers	Beverage bottles; baby milk bottles. Non-packaging uses for polycarbonate; compact discs; "unbreakable" glazing; electronic apparatus housings; lenses; automotive headlamps, riot shields, instrument panels

resin (bakelite type); powder resin (that can be melted and poured into various forms); semisolid resins (used as adhesives); and liquid resins (used for paints, varnish, polish, etc.). Phenol-formaldehyde resins are used as electrical insulators, wood varnishes, footwear, flooring, textile dressing, wood glues, leather glue, metal–metal glue, metal-rubber glue, paints, coatings, waterproof canvas and paper, phone manufacturing, etc. Phenol-formaldehyde resins are also used as core in foundries, as stands for chemical laboratories, and as surface sealers.

The manufacturing process of phenol-formaldehyde resins can be done with different catalysts. Novolac resins are produced in acidic conditions, resol resins are obtained in alkalinic conditions, and rezitole resins result when alcohols and acetone are used as catalysts.

Table 55.3
PG-1000 plastic and glues series

Index	Substance	Concentration
PG-1	Hydroquinone	1.0 pet
PG-2	Dibutyl phthalate	5.0 pet
PG-3	Phenyl salicylate (Salol)	1.0 pet
PG-4	Diethylhexylphthalate (Dioctylphthalate)	2.0 pet
PG-5	BHT/(2,6-Di-tertiary-butyl-4-cresol)	2.0 pet
PG-6	Drometrizole/(2(2-Hydroxy-5-methyl-phenyl)benzotriazole)	1.0 pet
PG-7	Benzoyl peroxide	1.0 pet
PG-8	4-tertiary-Butyl-catechol (PTBC)	0.25 pet
PG-9	Azodiisobutyrodinitrile	1.0 pet
PG-10	Bisphenol A	1.0 pet
PG-11	Tricresyl phosphate	5.0 pet
PG-12	Phenol formaldehyde resin (P-F-R-2)	1.0 pet
PG13	4-tertiary-Butyl-phenol formaldehyde resin	1.0 pet
PG-14	Triphenyl phosphate	5.0 pet
PG-15	Toluenesulfonamide formaldehyde resin	10.0 pet
PG-16	Resorcinol monobenzoate	1.0 pet
PG-17	2-Phenylindole	2.0 pet
PG-18	2-tertiary-Butyl-4-methoxyphenol (BHA)	2.0 pet
PG-19	Hydroabietyl alcohol/(Abitol)	10.0 pet
PG-20	4-tertiary-Butyl-phenol	1.0 pet
PG-21	2-Monomethylol phenol	1.0 pet
PG-22	Diphenylthiourea	1.0 pet
PG-23	2-*n*-Octyl-4-isothiazolin-3-one	0.1 pet
PG-24	Cyclohexanone resin	1.0 pet
PG-25	Triglycidyl isocyanurate	0.5 pet

To diagnose allergic skin conditions, patch tests can be performed with:

Resin (whole finished product)	5–10% pet
Bakelite	10% pet
Novolac	5% pet or 20% in ethanol
Resol	5% pet or 20% in ethanol
Formaldehyde	1–2% aq
Hexamethylenetetramine	1–2% pet
Furfural	5% aq
Phenols	2% aq
PTBP	1% pet (Chemo, Trolab)
2-MMP = mono-methylol-2-phenol	1% pet
4-MMP = methylol-*p*-phenol	1% in ethanol

Skin Problems

Formaldehyde is both irritating and sensitizing. Direct contact can produce contact dermatitis or contact urticaria. Airborne dermatitis was also described. Many people sensitized to formaldehyde resins do not have positive skin reactions to formaldehyde.

A case of a 49-year-old pediatrician was observed with severe widespread occupational allergic dermatitis caused by contact with formaldehyde textile resin from the hospital "greens" ("scrubs") and mask. In this case patch testing was performed with formaldehyde and ethyleneurea/melamine formaldehyde resin, not with the suspected offending fabric, which gives most often a false negative result (Donovan and Skotnicki-Grant 2007).

Solid resins are irritants not only through their phenol and formaldehyde derivatives (which have also sensitizing properties), but also through the fine traces of oil that remain from the manufacturing process or through the highly alkaline NaOH used to neutralize the uncured excess of phenol and formaldehyde.

Airborne particles from phenol-formaldehyde resins in powder can produce allergic contact dermatitis in 10% of exposed workers during the first year of work. Most affected areas are the face (periorbital area, eyelids), neck, presternal area, uncovered hands and feet. In 80% of cases the cause is formaldehyde or hexamethylenetetramine, but some dyes or zinc stearate can also be involved. Respiratory problems (including pharyngitis, bronchitis, asthma) were also described when working with phenol-formaldehyde resins containing methylol-phenol.

Bakelite in powder can induce irritating or allergic dermatitis (Fregert 1981). Phenols initially induce skin erythema and after prolonged contact ulcers that heal with skin hyperpigmentation, usually located on the hands, nose, and ear pavilions. These resins can induce allergic cross-reactions with colophony (rosin) and Peru balm.

2.1.2 *Para*-tertiary-Butyl-phenol-formaldehyde Resins

Para-tertiary-butyl-phenol-formaldehyde resins are widely used as adhesives (glues for footwear, leather, wood, wool, glass, stickers, door of the car upholstery, dental cement, brakes, textile starches, insulation) (See also: ➋ Chap. 52, "Contact Allergy to Phenol-Formaldehyde Resins"). Patch tests for diagnostic are using:

p-tertiary-butyl-phenol = PTBP	1–10% pet
Resin (whole finished product)	1–10% pet
Formaldehyde	1–2% aq

Skin Problems

P-tertiary-butyl-phenol is usually the sensitizer. The pathogenic allergic mechanism includes type I and type IV reactions. Not only skin is affected as there are cases reported with aphonia and bronchospasm (Kalimo et al. 1980) and allergic asthma. Contact with these resins can also produce skin depigmentation (occupational vitiligo). PTBP resins can also induce orthoergic contact dermatitis (especially on hands) and conjunctival irritation. Nonoccupational allergies can develop in persons using footwear containing PTBP resins.

2.1.3 Resorcinol-Formaldehyde Resins

Resorcinol-formaldehyde resins are used in the preparation of glues and adhesive solutions.

Resorcinol is a widely used chemical reagent present in some drugs (antiacne topical treatment – as keratolytic agent, antipruritic and antiseptic solutions; eye drops; suppositories), in synthetic resins (with formaldehyde), in cosmetics (hair dyes, defoliants), explosives, photographic and photocopying solutions, etc.

Patch test can be done using:

Resorcinol-formaldehyde resin (whole finished product)	20% in ethanol
Formaldehyde	1–2% aq
Resorcinol	2% pet

Skin Problems

Formaldehyde is the main sensitizer. Resorcinol can give cross-reactions with phenol and may induce allergic contact dermatitis. Resorcinol in contact with varnished nails turns them into brown-orange and in contact with hair gives it darker shades.

2.1.4 Sulfonamide-Formaldehyde Resins

Sulfonamide-formaldehyde resins combines d-sulfonamide with formaldehyde resulting in a liquid soluble in alcohol and acetone, much used in paint and varnish industry. When cellulose nitrate is added, the resin can be used as adhesive and gain in plasticity. These new properties expand the industrial uses to cosmetics (nail varnish) as toluene-sulfonamide-formaldehyde resin.

Patch test can be performed with:

Toluene-sulfonamide-formaldehyde resin	10% pet
Formaldehyde	1–2% aq

Skin Problems

Allergic lesions in fingers and nails lesions may occur.

2.1.5 Urea-Formaldehyde Resins

Urea-formaldehyde resins are thermoset-type resins. The condensation of formaldehyde (a major sensitizer) with urea (carbamide, $H_2N–CO–NH_2$) produces a liquid that is treated with pigments, zinc stearate, hexamethylenetetramine 10.5%, etc., for the finished product.

Urea-formaldehyde powder can be molded into containers for cosmetics, electrical fittings, refrigerators insulation, wall insulation, pipes, bottle caps, foam insulation, textiles starches (cotton, rayon), surface coatings, wood glues, lavatory seats, buttons, clock cases, etc. (Rusu 2009).

Patch tests are performed with:

Urea-formaldehyde resin	10% pet or 50% in ethanol
Uroformin (hardener)	55% pet

Skin Problems

Urea-formaldehyde resins are not sensitizers. Starches are generally only very rarely sensitizing excepting exposures that combines wet and warm or the use of chlorine or alkali, conditions for the formation of allergic dimethyl or urea compounds.

Dermatitis (including contact urticaria) from textiles on which urea-formaldehyde resin was used as starches is usually due to formaldehyde (Belsito 1997). Lesions are diffuse and occur in particular on the hands, face, neck, and torso.

Irritant contact dermatitis was induced in a patient by urea-formaldehyde fiber board containing resin (Vale and Rycroft 1988). Airborne irritancy to dust from urea-formaldehyde insulation was also reported (Dooms-Goossens et al. 1986). Persistent perionixis was described when using artificial nails made of urea-formaldehyde resins.

2.1.6 Melamine-Formaldehyde Resins

Melamine-formaldehyde resins are thermoset resins obtained through polycondensation of melamine (2,4,6-triamino-1,3,5-triazines) with formaldehyde. Melamine-formaldehyde resins are similar to urea-formaldehyde resins but have a higher resistance to water. Due to their resistance to water, heat and because they do not stain they are frequently used as coating for furniture (particularly kitchen), plates, and cups. Other common uses are for orthopedic and dental cement, as an aid in pulp paper, and synthetic textiles to make them waterproof.

Patch tests can be performed with:

Melamine-formaldehyde resin	50% in ethanol
Ethylene-urea + melamine-formaldehyde	5% pet
Formaldehyde (aq)	1–2% aq
Ethylene-urea	1% pet
Dicyandiamine (fireproof)	1% pet

Skin Problems

Melamine-formaldehyde resins are rarely sensitizing. However, contact dermatitis may occur, including purpuric type (Romaguera et al. 1989) in orthopedic casts (Ross et al. 1992), gypsum molds (Fregert 1981), or coatings of plastic tubes for cosmetics. Formaldehyde is the primary irritant and sensitizer.

The combination of melamine and ammonium chloride produces a resin used in adhesive bandages (ammonium chloride acts as sensitizer).

Aalto-Korte et al. described three cases of occupational allergic contact dermatitis from melamine formaldehyde resin without contact allergy to formaldehyde: one in the plywood industry, one in the production of melamine-laminated chipboard, and one in laboratory work (Aalto-Korte et al. 2003).

A 28-year-old female plywood worker developed eczema on the dorsal side of her hands and wrists after 2 years of occupational exposure. She tested positive to melamine-formaldehyde resin and negative to formaldehyde (which is usually responsible for most skin reactions to formaldehyde resins). Contact dermatitis due to melamine formaldehyde resin is rare and usually due to products that are not fully cured or to a close contact with by-products on the assembly line (García Gavin et al. 2008).

2.2 Furfuraldehyde Resins

Furfuryl alcohol (furfurol) and furfuryl aldehyde (furfural), both from the group of furan, are colorless liquid substances derived from agricultural waste: corn stalks, reeds, sawdust, sunflower seeds, etc. (Rusu 2009).

Furfurol is used as a solvent in refining of vegetable and mineral oils and as a reactive in many organic syntheses: plastic material, nylon, furan, and certain drugs.

Furfuraldehyde resins are produced by polymerization from the bark of barley treated with sulfuric acid. For industrial use they are combined with phenols, amines, ketones, or casein, and have the same uses as formaldehyde resins.

2.2.1 Skin Problems

Furfuraldehyde resins can induce skin and mucosal sensitization (especially respiratory allergy: allergic asthma). Systemic poisoning may also occur.

2.3 Polycarbonates

Polycarbonates are polymers containing carbonate groups (–O–(C=O)–O–). The main polycarbonate material is produced from bisphenol A (4,4′-dihydroxydiphenyl-2,2-propane) and phosgene ($COCl_2$). Other bisphenols than bisphenol A can also be used. Polycarbonate is a very durable material (resistant to sunlight, weather, scratches) and highly transparent to visible light (with better light transmission characteristics than many kinds of glass). Polycarbonates are thermoplastics but can undergo large plastic deformations without cracking or breaking (Rusu 2009). Polycarbonates are used for electronic applications due to the good electrical insulating characteristics (they can serve as dielectric in high-stability capacitors). Polycarbonates are also used in the construction industry (domelights and sound walls) and in the production of compact discs, DVDs, and Blu-ray discs. Due to their durability they are used as bullet-proof windows in automobiles and banks. The use of polycarbonate containers for food storage is controversial. In contact with water small quantities of bisphenol are released. Polycarbonate is dissolved by ammonia and acetone and can be cleaned (of oil and grease) with alcohol. Polycarbonates are relatively expensive.

2.3.1 Skin Problems

Polycarbonates rarely give orthoergic or allergic contact dermatitis (Bruze et al. 1988). Bisphenol A is an endocrine disruptor with weak estrogenic activity. Occupational contact dermatitis can be associated with Bisphenol A exposure. Most allergic contact dermatites occur in workers handling Bisphenol A products, such as plastic product workers, and those exposed to epoxy adhesive tapes, foams, and dental products (Kaddar et al. 2008).

2.4 Polyamide Resins

Polyamide resins are produced by polycondensation of adipic acid $-HOOC-(CH_2)_4-COOH$ with hexamethylenediamine $-H_2N-(CH_2)_6-NH-$ or of water with caprolactam.

Polymerization of hexamethylenediamine adipate generates nylon.

The main use of polyamides is in the textile industry (synthetic fibers). Polyamides are also used for transparent packaging (vacuum packaging of meat) and hospital wares with good stability at sterilization temperatures.

The sensitizers are the additives designed to improve the product, like dihydrochloric ethylenediamine – hardener (for patch test 1% pet), which releases formaldehyde.

2.4.1 Skin Problems

Polyamide resins rarely induce skin allergies or irritation. Allergy of the respiratory mucosa was also described (Bruze et al. 1988).

A group of eight workers who had been chronically exposed to high atmospheric caprolactam levels showed no evidence of systemic toxicity. All workers had a greater or lesser degree of skin change in the form of peeling and fissuring (Kelman 1986).

2.5 Allyl Resins

Allyl resins are formed by polymerization of a monomer resulted from the combination of allyl alcohol with diglyco-chloroform.

Allyl resins are thermostable, widely used in glass factories.

2.5.1 Skin Problems

Allyl resins are sensitizers (both as monomers and polymers). Allyl alcohol may be fatal if swallowed or inhaled, and when in direct contact with the skin, it causes burns. Inhalation may lead to severe irritation or burns.

2.6 Cellulose Resins (Cellulose Estheric Resins)

Cellulose resins are used for manufacturing spectacle frames, hearing aids, wheels, brushes, toothbrushes, different handles, pens and pencils, toys, cellophane, photographic film etc. (Rusu 2009).

Celluloid is made from cellulose nitrate and cellulose acetate, mixed with camphor, various solvents (ethanol, acetone, ethyl acetate, amyl acetate), and plasticizers (dimethyl-phthalate, dibutyl-phthalate, tricresyl-phthalate, triphenyl-phosphate), and used in paints and waterproof paper.

Patch tests for cellulose resins can be performed with (Jordan and Dahl 1971):

Cellulose-acetate (film or flakes)	As such or 10% in methyl-ethyl-ketone
Cellulose acetate propionate film	As such
Cellulose acetate butyrate film	As such
Resorcinol monobenzoate (rarely used today, it is UV-absorbent and gives cross-reaction with balm of Peru but not with Resorcinol!)	1% pet
2,2′-Dihydroxy-4, 4′-dimethoxybenzophenone	1% in methyl ethyl ketone
p-tertiary-Butyl-phenol	2% pet
Azo-pigments ("Black dye mixture")	1% pet
Carbon black	1% pet

Solvent Yellow 3 (Color Index No. 11 160)	1% pet
Solvent Red 26 (Color Index No. 26 102)	1% pet
Mono-ethyl ethylene glycol ether acetate	5% in methyl-ethyl-ketone
Potassium acid oxalate	0.5% aq
Dimethyl-phthalate	As such
Diethyl phthalate	As such
Tricresyl phosphate	5% pet
Triphenyl-phosphate	5% pet
Phenyl salicylate	2% pet

2.6.1 Skin Problems

Cellulose resins rarely act as sensitizers and this is mainly due to additives. One of those additives, *p*-tertiary-butyl-phenol, is a thermostabilizer acting as irritant and sensitizer. It can also induce skin hypopigmentation. Plasticizers like tricresyl phosphate and triphenyl phosphate are highly sensitizing, while dimethyl phthalate and diethyl phthalate only rarely sensitize.

Sodium-carboxymethyl-cellulose allergic contact dermatitis positive patch test to 2% pet. was reported in a baker (Hamada and Horiguchi 1978). It is an anionic cellulosic polymer synthesized from purified cellulose and sodium chloroacetate. It is used to increase viscosity in foods, cosmetics, and some drugs (laxatives, antiulcer drugs, antacids). The occurrence of contact dermatitis from *p*-tertiary-butyl-phenol and tricresyl ethyl phthalate was reported in a plastic nail adhesive (Burrows and Rycroft 1981).

Triphenylphosphate, the most commonly used flame retardant for cellulose acetate, exhibits low acute toxicity by dermal or oral contact (Svara et al. 2006).

2.7 Polyester Resins

Polyester resins are produced from unsaturated acids (maleic acid, fumaric acid, etc.) and di-alcohols (diethylene glycol and polyethylene glycol) (See also: ➋ Chap. 54, "Polyester Resins"). Their properties can be changed by adding colophony, dimethylalanine, diethylalanine, etc. Benzoyl peroxide is used as catalyst, methylenamine as accelerator, and cobalt naphthenate as desiccant.

Polyester resins are used in the manufacture of bathtubs, car covers, furniture, props, plaster, paint industry, aeronautics, and electric cable insulation.

Patch tests that can be performed for polyester resins include:

Unsaturated polyester resin	10–20% in acetone
Maleic acid	0.5% in acetone
Diethylene glycol	10% aq
Propylene glycol (sensitizer and irritating)	2–5% pet
Polyethylene glycol	10% aq
Colophony	20% pet or in acetone

Cross-link agents:

Methyl methacrylate	5% pet
Alpha-methylstyrene	1% pet
Styrene (vinyl-benzene – sensitizer and irritating)	1% in olive oil
Vinyl-toluene	1% in olive oil

Activators (accelerators):

Dimethylalanine	2% pet or 10% in alcohol
Diethylaniline	2% pet or 10% in alcohol
Cobalt-naphthenate (powerful sensitizer)	2–5% pet
Cobalt-octate (powerful sensitizer)	5% pet

Peroxide organic catalysts (powerful sensitizers):

Benzoyl peroxide	5% pet or 2% aq
Cyclohexanone peroxide	0.5% pet
Antimony-hydroperoxide	0.5% pet

UV absorbers:

Benzophenone	5% pet
Benzotriazole	1% pet

Inhibitors:

Hydroquinone	5% pet
Quinone	5% pet
p-tertiary-Butyl-catechol	1% in acetone

Consolidating agents:

Glass fiber	Highly irritating, do not test

Others:

Acetone	Irritant
Phthalic anhydride (also irritant)	1% in ethanol

2.7.1 Skin Problems

Occupational irritation to polyester resins is produced by contact with solvents and fibers.

Finished products such as polyester fibers (e.g., Dacron) and film (e.g., Mylar) have not so far caused dermatitis. Fibers may be, however, treated with oils, biocides, and antistatics that act as irritating agents and sensitizers. About 50% of all exposed and inadequately protected workers can develop occupational allergic contact dermatitis of the hands, arms, and neck after 2–4 months of exposure (Piper 1965).

2.8 Alkyd Resins

Alkyd resins are polyesters obtained by polycondensation of acid anhydrides or diacids (phthalic acid, maleic acid, etc.) with polyalcohols (dialcohols, trialcohols, ethylene glycol, propylene glycol, sorbitol, mannitol, etc.). The best known are the glycero-phtalic resins, the result of combining phthalic anhydride with glycerol.

There are simple alkyd resins and modified alkyd resins by the addition of vegetable oils (linseed oil or castor oil) – generating great flexibility. These oleoglycerophtalic resins are used in paints and lacquers for automotive, printing inks, and dressing for textiles (Martin-Scott 1966).

Combining alkyd resins with other resins (e.g., melamine-formaldehyde) enhances not only the quality of the products, but also the sensitizing properties. If glycocole, vinyl chloride, styrene, or glass fibers are added, the risk of skin and respiratory irritation is also higher.

Patch tests are performed with:

Alkyd resin	10% in acetone
Phthalic aldehyde	1% in ethanol
Diethylene glycol (DEG)	10% aq
Polyethylene glycol (PEG)	10% aq
Colophony	20% pet or acetone

2.8.1 Skin Problems

Alkyd resins can induce allergic contact dermatitis and irritation sometimes associated with respiratory irritation. Allergic lesions are most often generated by:

- Phthalic anhydride
- Colophony (traces) in the product
- Propylene or ethylene (as solvents)

2.9 Polystyrene (PS)

Polystyrene (PS) is a hard, transparent, thermoplastic resin, available in expanded form, film, foam, tablets or pellets, obtained by styrene polymerization (vinyl benzene, $CH_2{=}CH{-}C_6H_5$) with peroxide as initiator. As stabilizers benzotriazoles, benzophenones, and nickel organic compounds are used (Belsito 1997).

Hot cutting of large pieces of polystyrene and styrene monomers releases methyl chloride – a colorless and odorless gas which, if inhaled, in small doses can give intoxicating and narcotic effect (or ebrionarcotic syndrome: tiredness, confusion, weakness, drunken-type actions, memory loss, nausea, loss of appetite, and hearing and color vision loss) and in large quantities can induce dizziness, confusion, stupor, and even coma followed by death (Niculescu et al. 2003).

In the presence of expanded polystyrene granules, open fire sources should be avoided (the granules contain pentane – a flammable gas).

Polystyrene is used in the production of lacquers, molds, packaging film, disposable tableware, and some insulators. Some styrene cements (styrofoam) contain free molecules of styrene.

Polystyrene is used in compound polymers such as acrylonitrile-butadiene-styrene (ABS), styrene-acrylonitrile (SAN), or styrene-butadiene (SB). Those compounds are used in the manufacture of handles, toys, pipes, electric appliances, bags, household ustensils that can produce a metallic sound when dropped on a hard surface (Belsito 1997).

Styrene is also used in the manufacture of synthetic rubber and acrylic-alkyd resins. In nature it can be extracted from raspberries (as a result of enzymatic decarboxylation of *cis*-cinnamic acid) or from styrax balm. Styrax is used in the preparation of dyes, perfumes, and soaps and can be removed from the skin with acetone.

Methylstyrenes (vinyl-toluenes) occur as by-products in plastics manufacturing (Sjöborg et al. 1984).

Styrene can cross-react with epoxy resins and vinyltoluene resins.

Patch tests:

Styrax	2% pet
Styrene	1% in olive oil, 1–2% pet or 1% in butyrolactone
Styrene oxide	1% pet

2.9.1 Skin Problems

Styrene is a mild primary irritant (Kanerva et al. 1996), (Schmunes 1990) by destroying the protective lipid film of the skin surface. Cases of chemical skin burns caused by styrene have also been described (Bruze and Fregert 1994). Styrene acts only in rare situations as sensitizer. Styrene presumably functions as a pro-haptene that undergoes skin metabolization to styrene epoxide which acts as a true haptene (Belsito 1997).

There have been reports of immediate type I allergy to styrene (Sjöborg et al. 1984; Bourne and Milner 1963; Condé-Salazar et al. 1989; Moscato et al. 1987).

In one reported case, the patient which was allergic to styrene cross-reacted in patch testing with 2-, 3- and 4-vinyl-toluene (2-, 3-, and 4-methyl-styrene) and with its metabolites: styrene epoxide and 4-vinyl-phenol (4-hydroxy-styrene) (Belsito 1997).

2.10 Polyurethane Resins

Polyurethanes resins are defined by the presence of the urethane sequence –O–CO–NH– (See also: ➋ Chap. 53, "Polyurethane Resins").

Isocyanates with the generic formula $R\text{–}(N{=}CO)_n$ react with hydroxyl groups (–OH) of polyalcohols (polyols) to form polyurethanes:

- Polyols (polyesters or polyethers)
- Isocyanates (alkylic or arylic):
- 4,4′-Diisocyanate dicyclohexyl methane
- Methylene bis (4-cyclohexyl-isocyanate)
- Diphenyl-methane-4,4′-diisocyanate = MDI
- 1,6-Diisocyanate hexamethylene = HDI
- 3-Isocyanate-methyl-3,5,5-trimethyl-cyclohexyl-isocyanate = IPDI
- Polimethylene-polyphenyl isocyanate = PAPI
- Toluene-diisocyanates (2,4-TDI and 2,6-TDI) etc.

Polyurethanes can also be obtained from the reaction of glycol dichlor carbonic esters with diamines. In the technologic process, catalysts and amine curing agents are used such as triethylendiamine, ethylamine, methylamine, triethylamine, etc. Organostannic catalysts and blowing agents (dichloromethane, trichlorfluoromethane) are also used.

Polyurethanes are used for paints, lacquers, adhesives, binders for core castings, building materials (for sealing cracks and consolidation), synthetic fibers (duraspan, perlon U, gospan), fiber and cable insulators (as sprays with flexible and rigid foams). Polyurethanes are also used to impregnate textiles, paper, etc. Lacquers are applied with special guns, the ingredients being united automatically at application. In this case the aerosols are not detained by ordinary protection masks but only by milipores or activated carbon filter masks. Polyurethanes are widely used in microcellular foam seals and gaskets, durable elastomeric wheels and tires, automotive suspension bushings, high-performance adhesives, sealants. Polyurethane products are often called "urethanes" and also confused with the specific substance urethane (ethyl-carbamate). Polyurethanes are not produced from ethyl-carbamate and do not contain it.

Hexamethylene 1,6-diisocyanate (HDI) is found in lacquers, coatings, and spray paints, mainly composed of HDI trimers, but also containing larger oligomers and under 1% HDI monomers. HDI trimers occur as biuret, isocyanurate, and asymmetrical types (Aalto-Korte et al. 2010). Diisocyanates are used also as adjuvants in the rubber industry (Rusu 2009).

Isocyanates patch test battery I–1000 – Isocyanate series are listed in ➋ *Table 55.4*.

Patch test for polyurethanes can also include:

Table 55.4
I-1000 – isocyanate series

1. Toluene diisocyanate (TDI)	2% pet
2. Diphenylmethane-4,4-diisocyanate (MDI)	2% pet
3. Diamino-diphenyl-methane	0.5% pet
4. Isophorone-diisocyanate (IPDI)	1% pet
5. Isophorone-diamine (IPD)	0.1% pet
6. 1,6-Hexamethylene-diisocyanate (HDI)	0.1% pet

Isocyanates:	
Polymethyl-phenyl isocyanate (PAPI)	0.1% pet
Dicyclohexylmethane p,p′-diisocyanate (Desmodur W or WS) = Hylene W	1% pet
Methylene-bis (4-cyclohexyl-isocyanate)	1% pet

Amines:	
Dimethyl-3,3′-diamino-4,4′-diphenylmethane (classified as carcinogen, is proposed for banning)	0.5 pet
Methylene dianiline	0.1% in olive oil
Tri-isopropanol amine	0.5% pet
Ethylamine	2% aq
Methylamine	2% aq
Triethylamine	2% aq
Triethylene diamine (DABCO)	0.05–3% aq
m-Xylene-diamine (MXDA)	0.1% pet

Patch-test preparations of polymeric diphenylmethane diisocyanate (PMDI) are more stable than preparations of diphenylmethane-4,4′-diisocyanate (4,4′-MDI). It is recommended to use PMDIs with a monomer content of at least 35% in 2.0% pet, i.e., monomer patch test concentration approximately 0.7%. Reactions to 4,4′-MDI and PMDIs appear late and it is strongly recommended to repeat readings at least on days 3, 4, and 7. 4,4′-diaminodiphenylmethane (4,4′-MDA) was shown to be a good marker for 4,4′-MDI and patch testing with 4,4′-MDA in 0.25% pet can be used instead of PMDI. Concomitant reactions to 4,4′-MDI and 4,4′-MDA are probably not caused by conversion of 4,4′-MDI into 4,4′-MDA by reaction with water. Another explanation is a path of reactions leading to ureas and MDI conjugates with skin constituents, which are hydrolyzed into 4,4′-MDA (a complex process depending upon several factors and probably responsable for positive MDI reactions after up to 7 days) (Frick-Engfeldt et al. 2007).

2.10.1 Skin Problems

Of the two components of polyurethanes:

- Polyols (polyesters or polyethers) have a reputation of not being sensitizers
- Some of the isocyanates (alkyl or aryl) may induce sensitization

Allergic contact dermatitis from handling the finished resins are extremely rare, but resins manufacture can cause skin allergies and irritation, asthma, extrinsic allergic alveolitis, rhino-conjunctival and respiratory irritation.

Low molecular weight aliphatic isocyanates are volatile and act as intense respiratory sensitizers (causing allergic rhinitis, allergic asthma, and extrinsic alveolitis) but are weak skin sensitizers (face, neck, and V-shape area contact dermatitis is probably induced by airborne molecules). High molecular weight isocyanates (HDI, the "aromatics") are not as volatile and are far less sensitizing. However, catalysts – amino compounds (triethylamine, triethylene diamine), cobalt, or copper naphthenate – and other adjuvants can induce allergies.

MDI is used as aerosol and therefore involves especially respiratory risks and only seldom generates skin problems.

Dicyclohexylmethane-4,4′-diisocyanate (DMDI) is known to be a strong cutaneous sensitizer. A 27-year-old woman developed a severe eczematous eruption on the arms, trunk, and abdomen within 2 weeks of employment at a company using the product Chem-Dec 808 isocyanate (containing 40–70% weight per weight DMDI). Patch testing was performed with the North American screening series, an isocyanate series and 1% Chem-Dec 808 isocyanate. At day 7, a +++ reaction to Chem-Dec 808 isocyanate and a ++ reaction to the aromatic isocyanate diphenylmethane-4,4′-diisocyanate were observed (Donovan et al. 2009).

TDI (a strong irritant and a weak sensitizer) induces orthoergic and allergic contact dermatitis, extrinsic allergic alveolitis, asthma and respiratory irritation.

HDI (from polyester resins for textiles and paints) induces blepharoconjunctivitis, respiratory irritation and rarely allergic contact dermatitis or asthma. Four patients with allergic contact dermatitis from HDI-based polyisocyanates in polyurethane paints were diagnosed between 2000 and 2009 at the Finnish Institute of Occupational Health. None of the four patients tested positive to HDI monomer (Aalto-Korte et al. 2010).

Naphtalene-diisocyanate (NDI) eliminates noxious fumes when above 100°C. It is rarely used. Amine and organostannic catalysts can induce orthoergic or allergic contact dermatitis, allergies, and irritation of the respiratory tract (asthma, rhino-conjunctivitis).

First aid measures in contamination with isocyanates:

- Contaminated clothes should be removed quickly, preferably in an isolated shower in order not to contaminate the entourage.
- Immediate decontamination of the skin affected by the liquid monomer (which can cause an intense inflammatory reaction, with redness and swelling) by washing thoroughly with water and treating with isopropanol (isopropyl alcohol) 30%, followed by further washing with soap and water.

2.11 Polyolefins

Polyolefins are thermoplastic resins obtained by polyaddiction of olefins (unsaturated hydrocarbons).

2.11.1 Polyethylene

Polyethylene is produced by polymerization of ethylene (CH_2=CH_2), at low or high pressure, using initiators and catalysts, into chains of repeating unit –CH_2–CH_2–. Polyethylene is cheaper, lighter than water and widely used in the manufacture of protective gloves, film for packaging (bags, sacks), filters for air conditioning, plastic containers (PET), etc. Polyethylene production represents about 50% of the total output of plastics worldwide.

Polyethylenes can be divided into three groups:

- Low-density polyethylenes – soft, flexible, transparent, nontoxic (they have no plasticizers), used for food packaging, shopping bags, sacks
- Linear low-density polyethylenes – with better mechanical strength, used for coating of electric cables and wires, hoses, containers, jars, deep-freeze boxes and cases
- High-density polyethylenes – used for bottles, containers, pipes, shopping bags

2.11.2 Polypropylene

Polypropylene is a chain of repeating unit –CH_2–CH–CH_3, derived from propylene (CH_2=CH–CH_3). It is similar to high-density polyethylene, but harder and tougher. It is used in the manufacture of films, pipes, nonwoven products and carpets, home furnishings.

Skin Problems

Polyethylene is not a sensitizer in the form of the polymerized finite product.

Skin irritations and allergies may be due to incompletely cured resins, initiators, and catalysts.

Processing of polyolefin resins by sawing and grinding – under hot conditions – can induce the reaction of depolimerization and the release of ketones, aldehydes, acids, which can give itching airborne contact dermatitis (Thestrup-Pedersen et al. 1989).

Occupational contact dermatitis from irritating airborne molecules of polypropylene and polyethylene fibers from the filter of the air conditioning system in a hospital in Amsterdam was described in eight workers (Patiwael et al. 2005). Very low humidity contributed to the release of fibers from the polymer matrix under the influence of the air pressure column and precipitated skin irritations.

Sicca syndrome (reduction of exocrine secretions, especially tears) can be induced by polypropylene and polyethylene. Epidermal necrolysis was described in workers in contact with diethylphthalate and polyethylene.

Polyethylene airborne molecules derived from the mass of polyethylene polymer can induce respiratory disease from extrinsic allergic alveolitis to asthma. In a woman, extrinsic allergic alveolitis (confirmed by biopsy) was developed after 7 years of occupational contact with polyethylene flakes (Barroso et al. 2002). The exposure to polypropylene and polystyrene can modify color perception. In a group of 93 apparently healthy workers from two factories and three dry cleaning units, there was a significant color perception deficit compared with a control group of 56 unexposed persons (Kaur et al. 2004). The authors used Ishihara D-15 and Farnsworth Munsell 100 Hue tests. D-15 test revealed a sense of color deficiency in 28% of exposed persons (especially the yellow-blue line) and FM 100 Hue revealed a deficiency in 63% of exposed persons without identifying such deficits in the control group. The results were statistically significant. There have also been described:

- Smoke fever to polyethylene terephthalate resin (as in exposure to the smoke from polyester, cellulose resin, and polybutylene terephthalate resin)
- Asthma to polyethylene electrical insulation
- Bladder cancer in polyethylene exposure
- Colorectal cancer among workers exposed to polypropylene

2.11.3 Polyethylenglycol (PEG)

Polyethylenglycol (PEG) is a mixture of glycols. The glycols with molecular weights of 200–700 kDal are liquid, while those with molecular weights of 1,000–6,000 kDal are solid products.

Glycols are good solvents, being used as excipients for drugs, suppositories, shampoos, soaps, detergents, conditioners and other cosmetics, insecticides, toothpaste, contraception pills, nitrocellulose, epoxy resin hardeners, glues, etc. Polyethylene glycol ointment is a mixture of solid polyethylene glycol (molecular weight 4,000 kDal) with liquid polyethylene glycol (molecular weight 300 kDal). Carbowax is a polyethylene glycol waxy solid (molecular weight 1,500 kDal) used as lubricant and softener for textiles).

Skin Problems

PEG can induce both contact urticaria (Fisher 1978) and delayed type IV contact dermatitis (Braun 1969). There is no cross-reaction with propylene glycol. The sensitizing potential of PEGs is inversely proportional to their molecular weight, most allergens being in liquid forms with low molecular weight (200–400 kDal).

2.12 Polytetrafluoroethylene (PTFE)

PTFE is a synthetic thermoset fluoropolymer of tetrafluoroethylene accidentally invented by Roy Plunkett of Kinetic Chemicals in New Jersey in 1939 (Rietschel and Fowler 2008). PTFE is most well known by the DuPont brand name Teflon. Teflon coating consists of microscopic beads of Teflon co-deposited up to 20% with electroless nickel. Other polymers with similar composition are also known by the Teflon trade name:

- Perfluoroalkoxy (PFA)
- Fluorinated ethylene propylene (FEP)

PTFE is a fluorocarbon solid with high molecular weight, consisting entirely of carbon and fluorine. PTFE is hydrophobic and nonreactive due to the strength of carbon-fluorine bonds. Due to this property it is used in containers and pipework for reactive and corrosive chemicals. PTFE demonstrates a low friction coefficient against solids and it is used as a nonstick coating for pans and other cookware. PTFE is also used as a lubricant because it reduces friction, wear, and energy consumption of machinery (Funderburg 2000).

2.12.1 Skin Problems

Liquid PTFE is a skin irritant. Brief exposures may cause mild irritation. Frequent or prolonged contact may cause severe irritation, defatting of the skin and allergic dermatitis. Irritating and harmful fumes are released when PTFE is heated above 300°C (Rudnick 2009).

2.13 Other Rare Plastics

- Coumarone-indene polymers
- Cyclohexanone resins

2.13.1 Skin Problems

There have been cases of dermatitis reported from these types of resins, but it is unclear whether they were caused by monomers, impurities, or additives (Bruze et al. 1988; Heine and Laubstein 1990).

3 Occupational Diseases Induced by Plastics

- Orthoergic (irritative) contact dermatitis with different clinical forms: dry, cracked, desquamative, erosive (chemical burn)
- Allergic contact dermatitis, including contact dermatitis to airborne antigens that affects the face, neck, and the V-shape area
- Contact urticaria (with immunologic or nonimmunologic mechanism)
- Onixis and perionixis (perionichia) with nail dystrophy and onicholysis (in contact with cyanoacrylate resin)
- Epidermal necrolysis induced by cellulose acetate, polyesters, PVC, acrylonitrile-butadiene-styrene, polyethylene, and diethylphthalate (plasticizer) (Swan and Swan 2008)
- Occupational vitiligo induced by *p*-tertiary-butylphenol
- Altered chromatic perceptions from polypropylene and polystyrene
- Sicca syndrome in polypropylene and polyethylene workers
- Bladder cancer from polyethylene and acrylic resins
- Colorectal cancer in polypropylene workers
- Poisoning induced by organic solvents and developed as ebrionarcotic syndrome, neurological syndrome (neuropathy, coma), toxic hepatitis, hematological syndrome, renal failure, myocarditis, cardiac arrest, non-Hodgkin's lymphoma, etc. (Bucur and Bucur 2006)
- Allergic rhinitis
- Smoke fever when exposed to the fumes of polyester resins, cellulose resins, polyethylene terephthalate, and polybutylene terephthalate
- Asthma
- Allergic extrinsic alveolitis induced by exposure to isocyanates
- "Reactive Airways Dysfunctional Syndrome" (RADS) developed after exposure to cyanoacrylate

4 Primary and Secondary Prevention Measures in Exposure to Plastics

4.1 Primary Prevention

Judicious selection of masks and gloves, both in terms of cost-burst resistance report as in what concerns the chemical substances whose contact should be avoided and which must not penetrate the equipment. Changes in technological processes must be introduced whenever possible, in order to eliminate some low molecular weight volatile reagents. The replacement of some very harmful adjuvants with less dangerous ones is a good option. All workers should undergo proper health and safety instruction.

4.2 Secondary Prevention

Patients must receive valuable and useful recommendations from the medical team that treated the occupational skin disease. Unfortunately most patients will return to the previous jobs and their occupational exposure will resume. Several socioeconomic issues prevent improvements of working conditions and avoidance of the contact with hazards:

- Too expensive technological process changes.
- The impossibility to use protective equipment (gloves that do not allow performing of occupational gestures or block the leasions' healing; masks that hinder breathing; goggles that obscure the view).
- The ineffectiveness of protective equipment (airborne molecules that penetrate beneath the equipment, substances that penetrate the fabric of the equipment, etc.).
- Health and safety education of the patients: employees and their employers must come up with a deeper understanding and awareness of occupational hazards. Everyone should be involved in finding optimal solutions to improve working conditions in order to eliminate or at least minimize the number of occupational and work-related diseases.

References

Aalto-Korte K, Jolanki R, Estlander T (2003) Formaldehyde-negative allergic contact dermatitis from melamine-formaldehyde resin. Contact Dermatitis 49(4):194–196

Aalto-Korte K, Pesonen M, Kuuliala O, Alanko K, Jolanki R (2010) Contact allergy to aliphatic polyisocyanates based on hexamethylene-1,6-diisocyanate (HDI). Contact Dermatitis 63(6):357–363

Barroso E, Ibañez MD, Aranda FI, Romero S (2002) Polyethylene flock-associated interstitial lung disease in a Spanish female. Eur Respir J 20(6):1610–1612

Belsito DV (1997) The rise and fall of allergic contact dermatitis. Am J Contact Dermat 8(4):193–201

Björkner B (2000) Other plastics. In: Kanerva L, Elsner P, Wahlberg JE, Maibach HI (eds) Handbook of occupational dermatology. Springer, Berlin/Heidelberg, p 607

Bourne L, Milner FJ (1963) Polyester resin hazards. Br J Ind Med 20:100–109

Braun W (1969) Contact allergies to polyethylene glycols. Z Haut Geschlechtskr 44(11):385–389

Bruze M, Fregert S (1994) Chemical skin burns. In: Menne T, Maibach HI (eds) Hand eczema. CRC Press, Boca Raton, p 21

Bruze M, Boman A, Bergqvist-Karlsson A, Björkner B, Wahlberg JE, Voog E (1988) Contact allergy to cyclohexanone resin in humans and guinea pigs. Contact Dermatitis 18(1):46–49

Bucur L, Bucur G (2006) Probleme de toxicologie profesională dermatologică. Efecte generale apărute prin absorbţia cutanată a unor substanţe toxice de uz profesional. In: Bucur G, Bucur L, Sălăvăstru C, Tiplica GS (eds) Dermatoze profesionale. Niculescu, Bucharest, pp 349–358

Burrows D, Rycroft RJ (1981) Contact dermatitis from PTBP resin and tricresyl ethyl phthalate in a plastic nail adhesive. Contact Dermatitis 7(6):336–337

Condé-Salazar L, González MA, Guimaraens D, Romero L (1989) Occupational contact dermatitis from styrene. Contact Dermatitis 21(2):112

Donovan J, Skotnicki-Grant S (2007) Allergic contact dermatitis from formaldehyde textile resins in surgical uniforms and nonwoven textile masks. Dermatitis 18(1):40–44

Donovan JC, Kudla I, Dekoven JG (2009) Rapid development of allergic contact dermatitis from dicyclohexylmethane-4,4′-diisocyanate. Dermatitis 20(4):214–217

Dooms-Goossens AE, Debusschere KM, Gevers DM, Dupré KM, Degreef HJ, Loncke JP, Snauwaert JE (1986) Contact dermatitis caused by airborne agents. A review and case reports. J Am Acad Dermatol 15(1):1–10

Fisher AA (1978) Immediate and delayed allergic contact reactions to polyethylene glycol. Contact Dermatitis 4(3):135–138

Foussereau J, Benezra CJ (1970) Les Eczemas professionnels. Masson, Paris

Fregert S (1981) Formaldehyde dermatitis from a gypsum-melamine resin mixture. Contact Dermatitis 7(1):56

Frick-Engfeldt M, Isaksson M, Zimerson E, Bruze M (2007) How to optimize patch testing with diphenylmethane diisocyanate. Contact Dermatitis 57(3):138–151

Funderburg AC (2000) Making teflon stick. Invention and Technology Magazine, Summer 2000. 16(1)

García Gavin J, Loureiro Martinez M, Fernandez-Redondo V, Seoane MJ, Toribio J (2008) Contact allergic dermatitis from melamine formaldehyde resins in a patient with a negative patch-test reaction to formaldehyde. Dermatitis 19(2):E5–E6

Hamada T, Horiguchi S (1978) Allergic contact dermatitis due to sodium carboxymethyl cellulose. Contact Dermatitis 4(4):244

Heine A, Laubstein B (1990) Contact dermatitis from cyclohexanone-formaldehyde resin (L2 resin) in a hair lacquer spray. Contact Dermatitis 22(2):108

Jordan WP Jr, Dahl MV Jr (1971) Contact dermatitis to a plastic solvent in eyeglasses. Cross-sensitivity to ethyl acetate. Arch Dermatol 104(5):524–528

Kaddar N, Harthé C, Déchaud H, Mappus E, Pugeat M (2008) Cutaneous penetration of bisphenol A in pig skin. J Toxicol Environ Health A 71:471–473

Kalimo K, Saarni H, Kytta J (1980) Immediate and delayed type reactions to formaldehyde resin in glass wool. Contact Dermatitis 6(7):496

Kanerva L, Björkner B, Estlander T et al (1996) Plastic materials: occupational exposure, skin irritancy and its prevention. In: van der Valk PGM,

Maibach HI (eds) The irritant contact dermatitis syndrome. CRC Press, Boca Raton, p 127

Kaur S, Mursyid A, Kamaruddin A, Ariffin A (2004) Effect of petroleum derivatives and solvents on colour perception. Clin Exp Optom 87(4–5):339–343

Kelman GR (1986) Effects of human exposure to atmospheric ε-caprolactam. Hum Exp Toxicol 5(1):57–59

Martin-Scott I (1966) Contact textile dermatitis (with special reference to fire proof fabrics). Br J Dermatol 78(12):632–635

Moscato G, Biscaldi G, Cottica D, Pugliese F, Candura S, Candura F (1987) Occupational asthma due to styrene: two case reports. J Occup Med 29(12):957–960

Niculescu T, Todea A, Toma I, Pavel A, Niculescu R (2003) Intoxicaţia profesională cu stiren. In: Medicina muncii. Medmun, Bucharest, pp 210–211

Patiwael JA, Wintzen M, Rustemeyer T, Bruynzeel DP (2005) Airborne irritant contact dermatitis due to synthetic fibres from an air-conditioning filter. Contact Dermatitis 52(3):126–129

Piper R (1965) The hazards of painting and varnishing. Br J Ind Med 22(4):247–260

Rietschel RL, Fowler JF (2008) (Teflon). In: Rietschel RL, Fowler JF (eds.) Fisher's contact dermatitis, 6th edn., McGraw Hill, New York, p 335, 422, 542, 680, 688, 673

Romaguera C, Grimalt F, Vilaplana J (1989) Eczematous and purpuric allergic contact dermatitis from boots. Contact Dermatitis 21(4):269

Ross JS, Rycroft RJ, Cronin E (1992) Melamine-formaldehyde contact dermatitis in orthopaedic practice. Contact Dermatitis 26(3): 203–204

Rudnick M (2009) Material safety data sheets. Product name: Dry PTFE Lube (aerosol). Product number (s): 03044, 73044. CRC Industries: 670/670A. Revision Date: 07/22/2009

Rudzki E (1978) Dermatitis from epoxy resin, triethylentetramine and ethylendiamine. Contact Dermatitis 4:53–59

Rusu A (2009) Masele plastice. In: Cocârlă A (ed) Medicina ocupaţională, vol II. Medicală Universitară "Iuliu Haţieganu, Cluj-Napoca, pp 1399–1423

Schmunes E (1990) Solvents and plasticizers. In: Adams RM (ed) Occupational skin diseases, 2nd edn. WB Saunders, Philadelphia

Sjöborg S, Fregert S, Trulsson L (1984) Contact allergy to styrene and related chemicals. Contact Dermatitis 10(2):94–96

Svara J, Weferling N, Hofmann T (2006) Phosphorus compounds, organic. In: Ullmann's encyclopedia of industrial chemistry. Wiley-VCH, Weinheim

Swan SH (2008) Environmental phthalate exposure in relation to reproductive outcomes and other health endpoints in human. Environ Res 108(2):177–184

Thestrup-Pedersen K, Madsen JB, Rasmussen K (1989) Cumulative skin irritance from heat-decomposed polyethylene plastic. In: Frosch PJ, Dooms-Goossens A, Lachapelle J-M, Rycroft RJ, Scheper RJ (eds) Current topics in contact dermatitis. Springer, Berlin, p 412

Vale PT, Rycroft RJ (1988) Occupational irritant contact dermatitis from fibreboard containing urea formaldehyde resin. Contact Dermatitis 19(1):62

Williams LL (2002) Amino resins and plastics. In: Kirk-Othmer encyclopedia of chemical technology. Wiley, Hoboken

56 Plastic Composites

Kyllikki Tarvainen[1] · *Tuula Estlander*[2] · *Pirkko Pfäffli*[1] · *Katri Suuronen*[3]
[1]Helsinki, Finland
[2]Terveystalo Healthcare Oyj, Helsinki, Finland
[3]Occupational medicine, Finnish Institute of Occupational Health, Helsinki, Finland

Core Messages

- Plastic composites are combinations of a polymer *matrix* and a solid *reinforcement* material.
- Thermosetting and thermoplastic resins are used as matrices of plastic composites.
- Epoxy resins are the most common thermosetting resins in modern plastic composites.
- Dermatitis is a common occupational complaint in this industrial area.
- Skin hazards include irritant and allergic contact dermatoses and contact urticaria, as well as thermal or chemical burns.
- Epoxy resin compounds are the most common cause of allergic contact dermatitis from plastic composites.
- Man-made mineral fibers (MMMF) used for reinforcement are the main cause of irritant contact dermatitis in the manufacture of composite products.
- The development of occupational dermatitis depends on the materials (resins, reinforcements, and auxiliary substances), specific work tasks, working methods, workplace environment, and personal protection.

1 Introduction

Composites are combinations of two or more materials that are not dissolved or melted together. Plastic composites (PC) are manufactured by combining materials, at least one of which is plastic. In practice, they are combinations of a polymer *matrix* and a solid *reinforcement* (either plastic or another) material. A PC product may have a sandwich structure, having the matrix and the reinforcement material in layers, or it may be a mixture of un-oriented or oriented fibers or particles dispersed in the matrix. The purpose of the reinforcement is to increase the strength of the final product, while the matrix binds the fibers and protects them from corrosion, oxidation and from other degrading factors arising from the environment.

The PC matrices are either thermosetting resins, which are cured from a liquid state, or thermoplastics, which are processed through a melt-freeze cycle. Seventy percent of modern reinforced plastics contain thermosetting resins (➋ *Table 56.1*), while the use of thermoplastics, especially polyethylene, polypropylene, and polyamides as the matrix resin is increasing. Nonplastic reinforcement materials include glass fiber, other man-made mineral fibers (MMMF), metal particles, stone, cement, and silica; natural fibers are increasingly used in the manufacture of wood PCs (Ashori 2008). In dental composites, fine glass particles or silica are usually embedded in an acrylic polymer (Kanerva et al. 1989). The term composite also includes semifinished products called *prepregs*, which are reinforcing materials preimpregnated with resins.

The commercial PC industry began with glass-fiber-reinforced boats in the 1940s. Since then, PC products have increasingly been manufactured for the electrical, marine, aircraft, and aerospace industries. Thanks to their versatility, PCs are useful in construction, in the manufacture of corrosion-resistant equipment and in transport, as well as in a wide range of consumer goods, such as caravan bodies, pipes, bath tubes, roof panels, skis, racquets, and other sports equipment. Composite materials, especially advanced PCs, offer a number of advantages compared to other materials, the main advantages being their excellent strength and lightness. Reinforced PCs are also finding a place in corrosion repair, particularly in the gas and oil industry, thanks to their good corrosion resistance. Thus, due to the above-mentioned properties and their versatility, PCs are nowadays used in nearly all industrial areas.

People working in the manufacture and processing of PCs are exposed to matrix resins, resin precursors, reinforcing materials, such as glass fiber dust, plastic additives, and auxiliary chemicals used for assembling or finishing the products, as well as chemicals for cleaning purposes. Many of these compounds are skin sensitizers or have irritating potential (Midtgård and Knudsen 1994; Tarvainen and Kanerva 1999). Dermatoses from the manufacture of PCs have been reported since their production

T. Rustemeyer, P. Elsner, S.M. John & H.I. Maibach (eds.), *Kanerva's Occupational Dermatology*,
DOI 10.1007/978-3-642-02035-3_56,

Table 56.1
Polymers used in reinforced plastics composites

Thermosetting resins	Thermoplastic resins
Polyester resins	Polyphenylene sulfides (PPS)
Epoxy resins	Polyetheretherketones (PEEK)
Vinyl ester resins	Polyether sulfones (PES)
Phenol-formaldehyde resins	Polyvinyl chloride (PVC)
Polyurethanes	Polypropylene (PP), polyethylene (PE)
Polyimides	Polyamide

was started (Bourne and Milner 1963; Malten and Zielhuis 1964; Wehle 1966).

2 Plastic Composite Industry

The PC product industry is diverse and employs a wide variety of processing methods and materials. An enormous number of combinations can be made, depending on the design and cost of the final product. The manufacturer has the possibility to combine resin compounds, reinforcements, and various additives when making PCs, or to use preassembled material, such as prepregs, produced by specialist suppliers. The principal manufacturing process includes the molding of reinforcements and the matrix resin into the desired shape. Before the molding, resins are formulated by mixing them with solvents, curing agents, accelerators, fillers, mold releasers, dyes, fire retardants, and other additives needed for the desired properties. The cured composite pieces or ready products usually require finishing by sawing, drilling, sanding, or cutting with diamond-coated tools, lasers, or abrasive water jets (Rolston 1980; Bruze and Almgren 1989). During finishing operations, workers may be exposed to paints, coatings, glues, and various solvents, such as trichloroethylene, turpentine, methylene chloride, acetone, and toluene, as well as to woods, wood preservatives, and dust from the machining of the hardened product (Brigham and Landrigan 1985; Tarvainen and Kanerva 2000).

3 Fabrication of Plastic Composites

Contact molding, also called *hand lay-up* lamination, is the most commonly used open process method. Reinforcements and resins are laid down manually, using a roller, or sprayed over the mold in successive layers. In addition to wet hand lay-up methods, dry hand lay-up (prepregs) can also be used. Boats, caravan bodies, and many small articles are usually manufactured using the hand lay-up method. In *the filament winding method,* the reinforcements, wetted with the resin, are wound around a rotating mandrel or a work piece attached to a rotating mandrel by a machine, by robots or manually. The filament winding process originates from the aerospace industry, but is nowadays also used to manufacture pipes, tanks, and various poles. In the *injection method,* the products are made by feeding the matrix resin or resin-reinforced mix into a closed mold using a vacuum. In *pressure molding,* the resin is cast by means of pressure between heated matched male/female molds; these are the most widely used processes for large-scale production of composites, including domestic articles, cabinets, containers, and cab panels. *The pultrusion method* is a continuous process in which resin-impregnated fibers are drawn through a heated die, where the resin cures. The process is used in the production of structural elements, such as pipes and spade handles. Other molding methods include *resin transfer molding,* which is used to make small composite parts, such as boxes, seats, and benches, and *reaction molding,* which utilizes fast-reacting components. The methods of manufacturing PCs have been reviewed by Ehrenstein and Kabelka (2007).

While manual processes increase the risk of skin contact with harmful materials, pultrusion, centrifugal casting, resin transfer, compression molding, vacuum-bag molding, and prepregs are partly or totally automated working methods, where skin exposure is more easily avoided (Kelly 1994; Tarvainen and Kanerva 1999). However, even then the introduction of the resin into the mold may be done manually. Even in highly automated industries, workers may perform manual operations during assembly or repair work.

4 Matrices

4.1 Thermosetting Resins

The most widely used polymers in composite matrices are the thermosetting resins: unsaturated polyesters, epoxies, epoxy vinyl esters, phenolic resins, and polyurethane resins (Ilschner et al. 2007). More information on these resins can be found in other chapters of this book.

Unsaturated polyester resin (UPR, Chap. 54, "Polyester Resins") has been used extensively in the glass-fiber-reinforced plastics industry manufacturing products for transportation, construction, and marine applications. UPR is also used for coatings, finishes, lacquers, putties (Tarvainen et al. 1993b), and glues (Boenig 1964). Nowadays, in addition to boat building, there is a dynamic market for unsaturated polyester resins in wind turbine industries, where UPRs are used to produce rotor blades, engine housings, and gel coats in combination with epoxy resins and epoxy vinyl resins.

Polyesters are available in two different forms: saturated and unsaturated. UPRs are produced through esterification of organic acids or their anhydrides, e.g., maleic anhydride, phthalic anhydride (PA), or fumaric acid, with diols, e.g., diethylene glycol or 1,2-propylene glycol. The term "unsaturated" means that there are reactive double bonds within the resin that are able to form cross-links between the polymer chains. When a UP resin is manufactured, 10–50% styrene is added; the styrene serves both as a viscosity-reducing solvent and as a reactive monomer in cross-linking the linear polyester chains. In addition to styrene, vinyl toluene, methyl methacrylate, or diallyl phthalate can be used. Accelerators, such as cobalt naphthenate, cobalt octoate or tertiary amines such as dimethyl aniline, are necessary for the curing of plastic at room temperature. Hydroquinone is added to prevent premature cross-linking. Other additives include pigments, fillers, inhibitors, and light stabilizers. Halogenated monomers have been used as flame retardants in UPRs, and a new "flame-retardant polyester resin" with a copolymerized high concentration of phosphorus and fillers has also been developed. Polymerization of the UPR occurs after adding a polymer initiator, such as benzoyl peroxide or methyl ethyl ketone (MEK) peroxide.

Epoxy resin systems (➋ Chap. 51, "Epoxy Resins") are used especially in the manufacture of composites for sporting goods, boats, automobile, and transport industries, as well as for military, aerospace, and power production applications; for example, wind turbine systems and the aircraft industry commonly utilize epoxy composites (Pontén et al. 2004; Rasmussen et al. 2005). Epoxy resins are also used in the electrical industry, in the manufacture of circuit boards and covers for components (Isaksson and Bruze 2000; Kanerva et al. 1996). The epoxy resins used in the composites are commonly based on diglycidylether of bisphenol-A (DGEBA) epoxy resin or diglycidylether of bisphenol-F (DGEBF) epoxy resin, while other glycidyl derivatives, such as tetraglycidyl-4-4′-methylendianiline (TGMDA) and triglycidyl-*p*-aminophenol (TGPAP), have been used in special PCs. The most important hardeners of epoxy resins are the aromatic amines, including xylylene diamine and 4,4′-methylene dianiline, and aliphatic amines such as triethylenetetramine (TETA) and diethylenetriamine (DETA). Carboxylic acid anhydrides, e.g., hexahydrophthalic anhydride (HHPA) and methyltetrahydrophthalic anhydride (MTHPA) are used as latent hardeners in some epoxy resin PCs; in such products, the latent hardener activates only at elevated temperatures, and therefore heat is needed to cure them. The resins in prepreg PCs are most often epoxy compounds. The epoxy prepregs may contain DGEBA or DGEBF epoxy resin and diglycidyl ether of tetrabromo-bisphenol A (brominated DGEBA-epoxy resin); however, due to difficulties with their adherence to carbon or graphite fibers, the non-DGEBA epoxy resins 4-glycidyloxy-N,N-diglycidylaniline, TGMDA, TGPAP, and o-diglycidyl phthalate are often used (Kanerva et al. 2000). The most common fiber reinforcements are glass, graphite, and aramide (aromatic polyamide) fibers, whereas the particulate microcomposites and novel nanocomposites are usually reinforced with small silica or calcium carbonate particles.

Epoxy vinyl ester resins are used in products that are highly resistant to chemicals and corrosion. The epoxy vinyl ester resins (sometimes referred to as "vinyl esters resins") are also more resistant to moisture than, for example, standard UPRs. For this reason their use in boat building has increased. Epoxy vinyl esters are epoxy di(meth) acrylates (β-hydroxyester (meth)acrylates), which are obtained by reacting liquid DGEBA-epoxy resin or other epoxy resins with (meth)acrylic acid and diluted with styrene to 35–40% solvent by weight. Epoxy vinyl esters can be polymerized by electron beams, ultraviolet light, and by peroxides. The same cross-linker (styrene), hardeners (peroxides), and accelerators (cobalt) as for UPR, are used (Rolston 1980; Kanerva et al. 1989). *Dental composite resins* (➋ Chap. 143, "Occupational Contact Dermatitis in Dental Personnel") based on DGEBA-epoxy resin monomers and methacrylates or acrylates, e.g., BIS-GMA or BIS-GA, have been used since 1962 (Bowen 1962). In addition to the acrylic binders, dental composites contain inorganic reinforcements (also referred to as fillers), such as small glass particles or silica, and additives. The additives include (1) hardeners such as benzoyl peroxide, (2) activators such as tertiary aromatic amines, and (3) inhibitors such as hydroquinone.

Phenol-formaldehyde resins (PF resins, ➋ Chap. 52, "Contact Allergy to Phenol-Formaldehyde Resins") are polycondensation products of phenols and aldehydes, in particular, phenol, and formaldehyde. Phenol-formaldehyde resins are divided into *resols* that are self-curing in elevated temperatures and *novolacs* that require additional curing agents. PF resins have many industrial applications. Glues based on PF are used in the plywood industry, the building industry, and in boat building and also in aircraft construction. PF resins are also used as matrices for glass or mineral fibers in the production of various insulating materials and as binders of sand in foundry casting molds. PF resins are modified by fillers, e.g., minerals, graphite, cellulose, or wood particles, when needed (Zimerson 2006). PF resins are also used in prepregs with glass or carbon fiber reinforcements and processed by various automatic methods in the aircraft industry.

Polyurethane resins (PUR) are reaction products of di- or polyisocyanates and polyols (➋ Chap. 53, "Polyurethane Resins"). PURs are available in many forms. In addition to coatings, adhesives, and rigid and flexible foams, PURs are used also in advanced composite processes, such as pultrusion and filament winding. Many additives, such as fire retardants, fillers, coloring agents, and blowing agents, are needed. Urethane acrylates are used in dental composite and sealant applications and have the same role as BIS-GMA.

4.2 Thermoplastic Resins

The complete lists of applicable thermoplastics is extensive, and includes polypropylene (PP), polyethylene (PE), polystyrenes, polysulfones and polyvinyl chloride (PVC), acrylonitrile-butadiene-styrenes (ABS), acetals, acrylics, fluoropolymers, polyacrylsulfone, polycarbonates, thermoplastic polyesters, polyether ketone, polyether sulfones, and poly(phenylene sulfides).

Thermoplastics currently account for a relatively small proportion of the PC industry. They are solids and usually appear as pellets that are melted by applying heat and subsequently cast by application of pressure into the finished part. PP and PE are the most common thermoplastic resins in PCs. Chopped glass, carbon, aramid or metal fibers are usually used as reinforcements. For example, PP is used in the manufacture of packaging equipment and in plastic parts or fibers in the automotive and electrical industries. One of the most important applications is the glass-mat-thermoplastic, which is a thermoplastic laminate molded with a continuous glass-fiber-reinforced sheet and used in advanced aerospace industry applications and for the production of structural profiles and pipes (Björkner 2006). Polypropylene and polyethylene have been used for the manufacture of plastic boats in small series since the 1970s. *Rotation molding* and thermo-molding are the methods used in manufacturing thermoplastic boats.

5 Additives in Synthetic Polymers

Additives are used to modify the properties of plastics materials. Nearly 2,500 individual chemicals or mixtures are used as additives in polymer formulations, including synthetic polymers, biopolymers, composites, and biocomposites. Plastic additives are classified into three main groups: (1) additives that stabilize plastics against degradations involve antioxidants, light and heat stabilizers, (2) additives that affect the process include lubricants, mold release agents, and blowing agents, and (3) additives that impart new desirable qualities to plastics; these include flame retardants, fillers, dyes, pigments, antistatic agents, optical brighteners, and plasticizers. The concentration of additives varies greatly, from a few parts per million (ppm) to more than 50%. Plastics generally contain many additives, which either form an inherent part of the composite itself or are employed in a somewhat external manner. Resins commonly already contain additives when purchased from the manufacturers. Fillers and auxiliary substances are mixed with the resins at the workplace to improve its workability and the properties of the final product (IPCS 1997, Stepeck and Daoust 1983). Depending on the resin, additives may have different ways of functioning: for example, flame retardants can either bond covalently with the polymer molecules or be mixed into polymers (➋ *Table 56.2*). An additive may also have many functions: it can, for example, act as an antioxidant and stabilizer in the uncured resins, or as a flame retardant in the finished product. reviewed by Wolf and Kaul (2007).

5.1 Plasticizers

A plasticizer is a substance incorporated into a material to increase its flexibility or workability. Approximately 450 plasticizers are commercially available. The most commonly used are esters of carboxylic acids, phthalates, phosphates, adipates, and trimellitates. Other plasticizers are chlorinated paraffins, epoxidized vegetable oils, and adipate polymers. The principal use of plasticizers is in thermoplastic resins, and 80–85% of the world's production of plasticizers is used in PVC manufacturing. There are about 100 phthalates, but 14–15 are most frequently used (➋ *Table 56.3*). Adipates and other aliphatic diesters are used in low-temperature applications, while trimellitates are used for high-temperature applications. Methyl-, ethyl-, and butyl phthalates are more often used as solvents than as plasticizers in the plastics industry.

5.2 Fillers

When used in composite laminates, inorganic fillers may account for 40–65% of the composition. Calcium carbonate, kaolin (hydrous aluminum silicate), alumina trihydrate, and calcium sulfate can be used to improve

Table 56.2
Examples of flame retardants used in plastics (halogen compounds and organophosphates with a synergetic compound)

Commercial names of plastics	Flame retardant
Low-density polyethylene (LDPE)	Chlorinated paraffin with antimony trioxide (Sb_2O_3) as a synergic compound
LDPE, cross-linked	Brominated aromatic compounds
High-density polyethylene (HDEP)	Brominated aromatic compound
Polyolefins	Cycloparaffins, hexabromobenzene, tetrabromophthalic anhydride
Polypropylene	Tetrabromobisphenol A, bis(2,3-dibromopropyl ether) with Sb_2O_3
Unsaturated polyester	Chlorine- and bromine-containing organic compounds with Sb_2O_3 or $Al(OH)_3$, chlorendic anhydride, or chlorendic acid
Epoxy resin	Tetrabromobisphenol A, tetrabromodienes alone or with organophosphates
Polyamides	Brominated aromatic or cycloaliphatic compounds with Sb_2O_3, melamine
Polycarbonates	Tetrabromobisphenol A, brominated organic oligomers, sulfonate salts
Expandable polystyrene	Hexabromocyclododecane
High-impact polystyrene (HIPS)	Decabromodiphenyl ether, tetrabromobisphenol A with Sb_2O_3
Acrylonitrile-butadiene-styrene	Octabromodiphenyl ether, SB_2O_3, peroxides, brominated compounds
PVC	Chlorinated paraffin, phosphate ester with Sb_2O_3 or $Al(OH)_3$
Polyurethane foams	Organophospates, brominated organic compounds with $Al(OH)_3$
Polyurethanes	Polyols with a halogen, organophosphates, organophosphates with a halogen
Vinyl ester resin	Tetrabromobisphenol A, tetrabromodienes, organophosphates

Data from: (Stepeck and Daoust 1983), IPCS (1997) (International Programme on Chemical Safety) World Health Organization. Environmental Health Criteria, Geneva 1997, 133p.

Table 56.3
The most commonly used phthalate plasticizers

Diethylhexyl phthalate (DEHP) also called dioctyl phthalate (DOP)
Butyl benzyl phthalate (BBP)
Diisononyl phthalate (DINP)
Diisodecyl phthalate (DIDP)
Methyl-, ethyl-, butyl phthalate
Dialkyl (C6 C11) phthalate
Diethylhexyl adipate

mechanical properties. Fillers are used mostly in the manufacture of thermoplasts, such as PVC. Today, nanoparticles of various materials can also be used as fillers (Saarela et al. 2007)

5.3 Flame Retardants

Polymer materials are often flammable and thus require flame retardants, which may be inorganic compounds, halogenated organic compounds, organophosphorus compounds, or other organic substances. About 10% of all plastics (chiefly PVC, ABS, polystyrene, unsaturated polyesters, polypropylene, polyethylene, and polyurethanes) contain flame retardants (*Table 56.2*). Chlorine- and bromine-containing aliphatic, cycloaliphatic, and aromatic compounds are the most widely used. Others are antimony trioxide, aluminum hydrate, and chloroparaffins. A more fire-resistant epoxy resin can be produced by bromating bisphenol A in epoxy resins to form tetrabromobisphenol A.

5.4 Stabilizers

Special heat stabilizers are required for processing PVC. There are several kinds of stabilizers on the market. The most important of these contain lead, tin, calcium and zinc, or barium and zinc. Metal-free stabilizers are used in conjunction with metal-containing stabilizers. The principal epoxy stabilizers are epoxidized plant oils, chiefly soybean oil. Epoxidized oils and esters are also used. Diphenyltiourea is used as a heat stabilizer in PVC.

5.5 Antioxidants

Antioxidants prevent the autoxidation of polymers and minimize associated damage, e.g., discoloration. Examples of antioxidants are alkylated phenols and polyphenols (e.g., butylated hydroxytoluene (BHT) and 4-tertiary-bytylcathechol) and epoxidized soybean oil. Bisphenol A is used as an antioxidant in polyvinyl chloride plastics and corrosion-resistant unsaturated polyester resins.

5.6 UV-Light Absorbers

Radiation from the sun or fluorescent light degrades most plastics. Light stabilizers are mainly employed in plastics for outdoor services, e.g., garden furniture and automotive parts. The most widely used UV light absorbers belong to the following chemical classes: (1) benzophenones, (2) benzotriazoles, (3) salicylates, (4) acrylates, (5) organo-nickel derivates, (6) hindered amines, and (7) metal complexes with dialkyldithiocarbamate. The most common are 2-hydroxybenzophenones, 2-hydrocyphenyl-benzotriazoles, and 2-cyanodiphenylacrylate (Björkner 2006).

5.7 Biocides

Biocides are usually added to plastic products used in environments with high temperature and humidity, such as saunas and boats, since micro-organisms can cause discoloration and cracks in plastic materials. Especially PVC, polyurethane, silicon products, and fiber products based on polypropylene and polyamide are easily attacked by microorganisms. The most commonly used biocides are methyl- and octyl isothiazolinones and oxybisphenoxarsine (Björkner 2006).

5.8 Colorants (Dyes and Pigments)

Dyes and pigments are chosen from a wide range of organic and inorganic compounds. Inorganic pigments are insoluble in plastics, and due to the resulting stability, they are usually preferred. The most common inorganic pigments include titanium dioxide, zinc, iron oxide, chromium oxide green, lead chromate, and cadmium pigments. Organic pigments, although not as common, may be used either as such or in combinations with inorganic pigments. The chemical classes are numerous and include azo, phtalocyanide, and metal complex compounds.

5.9 Initiators

Polymer initiators must be used for starting the curing of UPRs and acrylic polymers. The curing agents are discussed under the heading *Thermosetting resins* and elsewhere in this book.

6 Reinforcements

Glass fibers, carbon fibers, and aramid fibers account for the majority of reinforcements found in PCs (Ehrenstein and Kabelka 2007). In the large-scale production of certain consumer products, hybrid composites are used, in which glass fibers are mixed with carbon or aramid fibers. The concentration of reinforcements in the composites ranges from less than 10% to over 80% by weight (Rolston 1980). Almost any inorganic fibers can be incorporated into a composite. Natural fibers such as cotton, jute, hemp, paper, and silk have been studied as reinforcements. However, the major problem is their susceptibility to fungal and insect attack and to degradation by moisture. Synthetic fibers, cellulosics, polyamides, polyvinyls, polyacrylonitrile, polyethylene, and polyesters have also found uses in composites.

Glass fibers belong to a group of inorganic man-made mineral fibers (MMMF). The main component in glass is silicon dioxide. The glass is usually in the form of continuous or chopped fibers in PCs (Tarvainen et al. 1994). The glass fibers are coated (sized) with chemicals to facilitate their binding to roving or to the matrix: they may be coated, for example, with polyvinyl polyacetate, chromium chloride, polyvinyl acetate, polyester silane, or epoxy silanes. Organic chromium compounds are used for coupling, and solid or liquid epoxies, polyesters, and polyvinyl acetate are useful for film forming. The lubricants and emulsifiers used in glass fibers are usually water-soluble oils or other mixtures containing surface-active agents (Rolston 1980).

Graphite and carbon fibers are generally prepared by the thermal decomposition of three fibrous organic precursors: polyacrylonitrile (PAN), rayon (cellulose), or pitch. The primary advantages of graphite over glass fibers are, among other things, its higher modulus and lower density. Graphite fibers are available in various forms: continuous, chopped, woven fabric, or mat. Hybrid fabrics with glass or aramid fibers are available. The carbon fibers usually intended for reinforcement are spun into rows and prepared for prepregs by impregnation with resins (Midtgård and Knudsen 1994).

Aramid fiber is a common name for aromatic polyamide fibers, which are fire-resistant and strong synthetic fibers. The fibers are produced as continuous filaments, and they are used primarily in high-temperature engineering thermoplastics, such as polyamides, polybutylene, terephthalate, and polycarbonate. Application areas include marine, aerospace, and military equipment.

Prepregs are materials that have been impregnated with a partially cured polymer matrix. Glass, carbon, graphite, and aramid fibers, in woven, roving, or in unidirectional tape form, are combined with specially formulated pre-catalyzed resin systems. Prepregs are provided as rolls, tapes, or precut squares, rectangles, and as laminates, and are used to produce composites that are faster and cleaner to apply than wet lay-up systems. Covered by a flexible backing paper, prepregs can easily be handled, molded, or laminated into the desired shape. Hardening of prepreg laminates is usually achieved by heating at elevated temperatures under pressure or by autoclave in accordance with the manufacturer's specification, resulting in activation of the curing system (Stewart 2009). Thermosetting prepregs are most often used in the aircraft industry, in the manufacture of boats, rotor blades, windmill parts, and various sporting and leisure goods. Thermoplastic resins, such as polypropylene and polyamides, are also used in prepregs. The working methods are the same as those used for thermosetting resin prepregs.

In addition to continuous fibers, other types of reinforcements are also used. These include particulate materials, such as graphite and glass in powder form, as well as silica and clay. The use of nanomaterials in PCs will, without doubt, increase in the future.

7 Dermatoses from Plastic Composites

In the PC industry, skin hazards include the following contact dermatoses: ACD, irritant contact dermatitis (ICD), and contact urticaria. The skin symptoms of occupational dermatitis usually appear on the hands, but also on other open skin areas, such as the wrists, flexures, face, legs, and ankles, which are exposed to workplace dusts and fumes. A finished PC product only occasionally causes contact allergy. Epidemiological studies have been conducted in the aircraft and boat building industries, in a factory manufacturing various glass-fiber-reinforced plastics, and in the manufacture of hat racks, ski poles, skis, and printed circuit boards (➋ *Table 56.4*) (Tarvainen and Kanerva 2000). Most of the reported dermatoses in PC manufacture have been case reports; these, together with the causes, are listed in ➋ *Tables 56.5* and ➋ *56.6*.

8 Allergic Contact Dermatitis

8.1 Epoxy Resins

Currently, epoxy resin compounds are the most common cause of ACD from PCs. The clinical picture of allergic epoxy dermatitis from composites may vary. Most cases of ACD caused by epoxy resin have been reported regarding DGEBA epoxy resins (see ➋ Chap. 51, "Epoxy Resins"). Epoxy resin hardeners, such as diethylenetriamine (DETA) and triethylenetetramine (TETA),

Table 56.4
Prevalence of occupational dermatoses in the plastic composite industry

Product	Methods	Number of workers	Prevalence of dermatoses (%)[a]	References
Aircraft	Clinical	30	6	Malten (1956)
Hat rack	Clinical	50	25	Malten and Zielhuis (1964)
Aircraft	Clinical	2137	5	Bord and Castellain (1967)
Ski poles	Clinical	101	15	Suhonen (1983)
Printed circuit boards	Clinical	79	22	Bruze and Almgren (1989)
Boats, pipes	Clinical	89	26	Tarvainen et al. (1993b)
Skis	Clinical	22	26	Jolanki et al. (1996)
Aircraft	Clinical	92	16	Bruze et al. (1996)
Boats	Questionnaire	151	25.6	Ruttenberg et al. (2001)
Boats, tanks	Questionnaire	148	58,8	Minamoto et al. (2002)
Wind turbines	Clinical	603	62.4	Rasmussen et al. (2005)

[a]Calculated from figures in the publications (Data from Tarvainen and Kanerva 2000)

Table 56.5
Causes of occupational allergic contact dermatitis and contact urticaria from plastic composite manufacture

Product	Cause	Dermatitis
Aircraft	DGEBA ER	ACD
	ER amine hardener	ACD
	Non-DGEBA epoxy resin	ACD
	UP resin	ACD
	Chromium (VI)	ACD
	Cyclohexanol peroxide	ACD
Boat	UP resin	ACD
	Cobalt	ACD
	Phenol formaldehyde resin	ACD
	Natural rubber latex	CU
Ski and ski poles	DGEBA ER	ACD, CU
	ER amine hardener	ACD, CU
	MTHPA	CU
	Polyester resin	CU
	Cobalt	ACD
Tennis rackets	ER IPDA hardener	ACD
TV cabinets	UP dust	ACD
	Rubber gloves	ACD
	MEK peroxide	ACD
Various	DGEBA	ACD
	UP resin	ACD
Dental composites	Methacrylates	ACD
Wind turbines	DGEBF	ACD

Data from: Tarvainen and Kanerva (1999)
ACD allergic contact dermatitis, *CU* contact urticaria, *DGEBA* diglycidylether of bisphenol-A, *DGEBF* diglycidylether of bisphenol-F, *UP* unsaturated polyester, *IPDA* isophoronediamine, *ER* epoxy resin, *MEK* methylethyl ketone

Table 56.6
Causes of irritant occupational contact dermatoses from plastic composite manufacture

Product	Cause
Aircraft	Glass fiber
	Mold releasers
	Prepregs
Boats	UP resin
	Glass fiber
	Styrene
Prepregs	Methylene dianiline
	Glass fiber
Skis and skipoles	Glass fiber dust
	DGEBA ER

Data from: Tarvainen and Kanerva (1999)
DGEBA diglycidylether of bisphenol-A, *UP* unsaturated polyester, *ER* epoxy resin

ethylenediamine, isophoronediamine (IPDA) (Lachapelle et al. 1978), or hexavalent chromate in an epoxy resin hardener, have also been reported to cause ACD. In the manufacture of carbon-fiber-reinforced composites, workers have been sensitized to non-DGEBA epoxy resins, including tetraglycidyl-4-4′-methylendianiline (TGMDA), triglycidyl-*p*-aminophenol (TGPAP), and 4-glycidyloxy-N,N-diglycidylaniline (Burrows et al. 1984; Mathias 1987; Lembo et al. 1989; Tarvainen et al. 1995; Jolanki et al. 1996). Not only workers manufacturing PC products but also cleaners have had delayed allergic reactions to a DGEBA epoxy resin used in ski poles (Suhonen 1983).

Six workers exposed to epoxy resin in a ski factory showed allergic reactions to the standard DGEBA epoxy resin as well as to a DGEBA epoxy resin used in the ski factory (Jolanki et al. 1996). Three of the workers reacted to reactive diluents (diethylene glycol diglycidyl ether DEGDGE) (➋ *Fig. 56.1*), phenyl glycidyl ether (PGE), and 1,4-butanediol diglycidyl ether (BDDGE). In a cross-sectional study of four facilities producing wind turbine systems in Denmark, clinically diagnosed dermatitis was found in 35.8% of 724 production workers; 61% were allergic to epoxy compounds and 37.9% to hardeners (Rasmussen et al. 2005). Epoxy resin compounds in prepregs are reported to cause ACD in workers in aircraft factories. In addition to ACD affecting the hands, patients also had airborne symptoms on the face when working in room where epoxy chemicals were handled (Kanerva et al. 2000).

Epoxy resins have been reported to cause skin sensitization more frequently than unsaturated polyester resins during simultaneous exposure to both resins. They are also suspected to be a concomitant factor in unsaturated polyester allergy (Wehle 1966).

8.2 Epoxy Vinyl Ester Resins

No cases of allergic or irritant contact dermatitis or contact urticaria caused by epoxy vinyl ester resins in industrial PCs have been reported. Sensitization from epoxy (meth)acrylates (BIS-GMA) has been reported in dental personnel (Aalto-Korte et al. 2003), and in connection with the use of the ultraviolet (UV) curing inks and anaerobic glues (Kanerva et al. 1989). Glycidyl methacrylate has been reported to cause a severe chemical burn after an accidental spill (Shimizu et al. 2008).

8.3 Unsaturated Polyester Resin

ACD caused by PCs were first reported in connection with unsaturated polyester resins by Lieber (1955), followed by Malten and Zielhuis (1964), who described five patients with contact eczema and positive patch tests to unsaturated polyester resins in a group of 30 workers in an airplane factory. ACD has been reported in connection with a limb prosthesis made from unsaturated polyester resin (Vincenzi et al. 1991). Cases of ACD caused by unsaturated polyester resin in lamination work, UV-light-cured inks, unsaturated polyester dust from reinforced plastic products, and automobile-repair putty have also been reported (Tarvainen et al. 1993a).

The small number of cases of ACD in the reinforced plastics industry is probably due to the low sensitizing capacity of unsaturated polyester resin (➲ Chap. 54, "Polyester Resins") (Bourne and Milner 1963; Tarvainen et al. 1993a, b; Tarvainen et al. 1995). The allergens in unsaturated polyester resins are often the auxiliary chemicals in the resin, such as cobalt naphthenate or cobalt octoate, phthalates, tricresyl phosphate, peroxide hardeners, or cross-linking monomers. Para-tertiary-butyl catechol used in the manufacture of styrene has caused contact allergy followed by vitiligo in workers in the PC industry (Bourne and Milner 1963; Malten and Zielhuis 1964; Horio et al. 1977).

The starting materials or intermediate substances in resin production, such as free or terminal maleic, fumaric, or adipic acids and their anhydrides, have also caused ACD (Minamoto et al. 2002). A macromolecule containing maleic ester, polyester methacrylate, or diethylene glycol maleate (DGM) (➲ *Fig. 56.2*) has also been reported as a cause of sensitization (Tarvainen et al. 1993a; Liden et al. 1984).

8.4 Polyurethane Resins

Fully cured polyurethane products do not generally cause dermatitis, but there are circumstances where skin problems can arise. Monomeric di-isocyanate may remain inside the product as a result of the slow curing process. Release of free isocyanate may then occur during heating, cutting, and sanding. Exposure to di-isocyanates may cause allergic or irritant dermatitis or urticaria. The main occupational hazards from polyurethanes are the di-isocyanates, which are well-known for their ability to cause rhinitis, asthma, and conjunctivitis (Estlander et al. 1992).

8.5 Phenol-Formaldehyde Resins

PF resins can cause chemical burns, irritant and allergic contact dermatoses, contact urticaria, and depigmentation. Residual raw materials and the intermediates and oligomers used in the formation of the resin have been reported as causative agents (➲ Chap. 52, "Contact Allergy to Phenol-Formaldehyde Resins"). ACD is possible, especially when handling fresh resins, for example, when cellulose or other prepregs are impregnated with phenol-

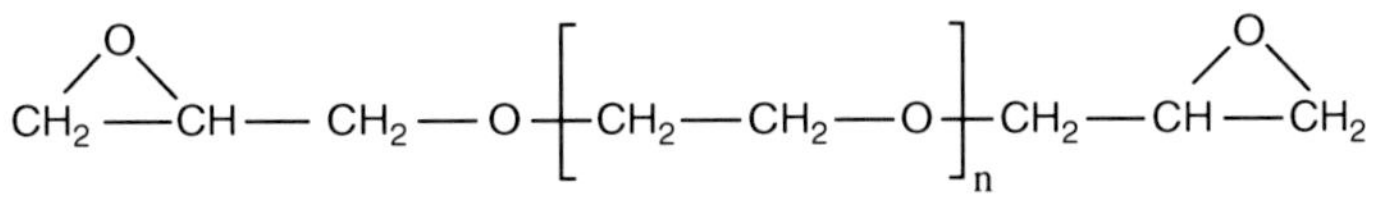

Fig. 56.1
Ethylene glycol diglycidyl ether (Quetol 651, *n* = 1) and diethyleneglycol diglycidyl ether (DEGDGE, *n* = 2)

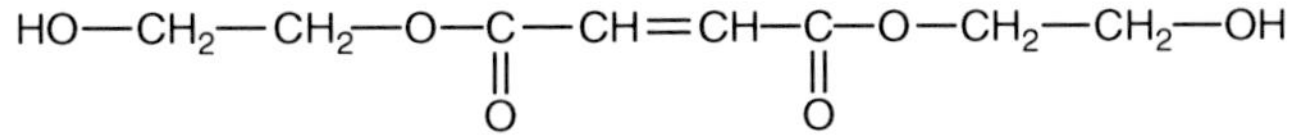

Fig. 56.2
Diethyleneglycol maleate (DGM)

formaldehyde resin or melamine-formaldehyde resin. Concomitant ACD caused both by phenol formaldehyde resins and melamine formaldehyde resins has been reported (Isaksson et al. 1999).

8.6 Polyethylene and Polypropylene

Cases of irritant and ACD caused by polyethylene and polypropylene are rare. Contact dermatitis may be caused by plastic additives such as catalysts and initiators. Heat, sawing, and other forming may cause degradation of the plastic and therefore release reactive chemicals into the air. Thus, airborne dermatitis is also possible in such operations (Björkner 2006).

8.7 Additives

ACD is reported in connection with various plastic additives (Björkner 2006), mostly in UPR and epoxy resins. Several allergic agents have been identified, although many of them are used only infrequently. Cases of ACD caused by dibutyl phthalate in a plastic watch strap, diethyl phthalate in spectacle frames, dimethyl phthalate in computer mice, and o-diglycidyl phthalate in aircraft production have been reported (Björkner 2006). ACD has also been found to be caused by bisphenol A in PVC gloves (Aalto-Korte et al. 2003).

8.8 Man-Made Mineral Fibers

ACD from glass fibers has been caused by sizing chemicals in MMMF production, such as epoxy resin of amine-functional methoxysilane (Sertoli et al. 2000) The risk of sensitization by contact with glass fibers is mainly due to professional exposure to the resins used for the finishing of glass fibers. ACD is reported in those who are in contact with uncured sizing resins, in particular epoxy and formaldehyde resins (Sertoli et al. 2000). Aramid fibers are not sensitizing.

9 Irritant Contact Dermatitis

Fiber reinforcements are the main cause of irritant contact dermatitis, both in the manufacture of PCs and in the finished products (➋ *Table 56.6*). Workers exposed to MMMF most frequently suffer itching without dermatitis, or rapidly healing papules and vesicles. Secondary lesions from scratching may lead to bacterial infections. Most workers will develop tolerance to MMMF itch within a few weeks of continuous exposure. However, not all workers become tolerant, and they may need to be transferred to another job. Of 28 patients who had been diagnosed with occupational dermatitis and had to change jobs, 21 patients were found to have irritant contact dermatitis caused by MMMFs (Sertoli et al. 2000; Tarvainen and Kanerva 2000). In addition, glass fibers in a school desk have caused irritant contact dermatitis (Eby and Jetton 1972).

The health hazards of carbon fiber handling are due to mechanical irritation and abrasion similar to that caused by glass fibers. Carbon fibers are easily broken by stretching, and the fibers can easily produce a fine dust during cutting. The particle size of the carbon fiber dust in the machining of PCs is considered to be too large to damage the respiratory system. Uncontrolled micro fibers have a potential to adhere to human skin or mucous membranes, causing irritation. Aramid fibers irritate the skin only in special situations. Rubbing of the fiber causes scaling into small, thin fibers which irritate the skin and may be inhaled deep into the respiratory organism (Saarela et al. 2007).

Although DGEBA epoxy resins are not strong irritants, cases of irritant contact dermatitis caused by DGEBA epoxy resins have been reported (Jolanki et al. 1996). Latent epoxy resin hardeners, namely, the carboxylic acid anhydrides may cause severe chemical burns when heated. On the sweating skin, anhydrides are hydrolyzed to the corresponding acids and may cause caustic dermatitis and burns (Jolanki et al. 2000). The hardener MTHPA has been reported to induce redness and hives on the skin (Kalimo et al. 1990). The irritant properties of unsaturated polyester resins and epoxy vinyl ester resins are most likely due to cross-linking styrene, or previously to diallyphthalate. Styrene is classified as a mild irritant, but repeated skin contact with styrene causes drying of the skin and may give rise to primary irritation, blisters, or even chemical burns (Bruze and Fregert 1994). However, skin resorption experiments with liquid styrene (Berode et al. 1985) have not caused skin symptoms in human volunteers. At levels of 50 ppm (215 mg/m), styrene vapor may irritate the conjunctivae and nasal mucous membranes. Some mold-releasing agents irritate the skin. For example, a patient packing thin composite bundles made of carbon fibers and DGEBA also used a mold-releasing agent containing 3% (wt./vol.) alkyl orthophosphate. The patient's hand dermatitis was located at the contact site of the bundles. Standard patch tests and the patient's own chemicals were negative, while according to the material data sheet, alkyl orthophosphate is a caustic chemical (Tarvainen et al. 1995).

Organic peroxides used as a 3–10% solution to initiate the curing reaction of unsaturated polyester, epoxy vinyl ester, and acrylic resins, have caused irritant dermatitis and blisters in workers in the PC industry (Bourne and Milner 1963). Reactive peroxide molecules in unhardened resin dust may cause stinging of uncovered skin areas during spray lamination. Acetone is used to clean equipment in the unsaturated polyester- and vinyl-ester-resin industries. On repeated contact, acetone defats the skin and has been reported to be a contributing factor for irritant dermatitis in the PC industry.

10 Contact Urticaria

Occupational allergic contact urticaria refers to the IgE-mediated, type I immediate contact reactions caused by exposure to substances in the work environment. Most cases of contact urticaria in PC manufacture have been caused by the natural rubber latex (NRL) proteins in protective rubber gloves. There are only a few reports of contact urticaria caused by the epoxy resin compounds used for PCs, including DGEBA epoxy resin and a polyamine hardener. On the other hand, IgE-mediated allergy and contact urticaria to carboxylic acid anhydrides (MTHPA, MHHPA and phthalic anhydride) in heat-cured epoxy resins and the starting materials of unsaturated polyester resin are reported more often, and they sometimes present in connection with generalized urticaria and/or upper respiratory symptoms. The processes have included lamination work, and the use of prepregs and sealants (Helaskoski et al. 2009; Tarvainen et al. 1995). Immediate allergy has been verified by an open skin test with 100% MHHPA and by positive skin scratch tests and radioallergosorbent tests (RASTs) using a human serum albumin (HSA)-conjugated test substance as the allergen (Helaskoski et al. 2009).

In a recent report, workers who experienced contact urticaria from acid anhydrides were working near the area for the curing of plastics, or mixing resin and hardener, cleaning the curing oven, repairing the curing area, or welding painted pipes. The principal route of exposure to acid anhydride was direct contact, or in a few cases airborne exposure. Airborne concentrations caused more widespread urticaria than direct skin contact. While IgE-mediated allergy to carboxylic acid anhydrides has been shown in many patients, it seems that allergic respiratory diseases, such as asthma and rhinitis, are more common than urticaria (Helaskoski et al. 2009).

11 Other Skin and Health Hazards

The use of machining equipment is associated with a risk of mechanical injuries, such as cuts or abrasions. Some processes operate at high temperatures and involve a danger of severe burns. A risk of fire and explosion is inherent to the nature of the raw materials used in industry. Styrene, acetone, and peroxides form flammable and explosive concentrations at normal room temperature. Certain chemical combinations are particularly hazardous, such as the mixture of organic peroxides and cobalt accelerators (Brigham and Landrigan 1985).

The health hazards in PC operations include respiratory hazards from exposure to toxic monomers, curing agents, solvents, dust, and fumes from thermal degradation products. Vapors of monomers and solvents are released into the ambient air during repair operations and during the curing of the resins. Solvent exposure is highest during degreasing and cleaning procedures and when using styrene-containing polyester resins (Midtgård and Knudsen 1994). Carboxylic acid anhydrides can cause IgE-mediated rhinitis and asthma. DGEBA epoxy resin has been considered to be responsible for IgE-mediated asthma. During open lamination, workers are exposed to styrene vapor (Eriksson and Wiklund 2004). The most common health problem related to styrene exposure is its neurotoxicity, resulting in symptoms of solvent encephalopathy. Symptoms include depression, concentration and memory problems, muscle weakness, fatigue, unsteadiness, and nausea. Exposure to styrene may also irritate the nose, throat, and eyes. Dermal absorption of styrene fumes has been shown to be low in humans compared with inhalation exposure (Riihimäki and Pfäffli 1978).

12 Diagnosis of Allergic Contact Dermatitis Caused by Plastic Composites

The cause of ACD in the handling of PC should be verified by patch tests. In the reported cases, standard patch-test trays have been used together with special epoxy resin test substances, other plastic chemicals, and chemicals from workplaces (Burrows et al. 1984; Mathias 1987; Lembo et al. 1989; Tarvainen et al. 1995; Jolanki et al. 1996). Safety data sheets (SDS) or product declarations on the chemicals are essential in choosing the correct patch test substances and concentrations. Care should be taken to prevent active sensitization through patch testing with test concentrations that are too high. The risk of active sensitization should be borne in mind, especially in testing prepregs, which are solid material and cannot be diluted. Prepregs may contain 10–25% by weight of uncured resin. Patch tests with samples cut from epoxy prepreg should only be performed on individuals already suspected on a clinical basis to be allergic (Mathias 1987).

Immediate allergy can be examined by skin-prick tests, scratch tests, or use tests, and determination of specific IgE antibodies in the patient's serum. Low-molecular-weight chemicals can be conjugated with HSA (Howe et al. 1983) before they are used in skin-prick tests or RAST examinations (Cesca and Lundgvist 1972).

Chemical analyses may be needed for the identification of new allergens and in order to find the allergens responsible for the patient's reactions to PC materials. These analyses may require liquid or gas chromatography coupled with spectroscopic methods, and they are often carried out in specialized laboratories. Thin-layer chromatography (TLC) can also be used in the separation of resin allergens, e.g., in unsaturated polyester resin and phenolformaldehyde resins (Tarvainen et al. 1993b)

Up-to-date knowledge about commercial raw materials, devices (equipment), and accessories can be found on the web sites of the companies and communities concerned. This knowledge may help both in the investigation of the causes of occupational disorders and in planning workplaces and working methods.

13 Prevention of Occupational Dermatitis

Irritant dermatitis and skin trauma often predispose individuals to ACD. In the PC industry, skin-irritating solvents, resins, and glass fibers predispose the skin to sensitization to resins, especially to epoxy resins. Exposure to epoxy chemicals may be low and of short duration before the appearance of dermatitis. Uncured chemicals on the surface of prepregs can easily cause sensitization (Estlander et al. 1992). Workers feeling only a slight tackiness of resin may not protect themselves sufficiently compared to the protection they would use during the handling of epoxy resin in its liquid form (Mathias 1987; Lembo et al. 1989; Tarvainen et al. 1995).

Even very small amounts of allergen can evoke dermatitis in previously sensitized subjects; this is also encountered in PC workers (Tarvainen et al. 1995). Thus, careful avoidance of any contacts with the allergens is needed in order to prevent skin manifestations. A small amount of the allergen in dust or in a finished product is sometimes enough to maintain or restore dermatitis, and in such cases, the sensitized person may have to change to another job. Discontinuing work with epoxy chemicals immediately after the diagnosis of contact allergy may also be beneficial in preventing respiratory problems. Dermatitis due to epoxy resin compounds is more severe when the exposure time to the causative agent has been long (Jolanki et al. 1996).

The use of protective gloves is essential in avoiding exposure to PC materials. Protective gloves are helpful in preventing dermatitis due to chemicals and glass fibers as well as mechanical, thermal, or chemical injuries or burns. Furthermore, workers who use gloves wash their hands less frequently, thus avoiding the drying effect of frequent hand washing (Tarvainen et al. 1993b). Chemical protective gloves suitable also for solvent work are often needed; general recommendations for the use of appropriate gloves are available in textbooks and from the glove suppliers. Rubber gloves do not necessarily offer enough protection against the solvents used in the PC industry and may cause sensitization to NRL or to rubber chemicals (➔ Chapter 65, "Rubber"). However, cotton under-gloves may prevent sensitization to NRL or to the rubber chemicals in protective gloves.

Incomplete protection has frequently been the cause of occupational PC dermatitis. Workers have been sensitized through epoxy resin splashes, uncured resin compounds in composite waste materials or through vapors, despite the use of protective gloves (Jolanki et al. 1996).

Good working practices and workplace hygiene are necessary, along with well-organized general and local ventilation, and automatic or closed processes should be used. These measures are important in the prevention of occupational dermatoses as well as respiratory and central nervous system symptoms. Workers should be aware of the best working techniques and the risks associated with the chemicals being handled. Workers need to be educated regarding the potential hazards when handling PCs and auxiliary chemicals, and they should be taught to use "no-touch" techniques when working with these materials, whether liquid or prepregs (Isaksson and Bruze 2000). Good skin care with emollients and rapid treatment of skin injuries also reduces the risk of allergic dermatitis.

References

Aalto-Korte K, Alanko K, Henriks-Eckerman ML et al (2003) Allergic contact demrtitis from bisphenol A in PVC gloves. Contact Dermatitis 49:202–205

Ashori A (2008) Wood-plastic composites as promising green-composites for automotive industries. Bioresour Technol 99:4661–4667

Berode M, Droz P-O, Guillemin M (1985) Human exposure to styrene. VI. Percutaneous absorption in human volunteers. Int Arch Occup Environ Health 55:331–336

Björkner B (2006) Plasticizers and other additives in synthetic polymers. In: Frosch PJ, Menné T, Lepoittevin JP (eds) Contact dermatitis, 4th edn. Springer, Berlin, pp 611–613

Boenig H (1964) Unsaturated polyesters: structure and properties. Elsevier, Amsterdam, pp 6–13

Bord A, Castellain P-Y (1967) Les dermatoses professionaelles dans l'industrie aéronautique. (Occupational dermatoses in the aircraft industry, in French). Rev Fr Allergol 7:85–91

Bourne L, Milner F (1963) Polyester resin hazards. Br J Ind Med 20:100–109

Bowen RL (1962) Dental filling material comprising vinyl silane treated fused silica and a binder consisting of reaction product of bisphenol and glycidyl acrylate. US Patent 3,066,112

Brigham CR, Landrigan PJ (1985) Safety and health in boatbuilding and repair. Am J Ind Med 8:169–182

Bruze M, Almgren G (1989) Occupational dermatoses in workers exposed to epoxy-impregnated fiberglass fabric. Dermatosen 37: 171–175

Bruze M, Fregert S (1994) Chemical skin burn. In: Menne T, Maibach HI (eds) Hand eczema. CRC Press, Boca Raton, pp 21–30

Bruze M, Edenholm M, Engström K, Svensson G (1996) Occupational dermatoses in a Swedish aircraft plant. Contact Dermatitis 34(5): 336–340

Burrows D, Fregert S, Cambell H et al (1984) Contact dermatitis from epoxy resins tetraglycidyl-4,4′-methylene dianiline and o-diglycidyl phthalate in composite material. Contact Dermatitis 11:80–82

Cesca M, Lundgvist U (1972) A new and simple radioimmuno assey method for determination of IgE. Immunochemistry 9:1021–1030

Eby CS, Jetton RL (1972) School desk dermatitis. Primary irritant contact dermatitis to fiberglass. Arch Dermatol 105:890–891

Ehrenstein G, Kabelka J (2007) Reinforced plastics. In: Ullmans encyclopedia of industrial chemistry, 7th edn. Wiley-VCH, Weinheim

Eriksson K, Wiklund L (2004) Dermal exposure to styrene in the fiberglass reinforced plastics industry. Ann Occup Hyg 48:203–208

Estlander T, Keskinen H, Jolanki R et al (1992) Occupational dermatitis from exposure to polyurethane chemicals. Contact Dermatitis 27:161–165

Helaskoski E, Kuuliala O, Aalto-Korte K (2009) Occupational contact urticaria caused by cyclic acid anhydrides. Contact Dermatitis 60:214–221

Horio T, Tanaka K, Komura J (1977) Depigmentation due to para-tertiary butylcatechol. Int Arch Occup Environ Health 39:127–133

Howe W, Venables KM, Topping MD (1983) Tetrachlorophthalic anhydride asthma: evidence for specific IgE antibody. J Allergy Clin Immunol 71:5–13

Ilschner B, Lees K, Dhingra A et al (2007) Composite materials. In: Ullmans encyclopedia of industrial chemistry, 7th edn. Wiley-VCH, Weinheim

IPCS (1997) International programme on chemical safety. World Health Organization, Environmental Health Criteria, Geneva, 133 pp

Isaksson M, Bruze M (2000) Aircraft Industry. In: Kanerva L, Elsner P, Wahlber JE, Maibach HI (eds) Handbook of occupational dermatology. Springer, Berlin/Heidelberg/New York, pp 805–807

Isaksson M, Zimerson E, Bruze M (1999) Occupational dermatoses in composite production. J Occup Environ Med 41(4):261–266

Jolanki R, Tarvainen K, Tatar T et al (1996) Occupational dermatoses from exposure to epoxy resin compounds in a ski factory. Contact Dermatitis 34:390–396

Jolanki R, Kanerva L, Estlander T (2000) Epoxy resins. In: Kanerva L, Elsner P, Wahlber JE, Maibach HI (eds) Handbook of occupational dermatology. Springer, Berlin/Heidelberg/New York, pp 570–590

Kalimo K, Liira K, Nordman H et al (1990) IgE-mediated allergy to methytetrahydrophthalic anhydride among workers producing electrical components. Contact Dermatitis 23:280

Kanerva L, Estlander T, Jolanki R (1989) Allergic contact dermatitis caused by epoxy diacrylate in ultraviolet-light-cured paint, and bisphenol A in dental composite resin. Contact Dermatitis 20:201–211

Kanerva L, Estlander T, Jolanki R (1996) Occupational allergic contact dermatitis caused by 2,4,6-tri-(dimethylaminomethyl)phenol, and a review of sensitizing epoxy resin hardeners. Int J Dermatol 35:852–856

Kanerva L, Jolanki R, Estlander T et al (2000) Airborne occupational allergic contact dermatitis from triglycidyl-p-aminophenol and tetraglycidyl-4,4′-methylene dianiline in preimpregnated epoxy products in the aircraft industry. Dermatology 201:29–33

Kelly E (1994) Applications of composites. In: Kelly E (ed) Concise encyclopedia of composite material. Pergamon/Elsevier, Oxford, pp 7–9

Lachapelle J-M, Tennstedt D, Dumont-Fruyntier M (1978) Occupational allergic contact dermatitis to isophoronediamine (IPDA) used as an epoxy resin hardener. Contact Dermatitis 4:109–112

Lembo G, Balato N, Baldo A et al (1989) Contact dermatitis to epoxy resin in composite material. In: Frosch P, Dooms-Goossens A, Lachapelle J-M, Rycroft RJG, Sheper RJ (eds) Current topics in contact dermatitis. Springer, Berlin/Heidelberg/New York, pp 377–380

Liden C, Löfström A, Storgårds-Hatam K (1984) Contact allergy to unsaturated polyester in a boat builder. Contact Dermatitis 11:262–264

Lieber EE (1955) Dermatitis- an industrial problem. Br Plastics 28:428–429

Malten KE, Zielhuis R (1964) Polyester resins. In: Malten KE, Zielhuis P (eds) Industrial toxicology and dermatology in the production and processing of plastics. Elsevier, Amsterdam, pp 71–84

Mathias CGT (1987) Allergic contact dermatitis from a non-bisphenol A epoxy resin in a graphite fiber reinforced epoxy laminate. J Occup Med 29:754–755

Midtgård U, Knudsen LE (1994) Fiber-reinforced plastic sand advanced polymer composites. Occupational hazards and toxicity of selected compounds. Nordic Council of Ministers and National Institute of Occupational Health, Copenhagen, pp 1–73

Minamoto K, Nagano M, Yonemitsu K et al (2002) Allergic contact dermatitis from unsaturated polyester resin consisting of maleic anhydride, phthalic anhydrid, ethylene glycol and dicyclopentadiene. Contact Dermatitis 46:62–63

Pontén A, Carstensen O, Rasmussen K et al (2004) Epoxy-based production of wind turbine rotor blades: occupational dermatoses. Contact Dermatitis 50:329–338

Rasmussen K, Carstensen O, Pontén A et al (2005) Risk of contact allergy and dermatitis at a wind turbine plant using epoxy resin-based plastics. Int Arch Occup Environ Health 78:211–217

Rolston JA (1980) Fiberglass composite materials and fabrication processes. Chem Eng 87:96–100

Ruttenberg D, Dryson E, Walls C, Curran N (2001) Hazards associated with the boat building industry in New Zealand: an OSH audit. N Z Med J 25:114(1132):225–226

Riihimäki V, Pfäffli P (1978) Percutaneous absorption of solvent vapours in man. Scand J Work Environ Health 4:73–85

Saarela O, Airasmaa I, Kokko J, Skrifvars M, Komppa V (eds) (2007) Kertamuovit (in Finish) Thermosetting plastics. Aramid fibers, prepregs. In: Komposiittirakenteet. Muoviyhdistys ry./ Hakapaino Oy, Helsinki, pp 35–51, 89,142–145

Sertoli A, Francalanci S, Giorgini S (2000) Fiberglass dermatitis. In: Kanerva L, Elsner P, Wahlber JE, Maibach HI (eds) Handbook of occupational dermatology. Springer, Berlin/Heidelberg/New York, pp 122–134

Shimizu A, Kamada N, Kamble N et al (2008) Chemical burn caused by glycidyl methacrylate. Contact Dermatitis 59:316–317

Stepeck J, Daoust H (1983) Additives for plastics, polymers/properties and applications, vol 5. Springer, New York, 243 p

Stewart R (2009) New prepreg materials offer versatility, top performance. Reinf Plast 53(5):28–33

Suhonen R (1983) Epoxy dermatitis in a ski factory. Contact Dermatitis 9:131–133

Tarvainen K, Kanerva L (1999) Occupational dermatoses from plastic composites. J Environ Med 1:3–17

Tarvainen K, Kanerva L (2000) Plastic composites. In: Kanerva L, Elsner P, Wahlberg JE, Maibach HI (eds) Handbook of occupational dermatology. Springer, Berlin/Heidelberg/New York, pp 611–621

Tarvainen K, Jolanki R, Forsman-Grönholm L et al (1993a) Exposure, skin protection and occupational diseases in the glass-fiber-reinforced plastics industry. Contact Dermatitis 29:119–127

Tarvainen K, Jolanki R, Estlander T (1993b) Occupational contact allergy to unsaturated polyester cements. Contact Dermatitis 28: 220–224

Tarvainen K, Estlander T, Jolanki R et al (1994) Occupational dermatoses from the manufacture of man-made-mineral fibers. Am J Contact Dermatitis 5:22–29

Tarvainen K, Kanerva L, Jolanki R et al (1995) Occupational dermatoses from the manufacture of plastic composite products. Am J Contact Dermatitis 6:95–104

Vincenzi C, Cameli N, Vassipoulou A et al (1991) Allergic contact dermatitis due to benzoyl peroxide in an arm prosthesis. Contact Dermatitis 24:66–67

Wehle U (1966) Arbeitsbedingte Eczeme durch polyester. (Occupational eczema from polyester, in English). Allerg Asthma 12:184–186

Wolf R, Kaul BL (2007) Plastics, additives. In: Ullmans encyclopedia of industrial chemistry, 7th edn. Wiley-VCH, Weinheim

Zimerson E (2006) Phenol-formaldehyde resins. Plasticizers and other additives in synthetic polymers. In: Frosch PJ, Menné T, Lepoittevin JP (eds) Contact dermatitis, 4th edn. Springer, Berlin, pp 600–603

57 Inks and Dyes

Christophe J. Le Coz
Cabinet de Dermatologie, Strasbourg, France
Unite Dermato–Allergologie, Hopitaux Universitaires de Strasbourg, Strasbourg, France
Laboratoire de Dermatochimie, Strasbourg, France

Core Messages

- CM1. Although seldom reported, contact dermatitis in printing industry seems frequent (in almost 50% of workers).
- CM2. Soaps, detergents, and solvents are mainly responsible for irritant contact dermatitis.
- CM3. Allergic contact dermatitis due to inks is mainly reported from (meth-)acrylic compounds in UV-curable inks and varnishes.
- CM4. Permanent hair coloring systems are frequent sensitizers in hairdressers, with dyes (*p*-phenylenediamine, toluene 2,5-diamine and *p*-aminophenol) and coupling agents (*m*-aminophenol).
- CM5. Textile dyes in industry can sensitize workers, mainly in emerging countries, during the fabrication, the mixing of dyes, and the tinting textile processes.
- CM6. Among textile dyes, the most frequent sensitizers are disperse dyes (anthraquinone and azo dyes), fiber-reactive dyes, and the coupling agent Naphthol AS.

1 Inks

1.1 Introduction

Inks are colored liquids (fluid or viscous) intended to be applied as thin layers on several media, in order to (re) produce information, message, image, or decoration. Inks can be employed in a domestic, leisure, or medical activity, but most frequently during an industrial process. Media may be paper, cardboard, wood, glass, textile, plastic, ceramics, metals, or even animal and human skin (FIPEC 2011; Castaing and Guilleux 2010).

Inks are more or less a complex and subtle mixture of coloring substance dispersed in a vehicle or binder. Coloring substances can be classified into dyes (generally soluble into the binder) and pigments (nonsoluble, but dispersed after crushing and mixing). The binders differ in the type of ink used: they can be fat binders (mixture of resins and oils), solvent-based, water-based, and can contain resins, oils and lubricants, UV-curing or electronic-curing systems, charges, and many additives like plasticizers, surfactants, stabilizers, (photo-) initiators, and preservatives.

Numerous allergens can be contained in classical inks, some of them being tested by the standard series like colophony or chromates (Meyer et al. 2000) but mostly at very low concentration. Printing industry is automated; some products like lead-based or chrome-based pigments are or will progressively be banned, and at least in occidental countries, occupational medicine highly contributes to prevention of allergies in workers, but direct skin contact with inks are frequent (constant) among workers. With the exception of UV-curable inks, occupational allergy to classical inks is now seldom reported, most cases being published before 1990 (Foussereau and Benezra 1970; Castelain et al. 1980; Foussereau 1991). Nevertheless, a recent study based on questionnaires reported a prevalence of skin complaints among 49% of 274 workers from contact with inks in the printing industry in the United Kingdom (Livesley et al. 2002).

1.2 Nonindustrial Inks

Some cases are reported, but rarely concern occupational activities; inks for stencils, bank checks, and stamps were reported (Braun 1975). *Aminoazotoluene and derivatives* contained in fountain pens and ballpoint pen inks were used in the 1950s (Foussereau and Benezra 1970; Cronin 1980).

Silver nitrate, at a 10% component of the ink contained in a skin marker used to mark patch testing, is a classical irritant but seems to be a rare allergen, with two cases reported in 1948 and due to marking patch tests (Özkaya 2009). It was tested 1% pet. and one patient also reacted to silver sulfadiazine cream.

1.3 Inks in Printing Industry

Different ways of application can be used for printing inks: direct application on the support (by writing or painting)

T. Rustemeyer, P. Elsner, S.M. John & H.I. Maibach (eds.), *Kanerva's Occupational Dermatology*,
DOI 10.1007/978-3-642-02035-3_57,

or a mechanical printing process like letterpress (the older process), flexography, photogravure, offset, silk-screen printing, digital printing, or roller coating. The main classes of inks depend on the type of application. Offset inks contain pigments (carbon, mineral, or organic type), resins, oils, and additives. Flexography and photogravure processes use solvent or water-based inks.

1.3.1 Composition of Inks

Solvent inks contain pigments, resins, solvents, and additives. Water-based inks include water (10–75%), pigments, resins, solvents, and additives: the binder is generally a blend of polymers like polyester-acrylics, polyurethane-acrylics, with surfactants, antifoam, and alcohols as additives. Some compositions are indicated in ➋ *Table 57.1*.

For silk-screen printing, the quality of the inks strongly depends on the medium: some are listed in ➋ *Table 57.2*.

Since industrial processes are – at least in occidental countries – highly automated, occupational skin contact with inks, and consecutive occupational dermatitis induced by such agents, seems more rarely reported than in earlier times. Most cases of dermatitis are described in

Table 57.1

Ingredients and compositions of some inks (Adapted from Castaing and Guilleux 2010), with indication of some irritant (*) allergenic (**) compounds

	Dyes and pigments *,**	Resins *,**	Solvents (for solvent inks)*	Oils *	Additives *,**
Offset	Carbon black	Hard resins:		Mineral oils	Siccatives: metal carboxylates like cobalt**or magnesium octoate
	Metals and metallic salts: titanium dioxide, calcium carbonate, zinc oxide* and sulfur, silicates*, iron oxides*, chromate oxides (III) and (VI) *,**, etc.,	Colophony and derivatives like gum ester*,**			
		Maleic (or fumaric-reacted) resins*,**		Vegetal oils: linen, tung, colza, soybean	Waxes: polyethylene, etc.
		Phenol-formaldehyde resins*,**			Antoxidants*,**: oximes (2-butanone oxime), BHT, hydroquinone, etc.
	Azo-dyes (mono- and di-azo)*,**	Alkyd resins: obtained by esterification of glycerol or pentaerythritol by phthalic anhydride and vegetal fatty acids*,**			Rheology modifiers*: silica, alcohols, triethanolamine, etc.
	Phthalocyanine dyes*,**				
	Dioxazin dyes *				
Flexography and photogravure solvent inks	Carbon black	Cellulosic resins (nitrocellulosic)	Alcohols: n-propanol, isopropanol, ethanol, etc.		Plasticizers: citrates, adipates, phthalates
	Metals and metallic salts: titanium dioxide, calcium carbonate, zinc oxide and sulfur, silicates, iron oxides *, chromate oxides (III) and (VI) **, etc.	Vinyl resins: polyvinyl acetate, polyvinyl chloride, etc.	Glycols and glycol ethers		Surfactants and antifoam
		Polyurethane resins (isocyanates based *,**) with polyfunctional aziridines **	Esters, ketons, hydrocarbons, etc.		Biocides: isothiazolinones*,**
		Acrylic resins*,**			
	Azo-dyes (mono- and di-azo) *,**	Other: polyamides, ketonic, maleic, polyester, urea-formaldehyde**, epoxy**, etc.			
	Phthalocyanine dyes*,**				
	Dioxazin dyes				

Table 57.2
Examples of inks used for silk-screen printing (Adapted from Castaing and Guilleux 2010)

Medium	Ink	Some special solvents and additives
Paper and cardboard	Nitrocellulosic, vinyl, acrylic, styrene-acrylic	Methoxypropanol, esters
Metals	Epoxy, polyester, nitrocellulosic	Butylglycol, hardening agents like diethylenetriamine
Plastics	Cellulosic, vinyl or acrylic	Mineral oils, ketones
Leather and textiles	Polyurethane	Isocyanates
	Plastisol (polymer within solvent)	Phthalates, PVC copolymers
Glass and china	Epoxy	Epoxy-silane, glycols
UV curable inks	(UV-curable) acrylic	Polyfunctional acrylates, primers

Table 57.3
Some components of UV-curable inks and overprint varnishes

Photo initiators	Acetophenone and alpha-hydroxyacetone derivatives
	Phosphine oxides
	Alpha-aminoketones
	Benzophenones
	Thioxanthone and derivatives
Monomers	Acrylates (A), diacrylates (DA), triacrylates (TA), etc.
	Monofunctional: isodecyl A, phenoxyethyl A, isobornyl A, etc.
	Bifunctional: 1,4-butanediol DA, 1,6-hexanediol DA, neopentylglycol DA, polyethyleneglycol DA, tripropyleneglycol DA, etc.
	Trifunctional: pentaerythritol TA, trimethylolpropane TA, glycerol TA, etc.
	Multifunctional: dipentaerythritol pentaacrylate, ditrimethylolpropane tetraacrylate, etc.
Prepolymers	Unsaturated polyesters
	Acrylated polyols: epoxy-acrylates, polyurethane-acrylates, polyester-or polyether-acrylates, etc.
Additives	Antioxidants: hydroquinone, hydroquinone monomethylether, etc.

people who make the inks, but are rare in the users. Moreover, pigments or dyes themselves are rarely the cause of dermatitis from inks.

1.3.2 Irritants Associated with Use of Inks

Workers using inks (mainly printers, typesetters, and press operators) are exposed to many irritants that include soaps and detergents, alcohols, solvents, greases and waxes, alkalis, and developers. Air contamination may induce respiratory symptoms. Washing hands, frictions, and use of irritants seem to be the main causes for skin symptoms due to contact with inks (Livesley et al. 2002).

1.3.3 Ultraviolet (UV)-Cured Printing Inks

UV-cured ink binders are composed by monomers, prepolymers, photoprimers, and additives. UV exposition will induce polymerization of the ink. Main compounds of dermatological interest are indicated in *Table 57.3.*

Sensitization to such inks has been reported at the end of the 1970s (Emmett and Kominsky 1977) and most reports of allergic contact dermatitis are due to inks used by silk-screen printers. Allergens include (meth)acrylic compounds, sometimes of epoxy type (epoxy (di)(meth)acrylates), isocyanates, and photoactivators (Emmett and Kominsky 1977; Björkner et al. 1980; Nethercott 1981; Malten and Seutter 1984; Nethercott et al. 1983; Aalto-Korte et al. 2009). It is important to test patients with their own products but a short screening series with EGDMA, DEGDA, 2-HPMA, and PETA could screen around 90% of patients occupationally sensitized to (meth-)acrylates (Aalto-Korte et al. 2010).

2-Hydroxyethyl methacrylate (*2-HEMA*) was pointed out in a silk-screen printer that had worked in the manufacture of circuit boards (Jolanki et al. 1994). Another bifunctional methacrylate, 2-hydroxypropyl methacrylate (*2-HPMA*) was reported (Björkner 1984) Several cases due to 2,2-bis[4-(2-hydroxy-3-acryloxypropoxy)phenyl]-propane (epoxy diacrylate, also named *Bis-GA*) were reported in silk-screen printers (Kanerva et al. 2000). One patient also reacted to DGEBA, and the other one to other acrylate compounds *like 2-phenoxyethylacrylate* and tripropylene glycol diacrylate (*TPGDA*). Patients sensitized to TPGDA, contained in UV-cured inks or in UV-curing overprint varnishes, generally react to several (di) (meth) acrylates (Aalto-Korte et al. 2009). TPGDA and a bifunctional aromatic methacrylate related to Bis-GMA, were responsible for dermatitis in a silk-screen maker also reacting to other resins *Bis-GMA* and ethyleneglycol dimethacrylate *EGDMA* (Goossens et al. 1998). TPGDA was reported as the only acrylate and sensitizer indicated on safety data sheet in a patient who reacted to several (meth) acrylates too (Skotnicki and Pratt 1998). In an advertisement and silk printing worker, sensitization was observed to bis-GA and diethyleneglycoldiacrylate (*DEGDA*) contained in a UV-curable silk print primer, and to *urethane acrylate* resins, and other acrylates as well (Aalto-Korte et al. 2009). Urethane acrylates and trimethylolpropane triacrylate (*TMPTA*) were reported in a series of six patients; three were also sensitized to pentaerythritol triacrylate (*PETA*), two to polyester acrylate, and two to Bis-GA (Björkner et al. 1980).

Polyfunctional aziridine hardeners are sensitizers (Garabrant 1985). Ink hardeners may contain 4,4′-diaminodiphenylmethane (Jolanki et al. 1994).

Triglycidyl isocyanurate (TGIC) was reported in a silk-screen printer on circuit boards (Jolanki et al. 1994).

Benzophenone-4 contained at 32–55% in printing lacquer was described as a sensitizer as well (Caruana et al. 2011)

1.3.4 Various Inks

Hybrid offset inks are formulated like offset inks, but also contain UV-curable components.

EB (electron beam) inks harden after use of an electron beam, and are sparingly used.

Overprint varnishes is a coating applied after a piece is printed. More than one type of overprint varnish may be used to create special effects. The overprint varnish may be applied as an all-over varnish or only to parts of the piece. Their composition can be close to offset inks (fat varnishes), acrylic type (water-based or solvent-based) or UV-curable (close to UV-curable inks).

2 Dyes

The most implicated dyes in (occupational) contact dermatitis are textile and hair dyes. Hair dyes frequently cause both irritation and sensitization in workers of hairdressing industry and consumers as well, but most cases of textile dyes dermatitis are claimed occurring in consumers.

2.1 Hair Dyes

They can be separated into "natural" (vegetal and metallic) and synthetic dyes (Le Coz 2007).

2.1.1 Vegetal and Metallic Dyes

Henna, also known as lawsonia inermis (extract from *Lawsonia inermis* L.), contains lawsone, a naphthoquinone that may be responsible for allergic contact dermatitis (Oztas et al. 2001) or immediate symptoms like urticaria, rhinitis, and asthma. On the other hand, "black henna" contains henna and synthetic dyes like aminobenzenes, aminotoluenes, and/or aminophenols. Contact allergy to lead acetate, still authorized in hair dyes, seems to be rare and not reported in hairdressers (Cronin 1980; Le Coz 2007).

2.1.2 Synthetic Dyes and Coupling Agents

The oldest synthetic permanent dye, *p*-phenylene diamine (PPD), remains the most frequent delayed-type occupational sensitizing dye in hairdressers, despite being less used than toluene-2,5-diamine. In a retrospective study of 729 hairdressers, 19% were sensitized to PPD (O'Connell et al. 2010). Toluene-2,5-diamine (sometimes named *p*-toluene diamine or PTD) is the most used permanent hair dye (100 tons in 2002), but stands second in terms of sensitization rate (Søsted et al. 2004). 2-Nitro-p-phenylene diamine, although less frequently used in permanent hair dyes, is often positive in hairdressers sensitized to PPD (Søsted 2007). Immediate-type reactions, including anaphylactic shock, have been reported in consumers.

Among aminophenols, *m*-aminophénol is a coupling agent, as *o*- and *p*-aminophenols are used as dyes. Resorcinol is a coupling agent widely used in permanent dyes, almost rarely positive in patch testing.

Other dyes (2-chloro-*p*-phenylene diamine) or coupling agents (2,7-Naphthalenediol or 2,7-dihydroxynaphthalene, pyrocatechol or 1,2-benzenediol) have not been reported in occupational sensitizations. Semipermanent or transient dyes like 3-nitro-*p*-hydroxyethylaminophenol, 4-amino-3-nitrophenol, 2-hydroxyethylamino-5-nitroanisole, Basic Blue 99, Basic Red 22, and HC yellow 7 were reported only in consumers (Le Coz 2007).

2.2 Textile Dyes

There are thousands of textile dyes, marketed under different names (up to 30 for some of them) and the Color Index (C.I.) does not contain all information about them. A final textile color often results from a subtle mixture of several dyes. Because of this, a priori unexpected dyes can be employed as yellow, red, or orange dyes, for black or blue garments, respectively. Moreover, a commercial dye often comprises one or two major components, and even impurities. For example, Disperse Blue 124 contains several dyes and traces of Disperse Blue 106, and "non-azo" impurities as ascertained by comparative thin layer chromatography. These impurities can also be responsible for sensitization. The manufacturing processes are complex and additional procedures such as bleaching can also lead to allergenic products. Skin metabolism may be responsible for transformation of dyes. For example, Disperse Orange 3 is degraded to *p*-phenylenediamine (PPD) and nitroaniline in the skin (➔ *Fig. 57.1*) (Le Coz 2011).

According to their chemical structures and the Color Index system, dyes can be classified into 17 groups: nitro dyes, triphenylmethane derivatives, xanthenes, acridine derivatives, quinoline derivatives, azines, anthraquinones, indigoid dyes, phthalocyanines dyes, oxidation bases, insoluble azo dye precursors, and azo dyes (classes XII to XVII). In practice, textile dyes are classified into different application classes: disperse, acid, basic, direct, vat, fiber-reactive, sulfur, premetallic, solvent dyes, and naphthols. Sensitization can occur from the dye itself, from intermediate products during the dyeing process or after-treatments, or from metabolites arising in the skin. This chapter focuses on textile dyes reported as occupational allergens only, but it is very likely that the majority of sensitizations, occurring in dyeing and textile industry of emerging countries, are not pointed out.

2.2.1 Disperse Dyes

Disperse dyes, partially soluble in water, are used to color synthetic fibers like polyester, acrylic, and acetate, and sometimes nylon, particularly in stockings. They are not employed for natural fibers.

Anthraquinone Dyes

These dyes consist of substituted anthraquinones. They are plastosoluble and used to stain synthetic fibers such as polyester, acetate, or nylon. Disperse Blue 7, structurally related to Disperse Blue 3, showed positive reactions in patients sensitized to Disperse Blue 106 contained in their occupational uniform (Mota et al. 2000).

Azo Dyes

Azo dyes are characterized by an R1-N = N-R2 chemical structure. They represent the majority of commercial colorants, enabling a broad spectrum of shades and fastness properties. They are suitable for coloring various substrates, including both synthetic and natural fibers. These molecules are trapped within the fibers in which they are formed during the dyeing process. Azo dyes, disperse type, are used in synthetic fibers. They are the molecules most often implicated in textile dye dermatitis, mainly in nylon stocking, socks, trousers, dresses, and underwear. Disperse Yellow 3, Disperse Orange 3, and Disperse Red 1 were the principal sensitizers until the 1980s. Today, Disperse Blue 124 and/or 106, Disperse Orange 3, Red 1, or Yellow 3 are frequently encountered.

The monoazoic compound Disperse Blue 124 has been responsible for occupational dermatitis in the textile industry (Soni and Sherertz 1996). It is closely related to another azo dye Disperse Blue 106, marketed since 1985 and formerly known as Disperse Blue 357. Five cases of occupational allergic dermatitis were reported among 200 employees wearing a working dark blue smock (Mota et al. 2000). Thin layer chromatography revealed that the uniform contained Disperse Blue 106 and Disperse Red 1. Two patients also reacted to anthraquinonic Disperse Blue 7, a third one with multiple reactions more likely due to an angry back.

Occupational airborne dermatitis has been reported in occupational plants (Manzini et al. 1996) and in workers who sewed and ironed clothes (Carretero Anibarro et al. 2000), for which reactive dyes and Disperse Blue 106 and 124 dyes were responsible, respectively.

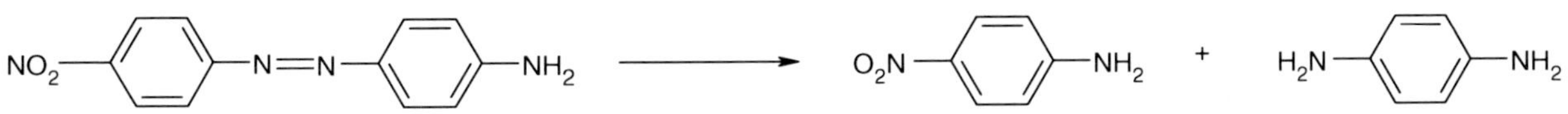

Fig. 57.1
Degradation of Disperse Orange 3 into nitroaniline and PPD

Disperse Orange 3 remains a frequent allergen, but sensitization seems in frequent cases acquired from hair dyes. With Disperse Yellow 3, they were reported as contact allergens in textile industry (Soni and Sherertz 1996).

2.2.2 Other Textile Dyes

Acid Dyes

These are used to color silk, wool, and other animal protein fibers, or nylon (polyamide) when high wet-fastness is needed. Such dyes include monoazoic, diazoic, triphenylmethane, and anthraquinone compounds. Acid Blue 158, an azo dye contained in suture material (Raap et al. 2008), was reported in two nonoccupational cases, although one of them was suspected to have been induced by toluene 2,5-diamine sensitization in a hairdresser (Hausen 2003).

Basic Dyes

These are mainly used to dye wool and silk, acrylic, modacrylic, nylon, polyester, and blends of these fibers with cotton. They can be applied to cotton with a mordant. Basic dyes comprise monoazoic, diazoic, and azine compounds. Basic Red 46, a monoazoic dye was implicated in occupational dermatitis (Chave et al. 2003). It seems to be an important cause of foot dermatitis, being a frequent allergen in acrylic socks (Opie et al. 2003).

Direct Dyes

These dyes are directly applied on fibers, most often cotton, wool, flax, or leather, in a neutral or alkaline bath. They have low wet-fastness and frequently need after-treatments.

Vat Dyes

Such water-insoluble dyes are applied in a reduced soluble form and then reoxidized to the original insoluble form once absorbed into the fiber. They have high wet-fastness and are used to dye cotton, flax, wool, and rayon fibers. Vat Blue 1 (synthetic indigo) is used to dye Levi Strauss 501 "shrink to fit" blue jeans. Vat Green 1, an anthraquinone derivative, has been reported as an occupational cause of contact dermatitis due to clothing, from navy-blue uniforms of nurses (Wilson and Cronin 1971).

Fiber-Reactive Dyes

Reactive dyes consist of a two-part, direct coloring agent. The first moiety is a chromophore with an azo, anthraquinone, or phthalocyanine derivative structure. This moiety is connected to a second reactive group, which is able to form covalent bonds with the amine or sulfhydryl groups of proteins in the textile fibers. Such dyes are used for coloring cellulosic fibers (cotton, silk), wool, or polyamides and are widely used for the production of clothes, most sources of sensitization being occupational. Sensitization can occur during occupational exposure, but reactive dyes should not be tested in nonoccupational patients, although the risk of active sensitization is theoretically of little consequence. Occupational airborne dermatitis has been reported in occupational plants (Manzini et al. 1996), and in workers who sewed and ironed clothes (Carretero Anibarro et al. 2000). Reactive dyes, and Disperse Blue 106 and 124 dyes were responsible, respectively.

Dye-Fixing and Dye-Coupling Agents

Naphthols are coupling agents, used for staining and dyeing. β-Naphthol (2-naphthol, Azoic coupling component 1, CAS [135-19-3]) is no longer used in textile industry. Naphthol AS (3-hydroxy-2-naphthoic acid anilide, Azoic Coupling Component 2), a coupling agent used for cotton dyeing, has replaced beta-naphthol because of a stronger affinity for cellulose. Naphthol AS first caused pigmented contact dermatitis in workers at a textile factory in Mexico in the 1970s, where it was widely used. It was reported as an agent of, sometimes, pigmented contact dermatitis in several patients (Roed-Petersen et al. 1990). Several other naphthols are used for textile dyeing, like Naphthol ASD (3-hydroxy-2naphthoic acid o-toluidine), Naphthol AS-E [2-naphtalenecarboxamide, 3-(acetyloxy)-*N*-(4-chlorophenyl)-, azoic Coupling Component 10], but they have not been reported as contact allergens.

2.3 Other Dyes

Except for textile and hair dyes, occupational contact allergy to dyes seems to be rare.

Food dyes are infrequently reported. Some cases concern asthma due to carmine (E120), a natural dye extracted from cochineal (Acero et al. 1998).

Solvent Yellow 33 (CI 47000), also known as D and C Yellow 11, caused occupational allergic dermatitis in an explosive factory (Noster and Hausen 1978), although the main cases reported with regard to this dye are due to the use of cosmetics, mainly lip cosmetics (Sasseville and Joncas 2009).

References

Aalto-Korte K, Jungewelter S, Henriks-Eckerman ML, Kuuliala O, Jolanki R (2009) Contact allergu to epoxy (meth)acrylates. Contact Dermatitis 1:9–21

Aalto-Korte K, Henriks-Eckerman ML, Kuuliala O, Jolanki R (2010) Occupational methacrylate and acrylate allergy – cross reactions and possible screening allergens. Contact Dermatitis 63:301–312

Acero S, Tabar AI, Alvarez MJ, Garcia BE, Olaguibel JM, Moneo I (1998) Occupational asthma and food allergy due to carmine. Allergy 53:897–901

Björkner B (1984) Contact allergy to 2-hydroxypropyl methacrylate (2-HPMA) in an ultraviolet curable ink. Acta Derm Venereol 64:264–267

Björkner B, Dahlquist I, Fregert S (1980) Allergic contact dermatitis from acrylates in ultraviolet curing inks. Contact Dermatitis 6:405–409

Braun WP (1975) Contact dermatitis from a stamp-ink of the German post office. Contact Dermatitis 1:189–190

Carretero Anibarro P, Gomez Breñosa B, Echechipia Madoz S, Garcia Figueroa BE, Aldunate Muruzabal MT, Lizaso Bacaicoa MT, Labarta Sanchez N, Tabar Purroy AI (2000) Occupational airborne allergic contact dermatitis from disperse dyes. Contact Dermatitis 43:44

Caruana DM, McPherson T, Cooper S (2011) Allergic contact dermatitis caused by benzophenone-4 in a printer. Contact Dermatitis 64: 183–184

Castaing G, Guilleux A (2010) Encres et vernis d'impression. Composition, risques toxicologiques et mesures de prévention. INRS ED 6069

Castelain PY, Pirious A, Raulot-Lapointe H, Robaglia JL (1980) Sensitization to abieto-formo-phenolic resın in printing ink. Contact Dermatitis 6:145–146

Chave TA, Nicolaou N, Johnston GA (2003) Hand dermatitis in a student caused by Basic Red 46. Contact Dermatitis 49:161–162

Cronin E (1980) Contact dermatitis. Churchill Livingstone, Edinburgh

Emmett EA, Kominsky JR (1977) Allergic contact dermatitis from ultraviolet-cured inks. Allergic contact sensitization to acrylates. J Occup Med 19:113–115

FIPEC (2011) http://www.fipec.org/afei

Foussereau J (1991) Guide de dermato-allergologie professionnelle. Masson Ed, Paris

Foussereau J, Benezra C (1970) Les eczémas allergiques professionnels. Masson Ed, Paris

Garabrant DH (1985) Dermatitis from aziridine hardener in printing ink. Contact Dermatitis 12:209–212

Goossens A, Coninx D, Rommens K, Verhamme B (1998) Occupational dermatitis in a silk-screen maker. Contact Dermatitis 39:40–42

Hausen BM (2003) Allergic contact dermatitis from colored surgical suture material: contact allergy to epsilon-caprolactam and Acid Blue 158. Am J Contact Dermat 14:174–175

Jolanki R, Kanerva L, Estlander T, Tarvainen K (1994) Concomitant sensitization to triglycidyl isocyanurate, diaminodiphenylmethane and 2-hydroxyethyl methacrylate from silk-screen printing coatings in the manufacture of circuit boards. Contact Dermatitis 30:12–15

Kanerva L, Estlander T, Jolanki R, Alanko K (2000) Occupational allergic contact dermatitis from 2,2-bis[4-(2-hydroxy-3-acryloxypropoxy) phenyl]-propane (epoxy diacrylate) in ultraviolet-cured inks. Contact Dermatitis 43:56–59

Le Coz CJ (2011) Clothing. In: Johansen JD, Frosch PJ, Lepoittevin JP (eds) Contact dermatitis, 5th edn. Springer, Berlin/Heidelberg

Le Coz CJ (2007) Les intolérances aux teintures capillaires et leur mise au point allergologique. Progrès en Dermato-Allergologie. John Libbey Eurotext, Paris, pp 99–129

Livesley EJ, Rushton L, English JS, Williams HC (2002) The prevalence of occupational dermatitis in the UK printing industry. Occup Environ Med 59:487–492

Malten KE, Seutter E (1984) Contact dermatitis from acrylated resins in UV Ebecryl printing inks. Contact Dermatitis 11:56–58

Manzini BM, Motoles A, Conti A, Ferdani G, Seidenari S (1996) Sensitization to reactive textile dyes in patients with contact dermatitis. Contact Dermatitis 34:172–175

Meyer JD, Chen Y, Holt DL, Beck MH, Cherry NM (2000) Occupational contact dermatitis in the UK: a surveillance report from EPIDERM and OPRA. Occup Med 50:265–273

Mota F, Silva E, Varela P, Azehna A, Massa A (2000) An outbreak of occupational textile dye dermatitis from Disperse Blue 106. Contact Dermatitis 43:235–236

Nethercott JR (1981) Allergic contact dermatitis due to an epoxy acrylate. Br J Dermatol 104:697–703

Nethercott JR, Jakubovic HR, Pilger C, Smith JW (1983) Allergic contact dermatitis due to urethane acrylate in ultraviolet cured inks. Br J Ind Med 40:241–250

Noster U, Hausen BM (1978) Berufsbedingtes Kontakteczem durch gelben Chinophthalonfarbstoff (Solvent Yellow 33: C.I. 47000). Hautarzt 29:153–157

O'Connell RL, White IR, Mc Fadden JP, White JML (2010) Hairdressers with dermatitis should always be patch tested regardless of atopy status. Contact Dermatitis 62:177–181

Opie J, Lee A, Frowen K, Fewings J, Nixon R (2003) Foot dermatitis caused by the textile dye Basic Red 46 in acrylic blend socks. Contact Dermatitis 49:297–303

Özkaya E (2009) A rare case of allergic contact dermatitis from silver nitrate in a widely used special patch test marker. Contact Dermatitis 61:120–122

Oztas MO, Onder M, Oztas P, Atahan C (2001) Contact allergy to henna. J Eur Acad Dermatol Venereol 15:91–92

Raap U, Wieczorek D, Kapp A, Wedi B (2008) Allergic contact dermatitis to Acid Blue 158 in suture material. Contact Dermatitis 59:192–193

Roed-Petersen J, Batsberg W, Larsen E (1990) Contact dermatitis from Naphthol AS. Contact Dermatitis 22:161–163

Sasseville D, Joncas V (2009) Allergic contact dermatitis from D 1 C Yellow 11. Contact Dermatitis 60:294–295

Skotnicki S, Pratt MD (1998) Occupational dermatitis to ultraviolet-cured acrylic-based inks in computer hard disc manufacturing. Am J Contact Dermat 9:179–181

Soni BP, Sherertz EF (1996) Contact dermatitis in the textile industry: a review of 72 patients. Am J Contact Dermat 7:226–230

Søsted H (2007) Allergic contact dermatitis to hair dye ingredients. Forum for Nordic dermato-venereology 12(Suppl 13):1–27

Søsted H, Basketter DA, Estrada E, Johansen JD, Patlewicz GY (2004) Ranking of hair dye substances according to predicted sensitization potency: quantitative structure-activity relationships. Contact Dermatitis 51:241–254

Wilson HTH, Cronin E (1971) Dermatitis from dyed uniforms. Br J Dermatol 85:67–69

58 Leather and Shoes

Johannes Geier · Holger Lessmann
Information Network of Departments of Dermatology (IVDK), Department of Dermatology, University of Goettingen, Goettingen, Germany

Core Messages

- Various allergens and irritants are used in the production and processing of leather and in the manufacture of shoes.
- Occupational skin disease is infrequently reported in these branches.
- The most important allergens are chromium salts, *p-tert*-butylphenol formaldehyde resin, rubber chemicals, and various biocides.
- Many possible allergens are not available for routine diagnostics, so sensitization may be overlooked.
- Residuals of allergens in leather or shoes also pose a risk for the consumer.

1 Introduction

Manufacturing leather is a process consisting of several subsequent steps which should be known in detail to the occupational dermatologist, because every step is characterized by a particular chemistry, adding up to a variety of exposures and possible skin hazards. Manufacturing shoes does not only involve leather and glues, but also various chemicals, of which several may cause a skin disease.

2 Manufacture of Leather

Leather is made from the dermis of animal hides. The subcutaneous tissue and the epidermis and hair are removed during the production process. Generally speaking, the production of leather includes three broad steps: (1) removal of all parts of the hide which are not needed, (2) improving physical resistance of the hide, stabilization of the collagen, and protection against biodegradation by tanning, and (3) processing of the tanned material in accordance with the desired qualities of the final product (Reich and Taeger 2009).

2.1 Pre-tanning Process

Bacterial degradation starts immediately after the removal of the hide from the animal corpse, so a temporary conservation is necessary. One simple possibility is air drying, but this is not applicable for thick hides (>2 mm) because the surface may be sealed by drying thus preventing water in deeper layers from evaporation which results in bacterial growth in the center of the hide. Only thin hides like sheep or goat skins can be air dried. Usually, the hides are protected with insecticides during this process. Salt curing by spreading sodium chloride between the piled hides is the most frequently applied curing method in modern commercial cattle hide production. This curing procedure takes about 20 days, and the required amount of salt is about 50% of the hide weight. Alternatively, the hides may be cured using saturated brine, usually with addition of bactericides. Further methods of curing have been established, e.g., application of disinfectants like quaternary amines, radiation sterilization, or refrigeration, but these are less frequently used. The cured hides are shipped from the slaughterhouse to the tannery (Heidemann 1990; Thorstensen 1995; Reich and Taeger 2009).

On arrival at the tannery, the hides are soaked in water, thus removing the salt, dirt, and manure. Bactericides and proteolytic enzymes are added to the soaking water. This procedure takes about 6 h.

Afterwards, the hides are trimmed and freed of flesh and subcutaneous tissue (fleshing), which is usually done by machines with rotating knives. For unhairing, the hides are then treated for 4–12 h with sodium sulfide (Na_2S or $NaSH$) and lime (calcium hydroxide). Under these alkaline conditions (pH 12), the disulfide bridges in the keratin proteins of the hair and epidermis are broken, the hair fiber structure is destroyed, and the hair can easily be removed mechanically together with the epidermis. Other methods of unhairing like the use of proteolytic enzymes, acids, or oxidizing agents are not frequently applied (Heidemann 1990; Thorstensen 1995).

After unhairing, the hides are again floated with lime, but without sulfide. This makes them swell, so an opening of the structure for the following tanning step takes place. In this state, the hide can be split into sheets of desired thickness.

As tanning requires acid conditions, the hides have to be "delimed" before further processing. By addition of

T. Rustemeyer, P. Elsner, S.M. John & H.I. Maibach (eds.), *Kanerva's Occupational Dermatology*,
DOI 10.1007/978-3-642-02035-3_58,

ammonium salts and acids, a neutral pH is achieved. Proteolytic enzymes are added to eliminate undesirable byproducts from the connective tissue and break down elastin in the hide (so-called "bating"), because elastin may make the leather too firm and stiff.

After removal of the degradation products, the bated hides are pickled, i.e., brought to acid conditions for tanning, which are reached by treating the hides again with acids and salts.

Pickled hides can be stored for a long time. However, mostly a continuous process of subsequent bating, pickling, and tanning is preferred, during which the hides remain in the same processing drum (Heidemann 1990; Thorstensen 1995; Reich an Taeger 2009).

2.2 Tanning

The most widely used tanning system is chrome tanning. Chrome tanning is usually done using basic chromium sulfate ($2Cr(OH)SO_4{\cdot}Na_2SO_4$), in which chromium is trivalent and forms a complex which penetrates the hide at pH <3. In the beginning of the process, the pH of the tanning solution usually is adjusted to 2.5. After the penetration of Cr(III) into the hide, the pH is raised to 3.5–4. Now the chromium complex is bound firmly to the collagen protein forming cross-links. The pH is raised further by adding sodium bicarbonate, thus transforming the chromium protein complexes into stable structures (Heidemann 1990; Thorstensen 1995; Reich and Taeger 2009).

Vegetable tanning has a far longer history than chrome tanning. Although it is more time consuming than chrome tanning, it is still done for special purposes, especially heavy leathers like in shoe soles, saddles, belts, etc. Vegetable tannins are polyphenolic compounds and can be classified into two groups: Hydrolyzable tannins can be regarded as derivatives of pyrogallol, condensed ones as derivatives of (pyro)catechol. The water molecules within the hide protein structures are replaced by the phenolic groups of the tannins. Subsequently, hydrogen bonds with the proteins are established (Heidemann 1990; Thorstensen 1995; Reich and Taeger 2009). Vegetable tanning agents coming from various sources (see ➔ *Table 58.1*) are brown, and they cause the typical odor of leather. Solutions of vegetable tanning agents contain residues from plants like sugar, salt, and proteins. Thus, growth of mold is promoted.

Synthetic tanning agents are sulfonated condensation products of formaldehyde and phenols. They have fungistatic properties, and are therefore used in combination with vegetable tannins.

Table 58.1
Vegetable tanning materials (Selection, modified from Haslam 1989; Hausen 1981; Reich and Taeger 2009)

Barks	Golden and Black Wattle (*Acacia* sp.), Oak (*Quercus* sp.), Spruce (*Picea* sp.), Hemlock (*Tsuga* sp.), Chestnut (*Castanea* sp.), Larch (*Larix* sp.), Birch (*Betula* sp.), Yellow Pine (*Pinus ponderosa*), Beech (*Fagus sylvatica*)
Woods	Quebracho (*Schinopsis lorentzii*), Redwood (*Sequoia sempervirens*), Oak (*Quercus* sp.), Chestnut (*Castanea* sp.), Red Cedar (*Thuja plicata*)
Leaves	American sumach (*Rhus* sp.), Gambier (*Uncaria gambier*)
Fruits, fruitpods	Myrobalans (*Terminalia chebula*), Valonea (*Quercus aegilopsis*)
Plant galls	Oak (*Quercus* sp.), Tamarisk (*Tamarix articulata*), Aleppo (*Quercus infectoria*)

Other, less frequently used tanning agents are salts of aluminum, iron, titanium, and zirconium. These tanning methods are often combined with chrome or vegetable tanning (Heidemann 1990; Thorstensen 1995; Reich and Taeger 2009).

Chrome tanned leather has a light blue color and tends to become stiff when dried. A lot of leather is sold and shipped semifinished as so-called wet blue. This is unsplit chrome tanned leather which is protected against mold by biocides, stacked in piles, and covered with plastic foil to prevent drying. The biocides in former or current use are mercury salts, mercaptobenzothiazole, DDT (dichloro diphenyl trichloroethane), HCH (hexachloro cyclohexane) (Foussereau et al. 1982), chloroacetamide (Jelen et al. 1989), octylisothiazolinone (Foussereau et al. 1984; Koch et al. 1996; Oleaga et al. 1992), quaternary ammonium salts, chlorinated cresols, and derivatives of benzothiazole (Koch et al. 1996), in particular 2-thiocyanomethyl benzothiazole (Nardelli et al. 2005). The use of the latter substances is said to be increasing due to the prohibition of pentachlorophenol, e.g., in Germany (Koch et al. 1996). However, "wet blue" is often produced in developing countries and sold to European or other tanneries for further processing, and the preservatives used in the production countries are mostly not known to the importing companies (Koch et al. 1996).

Usually, the leather is retanned using vegetable and/or synthetic tannins. This increases softness and makes the leather look more like vegetable-tanned leather ("natural look"). Furthermore, retanning improves the structure of those sites in the hide where chrome tanning has by accident not fastened the fiber structure sufficiently. Retanning with amino resins, i.e., oligomers constructed from urea, dicyanoamide, or melamine, results in a smooth leather. These resins, cationic under acidic conditions, improve the fixation of other anionic compounds like dyes. Polyacrylates and polymethacrylates are used for similar purposes (Heidemann 1990; Podmore 1995; Thorstensen 1995; Reich and Taeger 2009).

Formaldehyde and glutaraldehyde (syn. glutaral, glutaric dialdehyde) as well as some formaldehyde releasing substances are also used as cross-linking agents in tannery. While glutaraldehyde performs tanning properties under acidic conditions, formaldehyde requires a pH above 7. Glutaraldehyde is widely used in the production of upper shoe leather and formaldehyde in the production of white leathers (Rietschel and Fowler 1995). Both aldehydes are used for pretanning to accelerate vegetable tanning. Glutaraldehyde is also used for retanning after chrome tanning (Heidemann 1990; Rietschel and Fowler 1995; Thorstensen 1995). Glutaraldehyde or mixtures of glutaraldehyde and formaldehyde are used to improve colorfastness and washability of the final product (Koch et al. 1996).

2.3 Post-tanning Process

Almost every leather is dyed, mostly with synthetic organic colors. The majority of the dyes used are anionic azo dyes which bind to the cationic surface of the leather. For completion of the dyeing process, formic, acetic, or lactic acid is added. Afterward, basic dyes can be applied which give the leather a brilliant shade. Metal complex dyes are also widely used in the leather industry (Heidemann 1990; Thorstensen 1995). The manufacturers regard dyeing of leather as an art rather than as a technique. Therefore, combinations of dyes used are kept secret (Koch et al. 1996).

According to the final product, leather requires a certain softness which is achieved by application of fat. A fat content of 5% is essential; gloves, garments, and upholstery may contain up to 15%. So, after dyeing, the leather is oiled. For this process, called fatliquoring, oily fat is emulsified and applied to the leather in a warm bath. Coming into contact with the chrome tanned fibers of the leather, the emulsion breaks, and the fat remains on the leather. The oils used are sulfated or sulfonated plant, animal, or fish oils or synthetic products usually biocide preserved (Heidemann 1990; Podmore 1995; Thorstensen 1995; Reich and Taeger 2009).

As the leather has only little water resistance after all these processes, a hydrophobic treatment is necessary. For this purpose, silicones, organic chlorofluoropolymers, or water-in-oil-emulsions are used (Heidemann 1990).

The colored and fatliquored leather is dried, staked, and buffered. Staking and buffering are mechanical treatments to increase flexibility and softness and to achieve special surface aspects.

The last step is finishing, i.e., application of a protective and decorative coat. According to the purpose for which the leather will be used, the finishes should protect, e.g., against abrasion or water. Surface defects and irregularities in color should be leveled out. Usually, several layers of finishing are applied. Water-based latex finishes containing dyes or pigments may be applied first (Thorstensen 1995). Other base coats are polyacrylate dispersions which are often padded or brushed onto the leather surface. After application the leather is ironed, so thermoplastification and adhesion of the polymer to the leather fibers can take place. The second coating, often polyacrylate, polybutadiene, or polyurethan dispersions, usually containing pigments as well, is most important for the appearance of the leather. It is applied by spraying several times. After this, the leather is ironed again. The third layer is important for the feel and the rub resistance of the leather. Usually, a solvent-based nitrocellulose solution or water-based polyurethane or nitrocellulose emulsions are used (Heidemann 1990; Podmore 1995; Thorstensen 1995; Reich and Taeger 2009). Biocides are added to the finishing chemicals, if necessary (Podmore 1995).

Dimethylfumarate (DMF) is used as fungicide for mold prevention in finished leather products such as furniture (arm chairs, sofas), shoes, or handbags. DMF is added to siccative sachets placed inside the furniture or in the shoe box (Rantanen 2008; Williams et al. 2008; Giménez-Arnau et al. 2009; Lammintausta et al. 2009; Susitaival et al. 2010). At room temperature, DMF sublimates, thus impregnating the leather products with varying DMF concentrations. Alarmed by the epidemic of contact dermatitis, the use of DMF in consumer products is banned EU wide since May 2009 (Anonymus 2009). However, shoes contaminated with DMF have been reported by RAPEX, the EU rapid alert system for all dangerous consumer products, to be still on the European market even after this date (http://ec.europa.eu/consumers/safety/rapex/index_en.htm).

3 Occupational Dermatoses in the Leather Industry

Considering the variety of potentially sensitizing or irritating substances used, occupational dermatoses in the leather industry are infrequently reported (Dickel et al. 2001). This may be due to two facts: the increasing automation and the shift of hazardous works to developing countries where attention to occupational dermatoses is less than in industrialized ones (Cavelier and Foussereau 1995; Foussereau et al. 1982; Koch et al. 1996; Wardenbach et al. 1989).

A few decades ago, dichromate allergy was more frequently observed in the leather industry in Europe, too. Wagner and Wezel (1966) analyzed expert opinions on occupational dermatoses in the department of dermatology of the University of Kiel, Germany, from 1952 to 1962. Of the 598 patients, 36 worked in the leather industry. Among these, the most frequent contact allergens were: dichromate (19 patients), formaldehyde (8 patients), leather dyes (8 patients), and tanning agents (2 patients). Approximately until 1970, "occasionally" chromate sensitizations among tanners were observed in France (Cavelier and Foussereau 1995). Among 280 Swedish male patients with occupational contact allergy to chromate observed by Fregert (1975) from 1960 to 1969, 12% were tannery workers.

In contrast, an analysis of approved occupational diseases from 1978 to 1984 in Germany revealed that none of the 941 cases of allergic contact dermatitis due to chromium salts occurred in the leather industry (Wardenbach et al. 1989). A similar development in France was stated by Cavelier and Foussereau (1995). However, among 37 patients working in the leather and fur industry with an initial report of occupational skin disease recorded in the register of occupational skin diseases in Northern Bavaria, Germany, between 1990 and 1999, 10 cases of chromate sensitization were diagnosed, of which 8 were regarded occupationally relevant (Dickel et al. 2001). Sensitization to chromate due to exposure to leather also was a significant cause of occupational hand dermatitis in a Danish survey from 2001 to 2002 (Skoet et al. 2004).

As written above, tanning is done with trivalent chromium salts. Although it is known that trivalent chromium compounds penetrate the skin by far not as easily as hexavalent chromium compounds (Spruit and van Neer 1966), it has been shown by analysis of chromium in the urine that tanners, apart from absorption via the respiratory tract, may have a relevant chromium uptake via absorption through the skin (Bulikowski and Tyras 1976). Under alkaline conditions which may occur during the finishing process, trivalent chromium (Cr(III)) in leather can be oxidized to the hexavalent state (Cr(VI)) (Fregert 1981; Koch et al. 1996). In tanning, it happens that trivalent chromium salts are not completely bound to the collagen fibers or that excessive chromium is not washed out sufficiently. This can lead to a certain amount of free Cr(III) in the leather which under the a.m. circumstances is oxidized to the hexavalent state easily (Geier et al. 1995). In the epidermis, Cr(VI) is reduced to Cr(III) by methionine, cysteine, or glutathione, and subsequently Cr(III) binds to proteins forming the allergen (Cavelier and Foussereau 1995; Samitz and Katz 1964; Stein 1992). About one third of leather products bought in Denmark had a Cr(VI) content of 3.6 ppm to 14.7 ppm, while leachable Cr(III) was detected at levels of 430–980 ppm (Hansen et al. 2002). However, positive reactions to samples of these leather products were not in line with their Cr(III)/Cr(VI) content (Hansen et al. 2006b).

Although trivalent chromium rarely sensitizes, contact sensitization has been reported in tannery workers who had exclusively been exposed to Cr(III); on patch testing, they reacted to both Cr(III) and Cr(VI) salts (Estlander et al. 2000). Nygren and Wahlberg (1998) found small amounts (average 0.08%) of sweat leachable hexavalent chromium in both chromium- and vegetable-tanned leathers. Patch testing with samples of these leathers elicited allergic reactions in chromate-sensitized individuals. In a repeated open application test (ROAT) with a potassium dichromate solution containing 50 ppm Cr (VI) and 1% sodium lauryl sulfate (SLS), about half of the patients reacted positively. Twenty percent even reacted at 5 ppm Cr(VI) in the presence of 1% SLS (Basketter et al. 2001). The authors drew the conclusion that household products should not contain more than 5 ppm of Cr(VI). Recently, an increasing prevalence of chromate allergy due to leather goods has been reported from Denmark, which is plausible considering the mentioned amounts of Cr(VI) found in leather products (Thyssen et al. 2009). In chromate-sensitized patients, patch test elicitation threshold for Cr(III) was significantly higher than for Cr(VI) (Hansen et al. 2006a). The minimum concentration, to which at least 10% of the patients showed a positive reaction was 6 ppm for Cr(III) and 1 ppm for Cr(VI) (Hansen et al. 2003). For routine diagnostic purposes, i.e., for patch testing, potassium dichromate in which chromium is hexavalent is generally recommended (Cavelier and Foussereau 1995; Fuchs et al. 1996; Rietschel and Fowler 1995).

Vegetable tannins have not been reported as a cause of occupational contact dermatitis yet. Calnan and Cronin (1978) have seen a man suffering from allergic contact dermatitis due to a leather watch strap. In the patch test, he reacted to dichromate, Myrobalan extract powder, and Quebracho extract powder. Furthermore, some case reports on patients with dermatitis of the feet caused by contact allergy to vegetable-tanned shoe leather exist

(Cronin 1966; Minkin et al. 1971). The allergens in the vegetable tannins, however, have not been identified.

Also, occupational contact allergies to synthetic tannins in the leather industry have not been reported yet. However, Müller and Hausen (1994) described a patient with contact allergy to a synthetic tannin present in a tincture for topical dermatological therapy.

Azo dyes such as those used in the leather industry have a certain sensitizing capacity. Probably, p-phenylenediamine (PPD) is an intermediate or final product of the decomposition of some azo dyes in the skin. This might explain the high rate of concomitant patch test reactions to these azo dyes and PPD in up to 50–80% of patients allergic to PPD (Hausen 1997). Although PPD cannot be regarded as a perfectly reliable indicator of a contact allergy to azo dyes, it is often needed in this function because the incriminated dyes are unknown (Estlander et al. 1990).

Occasionally, metanil yellow (acid yellow 36) has been reported as a cause of contact allergy due to leather products. A young man suffered from a foot eczema after wearing industrial leather protective shoes. On patch testing he reacted to metanil yellow, which was present in the leather of the inners and stiffeners. He also reacted to the leather itself and p-aminoazobenzene, PPD, and some of its derivatives (Ancona et al. 1982). A woman working in a leather shop developed a contact allergy to metanil yellow, probably by contact to a brown leather portfolio. She also reacted to p-aminoazobenzene and p-aminodiphenylamine in the patch test (Hausen 1994).

A certain pattern of contact allergens in the leather industry may be expected from analyses of occupational dermatoses in this branch. Foussereau et al. (1982) mention potassium dichromate, dyes, and formaldehyde as the most frequent contact allergens in tanners. The authors cite a manual from 1947 in which nigrosine, chrysoidine, and dimethyl amino azobenzene are listed as sensitizing dyes, but they state that these substances are no longer or only rarely in use.

Koch et al. (1996) analyzed data of the Information Network of Departments of Dermatology in Germany (IVDK) on contact allergies in patients working in the leather and shoe industry. Of the 30,678 patients registered in the IVDK from 1990 to 1994, only 85 (0.3%) had an actual or former profession in this field. Compared to all other patients, increased rates of sensitizations to the following possibly occupational allergens of the standard series were noted: potassium dichromate, *p*-phenylenediamine, formaldehyde, *p-tert*-butylphenol formaldehyde resin (PTBP-F-R), mercaptobenzothiazole, and nickel sulfate. On patch testing with the leather industry series, allergic reactions were noted to glutaraldehyde, *p*-aminoazobenzene, Bismarck brown, octylisothiazolinone, disperse orange 3, 1,3-diphenylguanidine, and chloroacetamide. An additional analysis of contact allergies and their occupational relevance in the expert opinions from the department of dermatology at Homburg/Saar included in this study revealed a similar allergen spectrum. Although nickel is mentioned as allergen in shoes (buckles, trims) (Cronin 1980; Podmore 1995), the origin of the increased rate of allergies to nickel in the patients of this study remained unproved.

Polyfunctional aziridine (PFA) hardeners, which are used to harden surface coatings or finishes, have gained interest in occupational dermatology because they are potent sensitizers. Estlander reported cases of combined skin and respiratory sensitization to PFA in leather dyers (Estlander et al. 2001).

As far as clinical findings are concerned, there is no characteristic aspect, localization, or clinical course of occupational contact dermatitis in tanners (Foussereau et al. 1982). Adams (1990) mentioned callosities as occupational marks caused by mechanical trauma in leather buffers on the thumb, in cutters on the right index finger, and in glazers on the knuckles.

4 Production and Repairing of Shoes

Shoes are not only made of leather, but of a broad variety of materials. As shoes are subject to fashion, their design and the materials used change more or less rapidly. Shoes are produced in many countries of the world in different ways which makes it impossible to give a complete description of the occupational exposure of those working in the shoe industry. "It must be remembered that a modern shoe is so complex that the final assembler may not be aware of all of the chemicals that have been used to prepare each of the shoe's parts, because they may have come from all over the world to finally come together in a finished piece of footwear" (Rietschel and Fowler 1995).

Shoe uppers can be made of textiles, leather, rubber, or polyurethane. Outer and inner soles are made of rubber, polyurethane, polyvinylchloride, or Evaflex, a combination of ethyl vinyl acetate and rubber polymers (Podmore 1995). For insoles, fiberboard is also used. Fiberboard is made of wood or leather fibers, suspended in a mixture of rubber resins or acrylic resins, which are preserved with biocides, often copper-8-quinolinolate or sodium-*o*-phenylphenate (Podmore 1995). In wooden shoes, an insole may be present which has a cardboard-like appearance. This material is made from wood pulp, and tetramethylthiuram disulfide is added as an antimicrobial agent (Fogh and Pock-Steen 1992). Other parts like the reinforcements above the toes and around the heels are made of plastics or textile materials hardened with plastics, e.g., a nylon cloth to which rubber or polyurethane foam is flame-bonded or cotton material impregnated with various resins, e.g., formaldehyde resins (Cronin 1980; Grimalt and Romaguera 1975; Podmore 1995). The protective toe caps of industrial protective shoes are made of stainless steel, which may be coated with epoxy resin to increase the resistance of the metal to corrosion. The metal toe cap is protected by a synthetic foam padding (Foussereau et al. 1986). Linings can be made of polyvinylchloride or polyurethane.

Rubber boots may contain *N*-isopropyl-*N*′-phenyl-*p*-phenylenediamine (IPPD), chemically related compounds, and mercury compounds which are used for preservation of plasticizers (Cronin 1980; Koch and Nickolaus 1996; Nishioka et al. 1996). Occupational sensitizations to phthalates and coal tar were observed in a factory producing shoes from polyvinyl chloride granulate in former Yugoslavia. Both substances were present in the granulate (Vidovic and Kansky 1985).

In shoe production, urethane, neoprene, natural rubber, and hot melt adhesives are used. The latter ones are inert high molecular weight polymers which are melted and applied to heated material surfaces. They are used, e.g., for gluing of sole or heels, and are not known as a cause of contact allergy (Podmore 1995). Urethane adhesives are modified polyurethane solutions. Additives, e.g., isocyanates, epoxy resins, acrylic, or phenol formaldehyde resins, depend on the material to be glued (Podmore 1995). Further chemicals (catalysts, hardeners, plasticizers, etc.) such as triethylenediamine, 4,4′-diaminodiphenylmethane, or dibutyl tin which are used in the production of polyurethanes have not been reported as a problem in the shoe industry. However, Rietschel and Fowler (1995) emphasize that contact allergies to these substances may be underreported, and therefore recommend to keep these substances in mind for unclear cases of contact allergy. Neoprene glues may, in addition to neoprene itself, contain isocyanates, phenolic resins like PTBP-F-R, ethylene thiourea, dioctyl-*p*-phenylenediamine, tetramethylthiuram disulfide, di-*o*-tolyl guanidine, sodium dibutyldithiocarbamate, and zinc oxide, magnesium oxide, and silicates (Podmore 1995). Dodecyl mercaptan has been used to arrest polymerization in neoprenes and neoprene glues (Grimalt and Romaguera 1975). Natural rubber glues are water-based solutions of natural rubber, preserved with biocides, e.g., phenol, formaldehyde, or *p*-chloro-*m*-cresol. They may contain triethanolamine (Podmore 1995). Occasionally, colophony is used as a tackifier or in finishes in shoe production (Fisher 1991; Podmore 1995; Strauss and Wilkinson 2002).

In shoe manufactures, the different parts of the shoes are prepared and assembled. Uppers, toe-caps, quarters, linings, and insoles are cut and edged which includes folding, glueing, and sewing. The insoles and heels are also cut and glued. After assembly, the shoe is finished and trimmed. Possible occupational exposure covers a broad spectrum of allergens: preservatives, dyes, tanning agents, neoprene materials and neoprene glues, polyurethane materials and polyurethane glues, epoxy resins, diluents and epoxy resin glues, rubber materials and rubber glues, and acrylic resins (Mancuso et al. 1996). Podmore (1995) mentioned occupational exposure to the preservatives benzisothiazolinone, octylisothiazolinone, di-iodomethyl-*p*-tolylsulfone, 2-thiocyanomethyl benzothiazole, sodium-*o*-phenylphenate, copper-8-quinolinolate, and *N*-trichloromethyl thiophthalimide, and in some East Asian countries trichlorophenol and pentachlorophenol. Although occupational contact allergy due to dimethyl fumarate has not yet been reported, exposure to this highly allergenic fungicide should be considered in cases of occupational dermatitis due to leather contact.

5 Occupational Dermatoses in the Shoe Industry and in Shoe Repairers

"Shoes are manufactured from a vast range of potentially sensitizing chemicals" (Podmore 1995). The most frequent allergen in shoe makers is PTBP-F-R in neoprene-based glues (Foussereau et al. 1976, 1982; Mancuso et al. 1996). A sensitization to PTBP-F-R is probably due to intermediate products, but not to the resin itself or to the two basic chemicals, formaldehyde and PTBP (Bruze 1986; Geldof et al. 1989; Malten and Seutter 1985; Malten et al. 1983; Mancuso et al. 1996; Schubert and Agatha 1979; Zimerson and Bruze 2000, 2002a, b; Zimerson et al. 2002). Allergic contact dermatitis caused by PTBP-F-R often appears as hyperkeratotic eczema of the fingers and palms with fissures (Foussereau et al. 1982). Malten (1958) and Malten and van Aerssen (1962) describe allergic contact eczema due to PTBP-F-R containing neoprene glue in right-handed shoe repairers preferably being localized at the finger tips and finger sides of the left hand because the parts to be glued are held with the left hand while the glue is brushed on with the right hand.

Additionally, the face may be affected. Sometimes eczematic lesions are also seen on the thighs when the shoe repairer holds the shoe between his knees (Foussereau et al. 1982).

Mancuso et al. (1996) have studied occupational dermatoses in 246 shoe factory workers in Italy from 1992 to 1994: 20 suffered from irritant contact dermatitis, 16 from allergic contact dermatitis. Most frequently, occupational contact dermatitis occurred in the assembly department (20 out of 70 employees). Irritant occupational dermatitis was mostly caused by organic solvents (toluene, xylene, *n*-hexane) in adhesives and varnishes. Among those patients with occupational allergic contact dermatitis, five were sensitized to PTBP-F-R, three to mercaptobenzothiazole, two each to diphenylmethane-4,4′-diisocyanate, epoxy resin, potassium dichromate, tetramethylthiuram disulfide, and thiuram mix, and a single patient to Bismarck brown, carba mix, chloroacetamide, colophony, 4,4′-diaminodiphenylmethane, 1,3-diphenylguanidine, dodecyl mercaptan, ethylenediamine dihydrochloride, mercapto mix, nickel sulfate, *p*-phenylenediamine, phenyl glycidyl ether, phenylmercuric nitrate, and triethylenediamine. The authors give an extensive, detailed list of possible occupational allergens in this branch which is partly incorporated in the tables shown in ➋ Chap. 189, "Job Description: Shoe Manufacturers and Repairers."

The case history of an apprentice cobbler was reported. He was occupationally exposed to leather, rubber, plastic items, and several glues, and acquired a contact allergy to the major monomer of an ethyl cyanoacrylate glue (Bruze et al. 1995). Henschel et al. (2002) reported a case of occupational contact sensitization to propolis in bees wax that was used by a shoemaker for seams of handmade heavy boots.

Although under quite different local conditions (occlusion, sweat), patients with allergic contact dermatitis of the feet due to shoes have an exposure similar to those working in shoe production or repairing. These patients show a similar pattern of contact allergens including mercaptobenzothiazole and derivatives, *N*-isopropyl-*N*′-phenyl-*p*-phenylenediamine (IPPD) and other *p*-phenylenediamine derivatives, thiurams, *p*-phenylenediamine, azo dyes, *N*, *N*-dibutyl thiourea, PTBP-F-R, dodecyl mercaptan, colophony, potassium dichromate, 2-thiocyanomethyl benzothiazole, dimethyl fumarate, and formaldehyde (Angelini et al. 1980; Bajaj et al. 1991; Correia and Menezes Brandao 1986; Cronin 1980; Foussereau et al. 1986; Freeman 1997; Jung et al. 1988; Lynde et al. 1982; Oumeish and Rushaidat 1980; Romaguera 1987; Scutt 1966; Suurmond and Verspijck Mijnssen 1967; Strauss and Wilkinson 2002; Rani et al. 2003; Onder et al. 2004; Holden and Gawkrodger 2005; Nardelli et al. 2005; Teixeira et al. 2005; Corazza et al. 2006; Chowdhuri and Ghosh 2007; Oztas et al. 2007; Verma et al. 2007; Warshaw et al. 2007; Castanedo-Tardan et al. 2008; Giménez-Arnau et al. 2009). Ethyl butyl thiourea is mentioned as an allergen in a rubber adhesive (for neoprene/polychloroprene) used in athletic shoes (Roberts and Hanifin 1979). Cronin (1966) gives a very good synopsis of the historical development of the diagnostic in this field.

Nonallergic occupational dermatoses in the shoe industry were observed by Mancuso et al. (1996), too. Fifteen workers in the upper- and sole-cutting departments presented with hyperkeratosis and scaling of the fingertips, mechanically provoked by continuous trauma of the leather. A work-dependent localized itching of uncovered areas was reported by eight workers employed in the sole-cutting and scraping departments. This pruritus sine materia was probably caused by dust in the work place. Two workers who had been exposed to *p-tert*-butylphenol-based glues for a long time showed leucodermic lesions on the back of the hands. The depigmenting activity of *p-tert*-butylphenol has been described previously (Gellin 1990).

Some years ago, methyl ethyl ketone in glues has been accused to be the cause of polyneuropathy in shoe factory workers (Dyro 1978).

References

Adams RM (1990) Occupational skin disease, 2nd edn. WB Saunders, Philadelphia, 45, 662–663, 667–669

Ancona A, Serviere L, Trejo A, Monroy F (1982) Dermatitis from an azo-dye in industrial leather protective shoes. Contact Dermatitis 8:220–221

Angelini G, Vena GA, Meneghini CL (1980) Shoe contact dermatitis. Contact Dermatitis 6:279–283

Anonymus (2009) Commission decision of 17March 2009 requiring Member States to ensure that products containing the biocide dimethylfumarate are not placed or made available on the market (2009/251/CE). Official Journal of the European Union 20.3.2009. L 74/32. Available at: http://eur-lex.europa.eu/LexUriServ/LexUriServ.do?uri=OJ:L:2009:074:0032:0034:EN:PDF. Last accessed 25 March 2010

Bajaj AK, Gupta SC, Chatterjee AK, Singh KG (1991) Shoe dermatitis in India: further observations. Contact Dermatitis 24:149–151

Basketter D, Horev L, Slodovnik D, Merimes S, Trattner A, Ingber A (2001) Investigation of the threshold for allergic reactivity to chromium. Contact Dermatitis 44:70–74

Bruze M (1986) Sensitizers in PTBP-formaldehyde resins. Contact Dermatitis 14:132–133

Bruze M, Björkner B, Lepoittevin JP (1995) Occupational allergic contact dermatitis from ethyl cyanoacrylate. Contact Dermatitis 32:156–159

Bulikowski W, Tyras H (1976) Dermatological evaluation of occupational exposure of tanners to chromium compounds. Berufsdermatosen 24:132–137

Calnan CD, Cronin E (1978) Vegetable tans in leather. Contact Dermatitis 4:295–296

Castanedo-Tardan MP, Gelpi C, Jacob SE (2008) Allergic contact dermatitis to Crocs™. Contact Dermatitis 58:248–249

Cavelier C, Foussereau J (1995) Kontaktallergie gegen Metalle und deren Salze. Teil I: Chrom und Chromate. Dermatosen/Occup Environ 43:100–112

Chowdhuri S, Ghosh S (2007) Epidemio-allergological study in 155 cases of footwear dermatitis. Indian J Dermatol Venereol Leprol 73:319–322

Corazza M, Lauriola MM, Mantovani L, Virgili A (2006) Allergic contact dermatitis due to orthopedic shoes and a prosthesis for an amputated foot. Contact Dermatitis 55:115–117

Correia S, Menezes Brandao F (1986) Contact dermatitis of the feet. Derm Beruf Umwelt 34:102–106

Cronin E (1966) Shoe dermatitis. Br J Dermatol 78:617–625

Cronin E (1980) Contact dermatitis. Churchill Livingstone, Edinburgh, pp 68–76

Dickel H, Kuss O, Schmidt A, Diepgen TL (2001) Occupational relevance of positive standard patch-test results in employed persons with an initial report of an occupational skin disease. Int Arch Occup Environ Health 75:423–434

Dyro FM (1978) Methyl ethyl ketone polyneuropathy in shoe factory workers. Clin Toxicol 13:371–376

Estlander T, Kanerva L, Jolanki R (1990) Occupational allergic dermatoses from textile, leather, and fur dyes. Am J Contact Dermat 1:13–20

Estlander T, Jolanki R, Kanerva L (2000) Occupational allergic contact dermatitis from trivalent chromium in leather tanning. Contact Dermatitis 43:114

Estlander T, Kanerva L, Talola P, Jolanki R, Soini M (2001) Aziridine hardener – a new sensitizer in the dyeing of leather. Contact Dermatitis 44:107–109

Fisher AA (1991) Shoe dermatitis in a rosin-(colophony) sensitive individual. Am J Contact Dermat 2:209–210

Fogh A, Pock-Steen B (1992) Contact sensitivity to thiram in wooden shoes. Contact Dermatitis 27:348

Foussereau J, Cavelier C, Selig D (1976) Occupational eczema from para-tertiary-butylphenol formaldehyde resins: a review of the sensitizing resins. Contact Dermatitis 2:254–258

Foussereau J, Benezra C, Maibach HI (1982) Occupational contact dermatitis. Clinical and chemical aspects. Munksgaard, Kopenhagen, pp 256–259, 342–345

Foussereau J, Brändle I, Boujnah Khouadja A (1984) Allergisches Kontaktekzem durch Isothiazolin-3-on-Derivate. Derm Beruf Umwelt 32:208–211

Foussereau J, Muslmani M, Cavelier C, Herve Bazin B (1986) Contact allergy to safety shoes. Contact Dermatitis 14:233–236

Freeman S (1997) Shoe dermatitis. Contact Dermatitis 36:247–251

Fregert S (1975) Occupational dermatitis in a 10-year material. Contact Dermatitis 1:96–107

Fregert S (1981) Chromium valencies and cement dermatitis. Br J Dermatol 105(Suppl 21):7–9

Fuchs T, Geier J, Nickolaus G (1996) Ungewöhnliche Manifestation einer Chromatallergie. Allergo J 5:33 Sonderausgabe 1

Geier J, Nickolaus G, Fuchs Th (1995) Durch Lederschuhe provozierte Psoriasis pustulosa plantaris bei Chromatallergie. Allergologie 18:433–435

Geldof BA, Roesyanto ID, van Joost T (1989) Clinical aspects of para-tertiary-butylphenolformaldehyde resin (PTBP-FR) allergy. Contact Dermatitis 21:312–315

Gellin GA (1990) Pigmentary changes. In: Adams RM (ed) Occupational skin disease, 2nd edn. W B Saunders, Philadelphia, pp 21–25

Giménez-Arnau A, Silvestre JF, Mercader P, de la Cuadra J, Ballester I, Gallardo F, Pujol RM, Zimerson E, Bruze M (2009) Shoe contact dermatitis from dimethyl fumarate: clinical manifestations, patch test results, chemical analysis, and source of exposure. Contact Dermatitis 61:249–260

Grimalt F, Romaguera C (1975) New resin allergens in shoe contact dermatitis. Contact Dermatitis 1:169–174

Hansen MB, Rydin S, Menné T, Johansen JD (2002) Quantitative aspects of contact allergy to chromium and exposure to chrome-tanned leather. Contact Dermatitis 47:127–134

Hansen MB, Johansen JD, Menné T (2003) Chromium allergy: significance of both Cr(III) and Cr(VI). Contact Dermatitis 49:206–212

Hansen MB, Menné T, Johansen JD (2006a) Cr(III) reactivity and foot dermatitis in Cr(VI) positive patients. Contact Dermatitis 54:140–144

Hansen MB, Menné T, Johansen JD (2006b) Cr(III) and Cr(VI) in leather and elicitation of eczema. Contact Dermatitis 54:278–282

Haslam E (1989) Plant polyphenols. Vegetable tannins revisited. Cambridge University Press, Cambridge

Hausen B (1981) Woods injurious to human health. de Gruyter, Berlin

Hausen BM (1994) A case of allergic contact dermatitis due to metanil yellow. Contact Dermatitis 31:117–118

Hausen BM (1997) Lexikon der Kontaktallergene, 4. Ergänzungslieferung, ecomed Verlag, Landsberg/Lech

Heidemann E (1990) Leather. In: Elvers B, Hawkins S, Schulz G (eds) Ullmann's encyclopedia of industrial chemistry, vol A 15, 5th edn. VCH, Weinheim, pp 259–282

Henschel R, Agathos M, Breit R (2002) Occupational contact dermatitis from propolis. Contact Dermatitis 47:52

Holden CR, Gawkrodger DJ (2005) 10 years' experience of patch testing with a shoe series in 230 patients: which allergens are important? Contact Dermatitis 53:37–39

Jelen G, Cavelier C, Protois JP, Foussereau J (1989) A new allergen responsible for shoe allergy: chloroacetamide. Contact Dermatitis 21:110–111

Jung JH, McLaughlin JL, Stannard J, Guin JD (1988) Isolation, via activity-directed fractionation, of mercaptobenzothiazole and dibenzothiazyl disulfide as 2 allergens responsible for tennis shoe dermatitis. Contact Dermatitis 19:254–259

Koch P, Nickolaus G (1996) Allergic contact dermatitis and mercury exanthem due to mercury chloride in plastic boots. Contact Dermatitis 34:405–409

Koch P, Nickolaus G, Geier J (1996) Kontaktallergien bei Lederherstellern. Lederverarbeitern und in der Schuhindustrie. Fünf-Jahres-Analyse auf der Grundlage von Daten des Informationsverbundes Dermatologischer Kliniken. Dermatosen/Occup Environ 44:257–262

Lammintausta K, Zimerson E, Hasan T, Susitaival P, Winhoven S, Gruvberger B, Beck M, Williams JD, Bruze M (2009) An epidemic of furniture-related dermatitis: searching for a cause. Br J Dermatol 162:108–116

Lynde CW, Warshawski L, Mitchell JC (1982) Patch test results with a shoewear screening tray in 119 patients, 1977–80. Contact Dermatitis 8:423–425

Malten KE (1958) Occupational eczema due to para-tertiary butylphenol in a shoe adhesive. Dermatologica 117:103–109

Malten KE, Seutter E (1985) Allergenic degradation products of para-tertiary butylphenolformaldehyde plastic. Contact Dermatitis 12:222–224

Malten KE, van Aerssen RGL (1962) Kontaktekzeme durch Leime bei Schuhmachern und Schuhträgern. Berufsdermatosen 10:264–268

Malten KE, Rath R, Pastors PHM (1983) *p-tert*-Butylphenol formaldehyde and other causes of shoe dermatitis. Derm Beruf Umwelt 31:149–153

Mancuso G, Reggiani M, Berdondini RM (1996) Occupational dermatitis in shoemakers. Contact Dermatitis 34:17–22

Minkin W, Cohen HJ, Frank SB (1971) Contact dermatitis to east Indian leather. Arch Dermatol 103:522–523

Müller C, Hausen BM (1994) Contact allergy to a synthetic tannin in Tannosynt® liquid. Contact Dermatitis 31:185

Nardelli A, Taveirne M, Drieghe J, Carbonez A, Degreef H, Goossens A (2005) The relation between the localization of foot dermatitis and the causative allergens in shoes: a 13-year retrospective study. Contact Dermatitis 53:201–206

Nishioka K, Murata M, Ishikawa T, Kaniwa M (1996) Contact dermatitis due to rubber boots worn by Japanese farmers, with special attention to 6-ethoxy-2,2,4-trimethyl-1,2-dihydroquinoline (ETMDQ) sensitivity. Contact Dermatitis 35:241–245

Nygren O, Wahlberg JE (1998) Speciation of chromium in tanned leather gloves and relapse of chromium allergy from tanned leather samples. Analyst 123:935–937

Oleaga JM, Aguirre A, Landa N, Gonzalez M, Diaz-Perez JL (1992) Allergic contact dermatitis from Kathon 893. Contact Dermatitis 27:345–346

Onder M, Atahan AC, Bassoy B (2004) Foot dermatitis from the shoes. Int J Dermatol 43:565–567

Oumeish OY, Rushaidat QM (1980) Contact dermatitis to military boots in Jordan. Contact Dermatitis 6:498

Oztas P, Polat M, Cinar L, Alli M (2007) Shoe dermatitis from para-tertiary butylphenol formaldehyde. Contact Dermatitis 56:294–295

Podmore P (1995) Shoes. In: Rycroft RJG, Menné T, Frosch PJ (eds) Textbook of contact dermatitis, 2nd edn. Springer, Berlin/Heidelberg/New York, pp 516–526

Rani Z, Hussain I, Haroon TS (2003) Common allergens in shoe dermatitis: our experience in Lahore, Pakistan. Int J Dermatol 42:605–607

Rantanen T (2008) The cause of the Chinese sofa / chair dermatitis epidemic is likely to be contact allergy to dimethyl fumarate, a novel potent contact sensitizer. Br J Dermatol 159:218–221

Reich G, Taeger T (2009) Vom Kollagen tierischer Häute zum Werkstoff Leder. Chemikalien für die Lederherstellung. Chem Unserer Zeit 43:28–36

Rietschel RL, Fowler JF (1995) Fisher's contact dermatitis, 4th edn. Williams & Wilkins, Baltimore, pp 392–413

Roberts JL, Hanifin JM (1979) Athletic shoe dermatitis. JAMA 241:275–278

Romaguera C (1987) Shoe contact dermatitis. Int J Dermatol 26:532–535

Samitz MH, Katz SA (1964) A study of the chemical reactions between chromium and skin. J Invest Dermatol 43:35–42

Schubert H, Agatha G (1979) Zur Allergennatur der para-tert. Butylphenolformaldehydharze. Derm Beruf Umwelt 27:49–52

Scutt RWB (1966) Chrome sensitivity associated with tropical footwear in the royal navy. Br J Dermatol 78:337–343

Skoet R, Olsen J, Mathiesen B, Iversen L, Johansen JD, Agner T (2004) A survey of occupational hand eczema in Denmark. Contact Dermatitis 51:159–166

Spruit D, van Neer FCJ (1966) Penetration rate of Cr(III) and Cr(VI). Dermatologica 132:179–182

Stein G (1992) Chromatsensibilisierung durch Leder. Derm Beruf Umwelt 40:110–112

Strauss RM, Wilkinson SM (2002) Shoe dermatitis due to colophonium used as leather tanning or finishing agent in Portuguese shoes. Contact Dermatitis 47:59

Susitaival P, Winhoven SM, Williams J, Lammintausta K, Hasan T, Beck MH, Gruvberger B, Zimerson E, Bruze M (2010) An outbreak of furniture related dermatitis ("sofa dermatitis") in Finland and the UK: history and clinical cases. J Eur Acad Dermatol Venereol 24(4):486–489

Suurmond D, Verspijck Mijnssen GAW (1967) Allergic dermatitis due to shoes and a leather prothese. Dermatologica 134:371–378

Teixeira M, Machado S, Teixeira A, Silva E (2005) Severe contact allergy to footwear in a young child. Contact Dermatitis 52:159–160

Thorstensen TC (1995) Leather. In: Kroschwitz JI (ed) Kirk-Othmer encyclopedia of chemical technology, 4th edn. Wiley, New York, pp 159–177

Thyssen JP, Jensen P, Carlsen BC, Engkilde K, Menné T, Johansen JD (2009) The prevalence of chromium allergy in Denmark is currently increasing as a result of leather exposure. Br J Dermatol 161: 1288–1293

Verma GK, Sharma NL, Mahajan VK, Tegta GR, Shanker V (2007) Purpuric contact dermatitis from footwear. Contact Dermatitis 56:362–364

Vidovic R, Kansky A (1985) Contact dermatitis in workers processing polyvinyl chloride plastics. Derm Beruf Umwelt 33:104–105

Wagner G, Wezel G (1966) Art und Häufigkeit hautschädigender Berufsnoxen in Schleswig-Holstein. Berufsdermatosen 14:1–40

Wardenbach P, Henter A, Kollmeier H (1989) Kontaktekzeme und Krebserkrankungen durch Chrom, Nickel und deren Verbindungen. Eine Auswertung der BK-DOK 1978 bis 1984. Zbl Arbeitsmed 39:186–190

Warshaw E, Schram SE, Belsito DV, DeLeo VA, Fowler JF Jr, Maibach HI, Marks JG Jr, Mathias T, Pratt MD, Rietschel RL, Sasseville D, Storrs FJ, Taylor JS, Zug KA (2007) Shoe allergens: retrospective analysis of cross-sectional data from the North American Contact Dermatitis Group, 2001–2004. Dermatitis 18:191–202

Williams JD, Coulson IH, Susitaival P, Winhoven SM (2008) An outbreak of furniture dermatitis in the U.K. Br J Dermatol 159:233–234

Zimerson E, Bruze M (2000) Contact allergy to 5,5′-di-*tert*-butyl-2,2′-dihydroxy-(hydroxymethyl)-dibenzyl ethers, sensitizers in *p-tert*-butylphenol-formaldehyde resin. Contact Dermatitis 43:20–26

Zimerson E, Bruze M (2002a) Contact allergy to the monomers in *p-tert*-butylphenol-formaldehyde resin. Contact Dermatitis 47:147–153

Zimerson E, Bruze M (2002b) Low-molecular-weight contact allergens in *p-tert*-butylphenol-formaldehyde resin. Am J Contact Dermat 13: 190–197

Zimerson E, Sörensen Ö, Bruze M (2002) Contact allergy to trimers in *p-tert*-butylphenol-formaldehyde resin. Exog Dermatol 1:207–216

59 Adhesives and Glues

Jana Präßler[1] · *Matthias Gebhardt*[2] · *Peter Elsner*[2]
[1]Department of Dermatology and Allergology, Friedrich Schiller University, Jena, Germany
[2]Department of Dermatology, University Hospital Jena, Jena, Germany

Core Messages

- Exposure to adhesives and glues is common in occupation, leisure time, and household activities. There is a constantly growing group of occupational glues in which the adhesive is a polymerization product formed by a complex chemical reaction between the macromolecules.
- Phenol-formaldehyde resins have occupational relevance for shoemakers, in car manufacturing, in the wood industries, and in construction industries.
- Epoxy resins, used in a wide range of industries, penetrate regular gloves and may cause aerogenic contact dermatitis.
- While acrylic adhesives are less sensitizing than epoxy and colophony rosin, acrylates present with cross-reactions among each other, but not between methacrylates and cyanoacrylates.
- Colophony rosin is a natural material and also used in many occupational fields.
- Glues should be tested epicutaneously either using commercial patch-test substances or as is, but only after having completely dried in order to minimize the risk of active sensitization via patch testing.

1 Introduction

Exposure to adhesives and glues is common in occupation, leisure time, and household activities. Several types of glues and adhesives are in use, depending on the materials to be joined. Whereas a century ago only paper, wood, leather, and textiles could be glued, today almost any type of materials can be fixed to each other.

In the majority of glues, the action is simply due to removal of solvents, cooling, or crystallization. In these cases, it is not the action of the macromolecular molecules but rather the preservatives, detergents, and other additives added to the adhesive preparation that may cause dermatological problems, although this is rare. There is, however, a constantly growing second group of glues in which the adhesive is a polymerization product formed by a complex chemical reaction between macromolecules. This second group may cause many more irritant and allergic reactions on the skin (Malten 1984).

In this instance, two-component systems are common that react only after being mixed. Other ways to start the reaction include heating, UV irradiation, oxygen and air exposure, pressure-induced rupture of catalyst reservoirs, etc. The focus is mainly on this second group of adhesive chemicals and their occupational use.

2 Formaldehyde Resins

Phenol-formaldehyde resins resemble a group of chemicals that contain the formaldehyde structure but are not necessarily associated with formaldehyde allergy. Resols and novolacs are distinguished within that group. While the chemical curing of novolacs requires the presence of formaldehyde to react with the phenol terminate group, resols do not. Resols are intermediates, which, in turn, need heat to cure (Malten 1984). Para-substituted phenol resins do not cross-link but adhere readily under pressure. Among them, *para*-tertiary butylphenol-formaldehyde resin (PTBP-FR) is a well-known allergen with particular use as neoprene-based leather glue. Therefore it has occupational relevance for shoemakers. An Italian survey revealed PTBP-FR-containing neoprene adhesives to be the major allergens in a shoe factory (Manusco et al. 1996). Apart from PTBP-FR, mercaptobenzothiazole (MBT), two-component-polyurethane-, and epoxy resin-based glues were also found in the same study as relevant glue allergens with special applications each in shoe manufacture. PTBP-FR-based glues have also been reported for their use in car manufacture (Schubert and Agatha 1979).

Phenol-formaldehyde resin is used, for example, in glass microfiber production as a blend for the fiber to strengthen it (Sripaiboonkij et al. 2009). Exposure of the workers to the coated microfibers occurs via inhaling and direct contact. This leads besides respiratory, nasal, and eye symptoms also to skin symptoms with an exposure-response relation.

Mostly nonoccupationally relevant are foot dermatitis elicited by shoes, wrist dermatitis by watch straps, and by

T. Rustemeyer, P. Elsner, S.M. John & H.I. Maibach (eds.), *Kanerva's Occupational Dermatology*,
DOI 10.1007/978-3-642-02035-3_59,

other leather articles (Freeman 1997). Of 839 Finnish patients, 9 patch tested with a glue series reacted to PTBP-FR, which turned out to be the most common relevant glue allergen (Tarvainen 1995).

Despite the similar chemical nature, there is no evidence for cross-reactivity between phenol-formaldehyde resin and PTBP-FR (Geldof et al. 1989). Some authors have attributed test reactions to PTBP-FR to free formaldehyde; however, most patients are actually not allergic to formaldehyde. Schubert and Agatha (1979) performed patch-test studies with the chromatographically extracted ingredients of commercially available PTBP-FR. They found two linear condensates named 2-hydroxy-5-tert.-butylbenzylalcohol and 2,2′-dihydroxy-3,3-di-(2-hydroxy-5-tertiary butyl)-benzyl-5,5-ditertiary butyl-diphenylmethan to be the real allergens.

PTBP is used in the production of PTBP-FR. Formerly, PTBP has been added in excess, which might have caused concomitant reactions, whereas nowadays this is no longer relevant. PTBP and *para*-tertiary butylcatechol, both antioxidants in plastics, might cross-react. As PTBP-FR, they are also known for their toxic effects on skin. Toxic exposure to PTBP-FR may cause chemical burn and even toxic leukoderma. Vitiligo-like leukoderma on the hands of PTBP-FR-exposed shoe-manufacturing workers has been found in the above-cited Italian study. For patch-test purposes, PTBP-FR is available 1% in petrolatum by all well-known suppliers, either in a special plastic and glue or in the shoe series.

Urea-formaldehyde resin and melamine-formaldehyde resin are used as glues in the wood industries to make furniture press plates. Despite a low constant release of formaldehyde from these plates into the indoor air, the health effect for individuals living or working in the room is way overestimated in our opinion. Construction workers are also exposed to formaldehyde resins in modern building materials. Textile finishes are another use for these formaldehyde resins (Fowler et al. 1992). Even cosmetics may contain PTBP-FR as Angelini and others have shown (Angelini et al. 1993). Both resins are currently available from Chemotechnique, Sweden, urea-FR as a 10% petrolatum and melamine-FR as a 7% preparation in the textile color and finishes series.

If nail varnishes are considered to be adhesives, then toluene sulfonamide-formaldehyde resin (TS-FR) should be included in this chapter. A very common ingredient of nail lacquers and hardeners, it may be an occupational allergen for cosmetologists, beauticians, and, in a wider sense, those who use these products and who are in public service, such as bank clerks, office employees, and salespersons. Among patients with cosmetic-related contact dermatitis, TS-FR was found to be relevant in 12.6% of the cases, second only to skin care products (De Groot et al. 1988). Typically, TS-FR allergy involves the eyelids, lateral aspects of the neck, and, more seldom, the truly exposed periungual area. Because traces of the allergen are easily transferred to the eyelids, it has been included in the topical eye preparation series of several allergen providers. Almost all brands of nail polishes contain TS-FR (Hausen et al. 1995; Sainio et al. 1997). TS-FR has recently been included in most cosmetic patch-test trays. In addition to TS-FR, acrylates are gaining more and more importance in nail varnishes and lacquers. Chemotechnique provides a separate acrylic nail test series for this purpose.

3 Epoxy Resins

When used for industrial adhesive purposes, epoxy resins occur mostly in the construction industry, the assembly of cars, ships, and airplanes, the manufacturing of sports equipment, as well as in the optical and electronic industries. Much is similar between the chemistry of epoxy resins and acrylates. Both are (often) two-component systems. They are not sensitizing when fully cured but frequently contain an amount of remaining monomer, which is enough to booster a preexisting sensitization. Both penetrate regular gloves which makes skin protection a real problem, especially for sensitized people.

Epoxy resins are usually based on bisphenol A and epichlorohydrin, a highly reactive epoxy group which is responsible for the allergenicity of the compound. Many different chemicals may be added to improve or adapt the material to the required condition. Hardeners of the amine or acid anhydride type are cross-linking agents for the resin (White 1990). They are usually dissolved in organic solvents. Some of those additional chemicals, such as glycidyl ether, benzol, and toluol, are skin irritants, which may enhance the skin damage and thereby booster the induction or elicitation of an allergic reaction.

Workers in the electronics, optical, paint, and glue industries are most likely to acquire occupational allergy to epoxy resins (Richter 1974; Tosti et al. 1993). A Dutch survey among employees of several companies that specialize in epoxy resin-related work in the construction industry revealed hand eczema in 23 of 135 persons. Of these, 61% of the eczema population and 12% of the healthy skin group had positive patch-test reactions. Almost all positive patch-test reactions were due to epoxy resin. This shows the tremendous relevance of epoxy resin as occupational allergen (van Putten et al. 1984).

Epoxy resin coated fiberglass fibers have been reported as a cause of dermatitis in this particular field of industry (Holness and Nethercott 1989).

Occupational exposition to epoxy resin should be considered in patients with face dermatitis and proved sensitization to epoxy resin. The German information network of dermatology clinics reported higher rates of sensitization to epoxy resin especially in men with face dermatitis which correlates with the more frequent occupational (aerogenic) contact to epoxy resin, for example, in the production of cars, ships, machines, or in metal, chemistry, and construction industries (Schnuch et al. 2009).

There are frequent reports about nonoccupational cases of epoxy resin sensitivity too. Contact dermatitis due to the epoxy resin in textile label patches has been attributed to the epoxy containing adhesive (Fregert and Orsmark 1984). Limiting patch tests with epoxy chemicals to the standardized test series is recommended because of the danger of active sensitization. Once proven, epoxy resins should not be retested, in our opinion. When testing epoxy-exposed individuals, never forget to include chemical additives such as the broad range of hardeners.

Epoxy resins are in discussion to cause or trigger the onset of systemic sclerosis. There was also a description of a disease of skin sclerosis and muscle weakness after occupational exposition to vapor of epoxy resin (Yamakage et al. 1980). Animal and patient studies revealed that the most likely etiological agent in the epoxy resin is cyclohexylamine. Nevertheless, correlations between epoxy resin as a possible causer and sclerotic skin diseases are weak, not at last because of the low frequency of these diseases in comparison to the exposure rate to epoxy resins (Steen 1999).

4 Acrylates

Apart from their use in plastics, colors, lacquers, coatings, dental materials, orthopedic appliances, etc., acrylates are now increasingly used in adhesives (Kanerva and Alanko 1999; ➋ *Table 59.1*) because of their excellent properties, such as strong adhesion – even to metals, ceramics, glass, and other building0020materials – fast curing, and easy handling. Stickers, tapes, and office material may also be based on acrylic adhesives. An extensive list of ingredients in pressure-sensitive tapes was published in Fisher's Contact Dermatitis. The most common allergenic ingredient of those tapes is 2-ethylhexyl acrylate. Occupational problems can arise from workplaces where stickers and labels are put on the final products or, theoretically, in medicine. However, compared with epoxy and colophony rosin, which have been preferred in the past, acrylate-based tape adhesives are less sensitizing and reports are based on single cases. There are one- and two-component acrylic adhesive systems. Epoxy (meth)acrylates are a combination of epoxy resins or its raw materials bisphenol A and epichlorohydrin with acrylates and methacrylates. Positive patch-test results to epoxy (meth)acrylates are often not caused by a specific occupational exposure to these substances but due to a sensitization to diglycidyl ether of bisphenol A. This has relevance for various occupational fields (Aalto-Korte et al. 2009).

Table 59.1
Adhesives based on acrylates, methacrylates, and epoxy diacrylates according to Kanerva and Alanko (1999)

Anaerobic sealants
Cyanoacrylates
Ultraviolet-cured sealants
Methyl methacrylate
Metal and glass glues
Epoxy diacrylates (vinyl resins)
Acrylic dental bonding agents

Hazardous health effects on the skin are allergic sensitizations and irritation to several acrylates. Glue-induced adherence of contaminated skin (finger, eyelids) may be very difficult to separate. If possible, wait for spontaneous resolution; gentle teasing with repeated moistening of the skin may be applied in this otherwise harmless condition. Respiratory diseases like asthma, eosinophilic bronchitis, and rhinitis have often been reported when handling acrylics (Savonius et al. 1993; Kopferschmidt-Kubler et al. 1996; Quirce 2004).

As known from other fields of (meth)acrylate use (dental prostheses, daily plastic wear), allergy can only be initiated and elicited by uncured monomers. In contrast to plastic wear, monomers are always available when using glues. So the rate of sensitization could be rather high and similar to that of monomeric acrylate use in other occupational fields, such as dentistry. There is, however, only scanty data about real incidence of acrylate sensitivity caused by acrylic adhesives or glues in occupationally exposed individuals or even those within the normal population. Obviously there is (still) no major problem evolving from nonoccupational temporary use of these substances, although several reports on sensitization from an adhesive in an electrosurgical grounding plate were reported (Kanerva and Alanko 1999). In occupational medicine, acrylates are important sensitizers to keep in mind. Sometimes it may be hard to find suitable personal protective equipment for sensitized people because most acrylates do penetrate gloves easily.

Cyanoacrylates are among the most common ingredients of acrylate glues (Loctite is a well-known brand example). Eyelid eczema, nummular eczema on the hands, and periungual dermatitis and even allergic onycholysis (Kanerva 2000) are features of allergic contact dermatitis caused by cyanoacrylate glue used to fix artificial nails. Ethyl cyanoacrylate and methyl methacrylate were seen as allergens in these patients (Belsito 1987; Guin et al. 1998) as well as 2-hydroxy methacrylate, 2-hydroxpropyl methacrylate, and ethylene glycol dimethacrylate (Lazarov 2006). Aluminum test chambers should be avoided when testing cyanoacrylates, because they may contain catalysts for the polymerization process. The vehicle acetone further enhances the tendency to polymerize spontaneously (Bruze et al. 1995). Due to its excellent adhesive properties with various materials, cyanoacrylate glues may occur in many different occupations. When sticking something to glass, ceramics, or metal surfaces, 2-hydroxy ethyl methacrylate (2-HEMA), 2-hydroxy propyl methacrylate (2-HPMA), and (tri)ethylene glycol dimethacrylate (TEGDMA or EGDMA) are common ingredients of industrial adhesives (Kanerva et al. 1995). Methacrylates and cyanoacrylates do not cross-react.

Some acrylates have higher potential of sensitization then others. In workers with contact to a glue containing different acrylates some substances like tri- and diethylene glycol diacrylate showed a high number of positive tests while other ingredients like isobornyl acrylate did not obtain any reaction in patch testing (Kiec-Swierczynska et al. 2005).

For patch-test purposes, a test screening with several acrylates should therefore be carried out when suspecting acrylate allergy. Chemotechnique has the most diverse patch-test tray on methacrylates; however, other companies also provide a suitable screening composition. It was as early as 1975 when Jordan recommended that MMA alone is not a good screening for acrylate allergy (Jordan 1975). Aalto-Korte et al. (2008) recommended 2-hydroxyethyl methacrylate and ethylene glycol dimethacrylate as screeners for occupational contact allergy to anaerobic sealants and acrylic glues. Accelerators, inhibitors, and catalysts, which may be added to the acrylates, can also sensitize.

5 Colophony

Colophony rosin, a naturally occurring rosin from trees, is another natural base of glues and adhesives. Abietic acid, also available as patch-test allergen, and its oxidative derivatives are the causative allergens (Guin et al. 1995). It ranks high on hit lists of contact allergens because of widespread exposure reaching from occupational use in wood, paper, paint, electronics, metal, and cosmetics industries to household contacts to natural exposure (Sadhra et al. 1994). Some tackifiers for heel and toe stiffeners in shoes are based on colophony and may therefore be relevant allergens in shoe manufacturers (Freeman 1997). Contact dermatitis due to colophony has also been reported for musicians (Lombardi et al. 2003; Gambichler et al. 2004). This is of a special difficulty because the contact of the allergen to the skin cannot be avoided, for example, by using gloves, and the affected persons cannot change their work place/conditions easily.

Medical use of rosin derivatives on tapes, bandages, surgical and dental dressings, wart paints (Lachapelle and Leroy 1990), and hydrocolloid dressings has been reported (Sasseville et al. 1997). For several hydrocolloid dressings, the allergen is a modified ester of colophony, the pentaerythrite ester (Hausen and Kulenkamp 1998). Most patients with a sensitization to colophony report intolerance of brown-colored tapes. However, no report has been found of occupational contact dermatitis to medical colophony resin adhesives.

6 Others

A very special kind of biological adhesives are so-called fibrin tissue glues. They are two-component systems consisting of fibrinogen and factor XIII in one syringe and thrombin in the second syringe. By adding thrombin to the fibrinogen/factor-XIII mixture, there is a coagulation reaction. Tissue adhesives are used to recombine skin and organ cuts (liver, spleen, etc.), to seal wounds in surgically opened body cavities or vascular prostheses and to stop bleeding. There has been no report of either occupational contact dermatitis or immediate-type contact reactions to this product because skin contact to the medical person is always prevented by gloves worn for reasons of hygiene. Allergic reactions of the recipients are not the focus of this chapter, but it may be mentioned that moderate to severe anaphylactic reactions may appear after repeated instillations of fibrin sealants containing bovine aprotinin. Different surgical procedures in the dental, cardial, vascular, pulmonary, and other fields are described for this problem (Ockenfels et al. 1995; Wuethrich et al. 1996; Shirai et al. 2005; Kober et al. 2008). Aprotinin-specific IgG and IgE can be found in the affected recipients.

Table 59.2

Plastics and glue series as recommended by several distributors

	Miscellaneous	Chemotechnique	Brial	Almirall Hermal Trolab
1	**Abitol**	A-002		D 0915
2	**Abietic acid**	A-001	B 0328	D 2382
3	**Benzoyl peroxide**	B-007	B 0101	D 0201
4	Turpentine Oil		A 0701	D 2322
5	*o*-Cresyl glycidyl ether		C 0335	D 0917
6	**2,6-Ditert-butyl-4-cresol (BHT)**	D-006		D 0110
7	**2-tert-Butyl-4-methoxyphenol (BHA)**	B-022		
8	**Diphenyl thiourea**	D-025	C 0934	D 1021
9	**Cyclohexanone resin**	C-027		
10	**2-*n*-Octyl-4-isothiazolin-3-one**	O 004	E 1463	D 2427
11	*N,N*-Dimethyl-*p*-toluidine	D-016	B 0326	D 0963
Formaldehyde resins				
1	**Toluene-sulfonamide-formaldehyde resin**	T-010	0331	D 0908
2	***p*-tert-Butylphenol-formaldehyde resin**	B-024	A-0016/1	D 0030
3	**Resorcinol-formaldehyde resin**	P-005	B 0314	D 2865
4	**Para-tertiary butylphenol**	B-023	B 0318	D 0920
5	**2-Monomethylol phenol**	M-015		
Epoxies				
1	**Triethylenetetramine**	T-019	B 0316	D 0905
3	**4-4′-Diaminodiphenyl methane**	D-001	B 0313	0906
4	**Diethylenetriamine**	D-010		
6	**Isophoronediamine**	I-006	C 0332	D 0914
7	**Hexamethylenetetramine**	H-003	B 0909	D 2318
8	Cresylglycidylether			D 0917
9	**Epichlorhydrin, Epoxidharz**	E-002	A 0014/1	D 0021
10	**Triglycidyl isocyanurate**	T-028		
11	**Bisphenol A**	B-013	B 0327	D 0965
Plasticizer				
1	Diethylphthalate		B 0320	
2	Di-*n*-butylphthalate	D007	B 0916	D 0903
3	Tricresyl phosphate	T-015	B 0329	D 2511
4	Triphenyl phosphate	T-022	B 0323	D 0959
5	Dimethylphthalate		B 0311	D 0954
Plastic stabilizers				
1	2-Phenylindole	P-007		
Plastic inhibitors				
1	Azodiisobutyrodinitrile	A-018		
2	Hydroquinone	H-007	B 0304	D 0800
3	4-tert.Butylcatechol (PTBC)	B-030B	C 0338	D 2810
UV adsorbers in plastics				
1	2(2-Hydroxy-5-methylphenyl)benzotriazol	H-016	C 1416	D 0159

Table 59.2 (Continued)

	Miscellaneous	Chemotechnique	Brial	Almirall Hermal Trolab
2	Resorcinol monobenzoate			
3	Phenyl salicylate			
Isocyanates				
1	Diphenylmethane 4,4-diisocyanate	D-023	D 0336/1	
2	Phenylisocyanate		B 0322	
3	Toluenediisocyanate		E 0341	
Acrylates				
1	**(2-Hydroxyethyl) methacrylate (2-HEMA)**	H-010	C 2352	D 2477
2	**(2-Hydroxypropyl) methacrylate (2-HPMA)**	H-018	E 2356	
3	**2-Hydroxyethylacrylate**	H-009	E 2357	
4	**1,6-Hexanediol diacrylate**	H-004		
5	Tetrahydrofurfuryl methacrylate	T-027		
6	**Tetraethyleneglycol dimethacrylate**	T-029		
7	*N,N*-Dimethylaminoethyl methacrylate	D-045		
8	**Methyl methacrylate**	M-013	B 2308	D 1800
9	**Ethyleneglycol dimethacrylate**	E-007		D 1850
10	**Triethyleneglycol dimethacrylate**	T-018		D 1851
11	**Triethyleneglycol diacrylate**	T-017		
12	**BIS-GMA**	H-013	C 2353	D 1852
13	**BIS-MA**	M-007		
14	**Butylacrylate**		B 0205	
15	***n*-Butyl methacrylate**	B-021		
16	**2-ethylhexyl acrylate**	E-009	B 0206	
17	**Ethyl acrylate**	E-004		
18	**Ethyl methacrylate**	E-012		
19	Diurethane dimethacrylate		C 2354/1	D 2475
20	Urethandimethacrylat	U-004		

The plastic and glue series as provided by several suppliers is a mixture of glue and plastic ingredients as well as substances involved in the synthesis of these products. Substances relevant for glues and adhesives are marked in bold. Many of the above-mentioned substances are provided by all of the companies, but the ordering number is not mentioned. That is because the substance is not included in the glue and plastic series of this company. As an exception to this rule, Chemotechnique methacrylates have been included in this table because, in addition to the glue and adhesive series, they provide an extensive list of acrylic adhesives and acrylics for artificial nails which are therefore considered to be adhesives/glues

7 Patch Testing with Adhesives and Glues

The most important part of allergological diagnosis is to think about possible exposure to glues and adhesives. Optimally, one should only consider patch tests with possible allergenic glue ingredients when the chemical composition of the glue or adhesive is known. This can be determined by asking the manufacturer or, to a lesser extent, by looking at the material data safety sheets. In daily practice, however, this very often fails. Therefore, a glue-screening series makes good practical sense. *Table 59.2* includes information from three major European patch-test provider companies, namely, Chemotechnique, Almirall Hermal Trolab, and Brial. Their adhesive and glue series were combines in order to get an overview about available glue contact allergens. That not all substances in these trays are glue allergens is worth mentioning; many are plastic allergens such as phthalates, accelerators and inhibitors, or UV adsorbers. To make it easier the real glue allergens listed in the table are marked in boldface. Screening with the chemical subgroups after getting information about the basic glue composition, for example, epoxy, acrylic, and formaldehyde resin, is proposed.

Under special circumstances it is also recommended testing the glue itself. When the complete composition is known and the single allergenic ingredients are available, testing the native glue is avoidable. It is warned against testing unknown epoxy resin-based glues because of possible active sensitization. Active sensitization is also well known for acrylics and has been reported even after a single exposure. However, by leaving the glue exposed to air and letting it dry on the patch-test chamber, the risk of strong patch-test reactions is minimized.

The easiest way to patch test a patient's own products is using tapes and medical self-adhesive dressings. Simply cut a small piece and stick it to the skin for 24–48 h. For further information, the other chapters in this book that deal with acrylates and epoxy resins are referred to (see ❯ 62, "Coatings", ❯ 55, "Other Plastics", ❯ 206, "Polyvinyl Resins", and ❯ 51, "Epoxy Resins").

8 Other Tests

Since some of the mentioned allergens do not only cause type-VI-sensitizations with subsequent contact dermatitis but also allergic asthma, it seemed useful to find other methods then patch testing. Elms et al. (2005) tested serum samples for specific IgE antibodies against colophony which could be detected in colophony-exposed workers with symptoms of occupational asthma. The test is based on the production of a protein extract by monomac-6 cells after in vitro challenge with colophony extract.

Another method to determine exposure toward allergens is measuring components of allergens in body fluids. Jones et al. (2001) described the analysis of dehydroabietic acid in urine as a biomarker of colophony exposure. There was a detectable correlation of the levels of dehydroabietic acid in workers of a soldering factory to their colophony exposure.

In terms of contact dermatitis these tests are of course of lower interest but can give further information about the correlation of the present skin disease and the underlying workplace situation.

References

Aalto-Korte K, Alanko A, Kuuliala O, Jolanki J (2008) Occupational methacrylate and acrylate allergy from glues. Contact Dermatitis 58:340–346

Aalto-Korte K, Jungewelter S et al (2009) Contact allergy to epoxy methacrylates. Contact Dermatitis 61:9–21

Angelini E, Marinaro C, Carrozzo AM et al (1993) Allergic contact dermatitis of the lip margins from *para*-tertiary-butylphenol in a lip liner. Contact Dermatitis 28:146–148

Belsito DV (1987) Contact dermatitis to ethyl-cyanoacrylate-containing glue. Contact Dermatitis 17:234–236

Bruze M, Bjoerkner B, Lepoittevin JP (1995) Occupational allergic contact dermatitis from ethyl cyanoacrylate. Contact Dermatitis 32:156–159

De Groot AC, Bruynzeel DP, Bos JD et al (1988) The allergens in cosmetics. Arch Dermatol 124:1525–1529

Elms J, Fishwick D, Robinson E, Burge S, Huggins V, Barber C, Williams N, Curran A (2005) Specific IgE to colophony? Occup Med (Lond) 55(3):234–237

Fowler JF, Skinner SM, Belsito DV (1992) Allergic contact dermatitis from formaldehyde resins in permanent press clothing: an under diagnosed cause of generalized dermatitis. J Am Acad Dermatol 27:962–968

Freeman S (1997) Shoe dermatitis. Contact Dermatitis 36:247–251

Fregert S, Orsmark K (1984) Allergic contact dermatitis due to epoxy resin in textile labels. Contact Dermatitis 11:131–132

Gambichler T, Boms S, Freitag M (2004) Contact dermatitis and other skin conditions in instrumental musicians. BMC Dermatol 4:3

Geldof BA, Roesyanto ID, van Joost T (1989) Clinical aspects of paratertiary butylphenol formaldehyde resin (PTBP-FR) allergy. Contact Dermatitis 21:312–315

Guin JD (1995) Colophony (rosin). In: Practical contact dermatitis. McGraw-Hill, New York, pp 115–124

Guin JD, Baas K, Nelson-Adesokan P (1998) Contact sensitization to cyanoacrylate adhesive as a cause of severe onychodystrophy. Int J Dermatol 37:31–36

Hausen BM, Kulenkamp D (1998) Allergische kontaktdermatitis auf einem hydrokolloidverband bei kolophoniumallergikern. Aktuel Dermatol 24:174–177

Hausen BM, Milbrodt M, Koenig WA (1995) The allergens of nail polish. Contact Dermatitis 33:157–164

Holness DL, Nethercott JR (1989) Occupational contact dermatitis due to epoxy resin in a fiberglass binder. J Occup Med 31:87–89

Jones K, Garfit SJ, Calverley A, Channa K, Cocker J (2001) Identification of a possible biomarker for colophony exposure. Occup Med (Lond) 51(8):507–509

Jordan WP (1975) Cross-sensitization patterns in acrylate allergies. Contact Dermatitis 1:13–15

Kanerva L, Alanko K (1999) Allergic contact dermatitis from 2-hydroxy methacrylate in an adhesive of an electrosurgical grounding plate. Eur J Dermatol (in press)

Kanerva L, Estlander T (2000) Allergic onycholysis and paronychia caused by cyanoacrylate nail glue, but not by photobonded methacrylate nails. Eur J Dermatol 10(3):223–225

Kanerva L, Jolanki R, Leino T, Estlander T (1995) Occupational allergic contact dermatitis from 2-hydroxyethyl methacrylate and ethylene glycol dimethacrylate in a modified acrylic structural adhesive. Contact Dermatitis 33:84–89

Kiec-Swierczynska M, Krecisz B, Swiercynska-Machura D, Zaremba J (2005) An epidemic of occupational contact dermatitis from an acrylic glue. Contact Dermatitis 52(3):121–125

Kober BJ, Scheule AM, Voth V, Deschner N, Schmid E, Ziemer G (2008) Anaphylactic reaction after systemic application of aprotinin triggered by aprotinin-containing fibrin sealant. Anaesth Analg 107(2):406–409

Kopferschmidt-Kubler MC, Stenger R, Blaumeiser M et al (1996) Rev Mal Respir 13:305–307

Lachapelle JM, Leroy B (1990) Allergic contact dermatitis to colophony included in the formulation of flexible collodion BP, the vehicle of a salicylic and lactic acid wart paint. Dermatol Clin 8:143–146

Lazarov A (2007) Sensitization to acrylates is a common adverse reaction to artificial fingernails. J Eur Acad Dermatol Venereol 21:169–174

Lombardi C, Botello M, Caruso A, Passalacqua G (2003) Allergy and skin diseases in musicians. Eur Ann Allergy Clin Immunol 35(2):52–55

Malten KE (1984) Dermatological problems with synthetic resins and plastics in glues, part I. Dermatosen 32:81–86

Manusco G, Reggiani M, Berdondini RM (1996) Occupational dermatitis in shoemakers. Contact Dermatitis 34:17–22

Ockenfels HM, Seemann U, Goos M (1995) Allergy to fibrin tissue in dental medicine. Contact Dermatitis 32:363–364

Quirce S (2004) Eosinophilic bronchitis in the workplace. Curr Opin Allergy Clin Immunol 4(2):87–91

Richter G (1974) Zur epidemiologie des epoxidharzekzems. Dermatol Monatsschr 160:785–789

Sadhra S, Foulds IS, Gray CN et al (1997) Colophony uses, health effects, airborne measurement and analysis. Ann Occup Hyg 38:385–396

Sainio E-L, Engstroem K, Henriks-Eckerman M-L, Kanerva L (1997) Allergenic ingredients in nail polishes. Contact Dermatitis 37: 155–162

Sasseville D, Tennstedt D, Lachapelle JM (1997) Allergic contact dermatitis from hydrocolloid dressings. Am J Contact Dermat 8:236–238

Savonius B, Keskinen H, Tuppurainen M, Kanerva L (1993) Occupational respiratory disease caused by acrylics. Clin Exp Allergy 23:416–424

Schnuch A, Szliska C, Uter W (2009) Facial allergic contact dermatitis. Data from the IVDK and review of literature. Hautarzt 60:13–21

Schubert H, Agatha G (1979) Zur Allergennatur der para-tert. Butylphenolformaldehydharze. Dermatosen 27:49–52

Shirai T, Shimota H, Chida K, Sano S, Takeuchi Y, Yasueda H (2005) Anaphylaxis to aprotinin in fibrin sealant. Intern Med 44(10): 1088–1089

Sripaiboonkij P et al (2009) Respiratory and skin health among glass microfiber production workers: a cross sectional study. Environ Health 8:36

Steen VD (1999) Occupational scleroderma. Curr Opin Rheumatol 11(6):490–494

Tarvainen K (1995) Analysis of patients with allergic patch test reactions to a plastics and glue series. Contact Dermatitis 32:346–351

Tosti A, Guerra L, Vincenzi C, Peluso AM (1993) Occupational skin hazards from synthetic plastics. Toxicol Ind Health 9:493–502

van Putten PB, Coenraads PJ, Nater J (1984) Hand dermatoses and contact allergic reactions in construction workers exposed to epoxy resins. Contact Dermatitis 10:146–150

Wuethrich B, Bianchi Kusch E, Johansson SG (1996) Allergic urticaria and angioedema caused by a hemostatic sponge of bovine fibrin used in tooth extraction. Allergy 51:49–51

Yamakage A, Ishikawa H, Saito Y, Hattori A (1980) Occupational scleroderma-like disorder occurring in men engaged in the polymerization of epoxy resins. Dermatologica 161:33–44

Printed by Publishers' Graphics LLC